Water-Insoluble Drug Formulation

Third Edition

Water-Insoluble Drug Formulation

Third Edition

Edited by

Rong (Ron) Liu

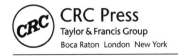

CRC Press
Taylor & Francis Group
Boca Raton London New York

CRC Press is an imprint of the
Taylor & Francis Group, an **informa** business

CRC Press
Taylor & Francis Group
6000 Broken Sound Parkway NW, Suite 300
Boca Raton, FL 33487-2742

First issued in paperback 2022

Printed on acid-free paper

ISBN-13: 978-1-498-72941-3 (hbk)
ISBN-13: 978-1-03-233921-4 (pbk)
DOI: 10.1201/9781315120492

Library of Congress Cataloging-in-Publication Data

Names: Liu, Rong, editor.
Title: Water-insoluble drug formulation / [edited by] Rong Liu.
Description: Third edition. | Boca Raton : CRC Press, [2018] | Includes bibliographical references and index.
Identifiers: LCCN 2017043052 | ISBN 9781498729413 (hardback : alk. paper) | ISBN 9781315120492 (ebook)
Subjects: LCSH: Solutions (Pharmacy) | Drugs--Solubility.
Classification: LCC RS201.S6 W38 2018 | DDC 615.1--dc23
LC record available at https://lccn.loc.gov/2017043052

Visit the Taylor & Francis Web site at
http://www.taylorandfrancis.com

and the CRC Press Web site at
http://www.crcpress.com

Contents

Preface to the First Edition

This book has its origin in a training course, "The Role of Drug Solubility in Formulation Development," offered by the American Association of Pharmaceutical Scientists, six years ago in Chicago. The course was designed to help young pharmaceutical scientists and pharmacy graduate students solve problems often encountered in dealing with water-insoluble drugs in their research and drug development programs, and it was chaired by Dr. Maureen Donovan from the University of Iowa College of Pharmacy, Iowa City, Iowa, with lectures by Dr. Steven Neau from University of Missouri-Kansas City College of Pharmacy, Kansas City, Missouri; Dr. Pramod Gupta from Abbott Laboratories, Chicago, Illinois; and myself, then working at American Cyanamid Company, New Jersey. Approximately one year after the course, I was approached by Interpharm Press to discuss the publication of a book on formulations of water-insoluble drugs.

As a pharmaceutical scientist working in the areas of drug discovery support, preformulation, and formulation at American Cyanamid and Abbott for a number of years, I have come to know the importance of utilizing solubilization techniques for solving drug insolubility problems in my daily work. I realize that the pharmaceutical industry has an urgent need for a collection of existing and up-to-date knowledge and techniques on the solubilization of water-insoluble drugs. The diligent work of all the contributors over the past years has made the book become a reality. I would like to thank them for all their hard work and sacrifices.

Many distinguished scholars in the fields of pharmaceuticals and related sciences have provided me with a lot of helpful discussion and valuable input during my editing of the book. I would like to take this opportunity to sincerely acknowledge these individuals for their much appreciated help:

> J.B. Cannon, PhD, Abbott Laboratories, Chicago, Illinois; P.P. Constantinides, PhD, Sonus Pharmaceuticals, Bothell, Washington DC; M.D. Donovan, PhD, University of Iowa, Iowa City, Iowa; J.L. Ford, PhD, Liverpool John Moors University, Liverpool, England; S.G. Frank, PhD, Ohio State University, Columbus, Ohio; J.K. Guillory, PhD, University of Iowa, Iowa City, Iowa; R.J.Y. Ho, PhD, University of Washington, Seattle, Washington; V. Kumar, PhD, University of Iowa, Iowa City, Iowa; M. Long, PhD, Abbott Laboratories, Chicago, Illinois; S.H. Neau, PhD, University of Missouri-Kansas City, Kansas City, Missouri; J.T. Rubino, PhD, American Home Products, Chicago, Illinois; A. Sinkula, PhD, West Pharmaceutical Services, West Whiteland Township, Pennsylvania; W.Q. Tong, PhD, Glaxo-Welcome, Inc., Brentford, UK; V.P. Torchilin, PhD, Northeastern University, Boston, Massachusetts; M.R. Violante, PhD, Medisperse; Y. Wei, PhD, R.P. Scherer; G. Zografi, PhD, University of Wisconsin, Madison, Wisconsin.

And last, but not the least, I would like to thank my wife, Ping Chen, my daughter, Catherine, and my son, Eric, for their love, understanding, support, and encouragement during my work on this book.

Rong (Ron) Liu

Preface to the Second Edition

It has been seven years since the book *Water-Insoluble Drug Formulation* was published in 2000. Both the publisher and I have received much positive feedback on the book from the readers since its publication. In the past decade, however, the field of water-insoluble drug delivery has seen much progress and advancement. Therefore, I felt obligated to the readers to update the book with the latest development in this field. In addition, I decided to broaden the scope of the book to include areas of the science encompassing pharmacokinetics, early development, regulations, manufacturing, and so forth in water-insoluble drugs, to make this book an even more complete and comprehensive tool for the users. It is for these reasons that I have decided to revise the book.

In the second edition of the book, chapters in the first edition have been updated (the chapter that described solid dispersion has been completely revised), and six new chapters have been added. The new chapters are as follows: "Water-Insoluble Drugs and Their Pharmacokinetic Behaviors;" "Regulatory Aspects of Dissolution for Low-Solubility Drug Products;" "Formulation Strategies and Practice Used for Drug Candidates with Water-Insoluble Properties for Toxicology, Biology, and Pharmacology Studies in Discovery Support;" "Emulsion, Microemulsion, and Lipid-Based Drug Delivery Systems for Drug Solubilization and Delivery in Oral Applications;" "Oral Modified-Release Drug Delivery for Water-Insoluble Drugs;" and "Scalable Manufacturing of Water-Insoluble Drug Products."

Besides acknowledging the critical review on various chapters by many distinguished scholars in the fields of pharmaceuticals and related sciences who were mentioned in the preface of the first edition, I would like to appreciate the following experts who have provided me with considerable amounts of helpful discussion and valuable input on the new chapters in the second edition: Parviz Mojaveria, PhD, FCP, Quintiles Inc., Durham, North Carolina; Ken Yamamoto, PhD, Pfizer Inc., New York; Marcus Brewster, PhD, Johnson & Johnson Company, New Brunswick, New Jersey; and Liang Dong, PhD, Johnson & Johnson Company, New Brunswick, New Jersey.

All the contributors and I hope the second edition will provide even more valuable information to the scientists who need help in dealing with water-insoluble drugs during their formulation development.

Rong (Ron) Liu

Preface to the Third Edition

In the year of 2000, the first edition of our book entitled *Water-Insoluble Drug Formulation* was published. Eight years later, in 2008, we provided the second edition of the book with updated information and additional six new chapters. We have continually received very positive feedback on our book during the last two decades. It gratified us to learn that this book has helped many scientists who are working on water-insoluble drugs either in industry or academia. Now another nine years have passed, new technologies have been invented, and new drug products containing water-insoluble drugs using advanced water-insoluble drug formulation technologies have been developed and launched in the marketplace. Meanwhile, the regulatory guidelines for the industry have also been advanced. Therefore, we decided to update this book again with the latest developments in this field.

In the third edition of this book, nearly all the chapters have been updated, especially Chapters 4, 10, 11, 13, 14, 17, 18, 20, and 22. New tables, figures, and the latest case studies were added. Chapter 20, "Pharmaceutical Powder Technology—ICH Q8 and Building the Pyramid of Knowledge," was almost completely rewritten with updated techniques.

Besides acknowledging all the contributors and review experts in the fields of pharmaceuticals and related sciences who were mentioned in the prefaces of the first two editions, I would like to appreciate the following experts who have provided great contributions to the update in the third edition: Joseph Boni, PhD, Pfizer Oncology; Isidoro Caraballo, PhD, University of Sevilla, Seville, Spain; Kun Cheng, PhD, University of Missouri-Kansas City, Kansas City, Missouri; Caly Chien, PhD, Janssen Research & Development, Raritan, New Jersey; Gerard M. Jensen, PhD, Gilead Sciences, Foster City, California; Peter Kleinebudde, PhD, Heinrich Heine University, Düsseldorf, Germany; Feng Qi, PhD, University of Missouri–Columbia, Columbia, Missouri; Robert G. Strickley, PhD, Gilead Sciences, Foster City, California; and Vicky Wang, PhD, Regeneron Pharmaceuticals Inc., Tarrytown, New York. I also highly appreciate Dr. Zhanguo Yue's contribution for coordinating with authors and the publishing company during preparation and publishing the third edition.

Finally, I would like to take this opportunity to express my gratitude and appreciation to my loving wife, Ping Chen, for her continuing support and understanding of my professional career. Also, to my family: my wife, Ping; my daughter, Catherine, and son-in-law, Dan; my son Eric; my lovely grandson, Sebastian; and my beautiful granddaughter, Elle; thank you so much for your love. I love you all very much!

All the contributors and I hope the third edition will continue to provide valuable information to the scientists who need help in dealing with water-insoluble drugs during their formulation development.

Rong (Ron) Liu

Editor

Rong (Ron) Liu, PhD, MBA, has been in the pharmaceutical industry for more than 25 years, presently leading AustarPharma LLC, Edison, New Jersey, and Guangzhou Bristol Drug Delivery Co., Ltd. Prior to his current role, Ron was employed at Bristol-Myers Squibb (BMS), New York, as a Director of Global Product Development for over 5 years. In his tenure, Ron has been responsible for pharmaceutical product development from exploratory development, preclinical, preformulation, drug delivery platform technologies, formulation, process, and scale-up manufacturing toward commercialization. Ron has led many successful commercial launches, including projects for which the R&D work was done in the U.S. R&D center. The fruits of these projects were transferred to BMS's Chinese Good Manufacturing Practice (GMP) facility in Shanghai for commercial manufacturing for the U.S. market. In addition, Ron worked closely with marketing staff and frequently participated in marketing activities. Through such activities, Ron received a sizeable amount of marketing experience. Prior to BMS, Ron also worked for Abbott Labs, Chicago, Illinois, as a manager in product development and represented Abbott to manage CMC-related activities for all projects of TAP (Taketa Abbott Pharmaceuticals). At Abbott, he has participated in several major commercial product developments, such as lansoprazole (Prevacid) and fenofibrate (TriCor). Ron has gained great experience in product life-cycle management. Previous to Abbott, Ron worked for Wyeth (previously Cyanamid and now Pfizer), where he contributed significantly from early development to full development. One of his key contributions was the development of injectable verteporfin liposomes (Visudyne), one of the several liposomal products approved by the FDA. Ron was the sole inventor of the patented liposomal technology for thus far the biggest (half a billion dollars in annual sales) liposomal product in the United States. During his years in the pharmaceutical industry, he has gained extensive experiences in drug delivery technologies and pharmaceutical dosage innovations. One aspect of his special expertise and research interests is water-insoluble drug delivery. He is the editor and author of the book *Water-Insoluble Drug Formulation*, published by CRC Press. Ron is an inventor for more than 15 issued and pending drug delivery technology and formulation patents. In addition, Ron has been a Grant Reviewer for NIH in Drug Delivery, Product Development and Manufacturing. Ron graduated with a PhD in Pharmaceutics from the University of Iowa, Iowa City, Iowa, in 1991 and an MBA in Marketing from Rutgers University, New Brunswick, New Jersey, in 2002.

Contributors

Gabriele Betz
Mozart Pharmacy
Mozartstr, Germany

John B. Cannon
University of South Carolina at Beaufort
Bluffton, South Carolina

Yisheng Chen
Novast Laboratories (China), Ltd.
Nantong, People's Republic of China

Rose-Marie Dannenfelser
Norvartis Pharmaceuticals
East Hanover, New Jersey

Jinquan Dong
Johnson & Johnson
Raritan, New Jersey

Silvia Kocova El-Arini
National Research Centre
Cairo, Egypt

M. Laird Forrest
Department of Pharmaceutical Chemistry
University of Kansas
Lawrence, Kansas

Stephen J. Franklin
Pfizer Essential Health R&D
Lake Forest, Illinois

Liangran Guo
AustarPharma, LLC
Edison, New Jersey

Pramod Gupta
Spectrum Pharmaceuticals
Irvine, California

Shanker L. Gupta
Pharmaceutical Research Branch
Developmental Therapeutics Program
Division of Cancer Treatment
Diagnosis National Cancer Institute
National Institutes of Health
Bethesda, Maryland

Simerdeep Singh Gupta
Teva Pharmaceuticals USA Inc.
Salt Lake City, Utah

Lian-Feng Huang
Johnson & Johnson
Raritan, New Jersey

Richard (Ruey-ching) Hwang
Pfizer, Inc.
Ann Arbor, Michigan

Michael J. Jozwiakowski
AMAG Pharmaceuticals
Waltham, Massachusetts

Shyam B. Karki
Johnson & Johnson
Raritan, New Jersey

Glen S. Kwon
Madison School of Pharmacy
University of Wisconsin
Madison, Wisconsin

Robert W. Lee
Pharmaceutical Development
Novavax, Inc.
Malvern, Pennsylvania

Sau Lawrence Lee
FDA Office of Generic Drugs
Derwood, Maryland

Hans Leuenberger
AMIFICAS Ltd.
Oviedo, Florida

Shaoling Li
Alza Corporation
Johnson & Johnson
Mountain View, California

Shoufeng Li
Norvartis Pharmaceuticals
East Hanover, New Jersey

Wei (William) Li
Guangzhou Bristol Drug Delivery Co., Ltd.
Guangzhou, China

Xiang (Lisa) Li
AustarPharma, LLC
Edison, New Jersey

Robert A. Lionberger
FDA Office of Generic Drugs
Derwood, Maryland

Rong (Ron) Liu
AustarPharma, LLC
Edison, New Jersey

Nikhil C. Loka
Ascent Pharmaceuticals
Central Islip, New York

and

Philadelphia College of Pharmacy
Philadelphia, Pennsylvania

Michelle A. Long
Abbvie Inc.
North Chicago, Illinois

James McShane
Pharmaceutical and Analytical Research and
    Development
Eisai Inc.
Research Triangle Park, North Carolina

Paul B. Myrdal
University of Arizona
Tucson, Arizona

Steven H. Neau
Philadelphia College of Pharmacy
Philadelphia, Pennsylvania

Sophia Y. L. Paspal
Halozyme Therapeutics, Inc.
San Diego, California

Nitin P. Pathak
Pfizer, Inc.
New York, New York

Xiaohong Qi
AustarPharma, LLC
Edison, New Jersey

Kalyan K. Saripella
Douglas Pharma US Inc.
Warminster, Pennsylvania

Pradeep Sathe
FDA Office of Generic Drugs
Derwood, Maryland

Abu T. M. Serajuddin
Novartis Pharmaceutical Corporation
East Hanover, New Jersey

J. Michael Shaw
Elan Pharmaceuticals Technologies
King of Prussia, Pennsylvania

Dinesh B. Shenoy
Formulation Development Novavax, Inc.
Rockville, Maryland

Yi Shi
Abbvie Inc.
North Chicago, Illinois

S. Esmail Tabibi
Pharmaceutical Research Branch
Developmental Therapeutics Program
Division of Cancer Treatment
Diagnosis National Cancer Institute
National Institutes of Health
Bethesda, Maryland

Wei-Qin (Tony) Tong
AustarPharma, LLC
Edison, New Jersey

Jay S. Trivedi
Patrin Pharma
Skokie, Illinois

Madhav Vasanthavada
Novartis Pharmaceuticals Corporation
East Hanover, New Jersey

Nuo (Nolan) Wang
AustarPharma, LLC
Edison, New Jersey

Hong Wen
U.S. Food and Drug Administration
Silver Spring, Maryland

Ray W. Wood
Pharmaceutical and Analytical Research and
    Development
Eisai Inc.
Research Triangle Park, North Carolina

Xiaobing Xiong
Wake Forest University School of Medicine
Winston-Salem, North Carolina

Lawrence X. Yu
FDA Office of Generic Drugs
Derwood, Maryland

Zhanguo Yue
AustarPharma, LLC
Edison, New Jersey

Di (Doris) Zhang
AustarPharma, LLC
Edison, New Jersey

Zhihong (John) Zhang
AustarPharma, LLC
Edison, New Jersey

Honghui Zhou
Global Clinical Pharmacology
Janssen Research and Development, LLC
Spring House, Pennsylvania

Hao Zhu
Office of Clinical Pharmacology
U.S. Food and Drug Administration
Silver Spring, Maryland

1 Introduction

Rong (Ron) Liu

"These new compounds, like rocks, never dissolve in water." It sounds so familiar to you, does it not? Product development scientists often encounter significant difficulties in solving the problem of poor water solubility of drug candidates in the development of pharmaceutical dosage forms (Sweetana and Akers, 1996; Yamashita and Furubayashi, 1998; Willmann et al., 2004; Di et al., 2006). Poor *drug-like* properties of lead compounds led to ineffective absorption in the site of administration, which has been designated as an important part of the high clinical failure due to poor pharmacokinetics (Caldwell et al., 2001; Kerns and Di, 2003; Hartmann et al., 2006). However, these kinds of compounds represent an increasing proportion of newly discovered drug candidates. It is commonly recognized in the pharmaceutical industry that on average more than 40% of newly discovered drug candidates are poorly water soluble. Recently, it was reported that the percentage could be as high as 90% for new chemical entities (Kalepu and Nekkanti, 2015) and 75% for compounds under development (Rodriguez-Aller et al., 2015). As a matter of fact, poorly soluble compounds represent 40% of the top 200 oral drugs marketed in the United States, and more than one-third of the drugs listed in the U.S. Pharmacopeia fall into the poorly water-soluble or water-insoluble categories (Pace et al., 1999; Takagi et al., 2006; Rodriguez-Aller et al., 2015).

Interpretations of the term *water-insoluble drug* can vary depending on an individual's definition. According to USP 40/NF 35, *slightly soluble* means that "one part of solute can be solubilized by 100 to 1000 parts of solvent." If water is the solvent, then the water solubility of a *slightly soluble* drug can range from 10 mg/mL down to 1 mg/mL. If the same assumption is applied, *very slightly soluble* and *practically insoluble or insoluble* can be translated to 1 mg/mL down to 100 μg/mL, and equal to or less than 100 μg/mL, respectively. Therefore, in the broader definition, the term *water-insoluble drug* in this book is defined as the aqueous solubility of a drug that falls into the range of *slightly soluble* and below (i.e., <10 mg/mL). In the narrower definition, the term *water-insoluble drug* in this book indicates that the aqueous solubility of a drug belongs to the category of *practically insoluble or insoluble* (i.e., <100 μg/mL).

In the past two decades, with the applications of genomics, high-throughput screening, robotics, combinatorial chemistry, computational modeling, informatics, and miniaturization to the drug discovery area, far more drug candidates than ever have been generated for development (Lipper, 1999; Hann and Oprea, 2004). However, as a result of the preferred pharmacological activity process of drug discovery, which attempts to maximize the activity, biopharmaceutical or *drug-like* properties of new drug candidates, including water solubility, tend to suffer (Yamashita and Furubayashi, 1998; Lipinski, 2000; Caldwell et al., 2001). Although the incompatible work partnership between the preclinical groups and the discovery groups has been improved in many companies in the recent years (Alanine et al., 2003), it is noteworthy that a compound with great receptor affinity and selectivity, but with poor *drug-like* properties for formulation or delivery, is still rarely regarded as ineligible to enter development. This viewpoint has prevailed in industry despite the potential for a compound's poor *drug-like* properties to be a major delay on the development timeline (Lipper, 1999; Kola and Landis, 2004). Compounds optimized solely on the basis of receptor-based potency, depending on the nature of the receptor, are usually hydrophobic or water insoluble. Therefore, many problems have recently been experienced in the early formulation development of drugs (Sweetana and Akers, 1996; Corswant et al., 1998; Pace et al., 1999; Di et al., 2006). Water insolubility can postpone or completely halt new drug development, and can prevent the much needed reformulation of currently marketed products (Pace et al., 1999; Caldwell et al., 2001; Hartmann et al., 2006).

Besides the newly discovered drug candidates, modification formulations of existing drugs are also gaining importance. Significant numbers of commercial insoluble drugs with improved formulations that provide for faster dissolution and enhanced bioavailability were filed as New Drug Applications (NDA) under 505(b)(2), which is relatively profitable strategy for pharmaceutical companies.

Through decades of diligent and intelligent research by pharmaceutical scientists, many techniques dealing with the formulation issues of water-insoluble drugs have been developed and accumulated in the pharmaceutical literature. A book that systematically described the techniques used for water-insoluble drug formulations could be a real benefit to development scientists. This was the primary motivation that led to the publication of *Water-Insoluble Drug Formulations* in 2000 and the updated second edition with additional content in 2008. During the last decade, various insoluble drug delivery technologies, especially nanoparticle-based technologies, bloomed in both academic and industrial settings, and several platforms were successfully adopted by many pharmaceutical companies. These developments have led to this updated third edition of *Water-Insoluble Drug Formulations*.

The aim of this book is to provide a handy reference for pharmaceutical scientists in the handling of formulation issues related to water-insoluble drugs. In addition, this book may be useful to pharmacy and chemistry undergraduate students, and to pharmaceutical and biopharmaceutical graduate students, to enhance their knowledge in the techniques of drug solubilization and dissolution enhancement. This book covers topics ranging from solubility theories, solubility prediction models, the aspects of preformulation, biopharmaceutics, pharmacokinetics, regulatory, and discovery support of water-insoluble drugs to various techniques used in developing delivery systems for water-insoluble drugs. In general, each chapter describing a solubilizing system starts with the brief theoretical background associated with the particular system, followed by practical discussions of industrial experiences, and concluded by examples or case studies.

The chapter "Solubility Theories" provides a systematic review of existing theories regarding the interactions between solutes and solvents. The chapter "Prediction of Solubility" may be helpful to those drug discovery chemists and pharmaceutical scientists who work in the discovery support area to design new drug candidates with improved aqueous solubility before they are synthesized. The chapters "Preformulation Aspects of Water-Insoluble Compounds" and "Water-Insoluble Drugs and Their Pharmacokinetic Behaviors" can be used by a formulator (especially an inexperienced one) to understand the particulars of the physicochemical, biopharmaceutical, and pharmacokinetic properties of a water-insoluble drug. When dealing with lead compounds with poor *drug-like* properties in early formulations, pharmaceutical scientists can refer to the chapter "Formulation Strategies and Practice Used for Drug Candidates with Water-Insoluble Properties for Toxicology, Biology, and Pharmacology Studies in Discovery Support" to obtain different formulation approaches to support the animal studies in toxicology, pharmacology, and pharmacokinetics. The chapter "Regulatory Aspects of Dissolution for Low Solubility Drug Products" provides some very useful guidelines for dissolution from the Food and Drug Administration (FDA) perspective. Some preformulation and exploratory solubilization experiments, guided by these chapters, are usually necessary before the design of a water-insoluble drug formulation.

For water-insoluble drugs with high permeability or Class II drugs in FDA's Biopharmaceutics Classification System (BCS), drug absorption in the gastrointestinal (GI) tract is primarily limited by drug dissolution rate (Amidon et al., 1995; McGilveray, 1996; Yu et al., 2002; Pepsin et al., 2016). Therefore, the formulation work of oral solid dosage forms for Class II compounds should focus on the enhancement of dissolution rate. Dissolution rate enhancement and related techniques for the development of oral solid dosage forms can be found in the chapters "Alteration of the Solid State of the Drug Substance: Polymorphs, Solvates, and Amorphous Forms," "Development of Solid Dispersions for Poorly Water-Soluble Drugs," "Particle Size Reduction," "Pharmaceutical Powder Technology—ICH (the International Conference on Harmonisation) Q8 and Building the Pyramid of Knowledge," "Prodrugs for Improved Aqueous Solubility," "Pharmaceutical Salts," "Applications of Complexation in the Formulation of Insoluble Compounds," "Liposomes in Solubilization," "Micellization and Drug Solubility Enhancement," and "Polymeric Micelles in Water-Insoluble Drug Delivery."

Both dispersion and solution systems can be used to formulate oral liquid dosage forms to enhance bioavailability for water-insoluble drugs (Pouton, 1997; Yamashita and Furubayashi, 1998; Porter and Charman, 2001; Wasan, 2001). These systems can also be used to develop solubilizing systems for parenteral dosage forms to deliver water-insoluble drugs (Sweetana and Akers, 1996; Corswant et al., 1998; Pace et al., 1999; Sarker, 2005). Formulation techniques used to enhance bioavailability for oral liquid dosage forms and to solubilize water-insoluble drugs for parenteral dosage forms can be found in the chapters "Solubilization Using Cosolvent Approach," "Micellization and Drug Solubility Enhancement," "Polymeric Micelles in Water-Insoluble Drug Delivery," "Liposomes in Solubilization," "Particle Size Reduction," "Emulsions, Microemulsions, and Lipid-Based Drug Delivery Systems for Drug Solubilization and Delivery (Parenteral and Oral Applications)," "Soft Gelatin Capsules Development," "Prodrugs for Improved Aqueous Solubility," and "Pharmaceutical Salts." The chapter "Oral Modified-Release Drug Delivery for Water-Insoluble Drugs" provides a systemic review on various controlled-release technologies, which may be suitable to be used on longer-lasting applications of water-insoluble drugs. Finally, the chapter "Scalable Manufacturing of Water-Insoluble Drug Products" provides some useful discussion in process development, especially for large scale-up manufacturing of finished dosage forms of water-insoluble drugs.

In many cases in drug development, the solubility of some leads is extremely low. Fast dissolution rate of many drug delivery systems, for example, particle size reduction, may not be translated into good GI absorption. The oral absorption of these molecules is usually limited by solubility (Willmann et al., 2004; Qiu et al., 2016). In the case of solubility limited absorption, creating supersaturation in the GI fluids for this type of insoluble drugs is very critical as supersaturation may greatly improve oral absorption (Tanno et al., 2004; Shanker, 2005; Taylor and Zhang, 2016). The techniques to create the so-called supersaturation in the GI fluids may include microemulsions, emulsions, liposomes, complexations, polymeric micelles, and conventional micelles, which can be found in some chapters in the book.

There are still some drug delivery strategies under wide investigation in academic settings, including mesoporous silica particles (Latify et al., 2017), graphene oxide (Liu et al., 2008), other inorganic particles (Yue et al., 2011), all kinds of sensitive organic particles (Guo and Huang, 2014), and targeted or intracellular delivery strategies (Mitragotri et al., 2014). However, these strategies still have a long way until clinic, with lots of challenges to be figured out. The related studies are discussed in this book.

It is the authors' hope that the concepts and techniques described in this book will lead to the development of improved dosage forms for water-insoluble drugs, and thus enhance the therapeutic advantage of this crucial class of drugs.

REFERENCES

Alanine, A., M. Nettekoven, E. Roberts, and A. W. Thomas. 2003. Lead generation—Enhancing the success of drug discovery by investing in the hit to lead process. *Combinatorial Chemistry & High Throughput Screening* 6: 51–66.

Amidon, G. L., H. Lennernas, V. P. Shah, and J. R. Crison. 1995. A theoretical basis for biopharmaceutic drug classification: The correlation of in vitro drug product dissolution and in vitro bioavailability. *Pharmaceutical Research* 12: 413–420.

Caldwell, G. W., D. M. Ritchie, J. A. Masucci, W. Hageman, and Z. Yan. 2001. The new pre-preclinical paradigm: Compound optimization in early and late phase drug discovery. *Current Topics in Medicinal Chemistry* 1: 353–366.

Corswant, C. V., P. Thoren, and S. Engstrom. 1998. Triglyceride-based microemulsion for intravenous administration of sparingly soluble substances. *Journal of Pharmaceutical Sciences* 87: 200–208.

Di, L., E. H. Kerns, S. Q. Li, and S. L. Petusky. 2006. High throughput microsomal stability assay for insoluble compounds. *International Journal of Pharmaceutics* 317: 54–60.

Guo, S. and L. Huang. 2014. Nanoparticles containing insoluble drug for cancer therapy. *Biotechnology Advances* 32(4): 778–788.

Hann, M. M. and T. I. Oprea. 2004. Pursuing the leadlikeness concept in pharmaceutical research. *Current Opinion in Chemical Biology* 8: 255–263.

Hartmann, T., J. Schmitt, C. Röhring, D. Nimptsch, J. Noller, and C. Mohr. 2006. ADME related profiling in 96 and 384 well plate format—A novel and robust HT-assay for the determination of lipophilicity and serum albumin binding. *Current Drug Delivery* 3: 181–192.

Kalepu, S. and V. Nekkanti. 2015. Insoluble drug delivery strategies: Review of recent advances and business prospects. *Acta Pharmaceutica Sinica B* 5(5): 442–453.

Kerns, E. H. and L. Di. 2003. Pharmaceutical profiling in drug discovery. *Drug Discovery Today* 8: 316–323.

Kola, I. and J. Landis. 2004. Can the pharmaceutical industry reduce attrition rates? *Nature Reviews Drug Discovery* 3: 711–715.

Latify, L., S. Sohrabnezhad, and M. Hadavi. 2017. Mesoporous silica as a support for poorly soluble drug: Influence of pH and amino group on the drug release. *Microporous and Mesoporous Materials* 250: 148–157.

Lipinski, C. A. 2000. Drug-like properties and the causes of poor solubility and poor permeability. *Journal of Pharmaceutical and Toxicological Methods* 44: 235–249.

Lipper, R. A. 1999. *E. pluribus* product. *Modern Drug Discovery* 2: 55–60.

Liu, Z., J. T. Robinson, X. Sun, and H. Dai. 2008. PEGylated nanographene oxide for delivery of water-insoluble cancer drugs. *Journal of the American Chemical Society* 130(33): 10876–10877.

McGilveray, I. J. 1996. Overview of workshop: In vitro dissolution of immediate release dosage forms: Development of in vivo relevance and quality control issues. *Drug Information Journal* 30: 1029–1037.

Mitragotri, S., P. A. Burke, and R. Langer. 2014. Overcoming the challenges in administering biopharmaceuticals: Formulation and delivery strategies. *Nature Reviews Drug Discovery* 13(9): 655–672.

Pace, S. N., G. W. Pace, I. Parikh, and A. K. Mishra. 1999. Novel injectable formulations of insoluble drugs. *Pharmaceutical Technology* 23: 116–134.

Pepsin, X. J., T. R. Flanagan, D. J. Holt, A. Eidelman, D. Treacy, and C. E. Rowlings. 2016. Justification of drug product dissolution rate and drug substance particle size specifications based on absorption PBPK modeling for Lesinurad immediate release tablets. *Molecular Pharmaceutics* 13(9): 3256–3269.

Porter, C. J. H. and W. N. Charman. 2001. In vitro assessment of oral lipid based formulations. *Advanced Drug Delivery Review* 50: S127–S147.

Pouton, C. W. 1997. Formulation of self-emulsifying drug delivery systems. *Advanced Drug Delivery Reviews* 25: 47–58.

Qiu, Y., Y. Chen, G. G. Zhang, L. Yu, and R. V. Mantri (Eds.). 2016. *Developing Solid Oral Dosage Forms: Pharmaceutical Theory and Practice*. London, UK: Academic Press.

Rodriguez-Aller, M., D. Guillarme, J. L. Veuthey, and R. Gurny. 2015. Strategies for formulating and delivering poorly water-soluble drugs. *Journal of Drug Delivery Science and Technology* 30: 342–351.

Sarker, D. K. 2005. Engineering of nanoemulsions for drug delivery. *Cancer Drug Delivery* 2: 297–310.

Shanker, R. M. 2005. Current concepts in the science of solid dispersion. *2nd Annual Simonelli Conference in Pharmaceutical Sciences*, June 9, Long Island University, Brookville, NY.

Sweetana, S. and M. J. Akers. 1996. Solubility principles and practices for parenteral drug dosage from development. *PDA Journal of Pharmaceutical Science & Technology* 50: 330–342.

Takagi, T., C. Ramachandran, M. Bermejo, S. Yamashita, L. X. Yu, and G. L. Amidon. 2006. A provisional biopharmaceutical classification of the top 200 oral drug products in the United States, Great Britain, Spain, and Japan. *Molecular Pharmaceutics* 3(6): 631–643.

Tanno, F., Y. Nishiyama, H. Kokubo, and S. Obara. 2004. Evaluation of hypromellose acetate succinate (HPMCAS) as a carrier in solid dispersions. *Drug Development and Industrial Pharmacy* 30: 9–17.

Taylor, L. S. and G. G. Zhang. 2016. Physical chemistry of supersaturated solutions and implications for oral absorption. *Advanced Drug Delivery Reviews* 101: 122–142.

Wasan, K. M. 2001. Formulation and physiological and biopharmaceutical issues in the development of oral lipid-based drug delivery systems. *Drug Development and Industrial Pharmacy* 27: 267–276.

Willmann, S., W. Schmitt, J. Keldenich, J. Lipert, and J. B. Dressman. 2004. A physiological model for the estimation of the fraction dose absorbed in humans. *Journal of Medicinal Chemistry* 47: 4022–4031.

Yamashita, S. and T. Furubayashi. 1998. In vitro–in vivo correlations: Application to water insoluble drugs. *Bulletin Technique Gattefossé* 91: 25–31.

Yu, L. X., G. L. Amidon, J. E. Polli, H. Zhao, M. U. Mehta, D. P. Conner, V. P. Shah, L. J. Lesko, M. L. Chen, and V. H. L. Lee. 2002. Biopharmaceutics classification system: The scientific basis for biowaiver extension. *Pharmaceutical Research* 19: 921–925.

Yue, Z. G., W. Wei, Z. X. You, Q. Z. Yang, H. Yue, Z. G. Su, and G. H. Ma. 2011. Iron oxide nanotubes for magnetically guided delivery and pH-activated release of insoluble anticancer drugs. *Advanced Functional Materials* 21(18): 3446–3453.

2 Solubility Theory

Steven H. Neau

CONTENTS

INTRODUCTION

Solubility is the concentration of the solute in a solution when equilibrium exists between the pure solute phase and the solution phase (Huang and Tong, 2004). At low concentrations, solubility is difficult to measure analytically, and at high concentrations, solubility is not an issue in the discovery process (Johnson and Zheng, 2006). If drug solubility is greater than 65 μg/mL, Lipinski et al. (1997) claimed that the absorption of the drug will not be limited by solubility, but a solubility of less than 10 μg/mL will introduce bioavailability issues. Knowledge of the solubility of a drug in water can be critical in formulating products, developing analytical methods, and evaluating drug transport or distribution problems. The approaches presented in this chapter are ideal solution theory, regular solution theory, and the Hansen solubility approach. Of these three, the only one that was developed to describe solutions involving polar species was the Hansen approach. As the reader will discover, however, the Hansen approach is principally based on regular solution theory, which, in turn, was derived from ideal solution theory. Thus, one cannot consider the Hansen solubility approach without some background in the previous theoretical discussions of solubility behavior.

This chapter begins with a description of ideal solution theory because ideal behavior is the reference point by which all other solution behavior is judged. Understanding the properties of real solutions relies on the ability to describe why particular behavior is nonideal. Regular solution theory best describes solution behavior of nonelectrolytes in nonpolar solvents where the enthalpy of mixing is not negligible. The Hansen approach opens up the possibility of describing enthalpic contributions resulting from interactions involving dipoles and hydrogen bonding. It can therefore be applied with some success to the description and prediction of solution behavior involving polar solutes in polar media.

IDEAL SOLUTIONS

THEORY

Entropy, which is a measure of disorder, is the driving force for mixing solutes and solvents to form solutions because there is an increase in the randomness of the molecules of both the solvent and the solute when they mix to form a solution. If the process is somewhat endothermic, a chemical will not readily dissolve if the available increase in the entropy contribution to the change in free energy does not exceed the enthalpy increase. The expression describing the ideal entropy of mixing for a binary system of a single liquid solute in a solvent, ΔS_{mix}, in terms of mole fractions in the solution, X, is:

$$\Delta S_{mix} = -R\left(n_1 \ln X_1^i + n_2 \ln X_2^i\right) \tag{2.1}$$

where the subscript convention is 1 for the solvent and 2 for the solute, the superscript i indicates that ideal conditions hold, n is the number of moles, and R is the ideal gas law constant (Lewis and Randall, 1961).

The derivation of this equation is based on the statistical mixing of the two components, and the assumptions of random molecular mixing, essentially equal molecular sizes of solute and solvent, no aggregation of solute molecules in solution, and no solvent penetration into the solute phase, that is, solvent molecules would not be found as components in the solute phase exposed to the solution. If the molar volumes of the solute and solvent are not equal, but there is sufficient thermal agitation to accomplish the maximum entropy of mixing, Equation 2.1 still holds (Hildebrand and Scott, 1950). Since the mole fractions must be less than 1, this change in entropy on mixing the solution is always positive and contributes to the spontaneity of solution formation. An interesting feature of ideal solutions involving liquids is that there is no volume change on mixing, the final solution volume being the sum of the volumes of the liquid components. For an ideal solution consisting of a solid dissolved in a liquid solvent, the final volume would equal the sum of the volume occupied by the solvent plus the volume that would be occupied by the mass of solid that has become solute when it has been supercooled to the solution temperature.

If we consider the partial molal entropy of solution with respect to the solute, Equation 2.1 becomes:

$$\Delta \bar{S}_{mix,2} = -R \ln X_2^i \tag{2.2}$$

In the event that the molar volumes of solute and solvent are not comparable, and the thermal agitation is not adequate to achieve maximum entropy of mixing, a nonideal entropy of mixing exists (Bustamante et al., 1989). Two equations that account for the nonideal entropy of mixing have been derived by considering the partial molal volume, $\bar{V}$, and the volume fraction, ϕ, occupied by each solution component. The first was developed by Flory and Huggins (Hildebrand, 1949; Kertes, 1965):

$$\Delta \bar{S}_{mix,2} = -R\left[\ln \phi_2 + \phi_1\left(1 - \frac{\bar{V}_2}{\bar{V}_1}\right)\right] \tag{2.3}$$

The second was introduced by Huyskens and Haulait-Pirson (1985):

$$\Delta \bar{S}_{mix,2} = -R\left[\ln \phi_2 + 0.5\phi_1\left(1 - \frac{\bar{V}_2}{\bar{V}_1}\right) - 0.5\ln\left(\phi_2 + \phi_1\frac{\bar{V}_2}{\bar{V}_1}\right)\right] \tag{2.4}$$

Either of these expressions can be substituted for the ideal partial molal entropy of mixing, as defined in Equation 2.2. The Flory–Huggins approach, for example, has been used to improve the prediction of the solubility of sulfamethoxypyridazine (Bustamante et al., 1989) and temazepam (Richardson et al., 1992) in a wide variety of solvents, including water.

If the interactions between solute and solute molecules are comparable in type and magnitude to those between solute and solvent molecules and between solvent and solvent molecules, the enthalpy of mixing is negligible. If the enthalpy of mixing a liquid solute in a solvent is negligible, and can be assumed to be zero, the solution is considered ideal, and the equation:

$$\Delta \bar{H}_{mix,2} = 0 \tag{2.5}$$

holds. If we are concerned with the partial molal changes on mixing with respect to the solute, the familiar Gibbs–Helmholtz relation:

$$\Delta G = \Delta H - T \Delta S \tag{2.6}$$

becomes:

$$\Delta \bar{G}_{mix,2} = \bar{H}_{mix,2} - T \bar{S}_{mix,2} \tag{2.7}$$

Substituting for the partial molal change in molar enthalpy of mixing with respect to the solute (Equation 2.5) gives:

$$\Delta \bar{G}_{mix,2} = - T \bar{S}_{mix,2} \tag{2.8}$$

and then substituting for the partial molal entropy of mixing with respect to the solute (Equation 2.2) gives:

$$\Delta \bar{G}_{mix,2} = R \ln X_2^i \tag{2.9}$$

By thermodynamic definition:

$$\Delta \bar{G}_{mix,2} = RT \ln a_2 \tag{2.10}$$

where a_2 is the activity of the solute in solution. It therefore follows from Equations 2.9 and 2.10 that the mole fraction equals the activity of the solute in solution when the solution is ideal.

Consider the case of an ideal solution involving a solute, a crystalline material at the solution temperature, that is now dissolved in a liquid solvent. Even though the partial molal enthalpy of mixing is still zero because it is an ideal solution, there is an enthalpy requirement to overcome the intermolecular forces of attraction in the crystal structure. The van't Hoff equation (Adamson, 1979) is:

$$\frac{\partial \left(\dfrac{\Delta G}{T} \right)}{\partial T} = - \frac{\Delta H}{T^2} \tag{2.11}$$

Using the superscript sc to refer to the transition from crystalline solid to supercooled liquid at a constant temperature, substituting:

$$\Delta \bar{G}_2^{sc} = - RT \ln a_2 \tag{2.12}$$

for ΔG, and acknowledging that the molar enthalpy of fusion is the change in enthalpy for this transition (Hildebrand and Scott, 1962) gives:

$$\frac{d \ln a_2}{dT} = \frac{\Delta \bar{H}_f}{RT^2} \tag{2.13}$$

Integration between the melting point, T_m, and the solution temperature, T (Kertes, 1965) gives:

$$\ln a_2 = -\frac{\bar{H}_f}{RT_m}\left(\frac{T_m - T}{T}\right) \tag{2.14}$$

The mole fraction solubility can be substituted for the activity, keeping in mind that this is acceptable with an ideal solution:

$$\ln X_2^i = -\frac{\bar{H}_f}{RT_m}\left(\frac{T_m - T}{T}\right) \tag{2.15}$$

Therefore, the mole fraction ideal solubility of a crystalline solute in a saturated ideal solution is a function of three experimental parameters: the melting point, the molar enthalpy of fusion, and the solution temperature. Equation 2.15 can be expressed as a linear relationship with respect to the inverse of the solution temperature:

$$\ln X_2^i = -\frac{\Delta \bar{H}_f}{RT} + \frac{\Delta \bar{H}_f}{RT_m} \tag{2.16}$$

where $(\Delta \bar{H}_f / RT_m)$ is assumed to be a constant.

The general rules regarding the influence of the melting point and the molar enthalpy of fusion are the greater the melting point, the lower the ideal solubility, and the greater the molar enthalpy of fusion, the lower the ideal solubility. In the case of a crystalline solute, the molar enthalpy of fusion determines the temperature sensitivity. One of the easiest ways to see this is to plot the mole fraction solubility as a log-linear function of the inverse of the solution temperature (Figure 2.1). This linear relationship is predicted in Equation 2.16. The slope, therefore, can be derived mathematically from the expression:

$$\frac{d \ln X_2^i}{d\left(\frac{1}{T}\right)} = -\frac{\Delta \bar{H}_f}{R} \tag{2.17}$$

Thus, it can be seen that the greater the molar enthalpy of fusion, the greater the increase in solubility as the solution temperature is increased, and a steeper slope would be evident in a plot such as Figure 2.1. Note that for a real solution, the enthalpy of solution, designated $\Delta \bar{H}_{sol'n}$, substitutes for the enthalpy of fusion in Equation 2.17. The enthalpy of solution includes the enthalpy of fusion and the enthalpy associated with mixing of the hypothetical supercooled liquid form of the solute mass with the solvent.

MOLAR HEAT CAPACITY

The molar enthalpy for the transition from a solid to a supercooled liquid is not a constant with respect to temperature. The heat capacity of the solid and of the supercooled liquid forms of the solute at constant pressure influence the magnitude of the molar enthalpy for this transition at temperatures below the melting point. The heat capacity at constant pressure, C_p, is the amount of energy in the form of heat, Δq, required to raise the temperature of a particular material by a particular amount, ΔT (Dave et al., 2014):

$$C_p = \frac{\partial q}{\partial T} \sim \frac{\Delta q}{\Delta T} \tag{2.18}$$

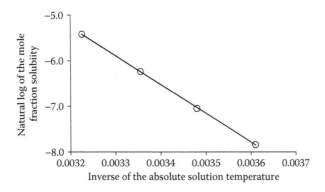

FIGURE 2.1   van't Hoff plot of ideal mole fraction solubility as a function of the inverse solution temperature.

The molar heat capacity at constant pressure, $\bar{C}_p$, would be the heat capacity divided by the amount of that material in moles, n, expressed as follows to show the relevance of the molar enthalpy of fusion:

$$\bar{C}_p = \left[\left(\frac{\partial \bar{H}_f}{\partial T} \right)_p \right] / n \tag{2.19}$$

It is frequently assumed that the heat capacity of the solid at constant pressure, $\bar{C}_{p,s}$, and the molar heat capacity of its liquid form at constant pressure, $\bar{C}_{p,l}$, are nearly constant, or that they change at the same rate with a change in temperature. In either case, the molar differential heat capacity, defined as:

$$\Delta \bar{C}_p = \bar{C}_{p,l} - \bar{C}_{p,s} \tag{2.20}$$

would be a constant. At these temperatures, then, the total enthalpy and entropy changes can be determined by simply acknowledging the contribution of the molar differential heat capacity to each of the solid to supercooled liquid thermodynamic parameters:

$$\Delta \bar{H}_2^{sc} = \Delta \bar{H}_f - \Delta \bar{C}_p \left(T_m - T \right) \tag{2.21}$$

$$\Delta \bar{S}_2^{sc} = \Delta \bar{S}_f - \Delta \bar{C}_p \ln \left(\frac{T}{T_m} \right) \tag{2.22}$$

Substitution into Equation 2.6 would then give:

$$\Delta \bar{G}_2^{sc} = \Delta \bar{H}_f - \Delta \bar{C}_p \left(T_m - T \right) - T \left[\Delta \bar{S}_f - \Delta \bar{C}_p \ln \left(\frac{T}{T_m} \right) \right] \tag{2.23}$$

If we consider the thermodynamic parameters at the melting point, Equation 2.6 becomes:

$$\Delta \bar{G}_f = \Delta \bar{H}_f - T_m \Delta \bar{S}_f \tag{2.24}$$

Fusion can be considered a reversible process at the melting point, and $\Delta \bar{G}_f$ as a result would be zero. Therefore, from rearrangement of Equation 2.24 comes the relationship:

$$\Delta \bar{S}_f = \frac{\Delta \bar{H}_f}{T_m} \tag{2.25}$$

Substituting this for the molar entropy of fusion in Equation 2.23, and rearranging, gives:

$$\Delta \bar{G}_2^{sc} = \Delta \bar{H}_f \left(\frac{T_m - T}{T_m} \right) - \Delta \bar{C}_p T \left[\left(\frac{T_m - T}{T} \right) + \ln \left(\frac{T}{T_m} \right) \right] \tag{2.26}$$

Substituting for $\Delta \bar{G}_2^{sc}$ using Equation 2.12 gives:

$$-RT \ln a_2 = \Delta \bar{H}_f \left(\frac{T_m - T}{T_m} \right) - \Delta \bar{C}_p T \left[\left(\frac{T_m - T}{T} \right) + \ln \left(\frac{T}{T_m} \right) \right] \tag{2.27}$$

Dividing through by $(-RT)$ and substituting the mole fraction solubility for the activity, which is acceptable since this is an ideal solution, one obtains:

$$\ln X_2^i = -\frac{\Delta \bar{H}_f}{RT_m} \left(\frac{T_m - T}{T} \right) + \frac{\Delta \bar{C}_p}{R} \left[\left(\frac{T_m - T}{T} \right) + \ln \left(\frac{T}{T_m} \right) \right] \tag{2.28}$$

which is a more exact expression for the ideal solubility of a crystalline material in a liquid solvent.

To simplify this expression, one of two assumptions is ordinarily made regarding the molar differential heat capacity. The first assumption is that $\Delta \bar{C}_p$ is negligible, and a practical approach is to set it equal to zero, which gives Equation 2.15:

$$\ln X_2^i = -\frac{\Delta \bar{H}_f}{RT_m} \left(\frac{T_m - T}{T} \right) \tag{2.15}$$

The second assumption is that $\Delta \bar{C}_p$ is essentially equal to the molar entropy of fusion, $\Delta \bar{S}_f$, which can be expressed in terms of the melting point and molar enthalpy of fusion, as in Equation 2.23. This second assumption results in the following expression:

$$\ln X_2^i = -\frac{\Delta \bar{H}_f}{RT_m} \ln \left(\frac{T_m}{T} \right) \tag{2.29}$$

The molar differential heat capacity at the melting point has proved to be negligible only for benzene and rigid, polyaromatic hydrocarbons, and a compilation of literature data indicates that $\Delta \bar{C}_p$ on the average is 80% of the molar entropy of fusion (Neau and Flynn, 1990). Although the first assumption has been applied in many studies, the second assumption gained favor in certain publications (Subrahmanyam et al., 1992; Claramonte et al., 1993; Yu et al., 1994).

NONIDEAL SOLUTIONS

It is unlikely that any real solution could possess the stringent qualifications that define the ideal solution. Indeed, the ideal solution exists only when a solute is dissolved in itself as the liquid solvent. The development of a theory for nonideality amounts to quantitatively estimating an activity coefficient for the solute in the nonideal solution. Irrespective of the nature of the nonideal solution,

$$a_2 = \gamma_2 X_2 \tag{2.30}$$

where γ is defined as the activity coefficient when solubility is expressed in mole fraction units. Note that the superscript i is not present on the mole fraction in Equation 2.30 because this equation applies to nonideal solutions. For a real solution, Equation 2.15 would be:

$$\ln\gamma_2 X_2 = -\frac{\Delta\bar{H}_f}{RT_m}\left(\frac{T_m - T}{T}\right) \tag{2.31}$$

Rearrangement gives:

$$\ln X_2 = -\frac{\Delta\bar{H}_f}{RT_m}\left(\frac{T_m - T}{T}\right) - \ln\gamma_2 \tag{2.32}$$

REGULAR SOLUTIONS

A molecule will most effectively mix with molecules that have the same cohesive energy density. Cohesive energy density is simply the sum of the interactive forces per unit volume; the customary units in regular solution theory are cal/cm^3. If there are substantial differences in the cohesive energy densities of the two species, the molecules with the greater cohesive energy density will prefer to interact with each other, perhaps even to the extent of excluding the molecules with the lower cohesive energy density. Immiscibility of the two species in whole or in part will result.

Hildebrand (1949) designated nonideal solutions as regular solutions if there was sufficient thermal agitation to overcome the segregating effect of unequal cohesive densities between the solute and the solvent. Thus, the maximum randomness in the final solution can still be achieved, and the ideal partial molal entropy of mixing, as defined in Equation 2.2, still holds. Assumptions were compiled and a quantitative relationship was developed to describe the behavior of nonelectrolytes in nonpolar solvents (Hildebrand, 1929; Scatchard, 1931, 1934). By the 1970s, the general equations that related solubility to the differences in cohesive energy densities between the solute and the solvent had been fully developed (Hildebrand and Scott, 1950, 1962; Hildebrand et al., 1970).

Because the cohesive energy density is a gross sum of the different types of forces that do not necessarily interact effectively, a similarity in cohesive energy density does not ensure miscibility. With this in mind, regular solutions have several characteristics caused by differences in cohesive energy density. The most significant difference between a regular solution and an ideal solution is a nonzero partial molal enthalpy of mixing. It is still assumed that the excess volume on mixing is negligible, although formation of a regular solution is usually accompanied by expansion and an increased entropy (Hildebrand, 1949); an essentially ideal entropy of mixing, derived from the statistical mixing of the components, holds; and the molar volumes of the solute and solvent are essentially equal.

When a solute is mixed with the solvent, one can assume that when both a solute–solute and a solvent–solvent interaction are broken there are two opportunities for solute–solvent interactions exist. Therefore, the enthalpy of mixing per mole of solute is assumed to be proportional to the differences in cohesive energy densities in this same 1:1:2 ratio:

$$\Delta\bar{H}_{mix,2} \alpha C_{11} + C_{22} - 2C_{12} \tag{2.33}$$

where C_{xx} refers to a cohesive energy density. C_{11} and C_{22}, then, represent the cohesive energy density of the solvent and solute, respectively (Nelson et al., 1970).

The cohesive energy density of the binary mixture, represented by C_{12}, cannot be easily predicted from the physicochemical properties of the solute and solvent. Instead, the cohesive energy density of the mixture is estimated using the geometric mean of the cohesive energy densities of the pure components:

$$C_{12} = \sqrt{C_{11}C_{22}} \tag{2.34}$$

Substituting into Equation 2.33 gives:

$$\Delta \bar{H}_{mix,2} \ \alpha \ C_{11} + C_{22} - 2\sqrt{C_{11}C_{22}} = \left(\sqrt{C_{11}} - \sqrt{C_{22}}\right)^2 \tag{2.35}$$

The square roots of the cohesive energy densities are given the designation δ, and have been labeled solubility parameters by Hildebrand (1949); Hildebrand and Scott, (1962). The typical units for this parameter in the early literature were $\sqrt{cal/cm^3}$, which have been labeled *hildebrands*; the SI unit is the MPa$^{1/2}$ where $1 \sqrt{cal/cm^3}$ equals 0.489 MPa$^{1/2}$. Substituting for the square root terms in Equation 2.35:

$$\Delta \bar{H}_{mix,2} \alpha \ \left(\delta_1 - \delta_2\right)^2 \tag{2.36}$$

The theoretical partial molal enthalpy of mixing resulting from mixing two compounds with different cohesive energy densities was estimated by:

$$\Delta \bar{H}_{mix,2} = \bar{V}_2 \phi_1^2 \left(\delta_1 - \delta_2\right)^2 \tag{2.37}$$

where ϕ_1 is the fraction of the solution volume occupied by the solvent (Hildebrand and Scott, 1950). For a dilute solution, ϕ_1 is essentially equal to unity.

The cohesive energy density of a pure compound can be estimated by different techniques (Scatchard, 1949; Hoy, 1970; Fedors, 1974). One method (Hildebrand et al., 1970) relates this parameter to the molar enthalpy of vaporization, $\Delta \bar{H}_v$, of the same chemical:

$$C_{22} = \frac{\left(\bar{H}_{v,2} - RT\right)}{\bar{V}_2} \tag{2.38}$$

where $\bar{V}_2$ is the molar volume of the liquid form of the solute in cm³/mole and $\Delta \bar{H}_v$ is in cal/mole. For liquids that do not have a reported molar enthalpy of vaporization, a convenient method of approximation is Hildebrand's empirical equation, based on the boiling point, T_b, in Kelvin units:

$$\Delta \bar{H}_{v,298 \, K} = 0.020 T_b^2 + 23.7 T_b - 295 \tag{2.39}$$

which yields the molar enthalpy of vaporization in cal/mole (Hildebrand and Scott, 1950). This equation cannot provide an accurate molar enthalpy of vaporization for liquids that are hydrogen bonded. Burrell (1955a, 1955b) found that a final correction can be added to the calculated solubility parameter to provide an estimate reliable enough for most practical applications. One should add 1.4 to the calculated solubility parameter for an alcohol, 0.6 for an ester, and 0.5 for a ketone that boils below 100°C. In other cases, no correction should be necessary.

Substituting Equation 2.37 for the partial molal enthalpy of mixing, along with Equation 2.2 for the partial molal entropy of mixing, which is still considered ideal, and Equation 2.10 for the free energy change in Equation 2.6, gives:

$$RT \ln a_2 = \bar{V}_2 \phi_1^2 \left(\delta_1 - \delta_2\right)^2 + RT \ln X_2 \tag{2.40}$$

which, from Equation 2.30, tells us that:

$$RT \ln \gamma_2 = \bar{V}_2 \phi_1^2 \left(\delta_1 - \delta_2\right)^2 \tag{2.41}$$

and the activity coefficient has been estimated for binary regular solutions involving a liquid solute. Rearranging the equation to the form:

$$\ln \gamma_2 = \frac{\bar{V}_2 \phi_1^2}{RT}(\delta_1 - \delta_2)^2 \tag{2.42}$$

allows inclusion of this term in Equation 2.32 to define the regular solution equation for a crystalline solute:

$$\ln X_2 = -\frac{\Delta \bar{H}_f}{RT_m}\left(\frac{T_m - T}{T}\right) - \frac{\bar{V}_2 \phi_1^2}{RT}(\delta_1 - \delta_2)^2 \tag{2.43}$$

It should be noted that $\bar{V}_2$ actually represents the partial molal volume of the liquid form of the solute at the solution temperature, and not the molar volume of the liquid. If the solution temperature is below the melting point of the solute, $\bar{V}_2$ would be estimated by the molar volume of a supercooled liquid form of the solute at temperature, T.

Equation 2.41 would be useful if the values of the solubility parameters and the partial molal volume of the supercooled liquid solute could be estimated. Additive procedures, based on functional groups found in the molecule, have been developed to estimate partial molal volumes and solubility parameters (Small, 1951; Hoy, 1970; Konstam and Feairheller, 1970; Fedors, 1974). Rathi (2010) presents the calculation of the Hildebrand solubility parameter for satranidazole (Consider Figure 2.2, Table 2.1) based on the group contribution values offered by Fedors (1974). Each functional group in the chemical is acknowledged not only by type but also by the number of times that functional group appears. The features of the chemical structure are also included, such as each time conjugation appears (represented by a series of double then single bonds) and each ring closure (such as the *N*-methyl imidazole ring). In Table 2.1, the sum of the entries in column D equals the estimated contributions to the cohesive energy density of satranidazole; the sum of the entries in column F equals the estimated molar volume of the supercooled liquid form of satranidazole at room temperature. The cohesive energy density for satranidazole therefore equals the sum of column D divided by the sum of column F that leads to:

$$\text{Satranidazole solubility parameter,} \delta = \sqrt{\frac{30580 \text{ cal/mole}}{235.6 \text{ cm}^3/\text{mole}}} = 11.4 \sqrt{\frac{\text{cal}}{\text{cm}^3}}$$

Another approach is to determine the solubility of the compound in a series of nonpolar solvents and use Equation 2.43 to estimate the solubility parameter of the solute by accounting for every other parameter in the equation. This has been somewhat successful for hydrocortisone (Hagen and Flynn, 1983) and for para-aminobenzoates (Neau et al., 1989). A plot of $\ln X_2$ as a function of the solubility parameter of the solvent, according to Equation 2.43, reveals a parabola for solubility data in reasonably nonpolar solvents (Figure 2.3). The maximum for the parabola occurs when the solvent solubility parameter equals the solute solubility parameter and the maximum represents the ideal solubility, as defined by Equation 2.15 or 2.29. It was shown that, by choosing a nonpolar solvent with a solubility parameter reasonably removed from that calculated for the solute, such as *n*-hexane ($\delta_1 = 7.27$) or:

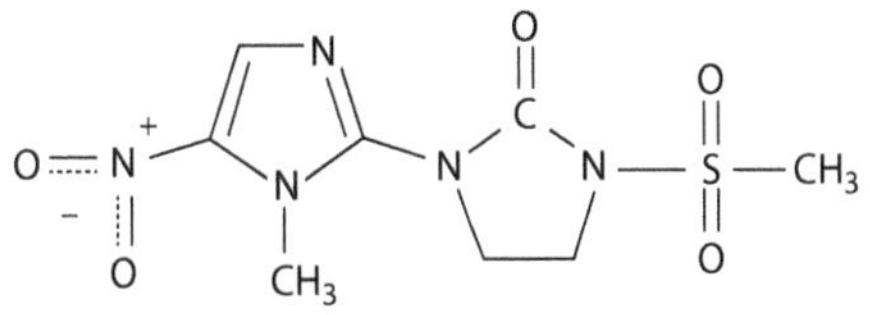

FIGURE 2.2   Chemical structure of satranidazole.

TABLE 2.1

Fedors Group Contribution Method (1974) Allows Calculation of the Solubility Parameter of Satranidazole

A	B	C	D	E	F
Functional Group or Feature	Number of Times[a]	Cohesive Energy (cal/mole)	Col B*Col C	Contribution to the Molar Volume[b]	Col B*Col E
$-CH_3$	2	1125	2250	33.5	67.0
$-CH_2-$	2	1180	2360	16.1	32.2
$=CH-$	1	1030	1030	13.5	13.5
$=C<$	3	1690	5070	6.5	19.5
$>N-$	3	2800	8400	5.0	15.0
$=N-$	1	2800	2800	5.0	5.0
$-NO_2$	1	3670	3670	32.0	32.0
$-SO_2$	1	3700	3700	23.8	23.8
Conjugation[c]	2	400	800	-2.2	-4.4
Ring closure	2	250	500	16.0	32.0
Sum			30580		235.6

[a] Indicates number of times that particular functional group or feature appears.
[b] Contribution to the molar volume by the particular functional group or feature.
[c] Conjugation indicates a series of double then single then double then single bonds.

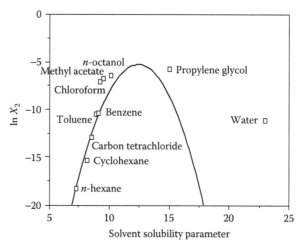

FIGURE 2.3 Regular solution theory plot for hydrocortisone solubility data. The curve presents the solubility predicted by Equation 2.43 using data from *n*-hexane, cyclohexane, carbon tetrachloride, toluene, and benzene to estimate the solubility parameter of hydrocortisone. (Data from Hagen, T. A., Physicochemical study of hydrocortisone and hydrocortisone n-alkyl-21-esters, PhD dissertation, University of Michigan, pp. 94–96, 1979. With permission.)

n-heptane ($\delta_1 = 7.50$), the solute solubility parameter for each para-aminobenzoate studied could be easily estimated using Equation 2.43 and the solubility in that nonpolar solvent (Neau et al., 1989). The solubility data associated with the nonpolar solvents is regressed as a quadratic equation in the solvent solubility parameter, acknowledging that the enthalpy of fusion term on the right-hand side of Equation 2.43 is a constant under these conditions, to estimate the solute solubility parameter.

EXTENDED HILDEBRAND SOLUBILITY APPROACH

Regular solution theory is largely limited to describing the solution behavior of nonelectrolytes in nonpolar solvents. The inadequacy, or inappropriate application, of the geometric mean assumption for the cohesive energy density of the solution is considered the reason why regular solution theory fails to describe other real solutions (Martin et al., 1985). It has been found that solutions that seemingly fit the criteria of regular solutions fail to yield a solubility predicted by regular solution equations. For example, solutions of benzene or simple substituted aromatics dissolved in alkane solvents were shown to deviate from behaviors predicted by literature solubility parameters and regular solution equations (Funk and Prausnitz, 1970; Hildebrand et al., 1970; Fung and Higuchi, 1971). Studies of these systems can frequently demonstrate that the deviation can be diminished by a correction factor applied to the geometric mean. Efforts have been made to generalize observed behaviors and to correct empirically for these deviations from predicted solubilities. In one method, the geometric mean is replaced with $k\delta_1\delta_2$, where k represents a constant (Walker, 1952). This has been applied with some success to pharmaceutical systems (Martin and Carstensen, 1981). It was found that the geometric mean rule could be relaxed empirically by inclusion of l_{12} (Funk and Prausnitz, 1970; Hildebrand et al., 1970) a binary constant that is small compared to unity:

$$C_{12} = \left(1 - l_{12}\right)\sqrt{C_{11}C_{22}} \tag{2.44}$$

such that Equation 2.42 would be rewritten as:

$$\ln \gamma_2 = \frac{\bar{V}_2\phi_1^2}{RT}\left[\left(\delta_1 - \delta_2\right)^2 + 2l_{12}\delta_1\delta_2\right] \tag{2.45}$$

An improvement in the prediction of androstanolone, nandrolone, and testosterone ester solubility in organic solvents was possible by including l_{12} in the calculations (James et al., 1976).

In the pharmaceutical literature, by far the most common means to account for the deviation from the geometric mean is the use of W, which is defined as follows:

$$W = K\delta_1\delta_2 \tag{2.46}$$

where K is a solute–solvent interaction factor that is not constant. The solubility equation used in this extended Hildebrand solubility approach (Adjei et al., 1980) is:

$$\ln X_2 = -\frac{\Delta \bar{H}_f}{RT_m}\left(\frac{T_m - T}{T}\right) - \frac{\bar{V}_2\phi_1^2}{RT}\left(\delta_1^2 - 2W + \delta_2^2\right) \tag{2.47}$$

This equation has been applied to data for caffeine (Adjei et al., 1980), theophylline (Martin et al., 1980), and satranidazole (Rathi, 2010) in a series of binary solvents consisting of water and dioxane; to data for testosterone in binary solvent systems consisting of chloroform and cyclohexane (Martin et al., 1982); and to polymorphs of mefenamic acid in a series of solvents involving ethanol and water or ethyl acetate and ethanol combinations necessary to cover a range of solvent solubility parameters (Romero et al., 1999). See Figure 2.4 for solubility data from Adjei et al. (1980). This approach is strictly empirical in that to assign values to W requires data for the solubility in a series of binary solvents consisting of two specific solvents in various proportions. The values of W for the solvent systems can be regressed as a power series in the solvent

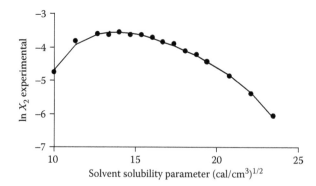

FIGURE 2.4 Caffeine solubility in dioxane-water binary solvents. The curve is an interpolation between calculated values. (From Adjei, A. et al.: Extended Hildebrand approach: Solubility of caffeine in dioxane-water mixtures. *Journal of Pharmaceutical Sciences.* 1980. 69. 659–661. Copyright Wiley-VCH Verlag GmbH & Co. KGaA. Reproduced with permission.)

solubility parameter, using the following equation to calculate the solvent solubility parameter for the binary solvent system:

$$\delta_{13} = \frac{\phi_1 \delta_1 + \phi_3 \delta_3}{\phi_1 + \phi_3} \tag{2.48}$$

where the subscripts 1 and 3 are assigned to the first and second solvent. The δ_{13} solvent solubility parameter would replace the δ_1 found in Equation 2.47. In the case of caffeine (Adjei et al., 1980), acetaminophen (Subrahmanyam et al., 1992), and mefenamic acid (Romero et al., 1999) in cosolvent–water systems, the W values were regressed as a fourth-order polynomial in the solvent solubility parameter to achieve a close fit to the experimental data (Figure 2.4). The fit can be excellent because it is possible to fit any data set using a polynomial if there are enough adjustable parameters (Grant and Higuchi, 1990). Each new term in the polynomial introduces another adjustable parameter.

Lin and Nash (1993) have proposed an equation to estimate the Hildebrand solubility parameter of a solute strictly from its mole fraction solubility in n different solvents and the corresponding solvent solubility parameter:

$$\delta_2 = \frac{\sum_{i=1}^{n} X_{2,i} \delta_{1,i}}{\sum_{i=1}^{n} X_{2,i}} \tag{2.49}$$

where $X_{2,i}$ refers to the mole fraction solubility of the solute in a particular solvent and $\delta_{1,i}$ is the solubility parameter of that particular solvent. This equation has been applied to benzoic acid, theophylline, and methylparaben data by Lin and Nash (1993) and to polymorphs of mefenamic acid data by Romero et al. (1999) with some success. The estimated solubility parameters for the two polymorphs of mefenamic acid were quite similar. This is to be expected since the solute interactions in solution would not depend on the solid characteristics defined by the polymorphic form. Indeed, it has been reported that the difference in solubility between different polymorphs is usually less than one order of magnitude (Huang and Tong, 2004) or might even be less than a factor of 2 (Pudipeddi and Serajuddin, 2005).

Grant and Higuchi (1990) noted that, although this approach can be used to correlate and condense data, its use as a predictive method is questionable. It would be more promising if W could be related to polar characteristics, but to date there is no means to estimate it based on the physicochemical properties of the solute or solvent (Adjei et al., 1980). The value of this approach is that the regression equation can be used to interpolate the magnitude of W for a binary solvent from the same system that has not been investigated experimentally. Therefore, it has a direct application in the investigation of solubility in cosolvent mixtures, as will be discussed later.

Hansen Approach

Attempts have been made to extend the solubility parameter approach to include polar systems. Compensation for hydrogen bonding (Burrell, 1955a, 1955b; Crowley et al., 1966; Karger et al., 1976) and polar contributions (Hildebrand and Scott, 1962; Blanks and Prausnitz, 1964; Harris and Prausnitz, 1969; Karger et al., 1976) refined the application, but a more successful approach was to acknowledge that the cohesive energy density is the sum of intermolecular forces consisting of dispersion forces (D), polar forces involving permanent dipoles (P), and hydrogen bonding (H) (Hansen, 1967). Each of these components can be represented in a three-dimensional solubility parameter:

$$\delta_T^2 = \delta_D^2 + \delta_P^2 + \delta_H^2 \qquad (2.50)$$

where δ_T is the one-dimensional solubility parameter, previously given the symbol δ and considered earlier in this chapter. Each of the component solubility parameters is expressed in the same units as the conventional solubility parameter. Three-dimensional solubility parameters have been the subject of much investigation, and tables of these solubility parameters, in particular for common solvents, are available (Beerbower and Dickey, 1969; Hansen and Beerbower, 1971; Hansen, 1972, 2007; Barton, 1983).

The solubility of the drug is determined in multiple solvents that possess different functional groups, both nonpolar and polar, to allow each of the three-dimensional solubility parameters to be estimated. A typical means to arrive at the values of the component solubility parameters is the use of multiple regression analysis (Thimmasetty et al., 2009). Alternatively, each of the three-dimensional solubility parameters can be estimated using group contribution methods, as described in the following paragraphs.

Tentatively, water was assigned $\delta_D = 7.0$, $\delta_P = 8.0$, and $\delta_H = 20.9$ hildebrands, which agrees with extrapolations for dispersion and polar components generated from the solubility and molar volume data for alcohols, and for the hydrogen-bonding contribution if one considers water as having two alcohol hydrogen atoms. Use of these values in calculations for organic solvent–water binary systems have met with success (Hansen, 1967). A recently reported set of parameters for water based on the energy of evaporation is still quite similar to those tentatively proposed: $\delta_D = 7.58$, $\delta_P = 7.82$, and $\delta_H = 20.7$ hildebrands (Hansen, 2007).

The dispersion solubility parameter can be estimated using the classical one-dimensional solubility parameter of a homomorph (Blanks and Prausnitz, 1964; Hansen, 1969; Barton, 1983). The homomorph of a polar molecule is defined as a nonpolar molecule having very nearly the same molecular size and shape. Alternatively, the dispersion contributions can be estimated using functional group contributions, $F_{D,i}$, and the formula:

$$\delta_D = \frac{\sum F_{D,i}}{V} \qquad (2.51)$$

The other components can also be estimated using additive functional group contributions, and tables of group contributions for dispersion, and polar and hydrogen-bonding contributions are available (Hansen and Beerbower, 1971; Van Krevelen and Hoftyzer, 1976; Barton, 1983; Hansen, 2007; Abbott and Hansen, 2010; Just et al., 2013). If we label the polar functional group contributions $F_{P,i}$, the polar contributions are summed in this fashion:

$$\delta_P = \frac{\sqrt{\sum F_{P,i}^2}}{V} \qquad (2.52)$$

The hydrogen-bonding cohesive energy contributions, $-U_{H,i}$, are also considered additive, and its component of the solubility parameter is estimated using:

$$\delta_H = \sqrt{\frac{\sum \left(-U_{H,i}\right)}{\bar{V}}} \tag{2.53}$$

Experimental results suggest that the hydrogen-bonding component is the most difficult to estimate by group contribution data (Barton, 1983). Nevertheless, the hydrogen-bonding component could be the most critical of the three components in determining solubility in water. Indeed, hydrogen-bonding potential has proved to be critical in recent computational chemistry approaches to prediction of drug solubility in water (Jorgensen and Duffy, 2002; Schaper et al., 2003; Raevsky et al., 2004) and of drug-excipient miscibility (Alhalaweh et al., 2014). By adding hydrogen bond donor strength to the computational model, the prediction of solubility in water improved substantially (Schaper et al., 2003; Raevsky et al., 2004).

The three-dimensional solubility parameters are substituted for the solubility parameters in Equation 2.42 to arrive at an expression describing the activity coefficient in these solutions:

$$\ln \gamma_2 = \frac{\bar{V}_2 \phi_1^2}{RT}\left[\left(\delta_{D1} - \delta_{D2}\right)^2 + \left(\delta_{P1} - \delta_{P2}\right)^2 + \left(\delta_{H1} - \delta_{H2}\right)^2\right] \tag{2.54}$$

If this activity coefficient term is applied to Equation 2.43, the mole fraction solubility can be shown to reach a maximum when δ_{D1} equals δ_{D2}, δ_{P1} equals δ_{P2}, and δ_{H1} equals δ_{H2}. Teas (1968) presented a triangular plot where the sides represent the three contributions to the solvent solubility parameter, f_D, f_P, and f_H, expressed as the percentage of the one-dimensional solubility parameter. For example, the dispersion force contribution would be:

$$f_D = 100\% \frac{\delta_D^2}{\delta_T^2} \tag{2.55}$$

and its value would be found on one side of the triangle. The other two sides would be the polar and the hydrogen-bonding contributions, and similar equations would define f_P and f_H as single values on those two triangle sides A solvent, then, would be represented by a single point in such a plot. From the solubility of testosterone propionate in various solvents, it was found that, in such a triangular plot, the maximum solubilities were in the vicinity of $f_D = 65$, $f_P = 20$, and $f_H = 15$ (James et al., 1976). Approximate component solubility parameters for testosterone propionate, suitable for solvent selection, were estimated using $\delta_T = 9.5 \sqrt{\text{cal/cm}^3}$ and equations similar to rearranged Equation 2.55, such as:

$$\delta_D = \sqrt{f_D \frac{\delta_T^2}{100}} = \sqrt{65 \frac{9.5^2}{100}} = 7.7 \sqrt{\text{cal/cm}^3} \tag{2.56}$$

Similar calculations yield $\delta_P = 4.2$ and $\delta_H = 3.7 \sqrt{\text{cal/cm}^3}$.

If the δ_D, δ_P, and δ_H values of two chemicals are each comparable in magnitude, those two chemicals will have high affinity for each other (Hansen, 2007). Similar δ_T values might not indicate this high affinity since δ_T is a mathematical combination of the three partial solubility parameters. The similarity of δ_T for ethanol and nitromethane has been noted, yet the two demonstrate markedly different physicochemical properties (Hansen, 1967). For example, ethanol is miscible with water; nitromethane is insoluble.

The Hansen approach has been expanded by acknowledging that δ_H represents the potential for interactions involving electron transfer, not limited to hydrogen bonding but also including Lewis acid–base interactions (Hansen, 1967; Thimmasetty et al., 2008). When acid–base interactions take place that obscure the hydrogen bonding effects, the acid and base interactions can be separated, using δ_a and δ_b instead of δ_H alone (Thimmasetty et al., 2008; Stefanis and Panayiotou, 2012), where:

$$\delta_H^2 = \delta_a^2 + \delta_b^2 \tag{2.57}$$

The following substitution in Equation 2.54 has been proposed (Thimmasetty et al., 2008):

$$\ln \gamma_2 = \frac{\bar{V}_2 \phi_1^2}{RT} \left[\left(\delta_{D1} - \delta_{D2} \right)^2 + \left(\delta_{P1} - \delta_{P2} \right)^2 + \left(\delta_{a1} - \delta_{a2} \right)^2 + \left(\delta_{b1} - \delta_{b2} \right)^2 \right] \tag{2.58}$$

This approach has not met with much interest, practical application, and published research because there are few compilations of the separate acid and base solubility parameters, especially in comparison to the number of published compilations for the hydrogen-bonding component solubility parameter (Stefanis and Panayiotou, 2012).

The three-dimensional solubility parameter has found application in the preparation of solid solutions, wherein the drug has been dispersed at a molecular level in a polymer carrier. The Hildebrand and the Hansen approaches to the calculation of solubility parameters were calculated for ibuprofen and for several polar chemicals for the purpose of identifying potential carriers for the preparation of solid dispersions of the drug. Although the one-dimensional solubility parameter approach was able to indicate a trend in the compatibility of carriers with the drug, the use of the three dimensional solubility parameter revealed incompatibilities with greater accuracy (Greenhalgh et al., 1999). The use of polar polymers is often observed as they can not only improve the disintegration and dissolution rate of the drug (Vasconcelos et al., 2007) but can also, in some cases, support a supersaturated solution of the drug at least on a transient basis (Curatolo et al., 2009; Ilevbare et al., 2013; Ozaki et al., 2013). (The reader is directed to reviews on drug-polymer dispersions by Serajuddin [1999] and Leuner and Dressman [2000].) An incompatibility between the polar polymer and a poorly soluble drug can be suggested by examining the differences in their three-dimensional solubility parameters (Greenhalgh et al., 1999).

EXTENSION OF THE HANSEN APPROACH

The Hansen equation has been extended (Martin et al., 1981, 1984; Wu et al., 1982; Beerbower et al., 1984; Thimmasetty et al., 2008) to acknowledge an empirical correction term, C_0, and empirical coefficients applied to each type of solubility parameter, C_i:

$$\ln \gamma_2 = \frac{\bar{V}_2 \phi_1^2}{RT} \left[C_0 + C_1 \left(\delta_{D1} - \delta_{D2} \right)^2 + C_2 \left(\delta_{P1} - \delta_{P2} \right)^2 + C_3 \left(\delta_{H1} - \delta_{H2} \right)^2 \right] \tag{2.59}$$

In the application of this expression to the estimation of the solubility parameters of benzodiazepines in various solvents, the expanded Hansen approach proved to be far superior to the Hansen approach (Verheyen et al., 2001). In a study of the solubility of temazepam in 29 solvents (Richardson et al., 1992), the predicted mole fraction solubility was always of the same

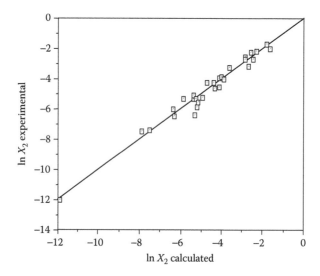

FIGURE 2.5 Extended Hansen solubility approach applied to the solubility of temazepam in solvents covering a wide range of polarities. The line represents equal calculated and experimental values. (Reprinted from *Int. J. Pharm.*, 78, Richardson, P. J. et al., Determination of three-component partial solubility parameters for temazepam and the effects of change in partial molal volume on the thermodynamics of drug solubility, 189–198. Copyright 1992, with permission from Elsevier.)

order of magnitude as the experimental value. When the Flory–Huggins correction was applied, a marked increase in overall predictive ability was observed. In the final analysis, a predicted solubility on the average was only off by 33% from the experimental solubility. The results are presented graphically in Figure 2.5. It should be noted that the estimated aqueous solubility was low by only 12%.

ADVANTAGES AND DISADVANTAGES

It has been noted that the regular solution expression, Equation 2.43, holds only with nonpolar systems (Claramonte et al., 1993), or in dilute systems where the solute–solvent and solvent–solvent interactions are limited to dispersion forces, that is, London forces (Hildebrand, 1949; Neau et al., 1989). The use of polar solvents introduces intermolecular forces in excess of London forces, with the consequence that there is an excess entropy of mixing that is not accounted for in regular solution theory (Hildebrand, 1949). This can be attributed to self-association of solute or solvent molecules, solvation of the solute by the solvent molecules, or complexation of solute species in solution (Martin et al., 1980; Grant and Abougela, 1984). The intermolecular interactions probably consist of hydrogen bonds, dipole interactions, charge-transfer complexation, and other types of Lewis acid–base interactions (Hildebrand, 1949; Martin et al., 1982, 1984, 1985; Grant and Abougela, 1984). Nevertheless, regular solution theory has successfully described the solution behavior of hydrocortisone in nonpolar solvents (Hagen and Flynn, 1983), steroids in homologous series of *n*-alkanes and *n*-alcohols (Gharavi et al., 1983), and naproxen in solvents used in the production of topical dosage forms (Claramonte et al., 1993).

The extensions of the Hildebrand and Hansen approaches are both empirical. After the solubility behavior has been evaluated in a series of solvent systems, regression analysis can be used to estimate the empirical coefficients, including the C_0 term of the extended Hansen approach, and then the solubility can be estimated in a solvent system which has not been included in the experimental portion of the study. The problem with acknowledging the predictive power of these equations is that the solubility in many solvents must be determined before being able to predict the solubility in the solvent of choice. It is probably easier to simply perform the solubility study in the solvent of choice and eliminate the prediction equation altogether. On the other hand, in a study of binary solvent systems consisting of water and a cosolvent appropriate to parenteral products, the solubility maximum in that series can be readily estimated by the mathematical expression finally achieved.

In addition, the theoretical equations in the Hildebrand and Hansen approaches can be effectively applied to predicting the solubility of a new chemical by employing the experimental solubility data of a structurally related chemical. The predicted values for the new chemical would be based on the experimental one- or three-dimensional solubility parameter of the structurally related chemical, and the group additivity principles would be applied to estimate the respective solubility parameter of the second chemical. Solubility parameters associated with the Hildebrand and Hansen approaches have proved useful in the selection of not only solvents, but also of other excipients found in formulations (Belmares et al., 2004).

This discussion has been largely limited to solubility parameter approaches that some consider to be of limited application since they have quantitative limits. It should be appreciated that these theoretical approaches and their applications have led to a deeper understanding of solubility behavior and of predictive approaches to solubility estimations. More to the point, extrapolations and interpolations dramatically extend the applicability of these approaches to the estimation, albeit a crude estimation, of the solubility of a new chemical in a well-studied solvent, or of a well-characterized chemical in a new solvent. In 1949, Hildebrand stated:

> The quantitative limitations set forth ... are not so serious as to prevent the theory from being qualitatively very serviceable. We seek qualitative and relative solubility data far more often than exact figures. We seek the best or sometimes the poorest solvent for a certain solute. We seldom want to know a solubility to, say, 1 per cent and, indeed, we seldom control temperature or purity to a corresponding degree. If we do need a solubility to that accuracy we must rely upon measurement ... to serve our purpose. (Reprinted with permission from Hildebrand, J. H., *Chem. Rev.*, 44, 37–45, 1949. Copyright 1949 by the American Chemical Society.)

REFERENCES

Abbott, S., and C. M. Hansen. 2010. *Hansen Solubility Parameters in Practice, Complete with Software, Data and Examples*, 3rd ed., v. 3.1. Book and software published by Hansen-Solubility.com.

Adamson, A. W. 1979. *A Textbook of Physical Chemistry*, p. 235. New York: Academic Press.

Adjei, A., J. Newburger, and A. Martin. 1980. Extended Hildebrand approach: Solubility of caffeine in dioxane-water mixtures. *J. Pharm. Sci.* 69:659–661.

Alhalaweh, A., A. Alzghoul, and W. Kaialy. 2014. Data mining of solubility parameters for computational prediction of drug-excipient miscibility. *Drug Dev. Ind. Pharm.* 40:904–909.

Barton, A. F. M. 1983. *Handbook of Solubility Parameters and Other Cohesion Parameters*. Boca Raton, FL: CRC Press.

Beerbower, A., and J. R. Dickey. 1969. Advanced methods for predicting elastomer/fluids interactions. *ASLE Trans.* 12:1–20.

Beerbower, A., P. L. Wu, and A. Martin. 1984. Expanded solubility parameter approach I: Naphthalene and benzoic acid in individual solvents. *J. Pharm. Sci.* 73:179–188.

Belmares, M., M. Blanco, W. A. Goddard, R. B. Ross, G. Caldwell, S.-H. Chou, J. Pham, P. M. Olofson, and C. Thomas. 2004. Hildebrand and Hansen solubility parameters from molecular dynamics with applications to electronic nose polymer sensors. *J. Comput. Chem.* 25:1814–1826.

Blanks, R. F., and J. M. Prausnitz. 1964. Thermodynamics of polymer solubility in polar and nonpolar systems. *Ind. Eng. Chem. Fund.* 3:1–8.

Burrell, H. 1955a. Solubility parameters, Part I. *Interchem. Rev.* 14:3–16.

Burrell, H. 1955b. Solubility parameters, Part II. *Interchem. Rev.* 14:31–46.

Bustamante, P., B. Escalera, A. Martin, and E. Sellés. 1989. Predicting the solubility of sulfamethoxypyridazine in individual solvents I: Calculating partial solubility parameters. *J. Pharm. Sci.* 78:567–573.

Claramonte, M. D. C., A. P. Vialard, and F. G. Vichez. 1993. An application of regular solution theory in the study of the solubility of naproxen in some solvents used in topical preparations. *Int. J. Pharm.* 94:23–30.

Crowley, J. D., G. S. Teague, and J. W. Lowe. 1966. A three-dimensional approach to solubility. *J. Paint Technol.* 38:269–280.

Curatolo W., J. A. Nightingale, and S. M. Herbig. 2009. Utility of hydroxypropylmethylcellulose acetate succinate (HPMCAS) for initiation and maintenance of drug supersaturation in the GI milieu. *Pharm. Res.* 26:1419–1431.

Dave, V. S., S. Hepburn, and S. W. Hoag. 2014. Physical states and thermodynamic principles in pharmaceutics. In A. K. Dash, S. Singh, and J. Tolman (Eds.), *Pharmaceutics: Basic Principles and Application to Pharmacy Practice.* New York: Academic Press, p. 40.

Fedors, R. F. 1974. A method for estimating both the solubility parameter and molar volumes of liquids. *Polymer Eng. Sci.* 14:147–154.

Fung, H.-L., and T. Higuchi. 1971. Molecular interactions and solubilities of polar nonelectrolytes in nonpolar solvents. *J. Pharm. Sci.* 60:1782–1788.

Funk, E. W., and J. M. Prausnitz. 1970. Thermodynamic properties of liquid mixtures: Aromatic-saturated hydrocarbon systems. *Ind. Eng. Chem.* 62:8–15.

Gharavi, M., K. C. James, and L. H. Sanderds. 1983. Solubilities of mestanolone, methandienone, methyltestosterone, nandrolone, and testosterone in homologous series of alkanes and alkanols. *Int. J. Pharm.* 14:333–341.

Grant, D. J. W., and I. K. A. Abougela. 1984. Solubility behavior of griseofulvin in solvents of relatively low polarity. *Labo-Pharma Probl. Technol.* 32:193–196.

Grant, D. J. W., and T. Higuchi. 1990. *Solubility Behavior of Organic Compounds.* New York: John Wiley & Sons.

Greenhalgh, D. J., A. C. Williams, P. Timmins, and P. York. 1999. Solubility parameters as predictors of miscibility in solid dispersions. *J. Pharm. Sci.* 88:1182–1190.

Hagen, T. A. 1979. Physicochemical study of hydrocortisone and hydrocortisone n-alkyl-21-esters. PhD dissertation, University of Michigan, Ann Arbor, MI, pp. 94–96.

Hagen, T. A., and G. L. Flynn. 1983. Solubility of hydrocortisone in organic and aqueous media: Evidence for regular solution behavior in a polar solvents. *J. Pharm. Sci.* 72:409–414.

Hansen, C. M. 1967. The three dimensional solubility parameter. Key to paint component affinities: I. Solvents, plasticizers, polymers, and resins. *J. Paint Technol.* 39:104–117.

Hansen, C. 1969. The universality of the solubility parameter. *Ind. Eng. Chem., Prod. Res. Develop.* 8:2–11.

Hansen, C. 1972. Solvents for coatings. *Chem. Technol.* 2:547–553.

Hansen, C. 2007. *Hansen Solubility Parameters: A User's Handbook*, 2nd ed. Boca Raton, FL: CRC Press, pp. 12, 13, 38.

Hansen, C., and A. Beerbower. 1971. Solubility parameters. In A. Standen (Ed.), *Kirk-Othmer Encyclopedia of Chemical Technology.* New York: John Wiley & Sons, pp. 889–910.

Harris, H. G., and J. M. Prausnitz. 1969. Thermodynamics of solutions with physical and chemical interactions. *Ind. Eng. Chem. Fund.* 8:180–188.

Hildebrand, J. H. 1929. Solubility. XII. Regular solutions. *J. Am. Chem. Soc.* 51:66–80.

Hildebrand, J. H. 1949. A critique of the theory of solubility of non-electrolytes. *Chem. Rev.* 44:37–45.

Hildebrand, J. H., and R. L. Scott. 1950. *The Solubility of Nonelectrolytes.* New York: Reinhold Publishing.

Hildebrand, J. H., and R. L. Scott. 1962. *Regular Solutions.* Englewood Cliffs, NJ: Prentice Hall.

Hildebrand, J. H., J. M. Prausnitz, and R. L. Scott. 1970. *Regular and Related Solutions.* New York: Van Nostrand Reinhold.

Hoy, K. L. 1970. New values of the solubility parameters from vapor pressure data. *J. Paint Technol.* 42:76–118.

Huang, L.-F., and W.-Q. Tong. 2004. Impact of solid state properties on developability assessment of drug candidates. *Adv. Drug Deliv. Rev.* 56:321–334.

Huyskens, P. L., and M. C. Haulait-Pirson. 1985. A new expression for the combinatorial entropy of mixing in liquid mixtures. *J. Mol. Liq.* 31:135–151.

Ilevbare, G. A., H. Liu, K. J. Edgar, and L. S. Taylor. 2013. Maintaining supersaturation in aqueous drug solutions: Impact of different polymers on induction times. *Cryst. Growth Des.* 13:740–751.

James, K. C., C. T. Ng, and P. R. Noyce. 1976. Solubilities of testosterone propionate and related esters in organic solvents. *J. Pharm. Sci.* 65:656–659.

Johnson, S. R., and W. Zheng. 2006. Recent progress in the computational prediction of aqueous solubility and absorption. *AAPS J.* 8:E27–E40.

Jorgensen, W. L., and E. M. Duffy. 2002. Prediction of drug solubility from structure. *Adv. Drug Deliv. Rev.* 54:355–366.

Just, S., F. Sievert, M. Thommes, and J. Breitkreutz. 2013. Improved group contribution parameter set for the application of solubility parameters to melt extrusion. *Eur. J. Pharm. Biopharm.* 85(3 Pt B):1191–1199.

Karger, B. L., L. R. Snyder, and C. Eon. 1976. An expanded solubility parameter treatment for classification and use of chromatographic solvents and adsorbents. *J. Chromatogr.* 125:71–88.

Kertes, A. S. 1965. Solubility and activity of high-molecular amine hydrochlorides in organic solvents. *J. Inorg.Nucl. Chem.* 27:209–217.

Konstam, A. H., and W. R. Feairheller. 1970. Calculation of solubility parameters of polar compounds. *AIChE J.* 16:837–840.

Leuner, C., and J. Dressman. 2000. Improving drug solubility for oral delivery using solid dispersions. *Eur. J. Pharm. Biopharm.* 50:47–60.

Lewis, G. N., and M. Randall. 1961. *Thermodynamics*, revised by K. S. Pitzer and L. Brewer, 2nd ed. New York: McGraw-Hill, p. 281.

Lin, H., and R. A. Nash. 1993. An experimental method for determining the Hildebrand solubility parameter of organic nonelectrolytes. *J. Pharm. Sci.* 82:1018–1026.

Lipinski, C. A., F. Lombardo, B. W. Dominy, and P. J. Feeney. 1997. Experimental and computational approaches to estimate solubility and permeability in drug discovery and development settings. *Adv. Drug Deliv. Rev.* 23:3–25.

Martin, A., and J. Carstensen. 1981. Extended solubility approach: Solubility parameters for crystalline solid compounds. *J. Pharm. Sci.* 70:170–172.

Martin, A., J. Newburger, and A. Adjei. 1980. Extended Hildebrand solubility approach: Solubility of theophylline in polar binary solvents. *J. Pharm. Sci.* 69:487–491.

Martin, A., P. L. Wu, A. Adjei, A. Beerbower, and J. M. Prausnitz. 1981. Extended Hansen solubility approach: Naphthalene in individual solvents. *J. Pharm. Sci.* 70:1260–1264.

Martin, A., P. L. Wu, A. Adjei, M. Mehdizadeh, K. C. James, and C. Metzler. 1982. Extended Hildebrand solubility approach: Testosterone and testosterone propionate in binary solvents. *J. Pharm. Sci.* 71:1334–1340.

Martin, A., P. L. Wu, and A. Beerbower. 1984. Expanded solubility parameter approach II: Naphthalene and benzoic acid in individual solvents. *J. Pharm. Sci.* 73:188–194.

Martin, A., P. L. Wu, Z. Liron, and S. Cohen. 1985. Dependence of solute solubility parameter on solvent polarity. *J. Pharm. Sci.* 74:638–642.

Neau, S. H., G. L. Flynn, and S. H. Yalkowsky. 1989. The influence of heat capacity assumptions on the estimation of solubility parameters from solubility data. *Int. J. Pharm.* 49:223–229.

Neau, S. H., and G. L. Flynn. 1990. Solid and liquid heat capacities of n-alkyl para-aminobenzoates near the melting point. *Pharm. Res.* 7:1157–1162.

Nelson, R. C., R. W. Hemwall, and G. D. Edwards. 1970. Treatment of hydrogen bonding in predicting miscibility. *J. Paint Technol.* 42:636–643.

Ozaki, S., I. Kushida, T. Yamashita, T. Hasebe, O. Shirai, and K. Kano. 2013. Inhibition of crystal nucleation and growth by water-soluble polymers and its impact on the supersaturation profiles of amorphous drugs. *J. Pharm. Sci.* 102:2273–2281.

Pudipeddi, M., and A. T. M. Serajuddin. 2005. Trends in solubility of polymorphs. *J. Pharm. Sci.* 94:929–339.

Raevsky, O. A., O. E. Raevskaja, and K.-J. Schaper. 2004. Analysis of water solubility data on the basis of HYBOT descriptors, part 3: Solubility of solid neutral chemicals and drugs. *QSAR Combinator. Sci.* 23:327–343.

Rathi, P. B. 2010. Determination and evaluation of solubility parameter of satranidazole using dioxane-water system. *Ind. J. Pharm. Sci.* 72:671–674.

Richardson, P. J., D. F. McCafferty, and A. D. Woolfson. 1992. Determination of three-component partial solubility parameters for temazepam and the effects of change in partial molal volume on the thermodynamics of drug solubility. *Int. J. Pharm.* 78:189–198.

Romero, S., B. Escalera, and P. Bustamante. 1999. Solubility behavior of polymorphs I and II of mefenamic acid in solvent mixtures. *Int. J. Pharm.* 178:193–202.

Scatchard, G. 1931. Equilibria in non-electrolyte solutions in relation to the vapor pressures and densities of the components. *Chem. Rev.* 8:321–333.

Scatchard, G. 1934. Non-electrolyte solutions. *J. Am. Chem. Soc.* 56:995–996.

Scatchard, G. 1949. Equilibrium in non-electrolyte mixtures. *Chem. Rev.* 44:7–35.

Schaper, K.-J., B. Kunz, and O. A. Raevsky. 2003. Analysis of water solubility data on the basis of HYBOT descriptors, part 2: Solubility of liquid chemicals and drugs. *QSAR Combinator. Sci.* 22:943–948.

Serajuddin, A. T. M. 1999. Solid dispersion of poorly water-soluble drugs: Early promises, subsequent problems, and recent breakthroughs. *J. Pharm. Sci.* 88:1058–1066.

Small, P. A. 1951. Some factors affecting the solubility of polymers. *J. Appl. Chem.* 3:71–80.

Stefanis, E., and C. Panayiotou. 2012. A new expanded solubility parameter approach. *Int. J. Pharm.* 426:29–43.

Subrahmanyam, C. V. S., M. S. Reddy, J. V. Rao, and P. G. Rao. 1992. Irregular solution behavior of paracetamol in binary solvents. *Int. J. Pharm.* 78:17–24.

Teas, J. P. 1968. Graphic analysis of resin solubilities. *J. Paint Technol.* 40:19–25.

Thimmasetty, J., C. V. S. Subrahmanyam, P. R. Sathesh Babu, M. A. Maulik, and B. A. Viswanath. 2008. Solubility behavior of pimozide in polar and nonpolar solvents: Partial solubility parameters approach. *J. Solution Chem.* 37:1365–1378.

Thimmasetty, J., C. V. S. Subrahmanyam, B. A. Vishwanath, and P. R. Sathesh Babu. 2009. Solubility parameter estimation of celecoxib by current methods. *Asian J. Res. Chem.* 2:188–195.

Van Krevelen, D. W., and P. J. Hoftyzer. 1976. *Properties of Polymers: Their Estimation and Correlation with Chemical Structure.* New York: Elsevier Science.

Vasconcelos, T., B. Sarmento, and P. Costa. 2007. Solid dispersion as strategy to improve oral bioavailability of poor water soluble drugs. *Drug Discov. Today* 12:1068–1075.

Verheyen, S., P. Augustijns, R. Kinget, and G. Van den Mooter. 2001. Determination of partial solubility parameters of five benzodiazepines in individual solvents. *Int. J. Pharm.* 228:199–207.

Walker, E. E. 1952. The solvent action of organic substances on polyacrylonitrile. *J. Appl. Chem.* 2:470–481.

Wu, P. L., A. Beerbower, and A. Martin. 1982. Extended Hildebrand approach: Calculating partial solubility parameters of solid solutes. *J. Pharm. Sci.* 71:1285–1287.

Yu, X., G. L. Zipp, and G. W. R. Davidson. 1994. The effect of temperature and pH on the solubility of quinolone compounds: Estimation of heat of fusion. *Pharm. Res.* 11:522–527.

3 Prediction of Solubility

Yisheng Chen, Xiaohong Qi, and Rong (Ron) Liu

CONTENTS

INTRODUCTION

Solubility has been conventionally attributed to the maximum thermodynamic activity of a solute (Higuchi, 1977, 1982). In pharmaceutical science, solubility is commonly related to the bioavailability of the compound of interest, especially for poorly soluble compounds. In general, a higher bioavailability is easier to achieve for a soluble compound than for an insoluble one. This relationship, together with the intestinal permeability of drug substances, has been extended to form the basis of the scientific framework of the Biopharmaceutics Classification System (BCS) to classify drug substances so as to set expectations for the *in vivo* performance of drug products (Amidon et al., 1995; FDA, 2000). According to the Food and Drug Administration (FDA) BCS guidance (FDA, 2000), solubility may be used as an important criterion to justify the waiver of bioequivalence study (BE) for drug product if the drug substance has high intestinal permeability and the product has a rapid *in vitro* dissolution rate. A high solubility and a successful waiver of BE study for any significant post-approval changes will lead to a significant reduction of regulatory burden for the pharmaceutical industry and FDA. A significant saving may also be realized for development of new chemical entities (NCEs), if the NCEs have adequate water solubility and do not require any special solubilization techniques to achieve some desired bioavailability, leading to a reduced cost for product development and a reduced time for drug product to reach patients. It is thus apparent that being able to predict the solubility is important in the design and development of pharmaceuticals.

Solubility can be studied by thermodynamic and structure–solubility relationship approaches. The thermodynamic approach solves solubility problems using exact theoretical equations to relate the activity of a chemical in solution to the Gibb's free-energy change for the dissolution process. Similar to many other material equilibrium processes, the dissolution process and hence the equilibrium solubility are governed by the Gibb's free-energy change for the process. For an isothermal process under constant pressure, the partial molal Gibb's free-energy change for a dissolution process, $\Delta \bar{G}_{d,2}$, can be written by the following equation:

$$\Delta \bar{G}_{d,2} = \Delta \bar{H}_{d,2} - T\Delta \bar{S}_{d,2} \tag{3.1}$$

where the subscript, d, denotes the dissolution process, 2 represents the solute as the second component in the solution system, $\Delta \bar{H}_{d,2}$ is the partial molal enthalpy change for the solute, T denotes the absolute temperature at which dissolution occurs, and $\Delta \bar{S}_{d,2}$ is the partial molal entropy change for the solute. A negative free-energy change is the driving force for the dissolution process. Thus, an exothermic process promotes dissolution, and an endothermic process inhibits dissolution.

On the basis of the thermodynamic expression, the Gibb's free-energy change for mixing in solution can in turn be related to the activity of a solute at equilibrium as described by Equations 3.7 through 3.10 in Chapter 2 of this book, namely,

$$\Delta \bar{G}_{mix,2} = RT \ln a_2 \tag{3.2}$$

where a_2 is the activity of the solute in the solution.

It is clear from Equations 3.1 and 3.2 that the activity of the solute at equilibrium can be calculated if the free-energy change can be determined. Indeed, this approach has been taken by Hildebrand to develop regular solution theory (Hildebrand et al., 1970). In regular solution theory, the enthalpy of mixing was approximated using a geometric rule, while the entropy of mixing was simplified using the entropy of mixing in an ideal solution. These approximations limit the theory to solutions in which no specific interactions occur. When hydrogen bonding occurs in molecular interactions, the enthalpy of mixing will deviate from the geometric rule, and the entropy of mixing will be smaller than the random mixing in an ideal solution. Therefore, new methods accounting the effects of specific molecular interactions in a solution will be useful for the study of solubility.

Alternatively, the structure–solubility relationship estimates solubility using equations that relate solubility to the molecular structures of solutes. The structure–solubility relationship is generally regarded as an empirical method. There is no doubt that an exact theoretical method is preferred over an empirical method for the study of solubility phenomena. However, owing to the very complicated nature of molecular interactions and the various simplifications used in the development of mathematical models, exact thermodynamic approaches may not always provide accurate results without an extensive study of the compound of interest. At the present time, both theoretical and empirical approaches result in similar accuracy, and can be used equally well in the estimation of solubility.

In this chapter, new approaches developed in recent years for the prediction of solubility of organic compounds in solutions, both theoretical and empirical, will be discussed. It is intended to update readers on the methods for prediction of solubility and to provide tools for the design and study of new molecules in pharmaceutical research and development.

MOBILE ORDER THEORY

Taking the specific interactions in solution into consideration, Ruelle et al. (1991) have developed a comprehensive equation for the calculation of solubility of nonelectrolytes. This equation was called the mobile order theory. The equation was developed partly on the basis of the perpetual moving nature of molecules. According to this theory, each molecule of a particular species in a solution is presented the same mobile environment. Spatial orientations of molecules in solution change constantly. Molecular movement in the solution is random, and the entropy of mixing is the same as that of an ideal solution if there is no preferential molecular interaction in the system. When preferential interactions such as hydrogen bonding occur, molecular orientation and movement in the solution are not random. Consequently, the entropy of solution decreases as compared to that of an ideal solution. The change in entropy as a result of preferential intermolecular interaction is then used to account for solubility. In this approach, solubility in a nonpolar solution system is predicted in a way similar to regular solution theory, while solubility in solutions with polar interactions is treated with specific interaction constants. Thus, this approach provides more accurate results for the estimation of solubility.

According to the mobile order theory, a general equation for the expression of volume fraction solubility, Θ_2, is given by

$$\ln \Theta_2 = -A_m + B - D - F + O - OH \tag{3.3}$$

Physical meaning and mathematical expression for each of the terms in Equation 3.3 are defined in the following paragraphs. Readers are referred to the original publications (Ruelle et al., 1991, 1992) for the derivation of each term. For comparison with other methods, one has to convert the unit of solubility from volume fraction to mole fraction.

A_m in Equation 3.3 is the fluidization term accounting for the hypothetical melting of a crystalline solute in the dissolution process. A_m takes the same expression for crystalline material used in the regular solubility equation, assuming that heat capacity is the same for both the crystalline and the hypothetical molten solute:

$$A_m = \frac{\Delta \bar{H}_m}{R} \left(\frac{T_m - T}{T_m T} \right) \tag{3.4}$$

where $\Delta \bar{H}_m$ represents the molar enthalpy of melting of a crystalline solute at its absolute melting point T_m, R is the gas constant, and T denotes the absolute temperature at which solubility is measured. In an ideal solution, Equation 3.4 is the expression for the solubility of a crystalline solute that has the same size as the solvent.

The B term in Equation 3.3 is an entropy correction term for any solutes with a molar volume different from solvent. In a conventional expression, the partial entropy of mixing for an ideal solution can be related to the mole fraction concentration of the species of interest by

$$\Delta \bar{S}_{mix,2} = -R \ln x_2^i \tag{3.5}$$

where x_2^i is the mole fraction concentration of the solute in an ideal solution. If the molar volumes of solvent and solute are different, entropy of mixing will deviate from Equation 3.5 (Bustamante et al., 1989). For the correction of such a deviation, several equations have been developed (Huyskens and Haulait-Pirson, 1985). Term B was derived from the corrected equation for entropy of mixing and is expressed as

$$B = 0.5 \Phi_1 \left(\frac{V_2}{V_1} - 1 \right) + 0.5 \ln \left(\Phi_2 + \frac{\Phi_1 V_2}{V_1} \right) \tag{3.6}$$

where V_1 and V_2 are the molar volumes of solvent and solute, respectively. The contribution of B to solubility becomes null if the molar volume is the same for solute and solvent. Note that solubility appears in both sides of the solubility equation when Equation 3.6 is substituted into Equation 3.3. Thus, an iterative procedure is needed for the calculation of solubility.

The D term in Equation 3.3 accounts for part of the effects of solution enthalpy. Enthalpy of mixing results when the solute–solvent interaction force is different from the solute–solute and the solvent–solvent interactions. Intermolecular forces can be further characterized as dispersion, dipolar, and hydrogen-bond forces. In the mobile order solubility approach, dispersion and dipolar forces were not separated. The effects of these two forces on solubility were expressed in terms of modified solubility parameters, δ_1' and δ_2'. The relationship between solubility and solubility parameters can be derived in the same manner as used in the regular solution equation described in Chapter 2 of this book, and can be written as

$$D = \frac{V_2 \Phi_1^2}{RT} \left(\delta_2' - \delta_1' \right)^2 \tag{3.7}$$

The modified solubility parameter, δ', in Equation 3.7 is different from the Hildebrand solubility parameters but is similar to the sum of the dispersion solubility parameter, δ_d, and the polar solubility parameter, δ_p, of the Hansen partial solubility parameters (Hansen, 1967). Values of the modified solubility parameters can be determined from the solubility of the solute in a nonpolar solvent. For example, pentane has been used as a solvent to determine the δ' of methylparaben (Ruelle et al., 1991).

The F term in Equation 3.3 describes the hydrophobic effects of solutes on the hydrogen-bonded solvent chain. The source of this term is the decrease in mixing entropy owing to the hydrogen bond formed among solvent molecules:

$$F = \Phi_1 \left(\frac{r_1 V_2}{V_1} - n_2 \right) \tag{3.8}$$

where n_2 represents the number of the amphiphilic OH sites on the solute molecule. The structural indicator of the solvent, r_1, has a value of zero for nonassociated solvents, 1 for alcohols, and 2 for water.

O accounts for the effects of solute–solvent hydrogen bonding. Intermolecular hydrogen bonding between solute and solvent results in a decrease of the Gibb's free energy and thus promotes mixing. Hydrogen bonding can occur in different modes, depending on the donor/acceptor structures of the solvent and solute. In this term, the effects of the hydrogen bond formed between the proton-donor solvent and the proton-acceptor solute are described. Mathematically, O is expressed as

$$O = \ln \left(\frac{K_{12} \Phi_1}{V_1} + 1 \right) \tag{3.9}$$

where K_{12} is the stability constant of the hydrogen bond between the proton-donor solvent and the proton-acceptor solute molecules.

When a solvent molecule possesses only proton-acceptor capability and a solute molecule possesses both proton-donor and proton-acceptor capabilities, competition among different molecular species for hydrogen bonding is inevitable. For such a system, the effects of the hydrogen bond between the solvent and solute can be described by the OH term in Equation 3.3. It is clear that bond stability for different species plays a significant role in the effect of hydrogen bonds. The larger the stability constant value, the stronger the hydrogen bond formed. Consequently, effects on solubility resulting from the formation of hydrogen bonds among solvent and solutes can be treated using bond stability constants as

$$\mathrm{OH} = \ln \left(\frac{K_{22}}{V_2} + 1 \right) - \ln \left(\frac{K_{OH} \Phi_1}{V_1} + 1 + \frac{K_{22} \Phi_2}{V_2} \right) \tag{3.10}$$

where K_{22} is the stability constant for hydrogen bonds between solutes and K_{OH} is the constant for the bonding between proton-donor solute and the proton-acceptor solvent.

A general equation for the calculation of solubility can then be obtained by substituting Equations 3.4 and 3.6 through 3.10 into Equation 3.3, as shown in the following equation:

$$\ln \Phi_2 = \frac{-\Delta \bar{H}_m}{R} \left(\frac{T_m - T}{T_m T} \right) + 0.5 \Phi_1 \left(\frac{V_2}{V_1} - 1 \right) + 0.5 \ln \left(\Phi_2 + \frac{\Phi_1 V_2}{V_1} \right) - \frac{V_2 \Phi_1^2}{RT} (\delta_2' - \delta_1')^2$$

$$- \Phi_1 \left(\frac{r_1 V_2}{V_1} - n_2 \right) + \ln \left(\frac{K_{12} \Phi_1}{V_1} + 1 \right) - \ln \left(\frac{K_{22}}{V_2} + 1 \right) + \ln \left(\frac{K_{OH} \Phi_1}{V_1} + 1 + \frac{K_{22} \Phi_2}{V_2} \right) \tag{3.11}$$

It is clear that Equation 3.11 is so far the most comprehensive equation ever developed for the calculation of solubility. Since hydrogen-bonding effects are accounted for by using stability constants, solubility is better represented and prediction results are more accurate. This approach is a step forward in dealing with intermolecular interactions. However, to use Equation 3.11, one needs to determine the modified solubility parameters and different types of hydrogen-bonding constants for both solute and solvent, as well as the melting point, enthalpy of melting, and the molar volumes of the solvent and the hypothetical molten solute. It is obvious that the determination of these specific binding constants and the modified solubility parameter is not straightforward. For this reason, one may have to use approximate values for the estimation of solubility. In addition, an iterative procedure is required for the calculation since solubility appears on both sides of the equation.

PARTITION THEORY

In the early 1980s, Yalkowsky and Valvani developed a partition theory (Yalkowsky and Valvani, 1980) for the estimation of solubility in aqueous solutions that could not be estimated using the regular solution equation owing to the dominant effects of hydrogen bonding in the aqueous solutions. In the partition theory, solubility was explained by the change of solute activity coefficient in the aqueous solution. Consequently, solubility in water was predicted using the oil/water partition coefficient, which was defined as the ratio of the activity coefficients of a solute in water and in octanol.

Conventionally, the activity of a solute in the solution can be described by the following equation:

$$a_2 = x_2 \gamma_2 \tag{3.12}$$

where a_2, x_2, and γ_2 are the activity, mole fraction concentration, and activity coefficient of a solute in solution, respectively. In an ideal solution, the activity coefficient is unity, and $a_2 = x_2^i$.

When a solution is equilibrated with a pure solute, the activity of the solute in the solution is the same as the activity of the pure solute substance. For a crystalline material in an ideal solution, solubility can be expressed by the following equation:

$$\log a_2 = \log x_2^i = \frac{-\Delta \bar{H}_m}{2.303R} \left(\frac{T_m - T}{TT_m} \right) \tag{3.13}$$

The ratio $-\Delta \bar{H}_m / T_m$ equals $\Delta \bar{S}_m$. At a given temperature of 25°C (298.2 K), and by using the value of $R = 1.987$ cal mol^{-1} K^{-1}, Equation 3.13 can be simplified to

$$\log x_2^i = \frac{-\Delta \bar{S}_m (\text{mp} - 25)}{1364} \tag{3.14}$$

where mp is the melting point (°C) of a crystalline solute.

In real solutions, the activity coefficient will deviate from unity owing to intermolecular interactions, especially when preferential hydrogen bonding and dipolar interactions occur. The effects of the activity coefficient on solubility can be accounted for by using Equation 3.12. Substituting Equations 3.13 and 3.14 into Equation 3.12, mole fraction solubility in water at 25°C can be written as

$$\log X_2 = \frac{-\Delta \bar{S}_m (\text{mp} - 25)}{1364} - \log \gamma_2 \tag{3.15}$$

Values of $\Delta \bar{S}_m$ can be measured. More interestingly, $\Delta \bar{S}_m$ can be estimated on the basis of the melting process as well as the molecular structure of a solute. When a crystalline material undergoes melting, molecules change from a highly ordered state in the immobilized crystalline lattice to a chaotic liquid state. During this transition process, entropy of solute increases in three subprocesses: rotation, translation, and internal molecular rotation. The total entropy change for the melting process is the summation of the entropy changes for the three subprocesses:

$$\Delta \bar{S}_m = \Delta \bar{S}_m^{rot} + \Delta \bar{S}_m^{tr} + \Delta \bar{S}_m^{intr} \tag{3.16}$$

where m designates melting, rot stands for molecular rotation, tr represents translation, and intr denotes internal molecular rotation resulting from the conformational change about flexible bonds.

Values for each term on the right-hand side of Equation 3.16 can be calculated by statistical mechanics, an approach that has been successfully used for an ideal gas (Levine, 1988). Alternatively, average values from experimental data can be used for estimation. In either case, some simplifications can be made based on the molecular structure and geometry. Specifically, $\Delta \bar{S}_m^{rot}$ is zero for spherical molecules, and $\Delta \bar{S}_m^{intr}$ is zero for rigid molecules. For many compounds, it has been found that $\Delta \bar{S}_m^{intr}$ is relatively constant, with an average value of 3.5 cal mol^{-1} K^{-1}. Similarly $\Delta \bar{S}_m^{rot}$ for a nonspherical molecule is approximately 10 cal mol^{-1} K^{-1}. Thus, entropy of melting for small, rigid, and nonspherical molecules can be estimated to be

$$\Delta \bar{S}_m = \Delta \bar{S}_m^{rot} + \Delta \bar{S}_m^{tr} = 13.5 \text{ cal mol}^{-1}\text{K}^{-1} \tag{3.17}$$

and, for rigid spherical molecules,

$$\Delta \bar{S}_m = \Delta \bar{S}_m^{tr} = 3.5 \text{ cal mol}^{-1}\text{K}^{-1} \tag{3.18}$$

In reality, almost all drug molecules are not spherical. Therefore, Equation 3.18 is rarely used.

The $\Delta \bar{S}_m^{intr}$ is determined by the increase in degrees of freedom for spatial conformation changes in the liquid state as compared to the crystalline state. In crystal lattices, spatial conformation change resulting from the rotation about a flexible bond is not permitted. Such a rotation, however, is possible in the liquid state. For each flexible bond, there are three possible conformations due to steric constrain. Thus, the probability of each conformation resulting from one single bond is one-third, and the probability of the fully stretched conformation is

$$p = \left(\frac{1}{3}\right)^{n-3} \tag{3.19}$$

Therefore, the entropy change due to the intramolecular rotation is

$$\Delta \bar{S}_m^{intr} = -R \ln p = -R \ln \left(\frac{1}{3}\right)^{n-3} = 2.2(n-3) \tag{3.20}$$

where n is the number of carbon and heteroatoms in a flexible chain, and $n - 3$ is the number of the twistable angles in the chain. $\Delta \bar{S}_m^{intr} = 0$ for $n \leq 3$. In practice, it was found (Yalkowsky and Valvani, 1980) that internal molecular rotation can be better approximated by

$$\Delta \bar{S}_m^{intr} = 2.5(n-5) \tag{3.21}$$

and $\Delta \bar{S}_m^{intr} = 0$ for $n \leq 5$.

On the basis of these approximations, ideal solubility can then be estimated on the basis of the structure of molecules. Using $\Delta \bar{S}_m = 13.5$ for rigid and nonspherical molecules as described in Equation 3.17, ideal solubility given by Equation 3.14 can be approximated by

$$\log x_2^i = -0.01(\text{mp} - 25) \tag{3.22}$$

For partially flexible molecules, the equation is

$$\log x_2^i = -[0.01+0.0018(n-5)](mp-25) \tag{3.23}$$

The next step in developing the solubility equation by partition theory is the estimation of the activity coefficient of solute γ_w in water solution. If an aqueous solution is equilibrated with octanol, then it can be shown that γ_w can be related to the octanol–water partition coefficient by

$$P = \frac{\gamma_w}{\gamma_o} \tag{3.24}$$

where P is the octanol–water partition coefficient and γ_o is the activity coefficient of the solute in octanol. Both γ_w and γ_o are expressed in mole fraction units.

When the cohesive energy of the solute is similar to that of octanol, the activity coefficient in octanol can be approximated as unity. As a result, the activity coefficient in water can be approximated using the octanol–water partition coefficient:

$$\log \gamma_w \approx \log P \tag{3.25}$$

Thus, solubility in water can be predicted using $\log P$ by substituting Equation 3.25 for $\log r_2$ in Equation 3.15.

The mole fraction partition coefficient given by Equation 3.24 can be replaced by the conventional concentration-based partitioning coefficient, PC, defined by

$$PC = \frac{c_o}{c_w} \tag{3.26}$$

where c_o is the molar concentration of the solute in the octanol phase in equilibrium with the water phase, and c_w represents the molar concentration of the solute in the aqueous phase in equilibrium with the octanol phase.

It can be shown that $\log P \approx \log PC + 0.94$, assuming that both solutions are dilute such that the solvent molarity is approximately 55 in the aqueous phase and 6.3 in the octanol phase. As a result, the mole fraction solubility for partially rigid molecules can be written as

$$\log x_2 = -[0.01+0.0018(n-5)](mp-25) - \log PC - 0.94 \tag{3.27}$$

Besides using the mole fraction scale for concentration, solubility in water can also be expressed in molar concentrations using S_w, which can be approximated as the product of x_2 and the molarity of water of 55, assuming the solution is dilute. Then, aqueous solubility at 25°C is

$$\log S_w = -[0.01+0.0018(n-5)](mp-25) - \log PC + 0.80 \tag{3.28}$$

For rigid molecules, in which internal molecular rotation is not permitted, Equation 3.28 reduces to

$$\log S_w = -0.01mp - \log PC + 1.05 \tag{3.29}$$

For substances that are liquid at 25°C, the solubility equation is further reduced to

$$\log S_w = \log PC + 1.05 \tag{3.30}$$

The partition approach is a relatively simple method that can be used to predict the solubility in a solution that involves complicated intermolecular interactions. In addition, the parameters used in the partition theory can be easily estimated. For example, partition coefficients can be estimated using many methods on the basis of the structure of solutes (Rekker, 1977; Dunn et al., 1986; Rekker and Mannhold, 1992; Mannhold et al., 1995). Thus, for a compound with a known chemical structure, solubility in water at 25°C can be calculated if the melting point and the octanol–water partition coefficient of the solute are known. This approach generally results in a satisfactory accuracy, as shown by Yalkowsky and Valvani (1980). More accurate results can be obtained if the solutes are classified according to their chemical structures. Yalkowsky and his coworkers estimated the solubility in water, $\log S_{est}$, of different classes of compounds, and compared the results with the experimental $\log S_{obs}$ (Yalkowsky and Valvani, 1980; Valvani et al., 1981). They have shown that, for polycyclic compounds, the estimated values were larger than the experimental values, as described by

$$\log S_{obs} = 0.944 \log S_{est} - 0.785 \tag{3.31}$$

A similar result was also found for halogen-substituted benzenes as

$$\log S_{obs} = 0.980 \log S_{est} - 0.32 \tag{3.32}$$

Equations 3.31 and 3.32 show that, for a particular class of compounds, predicted solubility using partition theory must be corrected by a unique value established by a comparison study. Otherwise, significant errors could result for some specific classes of compounds. Recently, Jain and Yalkowsky reevaluated the general solubility equation (GSE), proposed by Valvani and Yalkowsky in 1980, and revised the GSE equation. The revised GSE was validated on a set of 580 pharmaceutically, environmentally, and industrially relevant nonelectrolytes. The revised equation has a stronger theoretical background and provides a more accurate estimation of aqueous solubility (Jain and Yalkowsky, 2001). The applicability of the GSE was further extended to weak electrolytes. It was demonstrated that the GSE estimates the aqueous solubility of 949 compounds, including 367 weak electrolytes, with an AAE of 0.58. It was also shown that the intrinsic solubilities of weak acids for which the $pK_a + \log S(w) \le 0$ and for weak bases for which $pK_a + \log S(w) \le 14$ are within a factor of 2 of the total solubilities (Jain et al., 2006).

Example 3.1

Calculate the solubility of methylparaben in water at 25°C. The melting point of methylparaben is 131°C (Windholz and Budavari, 1983). The chemical structure of methylparaben is

SOLUTION

The octanol–water partition coefficient of methylparaben is estimated using a fragmental method as described by the following equation (Rekker, 1977):

$$\log PC = \sum_{i=1}^{n} f_i \tag{3.33}$$

where f is the fragmental partition coefficient of each of n molecular fragments. Using Equation 3.33 and the fragmental values determined by Rekker (1977), the partition coefficient of methylparaben is estimated to be

$$\log PC = f_{C_6H_4} + f_{OH} + f_{COO} + f_{CH_3} = 1.719 - 0.359 - 0.430 + 0.695 = 1.625 \tag{3.34}$$

Since the side chain backbone of methylparaben has less than five atoms, water solubility can be estimated using Equation 3.29. The result is

$$\log S_w = -0.01 \times 131 - 1.625 + 1.05 = -1.885$$

This result is translated into a molar solubility of 0.013 mol L^{-1}, which agrees well with the experimental values of 0.0196 mol L^{-1} (Windholz and Budavari, 1983) and 0.0158 mol L^{-1} (Manzo and Ahumada, 1990).

QUANTITATIVE STRUCTURE–SOLUBILITY RELATIONSHIPS

Previous discussions have shown that different theoretical equations can be derived for the prediction of solubility. Each of the equations may have unique advantages for certain applications. However, many of these equations are based on excessive assumptions and simplifications and hence have limitations. In addition, some of the physicochemical constants used in the equations are difficult to obtain. Alternatively, solubility can be estimated by the quantitative structure–solubility relationship (QSSR) approach. QSSR is an extension of the quantitative structure–activity relationship (QSAR), which was defined as an equation established using statistical techniques for expressing the biological potencies of a series of related compounds as a linear function of their physicochemical properties (Cramer et al., 1979). The QSAR technique was first developed in the early 1960s by Hansch et al. (1962) to correlate the bioactivity of phenoxyacetic acids with the Hammett constant and partition coefficient. Since then, QSAR has been widely used (Hansch, 1993), mostly in drug design, and has led to the identification and the development of potent drugs (Cramer et al., 1979; Gould et al., 1988). The QSAR technique has also been extended beyond the correlation of biological activities and has been used to correlate some physicochemical properties with others, such as the partition coefficient (Rekker, 1977; Seydel, 1985; Leo, 1993), a binding constant (Charton and Charton, 1985), chromatographic retention indices (Kaliszan and Höltje, 1982; Kaliszan, 1992), pharmacokinetic parameters (Schaper and Seydel, 1985; Herman and Veng-Pedersen, 1994), and, to our interests, solubility (Zhou et al., 1993; Sutter and Jurs, 1996). There are many such empirical methods developed for solubility prediction. However, the authors cannot include all methods here. In the remainder of this chapter, newly developed methods such as a molecular modeling approach (Bodor and Huang, 1992; Zhou et al., 1993), a group contribution approach (Wakita et al., 1986; Klopman et al., 1992; Kühne et al., 1995; Myrdal et al., 1995), and a frequently used linear free-energy relationship method (Taft et al., 1985; Lee, 1996) will be discussed.

MOLECULAR MODELING APPROACHES

Partial Atomic Charge Approach

One of the critical steps in developing an expression for solubility is the establishment of relationships for intermolecular interactions in the solution. Indeed, the treatment of intermolecular interactions has been the main challenge in the study of solubility. For nonpolar molecules, molecular interaction is mainly due to dispersion forces. For polar molecules, intermolecular interaction is complicated by the involvement of dipolar forces and hydrogen bonding in the solution. Apparently, the interaction energy can be calculated if the source and the strength of the interaction can be accurately expressed. It is well known that the polarity of a molecule is the result of uneven electron distribution within the molecule due to the differences in electronegativity of different atoms. Thus, the degree of electron localization within a molecule can be used to represent the polarity and hence the polar interactions. Atomic charges have been successfully used in correlations with permeability (Chen et al., 1993, 1996) and solubility in water (Bodor and Huang, 1992). The following sections present the use of partial atomic charges for the prediction of the solubility of polar compounds in a polar solvent, isopropyl alcohol.

According to Hildebrand et al. (1970), the simplified solubility equation (assuming the difference in heat capacity of the crystalline and the hypothetical molten forms of the solute is negligible) for a crystalline solute in a regular solution is

$$\ln x_2 = -\frac{\Delta \bar{H}_m}{R}\left(\frac{1}{T}-\frac{1}{T_m}\right)-\frac{v_2 \Phi_1^2}{RT}\left(E_1 + E_2 - 2E_{12}\right) \tag{3.35}$$

where v_2 is the molar volume of the hypothetical supercooled liquid solute, Φ_1 is the volume fraction of solvent in the solution at equilibrium, and E represents the cohesive or adhesive energy densities. The subscripts 1, 2, and 12 represent solvent, solute, and the solute–solvent interaction, respectively.

It is assumed that the E terms in Equation 3.35 are linear combinations of the polar and nonpolar interaction energies and can be rewritten as

$$E_1 + E_2 - 2E_{12} = \left(E_1^n + E_2^n - 2E_{12}^n\right)+\left(E_1^p + E_2^p - 2E_{12}^p\right) \tag{3.36}$$

where E^n is the nonpolar interaction energy, and E^p represents the polar interaction energy. Substituting Equation 3.36 into Equation 3.35, the solubility equation can be written as

$$\ln x_2 = -\frac{\Delta \bar{H}_m}{R}\left(\frac{1}{T}-\frac{1}{T_m}\right)-\frac{v_2 \Phi_1^2}{RT}\left[\left(E_1^n + E_2^n - 2E_{12}^n\right)+\left(E_1^p + E_2^p - 2E_{12}^p\right)\right] \tag{3.37}$$

The division of total cohesive energy into multicomponents has been successfully studied by Hansen (1967) and has been extended for solubility prediction for different compounds in separate cases (Martin et al., 1981; Bustamante et al., 1991; Richardson et al., 1992).

In this study, partial atomic charges were used as predictors to represent the effects of the polar portion of cohesive and adhesive energies. In this approach, a molecule was arbitrarily divided into polar and nonpolar parts on the basis of the elements constituting the chemical structure of the molecule. The polar portion of a molecule consisted of the following two classes of elements: (1) any oxygen and/or nitrogen atoms in the molecule and (2) any hydrogen and carbon atoms directly bonded to the oxygen and/or the nitrogen atoms. Any other remaining carbon atoms, together with their bonded hydrogens and/or halogens, were then defined as the nonpolar parts of a molecule. An example of this classification is given in Figure 3.1.

It can be seen from the structures shown in Figure 3.1 that the nonpolar parts of a molecule are essentially hydrocarbon fragments. Effects of the nonpolar parts of the molecular structure on solubility can be estimated using the regular solution equation, that is,

$$E_1^n + E_2^n - 2E_{12}^n = (\delta_1^n - \delta_2^n)^2 \tag{3.38}$$

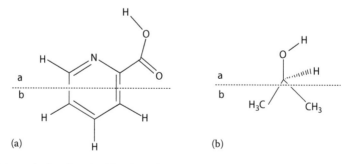

(a)   (b)

FIGURE 3.1 Schematic for the classification of polar and nonpolar portions of molecules. a: Polar; b: Nonpolar. (a) Picolinic acid; (b) Isopropyl alcohol.

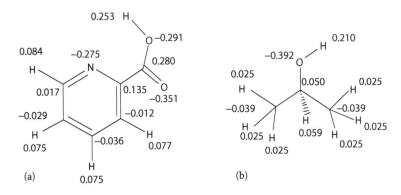

FIGURE 3.2 Examples of calculated partial atomic charges: (a) Picolinic acid; (b) Isopropyl alcohol.

where δ^n is the solubility parameter for the nonpolar portion. δ_1^n and δ_2^n can be estimated by the group contribution method (Barton, 1983) as defined by

$$\delta^n = \frac{\sum {}^z F_i}{\sum {}^z v_i}$$

(3.39)

where ${}^z F_i$ is the group molar attraction constant, and ${}^z v_i$ is the molar volume of the ith group.

The effects of the polar portion of a molecule can be related to the partial atomic charges. In this study, a molecular modeling computer software, SYBYL® (Tripos, 1992), was used to generate the molecular models. Atomic charges were then calculated using the Gast-Hück method in SYBYL.

Examples for the calculated atomic charges are shown in Figure 3.2. There are several different methods for estimating atomic charges. Different methods (Levine, 1988; Tripos, 1992) may result in different charge values, but the results for the correlation may be similar (Klopman and Iroff, 1981; Kantola et al., 1991; Cramer et al., 1993).

In this study, it was observed that only the atomic charges of nitrogen, oxygen, and polar hydrogen contribute significantly to the solubility in isopropyl alcohol. A polar hydrogen is empirically defined as any hydrogen atom with a charge value higher than 0.15 when the atom is not involved in intramolecular hydrogen bonding. For example, the hydrogen atoms in hydroxy, carboxylic acid, and amino groups may be polar hydrogens. On the basis of these observations, the charges of the solute were classified into three types, namely nitrogen, oxygen, and polar hydrogen. In the case of isopropyl alcohol, the charges were classified into two terms, oxygen and polar hydrogen (Figure 3.2b).

The regression equation for correlating the mole fraction solubility of solid compounds in isopropyl alcohol at 30°C with the selected parameters is

$$\log x_2 = -7.54 \times 10^{-3}(mp - 30) - 6.50 \times 10^{-5} MW(\delta_1^n - \delta_2^n)^2$$
$$- 4.12 \times 10^{-3} MW\left(\sum Q_{1i} + \sum Q_{2j}\right) + 5.08 \times 10^{-3} \times 2MW \sum \sqrt{Q_{2j}}$$

(3.40)

where x_2 is the mole fraction solubility in isopropyl alcohol at 30°C; MW represents the molecular weight of solute; δ_1^n denotes the solubility parameter of the nonpolar part of isopropyl alcohol, δ_2^n is the nonpolar solubility parameter of a solute; Q represents the absolute values of the sum of atomic charges of the polar hydrogen, Q_H, oxygen, Q_O, and nitrogen, Q_N, respectively. The last two parameters in Equation 3.40 are calculated by Equations 3.41 and 3.42:

TABLE 3.1

Experimental and Predicted Mole Fraction Solubility at 30°C in Isopropyl Alcohol and Selected Parameters

Compounds	MW	mp (°C)	δ''	Q_H	Q_O	Q_N	Exp. log x	Equation 3.40 log x	Residual	Equations 3.41 and 3.42 log x	Residual
4-Nitroimidazole	113.08	303	0.0	0.232	0.240	0.692	-3.4556	-2.9012	-0.5544	-2.958	-0.497
Imidazole	68.08	90	0.0	0.241	0.000	0.596	-0.3859	-0.6703	0.2843	-0.677	0.291
Benzimidazole	118.14	170	9.8	0.234	0.000	0.557	-1.0691	-1.2217	0.1526	-1.258	0.188
2-Methylbenzimidazole	132.17	176	8.4	0.232	0.000	0.565	-0.9681	-1.2141	0.2460	-1.225	0.257
2-Methyl-5-nitrobenzimidazole	177.16	223	8.1	0.229	0.232	0.689	-1.8752	-2.3534	0.4782	-2.336	0.460
2-Hydroxybenzimidazole	134.14	318	9.8	0.498	0.277	0.521	-2.4421	-2.7498	0.3077	-2.828	0.386
Indole	117.15	52	9.8	0.227	0.000	0.280	-0.2138	-0.2114	-0.0024	-0.200	-0.014
7-Nitroindole	162.15	94	9.8	0.225	0.230	0.402	-1.5654	-1.2712	-0.2942	-1.272	-0.293
2-Methylindole	131.18	61	8.7	0.226	0.000	0.274	-0.4383	-0.2225	-0.2158	-0.219	-0.219
2-Methylimidazole	82.11	142	6.3	0.237	0.000	0.565	-0.5445	-0.8926	0.3481	-0.874	0.330
2-Ethylimidazole	96.13	85	6.9	0.237	0.000	0.604	-0.2186	-0.4824	0.2638	-0.482	0.263
Ethyl 4-methyl-5-imidazolecarboxylate	154.17	204	6.3	0.237	0.651	0.568	-2.3883	-2.2523	-0.1354	-2.242	-0.096
Pyrazole	68.08	69	9.8	0.258	0.000	0.443	-0.2606	-0.3538	0.0932	-0.356	0.095
3,5-Dimethylpyrazole	96.13	107	6.8	0.248	0.000	0.475	-0.5573	-0.6069	0.0496	-0.620	0.063
1,5-Dimethyl-2-pyrrolecarbonitrile	120.16	54	7.8	0.000	0.000	0.616	-0.7200	-0.7598	0.0398	-0.772	0.052
2-Methyl-5-nitroimidazole	127.1	252	6.3	0.235	0.226	0.741	-2.4816	-2.2935	-0.1881	-2.339	-0.142
2-Aminopyrazine	95.11	119	0.0	0.312	0.000	0.806	-1.0482	-0.9770	-0.0712	-0.988	-0.060
7-Amino-2,4-dimethyl-1,8-naphthyridine	173.22	221	8.0	0.316	0.000	0.847	-2.0640	-1.5931	-0.4709	-1.578	-0.486
5-Chloro-3-pyridinol	129.55	160	10.5	0.251	0.325	0.307	-1.0605	-1.6464	0.5860	-1.636	0.575
3,5-Dichloropyridine	147.99	65	10.6	0.000	0.000	0.296	-0.9726	-0.9660	-0.0066	-0.981	0.008
Nicotinic acid	123.11	236	9.8	0.252	0.646	0.290	-2.3830	-2.2611	-0.1219	-2.235	-0.148
3-Aminopyridine	94.12	64	9.8	0.304	0.000	0.584	-0.2845	-0.3548	0.0703	-0.348	0.063
2-Aminopyridine	94.12	57	9.8	0.308	0.000	0.553	-0.3099	-0.2929	-0.0170	-0.292	-0.018
2-Methoxy-5-nitropyridine	154.13	108	9.8	0.000	0.539	0.410	-2.1175	-2.1415	0.0240	-2.121	0.004
2-Hydroxy-5-nitropyridine	140.1	188	9.8	0.249	0.551	0.410	-2.2700	-2.0919	-0.1781	-2.085	-0.185
2-Hydroxypyridine	95.10	106	9.8	0.251	0.315	0.274	-0.8165	-1.0290	0.2126	-1.024	0.207
3-Hydroxypyridine	95.10	129	9.8	0.251	0.325	0.307	-0.8477	-1.2025	0.3548	-1.219	0.372

(Continued)

TABLE 3.1 (Continued)
Experimental and Predicted Mole Fraction Solubility at 30°C in Isopropyl Alcohol and Selected Parameters

Compounds	MW	mp (°C)	δ^n	Q_H	Q_O	Q_N	Exp. log x	Equation 3.40 log x	Residual	Equations 3.41 and 3.42 log x	Residual
Picolinic acid	123.11	136	9.8	0.000	0.642	0.275	−1.7595	−1.9953	0.2358	−1.995	0.236
2-Amino-4-methylpyridine	108.14	98	8.1	0.308	0.000	0.564	−0.7206	−0.5409	−0.1797	−0.546	−0.174
2-Amino-4,6-dimethylpyridine	122.17	63	7.5	0.308	0.000	0.568	−0.3534	−0.2846	−0.0688	−0.277	−0.076
2-Amino-5-nitropyridine	139.11	188	9.8	0.302	0.228	0.696	−2.3820	−1.9122	−0.4698	−1.936	−0.446
2,4-Dihydroxypyridine	111.10	278	9.8	0.505	0.643	0.290	−2.4535	−2.3887	−0.0648	−2.453	−0.001
2,5-Pyridinedicarboxylic acid	167.12	256	9.8	0.252	1.284	0.269	−3.2840	−2.7647	−0.5193	−2.769	−0.515
6-Chloronicotinic acid	157.56	190	10.4	0.252	0.648	0.275	−1.5935	−2.1464	0.5529	−2.157	0.563
2-Amino-5-chloropyridine	128.56	136	10.4	0.308	0.000	0.552	−1.4023	−0.9582	−0.4441	−0.955	−0.447
6-Hydroxynicotinic acid	139.11	304	9.8	0.507	0.964	0.266	−3.2757	−2.7662	−0.5095	−2.729	−0.547
Benzoic acid	122.12	122	9.8	0.252	0.650	0.000	−0.6979	−0.8753	−0.1774	−0.879	0.181
Salicylic acid	138.12	158	9.8	0.503	0.986	0.000	−0.7553	−1.1001	0.3456	−1.109	0.354
3-Aminobenzoic acid	137.14	178	9.8	0.252	0.651	0.281	−2.0602	−1.8992	−0.1610	−1.913	−0.147
Phenol	94.11	43	9.8	0.248	0.333	0.000	−0.0250	−0.1443	0.1193	−0.136	0.110
4-Aminophenol	109.13	188	9.8	0.244	0.341	0.288	−2.1285	−1.7167	−0.4118	−1.693	−0.436
3-tert-Butylphenol	150.22	41	7.2	0.249	0.326	0.000	−0.1322	−0.0602	−0.0720	−0.048	−0.084
3-Hydroxybenzoic acid	138.12	202	9.8	0.500	0.982	0.000	−0.8804	−1.4259	0.5455	−1.448	0.568
4-Hydroxybenzoic acid	138.12	214	9.8	0.502	0.987	0.000	−0.8948	−1.5163	0.6214	−1.501	0.607
m-Nitrobenzaldehyde	151.12	58	9.8	0.000	0.588	0.122	−1.4763	−1.4867	0.0104	−1.507	0.031
4-Aminoacetophenone	135.17	106	8.6	0.304	0.385	0.279	−1.2757	−1.1351	−0.1406	−1.141	−0.135
4-tert-Butylbenzoic acid	178.23	164	7.2	0.253	0.637	0.000	−0.9893	−1.1616	0.1723	−1.162	0.173
Methylparaben	152.15	131	9.8	0.250	0.973	0.000	−0.7376	−1.0620	0.3276	−1.082	0.345
Ethylparaben	166.18	116	8.6	0.250	0.970	0.000	−0.6983	−0.9030	0.2047	−0.922	0.224
Isophthalic acid	166.13	348	9.8	0.504	1.300	0.000	−2.3205	−2.5848	0.2643	−2.633	0.312
4-Nitrobenzoic acid	167.12	242	9.8	0.252	0.877	0.125	−2.0636	−2.4252	0.3616	−2.447	0.384
4-Carboxybenzaldehyde	150.13	247	9.8	0.252	1.008	0.000	−2.0689	−1.9393	−0.1296	−1.962	−0.107
4-Chlorobenzyl alcohol	142.59	70	10.2	0.213	0.382	0.000	−0.5037	−0.4617	−0.0420	−0.451	−0.053
2-Amino-benzyl alcohol	123.16	83	9.8	0.212	0.385	0.285	−1.0240	−1.0394	0.0154	−1.033	0.009

(Continued)

TABLE 3.1 (Continued)

Experimental and Predicted Mole Fraction Solubility at 30°C in Isopropyl Alcohol and Selected Parameters

Compounds	MW	mp (°C)	δ''	Q_H	Q_O	Q_N	Exp. log x	Equation 3.40 log x	Residual	Equations 3.41 and 3.42 log x	Residual
m-Toluic acid	136.15	108	8.6	0.252	0.650	0.000	-0.7593	-0.7278	-0.0315	-0.726	-0.033
m-Anisic acid	152.15	106	9.8	0.252	0.970	0.000	-0.9050	-0.8744	-0.0306	-0.898	-0.007
3-Chlorobenzoic acid	156.57	155	10.2	0.252	0.650	0.000	-1.0378	-1.2052	0.1674	-1.207	0.169
4-Chlorobenzoic acid	156.57	239	10.2	0.252	0.650	0.000	-1.8124	-1.8387	-0.0263	-1.873	0.060
4-Aminobenzoic acid	137.14	188	9.8	0.556	0.658	0.279	-1.4845	-1.8079	0.3234	-1.837	0.353
p-Anisic acid	152.15	182	9.8	0.252	0.966	0.000	-1.8529	-1.4469	-0.4060	-1.448	-0.405
4-Acetoxybenzoic acid	180.16	191	8.6	0.252	1.230	0.000	-1.6047	-1.5217	-0.0830	-1.537	-0.068
4,7-Dichloroquinoline	198.05	93	10.6	0.000	0.000	0.296	-1.5670	-1.4147	-0.1524	-1.431	-0.136
8-Hydroxyquinaldine	159.19	72	8.7	0.000	0.328	0.299	-1.4486	-1.6543	0.2057	-1.664	0.215
8-Nitroquinoline	174.16	89	9.8	0.000	0.220	0.424	-2.2366	-1.9696	-0.2670	-1.983	-0.254
8-Aminoquinoline	144.18	66	9.8	0.156	0.000	0.571	-1.0701	-0.5583	-0.5118	-0.537	-0.533
2-Chlorolepidine	177.63	56	8.5	0.000	0.000	0.295	-0.9666	-0.9237	-0.0429	-0.907	-0.060
8-Nitroquinaldine	188.19	139	8.7	0.000	0.222	0.427	-2.6840	-2.3958	-0.2882	-2.397	-0.287
4-Aminoquinaldine	158.20	167	8.7	0.316	0.000	0.592	-1.1561	-1.1264	-0.0297	-1.146	-0.010
5-Nitro-8-hydroxyquinoline	190.16	181	9.8	0.000	0.564	0.421	-3.1713	-3.0758	-0.0955	-3.081	-0.090
5-Chloro-8-hydroxyquinoline	179.61	122	10.2	0.000	0.326	0.294	-2.2660	-2.3010	-0.0350	-2.293	0.027
4-Methoxy-2-quinolinecarboxylic acid	203.20	197	9.8	0.000	0.943	0.294	-3.0809	-3.3521	0.2712	-3.328	0.247
6-Quinolinecarboxylic acid	173.13	295	9.8	0.252	0.649	0.293	-3.0223	-2.9974	-0.0249	-2.967	-0.055
2-Quinolinecarboxylic acid	173.13	157	9.8	0.000	0.639	0.272	-2.0809	-2.6355	0.5546	-2.641	0.560
2-Hydroxy-4-methylquinoline	159.19	245	8.8	0.256	0.313	0.291	-2.4547	-2.2967	-0.1580	-2.260	-0.195
2,4-Quinolinediol	161.16	355	9.8	0.513	0.633	0.299	-3.3566	-3.2031	-0.1535	-3.284	-0.072
6-Aminoquinoline	144.18	117	9.8	0.302	0.000	0.581	-1.0013	-0.8072	-0.1941	-0.808	-0.193
5-Aminoquinoline	144.18	110	9.8	0.308	0.000	0.577	-1.0867	-0.7485	-0.3382	-0.753	-0.334
3-Aminoquinoline	144.18	91	9.8	0.302	0.000	0.575	-0.6925	-0.6088	-0.0836	-0.619	-0.074
2-Hydroxyquinoline	145.16	198	9.8	0.256	0.311	0.279	-2.2111	-1.9272	-0.2839	-1.961	-0.250
4-Hydroxyquinoline	145.16	200	9.8	0.258	0.316	0.316	-1.5317	-1.9720	0.4404	-2.005	0.473
6-Nitroquinoline	174.16	151	9.8	0.000	0.224	0.403	-2.5935	-2.4280	-0.1655	-2.424	-0.169

(Continued)

TABLE 3.1 (*Continued*)
Experimental and Predicted Mole Fraction Solubility at 30°C in Isopropyl Alcohol and Selected Parameters

Compounds	MW	mp (°C)	δ^b	Q_H	Q_O	Q_N	Exp. log x	Equation 3.40 log x	Residual	Equations 3.41 and 3.42 log x	Residual
5-Nitroquinoline	174.16	71	9.8	0.000	0.218	0.433	−1.4647	−1.7404	0.2757	−1.723	0.258
3-Quinolinecarboxylic acid	173.17	277	9.8	0.252	0.649	0.291	−2.8508	−2.8601	0.0093	−2.898	0.047
8-Quinolinecarboxylic acid	173.17	183	9.8	0.000	0.652	0.293	−2.9390	−2.8566	−0.0824	−2.856	−0.083
4-Quinolinecarboxylic acid	173.17	254	9.8	0.252	0.643	0.280	−2.8268	−2.6741	−0.1527	−2.656	−0.171
1-Isoquinolinecarboxylic acid	173.17	164	9.8	0.000	0.641	0.275	−2.6861	−2.6923	0.0062	−2.702	0.016
6-Methoxy-8-nitroquinoline	204.19	158	9.8	0.000	0.543	0.428	−3.1675	−3.0390	−0.1285	−3.020	−0.148
2-Methoxynaphthalene	158.20	73	9.8	0.000	0.321	0.000	−1.2697	−1.0309	−0.2388	−1.042	−0.228
1-Nitronaphthalene	173.17	59	9.8	0.000	0.222	0.127	−1.5899	−1.4287	−0.1612	−1.440	−0.150
1-Naphthoic acid	172.18	160	9.8	0.252	0.650	0.000	−1.4781	−1.2363	−0.2419	−1.241	−0.237
2-Naphthol	144.17	122	9.8	0.249	0.332	0.000	−0.5560	−0.7631	0.2071	−0.759	0.203
1,6-Dihydroxynaphthalene	160.17	138	9.8	0.501	0.662	0.000	−0.5881	−0.8865	0.2984	−0.883	0.295
4-Chloro-3-nitroacetophenone	199.50	99	8.3	0.000	0.608	0.122	−2.2700	−2.1572	−0.1128	−2.089	−0.181
Phenyl urea	136.15	145	9.8	0.590	0.391	0.452	−1.3110	−1.4623	0.1513	−1.449	0.138
Benzohydroxamic acid	137.14	126	9.8	0.470	0.657	0.163	−1.2472	−1.2674	0.0202	−1.264	0.017
Benzamide	121.14	128	9.8	0.362	0.385	0.300	−1.2959	−1.2791	−0.0168	−1.293	−0.003
2,4-Dimethyl-6-hydroxypyrimidine	124.14	198	6.8	0.257	0.309	0.535	−1.6716	−1.8626	0.1910	−1.836	0.165
Acridine	179.22	111	9.8	0.000	0.000	0.303	−1.3091	−1.3954	0.0863	−1.399	0.090
2-Quinoxalinol	146.15	271	9.8	0.258	0.305	0.526	−2.8665	−2.6195	−0.2470	−2.586	−0.281
1,2,4-Triazole	69.07	119	0.0	0.263	0.000	0.672	−0.7941	−0.8948	0.1008	−0.902	0.108
3-Amino-1,2,4-triazole	84.08	159	0.0	0.554	0.000	0.946	−1.4170	−1.1839	−0.2331	−1.179	−0.238
Nicotinamide	122.13	130	9.8	0.362	0.382	0.299	−1.2795	−1.2965	0.0170	−1.288	0.008
8-Hydroxyquinoline	145.15	75	9.8	0.000	0.328	0.299	−1.5171	−1.6192	0.1021	−1.604	0.087
Pyrazinecarboxylic acid	124.10	225	0.0	0.000	0.637	0.515	−2.7058	−3.0149	0.3091	−3.014	0.308

$$\sum Q_{2j} = Q_{2H} - Q_{2O} - Q_{2N} \tag{3.41}$$

$$\sum \sqrt{Q_{2j}} = \sqrt{Q_{2H}} - \sqrt{Q_{2O}} - \sqrt{Q_{2N}} \tag{3.42}$$

When Equation 3.40 is compared with Equation 3.37, it can be seen that molecular weight in Equation 3.40 is an estimation of molar volume, and the atomic charge terms represent the polar interaction energy. All the solutes studied were small and rigid molecules. A coefficient of 0.00754 for the melting point in Equation 3.40 is similar to the theoretical value of 0.00974 calculated using the experimental temperature of 30°C and an average entropy of melting of 13.5 cal mol^{-1} K^{-1}, noted by Yalkowsky and Valvani (1980). The similarity indicates that the effect of crystalline energy on solubility is correctly represented by Equation 3.40. Relative contribution analysis (Tripos, 1992) showed that other parameters in the model were also important for estimating solubility. Table 3.2 shows that the two atomic charges terms contribute a total of 60.1% to the model whereas melting point contributes only 36.2%. These results show that atomic charge is more important in the estimation of solubility of polar solutes in a polar solvent.

Regression statistics showed that 97.8% of the variation in $\log x$ for polar solutes in isopropyl alcohol was accounted for by Equation 3.40. The quality of Equation 3.40 was also evaluated by a cross-validation method (Myers, 1990; Tripos, 1992). In this study, the dataset was divided into two sets with an equal number of compounds in each. Fifty-two compounds in one of the datasets were used to generate a model. The resulting equation was used to predict the solubility of the other 52 compounds. The procedure was then repeated using the other set of data so that two equations were developed, and the solubility of each of the 104 compounds was predicted. The two models developed by cross-validation are

$$\log x_2 = -7.9 \times 10^{-3}(\mathrm{mp} - 30) - 6.0 \times 10^{-5}\mathrm{MW}(\delta_1^n - \delta_2^n)^2$$
$$- 4.5 \times 10^{-3}\mathrm{MW}\left(\sum Q_{1i} + \sum Q_{2j}\right) + 5.2 \times 10^{-3} \times 2\mathrm{MW}\sum \sqrt{Q_{2j}} \tag{3.43}$$

$$\log x_2 = -7.3 \times 10^{-3}(\mathrm{mp} - 30) - 7.0 \times 10^{-5}\mathrm{MW}(\delta_1^n - \delta_2^n)^2$$
$$- 3.8 \times 10^{-3}\mathrm{MW}\left(\sum Q_{1i} + \sum Q_{2j}\right) + 5.0 \times 10^{-3} \times 2\mathrm{MW}\sum \sqrt{Q_{2j}} \tag{3.44}$$

$$s_p = 0.272; \quad r_p^2 = 0.908; \quad F_p = 242; \quad n = 104$$

where the subscript p represents prediction.

Comparing Equations 3.40, 3.43, and 3.44, it can be seen that equation coefficients are not substantially changed when the number of compounds is reduced to half, indicating Equation 3.40 is robust. A prediction error of 0.272 in logarithmic scale for Equations 3.43 and 3.44 shows that, on the average, predicted values are accurate within a factor of 2.

Hydrogen bonding is an important interaction that controls solubility, partitioning, and transport of drugs, and is also an important force in drug–receptor interactions. Unfortunately, it is difficult

---

TABLE 3.2

Equation Coefficients, Normal Coefficients, and Relative Contributions for Predictors in Equation 3.40

Predictor	Equation Coefficient	Normal Coefficient	Relative Contribution (%)
$(\mathrm{mp} - 30)$	-7.53×10^{-3}	0.630	36.2
$\mathrm{MW}(\delta_1^n - \delta_2^n)^2$	-6.50×10^{-5}	0.063	3.6
$\mathrm{MW}(\sum Q_{1i} + \sum Q_{2j})^2$	-4.11×10^{-3}	0.248	14.2
$2\mathrm{MW}\sum \sqrt{Q_{2j}}$	5.08×10^{-3}	0.798	45.9

to quantify, and so inclusion of hydrogen-bonding descriptors into QSARs is often restricted to indicator variables. Ghafourian and Dearden devised readily accessible hydrogen-bonding descriptors by means of theoretical chemistry to use in QSAR studies. Because of the dominantly electrostatic nature of this bond, molecular-electrostatic potential (ESP) was considered and the highest ESP on the solvent accessible surface (ESP+) was used as the hydrogen-bonding-donor ability of the molecule. The ability of this descriptor to predict the measured hydrogen-bonding parameter of sigmalphaH2 was compared with that of the empirically derived atomic charges. The results suggested that ESP+ was superior to the atomic charge descriptor and that the use of this parameter as the hydrogen-bonding parameter in QSAR studies was successful (Ghafourian and Dearden, 2004).

Molecular Surface Area Approach

Molecular surface area is one of the other descriptors that can be derived using molecular modeling techniques for the estimation of solubility. Theoretically, the dissolution process can be carried out in four hypothetical steps: (1) melting of the crystalline solute, (2) separation of a solute molecule from the molten bulk, (3) creation of a cavity in the solvent for accommodation of a solute molecule, and (4) placement of the solute molecule into the cavity created. The energy required for these processes can be characterized using the enthalpy of melting, the cohesive energy of the solute and solvent, and the adhesive energy at the interface, which are directly proportional to the interfacial area. Hence, solubility can be related to the molecular surface area of a solute.

With the estimation of the molecular surface area available for specific and nonspecific interactions, the solubility in water of aliphatic compounds has been successfully related to molecular surface area by Equation 3.45 (Amidon et al., 1974, 1975; Valvani and Yalkowsky, 1976):

$$\log S_w = \theta_0 + \theta_1 HYSA + \theta_2 FGSA + \theta_3 IFG \tag{3.45}$$

where HYSA is the hydrocarbon surface area, FGSA represents functional group surface area, IFG is the functional group index (zero for hydrocarbons and one for monofunctional compounds), and θ denotes equation coefficients.

Similar to many other empirical relationships, the coefficients in Equation 3.45 are specific for different classes of solutes. The effect of functional group surface area on solubility would also vary for different functional groups. Hence, equations for the prediction of solubility in water will be different for compounds with different functional groups.

As discussed in the previous sections, molecular interaction can be classified into dispersion, polar, and hydrogen-bond interactions. It is clear that hydrogen bonding, as well as polarity of different functional groups, is electrostatic in nature. Atomic charges can be used as an alternative to represent the effect of different functional groups. Combining partial atomic charge and melting point, the molecular surface area approach has been extended in a simple equation for the prediction of the aqueous solubility of different classes of compounds (Zhou et al., 1993), using solubility data from the literature (Kamlet et al., 1987; Bodor and Huang, 1992). The aqueous solubility of 115 aromatic compounds, including the substituted benzenes, polycyclic aromatics, and heteroaromatic compounds with functional groups including alcohol, ketone, carboxylic acid, ether, ester, amine, nitro, and halogens, was related to atomic charges and molecular surface area by Equation 3.46. The experimental and calculated results are listed in Table 3.3.

$$\log S_w = 2.06 - 0.0290(PHOBSAc) + 4.41\left(\sum Q_i\right) - 0.0243(TSA) - 0.008(mp - 25) \tag{3.46}$$

$$s = 0.282; \quad r^2 = 0.970; \quad F = 876; \quad n = 115$$

where PHOBSAc is the hydrophobic contact surface area, TSA represents the total molecular surface area, mp is the melting point in °C, and $\sum Q_i$ denotes the sum of the absolute values of the negative charges of oxygen and nitrogen atoms of a solute.

TABLE 3.3
Parameters, Experimental and Calculated Water Solubility Using Equation 3.46

Compound	TSA	PHOBSAc	mp − 25	−Q_i	Exp. log S_w	Calc. log S_w	Residual
Benzene	91.71	45.26	0	0	−1.68	−1.49	−0.19
Toluene	110.70	50.54	0	0	−2.29	−2.10	−0.19
Ethylbenzene	130.69	58.33	0	0	−2.91	−2.81	−0.10
n-Propylbenzene	151.80	62.45	0	0	−3.30	−3.44	0.14
Isopropylbenzene	145.21	60.85	0	0	−3.38	−3.24	−0.14
n-Butylbenzene	172.64	69.09	0	0	−3.94	−4.14	0.20
t-Butylbenzene	165.89	65.89	0	0	−3.60	−3.89	0.29
2-Butylbenzene	162.16	65.21	0	0	−3.67	−3.78	0.11
Benzyl alcohol	121.91	46.19	0	0.38	−0.45	−0.57	0.12
Benzoic acid	129.17	37.48	97.13	0.36	−0.78	−1.36	0.58
Phenyl acetic acid	139.69	43.45	52	0.37	−0.91	−1.38	0.47
Styrene	123.95	57.6	0	0	−2.57	−2.63	0.06
Aniline	114.77	39.31	0	0.28	−0.41	−0.64	0.23
N-Methylaniline	132.71	51.69	0	0.27	−1.28	−1.48	0.20
N, N-Dimethylaniline	142.54	58.8	0	0.26	−2.04	−1.97	−0.07
Phenol	103.10	37.94	18	0.33	−0.08	−0.24	0.16
Benzaldehyde	114.84	40.69	0	0.37	−1.21	−0.28	−0.93
Acetophenone	140.89	53.28	0	0.38	−1.34	−1.24	−0.10
Bromobenzene	113.48	61.22	0	0	−2.55	−2.48	−0.07
Chlorobenzene	108.55	57.7	0	0	−2.35	−2.26	−0.09
Fluorobenzene	100.98	51.41	0	0	−1.87	−1.89	0.02
Iodobenzene	117.75	69.36	0	0	−2.78	−2.82	0.04
tert-Amylbenzene	171.07	68.42	0	0	−4.15	−4.09	−0.06
n-Propylbenzoate	181.74	65.55	0	0.36	−2.67	−2.67	0.00
Nitrobenzene	122.73	57.18	0	0.22	−1.80	−1.61	−0.19
Methyl benzoate	144.75	56.62	0	0.36	−1.53	−1.52	−0.01
Ethyl benzoate	160.80	59.12	0	0.36	−2.22	−1.98	−0.24
Anisole	126.31	55.61	12.3	0.32	−1.85	−1.31	−0.54
o-Xylene	134.35	56.95	0	0	−2.79	−2.86	0.07
m-Xylene	131.93	56.73	0	0	−2.86	−2.80	−0.06
p-Xylene	132.59	56.72	0	0	−2.83	−2.81	−0.02
m-Chloroaniline	131.21	51.75	0	0.28	−1.37	−1.40	0.03
o-Chloroaniline	128.15	51.85	0	0.28	−1.53	−1.33	−0.20
o-Toluidine	130.63	47.10	0	0.29	−0.82	−1.21	0.39
m-Toluidine	133.95	44.59	0	0.28	−0.85	−1.26	0.41
o-Cresol	123.84	47.56	5.9	0.34	−0.65	−0.88	0.23
m-Cresol	125.89	48.48	0	0.34	−0.71	−0.91	0.20
m-Dichlorobenzene	131.75	73.33	0	0	−3.08	−3.27	0.19
o-Dichlorobenzene	126.76	67.10	0	0	−2.98	−2.97	−0.01
p-Dichlorobenzene	128.55	70.57	28.0	0	−3.28	−3.34	0.06
p-Dibromobenzene	139.56	78.04	62.3	0	−4.01	−4.10	0.09
1,2-Difluorobenzene	108.52	57.11	0	0	−2.00	−2.24	0.24
1,2-Dibromobenzene	138.20	77.83	0	0	−3.50	−3.56	0.06
1,2-Diiodobenzene	150.14	91.27	2	0	−4.29	−4.26	−0.03
1,3-Dibromobenzene	141.17	80.09	0	0	−3.38	−3.70	0.32
1,3-Diiodobenzene	152.64	97.55	15.4	0	−4.55	−4.61	0.06

(Continued)

TABLE 3.3 (*Continued*)
Parameters, Experimental and Calculated Water Solubility Using Equation 3.46

Compound	TSA	PHOBSAc	mp − 25	−Q_i	Exp. log S_w	Calc. log S_w	Residual
1,4-Difluorobenzene	105.83	52.02	0	0	−1.97	−2.02	0.05
1,4-Diiodobenzene	148.10	94.32	106.5	0	−5.25	−5.13	−0.12
1-Fluoro-4-iodobenzene	125.17	72.97	0	0	−3.13	−3.10	−0.03
1-Chloro-2-fluorobenzene	116.57	61.69	0	0	−2.42	−2.57	0.15
1-Bromo-2-chlorobenzene	134.65	73.62	0	0	−3.19	−3.35	0.16
1-Bromo-3-chlorobenzene	137.60	77.49	0	0	−3.21	−3.53	0.32
1-Bromo-4-chlorobenzene	132.82	73.87	43	0	−3.63	−3.66	0.03
1-Bromo-4-iodobenzene	143.12	87.07	67	0	−4.56	−4.48	−0.08
1-Chloro-4-iodobenzene	138.42	83.34	32	0	−4.03	−3.98	−0.05
3-Nitrobenzene	143.50	64.29	0	0.22	−2.44	−2.33	−0.11
Dimethyl phthalate	228.68	55.10	0	0.72	−1.69	−1.92	0.23
Diethyl phthalate	220.88	72.29	0	0.72	−2.57	−2.23	−0.34
1-Bromo-2-ehtylbenzene	152.34	71.07	0	0	−3.67	−3.71	0.04
1,4-Dinitrobenzene	153.63	69.53	157	0.44	−3.33	−3.01	−0.32
1-Nitro-4-chlorobenzene	137.88	69.64	65	0.22	−2.85	−2.86	0.01
p-Nitrotoluene	145.72	63.40	35	0.22	−2.39	−2.63	0.24
1,3,5-Trimehtylbenzene	155.11	65.20	0	0	−3.40	−3.60	0.20
1,2,4-Trimehtylbenzene	145.30	59.26	0	0	−3.32	−3.19	−0.13
1,2,4,5-Tetramehtylbenzene	167.96	67.26	60	0	−4.34	−4.46	0.12
Pentamethylbenzene	178.58	70.25	29	0	−3.99	−4.55	0.56
Hexachlorobenzene	180.61	95.28	205	0	−6.78	−6.74	−0.04
1,2,4-Trichlorobenzene	147.21	79.98	0	0	−3.57	−3.84	0.27
1,2,3-Trichlorobenzene	143.16	77.44	28	0	−3.76	−3.89	0.13
1,2,4-Tribromobenzene	156.06	88.03	19.5	0	−4.50	−4.45	−0.05
1,3,5-Trichlorobenzene	146.57	77.96	38	0	−4.44	−4.07	−0.37
1,3,5-Tribromobenzene	157.87	90.29	97	0	−5.60	−5.17	−0.43
1,2,3,4-Tetrachlorobenzene	158.93	85.98	22	0	−4.47	−4.48	0.01
1,2,3,5-Tetrachlorobenzene	163.10	90.25	29	0	−4.77	−4.76	−0.01
1,2,4,5-Tetrafluorobenzene	119.73	59.04	0	0	−2.38	−2.57	0.19
1,2,4,5-Tetrachlorobenzene	164.73	89.85	114.5	0	−5.26	−5.47	0.21
1,2,4,5-Tetrabromobenzene	180.30	104.89	157	0	−6.98	−6.62	−0.36
Pentachlorobenzene	178.86	97.08	61	0	−5.57	−5.59	0.02
Biphenyl	169.71	69.96	46	0	−4.33	−4.46	0.13
Diphenylmethane	182.74	75.69	0.3	0	−4.70	−4.58	−0.12
Naphthalene	135.77	53.97	55.5	0	−3.62	−3.25	−0.37
2-Methylnaphthalene	151.44	60.61	9.6	0	−3.84	−3.46	−0.38
1,3-Dimethylnaphthalene	183.22	74.32	0	0	−4.30	−4.55	0.25
1,4-Dimethylnaphthalene	167.20	61.76	0	0	−4.16	−3.80	−0.36
2,3-Dimethylnaphthalene	171.23	64.96	80	0	−4.70	−4.63	−0.07
1-Ethylnaphthalene	168.76	66.11	0	0	−4.20	−3.96	−0.24
1-Methylnaphthalene	147.29	59.47	0	0	−3.70	−3.25	−0.45
1,5-Dimethylnaphthalene	167.43	64.28	57	0	−4.68	−4.33	−0.35
1-Chloronaphthalene	143.36	63.52	0	0	−3.86	−3.27	−0.59
2-Chloronaphthalene	158.91	73.69	36	0	−4.14	−4.23	0.09
2,6-Dimethylnaphthalene	177.53	72.95	83	0	−4.89	−5.04	0.15
1,4,5-Trimethylnaphthalene	192.31	73.42	39	0	−4.90	−5.06	0.16
Anthracene	164.15	64.94	190	0	−5.39	−5.34	−0.05

(Continued)

TABLE 3.3 (*Continued*)

Parameters, Experimental and Calculated Water Solubility Using Equation 3.46

Compound	TSA	PHOBSAc	mp − 25	−Q_i	Exp. log S_w	Calc. log S_w	Residual
9-Methylanthracene	203.10	79.10	56.5	0	−5.87	−5.63	−0.24
2-Methylanthracene	208.47	83.21	184	0	−6.75	−6.89	0.14
9,10-Dimethylanthracene	212.48	84.37	158	0	−6.57	−6.82	0.25
Phenanthrene	178.49	75.41	75	0	−5.15	−5.07	−0.08
1-Methylphenanthrene	201.70	83.66	84	0	−5.85	−5.94	0.09
Pyridine	86.70	36.60	0	0.3	0.47	0.21	0.26
3-Methylpyridine	112.74	46.65	0	0.3	0.04	−0.71	0.75
Quinoline	127.34	50.53	0	0.3	−1.30	−1.18	−0.12
Isoquinoline	133.68	51.21	1.5	0.3	−1.45	−1.37	−0.08
3-Methylisoquinoline	153.71	65.39	43	0.3	−2.19	−2.60	0.41
Benzoquinoline	175.96	68.58	68	0.29	−3.36	−3.47	0.11
Furan	76.90	36.58	0	0	−0.83	−0.87	0.04
Benzonitrile	118.69	41.18	0	0.33	−1.65	−0.57	−1.08
trans-1,2-Diphenyllethylene	203.50	86.17	98	0	−5.79	−6.17	0.38
1-Chloro-3-fluorobenzene	119.58	62.45	0	0	−2.35	−2.66	0.31
1-Bromo-2-fluorobenzene	118.30	62.92	0	0	−2.70	−2.64	−0.06
1-Bromo-3-fluorobenzene	125.52	68.73	0	0	−2.67	−2.99	0.32
1-Chloro-2-iodobenzene	138.10	57.12	0	0	−3.54	−2.96	−0.58
1-Chloro-3-iodobenzene	144.94	85.19	0	0	−3.55	−3.94	0.39
2-Chlorobiphenyl	182.38	79.82	9	0	−4.84	−4.76	−0.08
3-Chlorobiphenyl	188.40	81.49	0	0	−5.03	−4.89	−0.14
o-Bromocumene	163.04	75.42	0	0	−4.19	−4.09	−0.10

The charge on the oxygen is selected only when the unshared electron pairs of the oxygen atom are unconjugated. For example, the oxygen charges in the ketone and hydroxy groups are selected, while the charges of oxygen in the furan ring and the single-bonded oxygen in the carboxylic groups are not selected.

Regression statistics showed that Equation 3.46 was robust for different classes of compounds with a wide range of polarity. The predictive performance of Equation 3.46 was further evaluated by the prediction of the aqueous solubility of 48 new compounds, including substituted benzenes, pyridines, polycyclic aromatics, and steroids. These compounds were not included in the development of Equation 3.46. Results are listed in Table 3.4. The relationship between the experimental and predicted values is

$$\text{Exp. } \log S_w = 0.985 \text{ Pred. } \log S_w - 0.0057 \tag{3.47}$$

$$s_p = 0.355; \ r_p^2 = 0.983; \ F_p = 2583; \ n = 48$$

Equation 3.47 shows that the predicted results are remarkably close to the experimental values, since the slope in near unity and the intercept are essentially negligible. Once again, a molecular modeling approach is promising for predicting the solubility of different classes of compounds.

Using a semiempirical quantum-chemical method (AM1) in a separate study, the solubility of 331 organic liquids and solids was successfully calculated using molecular descriptors derived by molecular modeling without using melting points (Bodor and Huang, 1992). A combination of atomic charges, dipole moment, surface area, and other molecular descriptors has also been pursued for the prediction of aqueous solubility using a neural network approach (Sutter and Jurs, 1996).

TABLE 3.4
Predicted Water Solubility Using Equation 3.46

Compound	Exp. log S_w	Pred. log S_w	Residual
1,4-Dibromobenzene	−4.07	−4.29	0.22
1,2-Dichlorobenzene	−3.20	−3.10	−0.10
1,3-Dichlorobenzene	−3.09	−3.30	0.21
1,4-Dichlorobenzene	−3.21	−3.46	0.25
1,3-Difluorobenzene	−2.00	−2.30	0.30
Methyl p-aminobenzoate	−1.60	−1.46	−0.14
Ethyl p-aminobenzoate	−1.99	−1.95	−0.04
Propyl p-aminobenzoate	−2.33	−2.18	−0.15
Pentyl p-aminobenzoate	−3.35	−3.48	0.13
Hexyl p-aminobenzoate	−3.95	−3.82	−0.13
Heptyl p-aminobenzoate	−4.60	−4.37	−0.23
Dodecyl p-aminobenzoate	−7.80	−7.56	−0.24
Octyl p-aminobenzoate	−5.40	−5.02	−0.38
Nonyl p-aminobenzoate	−6.00	−5.49	−0.51
Ethyl paraben	−2.22	−1.71	−0.51
Propyl paraben	−2.59	−2.04	−0.55
Butyl paraben	−2.89	−2.60	−0.29
Indan	−3.03	−2.93	−0.10
Acenaphthene	−4.59	−4.33	−0.26
Fluorene	−4.92	−5.41	0.49
Pyrene	−6.18	−6.31	0.13
Fluoranthene	−5.90	−6.12	0.22
1,2-Benzofluorene	−6.68	−7.30	0.62
Chrysene	−8.06	−7.93	−0.13
Triphenylene	−6.73	−7.45	0.72
Naphthacene	−8.69	−8.59	−0.10
Naphthanthracene	−7.21	−7.33	0.12
Perylene	−8.80	−8.36	−0.44
3,4-Benzopyrene	−7.82	−8.01	0.19
2,3-Benzofluorene	−7.27	−7.79	0.52
Benzo[ghi]perylene	−9.02	−9.06	0.04
3-Methylchloanthrene	−7.97	−8.47	0.50
2-Aminopyrdine	1.05	0.36	0.69
2-Hydroxy-5-nitropyridine	−1.07	−1.46	0.39
2-Hydroxypyridine	1.00	0.69	0.31
Picolinic acid	0.66	−0.02	0.68
2-Chlorolepidine	−3.14	−3.14	0.00
4-Hydroxybenzoic acid	−1.27	−0.89	−0.38
4'-Aminoacetophenone	−1.24	−0.91	−0.33
3,5-Dichloropyridine	−2.04	−1.73	−0.31
2-Amino-4-methylpyridine	−0.23	−0.48	0.25
5-Nitroquinoline	−2.25	−2.01	−0.24
Progestrone	−4.42	−5.06	0.64
Testosterone	−4.08	−4.35	0.27
Deoxycorticosterone	−3.45	−3.61	0.16
11-a-Hydroxyprogestrone	−3.82	−3.84	0.02
Deoxycorticosterone acetate	−4.63	−5.10	0.47

Comparative Molecular Field Analysis

Comparative molecular field analysis (CoMFA) is another promising approach developed in recent years for QSAR study. CoMFA is a molecular modeling technique for the determination of molecular steric and electrostatic force fields (Tripos, 1992). It has been successfully used in deriving molecular descriptors for prediction of the bioactivity of steroids (Cramer et al., 1988), molecular flux through a polymer membrane (Liu and Matheson, 1994), and metabolism and cytochrome p450 enzyme activities (Long and Walker, 2003).

To compare the steric effects of different molecules in the CoMFA study, molecules must be displaced in space according to a set of specified rules (Cramer et al., 1988; Tripos, 1992; Liu and Matheson, 1994). In the study of predicting the solubility in isopropyl alcohol, the optimal molecular models for aromatic compounds were aligned in reference to the benzene molecule with assigned carbon atom positions according to the following rules:

1. For the monosubstituted compounds, the aromatic carbon atom connected to the functional group was selected as the prime atom and was assigned as position 1.
2. For multisubstituted compounds, the ring carbon atom connected to the functional group with the greatest effects on solubility, based on fragmental coefficients determined in a previous study (Hu, 1990), was selected as the prime atom and assigned as position 1.
3. All other six-membered rings were aligned with the reference benzene ring in the way as described earlier, with the added provision that alkyl groups and bulky groups were aligned in the direction of carbon atoms 4 and 5 on the reference molecule.

Following the fitting of each molecule to the reference benzene using the least squares method, electrostatic and steric fields of a molecule were calculated in a region ranging from -14.0 to $+14.0$ Å along the x- and y-axes and from -10 to $+10$ Å along the z-axis. A probe atom of sp^3 carbon with a charge of $+1$ was placed in the defined region, and the field energy was calculated with the probe atom moving in a spacing of 2 Å along the axes. The resultant steric and electrostatic field energies, together with the melting point (mp) and an intramolecular hydrogen-bond indicator (IHB), were then used for QSSR study, using a partial least squares (PLS) method in the SYBYL package. It should be noted that, owing to the nature of molecular field analysis, there would be hundreds or thousands of descriptors for the molecular steric and electrostatic force fields (Table 3.5), and it is inconvenient and unnecessary to write down the QSSR equation in a CoMFA study since these descriptors are generated and directly used to predict targeted properties using the same software package. Statistical results for the final models correlating the mole fraction solubility in isopropyl alcohol with the desired parameters for 60 aromatic and heteroaromatic crystalline compounds are $SD = 0.243$, $r^2 = 0.942$, and $F = 146$. The contribution of each parameter in the two CoMFA models is listed in Table 3.5. The experimental and calculated mole fraction solubilities by Model 2 using CoMFA, mp, and IHB as predictors are listed in Table 3.6.

TABLE 3.5
Relative Contribution of Predictors in CoMFA for Solubility

	Model 1		Model 2	
Predictors	Normal Coefficient	Contributions (%)	Normal Coefficient	Contributions (%)
CoMFA (864 vars) (Steric)	1.469	40.1	0.942	31.0
CoMFA (864 vars) (Electrostatic)	1.575	43.0	1.092	35.9
100/MP	0.622	17.0	0.656	21.6
1000*IHB			0.351	11.5

TABLE 3.6

Experimental and Calculated Mole Fraction Solubilities in Isopropyl Alcohol by CoMFA in Model 2 Using CoMFA, 100/MP, 1000*IHB as Predictors

Compounds	100/MP	Expt. log x	Cal. log x	Residual
Phenol	0.3185	−0.0250	−0.0317	0.0067
Benzoic acid	0.2528	−0.6979	−0.6610	−0.0386
3-Hydroxybenzoic acid	0.2105	−0.8804	−1.2841	0.4037
3-Tert-butylphenol	0.3145	−0.1322	−0.0267	−0.1055
4-Hydroxybenzoic acid	0.2105	−0.8948	−1.1456	0.2508
2-Hydroxy-5-nitropyridine	0.2162	−2.2700	−2.2887	0.0186
m-Nitrobenzaldehyde	0.3021	−1.4763	−1.6243	0.1480
4-Aminoacetophenone	0.2639	−1.2757	−0.9580	−0.3177
4-Tert-butylbenzoic acid	0.2278	−0.9893	−0.9893	−0.0000
3-Hydroxypyridine	0.2500	−0.8477	−1.1053	0.2576
3,5-Dichloropyridine	0.2950	−0.9726	−0.5225	−0.4401
3-Aminopyridine	0.3017	−0.2845	−0.2789	−0.0056
2-Aminopyridine	0.3008	−0.3099	−0.0783	−0.2316
2-Methoxy-5-nitropyridine	0.2621	−2.1175	−1.8728	−0.2447
2-Hydroxypyridine	0.2639	−0.8165	−0.7767	−0.0397
2,4-Dihydroxypyridine	0.1815	−2.4535	−2.4962	0.0428
2-Amino-4-methylpyridine	0.2688	−0.7206	−0.7493	0.0287
2-Amino-5-chloropyridine	0.2442	−1.4023	−1.1059	−0.2964
2-Amino-5-nitropyridine	0.2174	−2.3820	−2.3100	−0.0719
2,5-Pyridinedicarboxylic acid[a]	0.1916	−3.2840	−3.1436	−0.1404
3-Quinolinecarboxylic acid	0.1813	−2.8508	−2.7836	−0.0672
4,7-Dichloroquinoline	0.2793	−1.5670	−1.1765	−0.3905
8-Nitroquinoline	0.2755	−2.2366	−2.2387	0.0021
8-Hydroxyquinoline[a]	0.2890	−1.5171	−1.4499	−0.0067
8-Aminoquinoline[a]	0.2941	−1.0701	−1.2900	0.2200
5-Chloro-8-hydroxyquinoline[a]	0.2525	−2.2660	−2.1263	−0.1397
5-Nitro-8-hydroxyquinoline[a]	0.2198	−3.1713	−3.2861	0.1147
4-Methoxy-2-quinolinecarboxylic acid[a]	0.2128	−3.0809	−2.8765	−0.2044
6-Quinolinecarboxylic acid	0.1771	−3.0223	−2.8650	−0.1573
2-Hydroxy-4-methylquinoline	0.2020	−2.4547	−2.4130	−0.0417
6-Aminoquinoline	0.2558	−1.0013	−1.2423	0.2410
3-Aminoquinoline	0.2743	−0.6925	−1.3218	0.6293
2-Hydroxyquinoline	0.2121	−2.2111	−2.1970	−0.0142
4-Hydroxyquinoline	0.2110	−1.5317	−1.7020	0.1704
6-Nitroquinoline	0.2353	−2.5935	−2.6597	0.0662
8-Quinolinecarboxylic acid[a]	0.2174	−2.9393	−2.7353	−0.2040
4-Quinolinecarboxylic acid	0.1898	−2.8268	−2.5109	−0.3159
6-Methoxy-8-nitroquinoline	0.2315	−3.1675	−3.2908	0.1233
Ethylparaben	0.2564	−0.6983	−0.8481	0.1498
5-Chloro-3-pyridinol	0.2304	−1.0605	−1.4744	0.4139
Nicotinic acid	0.1959	−2.3830	−2.1697	−0.2133
6-Hydroxynicotinic acid	0.1745	−3.2757	−2.8374	−0.4384
Picolinic acid[a]	0.2439	−1.7595	−2.0545	0.2950
6-Choronicotinic acid	0.2119	−1.5935	−2.0052	0.4118

(*Continued*)

TABLE 3.6 (*Continued*)
Experimental and Calculated Mole Fraction Solubilities in Isopropyl Alcohol by CoMFA in Model 2 Using CoMFA, 100/MP, 1000*IHB as Predictors

Compounds	100/MP	Expt. log x	Cal. log x	Residual
8-Hydroxyquinaldine[a]	0.2894	−1.4486	−1.4640	0.0155
2-Chlorolepidine	0.3030	−0.9666	−0.8891	−0.0775
8-Nitroquinaldine	0.2421	−2.6840	−2.5881	−0.0959
4-Aminoquinaldine	0.2268	−1.1561	−1.3149	0.1588
6-Methoxyquinaldine	0.2976	−0.5146	−0.2470	−0.2676
2,4-Quinolinediol	0.1592	−3.3566	−3.2571	−0.0995
2-Amino-4,6-dimethylpyridine	0.2972	−0.3534	−0.3495	−0.0039
1-Isoquinolinecarboxylic acid[a]	0.2288	−2.6861	−2.6689	−0.0172
2,4-Dimethyl-6-hydroxypyrimidine	0.2119	−1.6716	−1.6693	−0.0024
Acridine	0.2621	−1.3091	−1.2955	−0.0136
2-Quinoxalinol	0.1837	−2.8665	−2.8543	−0.0121
Indole	0.3067	−0.2138	−0.3988	0.1850
2-Quinolinecarboxylic acid[a]	0.2320	−2.0809	−2.6499	0.5690
5-Aminoquinoline	0.2625	−1.0867	−0.7165	−0.3703
5-Nitroquinoline	0.2899	−1.4647	−1.4359	−0.0289
Methylparaben	0.2500	−0.7376	−0.9939	0.2564

[a] Compounds able to intramolecularly hydrogen bond.

To test the applicability of this approach, eight compounds were randomly removed. The remaining 52 compounds were used to develop a CoMFA model. The resultant model was then used to predict the solubility of the removed compounds. Results (Table 3.7) show that predicted values agree well with the experimental values.

Puri et al. (2003) applied the CoMFA method to three-dimensional-QSPR models for the fusion enthalpy at the melting point of a representative set of polychlorinated biphenyls (PCBs). Various alignment schemes, such as inertial, as is, atom fit, and field fit, were used to evaluate the predictive capabilities of the models. The CoMFA models have also been derived using partial atomic charges calculated from the ESP and Gasteiger–Marsili (GM) methods. The combination of atom fit alignment and GM charges yielded the greatest self-consistency ($r(2) = 0.955$) and

TABLE 3.7
Solubility in Isopropyl Alcohol Predicted Using CoMFA

Compounds	Exp. log x	Pred. log x	Residual
3-Quinolinecarboxylic acid	−2.8508	−2.9596	0.1088
2-Amino-4,6-diemthylpyridine	−0.3534	−0.1888	−0.1646
Acridine	−1.3091	−1.51	0.2009
4-Hydroxybenzoic acid	−0.8948	−1.1464	0.2516
2-Amino-5-nitropyridine	−2.382	−2.4363	0.0544
m-Nitrobenzaldehyde	−1.4763	−1.4609	−0.0154
Methylparaben	−0.7376	−0.9768	0.2392
8-Hydroxyquinoline	−1.5171	−1.2862	−0.2309

internal predictive ability ($r(cv)(2) = 0.783$). This CoMFA model was used to predict Delta(fus) H(m)(T(fus)) of the entire set of 209 PCB congeners, including 193 PCB congeners for which experimental values are unavailable. The CoMFA-predicted values, combined with previous estimations of vaporization and sublimation enthalpies, were used to construct a thermodynamic cycle that validated the internal self-consistency of the predictions for these three thermodynamic properties. The CoMFA-predicted values of fusion enthalpy were also used to calculate aqueous solubilities of PCBs using Mobile Order and Disorder Theory. The agreement between calculated and experimental values of solubility at 298.15 K, characterized by a standard deviation of ± 0.41 log units, demonstrates the utility of CoMFA-predicted values of fusion enthalpies to calculate aqueous solubilities of PCBs.

GROUP CONTRIBUTION METHOD

In group contribution methods, solubility is assumed to be an additive–constitutive property. That is, each fragment of a molecule possesses some intrinsic solubility. Thus, solubility of a molecule can be expressed as a summation of the solubility of all the groups as

$$-\log S_{\mathrm{w}} = \sum f_i \qquad (3.48)$$

where f_i is the fragmental solubility constant.

Fragmental solubility constants can be determined empirically from experimental solubility data using regression techniques. In 1986, Wakita et al. (1986) studied the solubility of a large number of nonhomologous compounds in water. In this study, fragmental solubility constants were determined in the following steps:

1. Liquid aliphatic hydrocarbons were used to derive the fragmental constants by regression for some primary groups consisting of hydrogen and carbon atoms.
2. Primary group constants from step 1 were then used to determine the constants of a variety of functional groups other than hydrocarbons for liquid aliphatic compounds.
3. The aliphatic fragmental values were used to calculate the aromatic fragmental values using the solubility data of liquid aromatic compounds.
4. On the basis of the above-mentioned values, the melting point contribution was then determined for solid compounds.

The aqueous solubility of 436 aliphatic and aromatic compounds, both liquid and solid, was calculated with Equation 3.48, using fragmental solubility constants (Wakita et al., 1986). Results are shown in Equation 3.49 and Figure 3.3:

$$\text{Exp.log} \frac{1}{S_{\mathrm{w}}} = 0.198 + 0.917 \, \text{Calc.log} \frac{1}{S_{\mathrm{w}}} \qquad (3.49)$$

$$s = 0.498; \quad r^2 = 0.956; \quad F = 10,050; \quad n = 463$$

In an approach similar to that discussed previously, Kühne et al. (1995) determined the fragmental solubility values of 58 structure fragments and melting points for the solubility (mol L^{-1}) of 694 compounds in water. Kühne compared the performance of different methods for the calculation of solubility in water, and showed that his fragmental method resulted in the smallest calculation error.

The group contribution method has also been pursued by other researchers. Klopman et al. (1992) defined contribution values to aqueous solubility for a large set of groups and determined solubility using Equation 3.50:

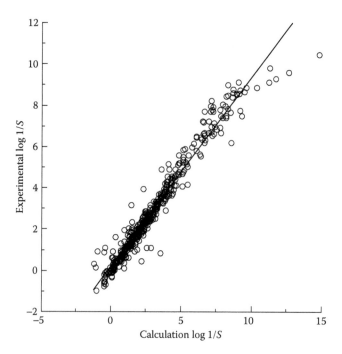

FIGURE 3.3 Experimental and calculated log 1/S using fragmental solubility constants. (Data from Wakita, K. et al., *Chem. Pharm. Bull.*, 34, 4663–4681, 1986.)

$$\log S = C_0 + \sum_{i=1}^{N} C_i G_i \tag{3.50}$$

where S is the % (w/w) solubility in water at 25°C, C_0 is a constant, and C_i is the contribution coefficient for the group G_i, which is an indicator for a functional group.

In Klopman's study (Klopman et al., 1992), functional groups of solutes in their database were defined in two different methods. The first definition method was more restrictive than the second method. For example, the hydroxy group, −OH, was either defined by a very restricted method as primary, secondary, or tertiary alcohols as well as five additional OH subgroups on the basis of the types of atoms to which the OH group connected, or defined by a less restrictive method as one group regardless of the chemical structural environment for the group. Apparently, the very restrictive definition of functional groups could result in more accurate results for the calculation of solubility in water than the less restrictive method. However, the reliability of the contribution coefficients was low for some of the functional groups defined by the very restrictive method owing to the insufficient occurrence of the functional groups in the dataset. On the basis of the different definitions of functional groups, two models (Model I and II) were developed for the calculation of solubility in water. A total of 45 group contribution coefficients were defined in Model I for the solubility of 469 compounds in water, and 33 different group contribution coefficients were defined in Model II for the solubility of 483 compounds, including the 469 compounds in Model I. As anticipated, the regression statistics in Klopman's study showed that the accuracy in the calculation of solubility using Model I was slightly higher than the accuracy using Model II. In the application of the models for the prediction of solubility, Model I was used when reliable contribution coefficients were available for all the functional groups defined by the very restrictive method. Otherwise, functional groups of a solute were defined by the less restrictive method, and solubility in water was predicted using Model II.

An outstanding characteristic of a fragmental approach is that the melting point of the solid solutes may not need to be included in the solubility equation. The elimination of the melting point makes it possible to predict the solubility without any measured physicochemical property. As long as the chemical structure for a compound is known, the solubility of the compound in water can be estimated. This may be one of the advantages of the empirical QSSR approach over the theoretical approach discussed in the first part of this chapter. Furthermore, the accuracy of the prediction using the fragmental approach is comparable with the accuracy of both the mobile order theory and the partitioning theory, as shown in Example 3.2.

Example 3.2

Estimate the solubility of naphthalene and methylparaben in water, using the group contribution method.

SOLUTION FOR NAPHTHALENE

The melting point of naphthalene is 80.2°C. Naphthalene contains eight hydrogen atoms (H) and 1.67 phenyl group (Ph). According to the constants determined by Wakita et al. (1986), the solubility fragmental coefficient value is 0.12 for each hydrogen, 1.08 for each phenyl group, and 1.43 for melting point normalized by. Using these values, the estimated solubility for naphthalene is

$$-\log S_{est} = \frac{1.43 \times (mp - 25)}{100} + 0.12 \times 8(H) + 1.08 \times 1.67(Ph) \tag{3.51}$$

$$-\log S_{est} = \frac{1.43 \times (80.2 - 25)}{100} + 0.12 \times 8 + 1.08 \times 1.67 = 3.55 \tag{3.52}$$

This value is translated into $S_{est} = 2.8 \times 10^{-4}$ mol L^{-1}. The experimental result is $S_{obs} = 2.7 \times 10^{-4}$ mol L^{-1} (Wakita et al., 1986).

SOLUTION FOR METHYLPARABEN

The melting point of methylparaben is 131°C. The chemical structure of methylparaben consists of one aromatic −OH, seven hydrogen atoms, one phenyl group, one aromatic ester CO_2, and one aliphatic carbon. The fragmental coefficients determined by Wakita et al. (1986) are as follows: 1.43 for melting point normalized by (mp − 25)/100, −1.50 for the aromatic −OH, 0.12 for each hydrogen atom, 1.08 for the phenyl group, −0.81 for the aromatic ester CO_2, and 0.37 for the aliphatic carbon. Using these values, the solubility of methylparaben can be calculated as

$$-\log S_{est} = \frac{1.43 \times (mp - 25)}{100} - 1.50(OH) + 0.12 \times 7(H) + 1.08(Ph) - 0.81(CO_2) + 0.37(C) \tag{3.53}$$

$$-\log S_{est} = \frac{1.43 \times (131 - 25)}{100} - 1.50 + 0.12 \times 7 + 1.08 - 0.81 + 0.37 = 1.50 \tag{3.54}$$

and $S_{est} = 0.032$ mol L^{-1}. The experimental solubility is 0.0145 mol L^{-1} (Wakita et al., 1986). As a comparison, $S_{est} = 0.0066$ mol L^{-1} by the partition theory and $S_{est} = 0.066$ mol L^{-1} by the mobile order theory.

LINEAR SOLVATION ENERGY RELATIONSHIPS

In studies of solvatochromic effects by Kamlet, Taft, and their coworkers, molecular interactions in solutions and polarity-related properties of molecules were characterized by the solvatochromic parameters, including a hydrogen-bond donor (HBD) acidity of α, a hydrogen-bond acceptor (HBA) basicity of β, and a polarity/polarizability of π^* (Kamlet and Taft, 1976; Taft and Kamlet, 1976; Kamlet et al., 1977). Values of these solvatochromic parameters were originally measured from the UV spectral shifts of pairs of probing molecules in a series of solvents with different polarities and hydrogen-bond capabilities. With careful selection of solutes and solvents, the UV spectral shifts of the probing solutes in different solvents were then assigned to the nonspecific polarity/polarizability effects and the specific hydrogen-bond effects of the solvents. The α values, the HBD acidities of the solvents, were the resultant spectral shifts normalized by the spectral shift value of methanol determined under the same conditions for the solvents (Taft and Kamlet, 1976). Similarly, the β values for solvents were the spectral shifts normalized by the spectral shift of hexamethylphosphoramine (Kamlet and Taft, 1976), and the π^* values were obtained from the slopes of the linear spectral relationship for a pair of molecular probes in a series of solvents (Kamlet et al., 1977). Other methods, such as the back calculation from hydrogen-bond formation constants, nuclear magnetic resonance (NMR) shifts, partition coefficients, high-performance liquid chromatography (HPLC) and GLC capacity factors, and from other polarity-related properties were also used to determine the solvatochromic parameters (Kamlet and Taft, 1976; Kamlet et al., 1987; Abraham, 1993).

Since solvatochromic parameters are derived from direct measurements of the energy resulting from intermolecular interaction, they can be used to predict solubility, which is determined by solute–solute, solvent–solvent, and solute–solvent interaction energies. For nonself-associated liquid aliphatic compounds with a weak or nonhydrogen-bond donor (Taft et al., 1985; Kamlet et al., 1986), the solubility in water at 25°C was related to molar volume ($\bar{V}$), hydrogen-bond basicity (β), and polarity/polarizability (π^*) by a linear solvation energy relationship (LSER), as in Equation 3.55:

$$\log S_w = 0.54 - 3.32 \frac{\bar{V}}{100} + 5.17 \beta + 0.46 \pi^*$$
(3.55)

$$s = 0.137; \quad r = 0.995; \quad n = 105$$

where $\bar{V}$ is defined as molecular weight divided by the liquid density of the solute. The $\bar{V}$ term in the equation represents the energy related to the creation of cavities in the solvent phase for accommodating solute molecules.

Equation 3.55 shows that solubility in water depends strongly on the solvatochromic parameters of the solutes. The small standard deviation of 0.137 on a log scale shows that the error of prediction using Equation 3.55 is in the same range as the experimental error in the measurement of solubility (Valvani et al., 1981). Compared with other methods, the LSER approach has resulted in the most accurate results for the solubility of nonself-associated, nonhydrogen-bonding, and weak hydrogen-bonding aliphatic liquids (Kamlet et al., 1986).

Similar to conventional QSAR, a specific LSER equation is limited for a specific set of compounds. In subsequent studies, Kamlet et al. (1987) found that dependency of solubility in water on polarity/polarizability is different for aromatic liquids than for aliphatic liquids. For liquid aromatic compounds with a hydrogen-bond acceptor and without hydrogen-bond donors, the LSER is

$$\log S_w = 1.44 - 3.17 \frac{\bar{V}}{100} + 4.05 \beta - 0.81 \pi^*$$
(3.56)

$$s = 0.150; \quad r = 0.990; \quad n = 31$$

It can be seen from Equation 3.56 that solubility of liquid aromatic compounds is still highly correlated to solvatochromic parameters. However, the intercept and the coefficients for β and π^*

in Equation 3.56 are substantially different from those in Equation 3.55. Indeed, the π^* term in Equation 3.56 has an improper sign (Kamlet et al., 1987) because the dependency of solubility on the solute–solvent dipolar interaction should be exoergic rather than endoergic. The improper sign for the π^* term was corrected when an intrinsic van der Waals molar volume, V_I, was used instead of the experimental molar volume. Interestingly, the π^* term was no longer significant in the equation when the V_I term was used, and the LSER for aromatic liquids became

$$\log S_{\mathrm{w}} = 0.44 - 5.33\frac{V_I}{100} + 3.89\,\beta \tag{3.57}$$

$$s = 0.166; \quad r = 0.987; \quad n = 31$$

Using a relationship developed by Yalkowsky and Valvani (1980), a melting point term was included in an LSER for the solubility of solid aromatic compounds, resulting in

$$\log S_{\mathrm{w}} = 0.54 - 5.60\frac{V_I}{100} + 3.68\,\beta - 0.0103\big(\mathrm{mp} - 25\big) \tag{3.58}$$

$$s = 0.238; \quad r = 0.987; \quad n = 39$$

The correlation coefficients are high for Equations 3.55 through 3.58. However, some important parameters are missing from the equations, in addition to the differences in the contributions of the solvatochromic parameters to aqueous solubility. As discussed in the section for the molecular surface approach, solubility is determined by the free-energy change resulting from the following four steps: (1) melting of the crystalline solute, (2) separation of the solute molecules from the bulk, (3) creation of a cavity in the solvent phase for accommodating the solute molecule, and (4) placement of the solute molecule into the cavity. The free-energy change in step 2 is contributed by the solute–solute interaction, and the free-energy change in step 4 is the result of the solute–solvent interaction, which consists of the hydrogen-bonding acidity effects as well as the polarity/polarizability and the hydrogen-bonding basicity effects in solutions. Both the solute–solute interactions and the hydrogen-bond acidity effects are missing in Equations 3.55 through 3.58, even though a large number of solutes in the dataset were hydrogen-bond donors. Kamlet et al. (1987) tried to account for the solute–solute interaction effects by adding the Hildebrand solubility parameter (δ) into the equations. To explain the missing δ term, Kamlet et al. (1986) hypothesized that the solute–solute and the solute–solvent interactions are not properly sorted out between δ and π^*. To explain the insignificant relationship between α and solubility, Kamlet and coworkers reasoned that alkanol solutes act only as hydrogen-bond acceptors in water.

In a recent study by Lee (1996), LSERs were combined with an extended Hildebrand solubility equation. From a comparison between LSER and the extended solubility parameter model, it has been found that the solute–solute interaction energy term is missing in the LSER equation. A new LSER equation with the supplementary interaction energy term has been proposed for the solvation process. The new LSER equation for both aliphatic and aromatic liquids is

$$\log S_{\mathrm{w}} = 0.25\big(\pm 0.17\big) + 0.15\big(\pm 0.15\big)R + 1.99\big(\pm 0.34\big)\pi^* + 4.64\big(\pm 0.80\big)\alpha$$

$$+ 4.78\big(\pm 0.17\big)\beta - 1.67\big(\pm 0.50\big)\frac{V_I}{100} - 3.34\big(\pm 0.58\big)U \tag{3.59}$$

$$s = 0.189; \quad r = 0.993; \quad n = 55$$

Equation 3.59 shows that the contributions of α and U to solubility are significant by a t-student test. With the inclusion of α and U, the solubility of either aliphatic or aromatic compounds can be expressed in a single LSER equation. The overall fit for Equation 3.59 is very good. However, the R term, which was intended to represent the dispersion energy (Abraham, 1993), is not statistically significant, as shown by the large standard error for the coefficient of the R term.

OTHER STATISTICAL METHODS AND PREDICTION MODELS

In modern drug discovery research, databases of drug-like properties, including partition coefficient, ionization constant, and aqueous solubility, are commonly established for a large number of compounds with diverse structures. Such databases can be utilized to develop models for predicting solubility by statistical methods. As more and more molecular descriptors are available, conventional regression methods are becoming less likely to be successful for modeling since the number of independent variables cannot be larger than the number of data points of the dependent variable for conventional regression analysis. For handling an unconventionally large number of descriptors, the following two statistical methods are particularly useful. These two methods are PLS and artificial neural network (ANN).

The method of PLS bears some relation to principal component analysis; instead of finding the hyperplanes of maximum variance, it finds a linear model describing some predicted variables in terms of other observable variables. It is used to find the fundamental relations between two matrices (X and Y), that is, a latent variable approach to modeling the covariance structures in these two spaces. A PLS model will try to find the multidimensional direction in the X space that explains the maximum multidimensional variance direction in the Y space.

Bergstrom et al. (2004) developed in silico protocols to predict aqueous solubility of drugs. They used the solubility data of 85 compounds covering the drug-like space as identified with the ChemGPS methodology. Two-dimensional molecular descriptors for electron distribution, lipophilicity, flexibility, and size were calculated by Molconn-Z and Selma. Monte Carlo simulations in macromodel were used to obtain global minimum energy conformers, and three-dimensional descriptors of molecular surface area properties were calculated by Marea. PLS models were obtained by using training and test datasets. Both a global drug solubility model and subset-specific models (after dividing the 85 compounds into acids, bases, ampholytes, and nonproteolytes) were generated. Furthermore, the final models successfully predicted the solubility values of external test sets taken from the literature. The results showed that homologous series and subsets could be predicted with high accuracy from easily comprehensible models, whereas consensus modeling might be needed for datasets with large structural diversity.

ANN is an interconnected group of artificial neurons that use a mathematical or computational model for information processing on the basis of a connectionist approach for computation. It is an adaptive system that changes its structure on the basis of external or internal information that flows through the network, as shown in Figure 3.4.

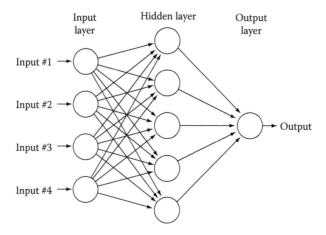

FIGURE 3.4 Schematic of the neural network structure.

ANN is capable of self-learning from the training data to maximize the prediction capability. This is particularly useful in applications where the complexity of the data or task makes the design of such a function by hand impractical (Haykin, 1999).

Goller et al. (2006) present an ANN model for the prediction of solubility of organic compounds in buffer at pH 6.5 to mimic the medium in the human gastrointestinal tract. The model was derived from consistently performed solubility measurements of about 5000 compounds. Semiempirical VAMP/AM1 quantum-chemical wave function-derived, HQSAR-derived log P, and topology-based descriptors were employed after preselection of significant contributors by statistical and data mining approaches. Ten ANNs were trained, each with 90% as a training set and 10% as a test set, and deterministic analysis of prediction quality was used in an iterative manner to optimize ANN architecture and descriptor space on the basis of Corina three-dimensional molecular structure and AM1/COSMO single point wave function. In production mode, a mean prediction value of the 10 ANNs was created, as was a standard deviation-based quality parameter. The productive ANN based on Corina geometries and AM1/COSMO wave function resulted in an r^2 cv of 0.50 and a root-mean-square error of 0.71 log units, with 87% and 96% of the compounds having an error of less than 1 and 1.5 log units, respectively. The model was able to predict permanently charged species, for example, zwitterions or quaternary amines, and problematic structures such as tautomers and unresolved diastereomers as well as neutral compounds.

Tantishaiyakul (2005) developed a model to predict aqueous solubility of benzylamine salts using multivariate PLS and ANN. Molecular descriptors, including binding energy and surface area of salts, were calculated by the use of Hyperchem and ChemPlus QSAR programs for Windows. Other physicochemical properties, such as hydrogen acceptors for oxygen and nitrogen atoms, hydrogen-bond donors, hydrogen-bond forming ability, molecular weight, and calculated log partition coefficient (clog P) of p-substituted benzoic acids, were also used as descriptors. In this study, the predictive ability of ANN, especially multilayer perceptron (MLP) architecture networks, was found to be superior to PLS models. The best ANN model derived, a 6-1-1 architecture, had an overall R^2 of 0.850 and root-mean-square error for cross-verification and test set of 0.189 and 0.185 log units, respectively. Since all the utilized descriptors are readily obtained from calculation, these models offer the advantage of not requiring experimental determination of some descriptors.

Jouyban et al. (2004) applied ANN to calculate the solubility of drugs in water–cosolvent mixtures, using 35 experimental datasets. The networks employed were feedforward back-propagation errors with one hidden layer. The topology of neural network was optimized in a 6-5-1 architecture. All data points in each set were used to train the ANN and the solubilities were back-calculated employing the trained networks. The difference between calculated solubilities and experimental values was used as an accuracy criterion and defined as mean percentage deviation (MPD). The overall MPD and its SD obtained for 35 datasets were 0.90% ± 0.65%. To assess the prediction capability of the method, five data points in each set were used as a training set and the solubility at other solvent compositions was predicted using trained ANNs, whereby the overall MPD (±SD) for this analysis was 9.04% ± 3.84%. When all the 496 data points from 35 datasets were used to train a general ANN model, the MPD (±SD) was 24.76% ± 14.76%. To test the prediction capability of the general ANN model, all data points with odd set numbers from 35 datasets were employed to train the ANN model, and the even numbered data were predicted with an overall MPD (±SD) of 55.97% ± 57.88%. When an ANN model was developed for a given cosolvent system, the overall MPD was smaller than 10%. When the ANN results were compared with those obtained from the most accurate multiple linear regression model, namely, the combined nearly ideal binary solvent/ Redlich–Kister equation, it showed that ANN was superior to the regression model.

Yan et al. (2004) developed several quantitative models for the prediction of aqueous solubility of organic compounds, on the basis of a diverse dataset with 2084 compounds, by using multilinear regression analysis and back-propagation neural networks. The compounds were described by two different structure representation methods: (1) with 18 topological descriptors and (2) with 32 radial distribution function codes representing the three-dimensional structure of a molecule and eight additional descriptors. The dataset was divided into a training and a test set on the basis of Kohonen's self-organizing neural network. Good prediction results were obtained for back-propagation neural network models: with 18 topological descriptors, for the 936 compounds in the test set, a correlation coefficient of 0.92 and a SD of 0.62 were achieved; with three-dimensional descriptors, for the 866 compounds in the test set, a correlation coefficient of 0.90 and a SD of 0.73 were achieved. The models were also tested by using another dataset, and the relationship of the two datasets was examined by Kohonen's self-organizing neural network.

In recent years, efforts were made to improve simulation efficiency and make use of readily available open-source software for solubility prediction. Sellers et al. (2016) extended various free-energy methodologies to determine the chemical potential of the solid and liquid phases of a fully flexible molecule using classical simulation. They outlined an efficient technique to find the absolute chemical potential and melting point of a fully flexible molecule using one set of simulations to compute the solid absolute chemical potential and one set of simulations to compute the solid–liquid free energy difference. With this combination, only a handful of simulations are needed, whereby the absolute quantities of the chemical potentials are obtained for use in other property calculations, such as the characterization of crystal polymorphs or the determination of the entropy. Using the LAMMPS molecular simulator, the Frenkel and Ladd and pseudo-supercritical path techniques are adapted to generate 3rd order fits of the solid and liquid chemical potentials. Results yield the thermodynamic melting point $T_m = 488.75$ K at 1.0 atm.

Conceptually, the simplest way to compute solubilities from simulation is to carry out *brute-force* direct coexistence simulations (Espinosa et al., 2016; Kolafa, 2016). While this method has the advantage of simplicity, it generally requires long simulations (in some cases up to microseconds) to achieve solubility equilibrium, even for highly soluble compounds. In order to develop a general method but make use of only readily available open-source software, Li et al. (2017) developed a methodology for universal solubility prediction. They developed a numerical method that enables convenient solubility estimation of general molecular crystals at arbitrary thermodynamic conditions where solid and solution can coexist. The methodology is based on standard alchemical free energy methods, such as thermodynamic integration and free energy perturbation, and consists of two parts: (1) systematic extension of the Einstein crystal method to calculate the absolute solid free energies of molecular crystals at arbitrary temperatures and pressures, and (2) a flexible cavity method that can yield accurate estimates of the excess solvation free energies. The results show that via classical Molecular Dynamic simulations, their approach can predict the solubility of OPLS-AA-based (Optimized Potentials for Liquid Simulations All Atomic) naphthalene in SPC (Simple Point Charge) water in good agreement with experimental data at various temperatures and pressures.

The Modified Separation of Cohesive Energy Density Model (MOSCED) is an efficient, analytic method to predict infinite dilution activity coefficients over a range of temperatures. Its predictability makes MOSCED an attractive engineering design tool. However, its use is limited. When trying to model a novel compound, reference data must first be available to regress the necessary MOSCED parameters. Here, Ley et al. (2016) proposed the use of molecular simulation to generate the reference dataset. In this fashion, MOSCED can be made a truly predictive engineering design tool. This combines the predictive strength of molecular simulation with the efficiency of MOSCED to create a powerful new tool. By adopting the melting point temperature and enthalpy of fusion of these compounds from available experimental data, they were able to predict equilibrium solubilities. Predictions using the new predictive MOSCED are in good agreement with available experimental solubility data for acetaminophen in non-aqueous solvents, as shown in Figure 3.5.

Cox et al. (2017) demonstrated for the solutes methylparaben, ethylparaben, propylparaben, butyl-paraben, lidocaine, and ephedrine how conventional molecular simulation free energy calculations or electronic structure calculations in a continuum solvent can instead be used to generate the necessary reference data, resulting in a predictive flavor of MOSCED. Adopting the melting point temperature and enthalpy of fusion of these compounds from experiment, they found the method is able to well

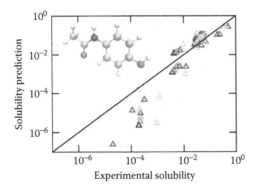

FIGURE 3.5 Prediction of solubility using the modified separation of cohesive energy density model MOSCED.

correlate the (mole fraction) equilibrium solubility in non-aqueous solvents over four orders of magnitude with good quantitative agreement. Phifer et al. (2017) applied MOSCED and compared a total of 422 non-aqueous and 193 aqueous experimental solubilities, and found the proposed method is able to well correlate the data. Their prediction work suggests that use of MOSCED in combination of molecular simulation could be an efficient tool for intuitive solvent selection and formulation.

SUMMARY

Solubility of an organic nonelectrolyte is largely determined by molecular interactions in solution and by the crystalline energy of the solute if the solute is a solid compound. Solubility can be estimated by either a theoretical or an empirical approach. However, the predictive power of an empirical equation usually depends on its limited application to a specific set of solutes or the limited domain of compounds used in the development of the equation, owing to the specific molecular interactions involved. In general, estimation of solubility is easier for a liquid compound than for a crystalline compound because crystalline energy is not a consideration for liquids. In addition, the solubility of molecules with nonspecific interactions is easier to predict than that of solutes that are capable of hydrogen bonding, owing to the complexity in the intermolecular or intramolecular interactions. Characterization of solute–solute, solvent–solvent, and solute–solvent molecular interactions is still the main challenge for the prediction of solubility.

Although solubility can be studied by either theoretical or empirical approaches, selection of a method might depend on the purpose of the study. An exact mathematical model is important in discerning the rules governing the molecular interactions in solutions. However, the utility of such an approach might be compromised in drug design if the model depends heavily on the measured data of existing materials, because there is usually no material available in the design stage. On the other hand, a structural relationship, such as the fragmental method, may seem crude, but yet may be very useful in predicting solubility, because one can design the chemical structure of a solute. At the present time, the accuracy of prediction is similar for theoretical models and the empirical QSSR equations. For these reasons, theoretical and empirical approaches are equally important in the study of solubility, and continuation of both efforts should be encouraged.

REFERENCES

Abraham, M. H. 1993. Physicochemical and biochemical processes. *Chem. Soc. Rev.* 22:73–83.

Amidon, G. L., H. Lennernaes, V. P. Shah, and J. R. Crison. 1995. A theoretical basis for a biopharmaceutic drug classification: The correlation of in vitro drug product dissolution and in vivo bioavailability. *Pharm. Res.* 12:413–420.

Amidon, G. L., S. H. Yalkowsky, S. T. Anik, and S. C. Valvani. 1975. Solubility of nonelectrolytes in polar solvents. V. Estimation of the solubility of aliphatic monofunctional compounds in water using a molecular surface area approach. *J. Phys. Chem.* 79:2239–2246.

Amidon, G. L., S. H. Yalkowsky, and S. Leung. 1974. Solubility of nonelectrolytes in polar solvents II: Solubility of aliphatic alcohols in water. *J. Pharm. Sci.* 63:1858–1866.

Barton, A. F. M. 1983. *Handbook of Solubility Parameters and Other Cohesion Parameters*, pp. 1–88. Boca Raton, FL: CRC Press.

Bergstrom, C. A., C. M. Wassvik, U. Norinder, K. Luthman, and P. Artursson. 2004. Global and local computational models for aqueous solubility prediction of drug-like molecules. *J. Chem. Inf. Comput. Sci.* 44:1477–1488.

Bodor, N. and M. J. Huang. 1992. A new method for the estimation of the aqueous solubility of organic compounds. *J. Pharm. Sci.* 81:954–960.

Bustamante, P., B. Escalera, A. Martin, and E. Selles. 1989. Predicting the solubility of sulfamethoxypyridazine in individual solvents I: Calculating partial solubility parameters. *J. Pharm. Sci.* 78:567–573.

Bustamante, P., D. V. Hinkley, A. Martin, and S. Shi. 1991. Statistical analysis of the extended Hansen method using the Bootstrap technique. *J. Pharm. Sci.* 80:971–977.

Charton, M. and B. Charton. 1985. The prediction of chemical, physical and biological properties of haloaromatic compounds. In *QSAR and Strategies in the Design of Bioactive Compounds*, J. K. Seydel (Ed.), pp. 398–402. Weinheim, Germany: VCH.

Chen, Y., P. Vayumhasuwan, and L. E. Matheson. 1996. Prediction of flux through polydimethylsiloxane membranes using atomic charge calculations: Application to an extended data set. *Int. J. Pharm.* 137:149–158.

Chen, Y., W. L. Yang, and L. E. Matheson. 1993. Prediction of flux through polydimethylsiloxane membranes using atomic charge calculations. *Int. J. Pharm.* 94:81–88.

Cox, C. E., J. R. Phifer, L. F. da Silva, G. G. Nogueira, R. T. Ley, E. J. O'Loughlin, A. K. P. Barbosa, B. T. Rygelski, and A. S. Paluch. 2017. Combining MOSCED with molecular simulation free energy calculations or electronic structure calculations to develop an efficient tool for solvent formulation and selection. *J. Comput. Aided Mol. Des.* 31(2):183–199.

Cramer, C. J., G. R. Famini, and A. H. Lowrey. 1993. Use of calculated quantum chemical properties as surrogates for solvatochromic parameters in structure–activity relationships. *Acc. Chem. Res.* 26:599–605.

Cramer, R. D., III, D. E. Patterson, and J. D. Bruce. 1988. Comparative molecular field analysis (CoMFA). 1. Effect of shape on binding of steroids to carrier proteins. *J. Am. Chem. Soc.* 110:5959–5967.

Cramer, R. D., III, K. M. Snader, C. R. Willis, L. W. Chakrin, J. Thomas, and B. M. Sutton. 1979. Application of quantitative structure-activity relationships in the development of the antiallergic pyranenamines. *J. Med. Chem.* 22:714–724.

Dunn, W. J., III, J. H. Block, and R. S. Pearlman. 1986. *Partition Coefficient Determination and Estimation*. New York: Pergamon Press.

Espinosa, J. R., J. M. Young, H. Jiang, D. Gupta, C. Vega, E. Sanz, P. G. Debenedetti, and A. Z. Panagiotopoulos. 2016. On the calculation of solubilities via direct coexistence simulations: Investigation of NaCl aqueous solutions and Lennard-Jones binary mixtures. *J. Chem. Phys.* 145(15):154111.

FDA. 2000. Waiver of *in vivo* bioavailability and bioequivalence studies for immediate-release solid oral dosage forms based on a biopharmaceutics classification system.

Ghafourian, T. and J. C. Dearden. 2004. The use of molecular electrostatic potentials as hydrogen-bonding-donor parameters for QSAR studies. *Farmaco* 59:473–479.

Goller, A. H., M. Hennemann, J. Keldenich, and T. Clark. 2006. In silico prediction of buffer solubility based on quantum-mechanical and HQSAR- and topology-based descriptors. *J. Chem. Inf. Model* 46: 648–658.

Gould, K. J., C. N. Manners, D. W. Payling, J. L. Suschitky, and E. Wells. 1988. Predictive structure–activity relationships in a series of pyranoquinoline derivatives. A new primate model for the identification of antiallergic activity. *J. Med. Chem.* 31:1445–1453.

Hansch, C. 1993. Quantitative structure–activity relationships and the unnamed science. *Acc. Chem. Res.* 26:147–153.

Hansch, C., P. P. Maloney, and T. Fujita. 1962. Correlation of biological activity of phenoxyacetic acids with Hammett substituent constants and partition coefficients. *Nature* 194:178–180.

Hansen, C. M. 1967. The three dimensional solubility parameter—Key to paint component affinities: I. Solvents, plasticizers, polymers and resins. *J. Paint Technol.* 39:104–117.

Haykin, S. 1999. *Neural Networks: A Comprehensive Foundation*. Upper Saddle River, NJ: Prentice Hall.

Herman, R. A. and P. Veng-Pedersen. 1994. Quantitative structure–pharmacokinetic relationships for systemic drug distribution kinetics not confined to a congeneric series. *J. Pharm. Sci.* 83:423–428.

Higuchi, T. 1977. Pro-drug, molecular structure and percutaneous delivery. In *Design of Biopharmaceutical Properties through Prodrugs and Analogs*, E. B. Roche (Ed.), pp. 409–421. Washington, DC: APhA.

Higuchi, T. 1982. *In vitro* drug release from ointment and creams. In *Dermal and Transdermal Absorption*, R. Brandau and B. H. Lippold (Eds.), pp. 90–100. Stuttgart, Germany: WBA.

Hildebrand, J. H., J. M. Prausnitz, and R. L. Scott. 1970. *Regular and Related Solutions, the Solubility of Gases, Liquids, and Solids*. New York: Van Nostrand Reinhold.

Hu, M. W. 1990. Prediction of the Diffusion Rate of Aromatic and Heteromatic Compounds in Polydimethylsiloxan Membranes. PhD Thesis. Iowa City, IA: The University of Iowa.

Huyskens, P. L. and M. C. Haulait-Pirson. 1985. A new expression for the combinatorial entropy of mixing in liquid mixtures. *J. Mol. Liq.* 31:135–151.

Jain, N. and S. H. Yalkowsky. 2001. Estimation of the aqueous solubility I: Application to organic nonelectrolytes. *J. Pharm. Sci.* 90:234–252.

Jain, N., G. Yang, S. G. Machatha, and S. H. Yalkowsky. 2006. Estimation of the aqueous solubility of weak electrolytes. *Int. J. Pharm.* 319:169–171.

Jouyban, A., M. R. Majidi, H. Jalilzadeh, and K. Asadpour-Zeynali. 2004. Modeling drug solubility in water–cosolvent mixtures using an artificial neural network. *Farmaco* 59:505–512.

Kaliszan, R. 1992. Quantitative structure–retention relationships. *Anal. Chem.* 64:619A–631A.

Kaliszan, R. and H. D. Höltje. 1982. Gas chromatographic determination of molecular polarity and quantum chemical calculation of dipole movements in a group of substituted phenoles. *J. Chromatogr.* 234:303–311.

Kamlet, M. J., J. L. Abboud, and R. W. Taft. 1977. The solvatochromic comparison method. 6. The π^* scale of solvent polarities. *J. Am. Chem. Soc.* 99:6027–6037.

Kamlet, M. J., R. M. Doherty, J. L. Abboud, M. H. Abraham, and R. W. Taft. 1986. Linear solvation energy relationships: 36. Molecular properties governing solubilities of organic nonelectrolytes in water. *J. Pharm. Sci.* 75:338–349.

Kamlet, M. J., R. M. Doherty, M. H. Abraham, P. W. Carr, R. F. Doherty, and R. W. Taft. 1987. Linear solvation energy relationships. 41. Important differences between aqueous solubility relationships for aliphatic and aromatic solutes. *J. Phys. Chem.* 91:1996–2004.

Kamlet, M. J. and R. W. Taft. 1976. The solvatochromic comparison method. I. The β-scale of solvent hydrogen-bond acceptor (HBA) basicities. *J. Am. Chem. Soc.* 98:377–383.

Kantola, A., H. O. Villar, and G. H. Loew. 1991. Atom based parametrization for a conformationally dependent hydrophobic index. *J. Comput. Chem.* 12:681–689.

Klopman, G. and L. D. Iroff. 1981. Calculation of partition coefficients by the charge density method. *J. Comput. Chem.* 2:157–160.

Klopman, G., S. Wang, and D. M. Balthasar. 1992. Estimation of aqueous solubility of organic molecules by the group contribution approach. Application to the study of biodegradation. *J. Chem. Inf. Comput. Sci.* 32:474–482.

Kolafa, J. 2016. Solubility of NaCl in water and its melting point by molecular dynamics in the slab geometry and a new BK3-compatible force field. *J. Chem. Phys.* 145(20):204509.

Kühne, R., R. U. Ebert, F. Kleint, G. Schmidt, and G. Schüürmann. 1995. Group contribution methods to estimate water solubility of organic chemicals. *Chemosphere* 30:2061–2077.

Lee, S. B. 1996. A new linear solvation energy relationship for the solubility of liquids in water. *J. Pharm. Sci.* 85:348–350.

Leo, A. J. 1993. Calculating log *Poct* from structures. *Chem. Rev.* 93:1281–1306.

Levine, I. N. 1988. *Physical Chemistry*. New York: McGraw-Hill.

Ley, R. T., G. B. Fuerst, B. N. Redeker, and A. S. Paluch. 2016. Developing a predictive form of MOSCED for nonelectrolyte solids using molecular simulation: Application to acetanilide, acetaminophen, and phenacetin. *Ind. Eng. Chem. Res.* 55(18):5415–5430.

Li, L., T. Totton, and D. Frenkel. 2017. Computational methodology for solubility prediction: Application to the sparingly soluble solutes. *J. Chem. Phys.* 146(21):214110.

Liu, R. and L. E. Matheson. 1994. Comparative molecular field analysis combined with physicochemical parameters for the prediction of polydimethylsiloxane membrane flux in isopropanol. *Pharm. Res.* 11:257–266.

Long, A. and J. D. Walker. 2003. Quantitative structure-activity relationships for predicting metabolism and modeling cytochrome p450 enzyme activities. *Environ. Toxicol. Chem.* 22:1894–1899.

Mannhold, R., R. F. Rekker, C. Sonntag, A. M. T. Laak, K. Dross, and E. E. Polymeropoulos. 1995. Comparative evaluation of the predictive power of calculation procedures for molecular lipophilicity. *J. Pharm. Sci.* 84:1410–1419.

Manzo, R. H. and A. A. Ahumada. 1990. Effects of solvent medium on solubility. V: Enthalpic and entropic contributions to the free energy changes of di-substituted benzene derivatives in enthanol:water and enthanol:cyclohexane mixtures. *J. Pharm. Sci.* 79:1109–1116.

Martin, A., P. L. Wu, A. Adjei, A. Beerbower, and J. M. Prausnitz. 1981. Extended Hansen solubility approach: Naphthalene in individual solvents. *J. Pharm. Sci.* 70:1260–1264.

Myers, R. H. 1990. *Classical and Modern Regression with Applications.* Boston, MA: PWS-KENT.

Myrdal, P. B., A. M. Manka, and S. H. Yalkowsky. 1995. AQUAFAC 3: Aqueous functional group activity coefficients; application to the estimation of aqueous solubility. *Chemosphere* 30:1619–1637.

Phifer, J. R., C. E. Cox, L. F. da Silva, G. G. Nogueira, A. K. P. Barbosa, R. T. Ley, S. M. Bozada, E. J. O'Loughlin, and A. S. Paluch. 2017. Predicting the equilibrium solubility of solid polycyclic aromatic hydrocarbons and dibenzothiophene using a combination of MOSCED plus molecular simulation or electronic structure calculations. *Mol. Phys.* 115:1286–1300.

Puri, S., J. S. Chickos, and W. J. Welsh. 2003. Three-dimensional quantitative structure–property relationship (3D-QSPR) models for prediction of thermodynamic properties of polychlorinated biphenyls (PCBs): Enthalpies of fusion and their application to estimates of enthalpies of sublimation and aqueous solubilities. *J. Chem. Inf. Comput. Sci.* 43:55–62.

Rekker, R. F. 1977. *The Hydrophobic Fragmental Constant.* New York: Elsevier.

Rekker, R. F. and R. Mannhold. 1992. *Calculation of Drug Lipophilicity, the Hydrophobic Fragmental Constant Approach.* Weinheim, Germany: VCH.

Richardson, P. J., D. F. McCafferty, and A. D. Woolson. 1992. Determination of three-component partial solubility parameters for temazepam and the effects of change in partial molal volume on the thermodynamics of drug solubility. *Int. J. Pharm.* 78:189–198.

Ruelle, P., M. Buchmann, H. Nam-Tran, and U. W. Kesselring. 1992. The mobile order theory versus UNIFAC and regular solution theory-derived models for predicting the solubility of solid substances. *Pharm. Res.* 9:788–791.

Ruelle, P., C. Rey-Mermet, M. Buchmann, H. Nam-Tran, U. W. Kesselring, and P. L. Huyskens. 1991. A new predictive equation for the solubility of drugs based on the thermodynamics of mobile disorder. *Pharm. Res.* 8:840–850.

Schaper, K. J. and J. K. Seydel. 1985. Multivariate methods in quantitative structure–pharmacokinetics relationship analysis. In *QSAR and Strategies in the Design of Bioactive Compounds*, J. K. Seydel (Ed.), pp. 173–189. Weinheim, Germany: VCH.

Sellers, M. S., M. Lísal, and J. K. Brennan. 2016. Free-energy calculations using classical molecular simulation: Application to the determination of the melting point and chemical potential of a flexible RDX model. *Phys. Chem. Chem. Phys.* 18(11):7841–7850.

Seydel, J. K. 1985. *QSAR and Strategies in the Design of Bioactive Compounds.* Weinheim, Germany: VCH.

Sutter, J. M. and P. C. Jurs. 1996. Prediction of aqueous solubility for a diverse set of heteroatom-containing organic compounds using a quantitative structure–property relationship. *J. Chem. Inf. Comput. Sci.* 36:100–107.

Taft, R. W., M. H. Abraham, R. M. Doherty, and M. J. Kamlet. 1985. The molecular properties governing solubilities of organic nonelectrolytes in water. *Nature* 313:384–386.

Taft, R. W. and M. J. Kamlet. 1976. The solvatochromic comparison method. 2. The α-scale of solvent hydrogen-bond donor (HBD) acidities. *J. Am. Chem. Soc.* 98:2886–2894.

Tantishaiyakul, V. 2005. Prediction of the aqueous solubility of benzylamine salts using QSPR model. *J. Pharm. Biomed. Anal.* 37:411–415.

Tripos. 1992. *SYBYL® Theory Manual.* St. Louis, MO: Tripos Associates.

Valvani, S. C. and S. H. Yalkowsky. 1976. Solubility of nonelectrolytes in polar solvents. VI. Refinements in molecular surface area computations. *J. Phys. Chem.* 80:829–835.

Valvani, S. C., S. H. Yalkowsky, and T. J. Roseman. 1981. Solubility and partitioning IV: Aqueous solubility and octanol-water partition coefficients of liquid nonelectrolytes. *J. Pharm. Sci.* 70:502–507.

Wakita, K., M. Yoshimoto, S. Miyamoto, and H. Watanabe. 1986. A method for calculation of the aqueous solubility of organic compounds by using new fragmental solubility constants. *Chem. Pharm. Bull.* 34:4663–4681.

Windholz, M. and S. Budavari. 1983. *The Merck Index, An Encyclopedia of Chemicals, Drugs, and Biologicals.* Rathway, NJ: Merck & Co.

Yalkowsky, S. H. and S. C. Valvani. 1980. Solubility and partitioning. I: Solubility of nonelectrolytes in water. *J. Pharm. Sci.* 69:912–922.

Yan, A., J. Gasteiger, M. Krug, and S. Anzali. 2004. Linear and nonlinear functions on modeling of aqueous solubility of organic compounds by two structure representation methods. *J. Comput. Aided Mol. Des.* 18:75–87.

Zhou, H., R. Liu, Y. Chen, and L. E. Matheson. 1993. A 3-dimensional molecular modeling approach for prediction of aqueous solubilities of aromatic compounds. *Pharm. Res.* 10:S261.

4 Preformulation Aspects of Insoluble Compounds

Wei-Qin (Tony) Tong and Hong Wen

CONTENTS

INTRODUCTION

Preformulation may be described as a stage of development during which the physicochemical and biopharmaceutical properties of a drug substance are characterized. Table 4.1 summarizes the material attributes of drug substance for consideration in drug development. A complete understanding of these physicochemical and biopharmaceutical properties is essential for the development of a robust, scalable formulation having desired bioavailability, and the most critical parameters are solubility, permeability (Burton and Goodwin 2010), and stability. Detailed reviews of pharmaceutical preformulation have been published (Fiese and Hagen 1986, Wells 1988, Ravin and Radebough 1990; Carstensen 2002, Marini et al. 2003, Lipinski et al. 2012).

TABLE 4.1
Material Attributes of Drug Substances

Physical Properties	Mechanical Properties[a]	Chemical Properties	Biological Properties
Appearance	Elasticity	Molecular structure	Partition coefficient
Particle size and shape	Plasticity	Molecular weight	Caco-2 permeability
Polymorphic form(s)	Viscoelasticity	pK_a	Biopharmaceutics classification
Crystallinity	Brittleness	Chemical stability	
Melting point	Strength		
Surface area	Bonding		
Density (bulk, tapped, and true) and flowability			
Hygroscopicity			
Solubility			
Dissolution rate			
Wettability			

[a] Mechanical properties are generally included in physical properties.

Compounds that have limited solubility (typically <0.1–1 mg/mL depending on the potency of compounds) in water and in common pharmaceutical solvents present unusual challenges. Although all the general principles of preformulation apply, there are certain preformulation aspects that are unique to insoluble compounds. These aspects need to be considered to ensure the successful development of formulations for these agents. The goals of this chapter are to discuss the theoretical and practical considerations for the preformulation of insoluble compounds; to review the experimental methods that are applicable to the characterization of insoluble compounds; and finally, to discuss how those preformulation considerations affect formulation design and process development.

ANALYTICAL METHODS DEVELOPMENT AND VALIDATION

A stability-indicating method must be developed and validated as early in the preformulation stage as possible. United States Pharmacopeia (USP) chapters, Food and Drug Administration (FDA) guidances, and International Conference on Harmonisation of Technical Requirements for Registration of Pharmaceuticals for Human Use (ICH) quality guidelines have provided very useful and comprehensive guidelines on analytical method development and method validation. Having an analytical method in place early on in the preformulation process is essential to ensure the quality of the preformulation results.

The first few batches of a drug substance in the hands of preformulation scientists may be not only very limited, but also impure. The compound itself may be unstable, or it may be unstable in solvents used in solubility studies. Furthermore, for insoluble compounds, methods development is often complicated by solubility limitations. Typically an organic solvent or some other solubilizing agents must be used for forced degradation studies and standards preparation. The effect of the solubilizing systems on the method should be considered as part of the methods development process. Additionally, should the need for different solubilizing agents arise, the method should be evaluated and modified accordingly so that these solubilizing agents do not interfere with the method.

SOLUBILITY AND DISSOLUTION

An understanding of the solubility behavior of a drug candidate can be regarded as one of the most important aspects of preformulation testing for poorly soluble compounds. For parenteral formulations, which are usually needed for preclinical and early clinical studies, the drug must be soluble in a pharmaceutically acceptable vehicle. For oral formulations, the drug must have an adequate solubility and dissolution rate to achieve suitable bioavailability. However, determining solubilities of these poorly soluble compounds and identifying solubilizing systems are not easy tasks. Special care must be taken and often special techniques must be applied to obtain desirable results.

For a drug to be called *soluble*, the FDA Biopharmaceutics Classification System (BCS) requires that the human dose of drug to be soluble in 250 mL throughout the gastrointestinal pH range of 1–7.5. For drugs with moderate permeability, when the projected doses are about 1 mg/kg, the effects of different solubility of drugs can be roughly estimated as in Table 4.2 (Chemical Sciences 2001).

TABLE 4.2
Solubility Data Interpretation

Solubility	Classification	Comments
≤20 µg/mL	*Low*	Will have solubility problems
20–65 µg/mL	*Moderate*	May have solubility problems
≥65 µg/mL	*High*	No solubility problem

THEORETICAL CONSIDERATIONS

The effects of various factors such as pH, the common ion effect, and temperature on solubility will have a greater impact on formulation development for insoluble compounds than for soluble ones. The general solubility theory has been extensively discussed. To afford better understanding of the solubility behavior of insoluble compounds, the pertinent solubility theory and its practical implications will be reviewed here.

Definition of Solubility

The simplest definition of solubility is that the solubility, S_T, of a substance is the molarity of that substance (counting all solution species) in a solution that is at chemical equilibrium with an excess of the undissolved substance. This implies that there must also be a uniform temperature throughout the system, because S_T is typically temperature dependent (Ramette 1981).

pH Effect on Solubility—pH-Solubility Profile

The equilibrium for the dissociation of the monoprotonated conjugate acid of a basic compound may be expressed by:

$$BH^+ + H_2O \xrightleftharpoons{K_a'} B + H_3O^+ \tag{4.1}$$

where BH^+ is the protonated species, B is the free base, and K_a' is the apparent dissociation constant of BH^+ which is defined as follows:

$$K_a' = \frac{[H_3O^+][B]}{[BH^+]} \tag{4.2}$$

Generally, the relationships drawn in Equations 4.1 and 4.2 must be satisfied for all weak electrolytes in equilibrium irrespective of pH and the degree of saturation. At any pH, the total concentration of a compound, S_T, is the sum of the individual concentrations of its respective species:

$$S_T = [BH^+] + [B] \tag{4.3}$$

In a saturated solution of arbitrary pH, this total concentration, S_T, is the sum of the solubility of one of the species and the concentration of the other necessary to satisfy the mass balance.

At low pH where the solubility of BH^+ is limiting, the following relationship holds:

$$S_{T,\,pH<pH_{max}} = [BH^+]_s + [B] = [BH^+]_s \left(1 + \frac{K_a'}{[H_3O^+]}\right) \tag{4.4}$$

where pH_{max} refers to the pH of maximum solubility and the subscript $pH < pH_{max}$ indicates that this equation is valid only for pH values less than pH_{max}. The subscript s indicates a saturated species. A similar equation can be written for solutions at pH values greater than pH_{max} where the free base solubility is limiting:

$$S_{T,\,pH>pH_{max}} = [BH^+] + [B]_s = [B]_s \left(1 + \frac{[H_3O^+]}{K_a'}\right) \tag{4.5}$$

Each of these equations describes an independent curve that is limited by the solubility of one of the two species.

The pH-solubility profile is non-uniformly continuous at the juncture of the respective solubility curves. This occurs at the precise pH where the species are simultaneously saturated, previously designated as the pH_{max}.

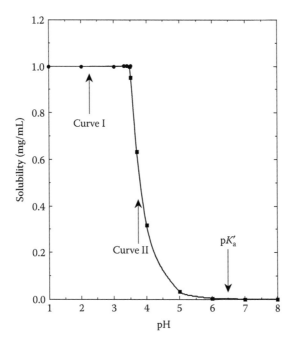

FIGURE 4.1   pH-solubility profile of an ideal compound BH^+Cl^-. Assuming $[BH^+]_s = 1$ mg/mL, $[B^+]_s = 0.001$ mg/mL, and $pK_a' = 6.5$. Note that at pK_a', $S_T = 2[B^+]_s$, $[BH^+] = [B]_s$.

In an uncomplicated system (as described in Equation 4.1), the theoretical pH-solubility profile can be generated using Equations 4.4 and 4.5, given the solubility of the salt, the solubility of the free base, and the apparent dissociation constant. Figure 4.1 is the pH-solubility profile for the hydrochloride salt of a free base (B) constructed by assuming that the solubilities of the hydrochloride salt and the free base are 1 mg/mL and 0.001 mg/mL, respectively, and that the pK_a' of the compound is equal to 6.5.

While the pK_a' does not determine the shape of the pH-solubility profile, it does fix the location of this profile on the pH coordinate. All other factors being equal, each upward or downward shift in the pK_a' is matched exactly by an upward or downward shift in pH_{max}. If the solubility of the free base is very small relative to that of the hydrochloride, the free base limiting curve (curve II) of the overall pH-solubility profile cuts deeply into the acidic pH range. Therefore, the solubility of the free base and the pK_a' basically determine the maximum pH at which formulation as a solution is possible, assuming the desired concentration exceeds the free base solubility (Kramer and Flynn 1972).

Solubility of Salts

General Considerations

Without assuming anything about the actual step-by-step mechanism of the solubility process, we may propose the following model for the equilibrium system of a 1:1 compound (e.g., a hydrochloride salt BH^+Cl^-) in contact with its saturated solution (Kramer and Flynn 1972, Ramette 1981):

$$BH^+Cl^-(s) \rightleftharpoons BH^+Cl^-(aq) \xrightarrow{K_s'} BH^+ + Cl^- \tag{4.6}$$

The *intrinsic solubility*, S_0, of the salt is simply the equilibrium quotient for the first step of this scheme:

$$S_0 = \frac{[BH^+Cl^-(aq)]}{X_{BH^+Cl^-(s)}} \tag{4.7}$$

If the solid is pure, then $X_{BH^+Cl^-(s)} = 1$ and

$$S_0 = [BH^+Cl^-(aq)] \tag{4.8}$$

The *dissociation constant*, K_s', can be defined as:

$$K_s' = \frac{[BH^+][Cl^-]}{[BH^+Cl^-(aq)]} = \frac{[BH^+][Cl^-]}{S_0} \tag{4.9}$$

The *solubility-product*, K_{sp}, is defined as the equilibrium expression that relates the concentrations of the final dissociated ions to the solid substance. It is an overall equilibrium quotient that reveals nothing about the concentrations of the intermediate species.

$$K_{sp} = \frac{[BH^+][Cl^-]}{X_{BH^+Cl^-(s)}} = [BH^+][Cl^-] \tag{4.10}$$

Saturated Solution with No Other Sources of Either Ion

The mass balance can be expressed in either of the two ways:

$$S_T = [BH^+Cl^-(aq)] + [BH^+] \tag{4.11}$$

or

$$S_T = [BH^+Cl^-(aq)] + [Cl^-] \tag{4.12}$$

where S_T is the total concentration of the compound, namely its solubility. Recognizing that $[BH^+Cl^-(aq)] = S_0$ and that $K_{sp} = [BH^+]^2 = [Cl^-]^2$ because $[BH^+] = [Cl^-]$, we find

$$S_T = S_0 + (K_{sp})^{1/2} \tag{4.13}$$

Saturated Solutions Containing Additional Common Ions

When the solution contains some other solute that can contribute Cl^- to the system, the dissociation of BH^+Cl^- will be partly depressed, the concentration of BH^+ and Cl^- will not be equal, the dissolution rate of the salt will be decreased (Li et al. 2005). The solubility-product itself, however, is still valid, and therefore, we may write:

$$[BH^+] = \frac{K_{sp}}{[Cl^-]_T} = \frac{K_{sp}}{[BH^+][Cl^-]_A} \tag{4.14}$$

where $[Cl^-]_T$ is the total concentration contributed both by the dissociation of BH^+Cl^- ($[BH^+]$) and by the second source of Cl^- ($[Cl^-]_A$). The solubility of the hydrochloride salt is inversely proportional to the equilibrium concentration of the Cl^-.

Saturated Solution in the Presence of Buffer Species

When the solubility of a salt, for example, the hydrochloride salt, is determined in buffer systems, the effect of the buffer species on the solubility must be taken into account. The anion of the buffer, L^-, for example, acetate, will compete with Cl^- to form a salt as illustrated in Equation 4.15.

$$BH^+Cl^- \text{ (solid)} \rightleftharpoons BH^+Cl^- \text{ (aq)} \rightleftharpoons BH^+ + Cl^-$$

$$K_s \Big\updownarrow +L^- \qquad (4.15)$$

$$BH^+L^- \text{ (solid)} \rightleftharpoons BH^+L^- \text{ (aq)}$$

where K_s is the dissociation constant of BH^+Cl^-(aq).

Case 1: If the salt formed with the anion of the buffer, L^- is less soluble than the hydrochloride salt, that is $K_{sp}(BH^+Cl^-) > K_{sp}(BH^+L^-)$, the compound is likely to precipitate out as BH^+L^-(s) provided the buffer concentration is high enough to meet the $K_{sp}(BH^+L^-)$. This means that solubility is controlled by the solubility of BH^+L^-(s).

Case 2: If the salt formed with the anion of the buffer, L^-, is more soluble than the hydrochloride salt, that is $K_{sp}(BH^+Cl^-) > K_{sp}(BH^+L^-)$, the compound will not likely precipitate out as BH^+L^-(s). If the formation of BH^+L^-(aq) is insignificant, the presence of the buffer species will not affect the solubility of the hydrochloride salt, assuming the effect of ionic strength is negligible.

Case 3: If the salt formed with the anion of the buffer, L^-, is more soluble than the hydrochloride salt, but the formation of BH^+L^-(aq) is significant, the solubility will be enhanced by the formation of the BH^+L^-(aq). The solubility, S_T, should account for all the species, as described in Equation 4.12.

$$S_T = S_0 + [BH^+] + [BH^+L^-(aq)] = S_0 + [BH^+] + \frac{[BH^+] \cdot [L^-]}{K_s} \qquad (4.16)$$

If S_0 is known, by plotting S_T versus $[L^-]$, K_s can be estimated:

$$K_s = \frac{\text{Intercept}}{\text{Slope}} \qquad (4.17)$$

In Situ Salt Screening Method

For ionizable compounds, pH adjustment is often one of the most important ways to improve solubility. For example, the diprotic nature of cosalane (NSC 658586) enabled a solubility enhancement of $>10^7$-fold by simple pH adjustment (Venkatesh et al. 1996). Most of the empirical methods for predicting solubility of salts require a melting point that is difficult to predict without actually preparing the salts. The *in situ* salt screening method provides a mean of obtaining solubility information without the need to make the individual salts (Tong and Whitesell 1998).

If free base (B) is added to a certain concentration of acid, the base will form the corresponding salt with the acid. If the acid concentration is chosen so that there is an excess amount of acid in the solution (ensuring that the pH of the solution is lower than pH_{max}), the solubility of the compound will be limited by the solubility of the salt ($[BH^+]$), as expressed in Equation 4.4. Knowing the amount of drug in solution, the volume of the solution, the solution pH and starting acid concentration, the K_{sp} and the solubility of the salt formed *in situ* can be calculated.

The amount of the compound precipitated, X_p can be calculated as follows:

$$X_p(\text{mg}) = X - S \cdot V \qquad (4.18)$$

where X (mg) is the added amount of solid base, S(mg/mL) is the solubility in the acid solution which is determined from solubility studies, and V(mL) is the volume of the solution.

The concentration of the acid remaining in solution, $[A_s]$ can then be calculated:

$$[A_s] = [A]\frac{X_p}{V \cdot \text{MW}} \quad (4.19)$$

where $[A]$ is the concentration of the acid used and MW is the compound's molecular weight.

Knowing the ionization constant of the acid, pK_a', and the pH of the saturated solution, the concentration of the acid in its ionized form, $[A_{\text{ionized}}]$, can be calculated based on Equation 4.2:

$$[A_{\text{ionized}}] = \frac{[A_s]}{1 + [\text{H}^+]/K_a'} \quad (4.20)$$

The molar concentration of the compound in solution is

$$[S] = \frac{S(\text{mg/mL})}{\text{MW}} \quad (4.21)$$

The K_{sp} of the salt can then be calculated:

$$K_{sp} = [S] \cdot [A_{\text{ionized}}] \quad (4.22)$$

Finally, the solubility of the salt, S_{salt} (mg/mL), is calculated as follows:

$$S_{salt} = (K_{sp})^{1/2} \cdot \text{MW} \quad (4.23)$$

Temperature Effect on Solubility

The heat of solution, ΔH_s, represents the heat released or absorbed when a mole of solute is dissolved in a large quantity of solvent. It can be determined by solution calorimetry or from solubility values for saturated solutions equilibrated at controlled temperatures over the range of interest. The working equation for determining ΔH_s is:

$$\ln S = \frac{\Delta H_s}{R}\left(\frac{1}{T}\right) + \text{constant} \quad (4.24)$$

where S is the molar solubility at temperature $T(K)$ and R is the ideal gas law constant. A semi-logarithmic plot of solubility *versus* reciprocal temperature is linear (van't Hoff plot), and ΔH_s is obtained from the slope. If ΔH_s is equal to 10 kcal/mol, which is typical for most organic compounds, S (25°C) over S (4°C) is about 3.6, suggesting a 3.6-fold decrease in solubility on refrigeration.

Very few systems follow ideality; most deviate significantly due to solute-solvent interaction. This is especially true for insoluble compounds in different solubilizing systems. The dependence of solubility on temperature will most likely change for different solubilizing systems, and therefore needs to be studied carefully.

For micellar systems, temperature changes may affect the micellar size and the degree of drug uptake, leading to a dependence of solubilization on temperature. An increase in temperature increases the aggregate size of polyoxyethylene nonionic surfactants by progressively dehydrating the ethylene oxide chains of the surfactant monomers (Elworthy et al. 1968). This change in micellar size typically leads to an increase in uptake of solute with increasing temperature for these types of surfactants. The extent of this increase will, of course, depend on the influence of temperature on the solution characteristics of the solubilized molecules and also on the micellar structure. There are, however, also cases reported where the solubility in certain surfactant systems decreases with increasing temperature. For example, the solubility of benzocaine in solutions of polyoxyethylene (23) lauryl ether and polysorbate 80 actually decreases as temperature increases over the temperature range of 30°C–70°C (Hamid and Parrott 1971).

For solubilizing systems containing complexing agents, because the standard enthalpy change accompanying the complexing process is generally negative, increasing temperature will reduce the degree of complexation (Szejtli 1982). Depending on the binding constants of complexes formed, this decreased binding can easily surpass the intrinsic solubility increase with increasing temperature, resulting in an overall solubility decrease in the presence of complexing agent with increasing temperature.

For co-solvent systems, because the heat of solution in different solvent systems is generally different, the temperature effect on solubility in these systems is also different. Detailed solubility mapping in the solvents of interest, including the effect of pH (for ionizable compounds), temperature, and co-solvent compositions is typically required in order to develop a robust formulation, such as a soft gel formulation.

DETERMINATION OF SOLUBILITY

The determination of solubility for insoluble compounds may be very challenging and time-consuming. Recognizing the advantages and limitations of various methods and choosing the proper method(s) or combination of methods for the specific preformulation requirement are essential to ensure the quality of the data. As solubility measurement is typically very labor-intensive and time-consuming, more and more high-through approaches have been developed for solubility measurement (Bard et al. 2008, Colclough et al. 2008, Heikkila et al. 2008, Alelyunas et al. 2009, Heikkilae et al. 2011, Wenlock et al. 2011).

Equilibrium Method

The equilibrium solubility of the drug candidate is obtained by equilibrating an excess of material in a vial with the solvent. The vial is shaken or stirred at constant temperature and the amount of drug determined periodically by analysis of the supernatant fluid. Generally, several samples should be assayed at different time intervals to determine if equilibrium has been achieved. When results from two successive samples are identical, equilibrium has most likely been reached. The residual solid from the solubility study should be checked to see if there are any crystal form changes.

For very insoluble compounds, using this method directly involves special difficulties, and therefore may not be practical (Higuchi et al. 1979). First of all, the analytical method may not be sensitive enough to quantitate the solubility. Secondly, the extremely low dissolution rate resulting from the low solubility may lead to difficulty in reaching equilibrium, leading to large errors in solubility results. For example, the reported solubility of cholesterol in water ranges from 0.025 to 2600 μg/mL (Madan and Cadwallader 1973).

There are several possible ways to improve the saturation rate. One reason for the delay in the attainment of equilibrium is the decrease in effective surface area during the dissolution process. This can be overcome by using a substantial excess of solid in the solubility sample (Higuchi et al. 1979). The surface area of the solid can also be increased by pre-processing the solubility samples. Both votexing after adding a small Teflon ball and sonication are very effective techniques for this purpose.

Another approach for enhancing the dissolution rate is the addition of a water-immiscible solvent in which the organic solute is more soluble, thereby increasing the effective surface area available for dissolution (Higuchi et al. 1979, Anderson et al. 1996). Since a small amount of non-aqueous solvent solubilized in water may change the solubility significantly, it is important to make sure that the water-immiscible solvent chosen is sufficiently immiscible in water so the solubility is not affected significantly. One way to check whether or not the effect of the solvent is significant is to determine solubilities in several different solvent-water systems. The solubility results should be rather independent of the solvents used. Some commonly used water-immiscible solvents include isooctane, octanol, and soy bean oil.

For a poorly water-soluble drug, when the equilibrated drug solutions are filtered, it is important to check the filter compatibility of the drug, and to make sure a suitable filter(s) that has low or no binding capacity for the drug has been selected. Because some filters may adsorb a small amount of the drug, the adsorption may affect the measured drug solubility, considering its poor aqueous solubility.

Intrinsic Dissolution Rate Method

The dissolution rate is directly proportional to the equilibrium solubility if the appropriate experimental conditions such as the ones used for intrinsic dissolution rate (IDR) measurements are selected. The rotating-disc method is the most useful and most widely used technique for measuring IDRs. The theoretical considerations and experimental details of this method will be considered later in this chapter in the discussion dealing with dissolution.

The IDR method is very useful where the equilibrium method cannot be used. For example, when one wishes to examine the influence of crystal habit, solvates and hydrates, polymorphism, and crystal defects on apparent solubility, the IDR method will usually avoid the crystal transitions likely to occur in equilibrium methods. However, crystal transitions can still occur at the surface, as in the case of anhydrous theophylline (De Smidt 1986) where the anhydrous form converts to the hydrate and the IDR changes over time. In these cases, the application of a fiber optical probe, which permits the detection of the drug concentration every few seconds, may prove to be very advantageous.

Non-Equilibrium Method

Any methods that do not contain steps to ensure the establishment of equilibrium can be considered non-equilibrium methods. Several methods commonly used for solubility measurements in the early discovery setting have been reported (Curatolo 1996, Pan et al. 2001), and these methods typically begin with dimethyl sulfoxide (DMSO) solutions or with amorphous material. Turbidity and ultraviolet detection are commonly used because they easily can be designed into high-throughput instrumentation.

The usefulness of the solubility data from these non-equilibrium methods often is questionable. Some pharmaceutical companies use these data as a first criterion to eliminate poorly solubility compounds. However, because the contribution of crystallinity to solubility is not controlled in non-equilibrium methods, the reliability of the data cannot be guaranteed. If experimental error is minimized, it is generally safe to assume that solubility can only be less when solid material is later used to determine equilibrium solubility. Therefore, the use of these solubility data as a gatekeeper seems to be justified. However, it is questionable whether data generated by these methods are any better for this purpose than those generated by computational methods. In addition, since for highly potent drug candidates the solubility requirement is dose-dependent, compounds whose solubility is in the microgram range may still be developable. Therefore, setting the right criteria to eliminate poorly soluble compounds may be challenging.

Estimation from the Partition Coefficient

For extremely insoluble compounds, the direct measurement of solubility may be impractical and unreliable. One possible way to obtain solubility information in these cases is through estimation from the partition coefficient (Higuchi et al. 1979). Typically, these very water-insoluble compounds are sufficiently soluble in a water-immiscible organic solvent to allow direct measurement. Once the solubility in some selected organic solvents is known, the solubility in water can be calculated from the directly measured or, more usually, the estimated partition coefficients. Based on the assumptions of the group contribution approach (Davis et al. 1974), the partition coefficient for a molecule can be predicted from the partition characteristics of its constituent parts by assuming that they are additive.

Another application of this method is the solubility estimation of drugs or prodrugs that are unstable in water (Beall et al. 1993). The synthesis of prodrugs is a commonly used approach for solubility and bioavailability enhancement. However, some prodrugs are unstable in water, making the direct measurement of their water solubility very difficult. The key to the success of this method is that partition coefficients can be determined very rapidly. By vigorous manual shaking of the two phases (about 10 s) and then allowing the two phases to separate by gravity for only 1 min, Beall et al. were able to determine the partition coefficients for hydrolytically unstable prodrugs such as 1-alkylcarbonyl-5-FU, prodrugs which exhibit a half-life of only about 7 min at pH 4.0 (Beall et al. 1993). They also discovered that octanol might not be a good solvent for this type of experiment. First of all, some prodrugs that are unstable in water may also be unstable in protic solvents such as octanol. Additionally, octanol tends to form emulsions upon vigorous shaking with an aqueous phase, making the required rapid separation impossible. Isopropyl myristate or similar esters have been found to separate quickly from the aqueous phases and were used successfully in these types of experiments (Beall et al. 1993).

Calculation Based on Melting Point and Octanol/Water Partition Coefficient

There are also empirical equations available that can be used for solubility estimation. Yalkowsky and Valvani (1980) developed the following equation by considering the transfer of a solute from the solid state to octanol followed by its transfer to the aqueous phase:

$$\log S_{aq} = -\log P_{o/w} - 0.01\text{MP} + 1.05 \tag{4.25}$$

where S_{aq} is the aqueous solubility of the drug, $P_{o/w}$ is the octanol/water partition coefficient, MP is the melting point. The equation was obtained by fitting the solubility data for 167 compounds as a function of their octanol/water partition coefficients and melting points.

Keep in mind that this is an empirical method; therefore it is realistic to expect that it may work well for certain compounds but not for others. When the method was used to estimate aqueous solubility of the very insoluble compound cosalane, the results were in fair agreement with those from the facilitated dissolution method (Venkatesh et al. 1996). However, when the method was used to estimate the solubility of a series of prodrugs of 5-FU, the calculated water solubilities were one to three orders of magnitude too high and did not accurately reflect trends in the series (Beall et al. 1993).

pH-Solubility Profile and Solubility of Salts

Solubility as a function of pH is traditionally determined by equilibrating an excess of solid in buffer solutions having different pH values. This can be problematic especially for insoluble compounds because of the effects buffer species have on solubility. Techniques using a pH-stat program with a titration system to control the pH may be more applicable and avoid the use of buffer systems (Todd and Winnike 1994). The compound is first equilibrated in HCl (for bases) or NaOH (for acids) solutions. The pH is then raised (or lowered) to the next desired value after the initial solubility is determined. For compounds whose solubility in HCl solutions is very low due to the low solubility of their hydrochloride salts, this method may not give a very informative pH-solubility profile. One way to overcome this is to combine the data with the results from the *in situ* salt screening. If the *in situ* salt screening is done before studying the solubility as a function of pH, the acid that gives the highest solubility can be chosen as the acid in the titration for the pH-solubility profile. An HCl solution can then be used to titrate the pH back to the acidic region. The resulting pH-solubility profile, especially drug solubility in simulated gastric fluid (pH 1.2) and simulated intestinal fluid (pH 7.5), contains information that is useful for both IV and oral formulation development.

Salt formation is often used to enhance the solubility of insoluble compounds. The very low intrinsic solubilities of these insoluble compounds coupled with weak basicity or acidity may make the solubility determination of these salts very difficult. For example, the water solubility of the phosphate salt of a very insoluble compound GW1818X was determined to be 6.8 mg/mL and the pH of the saturated solution was 5.0 (Tong and Whitesell 1998). The solubility at this pH was shown to be limited by the solubility of the base and did not adequately represent the solubility of the salt. One way to avoid this problem is to determine solubility in a diluted acidic solution using the same acid that formed the salt with the base. The solubility can then be estimated by correcting for the common ion effect from the acid. Keep in mind that it is only from a solubility experiment at a pH below pH_{max} that the solubility of the salt can be estimated.

SOLUBILIZATION

Various techniques for solubilization are discussed in other chapters in this book, and will not be considered individually here. When one particular technique does not give a satisfactory outcome, a combination of techniques should be considered. However, it is important to keep in mind that a combination of techniques may not always give a synergistic effect because of competitive mechanisms.

The commonly used solubilizing excipients for oral and injectable dosage forms include pH adjusters, water-soluble solvents, surfactants, water-insoluble organic solvents, medium-chain triglycerides, long-chain triglycerides, cyclodextrins, and phospholipids (Strickley 2004). Drug solubility in commonly used pharmaceutical solvents is often very useful in selecting suitable solubilization methods. Those solvents include, but are not limited to, ethanol, benzyl alcohol, Tween 80, PEG 400, propylene glycol, and glycerin.

Combining a cyclodextrin (CD) and a surfactant typically results in reduced solubilizing ability compared to each of these solubilizers used alone. This is due to the formation of an inclusion compound between the CD and the surfactant. On studying the effect of the presence of β-CD on the micellization process of sodium dodecyl sulfate or sodium perfluorooctanoate in water, Junquera et al. (1993) concluded that all the parameters directly related to the complexation process depend mainly on the hydrophobicity of the surfactant chain and its length, revealing that this is the part of the surfactant which is included into the CD cavity. Several other cases have also been reported. Methyltestosterone can be solubilized by HP-β-CD. However, when the micelle-forming excipient sodium deoxycholate is added, the drug is completely displaced from the cavity (Albers and Muller 1995). Both the nonionic surfactant Solutol HS 15 and β-CD increase the solubility of diazepam in water. However, a mixed solution of the two solubilizers does not increase diazepam solubility. Because of the high stability constant of the surfactant/β-CD, diazepam is displaced from its complex with β-CD (Kraus et al. 1991). Muller and Albers (1991) also reported that the combination of 1,2 propylene glycol and 2-HP-β-CD induced a decrease in the solubilizing capacity of the system as compared with 2-HP-β-CD alone.

DISSOLUTION

Dissolution of a drug substance is controlled by several physicochemical properties, including solubility, surface area, and wetting properties. For insoluble compounds, dissolution is often the rate-limiting step in the absorption process. Knowledge of the dissolution rate of a drug substance is therefore very useful for formulation development. The appropriate dissolution experiments can help to identify factors that contribute to bioavailability problems, and also assist in the selection of the appropriate crystal form and/or salt form. Dissolution tests are also used for other purposes such as quality control and assisting with the determination of bioequivalence (Dressman et al. 1998).

Experimentally for IDR measurement, a constant surface area is obtained by compressing powder into a disc of known area with a die and punch apparatus. Both rotating and static disks have been used extensively. Potential problems with this method are crystal form conversions during compression of powder into a pellet or during the dissolution experiment. Since many drug candidates are weak acids or bases, pH and common ion gradients at the solid-liquid interface can lead to erroneous conclusions, as discussed by Mooney and co-workers (Mooney et al. 1981a, 1981b).

Powder dissolution is another method that has been employed extensively. This method is particularly useful when the drug substances cannot readily be formed readily into disks by compression or when the particle size effect on dissolution needs to be studied. A variety of techniques for studying powder dissolution has been reported (Goldberg et al. 1965, Finholt 1974, Cakiryildiz et al. 1975, Lötter et al. 1983). Particles of hydrophobic substances tend to aggregate, and are often difficult to wet, causing a reduction in the effective surface area exposed to dissolution medium. For example, the dissolution rates of phenobarbital, aspirin, and phenacetin were found to increase unexpectedly with increasing particle size (Finholt 1974). This was attributed to the poor wettability of the drug substances. It was found that problems of flotation and aggregation of these drug substances could be overcome by adding 0.2% Tween 80 to the dissolution medium. The influence of aggregates on the dissolution process could also be eliminated effectively by deaggregating samples of insoluble drugs before they are introduced into the dissolution medium (Lötter et al. 1983).

The intrinsic dissolution and powder dissolution methods discussed earlier are typically used for the characterization of drug substances. For drug formulations, a USP apparatus such as the USP Apparatus 2 is more applicable. According to the Biopharmaceutics Classification Scheme (Amidon et al. 1995), drugs can be divided into four classes on the basis of their aqueous solubility and their ability to permeate the mucosa in the gut from the apical to the basolateral side. Low-solubility compounds are defined as those whose solubility in aqueous media is insufficient for the whole dose to be dissolved in the gastrointestinal (GI) contents under usual conditions. Since dissolution, for these substances, can depend on a wide variety of factors such surfactants, pH, buffer capacity, ionic strength, and volume available for dissolution, the media used for dissolution studies need to represent closely the prevailing conditions in the upper GI tract in order to achieve a meaningful *in vitro/in vivo* correlation.

Based on physiological parameters, media to simulate gastric and small intestinal conditions in the fed and fasted states have been suggested (Galia et al. 1996, Dressman et al. 1998). For many insoluble compounds, however, maintaining *sink* conditions may be very challenging. For ionizable compounds one may employ a totally aqueous medium by resorting to altering the pH. However, alternative strategies must be adopted for non-ionizable substances. Dissolution media containing solubilizing agents have been used to meet the requirement of *sink* conditions. However, one needs to be cautious in interpreting the results from these studies. A good *in vitro/in vivo* correlation needs to be established before the dissolution method can be used to predict the *in vivo* performance of drugs.

The addition of a co-solvent which increases the drug solubility in an aqueous-based dissolution medium has been widely employed to provide *sink* conditions for the dissolution of insoluble compounds (Poirier et al. 1981, Dodge et al. 1987, Corrigan 1991). When using this technique, the effects of the co-solvent on tablet disintegration and especially on the solubility and the dissolution rate of excipient(s) present in the dosage form need to be carefully considered to avoid anomalous release characteristics. Highly water-soluble excipients are often chosen for dosage forms containing insoluble compounds. Solubilities and dissolution rates of these water-soluble excipients, such as lactose, may decrease in the presence of co-solvents in sufficient concentration. Depending on the proportion of excipients in the formulation, drug dissolution in the co-solvent system may become controlled by the rate of dissolution of the less-soluble excipients. Theoretical models to predict the effect of co-solvent on the dissolution of a simple two-component drug-excipient compact are available in the literature (Corrigan 1991). Solubility and dissolution studies using Tolbutamide and lactose mixtures in water-ethanol mixtures provided results which were reasonably consistent with the theoretical models.

In developing dissolution method for poorly water-soluble drugs, besides selecting suitable pH in the dissolution medium, surfactants are often used to get suitable sink condition. However, special attention is needed in developing bio-relevant dissolution method with surfactants. Tang et al. (2001) used three different concentrations of sodium lauryl sulfate (SLS), 1%, 0.5%, and 0.25%, to execute dissolution for the formulations of a poorly water-soluble drug. In the 1% SLS-sink condition, the drug release from all the formulations was complete. However, the best bio-relevant dissolution condition was with 0.25% SLS, in which drug from all formulations could not release completely.

IONIZATION CONSTANT, pK_a

IMPORTANCE OF pK_a

Knowledge of the aqueous ionization constant, pK_a, of an ionizable drug candidate is very important because it can be used to predict solubility, lipophilicity, and permeability at different pH; therefore, help to improve drug adsorption by selecting suitable pH. Drugs in solution are distributed between their neutral and charged forms based on the pH and pK_a. Depending on whether drugs are acidic or basic compounds, pH lower or higher, respectively, than their pK_a will create more ionization, and make the drugs more soluble but less permeable.

If the pK_a of a drug substance is known in the early stage of the drug development process, the analytical assay method development, solubility and stability estimation as a function of pH can be accomplished with a minimum number of experiments, and it can guide formulation development for IV formulations.

TEMPERATURE EFFECT ON pK_a

The effect of temperature on ionization constants is related to the entropy change of the ionization process through the following equation (Perrin et al. 1981):

$$\frac{-d(pK_a)}{dT} = \frac{(pK_a + 0.052\Delta S^0)}{T} \tag{4.26}$$

Because the entropy change associated with ionization is different for different acids or bases, it is obvious that the effect of temperature on the ionization constants is highly structure dependent.

The pK_a values of common carboxylic acids vary only slightly with ambient temperature. For the ionization of organic bases little entropy change is involved because the number of ions and their charges do not change (ΔS^0 lies in the range of -17 Jdeg^{-1}mol^{-1}). Therefore the effect of temperature on the pK_a values of organic bases is given with acceptable accuracy by the following equations:

For monocations:

$$\frac{-d(pK_a)}{dT} = \frac{(pK_a - 0.09)}{T} \tag{4.27}$$

For dications:

$$\frac{-d(pK_a)}{dT} = \frac{(pK_a)}{T} \tag{4.28}$$

for temperatures near 25°C where T is in Kelvin.

For example, for a weak base with a pK_a of 7.0, every 10-degree increase in temperature will lower the pK_a by about 0.2 units.

When developing IV formulations for very insoluble weak bases, it is important to consider the temperature effect on the pK_a. If the pH values of these formulations are not low enough, the compound may precipitate out as the free base upon autoclaving. At elevated temperature, the pK_a of the compound may be shifted to such an extent that the solubility of the free base becomes limiting at the solution pH. The precipitated free base may take a very long time to redissolve due to its low solubility and slow dissolution rate, resulting in product failure (Tong et al. 1994).

SOLVENT EFFECTS ON pK_a

Solvent effects on pK_a values are also different for acids and bases. When acids ionize, two ions are generated for each neutral molecule that dissociates. This equilibrium is very sensitive to the dielectric constant of the medium. The pK_a increases markedly (the acid becomes weaker) in solvents of low dielectric constant. A shift of the pK_a value of up to 2 pH units is not uncommon (Rubino 1987).

On the other hand, the ionization of bases is an isoelectronic process, therefore the effect of solvent is much less; usually the pK_a decreases slightly (the base becomes weaker). For this type of equilibrium, measurements made in mixed solvents can usually be extrapolated to give values in aqueous solution, making the pK_a estimation of very insoluble compounds possible.

The direct implication of this solvent effect on pK_a is the effect co-solvents have on the action of pharmaceutical buffers. This is of particular interest in the formulation of parenteral products since many injectable formulations which contain co-solvents also contain a buffer system for the control of pH (Rubino 1987). Because of the shift in pK_a in the presence of co-solvents, buffer systems should be chosen based upon the pK_a values in the particular solvent system used in the vehicle. This is significant because for parenteral formulations that contain co-solvents, the buffer concentration that can be used is often limited by the solubility of the buffer. Choosing a buffer whose pK_a is close to the desired pH can certainly help in keeping the buffer concentration as low as possible while the buffer capacity is kept sufficiently high enough to achieve the desired goal.

In addition to considering an adjusted buffering range in mixed solvent systems, the effects of dilution on the pH of the formulation should also be considered (Rubino 1987). As formulations containing mixed solvent systems are diluted, the solvent effects on the pK_a will decrease. For example, the pK_a of the buffer acid will decrease as the formulation is diluted due to the dilution of the co-solvent. The consequences of these pK_a changes on the physicochemical stability of the active compounds should be carefully studied.

DETERMINATION OF pK_a

There are several well-established methods for pK_a determination (Albert and Serjeant 1984). However, not all the methods are suitable for insoluble compounds. Sometimes an estimation or prediction of the pK_a might be sufficient, depending on the need. Only some practical considerations pertinent to obtaining pK_a values for insoluble compounds are discussed here.

Phase Equilibria

The pK_a value can be calculated from the pH-solubility profile based on Equation 4.5, which can be rearranged to give Equation 4.29.

$$pK_a = pH + \log\left(\frac{S_T}{[B]_s} - 1\right) \tag{4.29}$$

For acids, a similar equation can be derived:

$$pK_a = pH - \log\left(\frac{S_T}{[A]_s} - 1\right) \tag{4.30}$$

where $[B]_s$ and $[A]_s$ are the solubility of neutral molecular species for the base and acid, respectively.

For some very insoluble compounds, the solubility of the neutral molecular species is too low to be measured accurately. In this case, the pK_a along with the solubility of the neutral species can still be estimated by determining solubilities at two pH values. If several solubility values can be measured along the rising part of the curve II in Figure 4.1, non-linear regression curve fitting can be used to estimate the pK_a and the solubility of the neutral species.

Spectrophotometry

The determination of ionization constants by UV or visible spectrophotometry may be particularly useful for insoluble compounds (Albert and Serjeant 1984). For many insoluble compounds, a solution with a concentration as low as 10^{-6} M may still give an analytically useful chromophore. The method depends upon the direct determination of the ratio of molecular species (neutral molecule) to ionized species in a series of non-absorbing buffer solutions. A wavelength, typically called the *analytical wavelength*, is chosen at which the greatest difference between the absorbances of the two species is observed (Albert and Serjeant 1984).

For acids, Equation 4.31 is used if A_I is greater than A_M, whereas Equation 4.32 is used if the reverse is the case.

$$pK_a = pH + \log \frac{A_I - A}{A - A_M} \tag{4.31}$$

$$pK_a = pH + \log \frac{A - A_I}{A_M - A} \tag{4.32}$$

where A_I and A_M are the absorbances of the ionized species and the neutral species, respectively. A is the observed absorbance at any particular pH.

For bases, Equation 4.33 is used if A_I is greater than A_M, and Equation 4.34 if the reverse is the case.

$$pK_a = pH + \log \frac{A - A_M}{A_I - A} \tag{4.33}$$

$$pK_a = pH + \log \frac{A_M - A}{A - A_I} \tag{4.34}$$

Potentiometric Titration

Potentiometric titration is a commonly used technique for pK_a determination (Albert and Serjeant 1984, Takacs-Novak et al. 1997, Glomme et al. 2005). The PCA101 chemical analyzer, developed and manufactured by Sirius Analytical Instruments Ltd., is the first commercial instrument designed specifically to determine ionization constants (Avdeef 1993).

To use the potentiometric titration method, the compound typically must have a solubility of at least 5×10^{-4} M. For insoluble compounds, a mixed solvent approach can be used (Avdeef 1993). Methanol is the most commonly used co-solvent for this purpose and its effect on pK_a has been studied extensively. Experimentally, several pK_a measurements need to be performed in mixed solvent solutions having various methanol-water proportions. The aqueous pK_a is deduced by extrapolation of the apparent pK_a values to zero methanol. Other co-solvents that can be used for this purpose and that are supported by the PCA101 include ethanol, ethylene glycol, DMSO, and 1,4-dioxane. Keep in mind that different co-solvents will have different effects on the pK_as and these effects are also different for acids and bases. Plots of apparent pK_a versus weight percent organic solvent (typically 0%–60%) show either a *hockey-stick* shape, or a *bow* shape, but rarely a straight line.

pK_a Prediction

Despite all the methods available for pK_a measurement, there are cases where the compounds are too insoluble or too unstable to measure. In the case of polyacids and bases, assigning experimental pK_a values to particular sites might be challenging. In some cases, only an estimation of a pK_a value is needed, such as in the early discovery stages. For these reasons, a method for a quick pK_a estimation may be very useful.

There are excellent reviews available for pK_a prediction (Fraczkiewicz 2006, Wan and Ulander 2006, Cruciani et al. 2009, Dearden 2012). A unique predictive algorithm has been established by *Advanced Chemistry Development* (1998), in which ACD/pK_a is a program that calculates pK_a values at 25°C and zero ionic strength in aqueous solution. It uses a structure fragment approach and takes into account electronic, steric, charge, tautomeric, vinylogy, and covalent hydration effects. Each calculation is provided with both its 95% confidence limits and a detailed report of how it has been carried out, including the Hammett-type equation(s), substituent constants, and literature references where available. The parameters on which the pK_a calculation is based are drawn from over 8900 structures in the scientific literature with over 23,000 experimental values at different temperatures and ionic strengths in purely aqueous solutions. The accuracy of calculations is usually better than 0.2 pK_a units except for very complex structures or poorly characterized substituents, where the accuracy is usually better than 0.5 pK_a units. Berger et al. (1997) determined the pK_a values for a total of 25 drugs representing a range of structures and liquid-phase properties using both experimental (potentiometric titration) and computational (ACD) methods, and most pK_a values fell well within the ±0.5 pK_a unit range.

LIPOPHILICTY AND PERMEABILITY

Lipophilicity of one drug is generally measured by checking its distribution between an aqueous and non-polar organic phase like *n*-octanol. The partition coefficient ($P_{o/w}$), a measurement of a drug's lipophilicity, is defined as the ratio of un-ionized drug distributed between the organic and aqueous phases at equilibrium.

$$P_{o/w} = \left(\frac{C_{oil}}{C_{water}} \right) \text{equilibrium} \tag{4.35}$$

It should be noted that the partition coefficient is a constant. The apparent partition coefficient of the protolytic forms of the drug substance, which obviously can vary as a function of pH, is defined as the distribution coefficient ($D_{o/w}$). Both log P and log D have been used widely as indications of lipophilicity of one drug.

Lipophilicity of one drug will affect its distribution in lipid membranes, protein binding, body fluids, and so on, thus affect many biopharmaceutical properties such as ADME (adsorption, distribution, metabolism, and excretion), plasma protein binding, toxicity, activity, plasma protein binding (Suzuki et al. 1970, Dressman et al. 1984, Wells 1988). Although partition coefficient/distribution coefficient data alone do not provide an understanding of *in vivo* absorption, they do provide a means of characterizing the lipophilic/hydrophilic nature of a drug. In general, log D of one drug ranges from 0.5 to 3 suggests that the drug has moderate lipophilicity and may have suitable GI tract adsorption (Chemical Sciences 2001).

Permeability of drugs is one of the most important biopharmaceutical properties (Varma et al. 2012, Hermens et al. 2013). For any drug by oral drug delivery systems, in order to reach systemic circulation from gastrointestinal (GI) tract, the drug must permeate the GI cellular barrier. After drug enters systemic circulation, some drugs still need to permeate through cell membrane to have its therapeutic effects. Permeation can occur through different routes, include active transport, efflux, and paracellular diffusion. However, most drugs mainly permeate through passive transcellular diffusion. To assess the passive diffusion of drugs, different artificial membranes, like phospholipids membrane, have been designed to measure permeation across the membrane from the donor side to the acceptor side. In pharmaceutical industry, the most commonly used methods in permeability measurements are Caco-2 cell membrane measurement and rat jejunal perfusion.

Considering the low solubility of those insoluble drugs, solubilizing excipients are often used to increase the drug concentration in permeability measurement. Sometimes, those solubilizing excipients may affect the drug permeability as well. Saha and Kou (2000) studied the effects of solubilizing excipients on Caco-2 transport for three poorly water-soluble compounds, Sch 56592, Sch-X, and Sch-Y. Caco-2 measurement showed that all three compounds have good permeability.

For Sch 56592, 1% Povidone could not only improve its solubility, but also improve its flux through Caco-2 membrane by 40%. Even though some other solubilizing excipients could also solubilize Sch 56592, they either did not change or even decrease its flux through the membrane. For Sch-X, 1% povidone, pluronic F68, Gelucire 44/14, and 3:2 propylene glycol/Tween-80 could significantly improve its solubility as well it flux through the membrane. The solubility of Sch-Y could be enhanced by quite a few solubilizing excipients, but only 1% pluronic F68 and PEG300 could increase its flux by 35%–50%. The study shows that for different drugs, solubilizing excipients may not enhance flux across Caco-2 membrane to the same extent as solubility enhancement, and some even decreased drug permeability. The effects of solubilizing excipients on oral drug adsorption will be determined by their contribution on both soluble drug concentration and transport parameters. Therefore, for insoluble drugs, solubilizing excipients should be carefully evaluated on drug permeation as well for developing bioavailable formulations.

MEASUREMENT OF PARTITION COEFFICIENTS

The methods commonly used for the measurement of partition coefficients include the traditional shake-flask method, HPLC, filter-probe, and pH-metric techniques (Dunn III et al. 1986, Avdeef 1993). Dearden and Bresnen (1988) gave *GLP* recommendations on experimental procedures. Hersey et al. (1989) presented a method selection guide. Additionally, several methods are available for partition coefficient calculations (Lipinski et al. 2012).

Shake Flask Method

The shake flask method is the most commonly used method for the measurement of partition coefficients (Leo et al. 1971). However, for many insoluble compounds, the solubility in the aqueous phase may be too low to be accurately determined. In these cases, an alternative method needs to be applied.

Potentiometric Titration

The determination of partition coefficients by the potentiometric method is part of the function of the Sirus PCA 101 (Avdeef 1993). Typically, a preacidified solution of a weak acid is alkalimetrically titrated to some appropriately high pH; the partition solvent such as octanol is then added, and the dual-solvent mixture is acidimetrically titrated back to the starting pH. Analysis of the two titration curves will yield two pK_as: pK_a and poK_a, where poK_a is the apparent constant derived from the octanol-containing segment of data. The partition coefficient is calculated from the following equations:

$$\text{For an acid: } P_{HA} = \frac{(10^{+(poK_a - pK_a)} - 1)}{r} \tag{4.36}$$

$$\text{For a base: } P_B = \frac{(10^{-(poK_a - pK_a)} - 1)}{r} \tag{4.37}$$

where

$$r = \frac{\text{Volume of the organic phase}}{\text{Volume of the aqueous phase}} \tag{4.38}$$

The converse of this technique is the partition-derived pK_a determination which may be very useful for the pK_a estimation for insoluble compounds. If log P data can be obtained by some alternative methods, a titration of a weak acid in the presence of octanol will give the apparent pK_a, poK_a. Equations 4.36 and 4.37 can be used to calculate the aqueous pK_a.

Chromatographic Hydrophobicity Index (CHI)

In reversed phase liquid chromatography, the lipophilicity of compounds governs their retention. The properly transformed retention data should reveal the lipophilicity of the compounds. Valko et al. (1997) converted a fast gradient reversed-phase retention time to a Chromatographic Hydrophobicity Index (CHI) using a set of test compounds to calibrate the HPLC system. CHI values have been found to correlate well with the log D well, suggesting that the CHI can serve as an alternative to log P or log D. Because no actual concentration needs to be determined, and organic solvents can be used to dissolve the compounds, the method is particularly suitable for compounds with poor aqueous solubility.

Partition Coefficient Prediction

Predictive software for the determination of log P is also available from *Advanced Chemistry Development* (ACD) (1998). ACD/log P calculates octanol/water partition coefficients for the neutral form of the molecule using a structure fragment approach with parameters derived from a large database. The accuracy of the predictive calculations is usually better than ± 0.3 log P units except for very complex structures or poorly -characterized substituents, where the accuracy is usually better than ± 0.5 log P units. In studies on 25 drugs (Berger et al. 1997), log P data generated by the shake-flask method, Sirius potentiometric method and computational (ACD) methods matched very well.

CHOICE OF PARTITIONING SOLVENT

As mentioned earlier, one of the most important uses of log P/log D is to correlate to the rate and extent of drug absorption as well as the biological response by offering a prediction of the tendency for a drug to move from an aqueous compartment into a biological membrane. Traditionally, the octanol–water partition coefficient was the most widely used to study the lipophilic character of drug molecules. In the octanol–water system, the partitioning of drug molecules in the neutral form is favored relative to the ionized form. In the membrane-water system, it has been found that partitioning of the ionized species is significantly enhanced over that shown in the octanol–water system (Miyazaki et al. 1992, Austin et al. 1995, Hellwich and Schubert 1995). Clearly, the octanol–water system is inadequate to account for certain critical characteristics of biological membranes, which are comprised of lipid bilayers consisting of amphipathic groups having strong electrostatic interactions (Schwarz 1996).

Rogers and Choi (1993) have shown that partition coefficients in liposome-water systems outperformed the oactanol-water system for the prediction of biological activities of certain classes of drugs. Dialysis (Formelova et al. 1991, Kuhnvelten 1991, Pauletti and Wunderli-Allenspach 1994) and ultrafiltration (Kuhnvelten 1991, Austin et al. 1995) methods have been used to measure liposomal membrane-water partition coefficients. Avdeef et al. (1998) successfully applied the pH-metric technique, an efficient and accurate way to determine liposomal membrane-water partition coefficients for ionizable drugs, and the results are consistent with those obtained from the ultrafiltration and dialysis methods. Despite the limitation of octanol as a solvent for predicting membrane partitioning, because of the enormous body of data that already exists and the ease of generating data, it undoubtedly remains the partitioning solvent of choice.

CACO-2 MEASUREMENT

The permeability of a drug can be determined in the Caco-2 Transwell polycarbonate filter cell culture system. The dose solution is prepared by dissolving the drug in DMSO and diluting the HBSS/HEPES to a suitable drug concentration. Sometimes, suitable amount of Tween 80 is added to the dose solution to ensure that the drug does not precipitate upon further dilution in the Caco-2 donor chamber. Three portions of this solution are dosed to Caco-2. Monolayer integrity was measured with an epithelia voltohmmeter, from which TEER (transepithelial electrical resistance) is calculated. Aliquot samples are taken from the receiver chamber over a period of 120 min and are analyzed by HPLC. The experiments are performed in both apical to basolateral (A->B) and basolateral to apical (B->A) directions under non-gradient pH conditions (pH7.4 on both sides) and pH-gradient conditions (pH5.5 apically, pH7.4 basolaterally) (Koljonen et al. 2006). Good recovery is important to determine drug permeability accurately.

Metoprolol, propranolol, and atenolol are commonly used as control in permeability measurement. Among them, metoprolol is generally used in manual method, and propranolol in automated method. If the apparent permeability coefficient (Papp) of one drug, in the apical (A) to basolateral (B) direction, is higher than that of metoprolol, the drug may have good permeability. If Papp of (B->A)/(A->B) is higher than 1, the drug may have efflux in the Caco-2 system.

RAT JEJUNAL PERFUSION

Under several conditions, it is preferred to measure drug permeability again with the rat jejunal perfusion method. For example, when drug recovery is low in Caco-2 measurement, the measured drug permeability data may not be accurate. When measured drug permeability is medium to low from Caco-2 study, it is important to confirm the drug permeability with the rat perfusion method. For insoluble drugs, the measured permeability from Caco-2 study may contain large experiment error, and rat perfusion study is often used to evaluate their intestinal adsorption. For several insoluble new chemical entities (NCEs) in clinical development, Caco-2 studies showed they have medium to low permeability, but rat perfusion studies confirmed they have high permeability. The rat perfusion measurements were consistent with the animal and human PK studies.

In one rat jejunal perfusion study, the jejunum was exposed via a midline incision from fasted rats (Swenson et al. 1994). The intestine was gently rinsed with 20 mL warm saline to remove residual contents, then securely fastened at both the proximal and distal incisions. The perfused segment was moistened with saline and covered with Parafilm. The solutions containing 0.25 mg/mL drug of interest, with some surfactants if needed, in isotonic pH6.5 sodium phosphate/sodium sulfate buffer was used to perfuse the intestine. The perfusion solution was kept at 37°C. Perfusate samples were collected over four 15 min intervals. An adsorption rate constant was calculated for each 15 min interval, based on the measured flow rate, the volume of the perfused intestinal segment, as well as the ingoing and outgoing drug concentration. Similarly, the reversibility experiments were executed, except that perfusion was carried out for 4 h, with perfusate collection in 15 min increments. GI stability study was executed at the same time to make sure that the drug did not degrade during the rat perfusion study. Overall, permeability data were average over 3 or 4 rats. The effective intestinal permeability (Peff) of drugs in jejunum will be compared with the value of metoprolol to see whether they have suitable permeability or not.

BIOPHARMACEUTICS CLASSIFICATION SYSTEM CLASSIFICATION

Biopharmaceutical classification depends on both the solubility and permeability of a given drug, and provides a basis for predicting the oral absorption of drugs. In the FDA's Biopharmaceutics Classification System (BCS) Guidance, a drug substance is considered *highly soluble* when the highest dose strength is soluble in <250 mL water over a pH range of 1–7.5, and is considered *highly permeable* when the extent of absorption in humans is determined to be >90% of an administered dose, based on mass-balance or in comparison to an intravenous reference dose. For oral dosage forms of BCS II drugs which have good permeability but poor solubility, the drug bioavailability is mainly limited by the dissolution process; however, the drug bioavailability of BCS IV drugs which have low permeability and poor solubility is limited by not only the dissolution process but also the adsorption process. Based on pH-dependent permeability and solubility, the BCS concepts

TABLE 4.3
Classification of Effective Permeability

Effective Permeability (Pe)	Classification	Comments
$\leq 0.1 \times 10^{-6}$ cm/sec	*Low*	Will have permeability problems
$0.1 - 1 \times 10^{-6}$ cm/sec	*Moderate*	May have permeability problems
$\geq 1 \times 10^{-6}$ cm/sec	*High*	No permeability problem

have been successfully extended in the Biopharmaceutics Drug Disposition Classification System (BDDCS) to explain the potential mechanism of drug clearance and understand the effects of uptake and efflux transporters on absorption, distribution, metabolism, and elimination (Varma et al. 2012).

In pharmaceutical industry, in both Caco-2 measurement and rat jejunal perfusion, if a drug has higher permeability than metoprolol, the drug is considered highly permeable. With permeability coefficient approximately 1×10^{-6} cm/sec, metoprolol has about 95% human adsorption fraction (Regardh et al. 1974, Kim et al. 2006). Even though the *in vitro* permeability measurement may not be exact the same as *in vivo* permeability data, many publications have shown that there exists good rank order relationship between true permeation rate constant with measured permeability from Caco-2 monolayer or rat jejunal perfusion (Polli and Ginski 1998, Winiwarter et al. 1998, Kim et al. 2006). Therefore, by comparing the measured drug permeability with the measured Metoprolol permeability in the same measurement system, it is possible to evaluate whether the drug has high permeability or not.

It is worthwhile to note that BCS was designed to evaluate whether or not clinical bioequivalence can be justified based on *in vitro* dissolution tests, especially for immediate release solid oral dosage forms. However, the criteria of high solubility and high permeability in the system are higher than actual drug developability. For example, some Class IV drugs with solubility and permeability just below the criteria are still good candidates in development to achieve desired bioavailability. With permeability about $0.1 \sim 0.3 \times 10^{-6}$ cm/sec, drugs like atenolol and a-methyldopa have about 50% absorption fraction (Walter et al. 1996, Kim et al. 2006). Combining the information about the permeability and absorption fraction of metoprolol, effective drug permeability can approximately be classified into three categories as shown in Table 4.3 (Chemical Sciences 2001). The table may provide more practical evaluation on drug permeability than does BCS evaluation.

STABILITY

Information about drug stability is important for drug synthesis, formulation, and storage to the final dosing in humans. In addition to chemical stability of drug substance reviewed in this section, physical stability will be reviewed in the section titled Solid State Properties. Table 4.4 illustrates some indicative stability studies (Chemical Sciences 2001). It is worthwhile to note that the stability of these insoluble compounds in the presence of solubilizing agents is very likely to be different from the stability in aqueous solutions. For this reason, stability in purely aqueous media may not be relevant at all and it may be difficult to determine because of the solubility limitation. Besides those solubilizing excipients, it is important to check whether the drug of interest is compatible with other excipients that may be used in formulation design and process development.

FORCED DEGRADATION STUDIES

Forced degradation studies are useful not only for checking the drug stability under different conditions, but also for analytical method development and method validation (Maheswaran 2012). In the forced degradation studies, the solubilized drug is exposed to extremes of acid, base, heat,

TABLE 4.4
Some Indicative Stability Studies

Stability Study	Relevance
Acid stability	Stomach
Base stability	Large intestine
Light stability	Lab and factory manufacturing
Heat and/or moisture stability	Accelerated storage conditions
Oxidative stability	Ambient environment as well as formulation
Plasma stability	Plasma

oxidation, and light. The typically experiment conditions are 0.1 N HCl, 0.1 N NaOH, water/heat, 3% H_2O_2, and light (1000 mW/cm^2 UV light and 500fc fluorescent light). To achieve the best compromise between time required for the studies and analytical accuracy, the desired degradation ranges are typically 5%–20%. In the HPLC method development, an optimal wavelength is critical to detect all important impurities and degradants, and sometimes, a dual wavelength detector can be used. A suitable solvent and mobile phase should be compatible with both the drug studied and their impurities/degradants. The chromatographic method should be tested to make sure that no impurities/degradants co-elute with the main peak of interest.

Finally, the developed HPLC method needs to have suitable mass balance based on major degradants.

Identifying the degradants is very important to understand the potential degradation pathways. LC-MS, LC-MS/MS, and LC-NMR are commonly used to help study the structures of the degradation products.

Scientists at GlaxoSmithKline (Sims et al. 2002) use an automated workstation for forced degradation studies. Conditions used are over a wide range of pH values, oxidative conditions, and thermally in solution. The system included an autosampler, a dilutor, a reaction station controlled by software, and an HPLC with UV detection and mass spectrometric detection. The automation process can not only save analysts' operating time, but also reduce the delay between sample preparation and analysis to a minimum. By combining mass detection with HPLC in the system, structural information about degradants along with kinetic data on the appearance and disappearance of degradants during forced degradation studies can also be collected. Overall, the increased knowledge about degradation reactions from the automated system should help scientists to focus more efficiently on the primary degradation processes.

pH-STABILITY PROFILE

For the purpose of stability prediction, the availability of a pH-rate profile for the drug is extremely valuable (Connors et al. 1986). In solution, many factors like pH, ionic strength, buffer species, and initial concentration can affect drug stability. However, studying the stability of insoluble compounds as a function of pH may be complicated due to the solubility limitation in certain pH regions, thus solubilizing agents may have to be used. On the other hand, even if the pH-rate profile can be generated in aqueous solutions, it may not be directly used to predict stability in the present of solubilizing agents. The activation energies and the effect of temperature on stability may be altered significantly by the presence of solubilizing agents such as co-solvents and surfactants. If buffers are used, their buffer capacities and solubility may also be affected by the presence of solubilizing agents. Careful consideration of these factors before obtaining the pH-stability profile is necessary for the generation of most meaningful and useful data.

EFFECT OF SOLVENTS, SURFACTANTS, AND COMPLEXING AGENTS ON STABILITY

For insoluble drugs, to achieve desirable bioavailability, many approaches have been used, such as pH control, cosolvents, surfactants, and complexing agents. Sometimes, several approaches can be used together to achieve the best solubilization effects. Ran et al. (2005) studied three combined techniques in solubilizing a poorly water-soluble anti-HIV drug, and achieved good stability as well. However, it is crucial to ensure that the solubilizing agents do not adversely affect the drug stability.

Effect of Solvents on Stability

Kearney and his colleagues (1994) studied the kinetics of degradation of PD144872, a dual-action hypoxic cell radiosensitizer in co-solvent systems containing 10% ethanol, varying amounts of propylene glycol (PG) (ranging from 0% to 30% v/v), and water. They found that increasing the percentage of PG from 0% to 10% had little to no effect on the stability of PD144872, whereas increasing the percentage of PG from 10% to 30% resulted in about a 1.3-fold increase in the degradation rate. They attributed this increased rate to changes in the apparent pH of the media and/or to a PG-induced increase in the apparent pK_a of PD144872. Similar changes of pK_a have been reported for other weak bases such as triethanolamine (Rubino 1987).

Ni et al. (2002) studied the stability of SarCNU (NSC364432) in water, ethanol, PG, Capmul PG, and DMSO, as well as their combinations over the temperature range of 25°C–60°C. The two cosolvents are an 80% PG: 20% ethanol mixture (PE), and a semi-aqueous vehicle (WPE) containing 50% water: 40% PG: 10% ethanol. The degradation mechanism in all the studied solvents is the same, and the stabilization by these vehicles follows the order of Capmul PG > Ethanol > PE > PE > PG > WPE > water, which is in agreement with their decreasing polarities.

Oxidative degradation is as important as hydrolysis in the stability evaluation of new drug substances. The oxygen concentration in solution is a factor in many cases and often depends upon the solvent employed. It was reported that ascorbic acid is more stable in 90% propylene glycol or in Syrup USP than in water, presumably because of the lower oxygen concentration in these vehicles (Ravin and Radebaugh 1990).

Effect of Surfactants on Stability

Many organic reactions have been found to be accelerated or inhibited in the presence of micellar media. The apparent reaction rates are altered in micellar solutions because of the distribution of substrate between the micellar and aqueous bulk phases in which different reaction rates occur (Fendler and Fendler 1975).

The effect of micelles on organic reactions can be attributed to both electrostatic and hydrophobic interactions (Rosen 1979). Electrostatic interaction is important because it may affect the transition state of a reaction or the concentration of reactant in the vicinity of the reaction site. The hydrophobic interactions are important because they determine the extent and the locus of solubilization in the micelle.

These principles have been demonstrated by a large number of reactions. The reader is directed to the excellent reviews by Fendler (1975) and Rosen (1979) for detailed discussions.

Effect of Complexing Agents on Stability

The stability of insoluble compounds will often change as a result of inclusion complex formation. This stability change may be the result of a microsolvent effect, hydrogen bonding, and/or a conformational effect (Szejtli 1982). The effect of CDs on the stability of a drug depends decisively on the geometry of the complex, as well as on the distance and relative orientation of the labile partial structure of the guest molecule with respect to the nucleophilic, catalytic center of CD (Albers and Muller 1995). In the case of ester hydrolysis, a nucleophilic attack at high pHs by one of the hydroxyl groups of the CD can accelerate the hydrolysis. Therefore, the closer the spatial approximation of ester groups to ionizable hydroxyl groups of the CDs is, the more drastic the increase of the hydrolysis rate will be, particularly when partial inclusion takes place. Inhibition of hydrolysis is expected when the ester function is included in the cavity protected from the attack of any reactive species.

Numerous examples of stability changes upon complexation have been reported in the literature (Albers and Muller 1995). However, because it is still rather difficult to predict the precise structure of the complexes, it is not possible at the current stage to predict how complexation should affect stability. For insoluble compounds that also have potential stability problems, a quick stability screening in the absence and presence of complexing agents may prove to be very useful. If complexing agents destabilize the compound, it will certainly make the complexation a less attractive option for solubilization.

SOLID STATE PROPERTIES

The solid state properties like crystallinity, polymorphism (crystal structure), shape (morphology), and particle size of drugs are important in the stability, dissolution, and processibility of drugs. Some commonly used methods in solid state studies include microscopy, hot stage microscopy with polarized light, X-ray powder diffraction (XRPD), thermogravimetric analysis (TGA), differential scanning calorimetry (DSC), FT-IR/Raman, and solid state NMR.

PARTICLE SIZE

It has been shown that dissolution rate, absorption rate, content uniformity, color, taste, texture, and stability depend to a varying degree on particle size and particle size distribution (Ravin and Radebaugh 1990). For poorly soluble drugs, bulk API having small particle size should be used to enhance *in situ* dissolution. In general, the particle size of API is recommended to reduce to 50% less than 10 μm and 90% less than 30 μm. From regulatory perspective, Sun et al. (2010) published a review on particle size specifications for solid oral dosage forms.

Particle size is very important because for most poorly soluble compounds, the absorption process is rate-limited by the dissolution rate in GI fluids. For example, digoxin exhibits a dissolution rate of limited absorption at particle sizes of greater than 10 μm in diameter because the poor driving force for dissolution supplied by the solubility, combined with the low surface area of drug at larger particle sizes, is insufficient to ensure timely dissolution (Dressman and Fleisher 1986). An increase in bioavailability with particle-size reduction also has been observed with griseofulvin. The extent of absorption of an oral dose increased 2.5 times when the surface area was increased approximately sixfold. Micronized griseofulvin permits a 50% decrease in dosage to obtain a satisfactory clinical response.

Because particle size reduction is often used as a mean of bioavailability enhancement, the effect of the micronization process on the physicochemical properties of the drug substance needs to be carefully studied. Increasing surface area by milling or other methods may lead to rapid degradation of a compound. Drug substances may also undergo polymorphic transformation during the milling process. Milling often causes crystalline material to convert, at least in part, to the amorphous form. The amorphous materials are frequently more hygroscopic and undergo more facile degradation reactions than their crystalline counterparts.

Besides stability concern from particle size reduction, the flowability of drug substances generally will decrease as particle size decreases, which makes it difficult to use direct compression in formulation design and process development. At high drug loading, the poor flowability from micronized API may also cause problems for both dry granulation and melt granulation. Considering the lipophilic property of insoluble drugs, even though reducing particle size can help improving dissolution rate, the sticking of API during compression may become a serious issue if using direct compression and dry granulation approaches.

Some of the most commonly used particle size determination methods in the pharmaceutical industry include sieving or screening, microscopy, sedimentation, stream scanning, and light scattering. The microscopic method measures the dimensions from two-dimension information, and the Malvern method measures the dimensions from three-dimension information. The measured particle size with different methods may be different sometimes; for example, for needle shape drug, the microscopic method gives larger API size than the Malvern method.

MOISTURE CONTENT AND HYGROSCOPICITY

The effects of moisture content in drug substances and finished dosage form have been widely studied. Static moisture content can be determined by many methods like Karl Fisher titration, loss on drying (LOD), and TGA. Dynamic hygroscopicity of a drug substance has been classified into four categories: non-hygroscopic, slightly-hygroscopic, moderately-hygroscopic and very-hygroscopic (Callahan et al. 1982). Hygroscopicity can be measured with DVS or VTI, by checking drug weight gain/loss at room temperature through at least two cycles of relative humidity gradient between 0% and 90%. At each incremental relative humidity, the drug sample needs to be suitable to ensure the moisture sorption/desorption near completion. For hygroscopic drugs, it is recommended to store them in hermetically sealed containers, with desiccators. A good point for insoluble drugs is that most of them are relative less hygroscopic.

For those drugs with both anhydrous and hydrous forms, they may hydrate/dehydrate during storage and processing. During dehydration, some drugs may convert to an amorphous form, and even have stability problems. Because of the significant solubility difference between the anhydrous and hydrous forms, the transformation may affect the therapeutic effects as well. Therefore, it is critical to study the relationship between the anhydrous and hydrous forms to avoid undesired crystal transformation for both drug substances and finished dosage during storage and processing.

SALT AND/OR POLYMORPH SELECTION

Salt selection may help to improve various properties of drug substance like bioavailability, stability, and manufacturability. Salt screen is often conducted in parallel to the polymorph screen in case a scalable crystallization process for the drug is not found. The importance of polymorphism in pharmaceuticals cannot be overemphasized. Some crystal structures contain molecules of water or solvents, known as hydrates or solvates, respectively, and they are also called as pseudopolymorphs. Identifying all relevant polymorphs and solvates at an early stage of development for new chemical entities has become a common practice in the pharmaceutical industry. For poorly soluble compounds, understanding their polymorphic behavior is even more important since solubility, crystal shape, dissolution rate, and bioavailability may vary with the polymorphic form. Conversion of a drug substance to a more thermodynamically stable form in the formulation can significantly increase the development cost or even result in product failure.

Preformulation should include rigorous studies to determine the number of polymorphs that exist, relative degree of stability of the various polymorphs, solubilities, method of preparation of each form, effect of micronization and tableting, and interaction with formulation ingredients. A conceptual approach to the characterization of pharmaceutical solids (Byrn et al. 1995), presented in the form of a series of decision trees, suggested a sequence for collecting data on a drug substance that will efficiently answer specific questions about solid state behavior in a logical order. These decision trees, although not a requirement by the FDA, should serve as a good strategic tool to organize the gathering of information early in the drug development process.

The importance of controlling the crystal form of a drug substance is also well recognized by the FDA. The FDA's guidance on abbreviated new drug applications (ANDAs) Pharmaceutical Solid Polymorphism states that *appropriate* analytical procedures should be used to detect polymorphic, hydrated, or amorphous forms of the drug substance. The guidance also states that it is the applicant's responsibility to control the crystal form of the drug substance, and if bioavailability is affected, to demonstrate the suitability of the control methods. Recently, the FDA has also finalized its guidance on co-crystals for the applicants of both new drug applications (NDAs) and ANDAs.

Besides regulatory importance, salts, polymorphs, and hydrates/solvates have clear novelty and patentability considering their different chemical compositions or distinguishable solid state (Von Raumer et al. 2006). Those new forms can affect not only their processibilities, like crystallization, filtration, and compression, but also their biological properties, like solubility and bioavailability. Besides those form themselves, the manufacturing processes for those forms are often innovative, thus patentable.

BULK DRUG STABILITY

Study on bulk drug stability at heat, moisture, and light is very important to recommend suitable storage, package, and shipping conditions for both API and finished dosage forms. Solid state stability of drugs was often studied at 40°C/75% RH, with the sample ampoules either open or closed (flame sealed). Based on the drug stability, sometimes drug needs to be stored at refrigerated conditions, with added desiccants, with protection from light, or in hermetically sealed containers.

PRODUCT-SPECIFIC ASPECTS

In addition to the general physical chemical evaluation of the insoluble compounds, there are certain considerations that are product specific. These are briefly discussed in the following four sections.

SOLID DOSAGE FORMS

Optimizing the dissolution profile is one of the most important aspects of solid dosage form development for insoluble compounds. Since particle size reduction is often used for improving dissolution rate, the effect of micronization on the powder properties and crystal form needs to be carefully studied. Flow properties and mixing efficiency are often adversely affected. Small particles with high static charge will present specific problems. If granulation is used to overcome the flow and mixing problem, the effect of granulation on the dissolution rate and crystal form also needs to be investigated. In early phase development of new chemical entities, solid dispersions are very commonly used to achieve higher dissolution rate, thus higher bioavailability. Even though a few drugs like tacrolimus have been successfully commercialized using solid dispersion, the physical stability of solid dispersion remains to be a significant challenge for drug development.

ORAL LIQUIDS

For oral liquids, taste masking becomes essential. The effects of solubilizing agents such as complexing agents and co-solvents on taste need to be evaluated. Preservatives such as sodium benzoate, sorbic acid, and methyl and propyl parabens have been used in liquid and semisolid dosage forms. There have been reports that the parabens have been inactivated when used in the presence of various surfactants. This loss of activity was thought to be due to the formation of complexes between the preservative and the surfactant. The interaction between polysorbate (Tween) 80 and the parabens has been demonstrated by a dialysis technique (Ravin 1990). It also has been shown that molecular complexes form when the parabens are mixed with polyethylene glycol (PEG) and methylcellulose. The degree of binding was less than that observed with Tween 80. Sorbic acid also interacts with Tweens but does not interact with PEGs. The quaternary ammonium compounds also are bound by Tween 80, which reduces their preservative activity.

Studies in which oral liquid formulations are diluted into simulated gastric fluid and subsequently into simulated intestinal fluid may be useful as an *in vitro* tool for formulation screening (Tong and Whitesell 1998). This is particularly important for compounds that are very insoluble in simulated gastric fluid. Information on how the compound precipitates in the stomach and how the precipitated material redissolves may assist in formulation selection for maximizing bioavailability.

SEMISOLIDS

Penetration enhancers are often needed for semisolid formulations of insoluble compounds for topical application. The effects of these penetration enhancers and the excipients on the crystal forms of actives need to be carefully studied. Certain semisolid excipients provide an ideal environment for crystal growth.

PARENTERALS

Specific problems exist with parenteral manufacture—the most obvious being the need to ensure sterility. It is necessary to assess the effect that a heat sterilization process will have on a drug (e.g., pK_a shift on heating) and on the formulation. Certain solubilization systems such as emulsions may not be suitable for autoclaving.

The implications of the addition of tonicity adjusters must also be considered, particularly with respect to ionic strength and common ion effects. Some additives may affect the solubility or form insoluble salts with the actives, resulting in formulation failure.

The potential of the compound precipitating upon injection needs to be evaluated. This is particularly important for formulations containing co-solvent systems or formulations where the compound is solubilized via pH adjustment. In these cases, the solubility of the compound changes non-linearly upon dilution and the compound may precipitate at the injection site (Yalkowsky and Roseman 1981). Several *in vitro* methods, including static serial dilution, dynamic injection, and dropwise dilution, have been successfully applied as a screening tool to detect the precipitation problem (Yalkowsky et al. 1983, Ward and Yalkowsky 1993, Ping et al. 1998). Details of these methods will be discussed in subsequent chapters.

SUMMARY

Preformulation testing for insoluble compounds has many unique aspects. Special techniques need to be applied to evaluate the physicochemical and biopharmaceutical properties, and to understand potential problems so that the correct foundations can be laid for a successful formulation and ultimately the finished products.

REFERENCES

Albers, E. and Muller, B. W. (1995). Cyclodextrin derivatives in pharmaceutics, *Crit. Rev. Ther. Drug Carrier Syst.*, 12(4): 311–337.

Alelyunas, Y. W., Liu, R., Pelosi-Kilby, L., and Shen, C. (2009). Application of a dried-DMSO rapid throughput 24-h equilibrium solubility in advancing discovery candidates, *Eur. J. Pharm. Sci.*, 37(2): 172–182.

Austin, R. P., Davis, A. M., and Manners, C. N. (1995). Partitioning of ionizing molecules between aqueous buffers and phospholipid vesicles, *J. Pharm. Sci.*, 84(10): 1180–1183.

Avdeef, A. (1993). *Applications and Theory Guide to pH-Metric pKa and log P Determination*, Sirius Analytical Instruments, Forest Row, UK.

Avdeef, A., Box, K. J., Comer, J. E. A., Hibbert, C., and Tam, K. Y. (1998). pH-metric logP 10. Determination of lopisomal membrane-water partition coefficents of ionizable drugs, *Pharm. Res.*, 15(2): 209–215.

Bard, B., Martel, S., and Carrupt, P.-A. (2008). High throughput UV method for the estimation of thermodynamic solubility and the determination of the solubility in biorelevant media, *Eur. J. Pharm. Sci.*, 33(3): 230–240.

Beall, H. D., Getz, J. J., and Sloan, K. B. (1993). The estimation of relative water solubility for prodrugs that are unstable in water, *Int. J. Pharm.*, 93: 37–47.

Burton, P. S. and Goodwin, J. T. (2010). Solubility and permeability measurement and applications in drug discovery, *Comb. Chem. High Throughput Screen.*, 13(2): 101–111.

Byrn, S., Pfeiffer, R., Ganey, M., Hoiberg, C., and Poochilian, G. (1995). Pharmaceutical solids: A strategic approach to regulatory considerations, *Pharm. Res.*, 12(7): 945–954.

Cakiryildiz, C., Methta, P. J., Rahmen, W., and Schoenleber, D. (1975). Dissolution studies with a multichannel continuous-flow apparatus, *J. Pharm. Sci.*, 64(10): 1692–1697.

Callahan, J. C., Cleary, G. W., Elefant, M., Kaplan, G., Kensler, T., and Nash, R. A. (1982). Equilibrium moisture content of pharmaceutical excipients, *Drug Dev. Ind. Pharm.*, 8(3): 355–369.

Carstensen, J. T. (2002). Preformulation, *Drugs Pharm. Sci.*, 121 (Modern Pharmaceutics (4th ed): 167–185.

Chemical Sciences. (2001, July). *Pharmaceutical Profiling User's Guide.* Version 1.0.

Colclough, N., Hunter, A., Kenny, P. W., Kittlety, R. S., Lobedan, L., Tam, K. Y., and Timms, M. A. (2008). High throughput solubility determination with application to selection of compounds for fragment screening, *Bioorganic Med. Chem.*, 16(13): 6611–6616.

Connors, K. A., Amidon, G. L., and Stella, V. J. (1986). *Chemical Stability of Pharmaceuticals, A Handbook for Pharmacists* (2nd ed.), John Wiley & Sons, New York.

Corrigan, O. I. (1991). Co-solvent systems in dissolution testing: Theoretical considerations, *Drug Dev. Ind. Pharm.*, 17(5): 695–708.

Cruciani, G., Milletti, F., Storchi, L., Sforna, G., and Goracci, L. (2009). In silico pK_a prediction and ADME profiling, *Chem. Biodivers.*, 6(11): 1812–1821.

Curatolo, W. J. (1996). Screening studies for transport properties, *Proceeding for 38th Annual International Industrial Pharmaceutical Research and Development Conference*, Merrimac, WI.

Davis, S. S., Higuchi, T., and Rytting, J. H. (1974). *Advances in Pharmaceutical Sciences*, Vol. 4, Bean, H. S., Beckett, A. H., and Carless, J. E. (Eds.), Academic Press, London, UK, pp. 73–261.

Dearden, J. C. (2012). Prediction of physicochemical properties, *Methods Mol. Biol.*, 929 (Computational Toxicology, Volume I): 93–138.

Dearden, J. C. and Bresnen, G. M. (1988). The measurement of partition coefficents, *Quant. Struct.-Act. Relat.*, 7: 133–144.

De Smidt, J. H., Fokkens, J. G., Grijseels, H., and Crommelin, D. J. A. (1986). Dissolution of theophylline monohydrate and anhydrous theophylline in buffer solutions, *J. Pharm. Sci.*, 75(5): 497–501.

Dressman, J. B. and Fleisher, D. (1986). Mixing-tank model for predicting dissolution rate control of oral absorption, *J. Pharm. Sci.*, 75: 109–116.

Dressman, J. B., Fleisher, D., and Amidon, G. L. (1984). Physicochemical model for dose-dependent drug absorption, *J. Pharm. Sci.*, 73(9): 1274–1279.

Elworthy, P. H., Florence, A. T., and Macfarlane, C. B. (1968). *Solubilization by Surface-Active Agents*, Chapman and Hall, London, UK.

Fendler, J. H. and Fendler, E. J. (1975). *Catalysis in Micellar and Macromolecular Systems*, Academic Press, New York, pp. 98–100.

Fiese, E. F. and Hagen, T. A. (1986). Preformulation, Chapter 8 in *The Theory and Practice of Industrial Pharmacy*, Lachman, L., Lieberman, H. A., and Kanig, J. L. (Eds.), Lea & Febiger, Philadelphia, PA.

Finholt, P. (1974). Influence of Formulation on dissolution rate, in *Dissolution Technology*, Lesson, L. J. and Carstensen, J. T. (Eds.), Washington, DC, Academy of Pharmaceutical Sciences, p. 106.

Formelova, J., Breier, A., Gemeiner, P., and Kurillova, L. (1991). Trypsin entrapped within liposomes. Partition of a low-molecular-mass substrate as the main factor in kinetic control of hydrolysis, *Coll. Czech. Chem. Comm.*, 56: 712–217.

Fraczkiewicz, R. (2006). In silico prediction of ionization, *Compr. Med. Chem. II*, 5, 603–626.

Glomme, A., Maerz, J., and Dressman, J. B. (2005). Comparison of a miniaturized shake-flask solubility method with automated potentiometric acid/base titrations and calculated solubilities, *J. Pharm. Sci.*, 94(1): 1–16.

Goldberg, A. H., Gibaldi, M., Kanig, J. L., and Shanker, J. (1965). Method for determining dissolution rates of multiparticulate systems, *J. Pharm. Sci.*, 54(12): 1722–1725.

Hamid, I. A. and Parrott, E. L. (1971). Effect of temperature on solubilization and hydrolytic degradation of solubilized benzocaine and homatropine, *J. Pharm. Sci.*, 60(6): 901–906.

Heikkila, T., Peltonen, L., Taskinen, S., Laaksonen, T., and Hirvonen, J. (2008). 96-Well plate surface tension measurements for fast determination of drug solubility, *Lett. Drug Des. Discov.*, 5(7): 471–476.

Heikkilae, T., Karjalainen, M., Ojala, K., Partola, K., Lammert, F., Augustijns, P., Urtti, A., Yliperttula, M., Peltonen, L., and Hirvonen, J. (2011). Equilibrium drug solubility measurements in 96-well plates reveal similar drug solubilities in phosphate buffer pH 6.8 and human intestinal fluid, *Int. J. Pharm.*, 405(1–2):132–136.

Hellwich, U. and Schubert, R. (1995). Concentration-dependent binding of the chiral b-blocker oxprenolol to isoelectric or negatively charged unilamellar vesicles, *Biochem. Pharmacol.*, 49(4): 511–517.

Hermens, J. L. M., de Bruijn, J. H. M., and Brooke, D. N. (2013). The octanol-water partition coefficient: Strengths and limitations, *Environ. Toxicol. Chem.*, 32(4): 732–733.

Hersey, A., Hill, A. P., Hyde, R. M., and Livingstone, D. J. (1989). Principles of method selection in partition studies, *Quant. Struct. -Act. Relat.*, 8: 288–296.

Higuchi, T., Shih, F. L., Kimura, T., and Rytting, J. H. (1979). Solubility determination of barely aqueous soluble organic solids, *J. Pharm. Sci.*, 68(10): 1267–1272.

Junquera, E., Tardajos, G., and Aicart, E. (1993). Effect of the presence of β-cyclodexdtrin on micellization process of sodium dodecyl sulfate or sodium perfluorooctanoate in water, *Langmuir*, 9, 1212–1219.

Kearney, A. S., Mehta, S. C., and Radebaugh, G. W. (1994). Preformulation studies to aid in the development of an injectable formulation of PD 144872, a radiosensitizing anticancer agent, *Int. J. Pharm.*, 102: 63–70.

Kim, J. S., Mitchell, S., Kijek, P., Tsume, Y., Hilfinger J., and Amidon, G. L. (2006). The suitability of an in situ perfusion model for permeability determinations: Utility for BCS class I biowaiver requests, *Mol. Pharm.*, 3(6): 686–694.

Koljonen, M., Hakala, K. S., Antola-Satila, T., Laitinen, L., Kostiainen, R., Kotiaho, T., Kaukonen, A. M., and Hirvonen, J. (2006). Evaluation of cocktail approach to standardize Caco-2 permeability experiments, *Eur. J. Pharm. Biopharm.*, 64: 379–387.

Kraus, C., Mehnert, W., and Fromming, K.-H. (1991). Interactions of β-cyclodextrin with Solutol HS 15 and their influence on diazepam solubilization, *Pharm. Ztg. Wiss.*, Nr. 1•4./136. Jahrgang, 11–15.

Kuhnvelten, W. N. (1991). Thermodynamics and modulation of progesterone microcompartmentation and hydrophobic interaction with cytochrome P450XVII based on quantification of local ligand concentrations in a complex multi-component system, *Eur. J. Biochem.*, 197: 381–390.

Leo, A., Hansch, C., and Elkins, D. (1971). Partition coefficients and their uses, *Chem. Rev.*, 71: 525–616.

Li, S., Doyle, P., Metz, S., Royce, A. E., and Serajuddin, A. T. M. (2005). Effect of chloride ion on dissolution of different salt forms of haloperidol, a model basic drug, *J. Pharm. Sci.*, 94(10): 2224–2231.

Lipinski, C. A., Lombardo, F., Dominy, B. W., and Feeney, P. J. (2012). Experimental and computational approaches to estimate solubility and permeability in drug discovery and development settings, *Adv. Drug Deliv. Rev.*, 64: 4–17.

Lötter, A. P., Flanagan, D. R., Jr., Palepu, N. R., and Guillory, J. K. (1983). A simple reproducible method for determining dissolution rates of hydrophobic powders, *Pharm. Technol.*, 4: 56–66.

Madan, D. K. and Cadwallader, D. E. (1973). Solubility of cholesterol and hormone drugs in water, *J. Pharm. Sci.*, 62(9): 1567–1569.

Maheswaran, R. (2012). FDA perspectives: Scientific considerations of forced degradation studies in ANDA submissions, *PharmTech*, 36(5): 73–80.

Marini, A., Berbenni, V., Bruni, G., Cofrancesco, P., Giordano, F., and Villa, M. (2003). Physico-chemical characterization of drugs and drug forms in the solid state, *Curr. Med. Chem. Anti-Infect. Agents*, 2(4): 303–321.

Miyazaki, J., Hideg, K., and Marsh, D. (1992). Interfacial ionization and partitioning of membrane-bound local anaesthetics, *Biochim. Biophys. Acta*, 1103: 63–68.

Mooney, K. G., Mintun, M. A., Himmelstein, K. J., and Stella, V. J. (1981a). Dissolution kinetics of carboxylic acids I: Effect of pH under unbuffered conditions, *J. Pharm. Sci.*, 70(1): 13–22.

Mooney, K. G., Mintun, M. A., Himmelstein, K. J., and Stella, V. J. (1981b). Dissolution kinetics of carboxylic acids II: Effect of buffers, *J. Pharm. Sci.*, 70(1): 22–32.

Muller, B. W. and Albers, E. (1991). Effect of hydrotropic substances on the complexation of sparingly soluble drugs with cyclodextrin derivatives and the influence of cyclodextrin complexation on the pharmacokinetics, *J. Pharm. Sci.*, 80: 599–604.

Ni, N., Sanghvi, T., and Yalkowsky, S. H. (2002). Solubilization and preformulation of carbendazim, *Int. J. Pharm.*, 244(1–2): 257–264.

Pan, L., Ho, Q., Tsutsui, K., and Takahashi, L. (2001). Comparison of chromatographic and spectroscopic methods used to rank compounds for aqueous solubility, *J. Pharm. Sci.*, 90: 521–529.

Pauletti, G. M. and Wunderli-Allenspach, H. (1994). Partition coefficients in vitro: Artificial membranes as a standardized distribution model, *Eur. J. Pharm. Sci.*, 1: 273–282.

Perrin, D. D., Dempsey, B., and Serjeant, E. P. (1981). *pKa Prediction for Organic Acids and Bases*, Chapman and Hall in association with Methuen, New York.

Ping, L., Vishnuvajjala, R., Tabibi, S. E., and Yalkowsky, S. H. (1998). Evaluation of in vitro precipitation methods, *J. Pharm. Sci.*, 87(2): 196–199.

Polli, J. E. and Ginski, M. J. (1998). Human drug absorption kinetics and comparison to Caco-2 monolayer permeabilities, *Pharm. Res.*, 15(1): 47–52.

Ran, Y., Jain, A., and Yalkowsky, S. H. (2005). Solubilization and preformulation studies on PG-300995 (an anti-HIV drug), *J. Pharm. Sci.*, 94(2): 297–303.

Ravin, L. J. and Radebaugh, G. W. (1990). Preformulation, Chapter 75: in *Remington's Pharmaceutical Sciences* (18th ed.), Gennaro, A. R. (Ed.), Mack Publishing Company, Easton, PA.

Regardh, C. G., Borg, K. O., Johansson, R., Johnsson, G., and Palmer, L. (1974). Pharmacokinetic studies on the selective bl-receptor antagonist metoprolol in man, *J. Pharm. Biopharm.*, 2(4): 347–364.

Rogers, J. A. and Choi, Y. W. (1993). The liposome partitioning system for correlating biological activities of imidazolidine derivatives, *Pharm. Res.*, 10(6): 913–917.

Rosen, M. J. (1979). *Surfactants and Interfacial Phenomena*, John Wiley & Sons, New York.

Rubino, J. T. (1987). The effect of cosolvents on the action of pharmaceutical buffers, *J. Parenter. Sci. Technol.*, 41: 45–49.

Saha, P. and Kou, J. H. (2000). Effect of solubilizing excipients on permeation of poorly water-soluble compounds across Caco-2 cell monolayers, *Eur J. Pharm Biopharm.*, 50(3): 403–411.

Sims, J. L., Roberts, J. K., Bateman, A. G., Carreira, J. A., and Hardy, M. J. (2002). An automated workstation for forced degradation of active pharmaceutical ingredients, *J. Pharm. Sci.*, 91(3): 884–892.

Strickley, R. G. (2004). Solubilizing excipients in oral and injectable formulations, *Pharm. Res.*, 21(2): 201–230.

Sun, Z., Ya, N., Adams, R. C., and Fang, F. S. (2010). Particle size specifications for solid oral dosage forms: A regulatory perspective, *Am. Pharm. Rev.*, 13(4): 68–73.

Suzuki, A., Higuchi, W. I., and Ho, N. F. (1970). Theoretical model studies of drug absorption and transport in the gastrointestinal tract I, *J. Pharm. Sci.*, 59(5): 644–651.

Swenson, E. S., Milisen, W. B. and Curatolo, W. (1994). Intestinal permeability enhancement: Efficacy, acute local toxicity, and reversibility, *Pharm. Res.*, 11(8): 1132–1142.

Szejtli, J. (1982). *Inclusion Compounds and Their Complexes*, Akademiai Kiado, Budapest, Hungary.

Takacs-Novak, K., Box, K. J., and Avdeef, A. (1997). Potentiometric pK_a determination of water-insoluble compounds: Validation study in methanol/water mixtures, *Int. J. Pharm.*, 151(2): 235–248.

Tang, L., Khan, S. U., and Muhammad, N. A. (2001). Evaluation and selection of bio-relevant dissolution media for a poorly water-soluble new chemical entity, *Pharm. Dev. Technol.*, 6(4): 531–540.

Todd, D. and Winnike, R. A. (1994). A rapid method for generating pH-solubility profiles for new chemical entities, *Pharm. Res.*, 11(10): S-271.

Tong, W. Q., Wells, M. L., and Williams, S. O. (1994). Solubility behavior of GF120918A, *Pharm. Res.*, 11(10): S-269.

Tong, W. Q. and Whitesell, G. (1998). In situ salt screening – A useful technique for discovery support and preformulation studies, *Pharm. Dev. Tech.*, 3(2): 215–223.

Varma, M. V., Gardner, I., Steyn, S. J., Nkansah, P., Rotter, C. J., Whitney-Pickett, C., Zhang, H. et al. (2012). pH-Dependent solubility and permeability criteria for provisional biopharmaceutics classification (BCS and BDDCS) in early drug discovery, *Mol. Pharm.*, 9(5): 1199–1212.

Venkatesh, S., Li, J. M., Xu, Y. H., Vishnuvajjala, R., and Anderson, B. D. (1996). Intrinsic solubility estimation and pH-solubility behavior of cosalane (NSC 658586), an extremely hydrophobic diprotic acid, *Pharm. Res.*, 15(10): 1453–1459.

Von Raumer, M., Dannappel, J., and Hilfiker, R. (2006). Polymorphism, salts, and crystallization: The relevance of solid-state development. *Chim. Oggi.*, 24(1): 41–44.

Walter, E., Janich, S., Roessler, B. J., Hilfinger, J. M., and Amidon, G. L. (1996). HT29-MTX/Caco-2 co-cultures as an in vitro model for the intestinal epithelium: In vitro–in vivo correlation with permeability data from rats and humans, *J. Pharm. Sci.*, 85(10): 1070–1076.

Wan, H. and Ulander, J. (2006). High-throughput pK_a screening and prediction amenable for ADME profiling, *Exp. Opin. Drug Metab. Toxicol.*, 2(1): 139–155.

Ward, G. H. and Yalkowsky, S. H. (1993). Studies in phlebitis VI: Dilution-induced precipitation of amiodarone HCL, *J. Parenter. Sci. Technol.*, 47: 161–165.

Wells, J. I. (1988). *Pharmaceutical Preformulation: The Physicochemical Properties of Drug Substances*, Ellis Horwood Limited, Chichester, UK.

Wenlock, M. C., Austin, R. P., Potter, T., and Barton, P. (2011). A highly automated assay for determining the aqueous equilibrium solubility of drug discovery compounds, *J. Lab. Autom.*, 16(4): 276–284.

Winiwarter, S., Bonham, N. M., Ax, F., Hallberg, A., Lennernaes, H., and Karlen, A. (1998). Correlation of human jejunal permeability (in vivo) of drugs with experimentally and theoretically derived parameters. A multivariate data analysis approach, *J. Med. Chem.*, 41(25): 4939–4949.

Yalkowsky, S. H. and Roseman T. J. (1981). Solubilization of drugs by cosolvents, in *Techniques of Solubilization of Drugs*, Yalkowsky, S. H. (Ed.), Marcel Dekker, New York.

Yalkowsky, S. H., Valvani S. C., and Johnson B. W. (1983). In vitro method for detecting precipitation of parenteral formulatrion after injection, *J. Pharm. Sci.*, 72: 1014–1017.

5 Water-Insoluble Drugs and Their Pharmacokinetic Behaviors

Honghui Zhou and Hao Zhu

CONTENTS

With the great advances in high-throughput chemical synthesis and bioactivity identification, more and more new chemical entities (NCEs) gush into the pharmaceutical pipelines in this postgenomic era. Many of these NCEs in the pipelines are water insoluble, and pose great challenges not only to the preformulation and formulation endeavors but also to the *in vivo* assessment of their pharmacokinetic characteristics.

On the basis of Biopharmaceutics Classification System (BCS), water-insoluble drugs fall into two broad categories: BCS Class II (low solubility and high permeability) and BCS Class IV (low solubility and low permeability). Given the inherent low aqueous solubility and slow dissolution rate of water-insoluble drugs, a large intersubject variability in their pharmacokinetics, sizable and sometimes unmanageable food effects, erratic absorption patterns, unfavorable oral bioavailability in high gastric pH environment, difficulties in development of sustained-release formulations, and serious hurdles in establishing IVIVC may be anticipated. Since the impact of poor water solubility on pharmacokinetics mostly occurs at the dissolution and absorption levels, this chapter focuses only on the absorption aspect. Other aspects of the pharmacokinetics, that is, distribution and elimination, are considered less important and thus are not covered in this chapter.

To help investigators overcome these hurdles, several case studies will be presented in this chapter from a pharmacokinetic perspective. Some pharmacokinetic strategies in the drug development will also be discussed to mitigate or overcome the inherent caveats of water-insoluble drugs.

BACKGROUND OF DRUG ABSORPTION

In 1937, the pioneering paper "Kinetics of Distribution of Substances Administered to the Body" was published (Teorell, 1937). Since then, pharmacokinetics has been well developed and matured as an independent discipline. Nevertheless, the characterization of drug absorption usually is assumed empirically and lacks sufficient physiological basis. Even to date, some absorption processes are still not well understood and adequately defined.

Most drugs on the market today are taken orally. As long as a drug is well absorbed, oral administration is considered as the safest and most economical way of delivering drugs and brings effective and convenient means for treating patients. Some disadvantages to oral administration include limited absorption of some drugs owing to their physicochemical characteristics (e.g., water solubility, pK_a), emesis as a result of irritation to the gastrointestinal (GI) mucosa, disintegration and destruction of some drugs by digestive enzymes or low gastric pH, irregularities in absorption or propulsion in the presence of food or other drugs such as gastric pH modulating agents, and necessity for cooperation on the patient's side (Goodman & Gilman's 10th ed., 2001). For some drugs that are insoluble or sparingly soluble in water, the oral absorption could be limited or erratic, and this in turn may give rise to inconsistent efficacy or impose safety concerns.

Hellriegel et al. (1996) observed a significant inverse linear relationship between the bioavailability of a drug and its coefficient of variation. An insoluble drug with very low oral bioavailability usually has a very large intersubject variability in its absorption pharmacokinetic parameters, which may result in a worrisome safety profile or unfavorable efficacy profile.

A number of insoluble NCEs may not survive long before they can enter clinical testing. Nevertheless, under some special situations, for example, if an NCE is first-in-class or first-in-therapy, even if it has unfavorably poor water solubility, its entrance into further clinical testing is not unimpossible.

FACTORS AFFECTING DRUG ABSORPTION

Absorption from the GI tract is governed by many factors. Broadly, it can be categorized into three classes: physicochemical properties, biopharmaceutical factors, and physiological and pathophysiological factors (Mojaverian et al., 1985, 1988; Nomeir et al., 1996). Since this chapter focuses on the pharmacokinetic perspectives, the main factors that could affect drug absorption are merely listed in the following, and will be discussed in detail in other chapters.

Physicochemical Properties of a Drug
- pK_a, solubility, permeability
- Crystal forms
- Rate of dissolution

Biopharmaceutical Factors of a Dosage
- Excipients
- Tablet compression parameters
- Coating and matrix

Physiological and Pathophysiological Factors
- GI transit and pH microenvironment
- Presystemic metabolism
- Transport mechanism/efflux
- Absorption window
- Diseases, demographics including gender, age, ethnicity, and so forth

A new drug application (NDA) can be approved primarily on the basis of the results from pivotal safety and efficacy studies conducted in the indicated patient population. The knowledge of drug absorption is necessary to ensure safe and effective use of an oral dosage form. As mentioned earlier, drug oral absorption and subsequently oral bioavailability can be impacted by many factors. It has been known for some time that the rate and extent of oral drug absorption can be influenced, and even significantly altered, by the presence of food (Welling, 1977) or coadministration with an agent that can alter the GI motility (Greiff and Rowbotham, 1994) or gastric pH (Yago et al., 2014; Zhang et al., 2014). It could become clinically significant if substantial interactions exist for an insoluble drug with narrow therapeutic window.

EFFECTS OF FOOD INTERACTIONS ON PHARMACOKINETICS OF INSOLUBLE DRUGS

Food–drug interaction mechanisms are variable and drug-specific (Toothaker and Welling, 1980; Welling and Tse, 1984). Better understanding of food–drug interactions for an insoluble drug is especially important for optimizing patient management and streamlining drug development.

The food–drug interactions for water-insoluble drugs usually manifest themselves either in alteration in absorption rate or in absorption extent. Herein several case examples are selected to further illustrate the food-drug interactions for water-insoluble drugs.

CASE STUDY 1

Compound A was developed for acute pain management. It has fascinating pharmacology, and was positioned as a first-in-class pain reliever under clinical development.

Compound A is insoluble in water over a wide pH range, and it has large molecular weight (>700). Numerous attempts had been made to improve its oral absorption and minimize its food effect through tedious preformulation and formulation works. However, no substantial improvement in terms of formulation performance and mitigated food effect had been achieved. Significant food interactions (about 2-fold) were observed in dog models, although different formulations were tested. When Compound A was moved into the clinical phase, food effect was the most outstanding pharmacokinetic concern, and the team recognized it could eventually hamper its further clinical development.

A food-effect cohort was incorporated into the first-in-human single ascending dose study to preliminarily evaluate food effect of Compound A. An approximately 5- to 8-fold increase in oral bioavailability under fed condition was observed when Compound A was ingested with a high-fat meal in this food-effect cohort with a small number of subjects. Realizing that such a significant food effect could be a great hurdle to the further clinical development for Compound A, the team decided to conduct a formal food-interaction study with both a Food and Drug Administration (FDA)–recommended high-fat meal and a low-fat meal. Intensive and identical pharmacokinetic samples were collected in each of the three study treatments (i.e., fasted, fed with a low-fat meal, and fed with a high-fat meal) in a crossover manner. A high-fat meal resulted in the highest mean plasma concentration profile of Compound A, followed by a low-fat meal, as shown in Figure 5.1. Consistent with the preliminary findings in the first-in-human study in a small number of subjects, an approximately 2- to 3-fold increase in oral bioavailability with the low-fat meal was observed, while an approximately 5-fold increase was observed with a high-fat meal. Apparently, the oral bioavailability enhancement was related to the percentage of fat content in the test meal, as illustrated in Figure 5.2 for

(Continued)

CASE STUDY 1 (*Continued*)

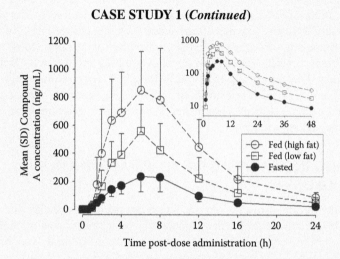

FIGURE 5.1 Mean (SD) concentration–time profiles for Compound A under fasted, fed with a high-fat meal, and fed with a low-fat meal.

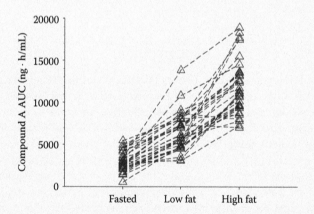

FIGURE 5.2 Compound A total exposure (AUC) increase under fed condition is fat content dependent in test meals.

AUC and Figure 5.3 for C_{max}. A similar observation was also found for another water-insoluble drug, griseofulvin (Ogunbona et al., 1985).

As anticipated, the oral bioavailability of Compound A can be significantly altered by food ingestion, and the extent of such food interaction was fat-content dependent. This degree of food effect did impose very high clinical development hurdles. The very low oral absolute bioavailability (<5%), due to its insolubility in water, resulted in very large intra- and interindividual variability, which might mask the inherent dose–response or exposure–response relationships. Since different meal types could give rise to variable oral bioavailability for Compound A, under Phases II and III settings, meal conditions could not be strictly controlled as in Phase I studies. Moreover, different geographic locations or regions may have vastly different meals (e.g., Japanese food versus American food). Thus, the food interaction for Compound A could become unmanageable in real clinical situations when it was used by large and diverse patient populations, which might have serious safety as well as efficacy implications.

(Continued)

CASE STUDY 1 (*Continued*)

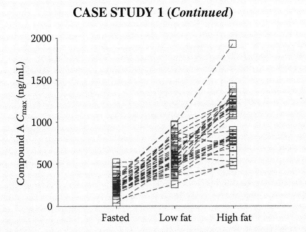

FIGURE 5.3 Compound A maximum exposure (C_{max}) increase under fed condition is fat content dependent in test meals.

Some strategies have been put in place to mitigate or minimize the risks that arise from such unmanageable food effects for Compound A. An extensive population pharmacokinetic–pharmacodynamic program had been designed for Phases II/III studies of Compound A: a number of biomarkers identified in the Phase I studies would be examined along with population pharmacokinetics in order to establish and define the exposure–response relationship; a number of covariates would be evaluated for their statistical and clinical relevancy on the pharmacokinetics of Compound A; and meal type was one of the most important covariates to be tested. The impact of food effect on pharmacokinetics, pharmacodynamics, and clinical outcome would be scrutinized and quantified (if at all possible) in the indicated patient population in Phases II/III trials, and optimized dose recommendation would therefore be proposed after the integrated considerations of efficacy, safety, pharmacokinetics, and pharmacodynamics of Compound A.

CASE STUDY 2

Itraconazole (Sporanox®), a potent and widely used anitfungal agent, is almost insoluble in water and dilute acid (<5 mg/L). It has very high lipophilicity (MLogP = 5.7), and its molecular weight is more than 700. Its absolute bioavailability is around 55% following oral administration.

Due to its very low water solubility, several food-interaction studies have been conducted for itraconazole in different formulations. It was found that a full meal could increase AUC of itraconazole by 63% (Lange et al., 1997). As a result, in its product labeling, it is indicated that the Sporanox capsule should be taken with a full meal to ensure maximal absorption. However, the food-effect study on Sporanox oral solution in healthy subjects observed that oral bioavailability of itraconazole actually decreased by 31% under fed condition (Van de Velde et al., 1996). Thus, in its product labeling, it is also indicated that Sporanox oral solution should be taken without a meal to ensure maximal absorption. Further, it is indicated that Sporanox oral solution and capsules should not be used interchangeably.

CASE STUDY 3

Lurasidone is an atypical antipsychotic drug approved for the treatment of schizophrenia and depressive episodes associated with bipolar I disorder. It has been on the U.S. market under the trade name of Latuda® since 2010. The starting dose for treating schizophrenia is 20 mg/day and the recommended dose is 40 mg to 160 mg/day. The starting dose and recommend dose for bipolar patients is 20 mg, and 20 mg to 120 mg/day, respectively (FDA, 2010; Citrome, 2012; Alamo et al., 2014; Bawa et al., 2015).

The solubility of lurasidone is low. Lurasidone is very slightly soluble in water, practically insoluble or insoluble in 0.1 N hydrochloride acid, slightly soluble in ethanol, sparingly soluble in methanol, practically insoluble or insoluble in toluene, and very slightly soluble in acetone. As anticipated, lurasidone's bioavailability is low. It is shown that only approximately 9%–19% of the dose is absorbed (FDA, 2010).

Food effect is substantial for lurasidone due to its low solubility. Preskorn et al. (2013) reported two pharmacokinetic trials aimed to assess food effect on lurasidone bioavailability. The two trials were both randomized, open-label, crossover trials conducted with stable patients. The first trial compared lurasidone exposure when lurasidone was given with three types of meals versus lurasidone was given under fasted condition. The three meals given to patients were a 100-kcal with medium-fat meal, a 200-kcal with medium-fat meal, and a 800–1000-kcal with high-fat meal. Lurasidone exposure under a high-fat, high-calorie meal (800–1000 kcal/high fat meal) was 2–3 times higher than that when lurasidone was given under fasted condition. Lurasidone exposure in patients under a 100-kcal/medium-fat meal and a 200-kcal/medium-fat meal was substantially lower than that in patients under a high-fat, high-calorie meal (800–1000 kcal/high fat). The second trial was conducted to further assess food effect on lurasidone bioavailability. Lurasidone was administered to patients either under fasted condition or with five different meal types (350 kcal/high fat, 500 kcal/low fat, 500 kcal/high fat, 800–1000 kcal/low fat, and 800–1000 kcal/high fat). The second trial confirmed the level of lurasidone exposure change in patients receiving a high-fat, high-calorie meal as compared to patients under fasted condition reported from the first trial. Furthermore, this trial showed that lurasidone exposure was similar in patients receiving lurasidone with meals containing 350–1000 kcal and independent from the fat content in the meals.

Based on the assessment of food effect, lurasidone is recommended to be administered with food containing at least 350 kcal to ensure adequate drug exposure, per the U.S. package insert of Latuda (FDA, 2010).

CASE STUDY 4

In 2015, palbociclib was approved under accelerated approval based on progression free survival and has been marked in the U.S. under the trade name of Ibrance®. Palbociclib is a kinase inhibitor and is indicated for the treatment of postmenopausal women with estrogen receptor (ER)-positive, human epidermal growth factor receptor 2 (HER2)-negative advanced breast cancer as initial endocrine-based therapy for their metastatic disease.

Palbociclib has a pK_a of 7.4 and 3.9, and its solubility changes significantly at different pH levels. Palbociclib is highly soluble below pH 4 and the solubility reduces significantly above pH 4 (FDA, 2015).

It has been shown that, at a population level, palbociclib exposures were similar when palbociclib was given under overnight fasting and with a high-fat, high-calorie meal (approximately

(Continued)

CASE STUDY 4 (*Continued*)

800–1000 cal with 150, 250, and 500–600 cal from protein, carbohydrate and fat, respectively), a low-fat, low-calorie meal (approximately 400–500 cal with 120, 250, and 28–35 cal from protein, carbohydrate and fat, respectively), or a moderate-fat, standard calorie meal (approximately 500–700 cal with 75–105, 250–350, and 175–245 cal from protein, carbohydrate, and fat, respectively). However, palbociclib absorption was very low in approximately 13% of the patient population under fasted condition. The reason for this observation is not clear since we cannot identify the study designed to understand the underlying mechanism in the public domain. It has been shown that food increased palbociclib exposure in this patient subgroup without altering that from the rest of other patients. Because food intake reduced the intersubject variability on palbociclib absorption, it is recommended that palbociclib be taken with food in the U.S. package insert of Ibrance (FDA, 2015).

EFFECTS OF GASTRIC ACID MODULATING AGENTS ON PHARMACOKINETICS OF INSOLUBLE DRUGS

Orally administered drugs with pH-dependent solubility, especially weak bases, may demonstrate altered drug absorption in patients with various gastric pH. Gastric pH can be affected by multiple factors, including physiological or pathological changes in patients (Haruma et al., 2000), acidic beverage (Malhotra et al., 2002), food (Lennard-Jones et al., 1968), and juice (Claytor et al., 1941). Gastric acid modulating agents are the other factor which significantly alters gastric pH. Three types of gastric acid modulating agents, including antacids, histamine H_2-antagonists (or H_2-blockers), and proton pump inhibitors (PPIs), are available. Antacids, such as calcium carbonate, magnesium hydroxide, and aluminum hydroxide, neutralize gastric acid resulting in a rapid increase in gastric pH with a relatively short duration. H_2-blockers, like famotidine and ranitidine, target histamine H_2 receptors in the gastric parietal cells and yield a reduced gastric acid secretion (FDA, 2014) with duration of approximately 12 h. Omeprazole and rabeprazole are examples of PPIs, which suppress gastric acid secretion by inhibition of the hydrogen/potassium adenosine triphosphatase system in the gastric parietal cell (FDA, 1989) for more than 24 h postdose. As anticipated, the exposure of drugs with pH-dependent solubility can be significantly different when a gastric acid modulating agent is given concomitantly. Hence it is suggested to assess this drug–drug interaction effect in the drug development to instruct safe and effective use of these drug products (Zhang et al., 2014).

CASE STUDY 5

Dasatinib is a kinase inhibitor that has been approved for the treatment of Philadelphia chromosome-positive chronic myeloid leukemia (Ph+ CML) in chronic, accelerated, myeloid or lymphoid blast phase, and Philadelphia chromosome-positive acute lymphoblastic leukemia (Ph+ ALL) since 2006 (FDA, 2006). It has been marked in the U.S. under the trade name of SPRYCEL®. The recommended starting dosages are 100 mg administered once daily for chronic phase CML, and 140 mg administered once daily for accelerated phase CML, myeloid or lymphoid blast phase CML, or Ph+ ALL, respectively.

Dasatinib is insoluble in water and slightly soluble in ethanol and methanol. As a weak base, dasatinib (pK_a = 3.1, 6.8, 10.8) demonstrates pH-dependent solubility change, with significantly reduced solubility as pH increasing from 1 to 6.5. Tsume et al. (2015) reported that

(*Continued*)

CASE STUDY 5 (*Continued*)

the saturated concentration of dasatinib at pH 4.0 was 3.6×10^{-2} mg/mL. At pH 6.3, the value dropped 5-fold. The dissolution profile of a 20-mg dasatinib tablet was determined with USP apparatus II (paddles). In 30 min, 80% of dasatinib was dissolved at pH 1.2; while less than 1% was dissolved at pH 6.5. A more prudent approach using mini-gastrointestinal simulator to assess dissolution change from pH 1.2 to pH 6.0 was also reported. Consistent with the findings from USP apparatus II, the amount of dissolved dasatinib significantly reduced (41.9% vs. 5.6%) from pH 1.2 to pH 4.0.

Gastric fluid secretion may be reduced in cancer patients while aging and/or concomitantly receiving gastric acid modulating agents. As expected, a large variability on dasatinib exposure was observed in patients. Wang et al. (2013) reported a population pharmacokinetic model of dasatinib established on the basis of more than 6000 dasatinib concentration observations obtained from approximately 1000 patients in 7 clinical trials. It has been shown that a linear two-compartment pharmacokinetic model adequately described the observed concentration data. The model assumed a random interindividual variability (IIV) on major pharmacokinetic parameters. Furthermore, an interoccasion variability (IOV) was included to account for the random changes on relative bioavailability for the same patient receiving dasatinib at various dosing occasions. It has been shown that a large proportion of overall variability for dasatinib exposure can be explained by the variability in relative bioavailability (IIV of 34.6% and IOV of 37.4%), contributing more than the variability in the apparent plasma clearance (IIV of 28.8%).

Dedicated clinical pharmacology studies were conducted in the development program to further assess the effect of gastric acid modulating agents on dasatinib exposure and to inform dosing instruction. Eley et al. (2009) reported a 3-period, 3-way crossover, drug–drug interaction study conducted in 24 healthy subjects receiving dasatinib, dasatinib in combination with famotidine (a H_2 blocker), and dasatinib in combination with aluminum/magnesium hydroxide (antacids). The study has shown that dasatinib exposure was reduced by 60% when famotidine was given 10 h prior to dasatinib dosing. In addition, a reduction of 55%–58% dasatinib exposure was observed when dasatinib was given together with aluminum/magnesium hydroxide; whereas no dasatinib exposure change was observed when alumimum/magnesium hydroxide was given 2 h before dasatinib dosing. One additional clinical pharmacology study was conducted to assess the effect of omeprazole (a proton pump inhibitor) on dasatinib exposure in 14 healthy subjects (FDA, 2006). About 40% reduction in dasatinib exposure was observed in patients receiving omeprazole at steady state. Based on the findings, the U.S. package insert of SPRYCEL indicates that concomitant use of dasatinib with an H_2 blocker or a proton pump inhibitor is not recommended. Simultaneous administration of dastinib with an acid-neutralizing antacid should be avoided. Rather, the use of antacids at least 2 h before or 2 h after the dosing of SPRYCEL should be considered.

Additional exploratory effort has been put to restore the reduction of dasatinib absorption due to hypochlorhydria. Yago et al. (2014) reported a three-treatment, three-way, crossover study. Healthy subjects received dasatinib, dasatinib after pretreatment with rabeprazole (a PPI), and simultaneous administration of dasatinib with betaine hydrochloride after pretreatment with rabeprazole. The study showed that rabeprazole reduced dasatinib exposure by 80%–90%. However, coadministration of betaine hydrochloride increased dasatinib C_{max} and AUC by 15- to 7.5-fold, restoring them to 105%–121% of the levels when dasatinib was given alone. The results suggested that simultaneous administration of betaine acid with dasatinib can be a potential strategy to ensure adequate absorption of dasatinib in patients with elevated gastric pH.

CASE STUDY 6

When a capsule formulation of intraconazole was used in AIDS patients, its oral absorption was lower compared with that in healthy subjects, presumably owing to the relative or absolute achlorhydria usually observed in AIDS patients. This assumption was confirmed by altering gastric pH. Under fasting conditions, when 8 oz. of cola was ingested along with itraconazole intake, its systemic exposure was greatly augmented (C_{max} was increased by 95% and $AUC_{0-24 h}$ by 75%) compared to those who received 8 oz. water and itraconazole intake. Interestingly, these effects were manifested in a totally opposite way for both Sporanox® capsule and Sporanox oral solution in healthy subjects. The underlying mechanism for this finding has not been fully elucidated.

With the pretreatment of ranitidine, an H_2-receptor blocker that could decrease the gastric acidity, it caused about 40% decrease in systemic exposure to itraconazole. The decrease in systemic exposure of itraconazole by ranitidine pretreatment could be offset by subsequent cola ingestion, which could increase the gastric acidity (Jaruratanasirikul and Sleepkaew, 1997).

EFFECTS OF GASTROINTESTINAL MOTILITY MODIFYING AGENTS ON PHARMACOKINETICS OF INSOLUBLE DRUGS

There are two classes of agents that can modify the GI motility. Both kinds are designated as GI motility modifying agents. One class, which can increase the rate of gastric emptying and also upper intestinal motility, is called GI prokinetic agents. Another class, which can delay the rate of gastric emptying, is called gastric emptying-slowing agents.

EFFECTS OF GASTROINTESTINAL PROKINETIC AGENTS

Several drugs or NCEs that can be categorized as GI prokinetic agents include (but are not limited to) metoclopramide (Lauritsen et al., 1990), cisapride (Bedford and Rowbotham, 1996), norcisapride (Gal, 2002), domperidone, prucalopride (Boeckxstaens et al., 2002), tegaserod (Degen et al., 2005), erythromycin (Bradley, 2001), and ranitidine (Mojaverian et al., 1990). By enhancing GI motility, this class of agents is anticipated to decrease total bioavailability of the coadministered drug by reducing GI transit or residence time that affects the amount of time that drug substance has to dissolve and be absorbed. Sometimes, however, a contrary effect can also be observed, and its underlying mechanism is not fully understood.

CASE STUDY 7

Griseofulvin, an antifungal agent, is insoluble in aqueous media. Its insolubility in water could be partly owing to its higher melting point (217°C–224°C). Numerous endeavors had been made to increase its water solubility and oral absorption, including size reduction through microsizing or ultramicrosizing (Bijanzadeh et al., 1990).

Owing to its insolubility in aqueous media, its oral absorption was slow, incomplete, and variable from the GI tract. For different formulations of griseofulvin, the effects of metoclopramide on pharmacokinetics of griseofulvin were different (Jamali and Axelson, 1977). The

(Continued)

CASE STUDY 7 (*Continued*)

pretreatment with metoclopramide decreased the systemic exposure by about a half, and shortened t_{max} by 2.7 h. However, for griseofulvin formulated in polyethylene glycol (PEG) 600, the pretreatment of metoclopramide could increase the systemic exposure to griseofulvin by approximately 2.5-fold. The underlying mechanism of the contrary results that were observed with different formulations of griseofulvin has not been well defined. The potential role of PEG 600 in facilitating the oral absorption of griseofulvin cannot be excluded.

CASE STUDY 8

Cyclosporine A, an immunomodulating agent, has poor water solubility (19 nM at 25°C). It has very large molecular weight (1203). Its oral absorption is incomplete and variable from the GI tract, and its absolute bioavailability was found to be less than 10% in liver transplant patients, but was more than 89% in some renal transplant patients. The pretreatment with metoclopramide could significantly shorten t_{max} of cyclosporine A owing to the increase in the absorption rate of cyclosporine A by metoclopramide. Meanwhile, its oral bioavailability was also enhanced by 29% with this GI prokinetic agent (Wadhwa et al., 1987).

EFFECTS OF GASTRIC EMPTYING-SLOWING AGENTS

Gastric emptying-slowing agents, another class of GI motility modifying agents, include (but are not limited to) opioids (such as morphine, pethidine [Wood, 1991]), anticholinergics, β-adrenoreceptor agonists, omeprazole (Cowan et al., 2005), and exenatide (Kolterman et al., 2003). This class of agents is anticipated to increase total bioavailability of a coadministered drug by decreasing its rate of absorption owing to decreasing gastric emptying.

One example is the examination of the effect of a gastric emptying-slowing agent, propantheline, on the bioavailability of ciglitazone (Cox et al., 1985). The coadministration of propantheline resulted in 20% increase in ciglitazone bioavailability, and this increase might be explained by the absorption window hypothesis. An increase in the residence time by a gastric emptying agent may have allowed more of the drug to dissolve at absorption sites. Though supported by very limited data, in theory, the increase in the residence time of a drug with poor water solubility by a gastric emptying agent may facilitate dissolution in the GI tract before absorption occurs, and subsequently augment its oral bioavailability (Zhou, 2003).

Although many effects reported in the literature are of limited clinical importance, they may be significant when prescribing a drug with a narrow therapeutic window, especially if it is absorbed poorly owing to its poor water solubility.

CHARACTERIZATION OF ABSORPTION PROCESSES VIA MODELING APPROACHES

Over the last several decades, modeling and simulation techniques have become more widely used to characterize the *in vivo* dissolution and subsequent absorption characteristics of orally administered drugs. These modeling and simulation approaches can help the formulation development and optimization for water-insoluble drugs. The understanding and characterization of the absorption kinetics is an important step in a successful absorption modeling endeavor.

TYPICAL ABSORPTION

In general, it is assumed that the oral absorption process follows first-order kinetics. This assumption appears to be valid for the majority of the drugs. The first-order process can also satisfactorily describe the oral absorption process of some drugs with very poor water solubility. Sometimes, the inclusion of the absorption time lag may appear to be needed to account for the lag time for the dissolution of the drug substance from the dosage form into the aqueous media in the GI tract. However, in some cases, the absorption patterns can't be readily characterized by the first-order kinetics with or without lag time; instead, they may be described by the following atypical or erratic absorption processes.

Zero-Order Absorption

For a typical drug with zero-order absorption, the concentrations after oral administration rise to a sharp peak and then quickly decline with no intermediate plateau. Examples of insoluble drugs whose absorption processes follow zero-order kinetics are cyclosporine (Grevel et al., 1986) and griseofulvin (Bates and Carrigan, 1975).

Erratic Absorption

Sometimes, absorption can be described by sequential zero-order and first-order absorption processes. Conceptually, if the first-order rate constant is linked to the zero-order input, the model can be postulated as the consequence of dissolution-limited absorption (Garrigues et al., 1991; Holford et al., 1992).

CASE STUDY 9

Apomine™, a biophosphonate ester, has poor water solubility (<0.1 µg/mL in water) and high lipophilicity (mLog $P = 6.8$). In the first single-dose study in healthy male subjects under fasting condition, it was observed that saturable absorption was occurring at a high dose (150 mg). This is consistent with the low solubility of apomine because it was anticipated that apomine's absorption would be dissolution rate limited, and that increasing the dose would eventually saturate the GI fluids (Bonate et al., 2004). A population pharmacokinetic modeling approach using NONMEM was applied to characterize the pharmacokinetics of apomine in healthy males and in male and female patients with solid tumors. Given the water-insoluble characteristics of apomine, two major modeling steps were adopted to well characterize its absorption process under both fasting and fed conditions:

Modeling of food effect on apomine's pharmacokinetics: It was expected that food would affect relative bioavailability ($F1$). Hence, three models had been tested:

$$\text{Model 1: } F1 = 1 - \frac{\text{Dose}}{D_{50} + \text{Dose}} \times (1 + \text{Food} \times \theta_{\text{Food}}) \tag{5.1}$$

$$\text{Model 2: } F1 = 1 - \frac{(\text{Dose})^n}{(D_{50})^n + (\text{Dose})^n} \times (1 + \text{Food} \times \theta_{\text{Food}}) \tag{5.2}$$

$$\text{Model 3: } F1 = [1 - \exp(-D_{50} \times \text{Dose})] \times (1 + \text{Food} \times \theta_{\text{Food}}) \tag{5.3}$$

(Continued)

CASE STUDY 9 (*Continued*)

where D_{50} is the dose that produces a 50% decrease in relative bioavailability, n is the shape factor, Food is a binary dummy variable indicating whether the dose was taken without (=0) or with food (=1), and θ_{Food} is the estimable parameter associated with a food effect. During the model selection process, Model 1 (Equation 5.1) was found to best describe the food effect on apomine's $F1$.

Modeling of absorption process of apomine: A simple first-order absorption model might not be applicable in this case. Thus, several absorption models were tested during model development process, including

- First-order absorption model with or without lag time
- Time-dependent absorption using a change-point model with or without lag time (Higaki et al., 2001)
- Time-dependent absorption using a Bateman function model with or without lag time (Higaki et al., 2001)
- Zero-order absorption
- Simultaneous first- (with and without lag time) and zero-order absorption
- First-order absorption (with and without lag time) treated as a mixture model

Of all the absorption models tested, the last absorption model (first-order model where the absorption rate constant and lag time were treated as a mixture model) fitted the data best. In 97% of the subjects, the population-estimated absorption rate constant was 1.77 h^{-1} with a lag time of 0.821 h, and in the remaining 3% of the subjects, the population-estimated absorption rate constant was 0.361 h^{-1} without a lag time (Bonate et al., 2004).

Besides the population-based pharmacokinetic modeling approach described in Case Study 9, recently, several other mechanistic modeling approaches have been used in describing and predicting absorption processes. For example, physiologically based pharmacokinetics (PBPK) modeling using commercially available software applications such as GastroPlus™ and SimCYP® have seen their increasing popularity in assisting formulation design and absorption optimization.

CONCLUSIONS

Drugs with very low aqueous solubility usually have sizeable inter- and/or intrasubject variability in their pharmacokinetics, which makes the study design and conduct of Phase I studies very challenging, makes the assessments of dose–response and exposure–response relationships more difficult, and makes the dose recommendation and optimization less feasible for NDA and product labeling.

Water-insoluble drugs usually have high propensity for drug interactions at absorption level, such as food interaction, interactions with GI prokinetic agents, effect of alteration in gastric pH with concomitant use of gastric pH modulating agents, especially if these drugs also have narrow therapeutic windows. Such hurdles and risks should be taken into consideration when a clinical drug development plan is put together. A risk/benefit reality check should be done at each critical stage gate, and if the risks are deemed too large, a tough call for termination of the program should be made. Early attention to absorption properties and close collaboration and communication between the Clinical Pharmacologists and Pharmaceutical Development scientists are crucial to ensure that the impact of formulation changes to address absorption challenges may not adversely affect the development timeline.

Owing to the inherent limitations of such drugs, more caution needs to be exercised and more resources may be warranted to make a sound assessment of their safety and efficacy profiles.

Similarly, testing may also pose significantly higher hurdles for bioanalytical sensitivity and reproducibility, as well as absorption evaluations of these drugs. To date, not many pharmacokinetic strategies are available to address such problems and eventually to assist in the dose regimen selection and optimization. For example, the growing popularity of the pharmacostatistical modeling approach (such as population exposure–response analyses in late-stage clinical development) may mitigate the negative impact arising from the low water solubility and associated disadvantages. The availability of emerging techniques and tools, such as positron emission tomography (PET), swallowable devices such as InteliSite® or IntelliCap® with real-time capsule localization achieved by gamma scintigraphy, or GI pH and temperature data may also shed more insight into the drug absorption process of these drugs. Moreover, the introduction of more and more validated and predictive surrogate markers or biomarkers early in the drug development stage may certainly help to overcome some (if not all) limitations of the current sole pharmacokinetics-based assessment of these water-insoluble drugs.

REFERENCES

Alamo, C., F. López-Muñoz, P. García-García, The effectiveness of lurasidone as an adjunct to lithium or divalproex in the treatment of bipolar disorder. *Expert Rev. Neurother.*, 2014; 14(6): 593–605.

Bates, T. R., P. J. Carrigan, Apparent absorption kinetics of micronized griseofulvin after its oral administration on single- and multiple-dose regimens to rats as a corn oil-in-water emulsion and aqueous suspension. *J. Pharm. Sci.*, 1975; 64: 1475–1481.

Bawa, R., J. R. Scarff, Lurasidone: A new treatment option for bipolar depression-a review. *Innov. Clin. Neurosci.*, 2015; 12(1–2): 21–23.

Bedford, T. A., D. J. Rowbotham, Cisapride. Drug interactions of clinical significance. *Drug Saf.*, 1996; 15: 167–175.

Bijanzadeh, M., M. Mahmoudian, P. Salehian, T. Khazainia, L. Eshghi, A. Khosravy, The bioavailability of griseofulvin from microsized and ultramicrosized tablets in nonfasting volunteers. *Indian J. Physiol. Pharmacol*, 1990; 34: 157–161.

Boeckxstaens, G. E., J. F. Bartelsman, L. Lauwers, G. N. Tytgat, Treatment of GI dysmotility in scleroderma with the new enterokinetic agent prucalopride. *Am. J. Gastroenterol*, 2002; 97: 194–197.

Bonate, P. L., S. Floret, and C. Bentzen, Population pharmacokinetics of APOMINE™: A meta-analysis in cancer patients and healthy males. *Br. J. Clin. Pharmacol*, 2004; 58: 142–155.

Bradley, C., Erythromycin as a gastrointestinal prokinetic agent. *Intens Crit Care Nurs*, 2001; 17: 117–119.

Citrome, L., Lurasidone in schizophrenia: New information about dosage and place in therapy. *Adv. Ther.*, 2012; 29(10): 815–825.

Claytor, F. W., W. L. Smith, E. L. Turner, The effect of orange juice on gastric acidity. *J. Natl. Med. Assoc.*, 1941; 33: 160–165.

Cowan, A., D. L. Earnest, G. Ligozio, M. A. Rojavin, Omeprazole-induced slowing of gastrointestinal transit in mice can be countered with tegaserod. *Eur. J. Pharmacol.*, 2005; 517: 127–131.

Cox, S. R., E. L. Harrington, V. J. Capponi, Bioavailability studies with ciglitazone in beagles: II. Effect of propantheline bromide and metoclopramide HCL on bioavailability of a tablet. *Biopharm. Drug Dispos.*, 1985; 6: 81–90.

Degen, L., C. Petrig, D. Studer, S. Schroller, C. Beglinger, Effect of tegaserod on gut transit in male and female subjects. *Neurogastroenterol Motil.*, 2005; 17: 821–826.

Eley, T., F. R. Luo, S. Agrawal, A. Sanil, J. Manning, T. Li, A. Blackwood-Chirchir, R. Bertz, Phase I study of the effect of gastric acid pH modulators on the bioavailability of oral dasatinib in healthy subjects. *J. Clin. Pharmacol*, 2009; 49(6): 700–709.

FDA. 1989. Nexium® U.S. Package Insert: http://www.accessdata.fda.gov/drugsatfda_docs/label/2014/022101s014021957s017021153s050lbl.pdf. Accessed October 3, 2015.

FDA. 2006. Sprycel® U.S. Package Insert: http://www.accessdata.fda.gov/drugsatfda_docs/label/2015/021986s016s017lbledt.pdf. Accessed October 3, 2015.

FDA. 2010. Latuda® U.S. Package Insert: http://www.accessdata.fda.gov/drugsatfda_docs/label/2013/200603s015lbl.pdf. Accessed October 3, 2015.

FDA. 2014. Pepcid® U.S. Package Insert: http://www.accessdata.fda.gov/drugsatfda_docs/label/2014/019462s038lbl.pdf. Accessed October 3, 2015.

FDA. 2015. Ibrance® U.S. Package Insert: http://www.accessdata.fda.gov/drugsatfda_docs/label/2015/207103s000lbl.pdf. Accessed October 3, 2015.

Gal, J., New single-isomer compounds on the horizon. *CNS Spectr.*, 2002; 7(Suppl 1): 45–54.

Garrigues, T. M., U. Martin, J. E. Peris-Ribera, L. F. Prescott, Dose-dependent absorption and elimination of cefadroxil in man. *Eur. J. Clin Pharmacol.*, 1991; 41: 179–183.

Goodman and Gilman's *The Pharmacological Basis of Therapeutics*, 10th ed., Hardman, J.G., Limbird, L.E., Gilman, A.G. (Eds.). New York: McGraw Hill, 2001.

Greiff, J. M., Rowbotham, D., Pharmacokinetic drug interactions with gastrointestinal motility modifying agents. *Clin. Pharmacokinet*, 1994; 27: 447–461.

Grevel, J., E. Nüesch, E. Abisch, K. Kutz, Pharmacokinetics of oral cyclosporine A (Sandimmun) in healthy subjects. *Eur. J. Clin. Pharmacol*, 1986; 31: 211–216.

Haruma, K., T. Kamada, H. Kawaguchi, S. Okamoto, M. Yoshihara, K. Sumii, M. Inoue, S. Kishimoto, G. Kajiyama, A. Miyoshi, Effect of age and Helicobacter pylori infection on gastric acid secretion. *J Gastroenterol Hepatol*, 2000; 15(3): 277–283.

Hellriegel, E. T., T. D. Bjornsson, W. W. Hauck, Interpatient variability in bioavailability is related to the extent of absorption: Implications for bioavailability and bioequivalence studies. *Clin Pharmacol Ther*, 1996; 60: 601–607.

Higaki, K., S. Yamashita, G. L. Amidon, Time-dependent oral absorption models. *J. Pharmacokinet. Pharmacodyn.*, 2001; 28: 109–128.

Holford, N. H., R. J. Ambros, K. Stoeckel, Models for describing absorption rate and estimating extent of bioavailability: Application to cefetamet pivoxil. *J. Pharmacokinet. Biopharm.*, 1992; 20: 421–442.

Jamali, F., J. F. Axelson, Influence of metoclopramide and propantheline on GI absorption of griseofulvin in rats. *J. Pharm. Sci.*, 1977; 66: 1540–1543.

Jaruratanasirikul, S., A. Sleepkaew, Influence of an acidic beverage (Coca-Cola) on the absorption of itraconazole. *Eur. J. Clin. Pharmacol.*, 1997; 52: 235–237.

Kolterman, O. G., J. B. Buse, M. S. Fineman, E. Gaines, S. Heintz, T. A. Bicsak, K. Taylor, et al. Synthetic exendine-4 (exenatide) significantly reduces postprandial and fasting plasma glucose in subjects with type 2 diabetes. *J. Clin. Endocrinol. Metab.*, 2003; 88: 3082–3089.

Lange, D., J. H. Pavao, J. Wu, M. Klausner, Effect of cola beverage on the bioavailability of itraconazole in the presence of H_2 blockers. *J. Clin. Pharmacol.*, 1997; 37: 535–540.

Lauritsen, K., L. S. Laursen, J. Rask-Madsen, Clinical pharmacokinetics of drugs used in the treatment of gastrointestinal diseases (Part I). *Clin. Pharmacokinet*, 1990; 19: 11–31.

Lennard-Jones, J. E., A. F. Cher, D. G. Shaw, Effect of different foods on the acidity of the gastric contents in patients with duodenal ulcer. *Gut.*, 1968; 9: 177–182.

Malhotra, S., R. K. Dixit, S. K. Garg, Effect of an acidic beverage (Coca-Cola) on the pharmacokinetics of carbamazepine in healthy volunteers. *Methods Find Exp. Clin. Pharmacol.*, 2002; 24(1): 31–33.

Mojaverian, P., P. K. Ferguson, P. H. Vlasses, M. L. Rocci Jr, A. Oren, J. A. Fix, L. J. Caldwell, C. Gardner, Estimation of gastric residence time of the Heidelberg capsule in humans: Effect of varying food composition. *Gastroenterology*, 1985; 89: 392–397.

Mojaverian, P., P. H. Vlasses, P. E. Kellner, M. L. Rocci Jr, Effects of gender, posture, and age on gastric residence time of an indigestible solid: pharmaceutical considerations. *Pharm. Res.*, 1988; 5: 639–644.

Mojaverian, P., P. H. Vlasses, S. Parker, C. Warner, Influence of single and multiple doses of oral ranitidine on the gastric transit of an indigestible capsule in humans. *Clin. Pharmacol. Ther.*, 1990; 47: 382–388.

Nomeir, A. A., P. Mojaverian, T. Kosoglou, M. B. Affrime, J. Nezamic, E. Rodwanski, C. C. Lin, M. N. Cayen, Influence of food on the oral bioavailability of loratadine and psuedoephedrine from extended-release tablets in healthy volunteers. *J. Clin. Pharmacol.*, 1996; 36: 923–930.

Ogunbona, F. A., I. F. Smith, O. S. Olawoye, Fat contents of meals and bioavailability of griseofulvin in man. *J. Pharm. Pharmacol.*, 1985; 37: 283–284.

Preskorn, S., L. Ereshefsky, Y. Y. Chiu, N. Poola, A. Loebel, Effect of food on the pharmacokinetics of lurasidone: results of two randomized, open-label, crossover studies. *Hum. Psychopharmacol*, 2013; 28(5): 495–505.

Teorell, T., Kinetics of distribution of substances administered to the body. *Arch. Intern. Pharmacodyn.*, 1937; 57: 205–240.

Toothaker, R. D., P. G. Welling, The effect of food on drug bioavailability. *Annu. Rev. Pharmacol. Toxicol.*, 1980; 20: 173–199.

Tsume, Y., S. Takeuchi, K. Matsui, G. E. Amidon, G. L. Amidon, In vitro dissolution methodology, mini-Gastrointestinal Simulator (mGIS), predicts better in vivo dissolution of a weak base drug, dasatinib. *Eur. J. Pharm. Sci.*, 2015; 76: 203–212.

Van de Velde, V. J., A. P. Van Peer, J. J. Heykants, R. J. Woestenborghs, P. Van Rooy, K. L. De Beule, G. F. Cauwenbergh, Effect of food on the pharmacokinetics of a new hydroxypropyl-beta-cyclodextrin formulation of itraconazole. *Pharmacotherapy*, 1996; 16: 424–428.

Wadhwa, N. K., T. J. Schroeder, E. O'Flaherty, A. J. Pesce, S. A. Myre, M. R. First, The effect of oral metoclopramide on the absorption of cyclosporine. *Transplantation*, 1987; 43: 211–213.

Wang, X., A. Roy, A. Hochhaus, H. M. Kantarjian, T. T. Chen, N. P. Shah, Differential effects of dosing regimen on the safety and efficacy of dasatinib: Retrospective exposure-response analysis of a Phase III study. *Clin. Pharmacol.*, 2013; 10(5): 85–97.

Welling, P. G., Influence of food and diet on gastrointestinal drug absorption: A review. *J Pharmacokinet Biopharm.*, 1977; 5: 291–334.

Welling, P. G., F. L. Tse, Factors contributing to variability in drug pharmacokinetics. I. Absorption. *J Clin Hosp Pharm.*, 1984; 9: 163–179.

Wood, M., Pharmacokinetic drug interactions in anesthetic practice. *Clin. Pharmacokinet.*, 1991; 21: 285–307.

Yago. M. R., A. Frymoyer, L. Z. Benet, G. S. Smelick, L. A. Frassetto, X. Ding, B. Dean et al., The use of betaine HCl to enhance dasatinib absorption in healthy volunteers with rabeprazole-induced hypochlorhydria. *AAPS J.*, 2014; 16(6): 1358–1365.

Zhang, L., F. Wu, S. C. Lee, H. Zhao, L. Zhang, pH-dependent drug-drug interactions for weak base drugs: Potential implications for new drug development. *Clin. Pharmacol. Ther.*, 2014; 96(2): 266–277.

Zhou, H., Pharmacokinetic strategies in deciphering atypical drug absorption profiles. *J. Clin. Pharmacol.*, 2003; 43: 211–227.

6 Regulatory Aspects of Dissolution for Low Solubility Drug Products

Pradeep Sathe, Robert A. Lionberger, Sau Lawrence Lee,
Lawrence X. Yu, and Di (Doris) Zhang

CONTENTS

INTRODUCTION

Despite recent progress in the use of combinatorial chemistry and high-throughput screening techniques to identify orally active drugs, the probability that poorly soluble compounds will make their way into development will likely remain in the foreseeable future (Yu 1999; Lipinski 2000). We have been relying heavily on formulation approaches to address issues relating to poor drug absorption of these compounds (Pinnamaneni et al. 2002; Pouton 2006). However, rational formulation design based on pharmaceutical properties of drugs is far from a reality. Among many factors, our lack of predictive dissolution testing *in vitro* often contributes to long and costly formulation development processes. In this chapter, we first describe roles of dissolution testing during drug development, manufacturing, and postapproval changes, followed by reviewing some important issues relevant to the Biopharmaceutics Classification System (BCS) classification and delivery of poorly soluble drugs. This chapter then proceeds with discussions on how to develop an appropriate dissolution test including classification and characterization of drugs, determination of appropriate medium, selection of dissolution apparatus and operating speed, and determination of dissolution acceptance criteria. Finally, we use several examples to illustrate the development of meaningful dissolution tests.

ROLES OF DISSOLUTION TESTING

Dissolution testing plays a key role during the drug product development and commercial manufacturing. During the development stages of a drug product, dissolution testing is used to evaluate the rate of drug release from formulations and assess their stability and formulation changes. In addition, it is employed to establish an *in vitro–in vivo* correlation (IVIVC) in order to predict bioavailability or bioequivalence of drug products. For release of drug products, dissolution testing is used to ensure manufacturing and product consistency. For instance, for an immediate-release (IR) product, a single-point release criterion is often used, such as, "*Q*" = 80% in 30 min. In certain circumstances, a complete dissolution profile comparison rather than a single-point assessment is used (Food and Drug Administration CDER 1997). Dissolution testing is also used in granting biowaivers of low strengths and for postapproval manufacturing changes. The BCS guidance (Food and Drug Administration CDER 2015) employs dissolution testing to demonstrate rapid dissolution of immediate-release solid oral dosage forms so that a biowaiver can be granted.

The continued use of dissolution as a quality control tool is based on the belief articulated by United States Pharmacopeia (USP) that the dissolution test is in general overly sensitive to formulation differences. As a result, dissolution tests used for quality control emphasize the selection of discriminatory media and conditions. In comparison, dissolution tests for predicting bioavailability/bioequivalence require the choice of biorelevant media and conditions. Although it is desirable to have a single dissolution test that can be applied for both evaluation of *in vivo* performance and assurance of product consistency, identifying such a dissolution test remains a significant challenge, particularly for dosage forms containing poorly soluble drugs (Brown et al. 2004; Zhang and Yu 2004).

FORMULATION OF LOW SOLUBILITY DRUGS

DEFINITION OF LOW SOLUBILITY

The U.S. Food and Drug Administration (FDA) issued a Guidance for Industry covering the BCS in August 2000 and revised it in May 2015 (Food and Drug Administration CDER 2015). The BCS is a scientific framework for classifying a drug substance on the basis of its equilibrium aqueous solubility and intestinal permeability (Amidon et al. 1995). When combined with the *in vitro* dissolution characteristics of a drug product, the BCS takes into account three major factors: solubility, intestinal permeability, and dissolution rate. These three factors govern the rate and extent of oral drug absorption for IR solid oral dosage forms (Food and Drug Administration CDER 2015). The BCS defines four classes of drug substances on the basis of their solubility and permeability characteristics.

	High Solubility	Low Solubility
High permeability	Class I	Class II
Low permeability	Class III	Class IV

From the BCS guidance, the criterion for high solubility uses the ratio of the highest strength to the minimum aqueous solubility in the pH range of 1–6.8 at 37°C ± 1°C. This ratio has a unit of volume and is referred to as the dose solubility volume. It is the volume needed to dissolve the strength across the entire pH range. If the dose solubility volume is ≤250 mL, the drug substance is considered highly soluble. However, if the dose solubility volume is >250 mL, the drug substance is considered poorly soluble. The volume estimate of 250 mL is derived from typical bioequivalence study protocols that prescribe administration of a drug product to fasting human volunteers with a glass (about 8 oz.) of water.

The permeability classification is based indirectly on the extent of intestinal absorption of a drug substance in humans and directly on measurements of the rate of mass transfer across the human intestinal membrane. A drug substance is considered highly permeable when the extent of intestinal absorption is determined to be 85% or higher. Otherwise, the drug substance is considered to be poorly permeable.

An IR drug product is characterized as a *rapidly dissolving* product when not less than 85% of the labeled amount of the drug dissolves within 30 min using USP Apparatus 1 at 100 rpm or USP Apparatus 2 at 50 rpm (at 75 rpm when appropriately justified) in a volume of 500 mL or less with each of the following media: (a) acidic media, such as 0.1 N HCl or USP-simulated gastric fluid (SGF) without enzymes; (b) a pH 4.5 buffer; and (c) a pH 6.8 buffer or USP-simulated intestinal fluid (SIF) without enzymes. Otherwise, the drug product is considered to be a slowly dissolving product.

We will use the BCS definition to define low solubility drugs. However, we recognize that the BCS definition is conservative because it is used to waive regulatory bioequivalence studies for Class I drugs (Yu et al. 2002). There are two reasons why the BCS definition for solubility is too conservative. The first reason is because of the need to show high solubility across the range of pH from 1.0 to 7.5. On the basis of the ionizable groups, the solubility of weak bases is higher in the stomach than that in the small intestine. A low solubility at high pH may not be a barrier to absorption of weak bases because the absorption may be complete before the drug enters the low solubility, high pH GI region. On the other hand, low solubility at low pH may not be a problem of weak acids as high solubility and high permeability at distal small intestine are sufficient for their complete absorption. For example, many nonsteroidal anti-inflammatory drugs, although classified as low solubility according to the BCS, have the bioavailability over 90% (Yazdanian et al. 2004).

The second reason is that for the low solubility drugs, the *in vitro* aqueous solubility is not reflective of the *in vivo* gastrointestinal (GI) tract solubility. The solubility of lipophilic drugs is generally better in an *in vivo* environment because of the presence of bile salts or lecithin micelles. Recent studies have shown that solubility in biorelevant medium can be 1.1–160 times greater than the aqueous solubility of BCS Class II drugs, ranging from griseofulvin to danazol (Takano et al. 2006).

FORMULATION OF LOW SOLUBILITY DRUGS

Some drugs classified as low solubility drugs on the basis of *in vitro* measures of aqueous solubility may have acceptable *in vivo* solubility because of either pH dependence or solubility in GI fluids. If these drugs with acceptable *in vivo* solubility are BCS Class II (Food and Drug Administration CDER 2015), they would then be expected to have acceptable oral bioavailability from standard solid oral dosage forms. For BCS Class II drugs that are shown to have low bioavailability owing to their poor solubility and inability to dissolve rapidly, the selection of formulation is often of great importance in developing a successful product for oral administration of Class II drugs. The bioavailability of these drugs can be improved by several formulation approaches. The most common method of increasing solubility (either a weak acid or weak base) is to induce salt formation. Even if the salt formation has no significant effect on the solubility, the salt dissolution rate will often be enhanced owing to the difference in the pH of the thin diffusion layer surrounding the drug particle. The dissolution rate can also be increased by reducing the size of solid drug particles, which leads to an increased surface area available for dissolution. A typical micronization method such as an air-jet mill can reduce the particle size to 2–5 μm. Further reduction requires the use of ball-milling media in aqueous suspension (Merisko-Liversidge et al. 2003). This technology can reduce the crystalline particle size to 100–250 nm, providing a considerable increase in dissolution rate.

Another method of improving bioavailability for these poorly soluble drugs is to prepare an amorphous formulation, since an amorphous form allows faster dissolution of the drug in comparison to its corresponding crystalline form. An amorphous formulation is prepared by incorporating the drug in its amorphous form into a carrier matrix (polyvinylpyrrolidone and polyethylene glycol) using various techniques such as spray drying and melt extrusion (Pouton 2006). However, it should be noted that amorphous solids are nonequilibrium solid phases and hence are generally less stable relative to their corresponding crystalline phases.

Lipid formulations are another option for solubilization of poorly soluble drugs. These formulations include oil-based systems, water-insoluble self-emulsifying drug delivery systems (SEDDS), water-soluble SEDDS, and systems that contain very little oil that disperses to form micellar solutions (Pouton 2006). The major advantage of the lipid delivery system is that the drug can be present in a stable liquid solution. This eliminates the time required to dissolve solid particles. Furthermore, the lipids used in the formulation may facilitate the transport of the drug substance across the intestinal membrane and further improve the absorption of drugs from lipid formulations (Pouton 2006). However, one possible concern associated with this type of formulation is drug precipitation on dilution as well as unexpected phase transformation to a more stable polymorphic form (Bauer et al. 2001).

In addition to the methods described earlier, the solubility of poorly soluble drugs can also be improved using solubilizing agents such as cyclodextrins. Cyclodextrins solubilize these poorly soluble compounds by forming water-soluble inclusion complexes with them. However, the dosage level can be limited by the use of this solubilizing agent, since there is a potential concern with regard to the toxicity of some commercially available cyclodextrins.

DEVELOPMENT OF DISSOLUTION METHOD

FDA is encouraging sponsors to use quality by design (QbD) in the development of their drug products. QbD means designing and developing formulations and manufacturing processes to ensure a predefined quality and understanding how formulation and manufacturing process variables influence product quality (Yu 2006). QbD consists of the following elements:

* Define target product quality profile.
* Design and develop product and manufacturing processes to meet the target product quality profile.
* Identify and control critical raw material attributes, process parameters, and sources of variability.
* Monitor and adapt processes to produce consistent quality over time.

Because *in vivo* drug dissolution and release is an essential step in delivering the drug to its site of action, it should be included in the target product quality profile of solid oral dosage forms. Under the QbD system, pharmaceutical quality is assured by understanding and controlling formulation and manufacturing variable, while end-product testing, including *in vitro* dissolution, confirms the quality of the product. In the context of dissolution, QbD implies establishing the relationships among raw material properties (such as particle size), formulation variables (excipient levels and grade), process parameters (such as compression force and blending time), and the target product quality profile. Efficient implementation of QbD requires a biorelevant dissolution test during product development. In a QbD system, product attributes such as particle size or polymorphic form that are previously monitored indirectly via a QC dissolution test are monitored and controlled through the design and control of the manufacturing process. Thus, under QbD, dissolution testing development should mainly focus on its clinical relevance.

The following steps are crucial for designing a dissolution test for poorly soluble drug products:

1. Classification and characterization
   - Measure solubility as a function of pH
   - Classify a drug substance according to BCS
   - Consider formulation factors
2. Determination of appropriate medium and volume
3. Selection of appropriate dissolution apparatus and operating speed
4. Determination of appropriate acceptance criteria

CLASSIFICATION AND CHARACTERIZATION

The first step is to know the BCS classification of the drug and use this information to help design formulations and evaluate the possibility of IVIVC. For a poorly soluble drug dosed in an immediate-release product, the disintegration of the dosage form is generally rapid and the oral drug absorption is mainly limited by dissolution rate and/or permeation rate (permeability), where permeation rate refers to the flux of drug across the intestinal membrane. The rate of dissolution and the uptake rate of permeation determine the concentration of drug in the GI tract. However, the concentration in the GI tract is also limited by the solubility of the drug. When the rate of dissolution is far more than the uptake rate of permeation, the drug concentration in the GI fluid approaches its solubility limit. Therefore, poor dissolution can be caused either by particle size (r) and/or solubility (C_s). To emphasize the importance of solubility, Yu (1999) referred to the dissolution/solubility-limited case as solubility-limited absorption. The dissolution/particle size-limited case is still called dissolution-limited absorption. As a result, permeability, solubility, and/or dissolution can limit the absorption of poorly absorbable drugs.

For poorly soluble drugs with dissolution-limited absorption, the formulation approach commonly used to overcome slow dissolution is to increase surface area by reducing the particle size. The *in vitro* dissolution testing can be predictive of evaluating the effect of particle size reduction. However, a very small particle size could complicate the development of a dissolution test as small particles can pass through filters and subsequently dissolve. In this situation, the use of small pore filters, centrifugation, ultracentrifugation, or high wavelength UV detection may be needed (Brown et al. 2004).

For poorly soluble drugs with solubility-limited absorption, possible formulation approaches are to use amorphous materials, lipid formulations, or one of the other technologies stated earlier. These formulation technologies and their potential failure modes will affect the selection of a dissolution test. In formulations using amorphous materials, a possible conversion of amorphous to crystalline state during the dissolution testing should be considered. An example of such an issue is the troglitazone data presented by Dressman and Reppas (2000). Troglitazone dissolution in the fasted state simulated intestinal fluid (FaSSIF) and fed state simulated intestinal fluid (FeSSIF) is predictive of the food effect observed in *in vivo* pharmacokinetic studies. However, the dissolution profile in FaSSIF demonstrates a maximum. This maximum is due to recrystallization of the drug substance during the dissolution process into a less soluble crystalline form. This peak was not seen in the FeSSIF dissolution medium, indicating the role of medium components on the rate of nucleation of the less soluble form.

For lipid-based formulations where the drug is in solution, dissolution testing is not used to evaluate drug dissolution. Instead, it is employed to measure product capsule disruption and possible drug emulsification or precipitation on dilution. Nevertheless, if *in vitro* sink condition is maintained, the precipitation that might occur *in vivo* will not be observed *in vitro*. Therefore, we need to be cautious when we develop dissolution testing for lipid-based formulations.

DISSOLUTION MEDIA

QUALITY CONTROL DISSOLUTION MEDIA

The choice of dissolution medium will depend on the purpose of the dissolution test. For batch-to-batch quality control testing, selection of the dissolution medium is based, in part, on the solubility data and the dose range of a drug product to ensure that sink conditions are met. However, under certain circumstances, a medium that fails to provide sink conditions may be justifiable (Brown et al. 2004). If the pH-dependent solubility indicates that the drug has a low solubility only in a particular pH range, the most likely media for an appropriate quality control dissolution test is an aqueous buffer at pH values that lead to high solubility. This approach becomes problematic when the pH with high solubility is greater than 6.8, because this condition is not relevant to *in vivo* dissolution. Nevertheless, in FDA OGD's dissolution database [http://www.accessdata.fda.gov/scripts/cder/dissolution/index.cfm], out of about 300 dissolution methods, 19 use a pH higher than 7.2 and 10 use pH greater than 6.8 but less than or equal to 7.2. The use of pH outside physiologically relevant pH should be strongly discouraged.

Surfactants can be used in a biorelevant manner by choosing a surfactant that matches solubility in more expensive simulated biological fluids. However, surfactants are more often used in a quality control setting for drugs whose solubility (even *in vivo* solubility) is too low to establish the sink condition. Noory et al. (2000) discuss some method development strategies and provide justification for the use of particular surfactants. Surfactants that have been used in the FDA-approved dissolution methods include Tween, CTAB, and Tris buffer, with SLS being by far the most commonly used surfactant. In general, it is desirable to use as little surfactant as possible to reach sink conditions. If too much surfactant is used, a dissolution test may not be able to detect changes in polymorphic form or particle size, as suggested in International Conference on Harmonisation of Technical Requirements for Registration of Pharmaceuticals for Human Use (ICH).

BIORELEVANT DISSOLUTION MEDIA

Although dissolution testing is currently used primarily for quality control, it is desirable to have a dissolution test that is predictive of *in vivo* performance. Therefore, there has been recent interest in developing biorelevant media whose properties match those of human gastric or intestinal fluids (Kalantzi et al. 2006). Vertzoni et al. (2005) proposed a fasted state simulating gastric fluid (FaSSGF), as shown in Table 6.1. The use of FaSSGF improves the predictability of dissolution for a weak base, but not for a neutral drug. Table 6.1 also describes Dressman's proposed biorelevant dissolution media that simulate intestinal fluid for the fasted state as well as fed state. A comparison of the *in vitro* dissolution data in biorelevant media with *in vivo* data shows that it is possible to simulate food effects and shows differences in absorption between products of the same drug with the physiologically relevant media (FaSSIF, FeSSIF, and milk) (Nicolaides et al. 1996).

TABLE 6.1
Biorelevant Media to Gastric and Intestinal Conditions

Ingredient	FaSSGF: Stomach (Fasted State)	FaSSIF: Small Intestine (Fasted State)	FeSSIF: Small Intestine (Fed State)
NaH$_2$PO$_4$ (mg/mL)	—	3.95	—
Acetic acid (mg/mL)	—	—	8.65
Pepsin (mg/mL)	0.1	—	—
Sodium taurochorate (mM)	0.08	3	15
Lecithin (mM)	0.02	0.75	3.75
NaCl (mM)	34.2	0.068 g	0.20

APPARATUS AND DISSOLUTION CONDITIONS

For immediate-release products, the most commonly used dissolution apparatus are the USP Apparatus 1 (basket) and USP Apparatus 2 (paddle). Usually, the Apparatus 1 is operated at 100 rpm and the Apparatus 2 at 50 rpm. However, it was suggested that the Apparatus 2 is operated at 75 rpm to reduce coning (Dressman 2005). By itself, the rotation speed would not be expected to affect the extent of dissolution of a low solubility drug because solubility is a thermodynamic property. However, once the solubility is addressed via selection of pH and surfactant, selection of the appropriate rotation speed raises similar issues to those found for higher solubility drugs. The rotation speed can be set on the basis of matching *in vivo* hydrodynamics, selecting the most sensitive speed, or selecting the speed that minimizes variability in the test method. In a recent article (Mirza et al. 2005), the effect of hydrodynamics on both low solubility and high solubility drugs were evaluated, and the low solubility drug was slightly more sensitive to perturbations. In this article, the low solubility drug was still able to dissolve greater than 90% in 45 min in a media of 1000 mL borate buffer, pH 8.0, containing 0.1% Tween® 80.

Other USP apparatus, the reciprocating cylinder (USP Apparatus 3) and the flow-through cell (USP Apparatus 4), are not commonly used for release testing but may be valuable for use in a biorelevant dissolution method during product development. The Apparatus 3 is believed to have hydrodynamic flow patterns that are more representative to those found *in vivo* (Yu et al. 2002). The flow-through cell allows removal of dissolved drug that would saturate media in other closed apparatus and thus gets much closer to the *in vivo* situation that a truly low solubility drug encounters.

ACCEPTANCE LIMIT

After dissolution conditions are identified for a dissolution test, the dissolution specification is not complete until an acceptance limit is set. Three categories of dissolution test acceptance limits for immediate-release drug products are described in the 1997 FDA Guidances for Industry for immediate-release (Food and Drug Administration CDER 1997) and sustained-release drug products (FDA Center for Drug Evaluation and Research 1997).

- *Single-point specifications*: As a routine quality control test (for highly soluble and rapidly dissolving drug products).
- *Two-point specifications*: For slowly dissolving or poorly water-soluble drugs (BCS Class II), a two-point dissolution specification, one at 15 min to include a dissolution range (a dissolution window) and the other at a later point (30, 45, or 60 min) to ensure 85% dissolution, is recommended to characterize the quality of the product.
- *Profile comparison.*

Although the FDA guidance for IR dissolution (Food and Drug Administration CDER 1997) suggests that a two-point limit be used for low solubility drugs, in practice almost all low solubility drugs in IR formulations have a single-point acceptance limit.

For regulatory approvals of new drug applications (NDAs)/abbreviated new drug applications (ANDAs) for solid oral dosage forms, sponsors are required to develop appropriate *in vitro* dissolution testing. For NDAs, the dissolution specifications are currently based on acceptable clinical, pivotal bioavailability, and/or bioequivalence batches. For ANDAs, the dissolution specifications are generally the same as that of the reference-listed drug (RLD). The specifications are then confirmed by testing the dissolution performance of the generic drug product from an acceptable bioequivalence study batch(es). If the dissolution of the generic product is substantially different from that of the RLD but the product is bioequivalent in an *in vivo* study, a different dissolution specification for the generic product may be set (Food and Drug Administration CDER 1997).

CASE STUDIES

CASE STUDY 1

Mebendazole is a broad-spectrum anthelmintic drug producing high cure rates in infestations by Ascaris, threadworms, hookworms, and whipworms. The drug is practically insoluble in water and has three polymorphic forms (A, B, and C) that have different solubility and therapeutic effects (Swanepoel et al. 2003). The USP dissolution method for mebendazole tablet is 0.1 HCl with 1.0% sodium lauryl sulfate (SLS). The acceptance criterion is >75% in 120 min. Swanepoel et al. (2003) used the USP method to determine the dissolution rate of powder for mebendazole forms A, B, and C. The percent dissolved at 120 min is more than 90% with 0.1 HCl containing 1.0% SLS for all three mebendazole forms A, B, and C (Figure 6.1). When SLS was removed from the dissolution medium, the dissolution profiles changed so that polymorph C dissolved faster (70% within 120 min) when compared to polymorph B (37% within 120 min) and polymorph A (20% within 120 min). This example suggests that excessive use of surfactant for BCS Class II drugs may make the dissolution testing insensitive to formulation changes such as polymorphic forms and particle size. As a result, this dissolution test will fail its objective of ensuring product quality and batch-to-batch consistency.

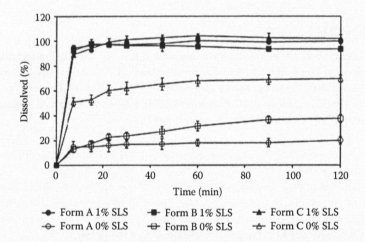

FIGURE 6.1 Powder dissolution profiles of mebendazole polymorphs in 0.1 M HCl (open symbols) and 0.1 M HCl containing 1% sodium lauryl sulfate (closed symbols). (Reprinted from *Eur. J. Pharm. Biopharm.*, 55, Swanepoel, E. et al., Quality evaluation of generic drugs by dissolution test: Changing the USP dissolution medium to distinguish between active and non-active mebendazole polymorphs, 345. Copyright 2003, with permission from Elsevier.)

CASE STUDY 2

Drug A is a large, peptide-like molecule (MW >700 g/mol) and is highly lipophilic and poorly water soluble. It is a BCS Class II drug. Its oral bioavailability in capsules and conventional tablet formulations is low, yielding practically undetected blood levels. A novel lipid formulation containing a solvent, a high HLB nonionic surfactant, and a fatty acid were developed with sufficient oral bioavailability for use in the clinic.

The dissolution testing was initially conducted in the following media using the USP Apparatus 2 at 50 rpm: pH 4.5 acetate buffer, 7.5 phosphate buffer, 0.1 N HCl, and 0.1 N HCl with 25 mM SLS. The dissolution results are shown in Figure 6.2.

Dissolution results at 30 min suggested further investigation of 25 mM SLS in 0.1 N HCl. In a second series of experiments, varying concentrations of SLS in 0.1 HCl were investigated, and the results are shown in Figure 6.3. Finally, the dissolution media of 5 mM SLS in 0.1 N HCl was chosen. The regulatory acceptance criterion was set at 80% in 30 min.

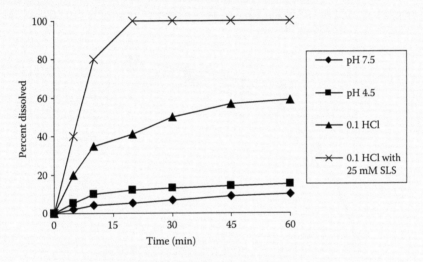

FIGURE 6.2 Dissolution of drug A lipid formulation in various dissolution media.

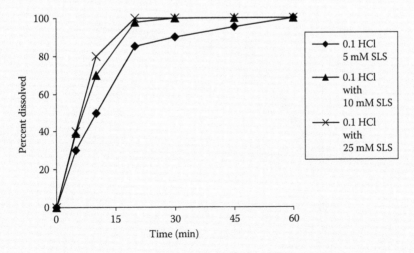

FIGURE 6.3 Dissolution of drug A lipid formulation in 0.1 N HCl with different levels of SLS.

CASE STUDY 3

Drug B is slightly soluble in water, and its water solubility is pH dependent with higher solubility at higher pH. Drug B has moderate permeability and is a BCS Class IV drug. The initial proposed dissolution method for drug B tablet was the USP apparatus 2 at 50 rpm in pH 6.8 phosphate buffer with the acceptance criterion of 80% in 30 min. However, during product development, three lots of products from the same formulation, but different manufacturing processes, were evaluated in bioequivalence/bioavailability studies. These three lots of products were bioequivalent, although Lot C failed to meet the dissolution acceptance criterion of 80% in 30 min and Lot B had to use S2 in order to pass the dissolution acceptance criterion. Therefore, the dissolution testing is more discriminating, as shown in Figure 6.4.

In order to establish an appropriate acceptance criterion, the additional dissolution studies with biorelevant dissolution media FaSSIF in Table 6.1 were conducted, and the results are shown in Figure 6.5. Figure 6.5 indicates that the dissolution rate has been uniformly increased, and all three lots pass the acceptance criterion of 80% in 30 min. On the basis of these biorelevant dissolution results along with the bioequivalence study data, the acceptance criterion was reduced to 70% in 30 min.

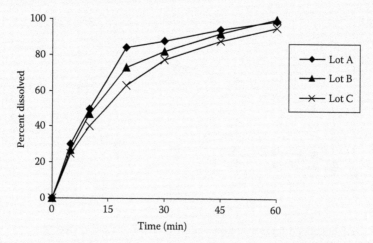

FIGURE 6.4   Dissolution of three lots of drug B tablet in pH 6.8 phosphate buffer.

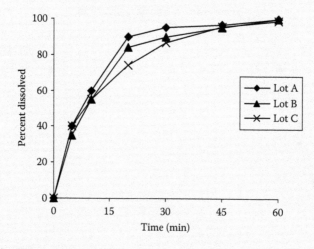

FIGURE 6.5   Dissolution of three lots of drug B tablet in pH 6.8 FaSSIF.

CONCLUSION

The need to develop predictive dissolution methods for low solubility drugs is growing. The use of surfactants in the dissolution media is widely accepted in quality control dissolution methods. Characterization of the drug solubility in SGF/SIF provides insight into whether the levels of surfactant are similar to the solubilization found *in vivo*. Examples are provided to illustrate the development of meaningful dissolution tests. Regulatory challenges include how to evaluate proposed dissolution methods that are used for both product quality control and *in vivo* performance prediction.

FUTURE DEVELOPMENT

Industry and regulatory scientists have made every effort in developing dissolution tests to meet at least two objectives: a quality control tool to assure batch-to-batch consistency and an *in vitro* surrogate for product performance that can guide formulation development and ascertain the need for bioequivalence tests. Since conditions that are optimum for the quality control purpose may not be applicable for establishing an IVIVC, it may be beneficial to develop and use two kinds of dissolution tests: one for quality control and the other for *in vivo* performance, to meet different objectives. The quality control test is sensitive enough to relevant product changes that ensure the high quality and consistent performance of products, while the dissolution test for IVIVC can predict *in vivo* performance of drug products and thus reduce unnecessary human studies, accelerate drug development, and hasten validation of postapproval changes.

Currently, the regulatory dissolution method is generally drug or drug product specific. Each drug product uses a different dissolution method, resulting in the development of IVIVC on a trial and error basis (Zhang and Yu 2004). Therefore, dissolution data gathered from thousands of dissolution tests can rarely be used to gain dissolution knowledge that helps to understand the *in vivo* performance of drug products. Furthermore, there is really no strong scientific and regulatory reason that immediate-release solid oral products of similar drugs cannot use a comparable dissolution method for predicting *in vivo* bioavailability and bioequivalence. Therefore, we should develop appropriate biorelevant dissolution testing methods, and academia, industry, and regulatory agencies should put more emphasis on devising predictive dissolution testing.

REFERENCES

Amidon, G. L., H. Lennernäs, V. P. Shah, and J. R. Crison. 1995. A theoretical basis for a biopharmaceutic drug classification: The correlation of *in vitro* drug product dissolution and *in vivo* bioavailability, *Pharm. Res.*, 12: 413.

Bauer, J., S. Spanton, R. Henry, J. Quick, W. Dziki, W. Porter, and J. Morris. 2001. Ritonavir: An extraordinary example of conformational polymorphism, *Pharm. Res.*, 18: 859.

Brown, C. K., H. P. Chokshi, B. Nickerson, R. A. Reed, B. R. Rohrs, and P. A. Shah. 2004. Acceptable analytical practices for dissolution testing of poorly soluble compounds, *Pharm. Technol.*, 28: 56–65.

Dressman, J. B. 2005. Dissolution tests—How they relate to drug product performance, FDA.

Dressman, J. B. and C. Reppas. 2000. *In vitro–in vivo* correlations for lipophilic, poorly water-soluble drugs, *Eur. J. Pharm. Sci.*, 11: S73.

FDA Center for Drug Evaluation and Research. 1997. Extended release oral dosage forms: Development, evaluation, and application of *in vitro/in vivo* correlations, FDA.

Food and Drug Administration CDER. 1997. Dissolution testing of immediate-release solid oral dosage forms.

Food and Drug Administration CDER. 2015. Guidance for industry: Waiver of *in vivo* bioavailability and bioequivalence studies for immediate-release solid oral dosage forms based on a biopharmaceutics classification system.

Kalantzi, L., K. Goumas, V. Kalioras, B. Abrahamsson, J. B. Dressman, and C. Reppas. 2006. Characterization of the human upper gastrointestinal contents under conditions simulating bioavailability/bioequivalence studies, *Pharm. Res.*, 23: 165.

Lipinski, C. A. 2000. Drug-like properties and the causes of poor solubility and poor permeability, *J. Pharmacol. Toxicol. Methods*, 44: 235.

Merisko-Liversidge, E., G. G. Liversidge, and E. R. Cooper. 2003. Nanosizing: A formulation approach for poorly water-soluble compounds, *Eur. J. Pharm. Sci.*, 18: 113.

Mirza, T., Y. Joshi, Q. J. Liu, and R. Vivilecchia. 2005. Evaluation of dissolution hydrodynamics in the USP, peak and flat-bottom vessels using different solubility drugs, *Dissol. Technol.*, 12: 11–16.

Nicolaides, E., E. Galia, C. Efthymiopoulos, J. B. Dressman, and C. Reppas. 1999. Forecasting the *in vivo* performance of four low solubility drugs from their *in vitro* dissolution data, *Pharm. Res.*, 16: 1876.

Noory, C., N. Tran, L. Ouderkirk, and V. Shah. 2000. Steps for development of a dissolution test for sparingly water-soluble drug products, *Dissol. Technol.*, 7: 3.

Pinnamaneni, S., N. G. Das, and S. K. Das. 2002. Formulation approaches for orally administered poorly soluble drugs, *Pharmazie*, 57: 291.

Pouton, C. W. 2006. Formulation of poorly water-soluble drugs for oral administration: Physicochemical and physiological issues and the lipid formulation classification system, *Eur. J. Pharm. Sci.*, 29: 278.

Swanepoel, E., W. Liebenberg, and M. M. de Villiers. 2003. Quality evaluation of generic drugs by dissolution test: Changing the USP dissolution medium to distinguish between active and non-active mebendazole polymorphs, *Eur. J. Pharm. Biopharm.*, 55: 345

Takano, R., K. Sugano, A. Higashida, Y. Hayashi, M. Machida, Y. Aso, and S. Yamashita. 2006. Oral absorption of poorly water-soluble drugs: Computer simulation of fraction absorbed in humans from a miniscale dissolution test, *Pharm. Res.*, 23: 1144.

Vertzoni, M., J. Dressman, J. Butler, J. Hempenstall, and C. Reppas. 2005. Simulation of fasting gastric conditions and its importance for the *in vivo* dissolution of lipophilic compounds, *Eur. J. Pharm. Biopharm.*, 60: 413.

Yazdanian, M., K. Briggs, C. Jankovsky, and A. Hawi. 2004. The high solubility definition of the current FDA Guidance on Biopharmaceutics Classification System may be too strict for acidic drugs, *Pharm. Res.*, 21: 293.

Yu, L. Implementing quality-by-design: OGD initiatives, Advisory Committee for Pharmaceutical Science, October 5, 2006. http://www.fda.gov/ohrms/dockets/ac/06/slides/2006-4241s1-index.htm (accessed December 1, 2006).

Yu, L. X. 1999. An integrated absorption model for determining causes of poor oral drug absorption, *Pharm. Res.*, 16: 1883.

Yu, L. X., G. L. Amidon, J. E. Polli, H. Zhao, M. U. Mehta, D. P. Conner, V. P. Shah et al. 2002. Biopharmaceutics classification system: The scientific basis for biowaiver extension, *Pharm. Res.*, 19: 921.

Yu, L. X., J. T. Wang, and A. S. Hussain. 2002. Evaluation of USP apparatus 3 for dissolution testing of immediate-release products, *AAPS Pharm. Sci.*, 4: E1.

Zhang, H. and L. X. Yu. 2004. Dissolution testing for solid oral drug products: Theoretical consideration, *Am. Pharm. Rev.*, 5: 26–31.

7 Formulation Strategies and Practice Used for Drug Candidates with Water-Insoluble Properties for Toxicology, Biology, and Pharmacology Studies in Discovery Support

Lian-Feng Huang, Jinquan Dong, and Shyam B. Karki

CONTENTS

INTRODUCTION

The advent of high-throughput screening technologies, combinatorial chemistry, computational modeling, and proteomics has resulted in many more targets and compounds during the drug discovery stage (Venkatesh and Lipper, 2000). However, many of these compounds are highly lipophilic and have a high molecular weight. This is because compounds with these properties tend to have high potency (*in vitro* binding activity) due to additional hydrophobic interactions with enzyme or receptor surface (Lombardino and Lowe III, 2004). These compounds are usually not drug-like because of their low water solubility, a major cause for poor pharmacokinetics (PK) and oral bioavailability. As a result, they may falter in further development, resulting in a higher attrition rate and lost productivity.

Because how the drug is delivered has a direct impact on the PK behavior and the availability of the compound in efficacy studies and toxicological studies, identification of an appropriate formulation is crucial for an accurate assessment of a compound's suitability for pharmaceutical development. Formulations in early stages of development face an additional set of challenges such as time and material limitation. Adding to the challenges is the requirement for superpharmacological exposures (and hence high doses) in toxicology studies. Therefore, it is important to have phase appropriate formulation strategies in order to balance formulation challenges, stringent timelines, and cost. Good formulations should aid the establishment of structure–activity relationships (SARs); maximize the efficacy of the compound, while minimizing side effects in an animal model; and enable identification of potential development challenges by evaluating biopharmaceutical properties.

FORMULATION NEEDS AND CHALLENGES IN DISCOVERY SETTING

In the early development stages, there are mainly three studies that require formulations: *in vivo* efficacy studies, PK studies, and toxicology studies. Because of the large numbers of compounds involved and the very low amounts of each compound available, several high-throughput formulation development platforms have been developed to enable efficient formulation development. For poorly water-soluble compounds, multiple formulation options often need to be evaluated. Depending on the study purpose, exotic vehicles sometimes have to be used without considering the commercial viability of the formulation. Typically, the materials from the medicinal chemistry laboratories tend to be less controlled and might vary from batch to batch with high impurity levels (Gardner et al., 2004); therefore, the physical parameters such as solid state form (Huang and Tong, 2004), morphology, and particle size are not optimized (Kerns and Di, 2002; Pritchard et al., 2003; Balbach and Korn, 2004; Chaubal, 2004). Solubility/dissolution rate of material with different quality may vary, which can result in variable PK performance.

FORMULATION STRATEGIES AND DRUG DELIVERY OPTIONS

Several recent publications reviewed the formulation development aspects of drug candidates at the discovery stage (Chen et al., 2006; Neervannan, 2006; Maas et al., 2007; Timpe and Forschung, 2007). Amidon et al. (1995) first developed a system that groups drug molecules on the basis of their different solubility and/or permeability, known as the Biopharmaceutics Classification System (BCS). This classification has been widely used as a guide to assess the formulation development challenge. However, lack of the dose information at this early stage makes the assessment difficult. This is because the minimum solubility requirement is dependent on dose and permeability (Lipinski, 2002). In addition, BCS does not account for drug metabolism, another important factor affecting drug bioavailability. The molecular parameters, such as H-bond donors, H-bond acceptors, molecular weight, and calculated log P (Clog P), can also serve as a guide to understand the challenge in formulation development (Lipinski et al., 1997). Lee et al. (2003) presented a high-throughput formulation decision scheme to support early discovery injectable formulation development to address the formulation development challenge presented at the discovery stage. Strickley (2004) summarized the solubilizing excipients used in commercially available solubilized oral and injectable formulations, providing a great reference in excipient selection. To ensure a rapid and efficient formulation development, a solubility classification for the selection of an appropriate formulation system for highly active compounds with good permeability ($P_{eff} > 10^{-6}$ cm/s) was introduced by Maas et al. (2007). This formulation system suggests that standard formulations can be applied for the compounds with the solubility greater than 100 μg/mL and only minimum effort is required. For the compounds with solubility greater than 10 μg/mL and less than 100 μg/mL, enabling formulation may be needed depending on dose. If the solubility is less than 10 μg/mL, enabling formulations are considered mandatory.

Several formulation technologies are discussed in the following. For detailed information, please refer to other chapters in this book.

pH Adjustment and Salt Formation

Two-thirds of all existing drug entities possess ionizable groups, and are weak electrolytes in aqueous solution (Stahl and Wermuth, 2002). The solubility of a compound in aqueous media is greater in the ionized state than in the neutral state (Sweetana and Akers, 1996). If ionizable groups are present within the molecule, adjusting the pH using HCl or NaOH or a buffer, such as citrate, acetate, phosphate, carbonate, or tris (hydroxymethyl) aminomethane (tris), can oftentimes increase the solubility of the drug in the dosing vehicle. For intravenous formulations, the pH should ideally be neutral (pH 7.4), but can reside within the range of pH 3–9, depending on an understanding of the tolerability of the vehicle and volume administered. For oral formulations, the pH should generally be within the range of 2–9.

For a compound with ionizable groups, its total solubility, S_T, is a function of the intrinsic solubility, S_o, and the difference between the molecule's dissociation constant, pK_a, and the solution pH. The intrinsic solubility is the solubility of the neutral molecular species. For a weak acid,

$$S_T = S_o \left(1 + 10^{pH - pK_a}\right)$$

and for a weak base,

$$S_T = S_o \left(1 + 10^{pK_a - pH}\right)$$

Weak acids can be solubilized at pHs above their acidic pK_a, and weak bases can be solubilized at pHs below their basic pK_a. It has to be noted that these equations neglect the effect of surfactant properties of the species, which can occasionally be significant on S_T.

For a weakly acidic compound at pH ≪ pK_a (e.g., by 2 units), the solubility is practically independent of pH and remains constant at S_o. At pH > pK_a, the solubility increases exponentially with pH, where the excess solid phase in equilibrium with the saturated solution is the free acid. At certain pH value, the log-linear relationship of solubility with pH abruptly ends, and the solubility plots enter a nearly constant range, where the excess solid phase is the salt. The pH value where the log-linear relationship ends and near constant solubility starts is the pH of maximum solubility pHmax. For compounds containing both acidic and basic functional groups, the solubility of zwitterion (internal salt pair) at the isoelectric point is typically the lowest over the entire pH range.

For formulation of a stable solution (oral or parenteral), the equilibrium solubility is more important than the rate of dissolution. During pH adjustment of a formulation, *in situ* salt formation with the free form and an appropriate counterion may provide the same advantage as using a salt. The solubility product of a salt, K_{sp}, needs to be taken into consideration in predicting the solubility of a salt in a particular environment that contains other salts with a common counterion.

A preliminary investigation of pH-solubility profile with different counterions provides an indication of the counterion best suited to maximize solubility (or optimize for pH based on stability and/or tolerability). Multiple counterions added in predetermined amounts so as not to exceed the solubility product K_{sp} of any salt, provided significantly higher solubility than any single counterion. The relevance of pHmax to solution formulations with acceptable pH for intravenous administration has been reported (Stahl and Wermuth, 2002).

However, salt formation is not feasible for compounds without ionizable groups. In addition, the formed salts may also converse to respective acid or base forms in the bloodstream or gastrointestinal tract (GIT). Since blood is a very efficient buffer (pH 7.4), this can result in potential precipitation of the drug at the injection site, leading to issues such as hemolysis, phlebitis, thromboembolism, and potential changes in drug distribution (Yalkowsky et al., 1998). The risk of precipitation is reduced by the efficiency of the compound to bind to blood proteins, by slow administration, by reducing the drug concentration in the vehicle, and by the relative buffering capacity if a buffer is used (Alvarez-Nunez and Yalkowsky, 1999). The propensity for precipitation has been evaluated using *in vitro* methods (Portmann and Simmons, 1995; Johnson et al., 2003). Similar issues are expected with water-insoluble acid drugs formulated as solutions with pH adjustment. When administered orally, the formulation is dispersed in the stomach's acidic environment. A potential problem is that the acid drug may precipitate out from the solution. Because the precipitation kinetics are highly dependent on local conditions and may require nucleation of the particle, they occur with high variability and, hence, may affect oral absorption in a variable manner, and result in poor bioavailability.

Drugs in solution formulations may be more susceptible to chemical reactions leading to degradation. The most common reactions are hydrolysis and oxidation. Usually, the reaction rate or type is influenced by pH. For example, the hydrolysis of acetylsalicylic acid (aspirin) is pH dependent, and its pH-rate profile shows a large and complex variation of k_{obs} due to four distinct mechanistic patterns (Alibrandi et al., 2001). Therefore, it is essential to monitor and understand the chemical stability of the drug in pH-adjusted formulations.

Cosolvents

A common practice in solubilizing water-insoluble compounds is to use water-miscible solvents. The use of cosolvents can enhance the solubility of nonpolar solutes by several orders of magnitude. Following the principle of *like dissolves like*, the polarity of water should be reduced by mixing with other less-polar hydrophilic substances and thus increasing the solubility of nonpolar, water-insoluble substances. For molecules without any ionizable group(s), which cannot be solubilized by pH adjustment, a cosolvent approach is often used. Solubility of a cosolvent system typically increases logarithmically with the linear increase in the fraction of organic solvent(s) (Rubino and Yalkowsky, 1987).

Assuming that the total free energy of the system is equal to the sum of the free energy of the individual components (Trivedi and Wells, 2000), the solubility of a compound in a binary mixture of water and an organic solvent can be described as

$$\log S_t = \log S_w + f(\log S_c - \log S_w)$$

where S_t is the total solubility in the cosolvent mixture, S_c is the solubility in pure organic solvent, S_w is the solubility in water, and f is the fraction of organic solvent in the cosolvent mixture.

If the cosolvent mixture contains more than two organic solvents (i.e., a ternary or higher cosolvent mixture), the total drug solubility can be approximated by a summation of solubilization potentials as

$$\log S_t = \log S_w + \Sigma(f_i(\log S_{ci} - \log S_{wi}))$$

Frequently, a simple approach of pH adjustment or cosolvent is not enough to achieve the target concentration. Cosolvents are often used in combination with pH adjustment to further enhance the solubility. Using this approach, Lee et al. (2003) observed that nearly 85% of Pfizer, Ann Arbor discovery compounds ($n > 300$) submitted for discovery and preclinical injectable formulation development in the year 2000 could be formulated by pH adjustment, cosolvent addition, or a combination of the two approaches. It was also observed that 11% of compounds were not formulatable using this approach, and another 32% of the formulation used more than 55% cosolvent. The high solvent content can limit the pertinent safety assessment of lead compounds. Therefore, the synergistic combinations of pH adjustment and cosolvent are not sufficient to develop commercially viable formulations for water-insoluble drugs. This leads to additional formulation technologies such as complexation, incorporation into micelles, nanosizing, and so forth, being employed in early discovery stages.

The most commonly used solvents for early-stage discovery formulation are polyethylene glycol 400 (PEG-400), propylene glycol, ethanol, glycerin, DMSO, dimethylacetamide (DMA), and N-methyl-2-pyrrolidone (NMP). PEG-400 has wide applications across several therapeutic areas for both oral and parenteral administrations. Higher molecular weight PEGs have melting points above room temperature and are viscous, while molecular weights lower than that of PEG-300&400 can be poorly tolerated in *in vivo* studies.

One of the disadvantages of cosolvent systems is their precipitation behavior when diluted with water or aqueous body fluids. Precipitation of drug could potentially occur during *in vivo* testing, which in turn could result in reduced bioavailability. In injectable formulation, this leads to drug precipitation at the injection site, causing injection site irritation. Although in the discovery phase it is preferable to use low volume, high-concentration cosolvent formulations to increase solubility and hence the amount of drug dosed, this practice have increased risks of hemolysis and tissue irritation when administered intravenously. Therefore, cautions need to be taken not to exceed the toxicity levels for the cosolvent. Based on vastly different physical and chemical properties of a wide range of new chemical entities, formulation scientists typically need to consider the molecular structure and consult with members of their therapeutic team to choose appropriate solvents for a particular pharmacokinetic/pharmacodynamic model. For example, high concentrations of ethanol may be unsuitable for CNS-related programs owing to its intoxicating effects. The hemolytic effect of propylene glycol (Krzyzaniak et al., 1997) might render it a liability for cardiovascular programs. Potent cosolvents, such as NMP and diethyleneglycol-monoethyl-ether (Transcutol), often display serious tolerability issues (e.g., drowsiness) in acute and/or chronic animal studies (Maas et al., 2007).

The water-immiscible solvents including the long-chain triglycerides such as peanut oil, corn oil, soybean oil, sesame oil, olive oil, hydrogenated vegetable oils, hydrogenated soybean oil, and the medium-chain triglycerides derived from coconut oil and palm seed, provide another approach to solubilize pharmaceutical compounds. These oily formulations are mainly for oral administration as oral solution or filled into soft-gelatin capsules. Surfactants may be needed for optimal performance of oil formulations.

COMPLEXATION

Complexation using cyclodextrins (CDs) is another approach that can be used for solubilization. CDs are a family of cyclic oligosaccharides, the most common α, β, and γ, consisting of 6–8 d-glucopyranosyl units, presenting a hydrophilic outer surface and a lipophilic cavity to which a hydrophobic guest molecule can complex (Szente and Szejtli, 1999). Different numbers of glucopyranose units lead to different cavity sizes. The inner diameter of the hydrophobic cavity is approximately 4.7–5.3, 6.0–6.5, and 7.5–8.3 Å for α-CD, β-CD, and γ-CD, respectively (Loftsson and Brewster, 1996). With lipophilic inner cavity and hydrophilic outer surface, CDs are capable of interacting with a large variety of guest molecules to form noncovalent inclusion complexes

(Challa et al., 2005). Natural CDs have limited application in solubilizing drug molecules owing to their limited aqueous solubility. Hydroxypropyl-β-cyclodextrin (HP-β-CD), a chemically modified β-CD obtained by treating a base-solubilized solution of β-CD with propylene oxide, has a much greater solubility than unfunctionalized β-CD. In addition, HP-β-CD is well tolerated and appears to be safe in clinical trials without observable renal toxicity as shown with β-CD (Irie and Uekama, 1997). Another commonly used cyclodextrin Captisol®, sulfobutylether of β-CD (SBE-β-CD), is a polyanionic β-cyclodextrin derivative with a sodium sulfonate salt separated from the lipophilic cavity by a butyl ether spacer group, or sulfobutylether. Both HP-β-CD and SBE-β-CD are widely used cyclodextrins for solubility-enhancing purpose.

If a drug molecule and CD complexing agent combine to form a 1:1 complex,

$$D + CD \overset{K}{\rightleftharpoons} D * CD$$

In the case of a 1:1 complex the total aqueous solubility of drug (S_t, mol/L) in the presence of a given total CD concentration (C_{CD}, mol/L) can be described as

$$S_t = S_w + [KS_w/(1 + KS_w)]C_{CD}$$

where K is the binding constant of the complex and S_w is the aqueous solubility of the compound in the absence of CDs. The magnitude of the binding constant, K in M^{-1}, between most pharmaceutical agents and CDs ranges from 0 to 100,000 (Rajewski and Stella, 1996). Therefore, the practicality of the CD approach depends on the binding constant K, the drug intrinsic solubility, S_w, the dose requirements of the formulation, and the maximum amount of CD that the formulation can accommodate (Rao and Stella, 2003).

Phase-solubility diagrams are frequently used to calculate stoichiometry of drug/CD complexes. A linear diagram (AL-type systems) indicates that the complexes are first order with respect to CD and first order with respect to the drug, that is, the complex usually contains a 1:1 mole ratio of drug to CD. Positive deviation from linearity (AP-type systems) indicates formation of complexes that are first order with respect to the drug but second or higher order with respect to CD, that is, the complex formed may have a drug/CD mole ratio greater than one. Negative deviation from linearity (AN-type systems) indicates solution artifacts or self-association of the CDs at high concentrations. Sometimes stoichiometry of drug/CD complexes cannot be derived from simple phase-solubility studies and drug/CD complexes can self-associate to form water-soluble aggregates, which then can further solubilize the drug through noninclusion complexation (Loftsson et al., 2002). Self-association through formation of water-soluble aggregates of several drug/CD complexes can further solubilize the drug through noninclusion complexation.

As dilution can be readily attainable on injection or in the stomach and intestinal contents, it reduces the percentage of the drug complex, releasing the free drug that can permeate through biological membranes. The ratio of free-to-complexed drug on dilution of a poorly water-soluble drug/CD complex depends on the phase-solubility behavior of the system. Precipitation on dilution is less likely than cosolvent formulation, when the relationship between drug solubility and CD concentration is linear, for example, in a 1:1 interaction of CD and drug. However, drug precipitation can still occur during dilution, when the relationship between drug solubility and CD concentration is nonlinear (Rajewski and Stella, 1996) or if another molecule preferentially forms complex.

Although CD complexes of unionized drugs usually have greater stability (based on K) than those of their ionic counterparts (Loftsson et al., 1993), the achieved total solubility (free-ionized drug + free-unionized drug + ionized drug complex + unionized drug complex) usually increases. Complexation with CDs and simultaneous salt formation can be successfully applied for improving the properties of ionic drugs, in particular for increasing their water solubility (S_w). The use of CD complexes can stabilize the stability of a compound, decrease irritant effects, improve rate and extent of absorption, and mask the taste. Complexation and simultaneous salt formation allow higher solubility in comparison with simple binary complexes (Redenti et al., 2000, 2001).

The combination of CD complexation and cosolvent has been reported extensively in the literature. In early 1990s, it was believed that cosolvents reduced the solubilization capacity of CDs. The solubility of testosterone with HP-β-CD was reported to be lower in the presence of 80% ethanol (Pitha and Hoshino, 1992). In aqueous CD solutions, the addition of propylene glycol or ethanol has been reported to reduce the solubility of testosterone and ibuprofen (Loftsson et al., 1993). However, in recent years, polymers have been reported to improve the solubilization capacity of CDs. A synergism between CDs and water-soluble polymers in solubilizing naproxen was observed (Faucci and Mura, 2001). The water-soluble polymers increased the complexation efficacy of CDs toward naproxen. Hydroxypropyl methylcellulose (HPMC) was observed to increase the solubilization effect of CDs. The amount of CD needed in the solid dosage form was significantly lower in the presence of HPMC (Savolainen et al., 1998). A mathematical model was developed to describe the combined effect of cosolvency and complexation on fluasterone solubilization (Li et al., 1999). Nandi et al. (2003) have observed that in solutions containing Trappsol HPB (HP-β-CD), at lower PEG-400 concentrations (<50%), the observed solubility was significantly greater than the expected solubility. In systems containing PEG-400 concentrations greater than 60%, the synergistic effect decreased, yielding observed solubilities close to the theoretical values. Overall, PEG-400 and Trappsol HPB showed a synergistic effect in improving progesterone solubility in water. In the case of systems containing Captisol, no synergism was observed in improving the solubility of progesterone. The observed solubility was less than the theoretical solubility. The author speculated that the synergistic effect of CD and PEG-400 could be attributed to additional breaking of hydrogen bonds in water's structure and a decrease in the dipole moment. At PEG-400 concentrations of 50% and higher, the synergistic effect diminished.

The application of CDs in formulation is by no means limited to solution formulations for parenteral and solution administrations. Solid dispersion of CD and drug has been studied extensively in the literature (Nagarsenker et al., 2000; Govindarajan and Nagarsenker, 2005). However, owing to the large molecular weight of CDs, this approach usually applies to drugs of high potency.

The pharmacokinetics of β-CD and HP-β-CD after intravenous administration have been assessed (Frijlink et al., 1990). As determined at doses of 25, 100, and 200 mg/kg in permanently cannulated rats, plasma levels of both CDs decreased rapidly upon injection. Within 24 h after administration, most of the doses were excreted unchanged via urine. There was no evidence for significant metabolism of the intravenously administered CDs. The pharmacokinetics and the tissue concentrations of methyl-β-cyclodextrin (MEBCD) and doxorubicin (DOX) in rabbits following administration of MEBCD and DOX, alone or in combination, were studied (Grosse et al., 1999). Results indicated that DOX did not modify MEBCD pharmacokinetic profile, but MEBCD reduced significantly the distribution half-life of DOX. Tissue determination showed that MEBCD did not enhance the cardiac accumulation of DOX.

The disadvantages of CD include (1) strict correlation between the structure of the guest molecule and the cavity size of the CD molecule; (2) limited solubility of CD in water, and thus limited the maximum concentrations this approach can achieve; and (3) CDs can significantly modify absorption-distribution-metabolism-excretion/elimination (ADME) parameters if the binding constant K is too high, and thus limited the amount of free drug for absorption (Miller et al., 2006).

SURFACTANTS AND MICELLES

There are mainly three reasons that surfactants are used in formulation: (1) to increase wetting of drugs, which in turn increase the dissolution; (2) to prevent drug precipitation from formulation; and (3) to increase solubilization through micellization.

Micelles are colloidal dispersions that form spontaneously, under certain concentrations, from amphiphilic or surface-active agents (surfactants), molecules of which consist of two distinct regions with opposite affinities toward a given solvent such as water (Torchilin, 2007). Micelles form when the concentration of these amphiphiles is above the critical micelle concentration (CMC). They consist of an inner core of assembled hydrophobic segments and an outer hydrophilic shell serving as a stabilizing interface between the hydrophobic core and the external aqueous environment. Micelles solubilize molecules of poorly soluble nonpolar pharmaceuticals within the micelle core, while polar molecules could be adsorbed on the micelle surface, and substances with intermediate polarity distributed along surfactant molecules in intermediate positions.

The total solubility of a drug in an aqueous surfactant solution can be described as

$$S_t = S_w + k(C_s - C_{cmc})$$

where k is the solubilizing capacity of micelles, C_s is the surfactant concentration, and C_{cmc} is the CMC of the surfactant. Usually, k increases with increase of the alkyl chain length, if the guest drugs are localized deep in the micelles (Kawakami et al., 2004).

Surfactant micelles form only above their CMC, and rapidly break apart on dilution, which can result in premature leakage of the drug and its precipitation *in situ*. Polymeric micelles are generally much more stable than surfactant micelles, exhibiting lower CMCs, slower rates of dissociation, and longer retention of loaded drugs (Kataoka et al., 1993; Francis et al., 2004; Gillies and Frechet, 2004).

Common surfactants used in micellar formulation are either amphoteric (e.g., Lecithin), nonionic (e.g., Tween-80, Cremophor EL, Solutol HS 15, TPGS), block copolymers (e.g., poloxamers), or ionic (e.g., sodium lauryl sulfate). The amphiphilic polyethoxylated castor oil derivative Cremophor EL is one of the most frequently used surface-active formulation ingredients in parenteral dosage forms. The surfactant is comparatively well tolerated on intravenous injection and has a high solubilizing potential for poorly water-soluble compounds. The plasma pharmacokinetics of Cremophor EL have been summarized by van Zuylen et al. (2001). Tween-80 (polyoxyethylene sorbitan monooleate) is another nonionic surfactant that is used as an ingredient in intravenous formulations of sparingly water-soluble compounds, such as lipophilic anticancer drugs. As with Cremophor EL, above its critical micelle concentration, Tween-80 exhibits micellar structures, potentially interacting with coadministered compounds (Shokri et al., 2001). In addition, Tween-80 modulates multidrug resistance *in vitro*, and is an even more potent *P*-glycoprotein (*P*-gp) inhibitor than Cremophor EL (Mountfield et al., 2000). An additional example of a surfactant that is tolerated intravenously at reasonably high concentration is Solutol HS 15, the main component of which is the PEG-660 ester of 12-hydroxystearate. Solutol HS 15 has a high solubilizing potential for a variety of different compounds (Bittner and Mountfield, 2002), but there is a lack of data on its pharmacokinetic profile in the literature. d-α-tocopherol polyethylene glycol 1000 succinate (TPGS) has been recognized as an effective oral absorption enhancer for improving the bioavailability of poorly absorbed drugs and as a vehicle for lipid-based drug delivery. TPGS is a potent inhibitor of an active efflux even at concentrations 10-fold below the CMC, suggesting that monomeric TPGS is capable of inhibiting the efflux mechanism. Therefore, TPGS improves *in vivo* performance not only by solubility-enhancing micelle formation but also by increasing the overall intestinal permeability via inhibiting an efflux mechanism (Wu and Hopkins, 1999). Overall, surface-active formulation ingredients may be suitable for preventing precipitation of coinjected, poorly water-soluble compounds.

The micelle formulation approach often possesses disadvantages such as its toxicity associated with surfactants even at relatively low concentrations. In general, nonionic surfactants have the least toxic effects. Cremophor EL produces hypersensitivity reactions in human and animals (Jonkman-de Vries et al., 1996). Tween-80 is also believed to cause acute hepatitis and renal failure (Uchegbu and Florence, 1996). On intravenous administration, owing to their surface activity, surfactant molecules have the potential to penetrate and disrupt biological membranes and can be hemolytic (Ten Tije et al., 2003). Often the absorption capacity of the micelle is too small and the extent of the solubilizing effect is too low. Therefore, frequently high surfactant concentrations are necessary, so that the liquid one-phase area is left under the formation of liquid-crystalline systems with high viscosity. Surfactants may also change the pharmacokinetic behaviors of coadministered compounds, which is mainly due to the delayed drug release because of the thermodynamic stability of the associated micelles. However, the many advantages of micellar formulations uniquely positioned them as one of the most useful drug delivery systems.

The combination of micelle with either cosolvent or complexation in formulation has been studied on a number of occasions. In general, this combination did not provide significant synergetic effects on solubilizing water-insoluble compounds, and the effects were dependent on the type and concentration of surfactants, complexing agents, and individual cosolvents. A mathematical model was developed to provide the quantitative basis for the combined use of surfactants and CDs (Rao et al., 2006). The addition of cosolvent modified the interaction between surfactant molecules as well as solution properties. In their study on the effect of the combination of Gelucire 44/14 (a semi-solid waxy material with 20% mono-, di-, and triglycerides, 72% mono- and di-fatty acid esters of PED 1500 adn 8% free PEG 1500) and cosolvent on the solubilization of Indomethacin and Phenytoin, Kawakami et al. (2004) found that the combined use offered only little advantage on solubility. Similar results were also observed for the combination of sodium dodecyl sulfate (SDS), Tween-80, and cosolvents (Kawakami et al., 2006).

EMULSIONS AND MICROEMULSIONS

Unlike micelles, an emulsion is a liquid system in which one liquid is dispersed in a second, immiscible liquid, usually in droplets, with emulsifiers added to stabilize the dispersed system. Conventional emulsions possess droplet diameters of more than 200 nm, and are therefore optically opaque or milky. Conventional emulsions are thermodynamically unstable, tending to reduce their total free energy by reducing the total area of the two-phase interface. In contrast, microemulsions with droplet diameters less than 100 nm are optically clear and thermodynamically stable. Unlike conventional emulsions that require the input of a substantial amount of energy, microemulsions are easy to prepare and form spontaneously on mixing, with little or no mechanical energy applied (Lawrence and Rees, 2000).

Emulsions are either oil phase dispersed in water phase, an oil-in-water (o/w) emulsion, or water phase dispersed in oil phase, a water-in-oil (w/o) emulsion. If a poorly water-soluble drug substance is soluble in oil, it can be solubilized in an emulsion where it partitions into the oil phase. The total solubility in an emulsion, S_t, is the summation of concentrations in the aqueous and oil phases (Strickley, 2004). The total solubility of the emulsion system is the sum of the drug concentration in the aqueous phase, S_w, and the concentration in the oil phase, which can be approximated by the product of the drug's solubility in the pure oil, S_{oil}, multiplied by the fraction of the oil in the emulsion, f_{oil}:

$$S_t = S_w + S_{oil} f_{oil}$$

Therefore, for compounds with good oil solubility, emulsion-based systems, especially lipid-based vehicles, can be used successfully.

Commercially available parenteral lipid emulsions, such as fat emulsion Intralipid®, usually contain 10%–20% oil phase, composed of long- or medium-chain fatty acids, lecithin, and glycerol.

Intralipid is approved for parenteral nutrition and is generally well tolerated upon intravenous administration (Li et al., 1998). Thus, large numbers of new drug candidates can be investigated without the need for intensive and time-consuming formulation development. In terms of reaching high dosing concentrations by prevention of precipitation of coadministered lipophilic nonionizable compounds, these vehicles are often superior to the formulation approaches such as pH adjustment, cosolvent, and micelles.

The formation of microemulsions usually involves a combination of oil, water, surfactant, and cosurfactant. The tendency toward a w/o (water-in-oil) or an o/w (oil-in-water) microemulsion is dependent on the properties of the oil and the surfactant, cosurfactant, the water-to-oil ratio, and the temperature. Nonionic surfactants are conveniently classified on an empirical scale known as hydrophilic–lipophilic balance (HLB), which (in practice) ranges from 1 to 20. In general, w/o microemulsions are formed using surfactants that have an HLB in the range of about 3–6 while o/w microemulsions are formed using surfactants that have an HLB value in the range of about 8–18. The role of the cosurfactant, usually a short-chain alcohol, is to increase the interfacial fluidity by penetrating into the surfactant film and consequently creating a disordered film owing to the void spaces among surfactant molecules (Leung and Shah, 1989). However, the use of cosurfactant in microemulsions is not mandatory. For maximum solubilization, it is desirable to have most of the surfactant at the interface between the oil and water, rather than dissolved in the oil or water phases. Increasing the interfacial area should also increase solubilization. The spontaneous formation of an emulsion upon drug release in the GIT presents the drug in a dissolved form, and the small droplet size provides a large interfacial surface area for drug absorption. For selecting a suitable self-emulsifying microemulsion vehicle, it is important to assess (1) the drug solubility in various components, (2) the area of self-emulsifying region in the phase diagram, and (3) droplet size distribution following self-emulsification (Kommuru et al., 2001). Self-emulsifying formulations have been assessed by simple dispersion tests in aqueous media coupled with particle size measurements to define the resulting dispersion. More recently, however, it has been suggested that additional assessment of the impact of lipid digestion on the solubilization capacity of a lipid-based formulation is required to more accurately explain the *in vivo* performance of lipid-based formulations (Dahan and Hoffman, 2006).

Microemulsion formulation process starts with the construction of pseudoternary phase diagram. The microemulsion phase was identified as the area in the phase diagram where clear and transparent formulations are obtained on the basis of visual inspection of many samples. One common approach to construct a ternary phase diagram considers two components as a single one, for example, the oil and surfactant or surfactant and cosurfactant. For the preparation of the drug-containing microemulsion, the following procedure was employed: the desired amount of the drug was first weighed out and then dissolved in the appropriate amount of oil phase. The oil phase containing the drug was subsequently added to the right amounts of the surfactant and cosurfactant mixture (Constantinides and Scalart, 1997).

Lipid emulsions have a significant impact on the pharmacokinetic profile of coadministered compounds. Depending on the time for the emulsion to circulate the system, the affinity of the drug to the oil phase, and the particle size of the oil droplets, intravenous emulsions are likely to affect the pharmacokinetics of the incorporated drug. In addition to the factors mentioned earlier, emulsion formulations for oral administration are also likely to affect the pharmacokinetics of the drug by the digestion of oil components *in vivo*. Cuine et al. (2007) reported that drug solubilization was markedly affected by lipase-mediated digestion, and a reduction in lipid (and an increase in surfactant) content resulted in increased drug precipitation. Consistent with these data, the bioavailability of Danazol decreased significantly when the lipid content in the formulations was reduced.

NANOSUSPENSIONS

A nanosuspension is a submicron colloidal dispersion of pure drug particles, which possess a large surface area for enhanced dissolution. Dissolution rate, depending on surface area and other factors, can be represented by the Noyes–Whitney equation:

$$\frac{\mathrm{d}C}{\mathrm{d}t} = \left(\frac{DS}{h} \right)(C_s - C)$$

where $\mathrm{d}C/\mathrm{d}t$ is the dissolution rate, D is the diffusion coefficient, S is the surface area, h is the diffusion layer thickness, C_s is the saturated solubility, and C is the concentration of the drug in bulk solution.

Water-insoluble drugs can be formulated as nanoparticles with high surface area and enhanced dissolution rates accompanied with reduced drug particles. Administering a compound as small particles of defined size may be superior to, for example, a cosolvent formulation. In the latter case, precipitation, particle size of the precipitate, and site of precipitation *in vivo* are difficult to control or predict from *in vitro* experiments (Pannuti et al., 1987). Assuming drug particles are in a near spherical shape, a reduction in particle size from 10 μm to 200 nm increases drug surface area by 50-fold, which may have a profound effect on drug absorption. For a drug with dissolution rate-limited bioavailability, particle size reduction can significantly improve the PK performance of the drug (Liversidge and Cundy, 1995).

Nanoparticles are typically produced by wet milling, homogenization, or precipitation techniques (Liversidge and Cundy, 1995; Merisko-Liversidge et al., 2003; Douroumis and Fahr, 2007). Nanosuspensions are thermodynamically metastable, being prone to particle regrowth and hence surface stabilizers are used to maintain particle size. The choice and concentration of stabilizers are selected to promote the particle size reduction process and generate physically stable formulations. To be effective, the stabilizer must be capable of wetting the surface of drug substance and providing a steric or ionic barrier to prevent the nanoparticle from aggregation. Many commonly used pharmaceutical excipients such as the celluloses, pluronics, polysorbates, and povidones are acceptable stabilizers for generating physically stable nanoparticle dispersions (Liversidge and Cundy, 1995). Celluloses increase aqueous viscosity and retard sedimentation of suspended drug, thereby improving dose uniformity. Common formulation includes vehicles containing dispersion agents such as hydroxylpropyl cellulose in the range of 1%–3% and surfactants such as Docusate Sodium (DOSS) in the range of 0.1%–1%.

Nanosuspensions have found wide use in recent years for oral, injectable, inhalation, and intrademeral applications (Merisko-Liversidge et al., 2003). The nanosuspension technology is extremely useful for conducting various screening studies with poorly water-soluble drugs at the preclinical stage. As the formulation does not contain high levels of excipients (cosolvents, surfactants), results of such studies can be more precisely correlated with the candidate molecule. The method has many formulation and therapeutic advantages, such as a relatively simple method of preparation, lower requirement for formulation excipients, reduction in the toxicity of the candidate drug, significant increase in the bioavailability leading to decrease in the optimal dose, decreased fed-fasted variability, and so forth (Rabinow, 2004; Wu et al., 2004; Dubey, 2006). One of the main applications of nanosuspension has been the formulation of pharmaceutical compositions that can be administered intravenously. For intravenous administration of a suspension, the particles in the suspension need to be less than 5 μm, which is the diameter of the smallest blood capillaries in the body. Intravenous administration of the nanosuspension may result in advantages such as no higher concentration of toxic cosolvents and improved therapeutic effect of the drug available as a conventional oral formulation. Nevertheless, several products are now available based on nanosuspension principles.

The nanosuspension technique usually does not work well for basic compounds with high pH-dependent solubility. When administered orally, nanoparticles of a basic drug may dissolve rapidly in stomach, but only to precipitate out in the small intestine as uncontrolled particles, thus defeating the purpose of nanosizing (Peagram et al., 2005). Some tend to agglomerate or increase in particle size owing to crystal growth (Neervannan, 2006). Another disadvantage is that not all compounds can form nanosuspensions.

AMORPHOUS SOLID DISPERSIONS

The amorphous state of drugs lacks an ordered structure and possesses higher free energy, the thermodynamic driving force that leads to higher apparent aqueous solubility and dissolution rate, which could eventually lead to improved oral absorption. The high free energy form frequently came with such disadvantages as poor physical and chemical stability. As a result, pure amorphous drugs are rarely used in formulation development. To take advantages of enhanced solubility and dissolution rate of the amorphous drugs, many amorphous solid dispersions (ASDs) have been developed. ASDs are dispersions of amorphous drug in a polymer matrix. Upon dosing, supersaturated solutions are formed, thus the flux across the intestinal membrane is greatly increased. The duration of supersaturation can last for as long as several hours, thus providing much-enhanced drug absorption. ASD technology has not only been used to drive high plasma exposures in toxicology studies with reduced variability, and to deliver challenging molecules in clinical studies (Verreck and Six, 2003; Vandecruys et al., 2007; Bikiaris, 2011), but it also has led to many successful commercial products as well (Baghel et al., 2016).

Polymers are critical components in ASDs because they act as carriers for the drug and inhibit crystallization in both the dosage form and *in vivo*. By remaining in an amorphous state during dissolution, the drug can achieve supersaturation and potentially greater absorption, when solubility is the limiting factor for absorption. In addition to *in vivo* performance considerations, polymer properties such as the glass transition temperature (Tg), solubility in organic solvents, and hygroscopicity are the key considerations in order to make the ASD stable and manufacturable. Polymers that are commonly used in ASD applications include hydroxypropyl methylcellulose (HPMC), hydroxypropyl methylcellulose acetate succinate (HPMC-AS), hydroxypropyl methylcellulose phthalate (HPMCP), polyvinylpyrrolidone (PVP), and methacylate-methacrylic acid copolymers (Eudragits). In addition to polymers, surfactants are often used as solubilizers or emulsifying agents in ASDs. The primary purpose of surfactants is to increase the apparent aqueous solubility and bioavailability of the drug. Common surfactants used in ASDs include Vitamin E-TPGS, polysorbate 20, polysorbate 80, sorbitan monostearate 60/80 (span 60/80), polyoxyl 40 hydrogenated castor oil (Cremophor RH 40), and so on.

Amorphous solid dispersions present a greater level of complexity, and require greater resources for formulation development and preparation of supplies for *in vivo* studies, when compared to the other formulation approaches that have been described in discovery support. Various amorphous solid dispersion techniques were reported in the literature. In discovery support to early phase preclinical studies, the methods of preparation typically include solvent cast, rotary evaporation, fusion, hot-melt extrusion, and spray drying.

Solvent Cast/Rotary Evaporation

Solvent-based ASD preparations enable molecular level mixing which is preferred to increase the solubility and stability of the product. Solid load is generally dictated by API/polymer/surfactant solubility in the solvent, and typically is 5%–25% by weight. This technique starts with dissolving the API and formulation components (polymers, surfactants) in a pharmaceutically acceptable solvent, followed by subsequent solvent removal. For solvent cast, the solution mixture is spread onto a mold, a scintillation vial, or a simple glass slide, and allowed to dry in a fume hood. Once dried, the film will then be collected for subsequent characterization. Preparation of ASDs by rotary evaporation is ideal for early stages (preclinical to Phase I) of drug development. After removal of the solvent, the resulting ASD is isolated, dried, and milled to the desired particle size. Secondary drying in a vacuum oven or tray dryer is often employed to remove any residual solvent that remains in the final ASD powder.

The main advantage of rotary evaporation is that the thermal decomposition of drug, surfactant and polymer can be prevented as low temperatures are typically required to evaporate organic solvents. Challenges of solvent cast/rotary evaporation method includes difficulty in finding suitable solvent systems for drug substance, surfactant and polymers, and slow rates of solvent removal often leads to drug-polymer phase separation.

Rotary evaporation is used to quickly prepare a large number of samples using mg quantities of material during early stage screening. Small samples allow for larger, more comprehensive screens to be carried out quickly while still providing enough material for meaningful characterization. Potential lead formulations can then be manufactured on a larger scale for further evaluation, including physical and chemical stability studies, *in vitro* release characterization, and *in vitro* studies in animals (Padden et al., 2011).

Spray Drying

ASD preparation by spray drying is also carried out by first dissolving the drug and formulation components (polymers, surfactants) in a pharmaceutically acceptable solvent. The total solids load in the feed solution is typically 5%–25% by weight, and this is generally dictated by API/polymer/surfactant solubility as well as viscosity of the solution. Spray drying converts a solution into a dry powder in a single step. Evaporation of solvent occurs at a very fast rate in spray drying, causing a sudden rise in viscosity that leads to the entrapment of drug molecules in the polymer matrix (Araujo et al., 2010). Because solvent evaporation time is extremely fast (on the order of seconds), spray drying is particularly advantageous for preparing ASDs of compounds with poor thermal stability. Drugs with poor aqueous solubility may be spray dried into very small particles provided that they are soluble in certain solvents suitable for spray drying. Challenges to employing spray drying during discovery and early stages of development include poor flow and compression properties due to the inherent small particle size of the resultant spray dried powder. In addition, the currently available lab scale spray dryers suffer from poor yield and generally cannot work on mg quantities of material (Padden et al., 2011).

Fusion/Hot-Melt Extrusion

The fusion method for ASD preparation involves heating a physical mixture of drug, surfactant, and polymer to form a molten mixture and then cooling and solidifying with rigorous stirring. The hot-melt extrusion method is the modern version of the fusion method in which intense mixing of the components is induced by the extruder. Compared with the traditional fusion method, melt extrusion offers the potential to shape the molten drug-polymer mixture into implants, pellets, or oral dosage forms (Patil et al., 2016). This method requires complete miscibility of the drug and polymer in the molten state. Hot-melt extrusion can be limited in the ability to process heat-sensitive and/or high melting point drugs and it is generally not amenable for manufacturing small quantities (mg to g) needed in preclinical development.

ASDs are inherently metastable systems. The chemical and physical stability of the solid dispersion formulation must be carefully evaluated to ensure that it possesses sufficient handling and storage characteristics for use in the desired study (Six et al., 2004; Vandecruys et al., 2007; Qian et al., 2010). Characterization should include analyses of both solid form and *in vitro* API release in aqueous media. Among numerous methods that are available for characterization of ASDs, polarized light microscopy (PLM), powder X-ray diffraction (pXRD), thermogravimetric analysis (TGA), and differential thermal analysis (DTA) are commonly utilized. Dynamic vapor sorption (DVS), solid-state NMR spectroscopy, Raman spectroscopy, infrared spectroscopy, and isothermal microcalorimetry are also widely employed in ASD characterization.

A simple method for drug release testing for ASD is performed by transferring a known mass of material into a known volume of biologically relevant dissolution medium (e.g., simulated gastric/intestinal fluid) under constant stirring. Solution concentrations are measured as a function of time to generate a concentration versus time release profile for the drug. Solution concentrations in significant excess of the equilibrium API solubility in the particular medium should be targeted to test the ability of the ASD to achieve and maintain supersaturation.

Accelerated stability studies on the ASDs should be conducted under stressed conditions (e.g., open dish at 40°C/75% RH, 60°C/75% RH, etc.) to understand both the physical stability of the ASD and any increased risk of chemical reactivity in the presence of excipients. Long-term stability of ASDs should be evaluated due to the increased risk of both physical and chemical instability associated with amorphous solids (Baghel et al., 2016).

PHASE APPROPRIATE FORMULATION CONSIDERATIONS

FORMULATION FOR PHARMACOKINETICS SCREENING *IN VIVO*

When an *in vitro* hit is identified, the analogous compounds are synthesized to explore the structure–activity relationships (SARs) for the structural family of compounds in an effort to maximize the desired activity and overcome the pharmacokinetic liabilities (Lombardino and Lowe, 2004). As the compounds are filtered through *in vitro* screens, selected compounds must be tested for pharmacokinetic properties *in vivo* to assess how well the *in vitro* data predict *in vivo* performance.

It is desirable to have a thorough understanding of the physicochemical properties of the drug candidate for the duration of the study, the Biopharmaceutics Classification System (BCS) class of the drug candidate, and the desired route of administration. However, at hit to lead stage, the major challenges for formulation development are limited availability of drug, short turnaround time, lack of physicochemical characterization, and unfavorable drug properties (Shah and Agnihotri, 2011).

To be able to rank order a series of compounds from discovery, it is desirable to identify standard vehicles for a particular compound series. It is also preferable to use solution formulation for the PK screening studies at this early stage as the use of the solution formulation can avoid the variability in the PK results caused by differences in dissolution rates of different crystallinities and particle sizes and provide the best performance for each compound. The most commonly used approaches include pH adjustment, cosolvents, complexation, oils, and surfactants.

If suspension formulations of the compounds are used in *in vivo* PK screening studies, it is very important to understand the impact of solid state form on PK performance before rank ordering the compounds. If 100 mg API is available, it is recommended to keep at least 5 mg of drug substance aside for possible solid state form assessment while performing *in vivo* PK screening studies. If a compound in suspension formulation gives a promising PK result, the solid state form of the compound should be evaluated by X-ray powder diffraction (XRPD), differential scanning calorimetry (DSC), and thermogravimetric analysis (TGA) to understand whether the high exposure of the compound is from a crystalline anhydrate, a solvate/hydrate, or an amorphous material. If the higher PK exposure of the molecule is the result of using more soluble amorphous material, a repeat PK study needs to be conducted using a crystalline material of the same compound. Only by doing this is the rank ordering of a series of compounds meaningful. At this early stage, most of the crystalline material can be obtained by simply slurrying amorphous material in different solvents. If the compounds in suspension formulations do not provide sufficient exposure, there is no need to conduct solid state characterization for those compounds.

Before any actual experiment, ACDLABS by Advanced Chemistry Development, Inc., or other software can be first utilized to calculate solubility, pK_a, and log P to assess the difficulty in formulation development for the compound. Glomme et al. (2005) compared the solubility generated by shake-flask method and software calculation and found that the solubility data seem to be sufficient for a first estimate of the solubility. The log P value can help us to understand if the water insolubility is caused by its high hydrophobicity or crystallinity; therefore, the appropriate solubilizing tools can be selected to enhance the solubility. For a highly hydrophobic compound, medium (mono-, di-) and long-chain triglycerides, surfactants, and oils can be used for improving solubility. If poor water solubility of the compound is caused by high crystallinity with high melting point, changing crystallinity by selecting a metastable form such as amorphous form, like amorphous solid dispersion, or switching to more soluble salts can increase the solubility.

Exotic formulation approaches such as 75% PG and 25% vitamin E TPGS, 100% PEG-400, and 50% Tween-80, 50% Imwitor 742 can also be used. The advantage of using the exotic formulation is that the compound availability is often limited and most compounds can be dissolved in these vehicles, providing a quick screening too. But these formulations are usually suitable for single dose or short-term use only. Rats are generally the species used.

Typically, in this first *in vivo* pharmacokinetic screening, both intravenous and oral formulations are administered to a rodent species, predominantly rats. If it is possible, the same formulation should be used for both intravenous and oral arms. Although in the discovery phase it is preferable to use low volume, high-concentration cosolvent formulations to increase solubility and hence the amount of drug dosed, it does have increased risks of hemolysis and tissue irritation when administered intravenously. Therefore, precaution needs to be taken not to exceed the toxicity levels for the cosolvent.

FORMULATIONS FOR PRECLINICAL PHARMACOLOGY STUDIES TO ASSESS EFFICACY

The primary objective of the early efficacy studies is to validate the pharmacology model with a compound that is known to interact with the desired receptor and develop the Pharmacokinetic–Pharmacodynamic (PK–PD) relationship for further screening during lead optimization (Neervannan, 2006). It is essential that the excipients selected for the vehicle do not interfere with the measured end points, especially for a disease-relevant animal model that has no clinically effective drugs to validate an animal model. In this situation, vehicles should be used as negative controls in the studies.

Before starting formulation development, some key factors, such as physicochemical properties of the compound, duration of action, duration of the study, and route of administration have to be considered. The easiest way to get this initial evaluation of efficacy may be to use solution formulations instead of suspensions, as solution formulations can eliminate the dissolution impact in the pharmacological end point and generally provide the best performance of the compound and, therefore, enable rank ordering of a series of compounds.

The formulation development strategies will not only depend on physicochemical properties, but also on duration of action and the desired route of administration. For a typical oral administration, formulation strategies are similar to that for *in vivo* PK screening. It is common to use supersaturated solutions in the early phase studies. However, the physical and chemical stabilities of the supersaturation systems should be well understood as the information provided will help formulation scientists to decide if the formulation needs to be prepared daily, weekly, or monthly. In general, a nucleation inhibitor should be considered to improve the stability of the supersaturated solutions. Pharmaceutical polymers, complexing agents, and surfactants have been used widely for this purpose (Brewster et al., 2007).

FORMULATION FOR PHARMACOKINETICS PROFILING AND BIOPHARMACEUTICAL ASSESSMENT

The goal of the formulation scientist at this stage is to support the candidate selection process by understanding key physicochemical properties and other factors that can affect the delivery and exposure of compounds. Well-designed and well-executed formulation support work helps to select drug candidates with appropriate physicochemical properties to ensure the suitability for pharmaceutical development. Insufficient plasma exposure after oral dosing usually results in the search for new, improved compounds, which is often combined with activities that identify the poor properties responsible for the low exposure.

At this stage, the formulation development must be considered as an interface between the drug substance and the drug product (Chassagneux, 2004). As most drugs are developed for oral administration of an eventual solid dosage form, it is often required to obtain initial data about the exposure of animals using a suspension formulation to gain information of the developmental prospects of a compound. This is particularly important for compounds with low aqueous solubility relative to expected doses. If it is possible, the most thermodynamically stable crystalline material should be used for the suspension dosing, as the most stable form of a water-insoluble compound usually gives the worst case exposures in animals. Unfortunately, the crystalline form for most of the compounds may not have been finalized at this stage. It is common to see different PK results due to batch-to-batch variations in crystalline form or particle sizes. The record about the crystal form and particle size used in the suspension formulations will facilitate better understanding of the solubility and dissolution rate impact on the PK results. The impact of solubility and dissolution rate of the solid drug substance on the rate and extent of oral drug absorption should, therefore, be evaluated and compared with the absorption achieved after oral administration with solution (or as an IV reference dosed in animals).

If absorption is solubility limited, solubility enhancement formulation techniques should be applied. The use of metastable form such as amorphous material can not only increase the solubility but also increase the dissolution rate, and the difference in apparent solubility between an amorphous and a crystalline form of a compound can be many orders of magnitude. The disadvantage of using amorphous material is the risk of form conversion from amorphous to crystalline material. Extensive physical stability studies have to be conducted before the amorphous material is selected for further development. For solubility-limited absorption, reduction of particle size will not have the desired effect of increased exposure. In contrast, for dissolution rate-limited absorption, any increases in the dissolution rate through formulation approaches, such as reduction of particle size of the solid drug or administration of a salt in the case of an ionizable compound, can lead to a profound effect on the rate and extent of drug absorption. Solution formulation, ultimately liquid filled or soft-gelatin capsule formulation, may be a choice to eliminate the dissolution step; however, it is crucial that the physical and chemical stability profiles of the solution formulation be evaluated thoroughly. Once the pharmacokinetic parameters of suspension and solution formulations of water-insoluble compounds become available, suitable formulation approaches can be evaluated, and these formulation approaches lay the foundation for future market formulation development. Hence, a proper design PK study can provide valuable information that is critical for the development risk assessment regarding the solubility as related to bioavailability. Different formulations will give different indications regarding the ability to formulate. Table 7.1 summarizes the four-tier formulation approaches and their formulation development implication proposed for animal PK studies (Huang and Tong, 2004). For instance, a traditional solid dosage formulation (tablet or capsule) could be a viable approach if the compound is having reasonable PK exposures from a suspension formulation. On the other hand, if a water-insoluble compound is showing poor bioavailability even from solution formulations, developing a traditional solid dosage form may be very challenging.

TABLE 7.1

Tier Formulation Approach for PK Studies and Its Implication for Future Formulation Development

Tier	Formulation	Formulatability Implication
1	Suspension (crystallinity and particle size monitored)	• Conventional dosage forms (capsule and tablet)
2	pH-adjusted solution	• Conventional dosage forms with salts • Most likely the best case for solubilization via a salt option
3	Nonaqueous solvents (e.g., PEG-400 and PG)	• Nonconventional dosage forms such as soft-gelatin capsule
4	Self-emulsifying lipid-based systems/microemulsions	• Nonconventional dosage forms such as soft-gelatin capsule • Many reduce bioavailability at low doses for drugs with solubility-limited absorption (drug partitioning into micelle, resulting in lower concentration of the *free* drug)
5	Nanomilling	• Best case: conventional dosage forms

Source: Huang, L. F. and Tong, W. Q., *Adv. Drug Deliv. Rev.*, 56, 321–334, 2004.

As indicated, the oral bioavailability of water-insoluble compounds can be greatly influenced by the formulation used. Occasionally, different solution formulations may provide significant differences in the animal exposure. One example by Quest Pharmaceutical Services showed that three formulations (methylcellulose [MC] suspension, PEG-400 solution, and glyceryl and PEG esters) were dosed orally to rats; both MC suspension and PEG-400 solution produced very low systemic exposure, while glyceryl and PEG esters vehicle provided approximately sevenfold greater bioavailability than the suspension or PEG solution (Aungst, 2006). Evidently, the compound dissolved in the vehicle precipitates out following dilution in the GIT to different extents. This can often lead to a confusing picture of oral bioavailability. During the formulation selection, it is important to perform precipitation studies for the solution formulation to understand the *in vivo* behavior of the formulation. Otherwise, a promising but poorly soluble lead compound might have been rejected on the basis of its initial animal pharmacokinetic results. The precipitation behavior for a given formulation in GIT can be evaluated using *in vitro* methods such as with simulated artificial media (SGF/SIF/FaSSIF/FeSSIF [Johnson et al., 2003]). Typically, the precipitation study can be carried out by adding 1, 2, 3, … , or 9 parts of SGF/SIF into 1 part of formulation, mixing well, and then monitoring the precipitation behaviors. The formulation that gives clear solution after dilution should be selected for future studies. If all the formulations show precipitation after dilution, formulation can be selected based on the precipitation behavior, such as time from dilution to precipitation, and solid state form and particle size of the precipitate.

At this stage, more precise determination of the aqueous solubility is necessary for designing appropriate formulation. These solubility measurements should ideally start with the solid compound, preferably crystalline, and the experiments should run for a long enough time, until the equilibrium is reached.

Regarding the use of beagle dogs, formulation scientists should be aware that, in case of testing weak base compounds, the dog's stomach typically has significantly higher pH values compared to human stomach pH as a nonbasal secreting species. Pretreatment of dogs with the pentapeptitide pentagastrin (a hormone gastric acid secretion stimulator [pH <2]) (Akomoto et al., 2000) with a 6 mg/kg i.m. (1 h before dosing) treatment regimen should give a pH-lowering effect from 0.5 to 1.5 h postdose (Timpe and Forschung, 2007).

Permeability is not a topic for this chapter. Poor permeability can cause poor absorption. Therefore, when several solution formulations do not give adequate animal exposure, we may be observing effects of other possible mechanisms of poor bioavailability such as permeability limitation, efflux, and metabolism.

Formulations for Preliminary Toxicological Studies

Before candidate selection, it is important to assess the preliminary toxicology of the compound as the part of the compound profiling. The primary goal of early toxicology studies is to find a dose that produces toxicity in one or more rodent or nonrodent species. The advantage at this stage is that the pharmacokinetic behavior of the molecule, as well as the compound physicochemical properties, is reasonably understood in the animal species of interest. However, the biggest challenge from a formulation perspective is that the highest desired toxicological doses can be two orders of magnitude greater than ED50 dose, and in cases where the compound does not elicit adverse effects, the doses are increased to a FDA-recommended maximum of 2 g/kg.

To avoid possible interferences of excipients with drug-related effects in long-term studies, it is preferred to dose with suspensions containing a surfactant at a level greater than the CMC with pH adjustment (e.g., 0.5%–1% HPMC or methylcellulose and 0.1% Tween-80 adjusted to pH 2–4 for bases or pH 7–9 for acids). This approach offers multiple means for solubilization, and in cases in which the solubility is very low, at a minimum, the compound will be well dispersed as a suspension in the medium, owing to the presence of HPMC. Since toxicology studies often include a wide range of doses, it is common in these studies that at lower doses, the compound is in solution, whereas at higher doses, suspensions are dosed in the same formulation. The suspension formulation often fails to provide dose-proportional increase in exposure because of poor solubility and inadequate dissolution in the GIT. To overcome the plateau effect (exposure does not increase as the dose increases), the goal of the formulation development is to maximize exposure of the molecule by enhancing solubility with formulation technologies. The use of a poor formulation in early toxicological studies can lead to an underestimation of the toxicity due to limited exposure resulting from low bioavailability.

It is desirable to keep clinical formulations in mind while developing toxicology formulations, and hopefully, the toxicology formulation can be directly used as the clinical formulation. Because of the high dose in the toxicology studies, quite often the toxicology formulation is rich in organic solvents (refer to the "Cosolvents" section in this chapter) that are not acceptable for clinical studies. It is common to develop several alternative formulations in parallel with different formulation approaches before the toxicology study, to ensure the high dose coverage. To better select the right formulations for the study, typically, formation PK screening in animals can be conducted in parallel to the *in vitro* dissolution testing.

Gad et al. (2016) summarized the comprehensive information of maximum tolerabilities for 65 single component vehicles used in 368 studies across multiple species (e.g., dog, primate, rat, mouse, rabbit, guinea pig, minipig, chick embryo, and cat) by multiple routes. The paper serves as a good reference for excipient selection in the toxicology formulation development.

Formulation Used in Preclinical Studies

A list of commonly used formulations in preclinical studies is provided in Table 7.2.

TABLE 7.2
Typical Formulation Used in Preclinical Studies

Oral

- Water with pH adjust (2–4 for bases, 7–9 for acids)[a]
- 20% HP-β-CD with and without pH adjustment[a]
- 40% Captisol® (SB-β-CD) with and without pH adjustment[a]
- 10% Cremophor EL, 10% EtOH[a]
- 10% Cremophor EL and up to 5% Tween-80
- 10% DMA, 10% EtOH, 20% propylene glycol[a]
- 100% PEG-400
- 40% PEG-400, 10% EtOH[a]
- 20% PEG-400, 10% Cremophor EL, 10% EtOH (with varying order of addition)[a]
- 0.5%–2% Cellulose derivative (methyl, hydroxypropyl methyl, hydroxypropyl, and carboxymethyl), up to 10% Tween-80, with or without pH adjustment[a]
- 0.5%–2% Cellulose derivative (methyl, hydroxypropyl methyl, hydroxypropyl, and carboxymethyl), up to 10% poloxamer (Pluronic F68 or Pluronic F108), with or without pH adjustment[a]
- 10%–50% DMSO[a]
- 25% Propylene glycol, 20% vitamin E TPGS in PEG-400[a]
- 25% Vitamin E TPGS and 75% propylene glycol
- 50% Imwitor 742 and 50% Tween-80
- Corn oil, soybean oil, or sesame oil with or without surfactant
- Oil suspension: corn oil, sesame oil, soybean oil with up to 30% surfactant
- Up to 30% Solutol HS 15 (polyethylene glycol/hydroxystearate) in water (w/w)[a]
- 20% Solutol HS 15, 30% PEG-400, with or without pH adjust or with or without surfactant
- 10% DMA, 20% propylene glycol, 40% PEG-400[a]
- 5% Labrasol in PEG-400[a]
- Up to 10% Tween-80 or 10% poloxamer
- 20% Vitamin E TPGS, 60% PEG-400, 5% PVP
- Milling/nanosuspension

Intravenous

- Up to 20% HP-β-CD with and without pH adjust (4–9)[a]
- Up to 40% Captisol (SB-β-CD) with and without pH adjust (4–9)[a]
- 10% Cremophor EL, 10% EtOH[a]
- 100% DMSO: single dose only[a]
- 10% DMA, 10% EtOH, 20% propylene glycol: single dose only[a]
- 20% Intralipid emulsion containing 5%–10% soybean oil, 1%–3% soy or egg lecithin and buffer[a]
- Solutol HS 15, up to 10%
- Up to 50% propylene glycol
- Up to 50% PEG-300
- Up to 50% PEG-400[a]
- Up to 40% DMA[a]
- Up to 40% NMP[a]
- Up to 40% glycerol[a]
- Up to 15% poloxamer[a]
- Up to 40% dimethylisosorbide[a]
- Nanosuspensions (90% particles <1 μm) with 1%–1.5% HPC-SL and 0.05%–0.1% docusate sodium (0.1% Tween-80 or 0.1% SLS can be substituted for docusate sodium)[a]

Notes: All formulations quantity sufficient (q.s.) to volume with aqueous component (except in cases where the excipient is at 100%). All vehicles dosed intravenously can also be dosed intraperitoneally.

DMA: Dimethylacetamide; DMSO: Dimethyl sulfoxide; HPC-SL: Hydroxypropyl cellulose, grade SL; PBS: Phosphate-buffered saline; SLS: Sodium lauryl sulfate; TPGS: α-Tocopheryl polyethylene glycol 1000 succinate.

[a] Neervannan, S., *Drug Metab. Toxicol.*, 2, 715–731, 2006.

ANIMAL SPECIES AND ROUTES CONSIDERATION

Since different animal species were used in various stages of compound evaluations, it is essential to understand the limitations of various animal species and dosing routes. Table 7.3 lists the typical dosing volumes for various routes and animal species.

FORMULATION STABILITY AND CHARACTERIZATION

For a drug to be absorbed from the GIT, the dose must dissolve or be in solution in the GI fluids during transit; hence, the compound has to be stable in GI fluids for at least 24 h. Typically, at an early stage, 24 h chemical stability of the compound in simulated intestinal fluid and simulated gastric fluid with and without light protection needs to be checked to ensure that the efficacy or PK profile is indeed generated by the compound and not by the degradation materials. Once there is enough drug substance available, the chemical stability studies should be conducted for all the formulations developed in supporting the *in vivo* studies. The duration of the stability study should cover the duration of the intended animal study. At this stage, daily preparation of the formulation is common; the instability issue can be usually resolved later through more lab-intensive formulation development and or salt selection.

TABLE 7.3
Typical Dosing Volumes of Formulations in Various Animal Species and through Various Routes of Administration

Animal Species	Nominal Weight (kg)	Route of Administration	Ideal Dose Volume	
			mL/kg	mL
Rat	0.25	Oral	10	2.5
		Intravenous (bolus injection)[a]	5	1.25
		Intravenous (slow injection)[b]	20	5
		Intraperitoneal	10	2.5
		Subcutaneous	5	1.25
Mouse	0.025	Oral	10	0.25
		Intravenous (bolus injection)[a]	5	0.125
		Intravenous (slow injection)[b]	25	0.625
		Intraperitoneal	10	0.25
		Subcutaneous	5	0.125
Dog	10	Oral	5	50
		Intravenous (bolus injection)[a]	1	10
		Intravenous (slow injection)[b]	5	50
		Intraperitoneal	1	10
		Subcutaneous	1	10
Monkey	4	Oral	5	20
		Intravenous (bolus injection)[a]	1	4
		Intraperitoneal	3	12
		Subcutaneous	1	4

Source: Diehl, K.-H. et al., *J. Appl. Toxicol.*, 21, 15–23, 2001; Neervannan, S., *Drug Metab. Toxicol.*, 2, 715–731, 2006.

[a] Bolus injection is typically defined as administration over a short period of time (~1 min).

[b] Slow injection is defined as administration over a course of 5–10 min.

It is important to characterize the physicochemical properties of the suspensions well, so that the PK data can be interpreted appropriately. Typical characterization of the drug substance includes purity, residual solvents, aqueous solubility profile (pH 2, FaSSIF), crystallinity (XRPD/DSC), particle size, pK_a, and log P. For solution formulations at various stages of discovery studies, dose analysis is essential, and for efficacy assessment and toxicology studies, chemical stability for the duration of study needs to be evaluated. For suspension formulations, the homogeneity can be determined by particle size and crystallinity using optical microscopy. Chemical stability and physical stability (for form conversion) need to be monitored for long-term studies such as efficacy assessments or toxicology studies.

REFERENCES

Akomoto, M., N. Furuya, A. Fukushima, K. Higuchi, F. Shohei, and T. Suwa (2000). Gastric pH profiles of beagle dogs and their use as an alternative to human testing. *Eur. J. Pharm. Biopharm.*, 49: 99–102.

Alibrandi, G., S. Coppolino, N. Micali, and A. Villari (2001). Variable pH kinetics: An easy determination of pH-rate profile. *J. Pharm. Sci.*, 90: 270–274.

Alvarez-Nunez, F. A. and S. H. Yalkowsky (1999). Buffer capacity and precipitation control of pH solubilized phenytoin formulations. *Int. J. Pharm.*, 185: 45–49.

Amidon, G. L., H. Lennernas, V. P. Shah, and J. R. Crison (1995). A theoretical basis for a biopharmaceutic drug classification: the correlation of *in vitro* drug product dissolution and *in vivo* bioavailability. *Pharm. Res.*, 12: 413–420.

Araujo, R., C. Teixeira, and L. Freitas (2010). The preparation of ternary solid dispersions of an herbal drug via spray drying of liquid feed. *Dry Technol.*, 28: 412–421.

Aungst, B. J. (2006). Optimising oral bioavailability of pharmaceutical leads. *AAPS Newsmagazine*, 9: 14–47.

Baghel, S., H. Cathcart, and N. J. O'Reilly (2016). Polymeric amorphous solid dispersions: A review of amorphization, crystallization, stabilization, solid-state characterization, and aqueous solubilization of Biopharmaceutical Classification System class II drugs. *J. Pharm. Sci.*, 105(9): 2527–2544.

Balbach, S. and C. Korn (2004). Pharmaceutical evaluation of early development candidates "the 100 mg-approach." *Int. J. Pharm.*, 275: 1–12.

Bikiaris, D. N. (2011). Solid dispersions, part I: Recent evolutions and future opportunities in manufacturing methods for dissolution rate enhancement of poorly water-soluble drugs. *Exp. Opin. Drug Deliv.*, 8(11): 1501–1519.

Bittner, B. and R. J. Mountfield (2002). Intravenous administration of poorly soluble new drug entities in early drug discovery: The potential impact of formulation on pharmacokinetic parameters. *Curr. Opin. Drug Disc. Dev.*, 5: 59–71.

Brewster, M., C. Mackie, M. Noppe, A. Lampo, and T. Loftsson (2007). The use of solubilizing excipients and approaches to generate toxicology vehicles for contemporary drug pipelines. In P. Augustijns and M. Brewster (Eds.), *Solvent Systems and Their Selection in Pharmaceutics and Biopharmaceutics*, New York: Springer, pp. 221–256.

Challa, R., A. Ahuja, J. Ali, and R. Khar (2005). Cyclodextrins in drug delivery: An updated review. *AAPS Pharm. Sci. Tech.*, 6: E329–E357.

Chassagneux, E. (2004). Preformulation and formulation development as tools for a good balance between time constraints and risks. *Business Briefing: Pharm Tech.*, 2004: 1–4.

Chaubal, M. V. (2004). Application of formulation technologies in lead candidate selection and optimization. *Drug Discov. Today*, 9: 603–609.

Chen, X.-Q., M. D. Antman, C. Gesenberg, and O. S. Gudmundsson (2006). Discovery pharmaceutics—Challenges and opportunities. *AAPS J.*, 8: E402–E408.

Constantinides, P. P. and J.-P. Scalart (1997). Formulation and physical characterization of water-in-oil microemulsions containing long- versus medium-chain glycerides. *Int. J. Pharm.*, 158: 57–68.

Cuine, J. F., W. N. Charman, C. W. Pouton, G. A. Edwards, and C. J. H. Porter (2007). Increasing the proportional content of surfactant (Cremophor EL) relative to lipid in self-emulsifying lipid-based formulations of Danazol reduces oral bioavailability in beagle dogs. *Pharm. Res.*, 24: 748–757.

Dahan, A. and A. Hoffman (2006). Use of a dynamic *in vitro* lipolysis model to rationalize oral formulation development for poor water-soluble drugs: Correlation with *in vivo* data and the relationship to intraenterocyte processes in rats. *Pharm. Res.*, 23: 2165–2174.

Diehl, K.-H., R. Hull, D. Morton, R. Pfister, Y. Rabemampianina, D. Smith, J.-M. Vidal, and C. van de Vorstenbosch (2001). A good practice guide to the administration of substances and removal of blood, including routes and volumes. *J. Appl. Toxicol.*, 21: 15–23.

Douroumis, D. and A. Fahr (2007). Stable carbamazepine colloidal systems using the cosolvent technique. *Eur. J. Pharm. Sci.*, 30: 367–374.

Dubey, R. (2006). Impact of nanosuspension technology on drug discovery & development. *Drug Deliv. Tech.*, 6: 65, 67–71.

Faucci, M. T. and P. Mura (2001). Effect of water-soluble polymers on naproxen complexation with natural and chemically modified β-cyclodextrins. *Drug Dev. Ind. Pharm.*, 27: 909–917.

Francis, M. F., M. Cristea, and F. M. Winnik (2004). Polymeric micelles for oral drug delivery: Why and how. *Pure Appl. Chem.*, 76: 1321–1335.

Frijlink, H. W., J. Visser, N. R. Hefting, R. Oosting, D. K. F. Meijer, and C. F. Lerk (1990). The pharmacokinetics of β-cyclodextrin and hydroxypropyl-β-cyclodextrin in the rat. *Pharm. Res.*, 7: 1248–1252.

Gad, S. C., C. B. Spainhour, C. Shoemake, D. R. S. Pallman, A. Stricker-Krongrad, P. A. Downing, R. E. Seals, L. A. Eagle, K. Polhamus, and J. Daly (2016). Tolerable levels of nonclinical vehicles and formulations used in studies by multiple routes in multiple species with notes on methods to improve utility. *Int. J. Toxicol.*, 25: 499–521.

Gardner, C. R., C. T. Walsh, and O. Almarsson (2004). Drugs as materials: Valuing physical form in drug discovery. *Nat. Rev. Drug Discov.*, 3: 926–934.

Gillies, E. R. and J. M. J. Fréchet (2004). Development of acid-sensitive copolymer micelles for drug delivery. *Pure Appl. Chem.*, 76: 1295–1307.

Glomme, A., J. Marz, and J. B. Dressman (2005). Comparison of a miniaturized shake-flask solubility method with automated potentiometric acid/base titrations and calculated solubilities. *J. Pharm. Sci.*, 94: 1–16.

Govindarajan, R. and M. S. Nagarsenker (2005). Formulation studies and *in vivo* evaluation of a flurbiprofen-hydroxypropyl β-cyclodextrin system. *Pharm. Dev. Technol.*, 10: 105–114.

Grosse, P. Y., F. Bresolle, P. Rouanet, J. M. Joulia, and F. Pinguet (1999). Methyl-β-cyclodextrin and doxorubicin pharmacokinetics and tissue concentrations following bolus injection of these drugs alone or together in the rabbit. *Int. J. Pharm.*, 180: 215–223.

Huang, L. F. and W. Q. Tong (2004). Impact of solid state properties on developability assessment of drug candidates. *Adv. Drug Deliv. Rev.*, 56: 321–334.

Irie, T. and K. Uekama (1997). Pharmaceutical applications of cyclodextrins. 3. Toxicological issues and safety evaluation. *J. Pharm. Sci.*, 86: 147–162.

Johnson, J. L. H., Y. He, and S. H. Yalkowsky (2003). Prediction of precipitation-induced phlebitis: A statistical validation of an *in vitro* model. *J. Pharm. Sci.*, 92: 1574–1581.

Jonkman-de Vries, J. D., K. P. Flora, A. Bult, and J. H. Beijnen (1996). Pharmaceutical development (investigational) anticancer agents for parenteral use—A review. *Drug Dev. Ind. Pharm.*, 22: 475–494.

Kataoka, K., G. S. Kwon, M. Yokoyama, T. Okano, and Y. Sakurai (1993). Block copolymer micelles as vehicles for drug delivery. *J. Control. Release*, 24: 119–132.

Kawakami, K., K. Miyoshi, and Y. Ida (2004). Solubilization behavior of poorly soluble drugs with combined use of gelucire 44/14 and cosolvent. *J. Pharm. Sci.*, 93: 1471–1479.

Kawakami, K., N. Oda, K. Miyoshi, T. Funaki, and Y. Ida (2006). Solubilization behavior of a poorly soluble drug under combined use of surfactants and cosolvents. *Eur. J. Pharm. Sci.*, 28: 7–14.

Kerns, E. H. and L. Di (2002). Multivariate pharmaceutical profiling for drug discovery. *Curr. Top. Med. Chem.*, 2: 87–98.

Kommuru, T. R., B. Gurley, M. A. Khan, and I. K. Reddy (2001). Self-emulsifying drug delivery systems (SEDDS) of coenzyme Q10: formulation development and bioavailability assessment. *Int. J. Pharm.*, 212: 233–246.

Krzyzaniak, J. F., D. M. Raymond, and S. H. Yalkowsky (1997). Lysis of human red blood cells 2: Effect of contact time on cosolvent induced hemolysis. *Int. J. Pharm.*, 152: 193–200.

Lawrence, M. J. and G. D. Rees (2000). Microemulsion-based media as novel drug delivery systems. *Adv. Drug Deliv. Rev.*, 45: 89–121.

Lee, Y.-C., P. D. Zocharski, and B. Samas (2003). An intravenous formulation decision tree for discovery compound formulation development. *Int. J. Pharm.*, 253: 111–119.

Leung, R. and D. O. Shah (1989). Microemulsions: An evolving technology for pharmaceutical applications. In M. Rossof (Ed.), *Controlled Release of Drugs: Polymers and Aggregate Systems*, New York: VCH, pp. 85–215.

Li, G.-X., J.-H. Che, B.-C. Kang, W.-W. Lee, J.-H. Ihm, J.-Y. Jung, B.-H. Yi, J.-S. Nam, J.-H. Park, and Y.-S. Lee (1998). Acute toxicity and four-week intravenous toxicity studies of intralipid. *J. Toxicol. Public Health*, 14: 443–452.

Li, P., L. Zhao, and S. H. Yalkowsky (1999). Combined effect of cosolvent and cyclodextrin on solubilization of nonpolar drugs journal of pharmaceutical sciences. *J. Pharm. Sci.*, 88: 1107–1111.

Lipinski, C. (2002). Poor aqueous solubility—an industry wide problem in drug discovery. *Am. Pharm. Rev.*, 5(3): 82–85.

Lipinski, C. A., F. Lombardo, B. W. Dominy, and P. J. Feeney (1997). Experimental and computational approaches to estimate solubility and permeability in drug discovery and development settings. *Adv. Drug Deliv. Rev.*, 23: 3–25.

Liversidge, G. G. and K. C. Cundy (1995). Particle size reduction for improvement of oral bioavailability of hydrophobic drugs: I. Absolute bioavailability of nanocrystalline danazol in beagle dogs. *Int. J. Pharm.*, 125: 91–97.

Loftsson, T. and M. Brewster (1996). Pharmaceutical applications of cyclodextrins. 1. Drug solubilization and stabilization. *J. Pharm. Sci.*, 85: 1017–1025.

Loftsson, T., A. Magnusdottir, M. Masson, and J. F. Sigurjonsdottir (2002). Self-association and cyclodextrin solubilization of drugs. *J. Pharm. Sci.*, 91: 2307–2316.

Loftsson, T., B. Olafsdottir, H. Fridriksdottir, and S. Jonsdottir (1993). Cyclodextrin complexation of NSAIDs: Physicochemical characteristics. *Eur. J. Pharm. Sci.*, 1: 95–101.

Lombardino, J. G. and J. A. Lowe III (2004). The role of the medicinal chemist in drug discovery—Then and now. *Nat. Rev. Drug Discov.*, 3: 853–862.

Maas, J., W. Kamm, and G. Hauck (2007). An integrated early formulation strategy—From hit evaluation to preclinical candidate profiling. *Eur. J. Pharm. Biopharm.*, 66: 1–10.

Merisko-Liversidge, E., G. G. Liversidge, and E. R. Cooper (2003). Nanosizing—A formulation approach for poorly water-soluble compounds. *Eur. J. Pharm. Sci.*, 18: 113–120.

Miller, L. A., R. L. Carrier, and I. Ahmed (2006). Practical considerations in development of solid dosage forms that contain cyclodextrin. *J. Pharm. Sci.*, 96: 1691–1707.

Mountfield, R. J., S. Senepin, M. Schleimer, I. Walter, and B. Bittner (2000). Potential inhibitory effects of formulation ingredients on intestinal cytochrome P450. *Int. J. Pharm.*, 211: 89–92.

Nagarsenker, M. S., R. N. Meshram, and G. Ramprakash (2000). Solid dispersion of hydroxypropyl-β-cyclodextrin and ketorolac: Enhancement of *in-vitro* dissolution rates, improvement in anti-inflammatory activity and reduction in ulcerogenicity in rats. *J. Pharm. Pharmacol.*, 52: 949–956.

Nandi, I., M. Bateson, M. Bari, and H. N. Joshi (2003). Synergistic effect of PEG-400 and cyclodextrin to enhance solubility of progesterone. *AAPS Pharm. Sci. Tech.*, 4: 1–5.

Neervannan, S. (2006). Preclinical formulations for discovery and toxicology: Physicochemical challenges. *Exp. Opin. Drug Metab. Toxicol.*, 2: 715–731.

Padden, B. E., J. M. Miller, T. Robbins, P. D. Zocharski, L. Prasad, J. K. Spence, and J. LaFountaine (2011). Amorphous solid dispersions as enabling formulations for discovery and early development. *Am. Pharm. Rev.*, 14(1): 66–73.

Pannuti, F., C. M. Camaggi, E. Strocchi, and R. Comparsi (1987). Medroxyprogesterone acetate plasma pharmacokinetics after intravenous administration to rabbits. *Cancer Chemother. Pharmacol.*, 19: 311–314.

Patil, H., R. Tiwari, and M. Repka (2016). Hot-melt extrusion: From theory to application in pharmaceutical formulation. *AAPS PharmSciTech.*, 17(1): 20–42.

Peagram, R., R. Gibb, and K. Sooben (2005). The rational selection of formulations for preclinical studies—An industrial perspective. *Bull. Tech. Gattefossé*, 98: 53–64.

Pitha, J. and T. Hoshino (1992). Effect of ethanol on formation of inclusion complexes of hydroxypropylcyclo-dextrins with testosterone or with methyl orange. *Int. J. Pharm.*, 80: 243–251.

Portmann, G. A. and M. Simmons (1995). Microscopic determination of drug solubility in plasma and calculation of injection rates with a plasma circulatory model to prevent precipitation on intravenous injection. *J. Pharm. Biomed. Anal.*, 13: 1189–1193.

Pritchard, J. F., M. Jurima-Romet, M. L. J. Reimer, E. Mortimer, B. Rolfe, and M. N. Cayen (2003). Making better drugs: Decision gates in non-clinical drug development. *Nat. Rev. Drug Discov.*, 2: 542–553.

Qian, F., J. Huang, and M. A. Hussain (2010). Drug-polymer solubility and miscibility: Stability consideration and practical challenges in amorphous solid dispersion development. *J. Pharm. Sci.*, 99(7): 2941–2947.

Rabinow, B. E. (2004). Nanosuspensions in drug delivery. *Nat. Rev. Drug Disc.*, 3: 785–796.

Rajewski, R. A. and V. J. Stella (1996). Pharmaceutical applications of cyclodextrins. 2. *In vivo* drug delivery. *J. Pharm. Sci.*, 85: 1142–1169.

Rao, V., M. Nerurkar, S. Pinnamaneni, F. Rinaldi, and K. Raghavan (2006). Co-solubilization of poorly soluble drugs by micellization and complexation. *Int. J. Pharm.*, 319: 98–106.

Rao, V. and V. J. Stella (2003). When can cyclodextrins be considered for solubilization purposes? *J. Pharm. Sci.*, 92: 927–932.

Redenti, E., L. Szente, and J. Szejtli (2000). Drug/cyclodextrin/hydroxy acid multicomponent systems. Properties and pharmaceutical applications. *J. Pharm. Sci.*, 89: 1–8.

Redenti, E., L. Szente, and J. Szejtli (2001). Cyclodextrin complexes of salts of acidic drugs. Thermodynamic properties, structural features, and pharmaceutical applications. *J. Pharm. Sci.*, 90: 979–986.

Rubino, J. T. and S. H. Yalkowsky (1987). Cosolvency and deviations from log-linear solubilization. *Pharm. Res.*, 4: 231–236.

Savolainen, J., K. Jarvinen, H. Taipale, P. Jarho, T. Loftsson, and T. Jarvinen (1998). Co-administration of a water-soluble polymer increases the usefulness of cyclodextrins in solid dosage forms. *Pharm. Res.*, 15: 1696–1701.

Shah, A. and S. A. Agnihotri (2011). Recent advances and novel strategies in pre-clinical formulation development: An overview. *J. Control. Release*, 156: 281–296.

Shokri, J., A. Nokhodchi, A. Dashbolaghi, D. Hassan-Zadeh, T. Ghafourian, and J. Barzegar (2001). The effects of surfactants on the skin penetration of diazepam. *Int. J. Pharm.*, 228: 99–107.

Six, K., G. Verreck, J. Peeters, M. Brewster, and G. Van Den Mooter (2004). Increased physical stability and improved dissolution properties of itraconazole, a class II drug, by solid dispersions that combine fast- and slow-dissolving polymers. *J. Pharm. Sci.*, 93(1): 124–131.

Stahl, P. H. and C. G. Wermuth (Eds.) (2002). *Handbook of Pharmaceutical Salts—Properties, Selection, and Use*, New York: Wiley-VCH.

Strickley, R. G. (2004). Solubilizing excipients in oral and injectable formulations. *Pharm. Res.*, 21: 201–230.

Sweetana, S. and M. J. Akers (1996). Solubility principles and practices for parenteral drug dosage form development. *PDA J. Pharm. Sci.*, 50(5): 330–342.

Szente, L. and J. Szejtli (1999). Highly soluble cyclodextrin derivatives: Chemistry, properties, and trends in development. *Adv. Drug Deliv. Rev.*, 36: 17–28.

Ten Tije, A. J., J. Verweij, W. J. Loos, and A. Sparreboom (2003). Pharmacological effects of formulation vehicles—Implications for cancer chemotherapy. *Clin. Pharmacokinet.*, 42: 665–685.

Timpe, C. and L. Forschung (2007). Strategies for formulation development of poorly water-soluble drug candidates—A recent perspective. *Am. Pharm. Rev.*, 10: 104–109.

Torchilin, V. P. (2007). Micellar nanocarriers: Pharmaceutical perspectives. *Pharm. Res.*, 24: 1–16.

Trivedi, J. S. and M. L. Wells (2000). Solubilization using cosolvent approach. In R. Liu (Ed.), *Water-Insoluble Drug Formulation*, Denver, CO: Interpharm Press, pp. 141–168.

Uchegbu, I. F. and A. T. Florence (1996). Adverse drug events related to dosage forms and delivery systems. *Drug Saf.*, 14: 39–67.

van Zuylen, L., J. Verweij, and A. Sparreboom (2001). Role of formulation vehicles in taxane pharmacology. *Invest. New Drugs*, 19: 125–141.

Vandecruys, R., J. Verreck, and M. E. Brewster (2007). Use of a screening method to determine excipients which optimize the extent and stability of supersaturated drug solutions and application of this system to solid formulation design. *Int. J. Pharm.*, 342(1–2): 168–175.

Venkatesh, S. and R. A. Lipper (2000). Role of the development scientist in compound lead selection and optimization. *J. Pharm. Sci.*, 3: 145–154.

Verreck, G. and K. Six (2003). Characterization of solid dispersion of itraconazole and hydroxypropylmethylcellulose prepared by melt extrusion—Part I. *Int. J. Pharm.*, 251(1–2): 165–174.

Wu, S. H.-W. and W. K. Hopkins (1999). Characteristics of d-α-tocopheryl PEG 1000 succinate for applications as an absorption enhancer in drug delivery systems. *Pharm. Tech.*, 23: 44–58.

Wu, W., A. Loper, E. Landis, L. Hettrick, L. Novak, K. Lynn, C. Chen et al. (2004). The role of biopharmaceutics in the development of a clinical nanoparticle formulation of MK-0869: A beagle dog model predicts improved bioavailability and diminished food effect on absorption in human. *Int. J. Pharm.*, 285: 135–146.

Yalkowsky, S. H., J. F. Krzyzaniak, and G. H. Ward (1998). Formulation-related problems associated with intravenous drug delivery. *J. Pharm. Sci.*, 87: 787–796.

8 Application of Complexation in Drug Development for Insoluble Compounds

Wei-Qin (Tony) Tong and Hong Wen

CONTENTS

INTRODUCTION

Despite significant effort and progress in improving the developability of drug candidates, poor aqueous solubility remains to be one of the major challenges to formulation scientists as nearly 40% of marketed drugs and 90% of molecules in the discovery pipeline are poorly water-soluble (Kalepu and Nekkanti 2015). As one of the most well-studied traditional solubilization techniques, complexation has also been used to increase drug stability, reduce gastrointestinal drug irritation, and so on (Szekely-Szentmiklosi and Tokes 2011). In the recent years, the increased applications of cyclodextrins (CDs), cyclic carbohydrates known to form complexes with hydrophobic drugs, and the successful approval of CD-containing products have resulted in increased interest in this technology. The objectives of this chapter are to discuss some theoretical and practical considerations in applying the complexation technique, and to review the recent applications of CD-based complexation.

BACKGROUND

DEFINITIONS

A complex is a species of definite substrate (S)-to-ligand (L) stoichiometry that can be formed in an equilibrium process, in solution, and also may exist in the solid state (Connors 1990). This definition can be expressed succinctly in the following chemical equation for the formation of a complex S_mL_n.

$$mS + nL \rightleftharpoons S_mL_n \qquad (8.1)$$

The distinction between substrate and ligand is arbitrary, and is made solely for experimental convenience. Normally, stoichiometric ratios are expressed in the order substrate: ligand, so that 1:2 stoichiometry denotes SL_2, 2:1 means S_2L, and so on.

TYPES OF COMPLEXES

Based on the type of chemical bonding, complexes can generally be classified into two groups (Connors 1990):

> *Coordination complexes*: These complexes are formed by coordinate bonds in which a pair of electrons is, in some degree, transferred from one molecule to the other. The most important examples are the metal-ion coordination complexes between metal ions and bases.
> *Molecular complexes*: These species are formed by non-covalent interactions between the substrate and ligand. Among the kinds of complex species included in this class are small molecule-small molecule complexes, small molecule-macromolecule species, ion-pairs, dimers and other self-associated species, and inclusion complexes in which one of the molecules, the *host*, forms or possesses a cavity into which it can admit a *guest* molecule.

The classification of complexes into various types is somewhat arbitrary. They can also be classified based on the types of species involved and the nature of interaction forces (Repta 1981). In addition to typical binary complexes, ternary complexes are supramolecular systems composed of three different molecular entities whose third component, as an auxiliary component, in conjunction with CD, further improves desired properties of a drug product (Lokamatha et al. 2010; Kurkov and Loftsson 2013). Most pharmaceutically useful systems are inclusion complexes and molecular complexes between small molecules. Therefore, these will be the topic of this chapter.

ADVANTAGES AND DISADVANTAGES OF COMPLEXATION

Solubilization by complexation is achieved through specific interactions rather than changes in bulk solvent properties as in other solubilizing systems such as co-solvents, emulsions and pH-adjustment. The dissociation is very rapid (Cramer et al. 1967; Hersey et al. 1986), quantitative, and therefore, predictable. Another significant advantage of the complexation technique is that some commonly used complexing agents such as hydroxypropyl-β-cyclodextrin (HP-β-CD) and sulfobutylether of β-CD (SBE-β-CD) are less toxic compared to other solubilizing agents such as surfactants and co-solvents. Since most complexes formed are 1:1 complexes of the A linear (AL) type, dilution of the complex will not result in a solution which is supersaturated with respect to substrate. This can be rather important for very insoluble compounds that may precipitate upon injection when solubilized by other systems such as co-solvents. Furthermore, complexation can be combined together with solid dispersion approaches to improve the bioavailability of water-insoluble drugs (Zoeller et al. 2012).

Another major advantage of CD complexation is the improvement in chemical stability of the guest, for example, resistance to oxidation, photolysis, or hydrolysis (Uekama et al. 1983b). Nagase et al. (2001) reported that SBE-β-CD significantly solubilized DY-9760e, a novel cytoprotective agent, through forming a drug-CD complex. It also markedly suppressed the photo-degradation of DY-9760e in aqueous solution and inhibited the adsorption of DY-9760e from solution to polyvinyl chloride (PVC) tubes. The stability enhancement by CD complexation is important not only to the chemical and physical stability of the products but also to the *in vivo* performance of the products.

Despite all the attractive advantages of complexation, there are several disadvantages. First of all the compound has to be able to form complexes with a selected ligand. For compounds with very limited solubility to start with, the solubility enhancement can be very limited. The second limitation is that for the complexes of A_p type, dilution of a system may still result in precipitation. This is also true for solubilization *via* combined techniques such as complexation with pH adjustment. Third, the potential toxicity issue, regulatory, and quality control issues related to the presence of the ligand may add complication and cost to the development process. Lastly, the complexation efficiency is often rather low, thus relatively large amount of CDs are typically required to achieve desirable solubilization effect (Loftsson et al. 1999).

STRUCTURES AND PHYSICOCHEMICAL PROPERTIES OF CYCLODEXTRINS

CDs are cyclic oligosaccharides consisting of a variable number of D-glucose residues attached by α-(1,4) linkages (Clarke et al. 1988). The three most important of these are α-, β-, and γ-CDs, which respectively consist of six, seven, and eight D-glucose units. Their conformation and numbering are presented in Figure 8.1. As a consequence of the $^4C_1$ conformation of the α-D-glucose residues and lack of free rotation about glycosidic bonds, the compounds are not perfectly cylindrical molecules, but are somewhat cone-shaped, with all of the secondary hydroxyl groups situated at one end of the annulus and the primary hydroxyl groups at the other. The cavity is lined by a ring of hydrogen atoms (bonded to C-5), a ring of D-glucosidic oxygen atoms, and another ring of hydrogen atoms (bonded to C-3), thus making the cavity relatively apolar. The shape of the molecule is stabilized by hydrogen bonds between secondary hydroxyl groups of adjacent α-D-glucose residues. The internal cavity diameters are approximately 5.7, 7–8, and 9.5 Å for α-, β-, and γ-CDs respectively. These structural features have been determined for the crystalline state (Hursthouse et al. 1982; Koehler et al. 1987; Vicens et al. 1988; Harata 1989) and are also retained in solution (Rao and Foster 1963; Glass 1965; Casu et al. 1970). Figure 8.2 shows the physical shape of the CD molecule.

Most of the CD derivatives presently in application are synthesized from β-CD. The main drawbacks, particularly in the case of β-CD, are related to parenteral toxicity and low aqueous

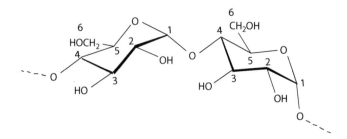

FIGURE 8.1   Conformation and numbering of the cyclodextrins (CDs).

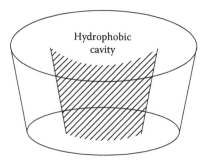

FIGURE 8.2   Physical shape of the cyclodextrin (CD) molecule.

solubility. The solubility of β-CD in water is only 1.85 g/100 mL, compared to 15 g/100 mL for α-CD and 23 g/100 mL for γ-CD. Suitable chemical modification leads to amorphous or at least partially crystalline CD derivatives with high aqueous solubility and considerable reduced parenteral toxicity, depending on the type, degree, and patterns of substitution. The two modi-fied CDs that have received the greatest attention are the HP-β-CDs and SBE-β-CDs, mainly as (SBE)7M-β-CD (Stella and Rajewski 1997; Ammar et al. 2006). The solubility of underivatized CDs generally increases with increasing temperature. On the other hand, the aqueous solubility of methylated CDs is inversely proportional to temperature. An increase in temperature may cause the dehydration of methylated CDs in a manner similar to nonionic surfactants (Uekama 1985).

The physical dimensions of inner cavity of HP-β-CD, that is, 7–8 Å, should be similar to those of its parent. The other dimensions such as height of the torus, diameter of the periphery, and effective volume of the cavity, can only be estimated to fall within a broad range, because of the freely rotating nature of the hydroxypropyl adducts. In the case of SBE-β-CDs, the long hydro-phobic groups with an ionic head in the substituent are expected to align themselves to reduce interactions with the aqueous environment similar to micellar formation, resulting in an extended hydrophobic cavity. Because the anionic sulfates repel each other, the opening of the cavity is still maintained.

CDs are fairly stable in alkaline media, whereas they are hydrolytically cleaved by strong acids to give linear oligosaccharides (Bender and Komiyama 1978). The acid-catalyzed ring-opening rate depends upon the cavity size; the larger the cavity, the greater the rate will be. The presence of guest molecules has been showed to decelerate the ring-opening rate of β-CD (Uekama et al. 1994). The authors attributed this to inhibition of access of catalytic oxonium ions to the glycosidic bond, because the CD cavity is occupied by guests.

METHODS FOR STUDYING COMPLEXATION

MEASUREMENT OF BINDING CONSTANTS IN SOLUTION

To find out if a drug (substrate) can form a complex with any potential ligand molecule and the stability of the complex, one will need to measure the binding constants of complexes. Generally speaking, any methodology, such as surface tension measurements (Baszkin et al. 1999), which can relate the changes in one or more properties of the system which are caused by intermolecular interaction, may be utilized. Several methods that are widely used in the pharmaceutical industry, including solubility measurement, UV spectroscopic analysis, kinetic method and titration calorimetry, are described in detail here.

Solubility Measurement

The solubility of a substance will change upon the formation of a complex with a second substance. The extent of solubility alteration directly relates to the binding affinity of the two compounds. Therefore, it is possible to evaluate equilibrium constants from solubility data (Higuchi and Connors 1965).

The heart of the solubility method is the solubility diagram which is constructed by plotting the total molar concentration of substrate (S_T) dissolved in solution against total ligand concentration (L_T). According to the solubility of the complex formed, phase solubility diagrams are generally classified into type A and type B diagrams as shown in Figure 8.3.

In type A diagrams, the formation of soluble complexes $(S_m L_n)$ results in an increase in the total amount of substrate in solution. If all complexes formed are first-order in L (i.e., if $n = 1$ in all species), then the solubility diagram will be linear as represented by A_L. The converse is not necessarily true, but a linear diagram is often taken as evidence for $n = 1$. If the slope is greater than unity, then at least one complex must exist for which m is greater than 1, for it is obviously impossible for one mole of L to take more than one mole of S into solution if the complex has 1:1 stoichiometry. On the other hand, a slope of less than unity does not necessarily mean that only a 1:1 complex is formed.

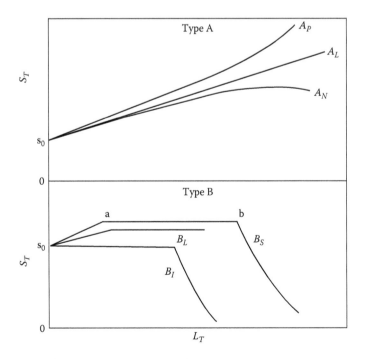

FIGURE 8.3   Phase-solubility diagrams of type A and type B systems.

A nonlinear plot with concave-upward curvature (A_P) implies that at least one complex is present having $n > 1$. A nonlinear plot with concave-downward curvature (A_N) may be evidence of nonideality effects (nonconstancy of activity coefficients) or of self-association by the ligand.

The second major class of phase-solubility diagrams, labeled type B diagrams, shows a characteristic plateau region representing a maximum value of S_T that additional quantities of ligand do not alter. The initial straight line portion is similar to that observed in type A diagrams, where the apparent solubility of S is increased due to soluble complex formation. Throughout the plateau region (a–b), the apparent solubility of the substrate remains constant due to precipitation of the complex with concomitant dissolution of solid substrate. When all of the solid substrate has been consumed (b), further addition of ligand results in depletion of substrate in the solution by complex formation and simultaneous precipitation of the complex. In some cases, the complex may be so insoluble that no initial rise in the apparent solubility of the substrate is observed (B_I). If L is not highly soluble, the break in the curve can be caused by saturation with respect to L (B_L). Just as complex formation of S with L increases the solubility of S, so it also increases the solubility of L. Normally, a stoichiometric ratio can be calculated in type B diagrams.

If a single 1:1 complex is formed, by combining the mass balance on substrate (S) and ligand (L) with the definition of the stability constant K, the stability isotherm is obtained:

$$S_T = s_0 + \frac{K_{11}s_0 L_T}{1 + K_{11}s_0} \tag{8.2}$$

where s_0 is the free substrate concentration and is constant because pure solid substrate is present in the system. Thus, a plot of S_T against L is linear. From this expression, the stability constant is given by:

$$K_{11} = \frac{\text{slope}}{s_0(1 - \text{slope})} \tag{8.3}$$

If a system exhibits multiple equilibria, a simple linear plot form without approximation cannot be obtained for the estimation of binding constants. Consider a system containing complexes SL, SL_2, ⋯, SL_n. Defining overall binding constants β_{1i}, where $i = 1$ to n, and substituting into the mass balance expression for substrate in the usual manner gives Equation 8.4.

$$S_T = s_0 + s_0 \sum_{i=1}^{n} \beta_{1i}[L]^i \tag{8.4}$$

The mass balance on ligand leads to Equation 8.5.

$$L_T = [L] + s_0 \sum_{i=1}^{n} i\beta_{1i}[L]^i \tag{8.5}$$

The most important case of this system is the $n = 2$ case, for which Equations 8.4 and 8.5 become:

$$S_T = s_0 + K_{11}s_0[L] + K_{11}K_{12}s_0[L]^2 \tag{8.6}$$

$$L_T = [L] + K_{11}s_0[L] + K_{11}K_{12}s_0[L]^2 \tag{8.7}$$

Several ways have been devised to obtain the stability constants from the S_T, L_T data for this case. An example is to rearrange Equation 8.6 to the linear plot form, Equation 8.8.

$$\frac{S_T - s_0}{[L]} = K_{11}s_0 + K_{11}K_{12}s_0[L] \tag{8.8}$$

It may be acceptable to make the approximation $[L] \approx L_T$, and then to plot $(S_T - s_0)/[L]$ against L_T. The binding constant can then be calculated from the slope and intercept.

Ultraviolet-Visible Spectroscopic Analysis

Many aromatic organic molecules show changes in their UV-visible absorption spectrum on inclusion by CDs (Cramer et al. 1967; Connors 1987) (Nagabhushanam et al. 2013). Generally, the spectral changes observed are similar to the effects caused by changes in solvent. These changes must be due to a perturbation of the electronic energy levels of the guest, caused either by direct interaction with the CD, by the exclusion of solvating water molecules, or by a combination of these two effects.

The stability constant of a complex can be determined from the analysis of a series of absorption spectra (Connors 1987). Consider the system in which a single 1:1 complex (*SL*) is formed, with the complex and free substrate (*S*) having significantly different absorption spectra. A wavelength is selected at which the molar absorptivity of substrate (ε_s) and complex (ε_{11}) are different. Then at a particular total concentration of substrate (S_T), in the absence of ligand, the solution absorbance is given by Equation 8.9,

$$A_0 = \varepsilon_s b S_T \tag{8.9}$$

where *b* is the cell path length. In the presence of ligand at total concentration L_T, assuming that Beer's law is followed by all species, the absorbance of a solution containing the same total substrate concentration can be expressed as Equation 8.10,

$$A_L = \varepsilon_s b[S] + \varepsilon_L b[L] + \varepsilon_{11} b[SL] \tag{8.10}$$

which, combined with the mass balances on *S* and *L*, gives:

$$A_L = \varepsilon_s b S_T + \varepsilon_L b L_T + \varepsilon_{11} b[SL] \tag{8.11}$$

where $\Delta\varepsilon_{11} = \varepsilon_{11} - \varepsilon_s - \varepsilon_L$, in which ε_L is the molar absorptivity of the ligand. By measuring the solution absorbance against a reference containing ligand at the same total concentration L_T, the measured absorbance becomes

$$A_L = \varepsilon_s b S_T + \varepsilon_{11} b[SL] \tag{8.12}$$

Combining Equation 8.12 with the stability constant definition, gives:

$$\Delta A = A - A_0 = K_{11}\Delta\varepsilon_{11}b[S][L] \tag{8.13}$$

When combined with the mass balance equation for *S*, Equation 8.14 is obtained which, when substituted back into Equation 8.13, gives Equation 8.15.

$$[S] = \frac{S_T}{1 + K_{11}[L]} \tag{8.14}$$

$$\frac{\Delta A}{b} = \frac{S_T K_{11}\Delta\varepsilon_{11}[L]}{1 + K_{11}[L]} \tag{8.15}$$

Equation 8.15 is the binding isotherm, which shows the hyperbolic dependence of absorbance on free ligand concentration.

By simple algebra, a double-reciprocal plot form, often called the Bensi-Hildebrand equation, can be derived.

$$\frac{b}{\Delta A} = \frac{1}{S_T K_{11}\Delta\varepsilon_{11}[L]} + \frac{1}{S_T\Delta\varepsilon_{11}} \tag{8.16}$$

The stability constant is evaluated from the linearized plot according to:

$$K_{11} = \frac{y\text{-intercept}}{slope} \tag{8.17}$$

Note that the reference solution contains the same total ligand concentration L_T as the sample solution. Even if the ligand does not absorb at the analytical wavelength, it is recommended to include it in the reference solution so that both the sample and reference have the same refractive index.

Both binding isotherm Equation 8.15 and double reciprocal plots Equation 8.16 are expressed as a function of free ligand concentration, which is not known. By means of the mass balance on ligand, L can be related to the known total ligand concentration L_T.

$$L_T = [L] = \frac{S_T K_{11}[L]}{1 + K_{11}[L]} \tag{8.18}$$

For multiple equilibria, consider a system containing only two complex states, namely, 1:1 (SL) and 1:2 (SL_2). Development following the lines of the treatment for the 1:1 system results in the following:

$$\frac{\Delta A}{b} = \frac{S_T(\beta_{11}\Delta\varepsilon_{11}[L] + \beta_{12}\Delta\varepsilon_{12}[L]^2)}{1 + \beta_{11}[L] + \beta_{12}[L]^2} \tag{8.19}$$

$$L_T = [L] = \frac{S_T(\beta_{11}[L] + 2\beta_{12}[L]^2)}{1 + \beta_{11}[L] + \beta_{12}[L]^2} \tag{8.20}$$

where $\beta_{11} = K_{11}$ and $\beta_{12} = K_{11}K_{12}$. By using nonlinear regression analysis, the parameters can be evaluated.

For multiple equilibria, spectroscopy is not in general a very useful tool. This is because the absorbance is not a direct measure of extent of binding, but rather is proportional to it. As a consequence, each stoichiometric state in the system adds two unknown parameters, a binding constant and a molar absorptivity, to the isotherm, so the number of parameters is twice the number of complex states.

Kinetic Method

The stabilization of S as the result of inclusion complex formation occurs non-covalently and may be the result of either a microsolvent effect, or of a conformational effect (Szejtli 1982). The kinetic method utilizes this reduction in rate of the reaction of S when L is present to obtain information about the nature of the complex. The basic assumption is that the decreased reactivity is the sole result of complexation, the complexed S being less reactive than free S. The kinetic scheme can be represented as below:

$$
\begin{array}{ccc}
S+L & \overset{K_{11}}{\rightleftharpoons} & SL \\
k_0 \downarrow & & \downarrow k_{11} \\
\text{Products} & & L + \text{Products}
\end{array}
$$

Kinetic scheme for a system in which a substrate degrades at a different rate inside the complex than the substrate alone, where k_0 is the rate constant for decomposition of uncomplexed S, k_{11} is the rate constant for the complex SL and K_{11} is the stability constant for complex formation. Assuming the degradation is under pseudo-first-order conditions, the theoretical rate equation is:

$$v = k_0[S] + k_{11}[SL] \tag{8.21}$$

and the experimental rate equation is:

$$v = k_{obs} S_T \tag{8.22}$$

where k_{obs} is the pseudo-first-order rate constant. Setting these equal and dividing through by S_T gives:

$$k_{obs} = k_0 f_{10} + k_{11} f_{11} \tag{8.23}$$

where f_{10} and f_{11} are the fractions of substrate present as S and SL, and can be expressed as Equation 8.24 and 8.25, respectively.

$$f_{10} = \frac{1}{1 + K_{11}[L]} \tag{8.24}$$

$$f_{11} = \frac{K_{11}[L]}{1 + K_{11}[L]} \tag{8.25}$$

The stability constant is combined with Equations 8.24 and 8.25, giving:

$$k_0 - k_{obs} = f_{11}(k_0 - k_{11}) \tag{8.26}$$

Defining:

$$\Delta k = k_0 - k_{obs} \tag{8.27}$$

$$q_{11} = 1 - \frac{k_{11}}{k_0} \tag{8.28}$$

Equation 8.26 can be rearranged as an expression of the binding isotherm.

$$\frac{\Delta k}{k_0} = \frac{q_{11} K_{11}[L]}{1 + K_{11}[L]} \tag{8.29}$$

A double reciprocal linear plot form can be easily derived.

$$\frac{1}{\Delta k} = \frac{1}{q_{11} k_{11} k_0 [L]} + \frac{1}{q_{11} k_0} \tag{8.30}$$

Equations 8.29 and 8.30 are identical in form with the isotherm and double reciprocal linear plot forms for optical spectroscopy Equations 8.15 and 8.16.

Titration Calorimetry

Titration calorimetry or thermometric titration calorimetry is a technique in which one reactant is titrated continuously into the other reactant, and either the temperature change or heat produced in the system is measured as a function of titrant added. In isoperibol titration calorimetry the temperature of a reaction vessel in a constant-temperature environment is monitored as a function of time (Figure 8.4) (Hansen et al. 1985; Winnike 1989). A single titration calorimetric experiment yields thermal data as a function of the ratio of the concentrations of the reactants.

Titration calorimetry depends on calculation of the extent of reaction from the quantity of heat evolved. Its successful application to a given system depends on (a) the equilibrium constant and the reaction conditions being such that the reaction occurs to a moderate extent (i.e., not to completion), and (b) the enthalpy of reaction being measurably different from zero.

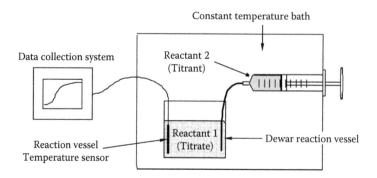

FIGURE 8.4 Simplified schematic of the major components of an isoperibol titration calorimetry system.

The conceptual basis of isoperibol solution calorimetry is that the reaction heat effect, Q_R, represents a quantitative measure of the amount of product formed, A_p, that is,

$$Q_R = A_p \cdot \Delta H^\circ \tag{8.31}$$

where ΔH° is the standard enthalpy change associated with the reaction.

For a one step reaction [Equation 8.32], given Equation 8.33 for the equilibrium system depicted in Equation 8.32, Equation 8.34 can be derived and SL_1 solved by for using the quadratic formula. The reaction heat can then be expressed as a function of moles of SL_1 produced [Equation 8.35].

$$S + L \underset{\Delta H_1^\circ}{\overset{K_{11}}{\rightleftharpoons}} SL_1 \tag{8.32}$$

$$K_{11} = \frac{[SL_1]}{[S][L]} \tag{8.33}$$

$$SL_1^2 - SL_1\left(S_T + L_T + \frac{\text{Vol}}{K_{11}}\right) + S_T L_T = 0 \tag{8.34}$$

$$Q_R = SL_1 \cdot \Delta H_1^\circ \tag{8.35}$$

where K_{11} and ΔH_1° are the binding constant and enthalpy change for the defined reaction, L_T is the amount of total ligand, L is the amount of free ligand, S_T is the amount of total substrate, S is the amount of free substrate, and Vol is the volume of solution in the reaction vessel.

The strategy for multiple step series reactions as defined in Equation 8.36 is the same. From mass balance, total ligand − total bound ligand − free ligand = 0, where *total bound ligand* is defined in Equation 8.37. Once the free ligand concentration is determined for the current K estimates, the moles of complex, SL_n, are calculated as defined by Equation 8.39. The reaction heat is then calculated for the current ΔH° estimates according to Equation 8.40.

$$S + L \underset{\Delta H_1^\circ}{\overset{K_{11}}{\rightleftharpoons}} SL_1 + L \underset{\Delta H_2^\circ}{\overset{K_{12}}{\rightleftharpoons}} \cdots \underset{\Delta H_n^\circ}{\overset{K_{1n}}{\rightleftharpoons}} SL_n \tag{8.36}$$

$$\text{total bound ligand} = S_T \cdot \frac{\sum_{i=1}^{n}\left(i[L]^i \prod_{j=1}^{i} K_{1j}\right)}{1 + \sum_{i=1}^{n}\left([L]^i \prod_{j=1}^{i} K_{1j}\right)} \tag{8.37}$$

$$S = \frac{S_T}{1 + \sum\limits_{i=1}^{n} \left([L]^i \prod\limits_{j=1}^{i} K_{1j} \right)} \tag{8.38}$$

$$SL_n = S[L]^n \prod\limits_{i=1}^{i} K_{1i} \tag{8.39}$$

$$Q_R = \Delta H_1^\circ (SL_1 + SL_2 \cdots + SL_n) + \Delta H_2^\circ (SL_2 \cdots + SL_n) + \cdots + \Delta H_n^\circ (SL_n) \tag{8.40}$$

ΔH° and K for the binding reaction can be simultaneously obtained by solving Equation 8.35 or 8.40 using a non-linear least squares curve fitting program. Once these values are known, other thermodynamic parameters can then be calculated from Equation 8.41.

$$\Delta G^\circ = -RT \ln K = \Delta H^\circ - T \Delta S^\circ \tag{8.41}$$

Since the thermal events observed calorimetrically contain both chemical and non-chemical components, all extraneous thermal effects must be subtracted from this composite of thermal events in order to obtain the relevant chemical reaction heat. Non-chemical thermal effects result from stirring, thermistor heating, heat transfer between the reaction vessel and the constant temperature bath, and titrant/titrate temperature mismatch. Chemical thermal effects result from evaporation, dilution of the reactants, and chemical reaction heat. Details of the data reduction and correction for extraneous heat effects are described by Winnike (1989).

Titration calorimetry has been successfully employed in the determination of thermodynamic parameters for complexation (Siimer et al. 1987; Tong et al. 1991). The technique has the advantage of employing direct calorimetric measurements and has been proposed as the most reliable method (Szejtli 1982). It should be noted that the information derived from multistep series reactions is macroscopic in nature. In contrast to spectrophotometric methods which provide information concerning only the equilibrium constant(s), titration calorimetry also provides information about the reaction enthalpy which is important in explaining the mechanism involved in the inclusion process.

Characterization of Complexes in Solid State

Several methods have been used to characterize complexes in solid state. Among the most commonly used methods are differential scanning calorimetry (DSC), X-ray powder diffraction (XRD), Fourier transform infrared spectroscopy (FTIR), X-ray crystallography, and nuclear magnetic resonance (NMR) (Demirel et al. 2011; Sravya et al. 2013; Zenget al. 2013; Kim et al. 2014).

Differential Scanning Calorimetry

DSC has been utilized by many to investigate inclusion complexes in the solid state. The melting endotherm of the substrate typically is changed as a result of complexation. The complex formed may have a different melting point, or no melting endotherm because of its amorphous nature. The physical mixture in most cases will still exhibit the melting endotherms of the substrate and the CD (if it is crystalline).

X-ray Powder Diffraction

XRD is a useful tool to study complexes in the solid state (Simon et al. 1981; Kim et al. 2014). The complex should give a different X-ray powder diffraction pattern compared to the physical mixture of the host and guest molecules. If the complex formed is crystalline, it is possible to get the single crystal X-ray pattern to elucidate the structure of the complex.

Fourier Transform Infrared Spectroscopy

Complex formation may be supported by IR spectroscopy either in the solid or the solution state in some cases, although the application of IR is limited to guests having characteristic absorption bands, such as carbonyl or sulfonyl groups. For example, the carbonyl stretching bands (*ca.* 1700 cm^{-1}) of parabens, are shifted about 40 cm^{-1} to a higher wave number by CD complexation since the intermolecular hydrogen bonding of the guests is ruptured, and the guests are dispersed in the CD cavity (Uekama et al. 1980). The band at 1690 cm^{-1}, characteristic of 4-biphenylacetic acid carbonyl stretching, appears as a lesser intensity band, also shifted to 1710 cm^{-1} in the inclusion complex sample with β-CD, due to the formation of a hydrogen bond between the secondary hydroxyl groups in β-CD and the carbonyl oxygen of the guest (Puglisi et al. 1990). In most cases, however, no change due to complex formation can be observed. Bands due to the included part of the guest molecule do shift or their intensities are altered, but since the mass of the guest molecule does not exceed 5%–15% of the mass of the complex, these alterations are usually obscured by the spectrum of the host. Therefore, no useful information can be obtained.

X-ray Crystallography

X-ray crystallography should be the ultimate tool for understanding crystalline complex structures. Many crystalline structures of complexes formed by natural CDs have been reported (Connors 1997; Caira and Dodds 1999). This technique is less useful for studying complexes formed with CD derivative since almost all the complexes formed with water-soluble CD derivatives are amorphous.

Nuclear Magnetic Resonance

NMR can be used in both solution and solid state. ^{1}H and ^{13}C-NMR have been used for studying space conformation of β-CD inclusion, and the formation of an inclusion complex can be evidenced by peak shifts of some of the drug protons and of the CD protons (Demirel et al. 2011). For the complexation between ketoconazole and β-CD, an upfield shift (0.082 ppm) in ^{1}H NMR spectroscopy of freeze-dried products confirmed that the aromatic groups of Ketoconazole were interacting with the β-CD.

COMPLEX FORMATION

Whether or not a compound can form inclusion complexes with CDs largely depends on the compound's size compatibility with the dimensions of the CD cavities. The stability of a complex also depends, however, on other properties of the guest molecule, such as its polarity. Compounds used medicinally usually are large molecules. Therefore, it is very commonly observed that the complexes form such that only certain groups or side chains penetrate into the carbohydrate channel.

The role of molecular dimensions is well demonstrated by complex formation with halogenated benzenes (Cohen and Lach 1963). 1:1 Complexes may be prepared from chloro-, bromo-, and iodobenzenes, but from chlorobenzene only with α-CD; from bromobenzene with α- and β-CDs, and from iodobenzene with β- and γ-CDs. A 1:2 (guest:CD) complex may be formed when the guest molecule is too large to find complete accommodation in one cavity and its other end is also amenable to complex formation. Some examples are the complexes of β-CD with prostaglandins, vitamin D3, and indomethacin.

Geometry, however, certainly is not the sole factor determining the stability of a complex. Antazoline and adiphenine should exhibit similar affinities for β-CD if only molecular dimension is considered. However, β-CD binds antazoline nearly twice as strongly as it does adiphenine. Cortisone acetate and testosterone also have common structural features. A similar affinity to β-CD would be expected, yet there is a definite preference for testosterone. The bulky side chain in cortisone acetate which encumbers the 17-hydroxyl group may be responsible for its low affinity for β-CD (Lach and Pauli 1966).

Certain chemical groups and substituents may greatly affect complex formation. There is, for example, a correlation between solubility and complexing ability of drugs, yet nitro-and amino-groups may alter this relationship (Lach and Pauli 1966). In the case of *p*-nitrophenol, methyl groups in positions 2 and 6 have no significant influence on the stability of the complex, but even one methyl group in the 3-position lowers the stability of the complex by about two orders of magnitude. 3,5-Dimethyl-4-nitrophenol fails to form a complex at all (Szejtli 1982).

The stability of the complex is proportional to the hydrophobic character of the substituents; thus a methyl or ethyl substituent will increase the stability. Hydroxyl groups hinder complex formation, and their hydrophilic effects decrease in the order *ortho* > *meta* > *para*. In the case of amine groups it is important whether they are present in their neutral form or ionized form. Ionic species usually do not form stable complexes (Szejtli 1982).

The importance of optimum matching of the cavity size and ligand size in determining the strength of binding is highlighted by the work of Cromwell et al. (1985). They studied the standard free energy change, $\Delta G°$, and standard enthalpy change, $\Delta H°$, for the interaction of adamantanecarboxylate with three CDs of varying cavity size to characterize structure/energetic relationships for complex formation. β-CD forms the strongest complex with adamantanecarboxylate and the reaction enthalpy change is negative ($\Delta H° = -4.85$ kcal/mol). They interpreted this favorable standard enthalpy change as indicating that the binding forces for this complex include a strong van der Waals interaction, due to the snug fit of adamantanecarboxylate into the β-CD cavity. The binding of adamantanecarboxylate to α-CD, with its smaller cavity, and to γ-CD, with its larger cavity, is poorer (140-fold lower binding constant for α-CD). They also found that the neutral carboxylic acid form of adamantanecarboxylate binds to CD better than does the carboxylate form.

A strong guest-size dependence is found for both the free energy change and enthalpy change for complex formation in a study of the effects of the variation in the size of alicyclic guests on CD inclusion complexation (Eftink et al. 1989). Thermodynamic parameters for the interaction of a congener series of alicyclic acids (e.g., adamantanecarboxylic acid) with α- and β-CDs in aqueous solution were determined. The side chains of these guests are roughly spherical and vary in carbon number from 11 to 5. With β-CD, it was found that 1:1 host:guest inclusion complexes were formed with all the guests at both low and high pH, with strong binding occurring at low pH, where the carboxylic acid forms of the guest predominate. With α-CD, 1:1 complexes are formed with the carboxylate forms of the guests, but 2:1 α-CD:guest complexes were formed, in a cooperative manner, with the carboxylic acid forms of the guests.

Although the neutral form of a drug generally forms a stronger complex with neutral CDs (α-, β-, γ-CD, and HP-β-CD), the effect of charge state of drug molecules on complexation is more complicated for anionic CDs such as SBE-β-CDs. Okimoto et al. (1995) reported that the anionic SBE-β-CD often exhibits 1:1 binding constants with neutral drugs that are comparable to or better than those observed for neutral HP-β-CD. The better binding was believed to be the result of the butyl micellar arms extending the hydrophobic cavity of the CD. For cationic drugs, SBE-β-CD was found to form much more stable complexes than HP-β-CD. For anionic drugs, however, the electrostatic repulsions may significantly affect the complexing ability of these molecules with SBE-β-CDs. The binding constant between the anionic warfarin molecule and SBE-β-CD, for example, is much lower than with HP-β-CD. There are cases, however, where the binding constants between anionic molecules and the anionic SBE-β-CD are almost equivalent to those observed for the neutral HP-β-CD, such as in the case of indomethacin and naproxen. These results suggest that the position of the charge in the drug and how it interacts with the charge in the CD may be important (Thompson 1997).

Although some correlation exists between the binding strength and a guest molecule's structural features or other physicochemical properties, the relationship is limited within certain groups of compounds. Despite some success in predicting binding constants of α-CD from the structures of guest molecules (Connors 1997), so far, no obvious correlation has been found between the physical or chemical properties of different families of guest molecules and complex forming ability with other CDs and their derivatives.

Connors (1997) summarized a collection of K_{11} values from CD literature. Treated as statistical populations, the complex stabilities appear to be reasonably described as normal distribution in log K_{11}, with the mean log K_{11} value equal to 2.11, 2.69, and 2.55 for α-β-, and γ- CDs, respectively.

THERMODYNAMICS OF COMPLEXATION

The standard free-energy decrease associated with formation of CD inclusion complexes is generally due to a negative standard enthalpy change ($\Delta H°$) accompanying the inclusion process. The standard entropy change ($\Delta S°$) can be either positive or negative, although the majority of guest molecules that have been studied appear to have negative $\Delta S°$ values.

Several intermolecular interactions have been proposed as being responsible for the formation of CD inclusion complexes in an aqueous solution (Matsui et al. 1985; Connors 1997). They are (a) hydrophobic interaction; (b) van der Waals interaction mainly induction and dispersion forces; (c) hydrogen bonding and dipole-dipole interactions; (d) the release of *high energy water* from the cyclodextrin cavity upon substrate inclusion; and (e) the release of conformational strain in a CD-water adduct, together with the formation of a hydrogen bonding network around the O(2), O(3) side of the CD macrocycle upon substrate inclusion.

Because the values of $\Delta H°$ and $\Delta S°$ for complex formation vary over such a wide range, it is reasonable to conclude that the various intermolecular interactions described earlier act simultaneously, and the extent to which these interactions contribute may largely depend on the nature of host and guest molecules.

For most other non-inclusion molecular complexes, the driving forces responsible for complex formation include London dispersion, dipolar (including hydrogen bonding), ionic, π-bonding, and hydrophobic effects (Higuchi and Connors 1965). Most small molecules that have been reported to form complexes exhibit molecular features that permit intermolecular hydrogen bonding. In addition, most molecules whose complex exhibits a substantial planar aromatic moiety, and data strongly suggest that such compounds stack together in a plane-to-plane configuration (Higuchi and Kristiansen 1970).

COMPLEXATION BY CYCLODEXTRINS

There are many examples to demonstrate the effect of CDs on the solubility, dissolution rates and the bioavailability of poorly water-soluble compounds (Uekama et al. 1985; Green and Guillory 1989; Szejtli 1994; Uekama et al. 1994; Thompson 1997; Emara et al. 2002; Patel et al. 2005; Lahiani-Skiba et al. 2006; Yao et al. 2014). Concerning bioavailability, both the rate and extent of absorption are typically enhanced: Not only is the blood concentration higher, with its peak occurring sooner, but the area under the curve is also larger. These results can be obtained, for example, after the oral administration of inclusion compounds of digoxin:γ-CD in the dog (Uekama et al. 1981), diazepam:γ-CD in the rabbit (Uekama et al. 1983c), and allobarbital, amobarbital, barbital, pentobarbital or phenobarbital:β-CD in the rabbit (Koizumi and Kidera 1977). A similar result is obtained following the oral administration in humans of the inclusion compounds salicylic acid:β-CD (Frömming and Weyermann 1973) or prednisolone: β-CD (Uekama et al. 1983a).

Many CDs have been successfully used to solubilize insoluble drugs, here are a partial list of CD derivatives reported in the literature: HP-β-CD, SBE-β-CDs, randomly methylated-β-cyclodextrin (RM-β-CD), 2,3,6-partially methylated-β-CD (PM-β-CD), glucosyl-β-CD (G1-β-CD), maltosyl-β-cyclodextrin (G2-β-CD), hydroxyethyl-β-cyclodextrin (He-β-CD), diethyl-β-cyclodextrin (DE-β-CD), O-carboxymethyl-O-ethyl-β-cyclodextrin (CME-β-CD), (2,6-di-O-methyl)-β-cyclodextrin (DOM-β-CD), 2-hydroxypropyl-γ-cyclodextrin (HP-γ-CD).

It is generally believed that the mechanism of bioavailability enhancement by CD complexation is through solubility and dissolution rate improvement. However, it should be also noted that CDs may also alter the lipid barrier of the absorption site, which may contribute to the enhanced drug absorption. This effect of CDs on the lipid barrier can be attributed to CDs' ability to form complexes with membrane components such as cholesterol, phospholipids and proteins (Nakanishi et al. 1992). Jambhekar et al. (2004) compared the solubilizing effects of β-CD, HP-β-CD and He-β-CD on indomethacin. They found that the three drug-CD complexes were bound similarly. The drug-CD complexes of HP-β-CD and He-β-CD were more soluble than β-CD complex in 0.1N HCl and distilled water. However, only capsules containing β-CD complex had a significantly higher bioavailability than other two complexes, suggesting that factors other than solubility and dissolution rate are contributing to the bioavailability.

Certain kinds of improvements are possible in almost every dosage form. Besides oral and injectable formulations, CD inclusion has been shown to improve bioavailability of compounds administered by other routes, including ocular, topical, nasal and rectal routes (Uekama et al. 1994; Marttin et al. 1998; Bary et al. 2001; Loftsson and Masson 2001; Rode et al. 2003). Some important applications particularly applicable for insoluble compounds are summarized in the following.

1. Solid Preparations:
   a. Oral bioavailability of poorly water-soluble drugs can be improved by enhancement of the dissolution rate and/or apparent solubility (via super-saturation in the GI fluids).
   b. Physical stability of compounds in their metastable forms (such as amorphous) can be enhanced by the inhibition or prevention of crystal-growth.
   c. Content uniformity of a small amount of a drug in bulky diluents can be ensured by an increase in dispersibility and fluidity.
   d. Shelf-life of drugs can be extended by increasing their stability.
2. Liquid Preparations:
   a. Solubility and/or stability of the drug in water can be improved.
3. Suspensions and Emulsions:
   a. Caking, creaming, and phase transitions can be suppressed by the protective sheath of CDs.
   b. Thixotropic nature of suspensions can be controlled.
   c. Physical stability of the dispersed system can be improved.
4. Semisolid Preparations:
   a. Topical bioavailability can be improved by the enhanced release of a drug from ointment or suppository bases.
   b. Water-absorbing capacity of oleaginous and water-in-oil bases can be improved by hydrophilic CDs.
5. Injectable Preparations:
   a. Solubility and/or stability of the drug in water can be improved.
   b. Drug-induced hemolysis and muscular tissue damage can be reduced.
   c. Solubilized products can be prepared by freeze-drying CD complexes if needed for enhanced stability.
   d. Suspensions for parenteral use can be prepared by reducing the drug to a fine powder containing the CD complex by use of ball milling.

It is worthwhile to mention that $(SBE)_{7\ m}$-β-CD also makes controlled drug delivery more feasible for water-insoluble compounds. It is well known that the release from controlled porosity osmotic pump tablets is limited due to its low aqueous solubility. However, Okimoto et al. (1999) successfully developed osmotic pump tablets for testosterone by using $(SBE)_{7\ m}$-β-CD. Because each $(SBE)_{7\,m}$-β-CD molecule has an average of seven negative charges and seven sodium ions, it can act as a osmotic pump agent in addition to solubilize insoluble drug through complexation. Furthermore, a sustained drug delivery system for a very lipophilic, water-insoluble antibacterial agent triclosan, was designed based on the ionic interactions between anionic SBE-β-CD and an anionic polymer, that is, hexadimethrine bromide (Loftsson et al. 2001).

FACTORS AFFECTING COMPLEXATION EFFECTIVENESS

To enhance the solubilization powder of complexation, many researchers have tried adding various agents in the complexation systems. Readers are directed to the recent review for six different types of ternary cyclodextrin complexes (Kurkov and Loftsson 2013). Water-soluble polymers, such as HPMC, PVP, and high-molecular PEGs, have been shown to enhance the drug dissolution rate of poorly water-soluble drugs in drug-CD complexes (Taneri et al. 2003; Duan et al. 2005; Ammar et al. 2006; Zoeller et al. 2012; Dahiya and Tayde 2013; Zaki et al. 2013). For example, addition of hydrophilic polymers (Soluplus® and two types of hydroxypropyl methylcellulose-Metolose® 90SH-100 and Metolose 65SH-1500) significantly increased solubilization capacity of HP-β-CD for carbamazepine (Djordje et al. 2015). The dissolution rate of the drug from these ternary systems was found to be highly dependent on polymer type and concentration. The optimum increase in dissolution rate of glimepiride was observed at a polymer concentration of 5% for PEG4000 or PEG6000 and at 20% for HPMC or PVP.

Some small molecules can also enhance the complexation of CDs with insoluble drugs. Basavaraj et al. (2006) studied the influence of a polyhydroxyl base, N-acetyl glucamine (also known as meglumine) on the complexation of DRF-4367, a poorly water-soluble molecule, with HP-β-CD. Phase solubility studies suggested that meglumine further enhanced the dissolution rate of drug through multiple factors, including specific hydrogen bonding and/or spatial alignment with the host. Other excipients like lysine, ascorbic acid and magnesium chloride have also been showed to enhance the solubilizing effects of HP-β-CD and randomly methylated-β-cyclodextrin (RM-β-CD) for several insoluble drugs (Duan et al. 2005). Using complexation with HP-β-CD as well as salt formation with arginine, the solubility and dissolution profiles for naproxen were significantly improved (Mura et al. 2005).

It is worthwhile to mention that the combined use of two solubilizing agents sometimes may result in a decreased solubilization capability. For example, the combined use of sodium lauryl sulfate (SLS) and $(SBE)_{7\,m}$-β-CD resulted in a much lower solubility for a insoluble drug, NSC-639829, than when either was used alone (Yang et al. 2004). In this case, the surfactant molecule acts as a competitive inhibitor in the solubilization of the drug by the complexing agent, and in turn the complexing agent makes surfactant unavailable for solubilizing the drug.

The effects of temperature on complexation are somehow complicated. In general, temperature has limited impact of complexation effectiveness. Although increase temperature can increase intrinsic solubility, higher temperature typically results in lower complexation binding constant due to a negative standard enthalpy change ($\Delta H°$) accompanying the complexation process. For example, this effect was seen with the complex formed between alfaxalone, a poorly water-soluble compound, and HP-β-CD (Peeters et al. 2002)

OTHER COMPLEXATIONS

In addition to the inclusion complexes formed by CDs, other types of molecular complexes also have been reported extensively (Murugan et al. 2014; Zhang and Isaacs 2014). For example, quaternized poly(propylene imine) dendrimer has been successfully used as a drug carrier for a poorly soluble drug nimesulide to enhance its solubility (Murugan et al. 2014). Devarakonda et al. (2005)

compared the solubilization of nicolsamide by complexing with polyamidoamine (PAMAM) dendrimers and CDs, and found the solubility of nicolsamide was significantly higher with PAMAM. However, the dissolution rate was lower with PAMAM compared to the CDs, which was due to the strong interaction between nicolsamide and PAMAM delayed the release of the drug from the complexes of dendrimers.

Chen et al. (1994) studied water-soluble vitamins, amino acids, and non-toxic pharmaceutical excipients as solubilizing agents for poorly water-soluble adenine (nucleic acid base), guanosine (nucleoside), and structurally related drugs (acyclovir and triamterene). A ligand pair (two ligands) consisting of ligands from the same class (Higuchi and Kristiansen 1970) was found to have additive solubility enhancement with respect to nucleosides and structurally related compounds.

Hussain (1978) discovered that 2-acetoxybenzoic acid formed a stable complex with nicotinamide or isonicotinamide. The complexes offer superior results over 2-acetoxybenzoic acid in pharmacokinetic studies. They permit 2-acetoxybenzoic acid to be released in a highly soluble and dissociated form, thus permitting extremely high blood levels to be obtained and yet, the complexing agent remains as a non-toxic moiety, which is metabolized into non-toxic by products.

p-Hydroxyphenylbutazone (p-HPB) contains two carbonyl groups which are able to associate with proton donating molecules through hydrogen bonding. Its complexes formed with many amine compounds are believed to be charge-transfer complexes (Marletti and Notelli 1976).

Some examples of molecular complexes reported in the literature are summarized in Table 8.1.

TABLE 8.1
Summary of Some Examples of Molecular Complexes Reported in the Literature

Drug	Ligand	Reference
Nimisulide	Quarternized poly(propylene imine) dendrimer	Murugan et al. (2014)
19 insoluble drugs	Cucurbit[n]urils	Zhang and Isaacs (2014)
Ibuprofen and Ketoprofen	N-methylglucamine	De Villiers et al. (1999)
N-4472	L-ascorbic acid	Itoh et al. (2003)
4-Sulfonic calix[n]arenes	Furosemide	Yang and De Villiers (2004)
Salicylaminde	Caffeine	Reuning and Levy (1968); Donbrow et al. (1976)
Hexamethylmelamine	Gentisic acid	Kreilgård et al. (1975)
p-Hydroxyphenylbutazone (p-HPB)	Amine compounds	Marletti and Notelli (1976)
Sulfonamides	Cyclic Polyether 180 Crown-6	Takayama et al. (1977b)
Aminobenzoic acids	N-Methyl-2-pyrrolidone (NMP)	Takayama et al. (1977a)
Acronine	Alkylgentisates	Repta and Hincal (1980)
Theophylline	Aliphatic diamines and aliphatic monoamines	Nishijo et al. (1982)
Heteroaromatic anti-cancer agents: Erythro-9-(2-hydroxy-3-nonyl) adenine, 3-deazauridine and thioquanine	Nicotinamide	Truelove et al. (1984)
Tolbutamide	Urea	McGinity et al. (1975)
Nifedipine	Substituted phenolic ligands	Boje et al. (1988)
p-Boronophenylalanine	Monosaccharides such as mannitol	Mori et al. (1989)

PRACTICAL CONSIDERATIONS

IDENTIFICATION OF USEFUL SYSTEMS

As shown in Equation 8.1, complexation is an equilibrium process. Most drugs (substrates) form 1:1 complexes with various ligands (e.g., CDs). These 1:1 complexes are defined by a binding constant, K_{11}. In solubility considerations, if S represents the solubility of a drug in the absence of any ligand, then the increase in solubility of a drug is largely driven by the product of K_{11} and [L], with [L] equal to [L_{total}] minus [SL]. Since most values of K_{11} are less than 20,000M^{-1} and [L_{total}] usually is less than 0.1–0.2 M, the maximum increases in solubility that can be expected from a 1:1 complexation are in the range of 1,000–2,000 times the intrinsic solubility (Stella and Rajewski 1997). This means that in order to solubilize a drug to the mg/mL range, the solubility of the drug in the absence of any ligand will have to be in the µg/mL range. For example, if the intrinsic solubility of the drug is 10 ng/mL, it is almost impossible to find a ligand which is capable of raising the solubility of this drug into the mg/mL range through just a 1:1 interaction. The only way to overcome this limitation is to increase the intrinsic solubility through other means such as pH adjustment. Although ionization of drug molecules may reduce the binding constants of complexes, an improvement in intrinsic solubility can often offset the binding constant decrease and the desired solubility can be achieved (Johnson et al. 1994).

While in some cases binding ability could be correlated with certain structure features (Tong et al. 1991a,b), no general rule is available to predict binding constants without carrying out an actual experiment. Fortunately it is relatively easy to determine whether or not certain ligands are capable of forming complexes with the compound of interest. A quick solubility screen of potentially useful ligands can provide a means of identifying the most useful system. For example, if 20% HP-β-CD and 40% SBE-β-CD do not improve solubility to the desirable levels, it is clear that solubility enhancement by these CDs will not be very successful.

In additional to the binding constant and safety considerations, economics and quality control issues also play a role in considering which ligands to use. Because of the difficulty in selectively derivatizing a specific hydroxyl or family of hydroxyls, most modified CDs of pharmaceutical interest are likely to be complex mixtures (Stella and Rajewski 1997). Methods to characterize these mixtures, therefore, need to be in place to assure lot to lot reproducibility. The costs of acute and chronic safety studies required to evaluate any new CD derivatives are very high, and this prohibits them from being widely evaluated for pharmaceutical applications.

PREPARATION OF COMPLEXES

Various methods have been reported for the preparations of complexes. The complexation effectiveness is dependent on the properties of the complexes formed and the preparation methods. The ability to consistently make the complexes with reproducible properties should be evaluated when developing methods for complex preparation.

In solution, the complexes can be formed at a diffusion-controlled rate by mixing solutions containing the host and the guest. The amount of the complex formed is dependent on the binding constant. Solid complexes can be prepared by co-precipitation (Celebi and Nagai 1988; Ficarra et al. 2002), neutralization (Celebi and Nagai 1988), kneading (Lengyel and Szejtli 1985), freeze-drying (Kurozumi et al. 1975; Fugioka et al. 1983; Pralhad and Rajendrakumar 2004), spray-drying (Tokumura et al. 1984; Fukuda et al. 1986; Miro et al. 2004) and coevaporation (Zugasti et al. 2009), grinding methods (Nakai et al. 1977, 1980; Lin et al. 1988; Mukne and Nagarsenker 2004; Mura et al. 2005). The melting method has been shown to be very effective in preparing solid complexes for some ternary systems of drug-CD and polymers like PEG6000 and PEG4000 (Lahiani-Skiba et al. 2006). The reader is directed to a recent review (Chordiya and Senthilkumaran 2012).

In the kneading method, the solid complex is formed by adding the substrate to a slurry of the ligand (e.g., CDs) and kneading until a paste is obtained. This material is dried and washed with a small amount of solvent to remove any free substrate. Aqueous solutions are typically employed in the freeze-drying and spray-drying methods. However, for water-insoluble compounds, these methods are not that useful unless organic solvents can be used. Organic solvents are also often utilized in the co-precipitation methods. One major problem with using organic solvents is that most organic solvents will compete for inclusion in the CD cavity, and thus inhibit complex formation. The neutralization method takes advantage of acidic or basic functional groups and is rather useful for insoluble compounds. It is important, however, to make sure that compounds are stable in the acidic or basic conditions. The absence of water in the grinding method makes it suitable for drugs which are unstable in aqueous solvents and/or at elevated temperatures.

Palmieri et al. (1997) studied the effect of preparation methods on the properties of solid inclusion complexes between methoxybutropate and β- and HP-β-CD. UV and HPLC analysis, DSC, XRD, and dissolution studies were carried out to characterize the complexes prepared by solid dispersion, kneading, and spray drying. Generally, it was found that for the complex with β-CD the spray drying preparation gave the best complexation effectiveness and dissolution rate, whereas for the complex with HP-β-CD, solid dispersion was the best method.

Fini et al. (1997) studied the feasibility of preparing β-CD-indomethacin (IM) complex by compacting a β-CD/IM mixture with low frequency ultrasound. Experimental results suggested that the material obtained by ultrasound had a dissolution rate comparable to that measured with the kneaded material. The use of ultrasound, however, can both reduce the production time and improve the homogeneity of the association between ID and β-CD. The proposed mechanism for this method is that in the absence of a solvent, ultrasound absorption by a solid promotes phase transition or disrupts the crystal lattice, resulting in a nearly amorphous state or, in the case of low melting compounds, can create the conditions for a low temperature fusion. In the case of the β-CD/IM complex, IM appears to be deposited on the β-CD particles as a melted film, creating an intimate contact between the two components.

Drug Release from Complexes

As mentioned earlier, complex formation is an equilibrium process and both the drug and ligand molecules are non-covalently bound. Also, it has been experimentally shown that the rates of complex formation and dissociation are very fast. It occurs at rates (> about $10^{-8} M^{-1} \cdot sec^{-1}$), and this is very close to diffusion controlled limits with the complexes being continually formed and broken down (Cramer et al. 1967; Thomason et al. 1990). Therefore, it is easy to picture the two major mechanisms that contribute to complex dissociation: dilution and competitive displacement (binding of drug and/or ligand molecule to other competing agents) (Stella and He 2008; Kurkov et al. 2012; Loftsson and Brewster 2013).

Consider a drug with an intrinsic solubility of 0.4 mM solubilized by 0.1M CD to 20 mM through a 1:1 complex with a binding constant of 610 M^{-1}, a dilution of 1:700 (assuming that 5 mL of the 20 mM solution was injected and the distribution volume for the complex is about 3.5 L). This will result in 92.1% dissociation of the complex (Stella and Rajewski 1997). The binding of drug and ligand molecule to other competing agents can be illustrated by the effect of *in vitro* dilution with plasma on the dissociation of HP-β-CD complexes of naproxen or flurbiprofen (Frijlink et al. 1991). Frijlink et al. found that only small fractions of the drugs remained bound to the CD in plasma. Albumin binding of the two drugs was able to compete effectively with CD binding. Displacement of the drugs from CD by a competing agent such as plasma cholesterol may have contributed to the low fraction of drug retained by the CD.

Based on an extensive review, Rajewski and Stella (1996) concluded that for parenteral delivery of complexes, except for local drug delivery where high concentrations of both drug and CDs can be maintained, drugs are qualitatively and quantitatively released from their inclusion complexes with little if any perturbation of the pharmacokinetics of the drug. For drug: CD complexes that have very strong binding constants (>10,000 M^{-1}), it will take a larger dilution to reduce the percentage of drug complexed to an insignificant level. The tendency for the drug to complex with plasma protein and to be replaced from the CD complex by endogenous lipids (e.g., cholesterol) will also be reduced (Mesens and Putteman 1991). As a result of these combined effects, the earlier time point pharmacokinetics may be perturbed (Frijlink et al. 1991). Similar statements should be applicable to other complexes based on the mechanism of the dissociation of all complexes. The reader is directed to the recent reviews for a summary of work that address the issue of CDs and drug pharmacokinetics (Palem et al. 2012; Kumar et al. 2013; Kurkov and Loftsson 2013).

Although most of the complexes dissociate upon dilution in the blood, Guo and his colleagues discovered that amphotericin B, a potential fungicidal agent, forms a very tight complex with sodium cholesteryl sulfate that does not readily dissociate after intravenous injection (Guo et al. 1991). The unique structure and tight association of the drug with this stable discoidal complex seem to prevent the incorporation of amphotericin B into the host tissues and cells. Both the toxic effects and the therapeutic index of the drug are significantly improved by using the complex.

For oral delivery, complexes will also dissociate rapidly upon dilution in the stomach and intestinal contents and it is generally believed that only the drug, and not the complex, is absorbed (Thompson 1997). Therefore, the primary function of complexes is to increase the dissolution rate and extent of drug dissolution. Other reported effects of CDs on oral absorption of drugs include enhancement of mucosal membrane permeation by CD as mentioned earlier in this chapter.

Ophthalmic, transmucosal, nasal, and transdermal products will be the most sensitive to the strength of binding (Abdul Rasool and Salmo 2012; Kumar et al. 2013; Juluri and Narasimha Murthy 2014; Kim et al. 2014). These routes of administration experience minimal dilution. However, this may not be a significant concern because the drug typically can also be displaced from the CD cavity at the delivery site by competing lipophiles at the delivery site, such as triglycerides, cholesterol, bile salts, and other hydrophobic compounds, which are often in much higher concentrations (Thompson 1997).

Safety Considerations

When a complex is used in a formulation, the toxicity of both the drug and the complexing agent must be evaluated. The presence of the complexing agent may alter the toxicity profile of the drug and *vice versa*. These factors need to be considered in designing toxicity studies.

Stella and He have reviewed the safety profiles of various CDs, and pointed out that human experience with CD derivatives, specifically SBE-β-CD and HP-β-CD, showed that these two CDs are well tolerated in humans and have no adverse effects on the kidneys or other organs following either oral or intravenous administration (Stella and He 2008). In summary, CDs are not absorbed upon oral administration and consequently exhibit a good oral safety profile (Thompson 1997). The main adverse effect observed with oral use occurs at very high doses and results from a secondary effect caused by removal of bile salts from enteroheptic recirculation. This effect is typically not observed at doses utilized in pharmaceutical formulations. It is expected to be less favorable to complex bile salts by anionic SBE-β-CD than by neutral CDs because the anionic charge on the bile salt may repel anionic CD.

Parent CDs α- and β-CD are not suitable for parenteral formulations because of renal toxicity, but nephrotic damage is not observed with γ-CD, HP-β-CD, or SBE-β-CD (Stella and He 2008). HP-β-CD is suitable for parenteral application because of its considerable solubility in water and low hemolytic activity (Dilova et al. 2004). Doses up to 2 g/kg body weight/day have been tested in animal safety studies for SBE-β-CD and human studies have been conducted for intravenous administration of 3 gm of HP-β-CD at an infusion rate of 100 mg/min. Because of the membrane-damaging effects of dimethyl-β-CD, it is probably suitable only as a penetration enhancer.

Regulatory Considerations

When a complex is formulated, the complexing agent is not considered a standard inactive ingredient. Currently there is no approval process in place for evaluating new excipients. Regulatory authorities are charged with evaluating and approving final commercial drug formulations, but they are not charged with approval of new excipients (Thompson 1997). In the U.S., the dossier on a new excipient must be filed by the excipient manufacturer as a drug master file (DMF)-Type 4. This data is then referenced when an investigational new drug application (IND), new drug application (NDA), or abbreviated new drug application (ANDA) is filed for a dosage form using the excipient. The existence of a DMF for a specific excipient, however, does not guarantee regulatory acceptance for the use of that excipient with a drug. The safety data for the excipient provided in the DMF needs to support the administration route, excipient dosing level and dosing frequency (Stella and Rajewski 1997). In addition, the regulatory document referencing the DMF will need to provide supporting safety data on the complexing agent/drug combination. Because of the additional problems associated with using a new excipient, when considering using the complexation technique in drug formulations, it is advisable to start the dialogue with the regulatory agents as early in the development process as possible so the expectations by the agents are clearly communicated.

DRUGS CONTAINING CYCLODEXTRINS

It is worthwhile to note that various CDs themselves have been used for different therapeutic indications as shown in clinicaltrials.gov, such as intravenous HP-β-CD for Niemann-Pick Type C1 Disease, oral α-CD on Fecal Fat Excretion, and oral α-CD for Decreasing Serum Chloesterol. According to clinicaltrials.gov, there are 32 clinical studies involving CD or CD complexation, and among them 11 studies are still recruiting study subjects or active but not recruiting. An important player in the field of CD complexation, CyDex Pharmaceuticals, Inc. was acquired by Ligand in 2011 and operates as a wholly-owned subsidiary of Ligand (http://www.ligand.com/cydex). In addition to approved drug products, CyDex is supporting drug development efforts with more than 40 companies, including developing a Captisol®-enabled IV formulation of Carfilzomib for refractory multiple myeloma for Onyx Pharmaceuticals (acquired by Amgen in 2013).

Chordiya and Senthilkumaran have summarized marketed drug products according to different CD derivatives (α-CD, β-CD, HP-β-CD, RM-β-CD, SBE-β-CD and HP-γ-CD), and most of the approved drugs are marketed in Europe and Japan, only a few in USA (Chordiya and Senthilkumaran 2012). The drugs approved in the United States and around the world utilizing SBE-β-CD (Captisol) include but not limited to Vfend® (voriconazole) and Zeldox®/Geodon® (ziprasidone mesylate) by Pfizer, ABILIFY (aripiprazole) by Bristol-Myers Squibb (https://notendur.hi.is/thorstlo/cyclodextrin.pdf), and Nexterone (amiodarone hydrochloride) of Baxter. The drugs approved in the United States and around the world utilizing HP-β-CD include but not limited to Sporanox (itraconazole) by Janssen, Idocid (indomethacin) by Chauvin, and MitoExtra (mitomycin) by Novartis. For Itraconazole (Sporanox), a broad-spectrum antifungal agent, based on HP-β-CD, Janssen developed different both oral (capsule) and oral (solution) formulations.

PATENT ISSUES

Applications of complexation agents especially modified CDs are heavily patented. The use of CD derivatives, for example, will typically involve certain royalty payment. However, this may also present opportunities for patent protection of new formulations containing complexes of new chemical entities (NCEs).

COST-OF-GOODS CONSIDERATIONS

The cost-of-goods is an important factor to consider in the current drug development environment. When complexation technology is used in a drug formulation, the cost of the complexing agents and the potential royalty payment associated with the technology may make the formulated products less attractive in a very competitive market. Additionally, the development cost with complex-containing formulations may be higher because of additional toxicity studies required, for example.

However, one should keep in mind that there are many potential issues associated with other solubilizing technologies that may not be so obvious in the early development stages, such as patient compliance issues with an injectable formulation that causes severe pain. Therefore, it is important in the early preformulation studies to carefully consider all the factors (pros and cons) before making a final commitment to complex technology.

SUMMARY

The use of complexation in overcoming pharmaceutical solubility problems has clear advantages over other means of solubilization. The advances in the area of CD research and commercialization will lead to lower costs and bulk production methods, making the technique even more attractive. The commercial viability of complex-containing drug formulations has been established with the marketing of many products. The high development cost associated with potential regulatory hurdles, loyalty payment and the cost-of-goods of complexing agents still remain as the major limitations for the wide utilization of this technique.

REFERENCES

Abdul Rasool, B. K. and H. M. Salmo. 2012. Development and clinical evaluation of clotrimazole-β-cyclodextrin eyedrops for the treatment of fungal keratitis. *AAPS PharmSciTech* 13(3): 883–889.

Ammar, H. O., H. A. Salama, M. Ghorab and A. A. Mahmoud. 2006. Implication of inclusion complexation of glimepiride in cyclodextrin-polymer systems on its dissolution, stability and therapeutic efficacy. *Int. J. Pharm.* 320(1–2): 53–57.

Bary, A. R., I. G. Tucker and N. M. Davies. 2001. An insight into how cyclodextrins increase the ocular bioavailability of poorly water-soluble compounds. *Proceedings–28th International Symposium on Controlled Release of Bioactive Materials and 4th Consumer & Diversified Products Conference*, San Diego, CA, June 23–27, 2001.

Basavaraj, S., V. Sihorkar, T. R. S. Kumar, P. Sundaramurthi, N. R. Srinivas, P. Venkatesh, M. Ramesh and S. K. Singh. 2006. Bioavailability enhancement of poorly water soluble and weakly acidic new chemical entity with 2-hydroxy propyl-β-cyclodextrin: Selection of meglumine, a polyhydroxy base, as a novel ternary component. *Pharm. Dev. Tech.* 11(4): 443–451.

Baszkin, A., A. Angelova and C. Ringard-Lefebvre. 1999. Host-guest complexation of water soluble and water insoluble drugs by cyclodextrins. *Book of Abstracts, 218th ACS National Meeting*, New Orleans, LA, August 22–26. COLL-011.

Bender, M. L. and M. Komiyama. 1978. *Cyclodextrin Chemistry*, Berlin, Germany: Springer-Verlag.

Boje, K. M., M. Sak and H. L. Fung. 1988. Complexation of nifedipine with substituted phenolic ligands, *Pharm. Res.* 5(10): 655–659.

Caira, M. R. and D. R. Dodds. 1999. Inclusion of nonopirate analgesic drugs in cyclodextrins. I. X-ray structure of a 1:1 beta-cyclodextrin-p-bromoacetanilide complex. *J. Incl. Phenom. Macrocycl. Chem.* 34: 19–29.

Casu, B., M. Reggiani, G. G. Gallo and A. Vigevanni. 1970. *Carbohydr. Res.* 12: 157–170.

Celebi, N. and T. Nagai. 1988. Improvement of dissolution characteristics of piromidic acid by dimethyl-β-cyclodextrin complexation. *Drug Dev. Ind. Pharm.* 14: 63–75.

Chen, A. X., S. W. Zito and R. A. Nash. 1994. Solubility enhancement of nucleosides and structurally related compounds by complex formation. *Pharm. Res.* 11(3): 398–401.

Chordiya, M. A. and K. Senthilkumaran. 2012. Cyclodextrin in drug delivery: A review. *Res. Rev. J. Pharm. Pharm. Sci.* 1(1): 19–29.

Clarke, R. J., J. H. Coates and S. F. Lincoln. 1988. Inclusion complexes of the cyclomalto-oligosaccharides. In *Advances in Carbohydrate Chemistry and Biochemistry*, R. S. Tipson and D. Horton (Eds.), San Diego, CA: Academic Press.

Cohen, J. and J. L. Lach. 1963. Interaction of pharmaceuticals with Schardinger Dextrins I interaction with hydroxybenzoic acids and p-hydroxybenzoates. *J. Pharm. Sci.* 52: 132–136.

Connors, K. A. 1987. *Binding Constants—The Measurement of Molecular Complex Stability*. New York: John Wiley & Sons.

Connors, K. A. 1990. Complex formation. In *Remington's Pharmaceutical Sciences*, 18th ed., A. R. Gebbaro (Ed.), London, UK: Mack Publishing Company.

Connors, K. A. 1997. The stability of cyclodextrin complexes in solution. *Chem. Rev.* 97: 1325–1357.

Cramer, F., W. Saenger and H. C. Spatz. 1967. Inclusion compounds. XIX. The formation of inclusion compounds of α-cyclodextrin in aqueous solutions. Thermodynamics and kinetics. *J. Am. Chem. Soc.* 89: 14–20.

Cromwell, W. C., K. Byström and M. R. Eftink. 1985. Cyclodextrin-adamantanecarboxylate inclusion complexes: Studies of the variation in cavity size. *J. Phys. Chem.* 89: 326–332.

Dahiya, S. and P. Tayde. 2013. Binary and ternary solid systems of carvedilol with 2-hydroxypropyl-β-cycllodextrin and Kollidon 30. *Bull. Pharm. Res.* 3(3): 128–134.

De Villiers, M. M., W. Liebenberg, S. F. Malan and J. J. Gerber. 1999. The dissolution and complexing properties of ibuprofen and ketoprofen when mixed with N-methylglucamine. *Drug Dev. Ind Pharm.* 25(8): 967–972.

Demirel, M., G. Yurtdas and L. Genc. 2011. Inclusion complexes of ketoconazole with beta-cyclodextrin: Physicochemical characterization and in vitro dissolution behaviour of its vaginal suppositories. *J. Incl. Phenom. Macrocycl. Chem.* 70(3–4): 437–445.

Devarakonda, B., R. A. Hill, W. Liebenberg, M. Brits and M. M. de Villiers. 2005. Comparison of the aqueous solubilization of practically insoluble niclosamide by polyamidoamine (PAMAM) dendrimers and cyclodextrins. *Int. J. Pharm.* 304(1–2): 193–209.

Dilova, V., V. Zlatarova, N. Spirova, K. Filcheva, A. Pavlova and P. Grigorova. 2004. Study of insolubility problems of dexamethasone and digoxin: Cyclodextrin complexation. *Bollettino Chimico Farmaceutico.* 143(1): 20–23.

Djordje, M., K. Kyriakos, D. Zorica and I. Svetlana. 2015. Influence of hydrophilic polymers on the complexation of carbamazepine with hydroxypropyl-b-cyclodextrin. *Eur. J. Pharm. Sci.* 78: 273–285.

Donbrow, M., E. Touitou and H. Ben Shalom. 1976. Stability of salicylamide-caffeine complex at different temperatures and its thermodynamic parameters. *J. Pharm. Pharmac.* 28: 766–769.

Duan, M. S., N. Zhao, I. B. Oessurardottir, T. Thorsteinsson and T. Loftsson. 2005. Cyclodextrin solubilization of the antibacterial agents triclosan and triclocarban: Formation of aggregates and higher-order complexes. *Int. J. Pharm.* 297(1–2): 213–222.

Eftink, M. R., M. L. Andy, K. Bystrom, H. D. Perlmutter and D. S. Kristol. 1989. Cyclodextrin inclusion complexes: Studies of the variation in the size of alicyclic guests. *J. Am. Chem. Soc.* 111: 6765–6772.

Emara, L. H., R. M. Badr and A. A. Elbary. 2002. Improving the dissolution and bioavailability of nifedipine using solid dispersions and solubilizers. *Drug Dev. Ind Pharm.* 28(7): 795–807.

Ficarra, R., S. Tommasini, D. Raneri, M. L. Calabro, M. R. Di Bella, C. Rustichelli, M. C. Gamberini and P. Ficarra. 2002. Study of flavonoids/β-cyclodextrins inclusion complexes by NMR, FT-IR, DSC, X-ray investigation. *J. Pharm. Biomed. Anal.* 29(6): 1005–1014.

Fini, A., M. J. Fernàndez-Hervàs, M. A. Holgado, L. Rodriguez, C. Cavallari, N. Passerini and O. Caputo. 1997. Fractal analysis of β-cyclodextrin-indomethacin particles compacted by ultrasound, *J. Pharm. Sci.* 86(11): 1303–1309.

Frijlink, H. W., J. F. Franssen, A. C. Eissens, R. Oosting, C. F. Lerk and D. K. F. Meijer. 1991. The effect of cyclodextrins on the disposition of introvenously injected drugs in the rat. *Pharm. Res.* 8: 380–384.

Frömming, K. H. and I. Weyermann. 1973. Release of active substance after oral application of β-cyclodextrin inclusion compound to humans. *Arzneim. Forsch. (Drg. Res.)* 23: 424–426.

Fugioka, K., Y. Kurosaki, S. Sato, T. Noguchi and Y. Yamahira. 1983. Biopharmaceutical study of inclusion complexes. I. Pharmaceutical advantages of cyclodextrin complexes of bencyclane fumarate. *Chem. Pharm. Bull.* 31: 2416–2423.

Fukuda, N., N. Higuichi, M. Ohno, H. Kenmochi, H. Sekikawa and M. Takada. 1986. Dissolution behavior of prednisone from solid dispersion systems with cyclodextrins and polyvinylpyrrolidone. *Chem. Pharm. Bull.* 34: 1366–1369.

Glass, C. A. 1965. Proton magnetic resonance spectra of D-glucopyranose polymers. *Can. J. Chem.* 43: 2652–2659.

Green, A. R. and J. K. Guillory. 1989. Heptakis (2,6-di-o-methyl)-β-cyclodextrin complexation with the antitumor agent chlorambucil. *J. Pharm. Sci.* 78: 427–431.

Guo, L. S. S., R. M. Fielding, D. D. Lasic, R. L. Hamilton, and D. Mufson. 1991. Novel antifungal drug delivery: Stable amphotericin B-cholesteryl sulfate discs. *Int. J. Pharm.* 75: 45–54.

Hansen, L. D., E. A. Lewis and D. J. Ratough. 1985. In *Analytical Solution Calorimetry*, J. K. Grime (Ed.), New York: John Wiley & Sons.

Harata, K. 1989. Crystal structure of the inclusion complex of hexakis(2,6-di-O-methyl)cyclomaltohexaose with 3-iodopropionic acid. *Carbohydr. Res.* 192: 33–42.

Hersey, A., B. H. Robinson and H. C. Kelly. 1986. Mechanisms of inclusion-compound formation for binding of organic dyes, ions and surfactants to α-cyclodextrin studied by kinetic methods based on competition experiments. *J. Chem. Soc. Faraday Trans.* 82: 1271–1287.

Higuchi, T. and H. Kristiansen. 1970. Binding specificity between small organic solutes in aqueous solution: Classification of some solutes into two groups according to binding tendencies. *J. Pharm. Sci.* 59: 1601–1608.

Higuchi, T. and K. A. Connors. 1965. *Advances in Analytical Chemistry and Instrumentation*, Vol. 4., C. N. Reilly (Ed.), New York: Interscience.

Hursthouse, M. B., C. Z. Smith, M. Thornton-Pett and J. H. P. Utley. 1982. The x-ray crystal structure of an ethyl cinnamate-β-cyclodextrin guest-host complex. *J. Chem. Soc., Chem. Commun.* (15): 881–882.

Hussain, A. A. 1978. Novel 2-acetoxybenzoic acid-nicotinamide complexes. United States Patent 4120958.

Itoh, K., Y. Tozuka, T. Oguchi and K. Yamamoto. 2003. Improvement of physicochemical properties of N-4472. Part III. VC/N-4472 complex formation and self-association in aqueous solution. *Chem. Pharm. Bull.* 51(1): 40–45.

Jambhekar, S., R. Casella and T. Maher. 2004. The physicochemical characteristics and bioavailability of indomethacin from β-cyclodextrin, hydroxyethyl-β-cyclodextrin, and hydroxypropyl-β-cyclodextrin complexes. *Int J. Pharm.* 270(1–2): 149–166.

Johnson, M. D., B. L. Hoesterey and B. D. Anderson. 1994. Solubilization of a tripeptide HIV inhibitor using a combination of ionization and complexation with chemically modified cyclodextrins. *J. Pharm. Sci.* 83(8): 1142–1146.

Juluri, A. and S. Narasimha Murthy. 2014. Transdermal iontophoretic delivery of a liquid lipophilic drug by complexation with an anionic cyclodextrin. *J. Control. Release* 189: 11–18.

Kalepu, S. and V. Nekkanti. 2015. Insoluble drug delivery strategies: Review of recent advances and business prospects. *Acta Pharm. Sin B.* 5(5): 442–453.

Kim, J.-E., H.-J. Cho and D.-D. Kim. 2014. Budesonide/cyclodextrin complex-loaded lyophilized micropar-ticles for intranasal application. *Drug Dev. Ind. Pharm.* 40(6): 743–748.

Koehler, J. E. H., W. Saenger and W. F. van Gunsteren. 1987. A molecular dynamics simulation of crystalline α-cyclodextrin hexahydrate. *Eur. Biophys. J.* 15: 197–210.

Koizumi, K. and Y. Kidera. 1977. Effect of α- and β-cyclodextrin on gastrointestinal absorption of barbituric acid derivatives. *Yakugaku Zasshi*, 97: 705–711.

Kreilgård, B., T. Higuchi and A. J. Repta. 1975. Complexation of parenteral solutions: Solubiliztion of cyctoxic agent hexamethylmelamine by complexation with gentisic acid species. *J. Pharm. Sci.* 11: 1850–1855.

Kumar, A. R., K. Ashok, B. Brahmaiah, S. Nama and C. B. Rao (2013). The cyclodextrins: A review. *Int. J. Pharm. Res. Bio-Sci.* 2(2): 291–304.

Kurkov, S. V. and T. Loftsson. 2013. Cyclodextrins. *Int. J. Pharm.(Amsterdam, the Netherlands)*, 453(1): 167–180.

Kurkov, S. V., D. E. Madden, D. Carr and T. Loftsson. 2012. The effect of parenterally administered cyclodex-trins on the pharmacokinetics of coadministered drugs. *J. Pharm. Sci.* 101(12): 4402–4408.

Kurozumi, M., N. Nambu and T. Nagai. 1975. Inclusion compounds of non-steroidal antiinflammatory and other slightly water soluble drugs with α- and β-cyclodextrins in powdered form. *Chem. Pharm. Bull.* 23: 3062–3068.

Lach, J. L. and W. A. Pauli. 1966. Interaction of pharmaceuticals with Schardinger dextrins VI. Interactions of β-cyclodextrin, sodium deoxycholate, and deoxycholic acid with amines and pharmaceutical agents. *J. Pharm. Sci.* 55: 32–38.

Lahiani-Skiba, M., C. Barbot, F. Bounoure, S. Joudieh and M. Skiba. 2006. Solubility and dissolution rate of progesterone-cyclodextrin-polymer systems. *Drug Dev Ind. Pharm.* 32(9): 1043–1058.

Lengyyel, M. T. and J. Szejtli. 1985. Menadione-gamma cyclodextrin inclusion complex. *J. Inclus.Phenom.* 3: 1–8.

Lin, S. Y., Y. H. Kao and J. C. Yong. 1988. Grinding effect on some pharmaceutical properties of drugs by adding β-cyclodextrin. *Drug Develop. Indus. Pharm.* 14: 99–118.

Loftsson, T. and M. E. Brewster. 2013. Drug solubilization and stabilization by cyclodextrin drug carriers. Drug Delivery Strategies Poorly Water-Soluble Drugs, 67–101.

Loftsson, T. and M. Masson. 2001. Cyclodextrins in topical drug formulations: Theory and practice. *Int. J. Pharm.* 225(1–2): 15–30.

Loftsson, T. and M. Masson. 2004. The effects of water-soluble polymers on cyclodextrins and cyclodextrin solubilization of drugs. *J. Drug Deliv. Sci. Technol.* 14(1): 35–43.

Loftsson, T., M. Masson, and J. F. Sigurjonsdottir. 1999. Methods to enhance the complexation efficiency of cyclodextrins. *STP. Pharma. Sci.* 9(3): 237–242.

Loftsson, T., N. Leeves, J. F. Sigurjonsdottir, H. H. Sigurosson and M. Masson. 2001. Sustained drug delivery system based on a cationic polymer and an anionic drug/cyclodextrin complex. *Pharmazie* 56(9): 746–747.

Lokamatha, K. M., A. Bharathi, S. M. Shanta Kumar and N. Rama Rao. 2010. Effect of PVP-K30 on complexation and dissolution rate of Nevirapine-β-cyclodextrin complexes. *Int. J. Pharm. Pharm. Sci.* 2(4): 169–176.

Marletti, F. and S. Notelli. 1976. Charge-transfer complexes of p-hydroxyphenylbutazone. *Il Farmaco, Ed. Sc.* 31: 665–670.

Marttin, E., J. C. Verhoef and F. W. H. M. Merkus. 1998. Efficacy, safety and mechanism of cyclodextrins as absorption enhancers in nasal delivery of peptide and protein drugs. *J. Drug Target.* 6(1): 17–36.

Matsui, Y., T. Nishioka and T. Fujita. 1985. Quantitative structure-reactivity analysis of the inclusion mechanism by cyclodextrins. *Top. Curr. Chem. (Biomimetic inorganic Chemistry).* 128: 61–89.

McGinity, J.W., A. B. Combs and H. N. Martin. 1975. Improved method for microencapsulation of soluble pharmaceuticals. *J. Pharm. Sci.*, 64: 889–890.

Mesens, L. J. and P. Putteman. 1991. Pharmaceutical applications of 2-hydroxypropyl-β-cyclodextrin. In *New Trends in Cyclodextrins and Derivatives*, D. Duchene (Ed.), Paris: Editions de Santé.

Miro, A., F. Quaglia, U. Sorrentino, M. I. La Rotonda, R. D'Emmanuele Di Villa Bianca and R. Sorrentino. 2004. Improvement of gliquidone hypoglycaemic effect in rats by cyclodextrin formulations. *Eur. J. Pharm. Sci.* 23(1): 57–64.

Mori, Y., A. Suzuki, K. Yoshino and H. Kakihana. 1989. Complex formation of p-Boronophenylalanine with some monosaccharides. *Pigment Cell Res.* 2: 273–277.

Mukne, A. P. and M. S. Nagarsenker. 2004. Triamterene-β-cyclodextrin systems: Preparation, characterization and in vivo evaluation. *AAPS PharmSciTech* 51(1): article 19: 142–150.

Mura, P., G. P. Bettinetti, M. Cirri, F. Maestrelli, M. Sorrenti and L. Catenacci. 2005. Solid-state characterization and dissolution properties of Naproxen-Arginine-Hydroxypropyl-β-cyclodextrin ternary system. *Eur. J. Pharm. Biopharm.* 59(1): 99–106.

Murugan, E., D. P. Geetha Rani and V. Yogaraj. 2014. Drug delivery investigations of quaternised poly(propylene imine) dendrimer using nimesulide as a model drug. *Colloids Surf B Biointerfaces* 114: 121–129.

Nagabhushanam, M. V., P. Radhika, M. V. Ramana and P. S. Surekha. 2013. Solubility enhancement of Naproxen by using cyclodextrin complexes. *Int. J. Invent. Pharm. Sci.* 1(6): 537–541, 535 pp.

Nagase, Y., M. Hirata, M., K. Wada, H. Arima, F. Hirayama, T. Irie, M. Kikuchi, and K. Uekama. 2001. Improvement of some pharmaceutical properties of DY-9760e by sulfobutyl ether β-cyclodextrin. *Int. J. Pharm.* 229(1–2): 163–172.

Nakai, Y., E. Fukuoka, S. Nakajima and K. Yamamoto. 1977. Effects of grinding on physical and chemical properties of crystalline medicinals with microcrystalline cellulose. I. Some physical properties of crystalline medicinals in ground mixtures. *Chem. Pharm. Bull.*, 25: 3340–3346.

Nakai, Y., S. Nakajima, K. Yamamoto, K. Terada and T. Konno. 1980. Effects of grinding on the physical and chemical properties of crystalline medicinals with microcrystalline cellulose V: Comparison with tri-O-methyl-β-cyclodextrin ground mixtures. *Chem. Pharm. Bull.*, 28: 1552–1558.

Nakanishi, K., T. Nadai, M. Masada and K. Miyajima. 1992. Effect of cyclodextrins on biological membrane II. Mechanism of enhancement on the intestinal absorption of non-absorbable drug by cyclodextrins. *Chem. Pharm. Bull.* 40: 1252–1256.

Nishijo, J., K. Ohno, K. Nishimura, M. Hukuda, H. Ishimaru and I. Yonetani. 1982. Soluble complex formation of theophylline with aliphatic di- and monoamines in aqueous solution. *Chem. and Pharm. Bull.* 30(3): 771–776.

Okimoto, K., R. A. Rajewski, J. A. Jona and V. J. Stella. 1995. The interaction of charged and uncharged drugs with a neutral (HP-β-CD) and anionically charged (SBE-β-CD) β-cyclodextrin. *Pharm. Res.* 12: S205.

Okimoto, K., R. A. Rajewski and V. J. Stella. 1999. Release of testosterone from an osmotic pump tablet utilizing (SBE)7m-β-cyclodextrin as both a solubilizing and an osmotic pump agent. *J. Control. Release.* 58(1): 29–38.

Palem, C. R., K. S. C. Chopparapu, P. V. R. S. Subrahmanyam and M. R. Yamsani. 2012. Cyclodextrins and their derivatives in drug delivery: A review. *Curr. Trends Biotechnol. Pharm.* 6(3): 255–275.

Palmieri, G. F., D. Galli-Angeli, G. Giovannucci and S. Martelli. 1997. Inclusion of methoxybutropate in β- and hydroxypropyl β-cyclodextrins: comparison of preparation methods. *Drug Dev. Ind. Pharm.* 23(1): 27–37.

Patel, R. P., K. K. Sawant, M. M. Patel and N. R. Patel. 2005. Enhancement of the dissolution properties of furosemide by inclusion complexation with β-cyclodextrin. *Drug Deliv. Technol.* 5(3): 62–66.

Peeters, J., P. Neeskens, J. Adriaensen and M. Brewster. 2002. Alfaxalone: Effect of temperature on complexation with 2-hydroxypropyl-β-cyclodextrin. *J. Incl. Phenom. Macrocycl. Chem.* 44(1–4): 75–77.

Pralhad, T. and K. Rajendrakumar. 2004. Study of freeze-dried quercetin-cyclodextrin binary systems by DSC, FT-IR, X-ray diffraction and SEM analysis. *J. Pharm. Biomed. Anal.* 34(2): 333–339.

Puglisi, G., N.A. Santagati, R. Pignatello, C. Ventura, F. A. Bottino, S. Mangiafico and G. Mazzone. 1990. Inclusion complexation of 4-biphenylacetic acid with β-cyclodextrin. *Drug Dev. Ind. Pharm.* 16: 395–413.

Rajewski, R. A. and V. J. Stella. 1996. Pharmaceutical applications of cyclodextrins. II. In vivo drug delivery. *J. Pharm. Sci.* 85: 1142–1169.

Rao, V. S. R. and J. F. Foster. 1963. On the conformation of the D-glucopyranose ring in maltose and in higher polymers of D-glucose. *J. Phys. Chem.* 67: 951–952.

Repta, A. J. 1981. Alteration of apparent solubility through complexation. In *Techniques of Solubilization of Drugs*, S. H. Yolkowsky (Ed.), New York: Marcel Dekker.

Repta, A. J. and A. A. Hincal. 1980. Complexation and solubilization of acronine with alkylgentisates. *Int. J. Pharm.* 5: 149–155.

Reuning, R. H. and G. Levy. 1968. Characterization of complex formation between small molecules by membrane permeation measurements. *J. Pharm. Sci.* 57: 1556–1561.

Rode, T., M. Frauen, B. W. Muller, H. J. Dusing, U. Schonrock, C. Mundt and H. Wenck. 2003. Complex formation of sericoside with hydrophilic cyclodextrins: Improvement of solubility and skin penetration in topical emulsion based formulations. *Eur. J. Pharm. Biopharm.* 55(2): 191–198.

Siimer, E., M. Kurvits and A. Kostner. 1987. Thermochemical investigation of β-cyclodextrin complexes with benzoic acid and sodium benzoate. *Thermochimica Acta* 116: 249–256.

Simon, K., A. Stadler and F. Hange. 1981. Investigation of cyclodextrin complexes by X-ray powder diffraction. *Proceedings of the First International Symposium on Cyclodextrins*, Budapest, Hungary, pp. 251–259.

Sravya, M., R. Deveswaran, S. Bharath, B. V. Basavaraj and V. Madhavan. 2013. Development of orodispersible tablets of candesartan cilexetil-β-cyclodextrin complex. *J. Pharm. (N.Y., NY, U.S.):* 583536/583531–583536/583514.

Stella, V. J. and Q. He (2008). Cyclodextrins. *Toxicol. Pathol.* 36(1): 30–42.

Stella, V. J. and R. A. Rajewski. 1997. Cyclodextrins: Their future in drug formulation and delivery. *Pharm. Res.* 14(5): 556–567.

Szejtli, J. 1982. *Cyclodextrins and Their Inclusion Complexes.* Budapest: Akademiai Kiadó.

Szejtli, J. 1994. Medicinal applications of cyclodextrins. *Med. Res. Rev.* 14: 353–386.

Szekely-Szentmiklosi, B. and B. Tokes. 2011. Characterization and molecular modelling of cyclodextrin/fluoroquinolone inclusion complexes. *Acta Med. Marisiensis* 57(2): 116–120.

Takayama, K., N. Nambu and T. Nagai. 1977a. Interaction of n-methyl-2-pyrrolidone with aminobenzoic acids in solution and in solid state. *Chem. Pharm. Bull.* 25(5): 887–897.

Takayama, K., N. Nambu and T. Nagai. 1977b. Interaction of sulfonamides with cyclic polyether 18-crown-6. *Chem. Pharm. Bull.* 25(10): 2608–2612.

Taneri, F., T. Guneri, Z. Aigner, I. Eroes and M. Kata. 2003. Improvement of the physicochemical properties of clotrimazole by cyclodextrin complexation. *J. Incl. Phenom. Macrocyclic Chem.* 46(1–2): 1–13.

Thomason, M. A., H. Mwakibete and E. Wyn-Jones. 1990. Ultrasonic and electrochemical studies on the interactions of the drug chlorocyclizine hydrochloride with α-cyclodextrin and surfactant micelles. *J. Chem. Soc. Faraday Trans.* 86: 1511–1515.

Thompson, D. O. 1997. Cyclodextrins-enabling excipients: Their present and future use in pharmaceuticals. *Crit. Rev. Ther. Drug Carrier Syst.* 14(1): 1–104.

Tokumura, T., H. Ueda, Y. Tsushima, M. Kasai, M. Kayano, I. Amada, Y. Machida and T. Nagai. 1984. Inclusion complex of cinnarizine with β-cyclodextrin in aqueous solution and in solid state. *J. Inclus. Phenom.* 2: 511–521.

Tong, W. Q., J. L. Lach, T. F. Chin and J. K. Guillory. 1991a. Structural effects on the binding of amine drugs with the diphenylmethyl functionality to cyclodextrin II: A molecular modeling study. *Pharm. Res.* 8: 1307–1312.

Tong, W. Q., J. L. Lach, T. F. Chin and J. K. Guillory. 1991b. Structural effects on the binding of amine drugs with the diphenylmethyl functionality to cyclodextrin I: A microcalorimetric study. *Pharm. Res.* 8: 951–957.

Tong, W.Q., T. F. Chin and J. K. Guillory. 1991. Microcalorimetric investigation of the complexation between 2-Hydroxypropyl-β-cyclodextrin and amine drugs with the diphenylmethyl functionality. *J. Pharm. Biomed. Anal.* 9: 1139–1146.

Truelove, J., R. Bawarshi-Nassar, N. R. Chen and A. Hussain. 1984. Solubility enhancement of some developmental anti-cancer nucleoside analogs by complexation with nicotinamide. *Int. J. Pharm.* 19: 17–25.

Uekama, K. 1985. Pharmaceutical applications of methylated cyclodextrins. *Pharm. Int.* 5: 61–65.

Uekama, K., T. Imai, T. Maeda, T. Irie, F. Hirayama and M. Otagiri. 1985. Improvement of dissolution and suppository release characteristics of flurbiprofen by inclusion complexation with heptakis(2,6-di-O-methyl)-β-cyclodextrin. *J. Pharm. Sci.* 74(8): 841–845.

Uekama, K., F. Hirayama and T. Irie. 1994. Application of cyclodextrins. In *Drug Absorption Enhancement*, A. G. de Boer. (Ed.), Chur, Switzerland: Harwood Academic Publishers.

Uekama, K., M. Otagiri, Y. Uemura, T. Fujinaga, K. Arimori, N. Matsuo, K. Tasaki and A. Sugii. 1983a. Improvement of oral bioavailability of prednisolone by β-cyclodextrin complexation in humans. *J. Pharmacobio-Dyn.* 6: 124–127.

Uekama, K., S. Narisawa, F. Hirayama and M. Otagiri. 1983b. Improvement of dissolution and absorption characteristics of benzodiazepines by cyclodextrin complexation. *Int. J. Pharm.* 16: 327–338.

Uekama, K., T. Fuginaga, F. Horayama, M. Otagiri, M. Yamasaki, H. Seo, T. Hashimoto and M. Tsuruoka. 1983c. Improvement of the oral bioavailability of digitalis glycosides by cyclodextrin complexation. *J. Pharm. Sci.* 72: 1338–1341.

Uekama, K., T. Fujinaga, F. Hirayama, M. Otagiri, H. Seo and M. Tsuruoka. 1981. *Proceedings of the First International Symposium on Cyclodextrins*, Budapest, p. 141.

Uekama, K., Y. Ikeda, F. Hirayama, M. Otagiri and M. Shibata. 1980. Inclusion complexation of *p*-hydroxybenzoic acid esters with α- and β-cyclodextrins: Dissolution behaviors and antimicrobial activities. *Yakugaku Zasshi*, 100: 994–1003.

Vicens, J., T. Fujiwara and K.-I. Tomita. 1988. X-ray structural studies of β-cyclodextrin inclusion complexes with racemic and S(-)methyl-p-tolylsulfoxides. *J. Incl. Phenom.* 6: 577–581.

Winnike, R. A., D. E. Wurster and J. K. Guillory. 1988. A solid sampling device for use in batch solution calorimetry. *Thermochimica Acta* 124: 99–108.

Yang, G., N. Jain and S. H. Yalkowsky. 2004. Combined effect of SLS and (SBE)7M-β-CD on the solubilization of NSC-639829. *Int. J. Pharm.* 269(1): 141–148.

Yang, W. and M. M. De Villiers. 2004. Aqueous solubilization of furosemide by supramolecular complexation with 4-sulphonic calix[n]arenes. *J Pharm Pharmacol.* 56(6): 703–708.

Yao, Y., Y. Xie, C. Hong, G. Li, H. Shen and G. Ji. 2014. Development of a myricetin/hydroxypropyl-β-cyclodextrin inclusion complex: Preparation, characterization, and evaluation. *Carbohydr. Polym.* 110: 329–337.

Zaki, R. M., A. A. Ali, S. F. El Menshawi and A. Abdel Bary. 2013. Effect of binary and ternary solid dispersions prepared by fusion method on the dissolution of poorly water soluble diacerein. *Int. J. Drug Deliv.* 5(1): 99–109.

Zeng, F., L. Wang, W. Zhang, K. Shi and L. Zong. 2013. Formulation and in vivo evaluation of orally disintegrating tablets of clozapine/hydroxypropyl-β-cyclodextrin inclusion complexes. *AAPS PharmSciTech* 14(2): 854–860.

Zhang, B. and L. Isaacs. 2014. Acyclic cucurbit[n]uril-type molecular containers: Influence of aromatic walls on their function as solubilizing excipients for insoluble drugs. *J. Med. Chem.* 57(22): 9554–9563.

Zoeller, T., J. B. Dressman and S. Klein. 2012. Application of a ternary HP-β-CD-complex approach to improve the dissolution performance of a poorly soluble weak acid under biorelevant conditions. *Int. J. Pharm. (Amsterdam, the Netherlands)* 430(1–2): 176–183.

Zugasti, M. E., A. Zornoza, M. d. M. Goni, J. R. Isasi, I. Velaz, C. Martin, M. Sanchez and M. C. Martinez-Oharriz. 2009. Influence of soluble and insoluble cyclodextrin polymers on drug release from hydroxypropyl methylcellulose tablets. *Drug Dev. Ind. Pharm.* 35(10): 1264–1270.

9 Solubilization Using Cosolvent Approach

Jay S. Trivedi and Zhanguo Yue

CONTENTS

INTRODUCTION

As the structural complexity of new compounds increases, typically solubility of the molecule is reduced dramatically. One of the first steps in the drug absorption process is the disintegration of a dosage form (e.g., tablet or capsule) followed by dissolution of the drug before any absorption can take place. Thus, dissolution is the rate-limiting step in the entire drug absorption process. At an early stage of the development (e.g., hit to lead or lead optimization), when physicochemical properties information is limited (e.g., crystallinity, solubility, dissolution, etc.), a solubilized formulation is highly desired to minimize dissolution limited absorption as well as to minimize interstudy variability. Often, these early stage formulations become the backbone for the later stage commercial formulations. Hence, the selection of an appropriate solubilizing technique is a tremendous challenge for a scientist.

Scientists have used numerous techniques, from pH manipulations to complexations with cyclodextrin to emulsions and microemulsions. All of these techniques are well described by our fellow authors in this book.

COSOLVENT

When the aqueous solubility of a drug is well below its therapeutic dose, a mixture of solvents is added to achieve sufficiently high solubility. Thus, a cosolvent is a water-miscible organic solvent that is used to increase the solubility of a poor water-soluble compound or to increase the chemical stability of a drug.

Cosolvents can increase the solubility of a nonpolar drug up to several orders of magnitude compared to its aqueous solubility. This is significant for a formulation where it may be necessary to increase substantially the solubility of a drug. Other methods such as complexation or micellization may not achieve the desired solubility for a necessary therapeutic dosage. Techniques such as complexation could suffer because identification of a suitable substance that will form a soluble complex with the drug may not be possible unless the drug conforms to certain structural requirements (Higuchi and Kristiansen 1970). The use of surface-active agents in drug formulations may result in toxicity problems, especially when given by the parental route (Attwood and Florence 1980). Even though methods such as prodrug and salt formation can result in an increase in solubility, it requires synthesis of new drug entities that results in additional animal studies to confirm their efficacy and toxicity. Thus, the advantages of using cosolvents are not only the dramatic increase in drug solubility but also its simplicity.

Another aspect of using cosolvents is that a change in solvent property can considerably change the rate and order of a reaction. In 1890, Menschutkin demonstrated the effect of various solvent media on the rate of reaction between triethylamine and iodoethane in 23 solvents (Menschutkin 1900). For drugs that may undergo hydrolytic degradation, an advantage of using a cosolvent is to reduce the degradation of the drug by reducing the concentration of water in the formulation and hence, increasing the chemical stability of the drug in its liquid state. Alternatively, a cosolvent may enhance the stability of a drug by providing a less suitable environment for the transition state of the reactants. This is provided the transition state is more polar than the reactants (Connors et al. 1979; Soni et al. 2014; Chen et al. 2015; Thakkar et al. 2016; Verma et al. 2016; Jouyban et al. 2017).

When delivered parentally or orally, a drug in solution is more rapidly bioavailable compared to a solid dosage form. The cosolvent approach also has some limitations as pointed out for other solubilization techniques. When solubilization of a drug is achieved by use of cosolvent, it must meet certain requirements, such as nontoxicity, compatibility with blood, nonsensitizing, nonirritating, and above all physically and chemically stable and inert. There is also some concern about whether cosolvents alter the affinity of a hydrophobic drug to its target (Senac et al. 2017). The biggest disadvantage of using a cosolvent is the toxicity of most of the water-miscible solvents that have a high potential for increasing drug solubility. The toxicological property of a solvent that may limit or eliminate its use in a formulation is its general toxicity, target organ toxicity, tissue irritation, or tonicity with respect to biologic membranes. Poor taste of a formulation is always a major consideration for a selection of a cosolvent intended for oral dosage formulation. There have been major efforts to mask a poorly tasted formulation with certain excipients such as corn syrup, citric acid, and fructose. The discussion on flavoring and taste masking of an oral formulation is outside the scope of this chapter, but those readers interested in that area may want to refer to review articles by Roy as a starting point (Roy 1990, 1992, 1994).

Under extreme time constraint for early phase animal studies, and availability of drug quantities to conduct appropriate solubility studies, it is very tempting to utilize various *exotic* excipients to solubilize the drug. However, one should be keenly aware that there is definite evidence of effect of formulation vehicles on metabolic enzymes, transporters, and distribution, and hence unintentional alteration of drug pharmacokinetic properties. Very little is known about drug–excipient interactions in blood through parenteral route, specifically low dosed compounds, biomarkers, and microdoses. Hence, drug–excipient interactions are very important in the drug development process, especially intended for parenteral route for *in vivo* animal pharmacokinetic studies or later for commercial dosage form. A formulator must avoid the use of some excipients unless the interaction is well understood.

In this chapter, the uses of cosolvents are discussed with some specific limitations. The discussion is limited to the cosolvent effects on solubility and stability, and their use in parenteral products. For information on the use of cosolvents in other dosage forms such as soft gelatin capsules, the reader is referred to the specific chapter in this book on the topic.

METHODS OF PREDICTING SOLUBILITY IN COSOLVENTS

THEORETICAL METHODS

Rubino (1984) has reviewed the progression of approaches for predicting solubility in cosolvents. One of the first advances beyond empirical trial-and-error was the use of the dielectric constant ($\in$) to optimize cosolvent systems. The dielectric constant is a dimensionless parameter because it is the ratio of the capacitance of a condenser filled with the material of interest versus a vacuum. Cosolvents that are more polar have larger dielectric constants. Much work has been done around the use of the dielectric constant for optimizing pharmaceutical cosolvent systems (Moore 1958; Paruta et al. 1962, 1964; Sorby et al. 1963, 1965; Gorman and Hall 1964; Paruta 1964, 1966a,b, 1969; Paruta and Irani 1965; Paruta et al. 1965a,b; Paruta and Sheth 1966; Kato and Ohuchi 1972; Amirjahed and Blake 1974, 1975; Neira et al. 1980; Chien, 1984; Ibrahim and Shawky 1984). Simply speaking, the optimal cosolvent system should have a dielectric constant analogous to the solute being dissolved. In general, it has been recognized that the $\in$ of a mixture of two or more solvents is directly proportional to the fraction of the individual solvents (Yalkowsky and Roseman 1981). In this method, to calculate $\in$ of a solvent mixture, one needs to know the $\in$ of the pure solvents. The $\in$ of a solvent mixture is calculated based on a simplified Onsager–Kirkwood equation shown in the following:

$$\text{D.C.} = \sum (\text{fraction of solvent } A \times \text{D.C. of solvent } A) \\ + (\text{fraction of solvent } B \times \text{D.C. of solvent } B)$$

(9.1)

The method of calculating $\in$ of complex mixtures using the above-mentioned equation would theoretically be correct only if the mixture behaves like an ideal solution. Since most solvent mixtures may exhibit a high degree of intermolecular association, a $\in$ of such systems would lead to a deviation from the experimental data. The simplified Onsager–Kirkwood equation provides only a good approximate dielectric constant for mixed solvent systems.

Owing to ease of use, volume/volume fraction system is used more frequently in mixing of two or more solvents over percent weight/weight fractions system. In case of percent volume/volume fraction system, one needs to recognize that the final volume of miscible solvents may not attain 100%. Sorby et al. (1963) have measured dielectric constant of mixtures containing water–ethanol–glycerin and water–ethanol–propylene glycol and compared them with the calculated dielectric constant of mixtures using Onsager–Kirkwood method. They observed large deviations for the measured values of dielectric constant from those calculated using Onsager–Kirkwood's simplified approach. They also noted that deviations of such a magnitude were also observed for binary systems. Another observation was noted that even though there was a poor agreement between calculated and measured dielectric constants, "the nature of the curves does indicate that dielectric constants in these systems are apparently some type of linear function of the concentration of the various components expressed on a volume basis; however, because of the various complexities of these systems, no simple relationship appears to exist between dielectric constants of the mixtures and those of the pure components, which would allow computation by the simplified form of the Onsager–Kirkwood equation." Furthermore, there was no advantage of using weight fractions over volume fractions.

Rubino (1984) cited the shortcoming of the dielectric constant as being the inability of this individual molecular polarity parameter to reflect the summation of all attractive forces that surround a molecule leading to an inability to predict solubilities in different solvent systems.

A better estimate of all attractive forces surrounding a molecule was found in the use of the solubility parameter, δ (Hildebrand 1916, 1919). Hancock et al. (1997) has reviewed the use of solubility parameters in pharmaceutical dosage form design. The solubility parameter is used as a measure of the internal pressures of the solvent and solute in nonideal solutions. Cosolvents that are more polar have larger solubility parameters. The square root of the cohesive energy density, that is, the square root of the energy of vaporization per unit volume of substance, is known as the solubility parameter and was developed from Hildebrand's regular solution theory in the Scatchard–Hildebrand equation (Hildebrand and Scott 1950, 1962):

$$-\log X_2 = \frac{\Delta H_f}{2.303RT}\left(\frac{T_m - T}{T_m}\right) + \frac{V_2\Phi_1^2}{2.303RT}(\delta_1 - \delta_2)^2 \tag{9.2}$$

where X_2 is the mole fraction of solute, ΔH_f is the heat of fusion of the solute, R is the gas constant, T is the absolute temperature of the solution, T_m is the melting point of the solid solute in absolute degrees, V_2 is the molar volume of the supercooled liquid solute, and Φ_1 is the volume fraction of the solvent. The second term to the right of the equal sign represents the decrease in solubility owing to intermolecular interaction differences of the solute and solvent molecules. Even though this represented advancement in the understanding of solubility (Gordon and Scott 1952; Chertkoff and Martin 1960; Restaino and Martin 1964), there are drawbacks to the regular solution theory. Rubino (1984) summarized these as being that the use of this equation is limited to one solute and one solvent, the equation is valid only for solutions where the solute and solvent are of comparable size, but most importantly, this equation is technically only applicable for solutions where the intermolecular forces between the solute and solvent consist of London dispersion forces.

Because of the need for better predictability in more aqueous cosolvent systems, the Scatchard–Hildebrand equation was modified into the Extended Hildebrand equation (Martin 1979, 1980):

$$-\log X_2 = \frac{\Delta H_f}{2.303RT}\left(\frac{T_m - T}{T_m}\right) + \frac{V_2\Phi_1^2}{2.303RT}(\delta_1^2 + \delta_2^2 - 2W)^2 \tag{9.3}$$

where W term is the potential energy or interaction energy between the solute and the solvent. While the Extended Hildebrand equation has been demonstrated in several cosolvent systems of varying polarity (Martin et al. 1979, 1980, 1981; Adjei et al. 1980; Martin and Miralles 1982), it suffers because calculation of the W term requires nonlinear regression of solubility data of the drug in the cosolvent system of interest. Therefore, it is not predictive.

To improve further on this equation, three-dimensional solubility parameters were proposed (Beerbower and Hansen 1971; Martin et al. 1981; Barton 1983) to account for more specific interactions that can occur, such as hydrogen bonding. The solubility parameter was divided into three components:

$$\delta_t^2 = \delta_d^2 + \delta_p^2 + \delta_h^2 \tag{9.4}$$

where δ_t^2 is the total cohesive energy density, δ_d^2 is the contribution to the cohesive energy density due to London dispersion forces, δ_p^2 is the contribution to the cohesive energy density due to polar interactions, and δ_h^2 is the contribution to the cohesive energy density due to hydrogen bonding. The cohesive energy density for dispersive forces can be calculated through a nonpolar homomorph or all three terms can be estimated through group contribution approaches (Martin et al. 1981).

The solubility parameter approach was subsequently expanded from three to four terms with the division of the hydrogen-bonding parameter into acidic and basic solubility parameters to quantify electron-donor and electron-acceptor properties (Beerbower et al. 1984; Martin et al. 1984). However, the expansion of these solubility parameter terms did not make the equation any easier to use for the *a priori* prediction of solubility in cosolvent systems.

Other attempts at characterizing the deviation from ideal solubility theory have been made. Anderson et al. (1980) showed that solubilities that could not be rationalized from the regular solution theory could be rationalized by assuming the formation of specific solute–solvent complexes. Yalkowsky et al. (1975) and Amidon et al. (1974) showed that the deviation from the ideal solubility equation could be expressed in terms of interfacial tension and surface area. In equation form,

$$-\log X_2 = \frac{\Delta H_f}{2.303RT}\left(\frac{T_m - T}{T_m}\right) + \frac{A\gamma_{12}}{2.303RT} \tag{9.5}$$

where A is the surface area of the solute and γ_{12} is the interfacial tension between the solute and solvent. Yalkowsky et al. (1976) expanded this concept further. The disadvantage to these equations is the fact that A, the surface area of the solute, must be known. The advantage of this approach is that the interfacial tension can be measured easily for compounds of different polarity when solubility parameters cannot be used. When interfacial tension is difficult to measure, for example, when polarities are low and very similar, the solubility parameter approach is more reasonable. Therefore, the two approaches are complementary.

Acree and Rytting (1982 and 1983) developed the nearly ideal binary solvent (NIBS) approach to predict solubilities. NIBS did show an increased ability to predict solubilities versus the Scatchard–Hildebrand equation. However, it is limited to use in systems only involving nonspecific interactions.

On the basis of excess Gibb's energy approach of Wohl (Wisniak and Tamir 1978), Williams and Amidon (1984a–c) predicted solubilities in aqueous cosolvent systems. This approach is based on expressing the solubility of a compound in a binary solvent system as the sum of the solubilities of the compound in each pure solvent plus any interaction terms resulting from solvent–solvent to solvent–solute interactions. This approach predicted solubilities fairly well, but included some simplifying assumptions about solute–solvent interactions that may not be applicable to all systems.

In Rubino's (1984) review of approaches to predicting solubility in cosolvent systems, Yalkowsky and Roseman (1981) proposed one of the simplest and most useful methods. Their equation,

$$\log S_\mathrm{m} = f \log S_\mathrm{c} + (1 - f) \log S_\mathrm{w} \tag{9.6}$$

where S_m is the solubility in the binary mixture, f is the volume fraction of cosolvent, S_c is the solubility of the drug in the pure cosolvent, and S_w is the solubility of the drug in water, predicts a log-linear increase in solubility with increasing cosolvent. This equation is based on the assumption that the total free energy of the system is equal to the sum of the free energies of the individual components. Rubino also pointed out that this equation is also only applicable to nonpolar compounds throughout the entire range of cosolvent concentration. For semipolar compounds that show a maximum in the solubility versus fraction cosolvent plot, this equation is useful for either the ascending or descending portions of the curve.

This equation can be further simplified into

$$\log S_\mathrm{m} = \log S_\mathrm{w} + f\sigma \tag{9.7}$$

where

$$\sigma = \log \mathrm{ac_w} - \log \mathrm{ac_c} \tag{9.8}$$

and $\mathrm{ac_w}$ and $\mathrm{ac_c}$ are the activity coefficients for the drug in water and cosolvent, respectively. In a given cosolvent–water system, σ will be constant. Therefore, if one plots $\log S_\mathrm{m}$ versus f, the slope will be σ. Comparing slopes for different cosolvent–water systems can easily be done by using σ as a measure of the solubilization potential of the cosolvent. This equation assumes there is no change in the melting point or enthalpy of fusion of the solute. This would not be the case if the solute precipitates as a different crystalline form (Bogardus 1983). Although this equation is not predictive *a priori*, knowing the solubility in water and in the pure cosolvent, one can estimate the solubility of a nonpolar solute at all other combinations of water and cosolvent at the given conditions.

Yalkowsky and Roseman (1981) investigated a through partition coefficients. Since partition coefficients are really activities of a compound in an organic phase, usually octanol, relative to an aqueous phase or other phase, the above-mentioned equation can be rewritten as

$$\sigma = \log \mathrm{PC_{o/w}} - \log \mathrm{PC_{o/w}} \tag{9.9}$$

where $\mathrm{PC_{o/w}}$ is the octanol/water partition coefficient and $\mathrm{PC_{o/c}}$ is the octanol/cosolvent partition coefficient. For nonpolar drugs, it has been shown that $\log \mathrm{PC_{o/c}}$ can be estimated to be less than and proportional to $\log \mathrm{PC_{o/w}}$ (Leo et al. 1971). This being true,

$$\sigma = S \log \mathrm{PC_{o/w}} + T \tag{9.10}$$

where S and T are constants for each cosolvent. Yalkowsky and Roseman (1981) showed that for the cosolvents of greatest interest in pharmaceuticals, the relative σ of propylene glycol/polyethylene glycols 200–500/ethanol/glycerin is 1:1:2:0.5.

Yalkowsky and Rubino (1985), Rubino et al. (1984, 1987), Rubino and Yalkowsky (1985), Li and Yalkowsky (1994) have further studied log-linear cosolvent solubilization. For organic solutes in propylene glycol–water mixtures, Yalkowsky and Rubino found that the following equation

$$\log \frac{S_m}{S_w} = (0.714 \log p_{o/w} + 0.174)f \tag{9.11}$$

gave an excellent prediction for solubility for almost 400 organic solutes (Yalkowsky and Rubino 1985). Therefore, knowing only compounds solubility in water and octanol/water partition coefficient, one can get a reasonable solubility estimate for any propylene glycol–water mixture.

Similarly, Li and Yalkowsky (1994) determined that for ethanol–water mixtures where the fraction of ethanol is less than 0.6, the following equation could be used to calculate solubility profiles of an organic solute:

$$\log S_m - \log S_w = (1.274 + 0.791 \, C \log P)f \tag{9.12}$$

where $C \log P$ is the calculated log of the partition coefficient for the compound through Hansch's fragment method.

Rubino et al. (1984, 1987), Rubino and Yalkowsky (1985) studied solubilization by cosolvents in binary and ternary systems. They determined that the solubility of poor water-soluble drugs was approximately described by the log-linear solubility equation as applied to multiple solvent systems:

$$\log \frac{S_m}{S_w} = \sum_{i=1}^{n} (\sigma_i f_i) \tag{9.13}$$

However, in all these investigations, deviations from exact log-linear behavior were seen.

Deviations, as mentioned earlier, can be seen when there is a change in the solid crystalline phase with a change in cosolvent concentration. Hydrate formation (Gould et al. 1989) decreases the solubility in primarily aqueous systems. Rubino and Thomas (1990) found that crystal solvation played a significant role in the solubility behavior of sodium salts in mixed solvent systems. Although the log-linear equation is not applicable to ionizable drugs, it still has been used in such cases. When doing so, one must remember that cosolvents can affect the ionization constant of compounds. In other words, the pH range where the compound is in its unionized state will be different with differing cosolvent amounts as compared to a totally aqueous system. Rubino (1987) has determined in general that for acidic species, cosolvents increase the pK_a, whereas for amines, cosolvents decrease the pK_a.

Deviations from log-linear behavior can still occur even if none of the previous explanations is valid for your system (Groves et al. 1984; Rubino and Yalkowsky 1987; Rubino and Obeng 1991; Tarantino et al. 1994). Deviations are typically at low and/or high concentrations of cosolvent. Typically, negative deviations are observed at low cosolvent concentrations and positive deviations are observed at high cosolvent concentrations. In Rubino and Yalkowsky's (1991) review of this topic, deviations could not be consistently attributed to physical properties of the cosolvent–water mixtures or alterations in the solute crystal. They concluded that changes in the structure of the solvent play a role in deviation from expected log-linear solubilities.

Yalkowsky and Roseman (1981) also discussed drug solubility in cosolvent systems where the drug is semipolar and polar. Typically, semipolar drugs have parabolic log solubility curves. The peak in these plots is where the best mixture of cosolvent and water is for greatest solubilization of the compound. Since the drug is semipolar, further addition of the more nonpolar cosolvent results in a decrease in the drug's solubility. Yalkowsky and Roseman (1981) proposed a semiempirical quadratic equation for application to semipolar drugs. For polar drugs, the addition of a less polar solvent tends to decrease the solubility of that compound. Therefore, their solubility curves show decreasing solubility with increasing cosolvent content.

Gould et al. (1984) studied the solubility relationships of polar, semipolar, and nonpolar drugs in mixed cosolvent systems. As expected, the nonpolar compound showed a log-linear increase in solubility with increasing cosolvent content. The semipolar compound showed parabolic log solubility curves. The polar compound showed a log-linear decrease in solubility with addition of cosolvent.

Comparisons between the Extended Hildebrand solubility approach and the log-linear solubility equation have been made (Martin et al. 1982; Wu and Martin 1983). However, the key to understanding when the log-linear solubility equation will apply is in understanding the relative polarities of the cosolvent(s) and solute.

Other methods of calculating solubility in cosolvent systems have included the UNIFAC group contribution method (Grunbauer et al. 1986) and the UNIQUAC local composition model (Grant and Higuchi 1990). In general, both approaches use the contributions of functional groups to estimate or predict the solubility of a nonelectrolyte in a cosolvent system. Both approaches require the use of tabulated parameters and at least one experimentally determined solubility of drug in pure water to predict a solubility profile. These are excellent methods for the computer-aided design of pharmaceutical dosage forms with increased solubility. The reader is referred to references for more details (Grunbauer et al. 1986; Grant and Higuchi 1990).

Rubino and Yalkowsky (1987) have reviewed cosolvency and cosolvent polarity. In this study, they related slopes, σ, of solubility plots, by means of linear or multiple linear regression, to indexes of polarity such as dielectric constant, solubility parameter, surface tension, interfacial tension, and octanol–water partition coefficients. Two other indexes were investigated: hydrogen-bond donor densities (HBD) and hydrogen-bond acceptor densities (HBA). These terms can be calculated by multiplying the number of proton donor groups for HBD or number of nonbonding electron pairs for HBA by the density of the cosolvent by 1000, then dividing by the molecular weight of the cosolvent. Those indexes that reflect the cohesive properties of the solvents, for example, solubility parameter and interfacial tension, resulted in the highest correlations with the slopes, σ. Therefore, these are better indexes for comparing polarity of compounds.

EMPIRICAL METHODS

The previous section discussed specific theoretical approaches to characterizing solubility in cosolvent systems. While this is extremely useful for understanding the theory behind solubilization, more empirical methods of characterizing the solubility of cosolvent systems can be utilized with the aid of statistical experimental design. Advantages to this approach are that one can add additional excipients, for example, surfactants, without having to consider assumptions used in the derivation of equations and their validity to the systems studied. Another advantage is that typically these studies provide very accurate predictions of solubilities within the design space studied. This allows determination of optimal mixtures of excipients for maximum solubility. Disadvantages to this approach are that it gives no scientific insight as to the mechanism of solubilization. Therefore, the scientist must still interpret the meaning behind data from such studies.

Although factorial designs are very useful for studying multiple variables at various levels, typically they will not be applicable to cosolvent solubility studies because of the constraint that all of the components must add to 100%. For this reason, mixtures of experimental designs are typically used. The statistical theory behind mixture designs has been extensively published (Scheffé 1957, 1963; Cornell 1975, 1990, 1991). There are also multiple examples of the use of mixture designs for solubility studies of pharmaceutical systems (Anik and Sukumar 1981; Moustafa et al. 1981; Belloto et al. 1985; Ochsner et al. 1985; Lewis and Chariot 1991; Vojnovic et al. 1995, 1996, 1997; Wells et al. 1996).

Before conducting a mixture study, some preliminary experimentation must be done to narrow down and select the cosolvents or other excipients to be used in the design. After selecting the appropriate excipients, the ranges to be studied must be determined. In doing so, one will usually want to stay within the ranges that have been previously used for marketed products. Another item for consideration is if a buffer will be used, and if so, what concentration and what pH or apparent pH will be used. In deciding the pH, one must select a pH or pH range that will ensure that the solid-state form of the compound does not change throughout the samples studied. Although this cannot be prevented with complete certainty, as simply changing cosolvent concentrations can induce such changes, selecting an apparent pH should help ensure against a change from the ionized to the unionized state for ionizable compounds.

STABILITY CONSIDERATIONS

INFLUENCE OF DIELECTRIC CONSTANT ON REACTION RATES

There are theoretical expressions for the effect of the solvent on the reaction rate using dielectric constant ($\in$) and viscosity parameters. Grissom et al. (1993) have reported the increase in photostability of Vitamin B-12 by addition of viscogens, such as glycerol and Ficoll. However, in this section the focus will be on the influence of the dielectric constant of the solvent.

The degradation rate of a drug can change with the $\in$ of the medium. As a general rule, for reactions leading to products that are less polar than the starting material, a less polar media may accelerate the reaction. On the other hand, reactions leading to products that are more polar than the starting material can proceed more rapidly in polar media.

From the Debye–Huckel theory for the potential (Ψ) in the vicinity of an ion, Scatchard (1932) derived an expression for the effect of dielectric constant of the solvent:

$$\psi = \frac{Z_i \varepsilon}{Dr} \frac{\exp^{[\chi(a_i - r)]}}{1 + \chi a_i} \tag{9.14}$$

In Equation 9.14, Z_i is the valance of the ith ion, ε is the electron charge, D is the dielectric constant of the solvent medium, a_i is the distance of the closest approach to the ith ion, r is the distance from the ion at where the potential is Ψ, and χ is the Debye kappa. The Debye χ is

$$\chi = \sqrt{\frac{4\pi\varepsilon^2}{DkT}} \sqrt{\sum n_i Z_i^2} \tag{9.15}$$

where k is the Boltzmann's gas constant, T is the absolute temperature, n_i is the number of the ith ion. The activity coefficient f_i of the ith ion is

$$\ln f_i = \frac{1}{kT \displaystyle\int_0^{Z_i\varepsilon} \psi d(Z_i\varepsilon)} \tag{9.16}$$

Substituting the value of Ψ from Equation 9.14 into Equation 9.16:

$$\ln f_i = \frac{Z_i^2 \varepsilon^2}{2DkT(1 + \chi a_i)r} \exp^{[\chi(a_i - r)]} \tag{9.17}$$

For the simple reaction

$$A + B \Leftrightarrow [G] \rightarrow \text{Products} \tag{9.18}$$

From Equation 9.17

$$\ln \frac{f_A f_B}{f_G} = \frac{[Z_A^2 + Z_B^2 - (Z_A + Z_B)^2]\varepsilon^2}{DkTr(1 + \chi a_i)} \exp^{[\chi(a_i - r)]} \tag{9.19}$$

where $(Z_A + Z_B)$ represents the total charge of intermediate G and

$$\frac{f_A f_B}{f_G} = \exp\left(-\frac{Z_A Z_B \varepsilon^2}{DkTr(1 + \chi a_i)}\right) \exp[\chi(a_i - r)] \tag{9.20}$$

and further simplifying by $\chi = 0$ in Equation 9.20:

$$\frac{f_A f_B}{f_G} = \exp\left(-\frac{Z_A Z_B \varepsilon^2}{DkTr}\right) \tag{9.21}$$

Applying the Bronsted (1922, 1925) approach for the reaction at zero ionic strength in Equation 9.5:

$$\frac{C_G^0 f_G}{C_A^0 f_A C_B^0 f_B} = K^0 \tag{9.22}$$

and also substituting in Equation 9.21:

$$\ln \frac{f_A f_B}{f_G} = \ln \frac{1}{K^0} \frac{C_G^0}{C_A^0 C_B^0} = -\frac{Z_A Z_B \varepsilon^2}{DkTr} \tag{9.23}$$

Taking the difference between the logarithmic term when the D.C. of the solvent is D and when the dielectric constant of the solvent is some standard reference value D' where the activity coefficients of solutes, reactants, and complex become unity:

$$\ln \frac{f_A f_B}{f_G} - \ln\left(\frac{f_A f_B}{f_G}\right)_+ = \ln\left(\frac{f_A f_B}{f_G}\right) = \ln \frac{C_G^0}{C_A^0 C_B^0} - \ln\left(\frac{C_G^0}{C_A^0 C_B^0}\right)_+$$

$$= \frac{Z_A Z_B \varepsilon^2}{DkTr} - \left(\frac{Z_A Z_B \varepsilon^2}{D'kTr}\right) = \frac{Z_A Z_B \varepsilon^2}{kTr}\left(\frac{1}{D'} - \frac{1}{D}\right) \tag{9.24}$$

Now using the Bronsted (1922, 1925) approach, the velocity constant $k_{\chi=0}$ for a reaction at absolute temperature T and zero ionic strength that is independent from electrostatic effects due to ions and charged reactants, a simplified equation is obtained:

$$\ln k'_{\chi=0} = \ln k_{\chi=0, D=D'} + \ln \frac{f_A f_B}{f_G} \tag{9.25}$$

$$= \ln k'_{\chi=0, D=D'} + \frac{Z_A Z_B \varepsilon^2}{kTr}\left(\frac{1}{D'} - \frac{1}{D}\right)$$

The term $k'_{\chi=0, D=D'}$ in Equation 9.25 represents the specific velocity constant that is corrected for the change of specific velocity due to a standard transfer of the reactants from the media of standard reference dielectric constant D' to a media of dielectric constant D. Thus, Equation 9.25 provides the change in the specific velocity constant at zero ionic strength for a reaction with changing dielectric constant of the solvent at a constant temperature, if the change in rate with changing dielectric constant (due to changing composition of solvent) is controlled primarily by electrostatic considerations.

As suggested by Amis (1949), Amis and LaMer (1939), if the standard reference state of dielectric constant is taken as infinity:

$$\ln k'_{\chi=0} = \ln k'_{\chi=0, D=D'} - \frac{Z_A Z_B \varepsilon^2}{kTrD} \tag{9.26}$$

Scatchard also used this approach to calculate the intermediate C_G in Equation 9.21. The r used in aforementioned equation is the radius of the intermediate and can be expressed as $r = r_A + r_B$ (Christiansen 1924). To react, this is the distance to which molecules A and B must approach. The Equation 9.26 demonstrates the relationship between rate of reaction and the dielectric constant of the medium.

In summary, an increase in the ϵ of the medium causes the increased reaction rate in the presence of ions with the same sign, and a decreased reaction rate when the ions have opposite signs. The rate of reaction between an ion and a neutral molecule will decrease as the dielectric constant of the solvent increases. The reader may want to consult further Reichardt's text for further theoretical discussions (Christian 2011).

EXAMPLES OF EMPIRICAL APPROACHES

A typical first step in the development for a new molecule is to check the aqueous solubility and the pH of the drug molecule. It is very important that intrinsic solubility is also measured for molecules with ionizable groups. It appears that Garrett (1956) was the first one to report the effect of vehicle on the stability of drugs (vitamins) in a formulation. Even though, Garrett's focus was on stability studies and Arrhenius correlation to predict the rate constants at a lower (room) temperature for these formulations, the degradation of d-pantothenyl alcohol in two formulations provides an excellent example for the effect of vehicle on the rate constant.

Garrett's two formulation vehicles consisted mainly of 60% sugar and 19% alcohol (Preparation A) and 36% sugar and 2.35% alcohol (Preparation B). The slopes of Arrhenius plots as well as heats of activation for the d-pantothenyl alcohol in preparations A and B are same, but the plots are not superimposable indicating that the actual rates at a given temperature are different (Figure 9.1). Garrett's assumption of a similar mechanism of degradation in both

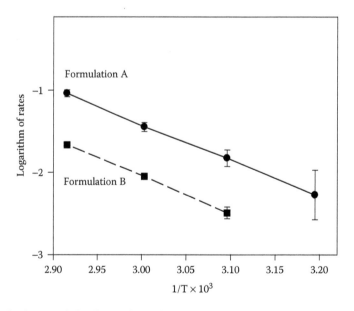

FIGURE 9.1 Arrhenius correlation for the first order rate constants for d-pantothenyl alcohol in Formulation A (60% sugar and 19% alcohol) and Formulation B (36% sugar and 2.35% alcohol). (Data replotted for Formulation A from *J. Am. Pharm. Assoc. Sci. Ed.*, 45, 470–473, 1956 (Table I) and for Formulation B, *J. Am. Pharm. Assoc. Sci. Ed.*, 45, 171–177, 1956 (Table II).)

preparations also leads to a conclusion that there may be a possible greater catalytic effect on the degradation in preparation A than the B. Since the main focus of Garrett's work was not to establish the individual effect of solvent component on the rate constant, it is difficult to conclude that the increase in degradation rate in preparation A is due to either higher sugar content or the alcohol content. Overall, these data indicate the effect of solvent vehicle on the degradation rate of *d*-pantothenyl alcohol.

Recently, a study on the effect of cosolvents on a degradation of zileuton has been reported (Trivedi et al. 1996). Under aqueous conditions, zileuton follows first order kinetics. In this study, authors have used a ternary solvent system consisting of water, ethanol, and propylene glycol to examine both the solubility and stability of zileuton.

Trivedi et al. showed that as the fraction of organic solvents was increased, the degradation rate of zileuton also increased (Figure 9.2). The increase in degradation was consistent with the decrease in the polarity (dielectric constant) of the solvent mixture.

Trivedi et al. utilized Sorby's experimental data for water–ethanol–propylene glycol and fitted to a complete second order polynomial model and performed a stepwise regression to arrive at following equation where x and y represent fractions of ethanol and propylene glycol, respectively:

$$\varepsilon = 81.25 - 77.5x - 42.9y + 19.2 \times 2 - 10.4y^2 \tag{9.27}$$

The authors further demonstrated a linear relationship between the degradation rate of zileuton and the $\in$ of solvent medium (Figure 9.3).

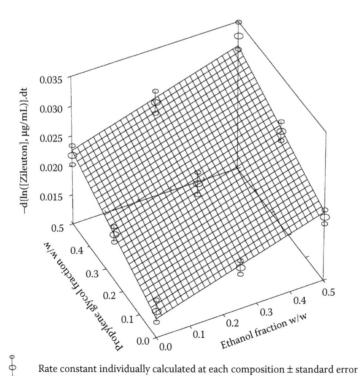

Rate constant individually calculated at each composition ± standard error

FIGURE 9.2 Pseudo-first-order degradation rate constant for zileuton as a function of water–ethanol–propylene glycol mixture composition.

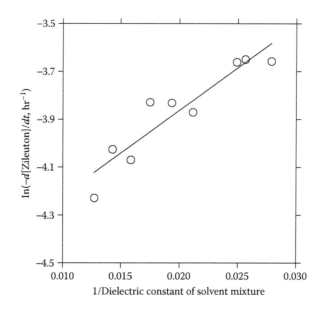

FIGURE 9.3 Effect of dielectric constant of water–ethanol–propylene glycol mixtures on the observed rate constant for zileuton.

Since the degradation of zileuton follows a hydrolytic degradation in aqueous environment, the increase in the rate of degradation in nonaqueous system (e.g., 50:50 ethanol:propylene glycol mixture exhibited the highest rate) was attributed to the solvent participation in the degradation mechanism, often referred as solvolysis. Patel et al. (1992) have reported that for their Drug 1 containing a carboxylic acid functional group, as compared to an aqueous medium, an increase in the rate of degradation was observed for the glycerin-containing medium.

COSOLVENTS IN ORAL COMMERCIAL PRODUCTS

Approximately 50% of the commercially available products are delivered through oral route. The majority of these products are formulated as either tablets or capsules. However, there is a significant amount of products still formulated as solutions, syrups, and elixirs. The primary role of the liquid dosage form is for pediatric and geriatric population who can swallow tablet or a capsule. In addition, solubilized formulations help overcome dissolution rate limited absorption issue. For an example, water-insoluble Digoxin when formulated with propylene glycol, ethanol with other excipients in Lanoxin Elixir, 70%–85% bioavailability is observed as a solubilized dosage (*Physician's Desk Reference* 2006). The solubilized formulations are also delivered through soft or hard gelatin capsules. In addition to solubilization, these capsule dosage forms have additional challenges such as cross-linking and compatibility. These are discussed in a separate chapter in this book and are not discussed further in this chapter.

A quick survey of the literature and pharmaceutical development report (PDR) suggests that the *most* commonly used water miscible cosolvents are dimethylacetamide (DMA), dimethyl sulfoxide (DMSO), ethanol, glycerin, polyethylene Glycol 300 and 400 (PEG), propylene glycol (PG), hydroxyl propyl-β-cyclodextrin (HP-β-CD), sulfobutyl-β-cyclodextrin (Captisol®), as well as surfactants such as Cremophor® (EL&RH), polysorbates (Tween® 20 and 80), *d*-∞-tocopheryl polyethylene glycol succinate (TPGS), Labrasol®, Labrafil®, Gellucire®, and Solutol HS 15®. Although, many of these surfactants at or above their critical micelle concentration (CMC) will self-assemble into micelles and may enhance solubilization process.

Table 9.1 is an alphabetical listing of commercially available solubilized formulations.

TABLE 9.1
List of Commercially Available Solubilized Oral Formulations

Molecule	Structure	Commercial Formulation	Excipients
Amprenavir		1. Soft gelatin capsule	1. PEG-400 (247, 740 mg), TPGS (280 mg), Propylene Glycol (19, 57 mg)
		2. Oral solution	2. PEG-400 (16%), TPGS (12%), propylene glycol (55%), sodium chloride, sodium citrate, citric acid
Bexarotene		Soft gelatin capsule	PEG-400, Polysorbate 20, Povidone and BHA
Calcitrol		1. Soft gelatin capsule	1. Fractionated coconut oil (medium-chain triglyceride)
		2. Oral solution	2. Fractionated palm seed oil (medium-chain triglyceride)

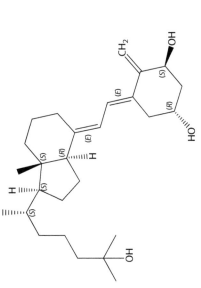

(Continued)

TABLE 9.1 (Continued)
List of Commercially Available Solubilized Oral Formulations

Molecule	Structure	Commercial Formulation	Excipients
Clofazimine		Soft gelatin capsule	Propylene glycol, oils, beeswax
Cyclosporin A		1. Soft gelatin capsule (Novartis)	1. Cremophor RH 40, glycerol, propylene glycol, DL-α-tocopherol, ethanol, corn oil-mono–di-triglyceride
		2. Oral solution (Novartis)	2. Cremophor RH 40, propylene glycol, DL-α-tocopherol, ethanol, corn oil-mono–di-triglyceride
Cyclosporin A		Hard gelatin capsule (Abbott)	Cremophor EL, polysorbate 80, propylene glycol sorbitan monooleate and ethanol
Cyclosporin A		1. Soft gelatin capsule (Novartis)	Corn oil, ethanol, Labrafil M2125 CS, glycerol
		2. Oral solution (Novartis)	Olive oil, ethanol, Labrafil M1944-CS

(Continued)

TABLE 9.1 (*Continued*)
List of Commercially Available Solubilized Oral Formulations

Molecule	Structure	Commercial Formulation	Excipients
Digoxin		1. Soft gelatin capsule 2. Elixir	PEG-400, propylene glycol, ethanol Ethanol, propylene glycol, citric acid, sodium phosphate, sucrose, flavor, methylparaben
Doxercalciferol		Soft gelatin capsule	Ethanol, medium-chain triglyceride
Dutasteride		Soft gelatin capsule	Mono- and diglyceride of caprylic/capric acid

(*Continued*)

TABLE 9.1 (*Continued*)
List of Commercially Available Solubilized Oral Formulations

Molecule	Structure	Commercial Formulation	Excipients
Etoposide		Soft gelatin capsule	PEG-400, glycerin, citric acid
Itraconazole		Oral solution	Propylene glycol, HP-β-CD

(*Continued*)

TABLE 9.1 (*Continued*)
List of Commercially Available Solubilized Oral Formulations

Molecule	Structure	Commercial Formulation	Excipients
Loratadine		Syrup	Propylene glycol, glycerin, citric acid, EDTA, sugar
Nifedipine		Soft gelatin capsule	PEG-400, glycerin, peppermint oil
Nimodipine		Soft gelatin capsule	PEG-400, glycerin, peppermint oil
Phenobarbital		Elixir	Glucose, ethanol, water, sodium saccharin

(Continued)

TABLE 9.1 (*Continued*)
List of Commercially Available Solubilized Oral Formulations

Molecule	Structure	Commercial Formulation	Excipients
Ritonavir		Soft gelatin capsule Oral solution	Cremophor EL, ethanol, BHT Cremophor EL, propylene glycol, ethanol
Sirolimus		Oral solution	Phosal 50 PG, Tween-80
Tretinoin		Soft gelatin capsule	Soybean oil, hydrogenated vegetable oil, beeswax, BHT, EDTA

Source: Adapted from Strickley, R. G., *Pharm. Sci Technol. Pharm. Res.*, 21, 201–230, 2004. With permission.

PARENTAL USE OF COSOLVENTS

As discussed earlier, cosolvents can be an effective way to alter the solubility and stability of compounds. In formulating a parenteral product, often these two parameters can be exploited to produce a commercially acceptable, elegant product. Often cosolvents can be used to concentrate a formulation to allow production of a dosage form for presentation as an ampule or vial. The concentrated ampule or vial is then diluted before administration to the patient. Nema et al. (1997) has reviewed excipient use, including cosolvents, in commercially available injectable products.

Even though use of cosolvents has its advantages in parenteral formulation, their use also brings up some additional issues that need to be addressed by the formulator.

Compatibility of cosolvent formulations with packaging components, for example, vials, ampules, stoppers, and plastic administration devices, for example, IV infusion sets and syringes, is something that must be thoroughly investigated (Motola and Agharkar 1992). In addition, one should be also keenly aware that there is definite evidence of effect of formulation vehicles on metabolic enzymes, transporters, and distribution and hence unintentional alteration of drug pharmacokinetic properties. Very little is known about drug–excipient interactions in blood through parenteral route, specifically low dosed compounds, biomarkers, and microdoses. Hence, drug–excipient interactions are very important in the drug development process, especially those intended for parenteral route for *in vivo* animal pharmacokinetic studies, and a formulator must avoid the use of some excipients unless the interaction is well understood.

More than likely, if a cosolvent is required for your parenteral product, there is the potential for precipitation on injection. Cosolvents are a mixed blessing in this regard. On the one hand, cosolvents can afford order of magnitude that increases in solubility. However, once diluted, with even the smallest amount of water, solubility usually exponentially decreases. Formulating cosolvent systems to prevent precipitation on injection has been reported by Yalkowsky and Valvani (1997, 1983). The key to remember is to include not only enough cosolvent to be above equilibrium solubility in the formulation but also enough to help prevent precipitation on injection. Figure 9.4 illustrates this point for a fictitious compound.

The dashed lines in Figure 9.4 represent the formulation dilution profiles of Formulation A and Formulation B. Both Formulations A and B have the same concentration of drug and both are well below the equilibrium solubility of the drug in either formulation because they are well below the solid equilibrium solubility line. However, because Formula B has more cosolvent, it has less area above the solid solubility limit line and therefore, should be less prone to precipitation on injection. *In vitro* methods of assessing precipitation on injections include static methods

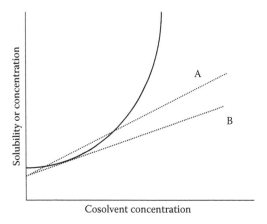

FIGURE 9.4 Dilution profile of two formulations containing same concentration of drug, but different concentration of cosolvent.

(Yalkowsky and Valvani 1977) and dynamic methods (Schroeder and DeLuca 1974; Yalkowsky et al. 1983; Cox et al. 1991; Davio et al. 1991; Irwin and Iqbal 1992). Static methods simply involve mixing of a formulation with another liquid, as opposed to injecting the formulation into a flowing stream of another liquid, that is, dynamic methods, to mimic more closely the actual injection process. These techniques allow formulation optimization to occur before animal testing is initiated.

One must also remember that precipitation can occur on dilution with other intravenous fluids. Investigation of dilution in common parenteral vehicles, for example, normal saline, 5% dextrose solution, or likely coadministered drug products, should be conducted for solubility and stability purposes before recommending such procedures. Phlebitis, hemolysis, and pain on injection are also issues for parenteral formulations containing cosolvents.

Hemolysis induced by cosolvents has been extensively studied (Cadwallader 1963; Banziger 1967; Oshida et al. 1979; Osigo et al. 1983; Fort et al. 1984; Howard and Gould 1985; Reed and Yalkowsky 1985, 1986; Cherng-Chyi Fu 1987; Obeng and Cadwallader 1989; Ward and Yalkowsky 1992; Krzyzaniak et al. 1996, 1997). In these references, various means of evaluating hemolysis are proposed. Reed and Yalkowsky (1985) used an *in vitro* method of determining hemolysis versus a reference formulation composed of 10% ethanol, 40% propylene glycol, and 50% water. They determined the LD_{50}, the concentration of cosolvent to induce hemolysis in 50% of healthy red blood cells, of various cosolvents. The measured LD_{50} values are expressed as total volume percent of cosolvent in whole blood. A higher LD_{50} indicates a relatively less hemolytic cosolvent. Reed and Yalkowsky determined LD_{50} values of 39.5% dimethyl isosorbide, 37.0% dimethylacetamide, 30.0% polyethylene glycol 400, 21.2% ethanol, 10.3% of the reference formulation, 5.7% propylene glycol, and 5.1% dimethyl sulfoxide. Therefore, although propylene glycol is commonly used in parenteral formulations, it is one of the more hemolytic cosolvents. Both Reed and Yalkowsky (1985) and Cadwallader (1963) have determined that the addition of sodium chloride to 40% propylene glycol solutions reduces or prevents hemolysis of red blood cells. On the basis of data summarized earlier by Reed and Yalkowsky (1985) and data by Fort et al. (1984), ethanol and polyethylene glycol 400 are less hemolytic alternatives to propylene glycol.

Muscle damage or myotoxicity is a concern when injecting cosolvents intramuscularly (Brazeau 1989a,b, 1990a,b, 1992). Brazeau and Fung (1989a) used an *in vitro* model to assess myotoxicity to see if there were any correlation with dielectric constant, apparent pH, surface tension, or viscosity. Aqueous mixtures of propylene glycol, ethanol, and polyethylene glycol 400 were studied. Muscle damage was assessed by release of creatine kinase. Brazeau and Fung (1989b) determined that no single property or combination of properties could predict the degree of muscle damage that occurred. They postulated that muscle damage might be due to complex interactions of a given cosolvent with the biochemical processes occurring in skeletal muscle. Further investigation by Brazeau and Fung (1990a) indicated that polyethylene glycol 400 in mixed cosolvent systems might have a protective effect on the myotoxicity generated by intramuscular injections. Studies where diazepam was injected intramuscularly in different cosolvent systems with varying degrees of producing muscle damage did not seem to affect the bioavailability of this compound.

Inflammation by subcutaneous injection of cosolvents has not been published on extensively. Radwan (1994) used an *in vivo* screening model to study the effect of various oils and cosolvents in oils on increasing skin fold thickness of rats after subcutaneous injection. With the exception of benzyl alcohol, ethyl oleate, and phospholipon 100, most excipients showed only minor inflammatory responses.

In multiuse parenteral products that require the use of a preservative system, studies have shown that preservative effectiveness can be influenced by the cosolvents. Darwish and Bloomfield (1995) determined that the presence of a cosolvent produced an increase in the preservative activity of methyl and propyl paraben because of the increase in solubility afforded by the presence of cosolvents. Further studies revealed that cosolvents also influence preservative efficacy by causing cell membrane damage in and of themselves (Darwish and Bloomfield 1997).

Since cosolvents can produce unwanted effects when used parenterally, investigation of other means of solubilizing compounds may be worthwhile if pain, inflammation, or phlebitis

TABLE 9.2
Examples of Solubilization Techniques and Limitations

Technique	Examples	Commercial Products (Radwan 1994)	Potential Drawbacks
Aqueous solution (physiological pH and osmolality)	Normal saline (0.9% NaCl)	pH 2–10 bolus	Precipitation
		pH 2–10 infusion (preferred pH range 4–9)	Pain
Cosolvent	Propylene glycol	≤68% bolus, ≤6% infusion	Precipitation
	Ethanol	≤20% bolus, ≤10% infusion	Pain/irritation
	PEG 300	≤50% bolus	Hemolysis
	PEG 400	≤9% bolus	Impact on PK properties
Surfactant	Cremophor EL	≤10% infusion	Precipitation
	Tween 80	≤4% bolus, ≤2% infusion	Pain/irritation
	Solutol HS 15	50%	Hemolysis
			Impact on PK properties
Complexing agent	HPBCD	20% Infusion	Precipitation
			Pain/irritation
			Hemolysis
Dispersed systems	Water + 10%–20% oil	(Lecithin + glycerol +	Impact on PK Profile
Emulsion/microemulsion (Darwish 1995, 1997)	Water + 5–20 mg/mL phospholipids	fatty acid) + buffer + isotonicifier + cholesterol	Sustained Release Instability
Liposome Nanosuspension	Water with stabilizer	Not yet marketed (Oner 1995)	Slow dissolution

are significant. Oner et al. (1995) determined that intravenous lorazepam formulations containing water miscible cosolvents were ten times more hemolytic than emulsion formulations. Al-Suwayeh et al. (1996) found that liposomal encapsulation of loxapine produced significantly less myotoxicity compared to the commercially available formulation containing propylene glycol and polysorbate 80. Stella et al. (1995a) determined that intramuscular injection of prednisolone in cosolvent mixtures produced significantly higher creatine kinase levels than when solubilized by SBE4-β-cyclodextrin, which was comparable to normal saline. Further work by this same team showed no change in pharmacokinetic parameters when methylprednisolone was injected intravenously as a cosolvent solution versus solubilized by SBE4-β-cyclodextrin, indicating that the drug was rapidly and quantitatively released from the cyclodextrin inclusion complex (Stella et al. 1995b). Table 9.2 shows the various techniques and the typical limitations one could potentially encounter.

COMMERCIAL INJECTABLE FORMULATIONS

When pH adjustment alone is not sufficient to achieve the desired level of solubility of a drug through parenteral route, a cosolvent approach using miscible organic solvent or a surfactant is the choice of method. Commonly used water miscible solvents and surfactants for parenteral formulations are propylene glycol 300 and 400, N-methyl-2-pyrrolidone (NMP), dimethyl sulfoxide (DMSO), dimethylacetamide (DMA), Solutol HS 15, and cremophors and polysorbates. Frequently, commercial formulations are formulated at much higher concentrations and diluted further at the point of care owing to various issues discussed previously. Table 9.3 lists the commercially available list of solubilized parenteral products in an alphabetical order (Strickley 2004).

TABLE 9.3
Commercially Available Aqueous-Based Solubilized Injectable Formulations

Molecule/Trade Name/Company/Indication	Chemical Structure	Formulation	Preparation	Administration	Solubilization Technique
Alprostadil (PGE$_1$)/ Edex/Schwarz/ Erectile dysfunction		Lyophilized powder 12–50 μg α-Cyclodextrin 400–1610 μg Lactose 56 mg pH 4–8	Reconstitute with 1.2 mL saline	Intracavernous	Cyclodextrin complexation 12:1 mole ratio CD:drug
Amiodarone HCl/ Cordarone/ Wyeth–Ayerst/ Antiarrhythmic, antianginal		Solution 50 mg/mL Polysorbate 80 at 10% Benzyl alcohol 2% pH 4.1	Dilute with D5W to <2 mg/mL	IV infusion	Weak base pH < pK_a, and cosolvent, micelles
Amphotericin B/ Ambisome/Gilead/ Antifungal		Lyophilized powder 50 mg HSPC 18 mg/mL Cholesterol 4 mg/mL α-Tocopherol 0.05 mg/mL Sucrose 75 mg/mL Disodium succinate 2 mg/mL pH 5.0–6.0	Reconstitute with WFI to a 4 mg/mL Dilute to 1–2 mg/mL with D5W	IV infusion	Liposome

(Continued)

TABLE 9.3 (*Continued*)

Commercially Available Aqueous-Based Solubilized Injectable Formulations

Molecule/Trade Name/Company/Indication	Chemical Structure	Formulation	Preparation	Administration	Solubilization Technique
Amphotericin B/ Abelcet/Elan/ Antifungal	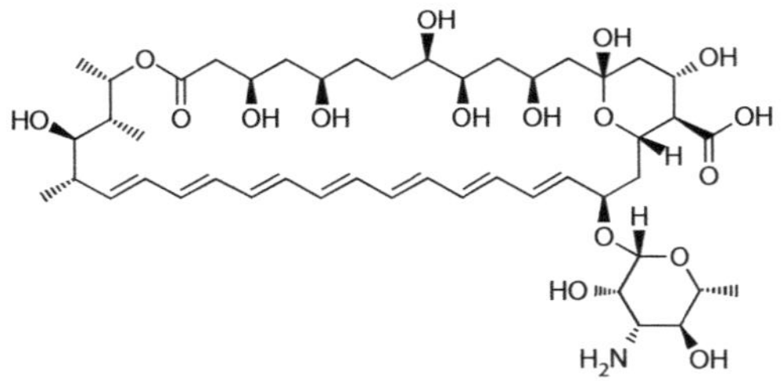	Solution 5 mg/mL DMPC 3.4 mg/mL DMPG 1.5 mg/mL Sodium chloride 9 mg/mL pH = 5–7	Dilute to 1–2 mg/mL with D5W	IV infusion	Lipid complex
Calcitriol/Calcijex/ Abbott/Management of hypokalcemia in patients undergoing chronic renal dialysis	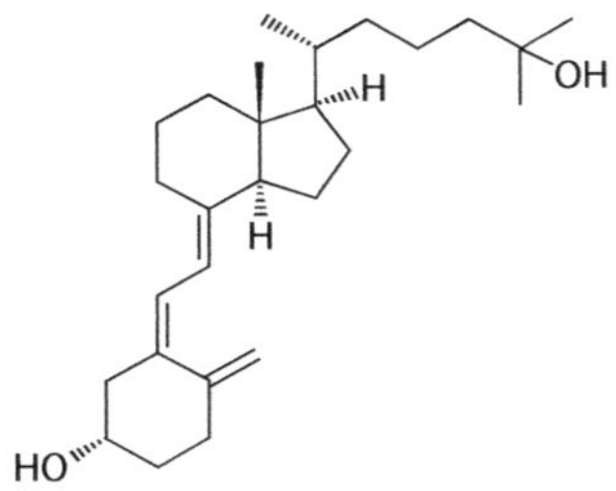	Solution 1–2 µg/mL Polysorbate 20 at 4 mg/mL Sodium ascorbate 10 mg/mL Sodium chloride 1.5 mg/mL EDTA 1.1 mg/mL Sodium phosphates 9.2 mg/mL pH 6.5–8.0	None	IV bolus	Micelles
Carmustine/BiCNU/ Bristol–Myers– Squibb/ Antineoplastic	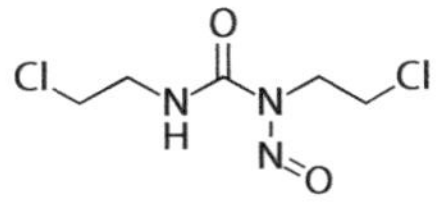	Lyophilized solid 100 mg pH 5–6	Reconstitute with 3 mL of ethanol, then further dilute with 27 mL WFI	IV infusion	Ethanol

(*Continued*)

TABLE 9.3 (Continued)

Commercially Available Aqueous-Based Solubilized Injectable Formulations

Molecule/Trade Name/Company/Indication	Chemical Structure	Formulation	Preparation	Administration	Solubilization Technique
Chloradiazepoxide HCl/Librium/ICN/ Tranquilizer	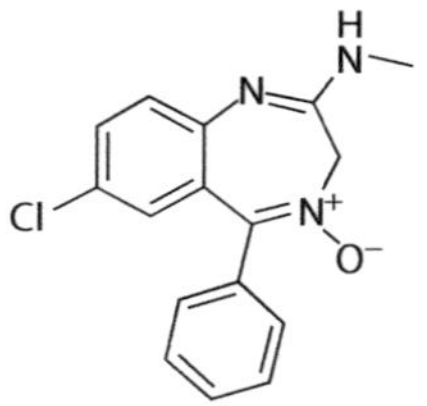	Powder 100 mg supplied diluent Propylene glycol 20% Tween 80 at 4% Benzyl alcohol 1.5% Maleic acid 1.6% pH = 3	Reconstitute with supplied diluent to 50 mg/mL for IM. Reconstitute with saline or WFI to 20 mg/mL for IV bolus	IM/Slow IV bolus over 1 min	Weak base pH < pK_a and cosolvent
Itraconazole/ Sporanox/ Orthobiotech and Janssen/Antifungal	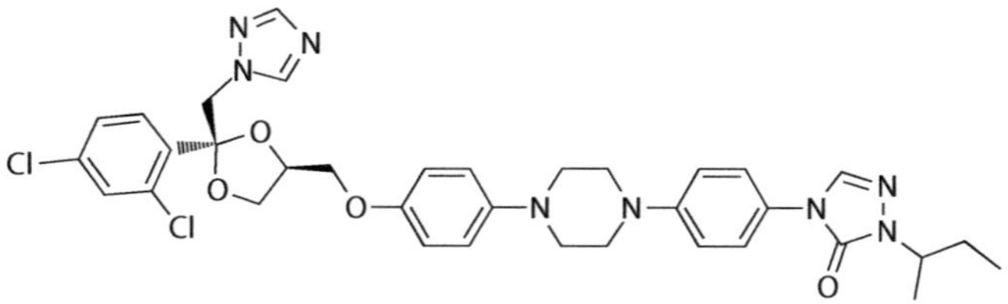	Solution 10 mg/mL HP-β-CD 40% Propylene glycol 2.5% pH 4.5	Dilute with saline to 5 mg/mL	IV infusion	Cyclodextrin complexation
Melphalan HCl/ Alkeran/ GlaxoSmithKline/ Antineoplastic, alkylating agent	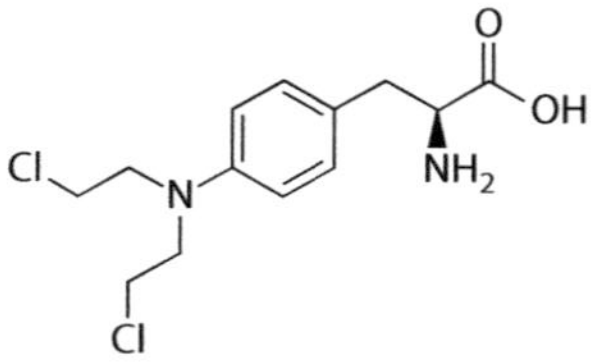	Lyophilized powder 50 mg Povidone 20 mg Provided 10 mL diluent: Water 35%, Propylene glycol 60% Ethyl alcohol 5% Sodium citrate 0.2 g pH 6.5–7.0	Reconstitute vigorously with provided diluent to 5.0 mg/mL, then further dilute with saline to 0.45 mg/mL	IV infusion over 15–20 min	Cosolvent

(Continued)

TABLE 9.3 (Continued)

Commercially Available Aqueous-Based Solubilized Injectable Formulations

Molecule/Trade Name/Company/ Indication	Chemical Structure	Formulation	Preparation	Administration	Solubilization Technique
Methocarbamol/ Robaxin/A.H. Robbins/Skeletal muscle relaxant	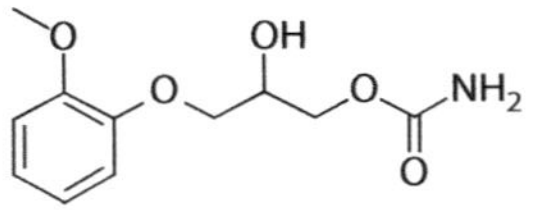	Solution 100 mg/mL PEG 300 50% pH = 4–5	None for IM or IV bolus. For IV infusion dilute with 250 mL saline or D5W	IM/IV bolus/IV infusion	Cosolvent
Oxytetracycline/ Terramycin/Pfizer/ Antibiotic	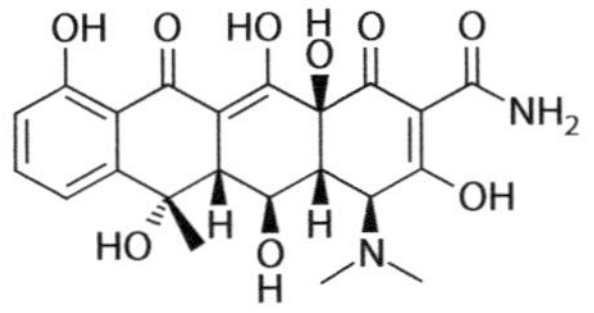	Solution 50–125 mg/mL Lidocaine 20 mg/mL Propylene glycol 67%–75% Monothioglycerol 10 mg/mL Magnesium chloride 25–60 mg/mL Ethanolamine 17–42 mg/mL Citric acid 10 mg/mL Propyl gallate 0.2 mg/mL pH–3	None	IM	Weak base < pK_a, and cosolvent
Paricalcitol/Zemplar/ Abbott/Treatment of secondary hyperparathyroidism associated with chronic failure	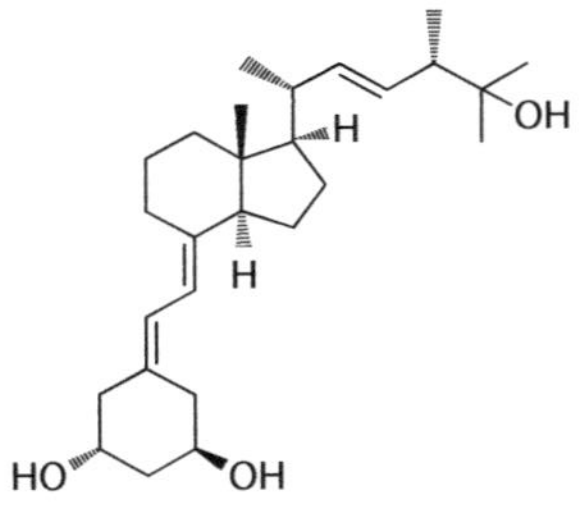	Solution 0.005 mg/mL Propylene glycol 30% Ethyl alcohol 20%	None	IV bolus	Cosolvent

(Continued)

TABLE 9.3 (*Continued*)
Commercially Available Aqueous-Based Solubilized Injectable Formulations

Molecule/Trade Name/Company/ Indication	Chemical Structure	Formulation	Preparation	Administration	Solubilization Technique
Pentobarbital sodium/ Nembutal/Abbott/ Anticonvulsant, sedative, hypnotic, anesthetic		Solution 50 mg/mL Propylene glycol 40% Ethyl alcohol 10% pH 9.5	None or dilute with saline, D5W or lactated Ringer's	IM/slow IV bolus	Weak acid > pK_a and cosolvent
Phenytoin sodium/ Dilantin/Elkins-Sinn/ Anticonvulsant		Solution 50 mg/mL Propylene glycol 40% Ethyl alcohol 10% pH 10–12.3	None	IM/IV bolus	Weak acids pH > pK_a and cosolvent
Phytonadione (Vitamin K_1) Aqua-MEPHYTON/ Merck/Vitamin K deficiency		Aqueous dispersion 2–10 mg/mL Polyoxyethylated fatty acid 70 mg/mL Dextrose 37 mg/mL Benzyl alcohol 0.9% pH 3.5–7	None for SC, IM or IV bolus. For IV infusion dilute with saline, D5W or lactated Ringer's	SC/IM/IV bolus IV infusion	Aqueous dispersion
Propofol/ Diprivan 1%/AstraZeneca/ Anesthetic, sedative		Emulsion, 10 mg/mL Soybean oil 100 mg/mL Glycerol 22.5 mg/mL Egg lecithin 12 mg/mL EDTA	None (shake well)	IV bolus/IV infusion	Emulsion

(Continued)

TABLE 9.3 (*Continued*)

Commercially Available Aqueous-Based Solubilized Injectable Formulations

Molecule/Trade Name/Company/ Indication	Chemical Structure	Formulation	Preparation	Administration	Solubilization Technique
Voriconazole/Vfend/ Pfizer/Antifungal		Lyophilized powder 200 mg Sulfobutylether-β-cyclodextrin 3200 mg	Reconstitute with water to 10 mg/mL Dilute with saline, D5W or lactated Ringers to ≤5 mg/mL	IV infusion	Cyclodextrin complexation
Ziprasidone mesylate/ Geodon/Pfizer/ Antipsychotic		Lyophilized powder 24 mg/par Sulfobutylether-β-cyclodextrin 350 mg	Reconstitute with 1.2 mL water to 20 mg/mL	IM	Cyclodextrin complexation

Source: Reprinted from Table IV of Strickley, R. G., *Pharm. Sci. Technol. Pharm. Res.*, 21, 201–230, 2004. With kind permission from Springer Science and Business Media.

CONCLUSIONS

For formulating poor water-soluble compounds, use of cosolvent(s) is one of the simplest and most common approaches. The approach is also widely used in the early development phase, as limited information is available for the molecule. The approach also allows overcoming dissolution rate limited drug absorption. In addition, solubilized formulations are greatly popular with pediatric, geriatric, and patients with swallowing difficulties.

There are several theoretical models to estimate the solubility of a solute in a solvent. However, use of dielectric constant is one of the oldest and simplest approaches and is very popular with the formulators. Fractional method to estimate the dielectric constant is the simplest approach and is not the most accurate. However, it offers a good starting point for the estimation. In addition, the solubility of a solute is dependent on the dielectric constant of a solvent mixture and not to the particular composition. Other approaches, such as solubility parameter method and UNIFAC group theory contributions are less frequently used by industry formulators.

There are certain limitations with cosolvent approach, as with any other approach, such as poor tasting cosolvent (PG), adverse physiological effects (e.g., alcohol), and potential of cosolvent on metabolic enzymes, transporters, and distribution, and hence unintentional alteration of drug pharmacokinetic properties. For solubilized parenteral application, choice of cosolvents is further limited by physiological acceptance, as well as precipitation on injection and pain on administration. However, the approach remains popular both for oral as well as parenteral application as demonstrated by numerous commercial products. In addition, application of newer cosolvents is increasing to overcome some of these barriers.

REFERENCES

Acree, W. E. and J. H. Rytting. 1982. Solubility in binary solvent systems I: Specific versus nonspecific interactions, *J. Pharm. Sci.*, 71: 201–205.

Acree, W. E. and J. H. Rytting. 1983. Solubility in binary solvent systems III: Predictive expressions based on molecular surface areas, *J. Pharm. Sci.*, 72: 292–296.

Adjei, A., J. Newburger, and A. Martin. 1980. Extended Hildebrand approach: Solubility of caffeine in dioxin–water mixtures, *J. Pharm. Sci.*, 69: 659–661.

Al-Suwayeh, S. A., I. R. Tebbett, D. Wielbo, and G. A. Brazeau. 1996. *In vitro–in vivo* myotoxicity of intramuscular liposomal formulations, *Pharm. Res.*, 13: 1384–1388.

Amidon, G. L., S. H. Yalkowsky, and S. Leung. 1974. Solubility of non-electrolytes in polar solvents II: Solubility of aliphatic alcohols in water, *J. Pharm. Sci.*, 63: 1858–1866.

Amirjahed, A. K. and M. I. Blake. 1974. Relationship of composition of nonaqueous binary solvent systems and dielectric constant, *J. Pharm. Sci.*, 63: 81–84.

Amirjahed, A. K. and M. I. Blake. 1975. Deviation of dielectric constant from ideality for certain binary solvent systems, *J. Pharm. Sci.*, 64: 1569–1570.

Amis, E. S. 1949. *Kinetics of Chemical Change in Solution*, New York: Macmillan, Chapter 4.

Amis, E. S. and V. K. LaMer. 1939. The entropies and energies of activation of ionic reactions, *J. Am. Chem. Soc.*, 61: 905.

Anderson, B. D., J. H. Rytting, and T. Higuchi. 1980. Solubility of polar organic solutes in nonaqueous systems: Role of specific interactions, *J. Pharm. Sci.*, 69: 676–680.

Anik, S. T. and L. Sukumar. 1981. Extreme vertexes design in formulation development: Solubility of butoconazole nitrate in a multicomponent system, *J. Pharm. Sci.*, 70: 897.

Attwood, D. and A. T. Florence. 1983. *The Surfactant Systems, Their Chemistry, Pharmacy and Biology*, New York: Chapman & Hall, Chapters 6 and 7.

Banziger, R. 1967. Hemolysis testing *in vivo* of parenteral formulations, *Bull. Parent. Drug Assoc.*, 21: 148.

Barton, A. F. M. 1983. *Handbook of Solubility Parameters and Other Cohesion Parameters*, Boca Raton, FL: CRC Press, pp. 85–87, 153–158.

Beerbower, A. and C. Hansen. 1971. Solubility parameters. *Encyclopedia of Chemical Technology*, Standen, E. A. (Ed.), New York: Interscience, pp. 889–910.

Beerbower, A., P. L. Wu, and A. Martin. 1984. Expanded solubility parameter approach I: Naphthalene and benzoic acid in individual solvents, *J. Pharm. Sci.*, 73: 179–188.

Belloto, R. J., A. M. Dean, M. A. Moustafa, A. M. Molokhia, M. W. Gouda, and T. D. Sokoloski. 1985. Statistical techniques applied to solubility predictions and pharmaceutical formulations: An approach to problem solving using mixture response surface methodology, *Int. J. Pharm.*, 23: 195.

Bogardus, J. B. 1983. Crystalline anhydrous–hydrate phase changes of caffeine and theophylline in solvent–water mixtures, *J. Pharm. Sci.*, 837–838.

Brazeau, G. A. and H.-L. Fung. 1989a. Physicochemical properties of binary organic cosolvent-water mixtures and their relationships to muscle damage following intramuscular injection, *J. Parent. Sci. Technol.*, 43: 144–149.

Brazeau, G. A. and H.-L. Fung. 1989b. Use of an *in vitro* model for the assessment of muscle damage from intramuscular injections: *In vitro–in vivo* correlation and predictability with mixed solvent systems, *Pharm. Res.*, 6: 766–771.

Brazeau, G. A. and H.-L. Fung. 1990a. Effect of organic cosolvent-induced skeletal muscle damage on the bioavailability of intramuscular [14C] Diazepam, *J. Pharm. Sci.*, 79: 773–777.

Brazeau, G. A. and H.-L. Fung. 1990b. Mechanisms of creatine kinase release from isolated rat skeletal muscles damaged by propylene glycol and ethanol, *J. Pharm. Sci.*, 79: 393–397.

Brazeau, G. A., S. S. Watts, and L. S. Mathews. 1992. Role of calcium and arachidonic acid metabolites in creatine kinase release from isolated rat skeletal muscles damaged by organic cosolvents, *J. Parent. Sci. Technol.*, 46: 25–30.

Bronsted, J. N. 1922. Solvent and solvent effects on the kinetics, *Z. Physik. Chem.*, 102: 169.

Bronsted, J. N. 1925. The effect of the hydrogen ion concentration on the rate of hydrolysis of glycyl glycine, glycyl leucine, glycyl alanine, glycyl asparagine and biuret base by Erepsid, *Z. Physik. Chem.*, 115: 337.

Cadwallader, D. W. 1963. Behavior of erythrocytes in various solvent systems, *J. Pharm. Sci.*, 52: 1175.

Charumanee, S., S. Okonogi, J. Sirithunyalug, P. Wolschann, and H. Viernstein. 2016. Effect of cyclodextrin types and co-solvent on solubility of a poorly water soluble drug, *Sci. Pharm.*, 84(4): 694–704.

Chen, X., H. M. Fadda, A. Aburub, D. Mishra, and R. Pinal. 2015. Cosolvency approach for assessing the solubility of drugs in poly (vinylpyrrolidone), *Int. J. Pharm.*, 494(1): 346–356.

Cherng-Chyi Fu, R., D. M. Lidgate, J. L. Whatley, and T. McCullough. 1987. The biocompatibility of parenteral vehicles—*In vitro/in vivo* screening comparison and the effect of excipients on hemolysis, *J. Parent. Sci. Technol.*, 41: 164–168.

Chertkoff, M. J. and A. N. Martin. 1960. The solubility of benzoic acid in mixed solvents, *J. Pharm. Sci.*, 49: 444–447.

Chien, Y. W. 1984. Solubilization of metronidazole by water-miscible multi-cosolvents and water-soluble vitamins, *J. Parent. Sci. Technol.*, 38: 32–36.

Christian R. 2011. Solvent effects on the rate of homogeneous reactions. In *Solvents and Solvent Effects in Organic Chemistry*, (2nd ed.), New York: Wiley-VCH Verlag GMBH, Chapter 5.

Christiansen, J. A. Z. 1924. Über die Geschwindigkeit bimolekularer Reaktionen in Lösungen, *Physik. Chem.*, 113: 35.

Connors, K. A., G. L. Gordon, and L. Kennon. 1979. *Chemical Stability of Pharmaceuticals*, New York: Wiley Interscience, pp. 39–42.

Cornell, J. A. 1975. Some comments on designs for cox's mixture polynomial, *Technometrics*, 17: 25.

Cornell, J. A. 1990. *Experiments with Mixtures: Designs, Models, and the Analysis of Mixture Data*, (2nd ed.), New York: Wiley.

Cornell, J. A. 1991. The fitting of Scheffé-type models for estimating solubilities of multisolvent systems, *J. Biopharm. Stat.*, 1: 303.

Cox, J. W., G. P. Sage, M. A. Wynalda, R. G. Ulrich, P. G. Larson, and C. C. Su. 1991. Plasma compatibility of injectables, *J. Phar. Sci.*, 80: 371–375.

Darwish, R. M. and S. F. Bloomfield. 1995. The effect of co-solvents on the antibacterial activity of paraben preservatives, *Int. J. Pharm.*, 119: 183–192.

Darwish, R. M. and S. F. Bloomfield. 1997. Effect of ethanol, propylene glycol, and glycerol on the interaction of methyl and propyl *p*-hydroxybenzoate with *Staphylococcus aureas* and *Pseudomonas aeruginosa*, *Int. J. Pharm.*, 147: 51–60.

Davio, S. R., M. M. McShane, T. J. Kakuk, R. M. Zaya, and S. L. Cole. 1991. Precipitation of the renin inhibitor ditekiren upon IV infusion, *Pharm. Res.*, 8: 80–83.

Fort, F. L., I. A. Heyman, and J. W. Kesterson. 1984. Hemolysis study of aqueous Polyethylene Glycol 400, propylene glycol, and ethanol combinations *in vivo* and *in vitro*, *J. Parent. Sci. Technol.*, 38: 82.

Garrett, E. R. 1956. Prediction of stability in pharmaceutical preparations III, *J. Am. Pharm. Assoc. Sci. Ed.*, 45: 171–177.

Gordon, L. J. and R. L. Scott. 1952. Enhanced solubility in solvent mixtures I. The system phenanthrene–cyclohexane–methylene iodide, *J. Am. Chem. Soc.*, 74: 4138–4140.

Gorman, W. G. and G. D. Hall. 1964. Dielectric constant correlations with solubility parameters, *J. Pharm. Sci.*, 53: 1017–1020.

Gould, P. L., M. Goodman, and P. A. Hanson. 1984. Investigation of the solubility relationships of polar, semi-polar and non-polar drugs in mixed co-solvent systems, *Int. J. Pharm.*, 19: 149–159.

Gould, P. L., J. R. Howard, and G. A. Oldershaw. 1989. The effect of hydrate formation on the solubility of theophylline in binary aqueous cosolvent systems, *Int. J. Pharm.*, 51: 195–202.

Grant, D. J. W. and T. Higuchi. 1990. Group contributions in prediction. *Solubility Behavior of Organic Compounds, Techniques of Chemistry*, Vol. 21, New York: John Wiley, Chapter 7.

Grissom, C. B., A. M. Chagovetz, and Z. Wang. 1993. Use of viscosigens to stabilize vitamin B12 solutions against photolysis, *J. Pharm. Sci.*, 82: 641–643.

Groves, M. J., B. Bassett, and V. Sheth. 1984. The solubility of 17 β-oestradiol in aqueous polyethylene glycol 400, *J. Pharm. Pharmacol.*, 36: 799–802.

Grunbauer, H. J. M., A. L. J. deMeere, and H. H. vanRooij. 1986. Local composition models in pharmaceutical chemistry. III. Prediction of drug solubility in binary aqueous mixtures, *Int. J. Pharm.*, 32: 187–198.

Gupta, S. L., J. P. Patel, D. L. Jones, and R. W. Partipilo. 1994. Parenteral formulation development of rennin inhibitor Abbott 72517, *J. Parent. Sci. Technol.*, 48: 86–91.

Hancock, B. C., P. York, and R. C. Rowe. 1997. The use of solubility parameters in pharmaceutical dosage form design, *Int. J. Pharm.*, 148: 1–21.

Higuchi, T. and H. Kristiansen. 1970. Binding specificity between small organic solutes in aqueous solution: Classification of some solutes into two groups according to binding tendencies, *J. Pharm. Sci.*, 59: 1601–1608.

Hildebrand, J. H. 1916. Solubility, *J. Am. Chem. Soc.*, 38: 1452–1473.

Hildebrand, J. H. 1919. Solubility III. Relative values of internal pressures and their application, *J. Am. Chem. Soc.*, 41: 1067–1080.

Hildebrand, J. H. and R. L. Scott. 1950. *Solubility of Nonelectrolytes*, New York: Reinhold Publishing.

Hildebrand, J. H. and R. L. Scott. 1962. *Regular Solutions*, Englewood Cliffs, NJ: Prentice-Hall, Chapter 7.

Howard, J. R. and P. L. Gould. 1985. The use of co-solvents in parenteral formulation of low-solubility drugs, *Int. J. Pharm.*, 25: 359–362.

Ibrahim, S. A. and S. Shawky. 1984. Solubility of acetazolamide and chlorthalidone in mixed aqueous solvent system, *Pharm. Ind.*, 46: 412–416.

Irwin, W. J. and M. Iqbal. 1992. Bropirimine formulation: The dynamic testing of injections, *Int. J. Pharm.*, 83(1–3): 241–249.

Jouyban, A., F. Martinez, and W. E. Acree. 2017. Correct derivation of cosolvency models and some comments on "Solubility of fenofibrate in different binary solvents: Experimental data and results of thermodynamic modeling," *J. Chem. Eng. Data*, 62(3): 1153–1156.

Kato, Y. and T. Ohuchi. 1972. Studies on solubilizing agents IV. Dielectric constant correlations with drug solubility in mixtures of glycols and their derivatives with water, *Yakugaku Zashi*, 92: 257–263.

Krzyzaniak, J. F., D. M. Raymond, and S. H. Yalkowsky. 1996. Lysis of human red blood cells 1: Effect of contact time on water induced hemolysis, *PDA J. Pharm. Sci. Technol.*, 50: 223–226.

Krzyzaniak, J. F., D. M. Raymond, and S. H. Yalkowsky. 1997. Lysis of human red blood cells 2: Effect of contact time on cosolvent induced hemolysis, *Int. J. Pharm.*, 152: 193–200.

Leo, A., C. Hansch, and D. Elkins. 1971. Partition coefficients and their uses, *Chem. Rev.*, 71: 525–616.

Lewis, G. A. and M. Chariot. 1991. Nonclassical experimental designs in pharmaceutical formulations, *Drug Dev. Ind. Pharm.*, 17: 1551.

Li, A. and S. H. Yalkowsky. 1994. Solubility of organic solutes in ethanol/water mixtures, *J. Pharm. Sci.*, 83: 1735–1740.

Martin, A. and M. J. Miralles. 1982. Extended Hildebrand solubility approach: Solubility of tolbutamide, acetohexamide, and sulfisomidine in binary solvent mixtures, *J. Pharm. Sci.*, 71: 439–442.

Martin, A., J. Newburger, and A. Adjei. 1979. New solubility equation, *J. Pharm. Sci.*, 68: IV.

Martin, A., J. Newburger, and A. Adjei. 1980. New solubility equation, *J. Pharm. Sci.*, 69: 487–491.

Martin, A., J. Newburger, and A. Adjei. 1981. Extended Hildebrand solubility approach: Methylxanthines in mixed solvents, *J. Pharm. Sci.*, 70: 1115–1120.

Martin, A., P. L. Wu, A. Adjei, A. Beerbower, and J. M. Prausnitz. 1981. Extended Hansen solubility approach: Naphthalene in individual solvents, *J. Pharm. Sci.*, 70: 1260–1264.

Martin, A., P. L. Wu, A. Adjei, R. E. Lindstrom, and P. H. Elworthy. 1982. Extended Hildebrand solubility approach and the log-linear solubility equation, *J. Pharm. Sci.*, 71: 849–855.

Martin, A., P. L. Wu, and A. Beerbower. 1984. Expanded solubility parameter approach II: *p*-hydroxybenzoic acid and methyl-*p*-hydroxybenzote in individual solvents, *J. Pharm. Sci.*, 73: 188–194.

Menschutkin, N. Z. 1890. Über die affinitätskoeffizienten der alkylhaloide und der amine, *Phys. Chem.*, 6: 41.

Menschutkin, N. Z. 1900. Zur Frage über den Einfluss chemisch indifferenter Lösungsmittel auf die Reaktionsgeschwindigkeiten, *Phys. Chem.*, 34: 157.

Moore, W. E. 1958. The use of approximate dielectric constant to blend solvent systems, *J. Am. Pharm. Assoc. Sci. Ed.*, 47: 855–857.

Motola, S. and S. N. Agharkar. 1992. Preformulation research of parenteral medications. In Avis, K. E., Lieberman, H. A., and Lachman, L. (Eds.), *Pharmaceutical Dosage Forms: Parenteral Medications*, Vol. 1, 2nd ed., New York: Marcel Dekker, pp. 158–163, Chapter 4.

Moustafa, M. A., A. M. Molokhia, and M. W. Gouda. 1981. Phenobarbital solubility in propylene glycol–glycerol–water systems, *J. Pharm. Sci.*, 70: 1172.

Neira, O. M. C., M. F. Jimenez, and L. F. Ponce de Leon. 1980. Influencia de la constante dielectrica in la solubilization del diazepam, *Rev. Colomb. Cien. Quim.-Farm.*, 3: 37–61.

Nema, S., R. J. Washkuhn, and R. J. Brendel. 1997. Excipients and their use in injectable products, *PDA J.Pharm. Sci. Tech.*, 51: 166–171.

Obeng, E. K. and D. E. Cadwallader. 1989. *In vitro* method for evaluating the hemolytic potential of intravenous solutions, *J. Parent. Sci. Technol.*, 43: 167–173.

Ochsner, A. B., R. J. Belloto, and T. D. Sokoloski. 1985. Prediction of xanthine solubilities using statistical techniques, *J. Pharm. Sci.*, 74: 132.

Oner, F., M. Yalin, and A. A. Hincal. 1995. Stability and hemolytic effect of parenteral lorazepam emulsion formulations, *FABAD J. Pharm. Sci.*, 20: 61–66.

Oshida, S., K. Degawa, Y. Takahashi, and S. Akaishi. 1979. Physico-chemical properties and local toxic effects of injectables, *Tohoku J. Exp. Med.*, 127: 301–316.

Osigo, T., M. Iwaki, and M. Kuranari. 1983. Relationship between hemolytic concentrations and physicochemical properties of basic drugs and major factors inducting hemolysis, *Chem. Pharm. Bull.*, 31: 4508.

Paruta, A. N. and S. A. Irani. 1965. Dielectric solubility profiles in dioxane–water mixtures for several antipyretic drugs, *J. Pharm. Sci.*, 54: 1334–1338.

Paruta, A. N. and B. B. Sheth. 1966. Solubility of xanthines, antipyrine and several derivatives in syrup vehicles, *J. Pharm. Sci.*, 55: 896–901.

Paruta, A. N. 1964. Solubility of several solutes as a function of dielectric constant of sugar solutions, *J. Pharm. Sci.*, 53: 1252–1254.

Paruta, A. N. 1966a. Solubility of parabens in syrup vehicles, *J. Pharm. Sci.*, 55: 1208–1211.

Paruta, A. N. 1966b. The solubility of succinic acid in binary mixtures as a function of the dielectric constant, *Am. J. Pharm.*, 138: 137–154.

Paruta, A. N. 1969. Solubility of the parabens in ethanol–water mixtures, *J. Pharm. Sci.*, 58: 364–366.

Paruta, A. N., B. J. Sciarrone, and N. G. Lordi. 1962. Correlation between solubility parameters and dielectric constants, *J. Pharm. Sci.*, 51: 704–705.

Paruta, A. N., B. J. Sciarrone, and N. G. Lordi. 1964. Solubility of salicylic acid as a function of dielectric constant, *J. Pharm. Sci.*, 53: 1349–1353.

Paruta, A. N., B. J. Sciarrone, and N. G. Lordi. 1965a. Dielectric solubility profiles of acetanilide and several derivatives in dioxane–water mixtures, *J. Pharm. Sci.*, 54: 1325–1333.

Paruta, A. N., B. J. Sciarrone, and N. G. Lordi. 1965b. Solubility profiles for the xanthines in dioxane–water mixtures, *J. Pharm. Sci.*, 54: 838–841.

Patel, M. S., F. S. S. Morton, H. Seager, and D. Howard. 1992. Factors affecting the chemical stability of carboxylic acid drugs in enhanced solubility system (ESS) softgel formulations based on polyethylene glycol (PEG), *Drug Dev. Ind. Pharm.*, 18: 1–19.

Medical Economic. 2006. *Physician's Desk Reference*, 60th ed., Montvale, NJ: Thomson Publishing.

Radwan, M. 1994. *In vivo* screening model for excipients and vehicles used in subcutaneous injections, *Drug Dev. Ind. Pharm.*, 20: 2753–2762.

Reed, K. W. and S. H. Yalkowsky. 1985. Lysis of human red blood cells in the presence of various cosolvents, *J. Parent. Sci. Technol.*, 38: 64–69.

Reed, K. W. and S. H. Yalkowsky. 1986. Lysis of human red blood cells. II. The effect of differing NaCl concentrations, *J. Parent. Sci. Technol.*, 40: 88.

Restaino, F. A. and A. N. Martin. 1964. Solubility of benzoic acid and related compounds in a series of *n*-Alkanols, *J. Pharm. Sci.*, 53: 636–639.

Roy, G. 1990. The applications and future implications of bitterness reduction and inhibition in food products, *Crit. Rev. Food Sci. Nutr.*, 29: 59–71.

Roy, G. 1992. Bitterness reduction and inhibition, *Trends Food Sci. Technol.*, 3: 85–91.

Roy, G. 1994. Taste masking in oral pharmaceuticals, *Pharm. Tech.*, 18(4): 84.

Rubino, J. T. 1984. Solubilization of some poorly soluble drugs by cosolvents, University of Arizona, PhD dissertation, Tucson, AZ.

Rubino, J. T. 1987. The effects of cosolvents on the action of pharmaceutical buffers, *J. Parent. Sci. Technol.*, 41: 45–49.

Rubino, J. T. and E. K. Obeng. 1991. Influence of solute structure on deviations from the log-linear solubility equation in propylene glycol: Water mixtures, *J. Pharm. Sci.*, 80: 479–483.

Rubino, J. T. and E. Thomas. 1990. Influence of solvent composition on the solubilities and solid-state properties of the sodium salts of some drugs, *Int. J. Pharm.*, 65: 141–145.

Rubino, J. T. and S. H. Yalkowsky. 1985. Solubilization by cosolvents III: Diazepam and benzocaine in binary solvents, *J. Parent. Sci. Technol.*, 39: 106–111.

Rubino, J. T. and S. H. Yalkowsky. 1987a. Cosolvency and cosolvent polarity, *Pharm. Res.*, 4: 220–230.

Rubino, J. T. and S. H. Yalkowsky. 1987b. Cosolvency and deviations from log-linear solubilization, *Pharm. Res.*, 4: 231–236.

Rubino, J. T., J. Blanchard, and S. H. Yalkowsky. 1984. Solubilization by cosolvents II: Phenytoin in binary and ternary solvents, *J. Parent. Sci. Technol.*, 38: 215–221.

Rubino, J. T., J. Blanchard, and S. H. Yalkowsky. 1987. Solubilization by cosolvents IV: Benzocaine, diazepam and phenytoin in aprotic cosolvent–water mixtures, *J. Parent. Sci. Technol.*, 41: 172–176.

Scatchard, G. 1932. Statistical mechanics and reduction reaction rates in liquid solutions, *Chem. Rev.*, 10: 229.

Scheffé, H. 1957. Experiments with mixtures, *J. R. Statist. Soc.*, B20: 344.

Scheffé, H. 1963. The simplex-centroid design for experiments with mixtures, *J. R. Statist. Soc.*, B25: 235.

Schroeder, H. G. and P. P. DeLuca. 1974. A study on the in vitro precipitation of poorly soluble drugs from nonaqueous vehicles in human plasma, *Bull. Parent. Drug Assoc.*, 28: 1–14.

Senac, C., P. Fuchs, W. Urbach, and N. Taulier. 2017. Does the presence of a co-solvent alter the affinity of a hydrophobic drug to its target? *Biophys. J.*, 112(3): 493a.

Soni, L. K., S. S. Solanki, and R. K. Maheshwari. 2014. Solubilization of poorly water soluble drug using mixed solvency approach for aqueous injection, *Br. J. Pharm. Res.*, 4(5): 549–568.

Sorby, D. L., R. G. Bitter, and J. G. Webb. 1963. Dielectric constants of complex pharmaceutical solvent systems. I. Water–ethanol–glycerin and water-ethanol-propylene glycol, *J. Pharm. Sci.*, 52: 1149–1153.

Sorby, D. L., G. Liu, and K. N. Horowitz. 1965. Dielectric constants of complex pharmaceutical solvent systems II, *J. Pharm. Sci.*, 54: 1811–1813.

Stella, V. J., H. K. Lee, and D. O. Thompson. 1995a. The effect of SBE4-β-CD on I.M. prednisolone pharmacokinetics and tissue damage in rabbits: Comparison to a co-solvent solution and a water-soluble prodrug, *Int. J. Pharm.*, 120: 197–204.

Stella, V. J., H. K. Lee, and D. O. Thompson. 1995b. The effect of SBE4-β-CD on I.V. methylprednisolone pharmacokinetics in rats: Comparison to a co-solvent solution and two water-soluble prodrugs, *Int. J. Pharm.*, 120: 189–195.

Strickley, R. G. 2004. Solubilizing excipients in oral and injectable formulations, *Pharm. Sci. Technol. Pharm. Res.*, 21: 201–230.

Tarantino, R., E. Bishop, F.-C. Chen, K. Iqbal, and A. W. Malick. 1994. *N*-Methyl-2-pyrrolidone as a cosolvent: Relationship of cosolvent effect with solute polarity and the presence of proton-donating groups on model drug compounds, *J. Pharm. Sci.*, 83: 1213–1216.

Thakkar, V. T., R. Dhankecha, M. Gohel, P. Shah, T. Pandya, T. Gandhi, and V. Thakkar. 2016. Enhancement of solubility of artemisinin and curcumin by co-solvency approach for application in parenteral drug delivery system, *Int. J. Drug Del.*, 8(3): 77–88.

Trivedi, J. S., W. R. Porter, J. J. Fort. 1996. Solubility and stability characterization of zileuton in a ternary solvent system, *Eur. J. Pharm. Sci.*, 4: 109–116.

Verma, M., S. S. Gangwar, Y. Kumar, M. Kumar, and A. K. Gupta. 2016. Study the effect of cosolvent on the solubility of a slightly water-soluble drug, *J. Drug Dis. Ther.*, 4(37).

Vojnovic, D. and D. Chicco. 1997. Mixture experimental design applied to solubility predictions, *Drug Dev. Ind. Pharm.*, 23: 639–645.

Vojnovic, D., M. Moneghini, and D. Chicco. 1996. Nonclassical experimental design applied in the optimization of a placebo formulation, *Drug Dev. Ind. Pharm.*, 22: 997.

Vojnovic, D., M. Moneghini, and F. Rubessa. 1995. Experimental design for a granulation process with "priori" criterias, *Drug Dev. Ind. Pharm.*, 21: 823.

Ward, G. H. and S. H. Yalkowsky. 1992. The role of effective concentration in interpreting hemolysis data, *J. Parent. Sci. Technol.*, 46: 161–162.

Wells, M. L., W.-Q. Tong, J. W. Campbell, E. O. McSorley, and M. R. Emptage. 1996. A four-component study for estimating solubilies of a poorly soluble compound in multisolvent systems using a Scheffé type model, *Drug Dev. Ind. Pharm.*, 22: 881–889.

Williams, N. A. and G. L. Amidon. 1984a. An excess free energy approach to the estimation of solubility in mixed solvent systems, *J. Pharm. Sci.*, 73: 9–12.

Williams, N. A. and G. L. Amidon. 1984b. An excess free energy approach to the estimation of solubility in mixed solvent systems II: Ethanol–water mixtures, *J. Pharm. Sci.*, 73: 14–18.

Williams, N. A. and G. L. Amidon. 1984c. An excess free energy approach to the estimation of solubility in mixed solvent systems III: Ethanol–propylene glycol–water mixtures, *J. Pharm. Sci.*, 73: 18–23.

Wisniak, J. and A. Tamir. 1978. *Mixing and Excess Thermodynamic Properties*, New York: Elsevier Scientific, pp. IX–XXXXVIII.

Wu, P. L. and A. Martin. 1983. Extended Hildebrand solubility approach: *p*-hydroxybenzoic acid in mixtures of dioxane and water, *J. Pharm. Sci.*, 72: 587–592.

Yalkowsky, S. H. and T. J. Roseman. 1981. Solubilization of drugs by cosolvents. In *Techniques of Solubilization of Drugs*, Yalkowsky, S. H. (Ed.), pp. 91–134. New York: Marcel Dekker, Chapter 3.

Yalkowsky, S. H. and J. T. Rubino. 1985. Solubilization by cosolvents I: Organic solutes in propylene glyol–water mixtures, *J. Pharm. Sci.*, 74: 416–421.

Yalkowsky, S. H. and S. C. Valvani. 1977. Precipitation of solubilized drugs due to injection or dilution, *Drug. Intell. Clin. Pharm.*, 11: 417–419.

Yalkowsky, S. H., G. L. Amidon, G. Zografi, and G. L. Flynn. 1975. Solubility of nonelectrolytes in polar solvents III: Alkyl *p*-aminobenzoates in polar and mixed solvents, *J. Pharm. Sci.*, 64: 48–52.

Yalkowsky, S. H., S. C. Valvani, and G. L. Amidon. 1976. Solubility of nonelectrolytes in polar solvents IV: Nonpolar drugs in mixed solvents, *J. Pharm. Sci.*, 65: 1488–1494.

Yalkowsky, S. H., S. C. Valvani, and B. W. Johnson. 1983. *In vitro* method for detecting precipitation of parenteral formulations after injection, *J. Pharm. Sci.*, 72: 1014–1017.

10 Emulsions, Microemulsions, and Lipid-Based Drug Delivery Systems for Drug Solubilization and Delivery— Part I: Parenteral Applications

John B. Cannon, Yi Shi, and Pramod Gupta

CONTENTS

INTRODUCTION

Over the past several decades, emulsion formulations have been explored for resolving a variety of drug delivery challenges. Unlike solutions for oral or parenteral administrations, which are usually homogeneous one-phase systems or molecular dispersions, emulsions are colloidal dispersions of at least two immiscible phases stabilized with the aid of a third component generally referred to as the emulsifying agent. Most of the advantages of emulsion systems over conventional dosage forms such as oral solutions and liquid injectables can be attributed to this stable heterogeneity, and their ability to deliver immiscible phases in a reliable and reproducible manner. This chapter focuses on demonstrating the usefulness of emulsion systems for the delivery of water-insoluble compounds for parenteral administration. Following some basic definitions and general properties of emulsions, their potential utility for parenteral delivery of lipophilic compounds is rationalized. Wherever possible, examples of experimental and clinical use of emulsion formulations for parenteral delivery of water-insoluble compounds are provided. The challenges encountered in development of these formulations are also discussed. Finally, the utility of this approach is compared with other pharmaceutical techniques of drug solubilization.

EMULSIONS AS PHARMACEUTICAL DOSAGE FORMS

DEFINITIONS

An emulsion can be defined as a mixture of two immiscible phases (namely, water and oil) with an emulsifier added to stabilize the dispersed droplets (Davis et al., 1987). As conventionally defined, emulsions will have droplet diameters of more than 100 nm (up to 50 μm), and thus are opaque or milky in appearance. In addition, they are thermodynamically unstable by nature, that is, on standing they will eventually separate into two phases. However, proper choice of emulsifier (generally 1%–5%) and preparation conditions can delay this separation and thus lead to nominal shelf lives of more than 2 years, as typically required for pharmaceutical products. An emulsion can be characterized as oil-in-water (o/w) (containing up to 40% oil) or water-in-oil (w/o), depending on the identity of the dispersed and continuous phases. Multiple (e.g., w/o/w) emulsions can also be prepared, but these are less widely used in pharmaceutical applications.

In contrast to the conventional emulsions or macroemulsions described earlier are the disperse systems currently termed microemulsions. The term was first introduced by Schulman in 1959 to describe a visually transparent or translucent thermodynamically stable system, with much smaller droplet diameter (6–80 nm) than conventional emulsions. In addition to the aqueous phase, oily phase, and surfactant, they have a high proportion of a *cosurfactant*, such as an alkanol of 4–8 carbons or a nonionic surfactant. Whereas microemulsions have found applications in oral use (as described in the next chapter), parenteral use of microemulsions has been less common owing to toxicity concerns (e.g., hemolysis) arising from the high surfactant and cosolvent levels. In one example, microemulsions composed of polyethylene glycol (PEG)/ethanol/water/medium-chain triglycerides/Solutol® HS15/soy phosphatidylcholine have been safely infused into rats at up to 0.5 mL/kg. On dilution into water, the microemulsion forms a o/w emulsion of 60–190 nm droplet size (Von Corswant et al., 1998).

Typically, emulsions for parenteral use should have droplet size less than 1 μm (generally 100–1000 nm), and hence are often called *submicron emulsions*, or (less properly) *nanoemulsions*. Use of the latter term is unfortunate and can lead to confusion, since their droplet size is actually larger than the microemulsion systems described earlier. The term *nanoemulsion* has been proposed to include metastable emulsions ≤100 nm as well as thermodynamically stable microemulsions (Sarker, 2005). Manufacture of submicron emulsions require special homogenization equipment will be described later.

COMPONENTS OF EMULSIONS USED FOR PARENTERAL APPLICATIONS

A typical parenteral o/w emulsion is composed of lipid droplets (10–20%), emulsifier, and osmotic agent; it is administered by either intravenous (IV) bolus or IV infusion. In addition, when an emulsion formulation is packaged in a multidose container, antimicrobial agents should be included in the formulation to prevent the growth of microorganisms.

LIPIDS

The classical operational definition of lipids are those components of biological material that are water insoluble but soluble in organic solvents such as methylene chloride. An alternative definition sometimes preferred by pharmaceutical scientists is that lipids are fatty acids and their derivatives, and substances related biosynthetically or functionally to these compounds (Christie and Han, 2010). Lipids can thus encompass not only naturally occurring lipophilic materials but also those easily derived from lipids that occur naturally. Table 10.1 summarizes the lipids most commonly used in parenteral emulsions. Long- and medium-chain triglycerides (LCT and MCT, respectively), either alone or in combination, are used in commercial parenteral emulsions owing to their long history of safety. LCT are derived from vegetable sources such as soybean oil, safflower oil, sesame oil, and cottonseed oil, whereas MCT are obtained by re-esterification of fractionated coconut oil (mainly caprylic and capric fatty acid). Other lipids have also been investigated for use in parenteral emulsions. Ethyl oleate can be used as the oil phase in emulsions for intramuscular or subcutaneous administration. Oleic acid has been used experimentally for parenteral emulsions; it is used in a number of commercial oral products. d-α-Tocopherol (vitamin E) has been recently investigated as a novel lipid for parenteral emulsions (Constantinides et al., 2004). A study has shown that d-α-tocopherol was well tolerated in patients receiving a daily IV administration of d-α-tocopherol at doses up to 2300 mg/m^2 for 9 consecutive days (Helson, 1984), but the safety of higher doses or chronic use of d-α-tocopherol needs to be further evaluated. Recently, marine oils containing large quantities of long-chain omega-3 polyunsaturated fatty acids have drawn lots of attention because of their health benefits. Parenteral emulsions prepared from marine oils have also been reported (Ton et al., 2005; Cui et al., 2006).

TABLE 10.1
Lipids Approved for Clinical Use in Parenteral Lipid-Based Formulations

Class	Trade or Common Name	Chemical name
Long-chain triglycerides	Triolein	(Z)-9-Octadecenoic acid 1,2,3-propanetriyl ester
	Soybean oil	
	Safflower oil	
	Sesame oil	
	Cottonseed oil	
	Castor oil	
Medium-chain triglycerides	Fractionated coconut oil	Medium-chain triglycerides
	Miglyol®, 810, 812	
	Neobee® M5	
	Captex® 300	
Fatty acids and derivatives	Oleic acid	(Z)-9-Octadecenoic acid
	Ethyl oleate	(Z)-9-Octadecenoic acid, ethyl ester
Novel lipids	Vitamin E	D-α-tocopherol

TABLE 10.2

Surfactants Used in Parenteral Emulsions

Chemical or Common Name	Trade Name	HLB	Recommended Concentration
Polyoxyl 35 castor oil	Cremophor® EL	12–14[a]	10%
Polyoxythylene-660-hydroxystearate	Solutol® HS15		
Polyoxyethylene sorbitan monolaurate	Polysorbate 20 (Tween® 20)	16.7[a]	
Polyoxyethylene sorbitan monolaurate	Polysorbate 40 (Tween® 40)	15.6[a]	
Polyoxyethylene sorbitan monolaurate	Polysorbate 80 (Tween® 80)	15.0[a]	
Sorbitan monolaurate	Span® 20	8.6[a]	0.01%–0.05%[a]
Sorbitan monopalmitate	Span® 40	6.7[a]	0.01%–0.05%[a]
Sorbitan monooleate	Span® 80	4.3[a]	
Sorbitan trioleate	Span® 85	1.8[a]	0.01%–0.05%[a]
Polyoxyethylene-polyoxypropylene block copolymer	Poloxamer 188 (Pluronic® F68)	29[b]	0.3%[a]
7-desoxycholic acid sodium	Bile salt	26	
Phosphatidylcholine	Phospholipon® 90		1%–3%

[a] Reference from *Handbook of Pharmaceutical Excipients*.
[b] Reference from vendor information.

SURFACTANTS

Surfactants are commonly used to stabilize the emulsion by reducing interfacial tension between the oil and the water phases. Although a variety of surfactants are available, only a few are used in approved parenteral emulsion products. The most commonly used surfactant in parenteral products is phosphatidylcholine (PC). PC is a natural emulsifying agent derived from egg yolk or soybean. PC is commonly called *lecithin*, but this term is also applied to the crude product that contains not only PC but also phosphatidylethanolamine and other phospholipids. Sodium deoxycholate (bile salt) is also a natural surfactant that has been used in marketed parenteral products (e.g., Fungizone®). Other surfactants that have been used in parenteral products are synthetic nonionic surfactants including Cremophor® EL (Polyoxyl-35 castor oil), Solutol HS-15 (polyoxyethylene-660-hydroxystearate), Tween® 20, 40, and 80, Span® 20, and Poloxamer 188. Poloxamer 188 has been shown to be superior in stabilizing emulsion during autoclaving compared to other surfactants (Jumaa and Muller, 1998). However, large volume or long-term administration of Poloxamer 188 need to be evaluated. The allowed concentration (after dilution) for administration for each of the surfactants is listed in Table 10.2.

HLB CLASSIFICATION SYSTEM AND REQUIRED HLB

The hydrophilic–lipophilic balance (HLB) classification system was first introduced by Griffin (1949) to characterize the relative affinity of a surfactant to the aqueous and oil phase. A HLB value is an empirical numerical value in the range of 1–30. The higher the HLB value, the more hydrophilic the surfactant is; and in turn, the lower the HLB value, the more lipophilic the surfactant is. As a result, surfactants with higher HLB values (>8) are favorable for formation of o/w emulsions, while surfactants with lower HLB values (3–6) are more suitable for the formation of w/o emulsions. The HLB values of the surfactants used in parenteral emulsions are listed in Table 10.2.

The HLB value of surfactants that provides the lowest interfacial tension between the oil and water phases for a given lipid mixture is called the required HLB. Each of the lipophilic ingredients used in an o/w emulsion has a required HLB value (e.g., 6–7 for cottonseed oil and 14 for castor oil). An emulsion is most stable when a surfactant or combination of surfactants has a HLB value close to that required HLB value of the oil phase.

OTHER COMPONENTS

As is being discussed, antioxidants may need to be included in a parenteral emulsion product if unsaturated lipids are present. Agents such as glycerol are also typically added to adjust tonicity. As bacteria can grow in the aqueous phases of emulsions, an adequate concentration of an antimicrobial preservative agent should be added. To achieve antimicrobial effect, the levels of antimicrobial agents with relatively high affinity to the oil phase of an emulsion (e.g., benzyl alcohol and parabens) will be higher than those that would be needed in single-phase liquid formulations. The antimicrobial agents should also be nonionized and not bound to other components of the emulsion to penetrate the bacterial membrane. Some hydrophilic antimicrobial agents (e.g., benzoic acid and ascorbic acid) are effective only at acidic pH, owing to formation of ionic forms at basic pH. The effects of these antimicrobial agents on the stability of the emulsion should also be considered during formulation development.

MARKETED EMULSION PRODUCTS

Topical medications have been formulated as o/w or w/o emulsions (e.g., lotions and ointments) for centuries and marketed by pharmaceutical companies for many decades. These applications are beyond the scope of this chapter, since the purpose of using an emulsion in topical formulations is generally to aid in spreading and penetration properties rather than for drug solubilization. Emulsions have also been used for some time as IV nutritional mixtures (total parenteral nutrition) to supply high-caloric lipids. These are generally emulsions of soybean, sesame, or safflower oil (10%–20%) emulsified with phospholipids, for example, egg lecithin containing 60%–70% PC. Liposyn® and Intralipid®, manufactured by Hospira and Kabi Vitrum, respectively, are two examples of the most widely used total parenteral emulsions; they contain 10%–20% soybean oil (Intralipid) or safflower oil (Liposyn), 1.2% egg phosphatides as emulsifier, and 2.5% glycerol. Another example is Lipofundin® (Braun), which contains 10%–20% soybean or cottonseed oil, 0.75% soybean phosphatides, 5% xylitol or sorbitol, and 0%–0.6% α-tocopherol. Other examples are Trive 1000® (Egic), Nutrafundin® (Braun), as well as Intralipid-type products marketed by Travenol, Green Cross, and Daigo (Hansrani et al., 1983). Parenteral nutrition emulsions such as Liposyn and Intralipid have recently been used in clinical therapy to treat drug and toxicity in cases of overdosage of a variety of lipid-soluble drugs such as anesthetics, antipsychotics, antidepressants, anti-arrhythmics, and calcium channel blockers (Cave et al., 2014; Muller et al. 2015); the proposed mechanism of action is sequestration of the drugs into an intravascular *lipid sink* of the emulsion to reduce to free drug concentration (Waring, 2012; Clark et al. 2014).

Development of drug-containing emulsions for parenteral use have been much less common. Drug-emulsion formulations marketed in Japan, Europe, and the United States for IV use are given in Table 10.3. The drug in these formulations (diazepam; propofol; prostaglandin E1; etomidate; vitamins A, D, E, and K; dexamethazone palmitate; flubiprofen; perflurodecalin; docetaxel; and cyclosporine) are all poorly water soluble, rationalizing use of an emulsion system for solubilization and improved delivery. In the blood substitute Fluosol-DA product, the *drug* is actually the oil phase of the emulsion that solubilizes oxygen. In 2008, an emulsion formulation of clevidipine (Cleviprex®), was approved for treatment of hypertension. Clevidipine is a calcium channel blocker that is practically insoluble in water; it is solubilized in a soybean oil/egg phospholipid/oleic acid emulsion for injection (Erickson et al. 2010). Ciclomulsion® is an cyclosporine emulsion formulation in which the drug is solubilized in a soybean oil/MCT/egg lecithin/sodium oleate emulsion. In development by NeuroVive Pharmaceutical, it is in Phase III clinical trials for the treatment of

TABLE 10.3

A Representative List of Parenteral Marketed Emulsion Products Containing Water-Insoluble Drugs

Drug	Product Name	Company	Route	Drug Activity	Product Status	References
Diazepam	Diazemuls® Diazepam®-Lipuro	Braun Melsungen	I.V.	Sedation	Marketed in Europe, Canada and Australia	Collins-Gold et al. (1990)
Etomidate	Etomidat®-Lipuro	Braun Melsungen	I.V.	Anesthesia	Marketed in Europe	Hippalgaonkar et al. (2010)
Prostaglandin E1	Liple	Green Cross	I.V.	Vasodilator	Marketed in Japan	Collins-Gold et al. (1990);Yamaguchi et al. (1994)
Propofol	Diprivan®	AstraZeneca	I.V.	Anesthesia	Marketed worldwide	Collins-Gold et al. (1990); dailymed. nlm.nih.gov
	Propofol®-Lipuro	Braun	I.V.	Anesthesia	Marketed in Europe	Kam et al. (2004)
Vitamins A, D, E and K	Vitalipid®	Kabi	I.V.	Nutrition	Marketed in Europe	Collins-Goldet al. (1990)
Clevidipine	Cleviprex®	The Medicines Co.	I.V.	Anti-hypertensive	Marketed in USA	Erickson et al. (2010); dailymed.nlm. nih.gov
Dexamethasone palmitate	Limethason (Lipotalon)	Green Cross Merckle	I.V.; Intra-articular	Cortico-steroid	Marketed in Japan and Germany	Yamaguchi et al. (1994)
Flurbiprofen	Lipfen®	Green Cross	I.V.	Analgesia	Marketed in Japan	Yamaguchi et al. (1994)
Perfluorodecalin + perfluro-tripropylamine	Fluosol-DA	Green Cross; Alpha	intracoronary	Blood substitute	Marketed worldwide until 1994	Yamaguchi et al. (1994); Physicians Desk Reference, p. 593 (1993)
Cyclosporine A	Restasis™	Allergan	Ophthalmic	Immunomodulator	Marketed in USA	dailymed.nlm.nih.gov
Alprostadil	Liple	Green Cross	I.V.	Peripheral vascular disorders	Marketed in Japan	Hippalgaonkar et al. (2010)
Lipo-NSAID	Flurbiprofen axetil	Kaken	I.V.	Post-operative and cancer pain	Marketed in Japan	Hippalgaonkar et al. (2010)
Docetaxel	Docetaxel non-alcohol formula	Eagle/Teikoku Pharma	I.V.	Cancer	Marketed in USA	dailymed.nlm.nih.gov

reperfusion injury in myocardial infarct patients, as an alternative to the current Cremophor EL containing products which can cause hypersensitivity reactions (Ehinger et al. 2013). In 2015 a docetaxel injection formulation containing 2.5% soybean oil, 42% PEG 300, 55% Tween 80 was approved for use in breast cancer, non-small cell lung cancer, prostate cancer, gastric adenocarcinoma, and head and neck cancer. The non-alcohol formulation was developed in response to concerns that docetaxel may cause symptoms of alcohol intoxication after treatment.

The brevity of the list illustrates the historical reluctance of the pharmaceutical industry to use emulsions as a formulation tool in the parenteral drug delivery areas, perhaps owing to parenteral safety concerns, difficulty in manufacturing, perceived lack of patient acceptability, or other concerns. This should hopefully change on the basis of recent experience with emulsions, some of which are outlined in this chapter.

PREPARATION OF EMULSIONS

Preparation of an emulsion requires mixing the two immiscible phases with the surfactant(s) and applying energy (generally mechanical) to create shear forces to deform the interface and form droplets, using sufficient force and time to achieve the required droplet size. There are a variety of devices that will accomplish this in either batch or continuous modes of operation. The forces involved in the emulsification process are not completely understood, but the methods can be classified according to three mechanisms. Laminar flow can be envisioned as the moving together of layers of the two phases, with resultant viscous forces leading to droplet formation and size reduction. Pipe flow devices, colloid mills, and ball and roller mills are based on laminar flow mechanisms. Turbulence, on the other hand, forms eddies or swirls, and the resulting inertial forces contribute to the emulsification process; shaking or injection can achieve the required turbulence. Cavitation involves the transient formation of small vapor bubbles that collapse extremely fast, and the resulting shock waves cause droplet formation and disruption; ultrasonic devices emulsify by this mechanism, along with turbulence. Rotor-stator and similar stirring devices emulsify by combination of turbulence and laminar flow mechanisms, while high-pressure homogenizers emulsify by combination of all three mechanisms. While most of the methods can be adapted for laboratory use, only rotor-stator stirrers, colloid mills, high-pressure homogenizers, and ultrasonic devices are practical for large-scale production (Walstra, 1983).

Since nutritional emulsions (e.g., Liposyn and Intralipid) have been in widespread use for several decades, procedures for large-scale manufacture of pharmaceutically acceptable o/w emulsions are now fairly well developed. Typically, the surfactant is dispersed in the aqueous phase along with any water-soluble components (e.g., glycerol for adjustment of tonicity) by stirring and heating as necessary until a homogenous mixture is formed. The oil phase is then added with stirring or shaking to form a *premix* with large (>10 μm) droplets, which is then subjected to a high-energy mechanical homogenization using one of the methods described earlier. The final droplet size depends on the formulation composition as well as the operating conditions (e.g., temperature, homogenization pressure, and duration of homogenization) (Collins-Gold et al., 1990).

Several apparati are available for the manufacture of pharmaceutical emulsions: the Gaulin® and Rannie® homogenizers are the most commonly used devices for large-scale manufacture; the Microfluidizer® and Five Star® Technologies Homogenizer are adaptable for laboratory or pilot scale preparations. Whatever device is used, procedures must be developed for validation of good manufacturing practice (GMP)-related issues such as drug losses owing to shear forces, product sterility, equipment cleaning, and product contamination from earlier uses.

When an emulsion is used for drug delivery, depending on the drug properties, one can envision several avenues by which the drug can be introduced into the emulsion. The simplest case would be if the drug is sufficiently lipophilic so that it can be readily dissolved in the oil phase before premix formation. Examples of *de novo* preparations shown in Table 10.3 are an emulsion containing Prostaglandin E1 (PGE1) and Vitalipid®, an emulsion containing oil-soluble vitamins. Similarly, penclomedine is soluble up to 100 mg/mL in soybean oil, allowing preparation of an emulsion with 10% soybean oil and 4.7 mg/mL final drug concentration (Prankerd and Stella, 1990). In some cases, an oil-soluble drug can be added directly to an already-prepared emulsion (e.g., Liposyn or Intralipid) and the drug preferentially partitions into the oil phase. In general, drugs that are liquid at room temperature are most amenable for these extemporaneously prepared emulsions, since the dissolution and required partitioning may be too slow for a solid drug. Anesthetics often meet this criteria. Examples are halothane and propofol: the latter is marketed as Diprivan®, an Intralipid/Liposyn–type emulsion containing 1% propofol and 10% soybean oil.

If a drug has sufficient water solubility, one can dissolve it into the aqueous component of the emulsion before formation of the premix for *de novo* emulsion preparation, or add the drug to a pre-formed emulsion for extemporaneous preparation. In these cases, knowledge of the oil–water partition coefficient is important to predict the final distribution of drug within the oil phases. Sila-On et al. (2008) examined the effect of incorporation method (*de novo* preparation vs. extemporaneous addition) into soybean-PC emulsions for four lipophilic drugs: alprazolam, clonazepam, diazepam, and lorazepam. The most lipophilic drug, diazepam, was readily incorporated into the oil phase regardless of preparation method. The other three, less lipophilic drugs, were preferentially localized in the phospholipid-rich region of the emulsion, and thus more efficiently solubilized in the *de novo* emulsions. If the drug is ionizable, one may be able to incorporate the drug by pH adjustment, that is, add the drug to the aqueous phase at a pH at which it is ionized and thus more water soluble, and then adjust the pH to a region in which it is nonionized and thus more hydrophobic, favoring partitioning into the oil phase.

Unfortunately, there are many drugs that have little or no solubility in either water or oil. In such a case, the final locale of drug would usually be the interface of the emulsion droplet, and emulsion preparation may be problematic. Nevertheless, several strategies have been devised for successful preparation of emulsions containing drugs in this category. Probably the most commonly used approach is the use of a cosolvent in which the drug is highly soluble; the drug solution can then be added extemporaneously to an emulsion, or to the oil phase before premix formation in a *de novo* preparation. Suitable pharmaceutically acceptable cosolvents include ethanol, propylene glycol (PEG), PEG 300, dimethylacetamide, triacetin, and mixtures of these solvents. However, the effect of cosolvent on chemical stability, emulsion droplet size, and drug partitioning must be carefully assessed. Diazemuls® is a diazepam (Valium®) emulsion marketed in Denmark; it contains 5% acetylated monoglycerides as the cosolvent along with 15% soybean oil, 1.2% egg phospholipids, and 2.25% glycerol (Collins-Gold et al., 1990). Amphotericin B emulsions have been prepared by a similar technique, wherein the drug is dissolved in dimethylacetamide to introduce the drug into the emulsion (Kirsch and Ravin, 1987). Similarly, triacetin allows preparation of a paclitaxel emulsion (Tarr et al., 1987), and addition of a solution of the chemotherapeutic agent Perilla ketone in 10% ethanol/40% propylene glycol/50% water to Intralipid results in a 1 mg/mL drug formulation (Collins-Gold et al., 1990). The same solvent mixture has been used to prepare an emulsion of Rhizoxin in 10% Intralipid (Prankerd and Stella, 1990). If the cosolvent is volatile, one can effect its removal following emulsion preparation. Such was the case for an amphotericin B emulsion, wherein methanol was used to introduce the drug and then allowed to evaporate from the formulation before emulsification with the oil (Forster et al., 1988). A similar approach involves the use of lipophilic counterions to increase the solubility of the drug in oil, allowing extemporaneous or *de novo* preparation of the emulsion. In this manner, clarithromycin was dissolved in a fatty acid/oil mixture (e.g., oleic acid/soybean oil or capric (decanoic) acid/Neobee® MCT oil) that was then formulated to obtain an o/w emulsion (Lovell et al., 1994). A flow diagram showing the composition and processing with the Microfluidizer for size reduction is shown in Figure 10.1. Another approach would be to solubilize the drug with an appropriate detergent and add this to an emulsion. For example, amphotericin B emulsions for clinical use have been prepared by dispersing lyophilized Fungizone into Intralipid 20% rather than into dextrose as is the standard practice; the presence of the deoxycholate in Fungizone apparently allows solubilization of the drug and partitioning into the

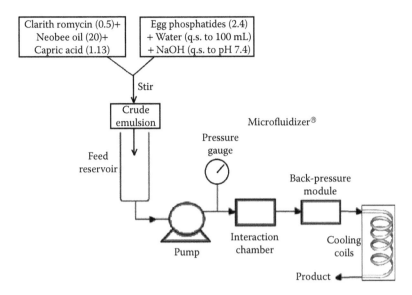

FIGURE 10.1   Flow diagram with composition for manufacture of a clarithromycin/capric acid/Neobee® MCT oil/egg phosphatide o/w emulsion using the Microfluidizer®. Amounts shown are in grams, to make 100 mL of emulsion. (From Lovell, M.W. et al., *Int. J. Pharm.*, 109, 45–57, 1994.)

emulsion droplet (Caillot et al., 1992). However, the validity of this approach has been questioned, since undissolved amphotericin B has been detected in such preparations (Davis, 1995).

If phospholipid dispersions (liposomes) of the drug can be prepared, one can envision addition of the oil phase to the drug liposomes, followed by emulsification, to give a drug emulsion, as was done to prepare an amphotericin B emulsion (Davis et al., 1987; Forster et al., 1988). If the drug is present in the lipid bilayer of the original liposomes, it will probably remain at the interface of the resulting emulsion. A simpler approach was used to prepare an emulsion of Almitrine, whereby a drug-phospholipid solution in chloroform/methanol solution was rotary evaporated to form a drug-lipid film (the first step in the classical method for liposome preparation), which was then hydrated with 10% Intralipid to form an emulsion. However, it was reported that drug crystals formed within several weeks of the preparation of this emulsion (Van Bloois et al., 1987).

Recently a solvent-free approach (SolEmuls®) using high-pressure homogenization to incorporate poorly soluble drugs in parenteral emulsions has been reported by Muller et al. (2004). Powdered drug or finely milled drug suspension is added to a commercial emulsion (e.g., Lipofundin or Intralipid) by stirring. Alternatively, the drug can be admixed during the *de novo* production of emulsion. The obtained dispersion containing oil droplets and drug particles is then subjected to high-pressure homogenization. The high-streaming velocities lead to drug dissolution and partitioning into the interfacial layer. Stable emulsion formulations of several poorly soluble drugs including ketoconazole, itraconazole, carbamazepine, and amphotericin B have been prepared using these methods. A 1 mg/mL itraconazole emulsion with mean particle size of 255 nm has been shown to be stable at room temperature for 9 months and no drug crystal was observed under microscopic examination (Akkar et al., 2004). As the interfacial layer could only solubilize a certain amount of drug, exceeding the saturation concentration of the drug at the interfacial layer, hybrid dispersions consisting of drug-loaded oil droplets and drug nanocrystals could form. Tiny crystals were found in a 2 mg/mL amphotericin B emulsion using a polarized microscope (Müller et al., 2004).

In the case of parenteral emulsions, insuring the sterility of the product is crucial. The preferred method for sterilization is generally terminal autoclaving. The nutritional emulsions such as Intralipid and Liposyn can be sterilized by autoclaving without phase separation or other stability problems (Washington et al., 1993). However, autoclaving has been found to cause some hydrolysis of lipids and lecithins, resulting in liberation of free fatty acids, which lowers the pH of the emulsions. To counter the pH dropping during autoclaving, it is suggested to adjust the pH of the emulsion to slightly alkaline pH (8.0) before autoclaving (Floyd, 1999). If the components of a particular drug-emulsion formulation preclude autoclaving owing to stability problems, sterile filtration of the product may be a viable alternative, requiring that the emulsion droplets pass through a 0.22 μm pore (Lidgate et al., 1992). There are also some reports of emulsions being successfully lyophilized; for example, an HIV protease inhibitor, AG1284, was solubilized in an Imwitor® 742/Tween 80/Span 80 emulsion, which could be lyophilized and reconstituted without loss of viability and potency (Chiang et al., 1995).

CHARACTERISTICS OF EMULSIONS

There are a number of physicochemical properties of emulsions that are important to consider when developing an emulsion formulation for a drug. These include, but are not limited to, particle (droplet) size, viscosity, osmolarity, and zeta potential, which are used to monitor the physical stability of emulsions. Assays of potency and degradant levels are used to monitor the chemical stability of emulsions.

> *Particle (droplet) size.* An important parameter is the particle (droplet) size of the emulsion. A variety of instruments and techniques exist for monitoring particle size. The most widely used techniques rely on laser light scattering, as reviewed by Tadros et al. (2004). Instrument manufacturers include Nicomp, Coulter, Horiba, Sympatec, and Malvern. Electron microscopy has also been used, but artifacts introduced by fixing techniques should be carefully controlled. Typically, emulsions produced by the methods described earlier yield particle sizes of 100–1000 nm; particle sizes less than 200 nm are generally required for emulsions used intravenously.
>
> *Viscosity.* This parameter can be monitored by standard rheological techniques. The rheological properties of emulsions, reviewed by Sherman (1983), can be complex, and depend on the identity of surfactants and oils used, ratio of disperse and continuous phase, particle size, and other factors. Flocculation will generally increase viscosity; thus, monitoring viscosity on storage will be important for assessing shelf life.
>
> *Osmolarity.* Osmolarity of a conventional emulsion is largely determined by components of the continuous phase, and the disperse phase may contribute little to the osmolarity. Thus, water-soluble excipients such as glycerol are frequently added to adjust tonicity of emulsions intended for parenteral use. Conventional techniques can be used for monitoring osmolarity. Owing to possible changes in emulsion structure on freezing, instruments that rely on vapor pressure lowering are more suitable for monitoring osmolarity of emulsions than those based on freezing point depression.
>
> *Zeta potential.* Zeta or electrokinetic potential is related to the surface charge of the emulsion droplets and it is generally measured by electrophoretic techniques. The zeta potential is highly dependent on the surfactants used. Yamaguchi et al. (1995) compared the properties of otherwise identical 10% soybean oil emulsions prepared from two different sources of lecithin: one containing 99% PC and the other containing only 70% PC, with phosphatidyl ethanolamine (PE) comprising much of the remaining phospholipid. At pH 4, 5, 6, and 8, the purified (99%) lecithin emulsion had zeta potentials of 5, −3, −8, and −30 mV, respectively, reflecting the zwitterionic nature of PC. In contrast, the crude (70%) preparation had zeta potentials of −15, −30, −45, and −60 mV, respectively, at the same pH values, reflecting the ionization properties of the free amino group of the PE (Yamaguchi et al., 1995). A charged drug molecule at the interface will also affect the zeta potential.
>
> *Chemical stability.* Certain emulsion components, especially those derived from unsaturated lipids, can give rise to undesirable degradation products on storage. These can include

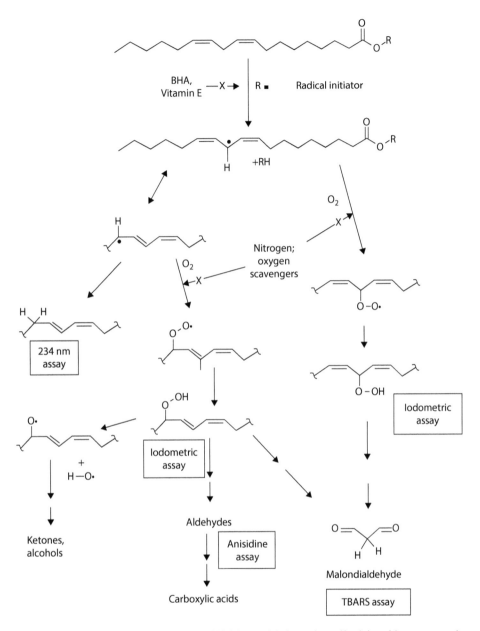

FIGURE 10.2 Schematic of the mechanisms of lipid peroxidation using a linoleic acid ester as a substrate.

oxidative products (e.g., lipid hydroperoxides and aldehydes), which may impair drug stability. Figure 10.2 shows a schematic of lipid peroxidation, using a linoleic acid ester (e.g., a glyceride) as an example.

The process is quite complex; a variety of pathways can ensue, giving a multitude of products and a number of assays that can be used to monitor lipid peroxidation. Lipid peroxidation is a radical initiated reaction; the radicals can initially arise from trace quantities of metal ions or other impurities, from peroxides present in PEG-based surfactants in the formulation, or from exposure to light that can generate singlet oxygen. The methylene group between two α, δ diene double bonds (present in linoleic and linolenic acids) is particularly susceptible to abstraction by radicals due to resonance stabilization of the product.

The lipid radical initially formed can react with oxygen to give a peroxy radical, propagating the radical pathway by abstracting a hydrogen from unreacted lipids to form a lipid hydroperoxide, which can be measured by an iodometric assay (Porter, 1984). This lipid hydroperoxide can decompose to give malondialdehyde (absorbance at 532 nm) and other products; thiobarbituric acid, which forms a colored product with malondialdehyde, can be used to quantitate these and similar products in the thiobarbituric acid reactive substances (TBARS) assay (Abuja and Albertini, 2001). Alternatively, and more likely, the initially formed radical from the α, δ diene can react through the alternate resonance form to form a conjugated diene, in this case 9-(cis)-11-(trans)-octadecenoic acid (detectable by its UV absorbance at 230–235 nm) (Antolovich et al., 2002), or react with oxygen to form conjugated lipid hydroperoxides. These can either decompose to give the highly reactive hydroxyl radical (with the remaining lipid fragment giving rise to ketone and alcohol products), or decompose to short-chain aldehydes (e.g., hexanal, butanal), which can be quantitated using the anisidine assay (Antolovich et al., 2002). Aldehydes themselves can be oxidized to short-chain carboxylic acids (e.g., butyric acid). These carbonyl products are responsible for the disagreeable odor associated with rancidity of lipids, and more importantly, can give rise to drug instability (Cannon, 2007; Stella, 2013).

As shown in the diagram, several different assays have been used in the past to monitor the lipid peroxidation process (Lang and Vigo-Pelfrey, 1993). Because of the complexity of the process, it is difficult to predict the ultimate pathway. Thus, using a single assay to quantitate the extent of lipid peroxidation may not be representative of the overall level of degradation. For example, the TBARS assay is reported to be unspecific and prone to artifacts (Abuja and Albertini, 2001), while the iodometric assay may not be reflective of the overall extent of peroxidation if lipid hydroperoxides do not build up and instead decompose (Antolovich et al., 2002). A method that monitors the overall peroxidation process by measuring the increase in conductivity and the associated induction time is the Rancimat method (Laubli and Bruttel, 1986; Halbaut et al., 1997). If it is suspected that lipid peroxidation could be a problem for drug instability or formulation properties, it may be more meaningful to monitor specific types of agents (e.g., high-performance liquid chromatography [HPLC] assay of aldehydes).

More importantly, lipid peroxidation can be controlled or minimized by design of formulation. While saturated lipids (e.g., medium-chain triglycerides, or MCTs) will themselves not be susceptible to peroxidation, they may contain sufficient unsaturated impurities to be problematic. Similarly, monounsaturated lipids (e.g., oleic acid glycerides) are much less susceptible to peroxidation. The relative rates of peroxidation of oleic, linoleic, and linolenic acids are 6:64:100, respectively (Swern, 1995). Monounsaturated lipids may, however, contain polyunsaturated impurities, which will catalyze the oxidation of the monounsaturated components (Swern, 1995). Surfactants, particularly those based on PEG, may contain peroxides that can promote lipid peroxidation; thus, particular attention should be paid to the purity and source of all formulation components.

The other important factor in retarding and controlling lipid peroxidation is the use of appropriate antioxidants, which can inhibit the pathway at various points and stabilize lipids. The most useful are phenol-based antioxidants, for example, butylated hydroxytoluene (BHT), butylated hydroxyanisole (BHA), propyl gallate, and vitamin E (α-tocopherol). All of these form stable free radicals, thus acting as radical scavengers and chain terminators. When using vitamin E, it is important to remember that only the free phenol is active as an antioxidant; derivatives such as vitamin E acetate or tocopherol polyethylene glycol (TPGS) will not inhibit lipid peroxidation until metabolized. Other antioxidants (e.g., ascorbic acid, ascorbyl palmitate) act as oxygen scavengers, which will prevent formation of lipid hydroperoxides but not conjugated dienes. The two types of antioxidants, by acting at different points in the pathway, can act synergistically if used together (*Handbook of*

Pharmaceutical Excipients, 1994). It should be noted that ascorbic acid derived oxygen scavengers are also reducing agents, and in fact can promote rather than retard peroxidation if metal ions are present (Sevanian and Ursini, 2000); inclusion of a chelating agent such as ethylene diamine tetraacetic acid (EDTA) in the formulation will prevent this and enhance the antioxidant activity of ascorbates. Use of ascorbates with drugs sensitive to reducing agents should be avoided. Use of a nitrogen atmosphere for formulation manufacture is another, but less convenient, method for excluding oxygen.

Hydrolysis is the other important mechanism for some lipids (glycerides and phosphoglycerides) to degrade. Lowering of pH can arise from both hydrolysis and lipid peroxidation (Arakane et al., 1995), as both processes can give acid products. It has also been reported that hydrolysis and peroxidation can act in synergy with one another in liposome bilayers (Swern, 1995), but it is uncertain whether this can happen for other structures since different mechanisms are operative for emulsified lipids and bulk lipids (Antolovich et al., 2002). Hydrolytic products (e.g., free fatty acids, mono- and diglycerides, and lyso-phospholipids) can form that can alter the surface properties and zeta potential of the emulsion and distribute into the aqueous phase (Herman and Groves, 1992, 1993). Fatty acid formation can also decrease the pH and increase the conductivity of the emulsion (Santos-Magalhaes et al., 1991). Hence, these two parameters should be monitored to aid stability evaluation. The emulsion excipients (namely, oils, surfactants, and cosolvents) should be monitored by periodic assays to insure no loss of excipient concentration.

Physical stability. As indicated earlier, conventional emulsions are inherently unstable from a physical standpoint. Poor physical stability is ultimately exhibited by phase separation, which can be visually monitored. Certain properties of the emulsion will start to change long before this separation is visually apparent. An increase in particle size is particularly indicative of physical instability, since this monitors the coalescence or flocculation that is part of the process involved in ultimate phase separation. Increases in viscosity (due to flocculation) and changes in zeta potential (arising from a decrease in droplet surface area) are both indicative of poor physical stability. The presence of drug and cosolvents can potentially hasten the phase separation.

From a theoretical standpoint, physical stability is probably the most complex property of emulsions. The key factor in determining the stability of an emulsion is believed to be the interfacial tension between the two phases, and lower interfacial tension (primarily governed by the surfactant) will increase the stability (Collins-Gold et al., 1990). Very low interfacial tension is thought to be the primary factor leading to the stability of microemulsions. A number of models allowing prediction of the stability of emulsions have been put forth. One of the most useful approaches is the so-called DLVO theory, developed over 50 years ago by Derjaguin and Landau (1941) and Verwey and Overbeek (1948). According to this theory, the stability of an emulsion depends on a balance of electrostatic repulsive forces and London-type Van der Waals attractive forces. Thus, higher surface charge (characterized by high absolute values of the zeta potential) will generally tend to stabilize emulsions due to the higher repulsion of the droplets from one another. For example, a 70% PC emulsion had a higher overall physical stability than a 99% PC emulsion, reflecting the latter's lower surface charge (Yamaguchi et al., 1995). An overabundance of electrolytes will generally tend to destabilize emulsions due to a lowering of the surface charge, leading to a so-called salting out effect, wherein the emulsion will undergo flocculation and phase separation at sufficiently high electrolyte concentration. Calcium and other divalent ions are particularly destabilizing. A parameter can be derived known as the *critical flocculation concentration* (CFC), which is the electrolyte concentration at which flocculation begins. For the PC emulsions described earlier, the CFC's for $CaCl_2$ were 0.4 mM for 99% PC and 1.2 mM for 70% PC (Yamaguchi et al., 1995).

DRUG SOLUBILIZATION AND DELIVERY USING EMULSIONS

RATIONALE

Various formulation approaches can be used for solubilization and delivery of pharmaceutical compounds. If the compound has ionizable groups, salt formation is often the first strategy used to improve solubility. Otherwise, use of cosolvents is perhaps the most common alternative for solubilization of compounds, probably owing to the high efficiency and ease of use of cosolvents to solubilize drug. However, the use of cosolvents has the potential to cause problems like drug precipitation on dilution, and pain and/or tissue damage on parenteral administration. Emulsion formulations have the potential to avoid precipitation after injection. Other approaches include prodrugs, surfactant (micellar) systems, complexation, and liposomes. Combined approaches of emulsions with one of the other formulation strategies may also be used to advantage. As mentioned earlier, cosolvents are frequently used to incorporate drugs into an emulsion. Similarly, use of a lipophilic counterion to increase drug affinity to an emulsion may be considered an approach combining salt formation and emulsion strategies. There have been several reports of lipophilic prodrugs having higher affinity to and retention within the oil phase of an emulsion relative to the parent drug. Incorporation of palmitoyl rhizoxin into an emulsion protected the drug from degradation in plasma (Kurihara et al., 1996). Similar prodrug emulsion examples include a prostaglandin E1 prodrug (Matsuo, 1998), etoposide oleate (Azevedo et al., 2005), and paclitaxel oleate (Rodriguez et al., 2005).

Emulsions are an attractive alternative for drug solubilization. If the drug has moderate solubility in bioacceptable oils, emulsion systems could offer several benefits apart from drug solubilization that are rarely achievable with other formulation systems. Some of these include improvement in drug toxicity, sustained drug release *in vivo*, reduction in pain, irritation and tissue damage after parenteral delivery. For example, emulsion formulation of amphotericin B has been shown to cause significantly less damage to red blood cells (RBCs) than the commercial product, Fungizone (Forster et al., 1988). Emulsions have also been shown to reduce the toxicity of drug (e.g., miconazole) (Levy et al., 1995). Other examples of emulsions for reduction in adverse effects after parenteral dosing will be mentioned in subsequent sections.

Use of an emulsion formulation for pharmaceutical drug delivery generally mandates that the drug be present in the internal (i.e., dispersed) phase and/or at the interface. This means that the process meets one of the following criteria:

1. Drug has a high log P value, that is, the drug prefers to partition into lipophilic versus aqueous media. For example, an O-alkyl-N-aryl thiocarbamate has poor solubility in water or water containing cosolvents; however, its solubility is 2–3 orders of magnitude higher in oils, expediting emulsion preparation (Strickley and Anderson, 1993).
2. Drug is marginally soluble in oils; however, it can be improved with the aid of excipients. For example, the oil solubility of clarithromycin has been increased with the aid of counterions like hexanoic and oleic acid (Lovell et al., 1994).
3. Drug is soluble in neither oil nor water; however, it can be retained at the interface of an emulsion. Thus, if a liposomal preparation can be made in which the drug resides in the lipid bilayer, or if it can be solubilized into micelles by an appropriate detergent, an emulsion can probably be made wherein the drug resides at the interface.

Conformance to one or more of the above-mentioned criteria generally qualifies development of an emulsion formulation for drugs that otherwise cannot be successfully administered parenterally as a solution. Hence, emulsions have been explored for improved drug efficacy after oral, topical and parenteral administration, and for improved patient compliance (e.g., reduced pain or irritation after parenteral administration, and improved palatability after oral delivery).

In addition, the formulations should meet the following two requirements:

1. The drug is retained in the dispersed phase or at the interface over time under normal handling and storage conditions.
2. Drug solubilization and delivery using emulsions does not lead to undesirable changes in its chemical stability, efficacy, or toxicity.

Examples of studies supporting use of emulsions for a variety of drug delivery needs are listed in Table 10.4. Some of the advantages conferred by emulsion formulations may be mediated by an improved solubilization of the drug. There is also a growing list of studies suggesting use of emulsions for drug solubilization *per se*; these are summarized in Table 10.5.

TABLE 10.4
A Representative List of Compounds Tested for Delivery as an Emulsion

Rationale for Emulsion Formulation	Compound(s) Tested	Reference(s)
Pain on Injection and Venous Irritation	Etomidate	Doenicke et al. (1990)[a]; Kulka et al. (1993)[a]
	Diazepam	Von Dardel et al. (1983)[a]
	Clarithromycin	Lovell et al. (1994, 1995)
	Vinorelbine	Li et al. (2013)
	Diallyl trisulfide	Mao et al. (2010)
	Cinnarizine	Shi et al. (2009)
	Tirilazad	Wang et al. (1999)
Thrombophlebitis	Etomidate	Doenicke et al. (1990)[a]; Kulka et al. (1993)[a]
Reduced Toxicity	Cyclosporine	Tibell et al. (1993); Venkatraman et al. (1990); Ehinger et al. (2013)[a]; Suzuki et al. (2004)
	Amphotericin B	Forster et al. (1988); Lamb et al. (1991); Sundar et al. (2008)[a]; Sundar et al. (2014)[a]
	Vincristine	Junping et al. (2003)
	Triptolide	Li et al. (2015)
	α-asarone	Ma et al. (2013)
	Paclitaxel	Lundberg et al. (2003); Jing et al. (2014);
Improved Stability	Sodium Phenobarbital	Dietz et al. (1988)
	Oxathiin Carboxanilide	Oh et al. (1991)
	Physostigmine	Pathak et al. (1990)
	Perilla Ketone (NSC 348407)	Paborji et al. (1988)
	Ligustrazine	Wei et al. (2012a)
	Breviscpine	Wei et al. (2012b)
	Tetrazepam	Jumaa and Muller et al. (2001)
	Etoposide	Tian et al. (2007)
Prolonged Activity	Peptides	Gasco et al. (1990)
	Somatotropin	Tyle and Cady (1990)
	Physostigmine	Benita et al. (1986)
	Etoposide	Reddy and Venkateswarlu (2005)
	Nystatin	Marín-Quintero et al. (2013)
	Cinnarizine	Shi et al. (2010)
	Nalbuphine	Wang et al. (2006)
Drug Targeting	Bleomycin	Tanigawa et al. (1987)[a]
	Titanocene Dichloride	Muller et al. (1991)
	Mitomycin C	Nakamoto et al. (1975)
	Triptolide	Xiong et al. (2010)
Vaccine Adjuvants	Muramyldipeptide	Lidgate et al. (1989)

[a] Describe clinical studies.

TABLE 10.5

A Representative List of Experimental Studies Exploring Emulsion System for Drug Solubilization

Drug	Reference(s)	Application/Result
Oxathiin Carboxanilide (NSC 615985)	Oh et al. (1991)	Solubilization in emulsion for tox studies.
Anticancer agent NSC 278214	El Sayed and Repta (1983)	Enhanced stability (100-fold) in emulsions relative to aqueous systems.
Hexamethylmelamine	Ames and Kovach (1982)	Emulsion reduces local irritation and venous thrombosis after IV injection.
Etoposide & Teniposide derivatives	Lundberg (1994)	Enhanced solubilization, cellular uptake, and cytotoxic activity of lipophilic prodrugs.
Penclomedine	Prankerd et al. (1988)	Emulsion formulation was more active and less toxic in mouse tumor model.
Paclitaxel	Tarr et al. (1987)	Triacetin emulsion to solubilize drug, alternative to surfactants and cosolvents.
Paclitaxel	Jing et al. (2014)	Same cytotoxicity against HeLa cells as Taxol®, with better therapeutic index.
Halothane	Johannesson et al. (1984); Biber et al. (1984)	IV administration of emulsion formulation induced anesthesia similar to inhalation route.
Pregnanolone	Hogskilde et al. (1987a, 1987b)	Good anesthetic affect from emulsion, avoids allergic reaction from Cremphor EL.
Rhizoxin (NSC 332598)	Stella et al. (1988)	Solubilization in emulsion formulation for slow infusion.
Anti-HIV: NSC 629243	Strickley and Anderson (1993)	Emulsion formulation enhanced solubilization and stabilization.
Testosterone and its esters; Progesterone; Medroxyprogesterone acetate	Malcolmson and Lawrence (1993)	Solubilization of steroids in emulsions; high drug loading achievable depending on log Po/w.
Clarithromycin	Lovell et al. (1994)	Emulsion formulation decreased pain on injection.
All-trans retinoic acid (ATRA)	Hwang et al. (2004)	Emulsion formulation enhanced drug solubilization and stabilization; maintained anti-tumor activity.
All-trans retinoic acid	Chansri et al. (2006)	Higher uptake in liver in mice, and mouse survival prolonged in liver metastasis model.
Prostaglandin: TEI-9826	Fukushima et al. (2000)	Emulsion formulation retarded tumor growth in mouse and rat models with sustained infusion.
Flurbiprofen	Park et al. (1999)	Solubilization in emulsion formulation reduces volume required for parenteral delivery.
Docetaxel	Gao et al. (2008)	Higher AUC and C_{max} in rats compared to micellar solution.
Triptolide	Li et al. (2015)	Increased distribution to pancreas and improved therapeutic efficacy for cancer in mice.
Cyclopamine	You et al. (2015)	Higher antitumor cytotoxicity (4- to 8-fold reduction in IC_{50}) compared to free drug
α-asarone	Ma et al. (2013)	Improved efficacy in vivo.
Ligustrazine	Wei et al. (2012a)	Improved bioavailability: 1.6-fold higher AUC compared to currently available product.
Breviscapine	Xiong et al. (2010)	Higher distribution to heart in mice.
Cinnarizine	Shi et al. (2010)	Higher AUC, lower clearance, and lower distribution volume than those of solution form.

(Continued)

TABLE 10.5 (*Continued*)
A Representative List of Experimental Studies Exploring Emulsion System for Drug Solubilization

Drug	Reference(s)	Application/Result
All-trans retinoic acid	Chansri et al. (2006)	Higher uptake in liver in mice, and mouse survival prolonged in liver metastasis model.
Diclofenac	Ramreddy et al. (2012)	Improved pharmacokinetics, higher AUC, and higher-elimination half-life in rats compared to solution.
Nalbuphine	Wang et al. (2006)	Improved analgesic duration and potency in rodents.
Paclitaxel oleate (paclitaxel prodrug)	Lundberg et al. (2003)	Greater AUC, higher Cmax, lower systemic clearance, and lower distribution volume in rabbits compared to Cremophor EL formulation.
Etoposide oleate	Azevedo et al. (2005)	Incorporation of drug into cholestrol-rich microemulsion led to 4-fold increase in uptake in malignant ovarian tissues in 4 patients relative to normal ovarian tissue.
Aclacinomycin A	Wang et al. (2002)	Higher AUC, lower toxicity, and higher antitumor effect in tumor-bearing mice.
Aclacinomycin A	Shiokawa et al. (2005)	Incorporation into folate-linked microemulsions led to greater in vitro cytotoxcity, 2.6-fold higher accumulation in tumors *in vivo*, and greater tumor growth inhibition than free drug.

MECHANISM OF DRUG RELEASE AND DRUG ABSORPTION

On introduction of a drug-containing emulsion into the biological milieu (into plasma by IV administration), drug diffusion out of the emulsion droplet occurs. To some extent, the kinetics of this process are governed by such properties as the distribution coefficient of drug between the emulsion oil phase, interface and external aqueous phase. Yamaguchi et al. (1994) examined the release of PGE1 from an o/w emulsion by equilibrium dialysis, and showed that 93% of the drug diffuses into the buffer, and all but 0.2% of the remainder is located at the interface. The process was suggested to be controlled by Fickian diffusion. In another study, a *reverse dialysis* technique was used to measure the *in vitro* release properties of clofibride from an emulsion formulation, whereby 1 mL of the emulsion was added to 500 mL of a buffer sink, along with a dialysis sack containing buffer alone (Santos-Magalhaes et al., 1991). Measurement of the rate of appearance of drug in the dialysis sack allowed calculation of the kinetics of drug release from the emulsion droplets. The results were comparable to those from an ultrafiltration method utilizing microcentrifuge filters. Both methods were indicated to be superior to standard dialysis techniques (i.e., where the emulsion is placed inside the dialysis sack), because diffusion of drug across the dialysis membrane can be the rate limiting step in standard techniques. Lundberg (1994) monitored leakage of the anticancer drugs etoposide oleate and teniposide oleate from emulsion droplets using gel permeation chromatography.

The quantitation of release of drug from an emulsion in the presence of serum is significantly more complex because of binding of drug and emulsion components to plasma proteins as well as plasma metabolism of emulsion lipids. Phospholipids of Liposyn/Intralipid-type emulsions are known to bind to plasma lipoproteins, especially high-density lipoprotein (HDL) (Williams and Tall, 1988). Minagawa et al. (1994) developed a technique for monitoring release of an antithrombic drug, TEI-9090, from emulsion droplets in serum by incubation of the test emulsion/serum mixtures with polydimethyl siloxane glass beads in the presence of sodium dodecyl sulfate (SDS). The latter displaced drug bound to serum albumin, and the beads selectively adsorbed the free drug. *In vivo*, the situation is even more complicated because of the tendency of emulsions to be taken up by the phagocytic cells of the reticuloendothelial systems (RES). Phospholipid-oil based emulsions resemble chylomicrons, which are rapidly cleared by liver: 65% of exogenously injected chylomicrons are recovered in the liver within 30 minutes after injection (Van Berkel et al., 1991). Triglycerides are removed and digested by lipoprotein lipases present in capillary endothelium, and the remnant emulsion droplets are almost completely taken up by the liver within a few hours (Handa et al., 1994). Thus, these factors could have a significant impact on the pharmacokinetics and biodistribution of the drug. If the diffusion of drug from the emulsion is slow, then a high uptake of drug by the RES cells will be expected. This may be desirable in some cases where liver and spleen are the therapeutic targets, and where subsequent slow release of drug from these sites is desirable, and where toxicity of drug to sites of low emulsion uptake would otherwise be a problem. On the other hand, if diffusion of drug out of the emulsion is rapid compared to the metabolism and clearance of the emulsion droplets, then the pharmacokinetics and distribution of the drug will be little different from those of aqueous formulations. In studies using a rat liver perfusion system comparing emulsions with mean diameters of 252 and 85 nm containing [^{3}H] retinoic acid (log $P_{o/w} = 6.6$) and [^{14}C] cholesterol oleate (calculated log $P_{o/w} = 18$), the rates of RES uptake and plasma release were shown to depend on the emulsion size and drug partition coefficient (Takino et al., 1995). It has been suggested that drugs with a log $P_{o/w} > 9$ will be retained in the lipid phase regardless of the emulsion's composition and particle size (Kawakami et al., 2000).

On the basis of these considerations, formulation of a drug may or may not have a significant impact on the pharmacokinetic properties of the drug, and there have been a number of studies comparing emulsion and aqueous-based formulations with regard to this question. Cyclosporine (Sandimmune®), is normally formulated for IV use with Cremophor EL, a solubilizer, which is known to cause nephrotoxicity. When formulated as a 1.2% phospholipid/10% soybean oil emulsion incorporating 2–3 mg/mL drug, the nephrotoxicity in rats was decreased (Tibell et al., 1993) without changes in systemic clearance, volume of distribution, or elimination half-lives in rats and pigs. Hence the two formulations were considered bioequivalent (Tibell et al., 1995). Another study compared cyclosporine formulated as liposomes and as an emulsion (with 10 mg/mL cyclosporine in 20% Intralipid) with Sandimmune. All three formulations showed similar elimination half-lives, but Sandimmune showed significantly higher area-under-the-curve (AUC) values and lower volume of distribution than the other 2 formulations (Venkatraman et al., 1990). The binding of cyclosporine to lipoproteins was suggested as one reason for the differences in the *in vivo* behavior among the formulations. Similar contrasting results have been obtained with diazepam. Earlier reports indicated significantly lower plasma diazepam levels with Diazemuls emulsion than Valium injectable solution (5 mg/mL diazepam in 10% ethanol/40% propylene glycol) (Fee et al., 1984); however, later studies were unable to find a significant difference (Naylor and Burlingham, 1985).

An emulsion formulation of hexamethylmelamine in 20% Intralipid resulted in peak plasma drug concentrations and rates of elimination similar to those from a pH 2–3 aqueous formulation of the hydrochloride salt; however, the emulsion alleviated the vein irritation in rabbits (Ames and Kovach, 1982). This suggests that drug remains associated with the emulsion long enough to reduce local tissue irritation, but diffuses rapidly into serum at sites distal from the injection site. In the case of propofol emulsion (Diprivan), an anesthetic, the drug molecule distributes rapidly from blood to tissues, with a blood-brain equilibration time of only 2–3 min. No difference in pharmacokinetics has been observed between healthy patients and those with liver cirrhosis (Dundee and Clarke, 1989). These observations suggest that the emulsion has little effect on the distribution of propofol, which is not surprising, based on the low molecular weight of the drug.

The antifungal drug amphotericin B (AmB) is currently marketed for IV administration as a colloidal dispersion with sodium deoxycholate as a solubilizer (Fungizone). The formulation has hemolytic and nephrotoxic effects that are believed to arise from membrane damaging effects. Hence, alternate formulations (e.g., liposomes) (Lopez-Berestein, 1988; Gates and Pinney, 1993) and emulsions have been actively explored to alleviate these effects. *De novo* PC/oil AmB emulsions have shown reduced toxicity in cell culture and animal studies (Davis et al., 1987; Kirsch and

Ravin, 1987; Forster et al., 1988; Collins-Gold et al., 1990; Lamb et al., 1991). These results imply an altering of the distribution of the drug away from sensitive membranes. The RES uptake of AmB emulsion has been suggested as a possible reason for its therapeutic advantage (Collins-Gold et al., 1990).

In cases where distribution of emulsion to the RES cells is undesirable, strategies similar to those used for extending the circulating half-lives of liposomes by incorporating PEG or sialic acids into the lipid bilayer could be used (Allen et al., 1989; Woodle and Lasic, 1992). *Long-circulating emulsions* have been described by Liu and Liu (1995), wherein a PEG-derivatized phospholipid has been incorporated into the outer layer of an emulsion. At 30 min after injection, only 30% of a conventional emulsion remained in the blood with 50% distributed to the liver, compared to 65% in blood and only 15% in liver at the same time point for the PEG-based emulsion. The apparent reason for this difference is the higher surface hydrophilicity, leading to reduced opsonization and phagocytosis by the RES cells (Liu and Liu, 1995). A similar approach has been used to deliver ibuprofen octyl ester in a poloxamer 338/oil emulsion. This emulsion reduced RES uptake compared to a PC/oil emulsion. The higher hydrophilicity of the poloxamer 338 was hypothesized to reduce the uptake of the emulsion by the RES cells (Lee et al., 1995). Use of more hydrophilic oils such as triacetin to increase dissolution has also been proposed as a strategy to decrease RES uptake of emulsions (Tarr et al., 1987). Incorporation of sphingomyelin into the surface of 100 nm emulsions prolonged their circulation (Takino et al., 1994).

There are fewer reports on other parenteral routes of administration of emulsions such as intramuscular, subcutaneous, and intraperitoneal. Water-in-oil and w/o/w emulsions of bleomycin, mytomycin C, and 5-fluorouracil have been administered by these routes, apparently resulting in increased regional lymphatic uptake, hence the term *lymphotropic emulsions* (Davis et al., 1987). Gasco et al. (1990) developed a w/o emulsion of an LHRH analog; measurements of testosterone levels after intramuscular administration to rats suggested that the formulation led to prolonged release of the drug.

EXAMPLES OF EMULSION FORMULATIONS OF WATER-INSOLUBLE DRUGS

EXPERIMENTAL CASE STUDIES

Lipophilic properties of halothane have been utilized for its parenteral delivery through an emulsion formulation. In one study, 0.3 mL of a 5% halothane in fat emulsion (Intralipid), prepared *de novo* immediately before testing, was injected through the rat tail vein. The emulsion formulation allowed short-lasting (30–100 s), potent analgesia with reduced adverse effects. All major organs of the animals (e.g., lung, kidney, heart, brain, and liver) demonstrated normal histology over a 29-day test period after dosing. Although some animals died in this test after dosing the emulsion formulation (probably due to nonoptimized injection rates), this formulation was found to be superior to injections of regular halothane, which has been shown to cause serious damage to the lung tissue (Johannesson et al., 1984).

Cyclosporine A (CsA) is a potent immunosuppressant indicated for the prevention of transplanted organs. However, it is known to cause dose-dependent nephrotoxicity when administered in the conventional formulation containing Cremophor EL; this solubilizing agent itself is reported to be nephrotoxic and allergic to some patients. Hence, feasibility of parenteral delivery of CsA as an emulsion with reduced adverse effects has been assessed (Venkatraman et al., 1990). The test formulation was prepared extemporaneously by adding drug to 20% Intralipid and mixing the contents until the powder was dispersed. Its performance was tested in rabbits and compared with the marketed IV product, Sandimmune. Whereas the terminal half-life of drug delivered through emulsion formulation was comparable to that of Sandimmune, some distribution parameters changed as a result of reformulation. The area under the blood drug concentration versus time curve (AUC) was significantly lower with the emulsion formulation than that with Sandimmune (7397 $\pm$ 2223 versus 13075 ± 224 μg*hr/mL, respectively; mean $\pm$ SD, $N = 4$ ($P = 0.002$). However, the lower bioequivalence of the emulsion was perceived as an advantage because of possible preferential liver distribution, along with lower drug concentrations in blood immediately after dosing. The emulsion formulation demonstrated *in vivo* mean residence time (MRT) of 462 ± 173, which was almost two-fold higher than that with Sandimmune (214 ± 17, $P = 0.029$), indicating that the emulsion system may offer improved efficacy over the commercial product. Hence, the emulsion formulation of CsA was shown to alleviate adverse effects associated with Sandimmune without compromising the efficacy (Venkatraman et al., 1990).

Several compounds are known to cause pain, irritation and local tissue damage following parenteral administration. Some of these compounds are water-insoluble. Although the exact mechanism of these adverse reactions is not well understood, drug solubilization and its encapsulation in oil droplets of o/w emulsion has been hypothesized to reduce the degree of these unacceptable events. For example, the IV administration of the standard diazepam formulation, a 5 mg/mL drug solution in a vehicle composed of 40% propylene glycol, 10% ethanol and water (Valium) is frequently known to cause pain and venous sequelae (i.e., change in color and/or thickness of injected vein along with erythema, edema, necrosis, and inflammation of the surrounding tissue). In one study, 0.3 mg/kg diazepam was injected through the ear vein of rabbits as a 5 mg/mL o/w emulsion or 5 mg/mL hydroalcoholic solution, with ~0.18 mL injected over 30 seconds. The results of the induction of venous sequelae were compared using saline as a negative control. The emulsion was found to cause significant reduction in local tissue reactions as compared to the hydroalcoholic formulation of diazepam ($P < 0.05$) (Figure 10.3). No statistical difference was observed in local tissue reaction with saline and the emulsion formulation. The scoring results were confirmed pathologically. Overall, the results suggested that avoidance of irritating solubilizing agents in the formulation and minimization of drug precipitation *in vivo* may reduce local tissue reactions (Levy et al., 1989).

To decrease the IV pain on injection of clarithromycin, the feasibility of emulsion formulation was evaluated. A 5 mg/mL emulsion formulation was developed using oleic and hexanoic acids as lipophilic counterions (Lovell et al., 1994). The degree of reduction in pain was assessed using various animal models, for example, mouse scratch test, rat-paw lick test, rabbit ear vein irritation test

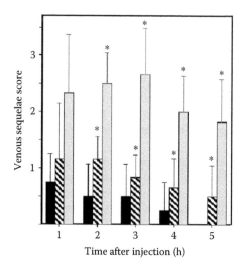

FIGURE 10.3 Mean venous sequalae scores after IV injection of saline (■), diazepam emulsion (◪), and hydroalcoholic solution of diazepam (□) to rabbits. Bar represents SD of 4–6 animals per group; (*) indicates significant difference of $P = 0.05$. Note the increase in score is indicative of increased severity of inflammation and/or drug reaction. (Adapted from Levy, M.Y. et al., *Pharm. Res.*, 6, 510–516, 1989. With permission.)

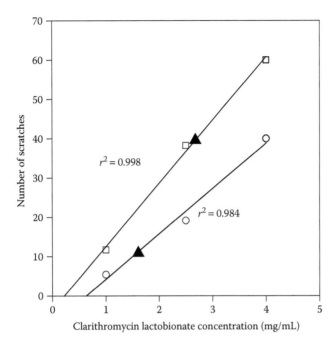

FIGURE 10.4   Dose response curves in mouse scratch model over the first 5 min (O) and the first 10 min (□) after injection of 1, 2.5, and 4 mg/mL of clarithromycin lactobionate solution to mouse. The scratches with 5 mg/mL clarithromycin are shown by symbol (▲) for comparison. (Adapted from Lovell, M.W. et al., *Int. J. Pharm.*, 109, 45–57, 1994. With permission.)

and rat tail vein irritation test. In the mouse scratch test, pain with 5 mg/mL emulsion formulation was found to be comparable to 1.6–2.7 mg/mL drug solution (Figure 10.4). In the rat paw lick test, only 70% of the animals receiving emulsion were found to respond to pain as opposed to 100% animals responding to pain after the injection of drug solution. The degree of paw lick (i.e., number of licks per rat and total licking time) was reduced by >50%. In vein irritation tests in rabbits and rats, the extent of adverse reactions at the site of injection was significantly lower with the emulsion than that with the drug solution. In addition, the emulsion formulation did not alter plasma drug distribution, toxicity, and efficacy of the drug (Lovell et al., 1994).

Several studies have examined targeted drug delivery aspects of emulsion formulations. Cancer cells have a much higher expression of LDL receptors on their surface compared to normal cells, and cholesterol-rich emulsions are taken up by these receptors. Uptake levels of paclitaxel oleate delivered in mice through such an emulsion were fourfold higher in tumor tissue than in adjacent normal tissues, and the lethal dose (LD50) of the emulsion was 9-fold that of the commercial (Cremophor EL) formulation (Rodriguez et al., 2005). Similar results were obtained in animals for cholesterol-rich emulsions delivering daunorubicin (Dorlhiac-Llacer et al., 2001), carmustine (Teixeira et al., 2004), and etoposide (Valduga et al., 2003). These studies demonstrate the potential of emulsions to increase the therapeutic index of cancer chemotherapeutic agents.

CLINICAL CASE STUDIES

Despite immense interest in the use of emulsions for pharmaceutical drug delivery, limited human data has been published with this delivery system beyond the marketed products listed in Table 10.3. In general, following IV administration, emulsion formulations demonstrate plasma profiles similar to those obtained with other solubilized formulations (e.g., micelles and cosolvent systems), but pain on injection or toxicity can be improved. The following examples demonstrate the utility of emulsions:

- Amphotericin B has been formulated as an emulsion by addition of Fungizone to Intralipid 20% and examined clinically. Several reports indicate that the emulsion reduces renal toxicity while maintaining efficacy (Caillot et al., 1992; Chavanet et al., 1992). However, one case report described a patient who had acute renal failure after administration of amphotericin B emulsion (Alford et al., 1994), perhaps due to incomplete incorporation of the drug into the emulsion droplets and precipitation of drug (Davis, 1995).
- Pregnanolone (eltanolone) is a water-insoluble anesthetic that has been in clinical trials as an emulsion developed by Kabi Pharmacia, Sweden. In a clinical study, pregnanolone emulsion appears to induce general anesthesia reliably and smoothly in 13 healthy volunteers, with cardiorespiratory effects similar to other anesthetics (Gray et al., 1992). EEG monitoring indicated the dose inducing 50% of the maximal central nervous system (CNS) depressant effect to be about 0.57 µg/mL (Hering et al., 1995). In a pharmacokinetic and pharmacodynamic study in 6 volunteers, the elimination half-life of pregnanolone was found to be between 0.9 and 1.4 h; hemodynamics and ventilation were only slightly affected (Carl et al., 1990).
- Intraiodol® is an iodinated lipid emulsion taken up by RES tissues, which has led to its clinical examination in 15 patients as a diagnostic agent for computed tomography (CT) of liver (Ivancev et al., 1989).
- Emulsions of perfluorooctyl bromide (perflubron, Imagent®) have been developed by Alliance Pharmaceutical Corp. for imaging of liver by both CT and sonography (Behan et al., 1993). They have also been used as contrast agents for lymph node imaging; subcutaneous dosage of perflubron emulsion into the hands of 18 volunteers led to a dose-related enhancement of CT images of axillary lymph nodes (Hanna et al., 1994). A similar perflubron emulsion, Oxygent®, has been tested clinically as a temporary oxygen carrier at relatively low (1.35–1.8 g perflubron/kg) doses in 57 conscious volunteers and 30 anesthetized surgical patients (Keipert, 1995). Oxygent can be considered a second-generation analog of Fluosol-DA (Table 10.3).
- An emulsion formulation of lipophilic prostaglandin E1 prodrug (AS-013) was evaluated in a clinical study with 10 patients with chronic peripheral aterial occlusive disease (PAOD). The stability of the prodrug was improved relative to the parent drug; the emulsion had acceptable efficacy, and no adverse effects were observed (Matsuo, 1998).

As indicated in Table 10.4, several studies have examined emulsions in decreasing thrombophlebitis and pain on injection of etomidate and diazepam (Von Dardel et al., 1983; Doenicke et al., 1990; Kulka et al., 1993). Intratumoral injection of a bleomycin emulsion has been used in treatment of cystic hygroma and lymphangioma in 27 patients with satisfactory results (Tanigawa et al., 1987).

TOCOSOL® Paclitaxel is a tocopherol emulsion formulation of paclitaxel currently in Phase III clinical trial for the treatment of cancers (Constantinides et al., 2004). The tocopherol-based paclitaxel formulation is prepared by dissolving 10 mg/mL paclitaxel in vitamin E and homogenizing with water and surfactants consisting of TPGS and Poloxamer 407 to yield an emulsion with mean particle size of approximately 100 nm. The use of tocopherol reduces the severe adverse effects related to the use of Cremophor EL in Taxol® (paclitaxel, Bristol-Myers Squibb). The tocopherol-based paclitaxel formulation can be easily administered to patients in a short 15-min infusion compared to 3-hr infusion required by Taxol. Antitumor activity of the formulation has been demonstrated clinically in bladder, ovarian, and non-small cell lung cancers (Hanauske et al., 2005). Paclitaxel is currently marketed as either a solubilized formulation containing polyoxyl 35 castor oil (Cremophor EL) and ethanol, or as a nanosuspension formulation (Abraxane®) containing human albumin.

An emulsion composed of MCTs with 2% propofol is being developed (Insoluble Drug Delivery-Microdroplet, IDD-D™) as an alternative to the 1% propofol emulsions based on LCTs (e.g., Diprivan) to avoid elevated triglyceride levels normally seen with Diprivan. In a Phase I clinical study, the 2% propofol IDD-D emulsion had similar propofol plasma concentrations, anesthesia induction times, and anesthesia emergence times to Diprivan. Since MCTs are metabolized more rapidly than LCTs, and since the oil content of the IDD-D was lower than that of Diprivan (4% vs. 10%), it was concluded that the MCT-based emulsion could avoid the hyperlipidemic effect and bacterial growth common for the LCT-based emulsions (Ward et al., 2002).

A Phase I clinical study was carried out in four ovarian cancer patients to exploit the drug targeting ability of cholesterol-rich emulsions to LDL receptors of tumor cells. Uptake of [^{3}H] etoposide oleate and [14C] cholesterol oleate were 4.1 and 4.9 times, respectively, greater than that in contralateral normal ovaries. This indicates that most of the etoposide is retained in the emulsion before its internalization by the tumor cells and shows the ability of the cholesterol-rich emulsions to concentrate in ovarian carcinomas (Azevedo et al., 2005).

CHALLENGES WITH EMULSION FORMULATIONS FOR DRUG SOLUBILIZATION AND DELIVERY

PHYSICAL STABILITY

As mentioned earlier, physical stability of an emulsion is perhaps one of the most important characteristics, which governs its commercial success. Being a heterogeneous system, and thermodynamically unstable, this pharmaceutical dosage form has a significantly higher tendency to lose its physical stability than other dosage forms. The assessment of physical stability of disperse systems, including emulsions, is important to allow rejection of unacceptable formulations, provides a basis to estimate long-term stability and expiration dates, allows understanding of mechanism(s) of instability, and provides a basis for setting specifications.

Physical instability of emulsions usually begins with creaming, that is, slow floatation of lipid droplets on more dense aqueous phase, which is usually reversible by shaking. This leads to flocculation and coalescence, that is, aggregation of lipid droplets, which is not reversible by mere agitation. The next stage is creaming of coalesced droplets, which ultimately results in separation of oil and aqueous phases. Owing to this thermodynamic instability, almost all emulsions exhibit increase in droplet size on storage. The extent of this process depends on the characteristics of formulation and its storage condition (Figure 10.5). Whereas an optimized emulsion formulation may undergo limited change in particle size, a poorly formulated emulsion has a large probability of particle coalescence and irreversible phase separation in a short time. In fact, wherever possible, particle coalescence in emulsion should be minimized as it is known to affect the rate of oral drug absorption and perhaps the efficacy of delivered drug (Toguchi et al., 1990).

Some of the factors that affect the physical stability of emulsions include the type and concentration of surfactant used to stabilize the emulsion, the phase volume ratio (i.e., ratio of oil to aqueous phase), droplet size, compatibility of drug and excipients with the emulsion, and storage condition of the emulsion.

Use of the appropriate emulsifying agent improves the physical stability of an emulsion by one or more of the following mechanisms: reducing interfacial tension, preventing coalescence (by the emulsifying agent being adsorbed around the droplets), imparting electrical potential on the droplets (which favors their repulsion), and/or increasing viscosity (which minimizes droplet interaction). Whereas an inadequate concentration of surfactant will do little to prevent coalescence, undue increase in its concentration often leads to problems like increased drug instability and difficulty in administration. Excess surfactant molecules will tend to self-associate, forming micellar or lamellar structures, which may compromise the effectiveness of the emulsion.

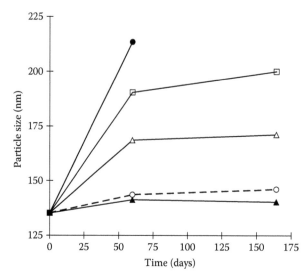

FIGURE 10.5 Effect of storage temperature on the change in particle size of clarithromycin emulsion over 165 days. The initial pH of the emulsion was 7.5. Key: (▲) 5°C; (O) 30°C; (△) 40°C; (□) 50°C; and (●) 60°C. (Adapted from Lovell, M.W. et al., *Int. J. Pharm.*, 118, 47–54, 1995. With permission.)

In general, the reduction in the concentration of dispersed phase increases the physical stability of emulsions. Lower dispersed phase concentration translates to a lower number of specific size droplets per unit volume of emulsion. This in turn reduces the degree of droplet interaction, coalescence, and hence phase separation. In general, the dispersed phase concentrations of <40% by volume of total emulsion are acceptable, and <20% desirable.

The compatibility of drug and excipients with emulsion components is important. The chemical properties as well as the amount of excipients can affect their physical stability. For example, increase in drug concentration in the oil phase may seem advantageous from the standpoint of being able to use smaller processing vessels, reduction in dose volume and reduction in the size of packaging commodities; however, increase in drug concentration beyond a certain level may lead to drug precipitation in the surrounding aqueous environment. Hence, the use of counterions to aid dissolution of drug in the oil phase could be evaluated from the standpoint of improving physical stability. Extemporaneous addition of drug to emulsions is also known to induce physical instability (Collins-Gold et al., 1990).

Sudden changes in the storage condition of an emulsion is usually detrimental to its physical stability. Whereas slight changes in temperature may be acceptable, large changes in temperature may cause phase inversion, that is, conversion from o/w to w/o and vice versa. The temperature at which this process occurs is called the phase inversion temperature. Usually, emulsions should be stored at least 20°C below the phase inversion temperature (Attwood and Florence, 1985).

CHEMICAL STABILITY

Once good physical stability of an emulsion is insured, its commercialization mandates chemical stability of the incorporated drug and other essential components for at least 18 months. Key factors that affect the chemical stability of pharmaceutical emulsions include drug stability in oil, drug stability in aqueous media, drug concentration in oil and emulsion, phase volume ratio, droplet size, presence of excipients, and presence of air and/or peroxide radicals. As mentioned earlier, choice of appropriate antioxidant is important.

Knowledge of the stability of a drug in different pharmaceutically approved oils and aqueous media is usually helpful in selecting appropriate formulation ingredients. Differences in the fatty acid composition of various oils can often contribute to different degrees of drug instability. Information on the relative stability of a drug in oil versus aqueous media may help make a decision if an emulsion is the preferred dosage form for drug delivery. Implicitly, an emulsion formulation can be developed only if the drug is stable in the oil selected for the emulsion.

Frequently, the hydrophobic environment of the emulsion droplet will retard hydrolysis of susceptible bonds in the drug molecule, gaining a stability advantage over aqueous formulations. For example, formulation of an antineoplastic drug NSC 278214 in a Liposyn or Intralipid emulsion rendered the drug about 100-fold more stable than in simple aqueous solution (El Sayed and Repta, 1983). Similar results have been reported by several other workers (Dietz et al., 1988; Paborji et al., 1988; Pathak et al., 1990; Oh et al., 1991). In this situation where the drug is more stable in oil than aqueous media, use of a higher fraction of oil may be advantageous, which translates to a lower drug concentration in oil. This may also improve the physical stability of the formulation, particularly if the drug concentration in oil is close to its solubility limit.

The role of droplet size on drug stability stems from the correlation between droplet size and surface area, and between surface area of droplets and exposure of drug to the aqueous media. If the drug is relatively insensitive to aqueous media, this may not be a major issue; however, for the converse situation, development of emulsions with relatively coarser droplet size may offer improved drug stability. Nonetheless, this should be balanced with physical stability of the emulsion as well as the efficiency of drug absorption after oral administration (Toguchi et al., 1990).

In other cases, however, the presence of certain emulsion components may be problematic for drug stability. In particular, lipid hydroperoxides present in the original lipid and/or surfactant components may destabilize drugs susceptible to oxidative degradation. For example, an anti-HIV drug NSC 629243 containing a thiocarbamate group was oxidatively degraded when formulated in an emulsion owing to the presence of peroxides in the oil. The degradation t_{90} was found to vary from less than 1 to more than 100 days depending on the age and supplier of the oil (Strickley and Anderson, 1993). Whereas peroxides may not directly interact with drugs, they serve as initiators of the oxidation process. Too low a drug concentration in oil phase may also lead to undesirable levels of drug degradation in the emulsion owing to peroxide triggered oxidation. Hence, emulsion formulations may require addition of oil-soluble antioxidants such as thioglycolic acid (Figure 10.6) (Strickley and Anderson, 1993). If the drug is sensitive to both hydrolytic (aqueous phase) and oxidative (lipid phase) processes, such factors as drug concentration, phase ratio and dose volume may have to be carefully balanced to achieve an optimum formulation.

The extent of pH reduction of emulsions owing to hydrolytic formation of fatty acids depends on the formulation and its storage condition. As can be anticipated, higher storage temperatures will increase the rate of hydrolysis and lead to a greater reduction in pH. While the rate of hydrolysis is generally low at ambient conditions, it could be sufficient to cause 0.05–0.08 units decrease in pH per month (Figure 10.7; Lovell et al., 1995). If the incorporated drug is unusually sensitive to pH changes, the hydrolysis of emulsion should be carefully monitored and, if necessary, controlled by addition of buffer or sodium hydroxide to the initial preparation.

Determination of drug potency in the presence of other emulsion components may require development of special analytical techniques; for example, oils may interfere with standard reverse phase HPLC assays, requiring extraction techniques or the development of normal phase assays. Similarly, bioassays may give erroneous results when the drug is presented in an emulsion form. Hence, adequate controls and/or extraction techniques must be developed to give reliable values from the bioassay.

The assessment of the shelf life (both chemical and physical stability) of an emulsion formulation is always a complex issue. Often, the data collected using accelerated conditions does not provide a good estimate of shelf life because the physical stability of an emulsion may change dramatically with changes in temperature. This alters the relative solubility, partitioning and interaction of drug within the two phases of the emulsion. Sometimes, this can alter the mechanism(s) governing the loss of drug over time. For example, the real-time analysis of clarithromycin o/w emulsion after

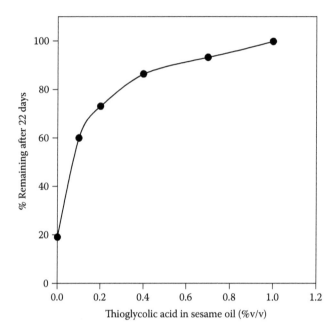

FIGURE 10.6 Effect of thioglycolic acid on the stability of *O*-alkyl *N*-aryl-thiocarbamate in sesame oil at 50°C. (Adapted from Strickley, R.G. and Anderson, B.D., *Pharm. Res.*, 10, 1076–1082, 1993. With permission.)

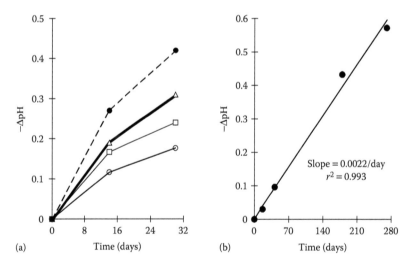

FIGURE 10.7 (a) Effect of initial pH of clarithromycin emulsion on its pH reduction (ΔpH) as a function of time at 40°C. Key: (○) pH 6.5; (□) pH 7.0; (Δ) pH 7.5; and (●) pH 8.0. (b) Effect of long-term storage of clarithromycin emulsion on its pH reduction (−ΔpH) at 30°C. The initial pH was 7.5. (Adapted from Lovell, M.W. et al., *Int. J. Pharm.*, 118, 47–54, 1995. With permission.)

1 year at 5°C indicated the presence of 90%–101% drug; however, the shelf life of this emulsion at 5°C, projected using the data collected at 40°C–60°C, was found to be much lower than that actually monitored at 5°C and did not follow Arrhenius kinetics (Lovell et al., 1995). Similar complications in the assessment of shelf life of emulsion formulations has also been reported by other workers (Pathak et al., 1990).

Dose Volume

As mentioned earlier, the use of emulsions as a dosage form stems from the fact that drugs can be solubilized in oils. However, depending on the dose of drug, intrinsic solubility of drug in oil, physical stability, and chemical stability, an emulsion with limited drug concentration may not be commercially viable especially when an emulsion formulation is intended for subcutaneous (SC) or intramuscular (IM) administration. Ideally, drug concentration in an emulsion will be in the range that is practical for dosing (e.g., dosing volume ≤1 mL for SC or ≤5 mL for IM administration). However, for large dose compounds, emulsion formulation may require administration of inconveniently large volumes. Hence, this issue should be kept in mind during the development of this dosage form. For drugs requiring IV dosing, the administration volume is generally a less critical issue.

Toxicity

If an emulsion formulation utilizes excipients within limits approved for human use, then the toxicity of the formulation is unlikely to be higher than that of the drug. However, if unapproved excipients are being considered (e.g., to increase drug solubility) or if excipients are used in quantities much larger than those approved for human use, extensive toxicity testing is required before investigation in humans, and large regulatory hurdles must be overcome in partnership with suppliers of the proposed excipients. A recent example of approval of a new excipient for use in parenteral emulsions is provided by Solutol HS-15 (polyoxythylene-660-hydroxystearate) which showed improved safety compared to Cremophor EL (Velagaleti and Ku, 2010). On the other hand, there may be cases where formulating in an emulsion will decrease toxicity (e.g., cyclosporine and amphotericin B) (Table 10.4).

FORMULATION AND PROCESS OPTIMIZATION

Optimization of an emulsion formulation is perhaps one of the most challenging aspects of its development program. Promising results with preliminary formulations often warrant improvements, for example, with regard to stability, toxicity, and processing time. However, once a parameter is altered to meet an intended goal, it often leads to loss of some other desirable characteristic. For example, an increase in drug concentration to reduce dose volume may induce physical instability (Davis, 1995). Alternatively, an increase in the oil fraction to aid drug solubilization and/or reduce pain or irritation on injection may also induce physical instability. The complexity of this issue can be appreciated by reviewing the effects of changing some obvious variables as listed in Table 10.6. However, it does not imply that emulsion formulations cannot be optimized. In fact, if formulation optimization is necessary for the life of the development program, it should be pursued using statistical experimental protocols. If chemical stability of drug is critical, then the conclusions regarding reformulated or optimized formulations should be made using the real-time data.

It should be realized that if emulsions are used strictly to solubilize drug, the use of this formulation approach brings the following challenges:

1. Their use as a delivery system may change the biodistribution of parenterally administered drug. Emulsion systems have indeed been investigated for preferential drug localization and altered *in vivo* distribution after parenteral administration (see Table 10.4). The kinetics of efflux from the emulsion droplets and binding to plasma proteins versus uptake by the reticuloendothelial systems should be understood.
2. Their use as an injectable warrants assurance of product sterility. Whereas the Food and Drug Administration (FDA)-preferred heat-sterilization process is acceptable for total parenteral nutritional (TPN) emulsions, it could affect chemical as well as physical stability of

TABLE 10.6

Probable Effect of Different Variables on the Properties of Emulsion Formulation

Variable	Probable Effect
Increase in drug concentration	(a) Physical/chemical instability
	(b) Pain/irritation upon injection
Increase in oil concentration	(a) Increase in particle size and viscosity
	(b) Difficulty in filter sterilization
	(c) Physical/chemical instability
	(d) Reduced pain/irritation upon injection
Presence of excipients	(a) Altered physical/chemical stability
	(b) Altered toxicity
Increase in surfactant concentration	(a) Decrease in particle size
	(b) Improved physical stability
	(c) Increase in pain/irritation upon injection
	(d) Increase in non-emulsion components (viz., micelles, liposomes)
Increase in formulation pH	(a) Improved physical stability
	(b) Alteration in drug solubility in oil
	(c) Alteration in chemical stability
	(d) Increased container/closure incompatibility
Increase in processing temperature	(a) Decrease in particle size and viscosity
	(b) Improved drug solubility in oil
	(c) Increased probability of drug degradation
	(d) Increased likelihood of drug precipitation upon cooling
Increase in processing pressure	(a) Narrower particle size distribution
	(b) Increased probability of drug degradation

emulsions containing therapeutic agents. Recently, data supporting the filter sterilization of emulsions have been published.

3. The manufacturing process of emulsions is apparently more cumbersome and time-consuming than that for the conventional formulations. This adds to the cost of the product.
4. To maintain good physical and chemical stability, emulsion formulations may warrant storage at 5°C. This limits the manufacturing volume as well as product storage in distribution centers.

At times, extemporaneous addition of drug to a ready-to-use emulsion (e.g., Liposyn), may not be the preferred way of developing formulations. This can be explained in view of the following reasons:

1. It may require use of an organic solvent. For example, drug is often solubilized in pure cosolvent (e.g., ethanol, dimethylsulfoxide, dimethylacetamide, or N-methyl pyrrolidone) which is then added to the emulsion. As mentioned earlier, this bears toxicological/safety concerns.
2. Extemporaneous addition of drug, alone and/or in solvent, has the tendency to damage emulsion droplets, sometimes resulting in permanent loss of its physical stability.
3. Incomplete solubilization or re-precipitation of extemporaneously added drug cannot be easily ruled out.
4. This process has a tendency to compromise the sterility of the emulsion.

Hence, due to the above-mentioned considerations, *de novo* emulsification of oil containing drug is generally the method of choice for the preparation of drug emulsions wherever possible.

FUTURE PERSPECTIVES

As can be appreciated from the review of the literature covered in this chapter, emulsion formulations offer an appealing alternative for the administration of water-insoluble compounds. From the development scientists' standpoint, drug dose and physical stability of formulation in the presence of drug represent the two most challenging aspects of this drug delivery technology. However, these complications are usually compensated by the effectiveness of emulsion formulations for increased drug solubilization, improved chemical stability, and reduced toxicity. For parenteral applications, an additional benefit may be improved patient acceptance arising from reduced adverse effects (such as pain or irritation).

Owing to the growing number of water-insoluble drugs coming from drug discovery programs, the scope of pharmaceutical emulsions is likely to grow in the future. This is likely to stimulate development of newer *oil-like* synthetic liquids and emulsifying agents. In addition, the industry will continue to improve techniques for efficient commercial production of these formulations. Overall, these changes will result in greater choices for the development of emulsion formulations of difficult compounds, with perhaps fewer drug solubility and physical stability problems currently encountered owing to limited choice of excipients. Another promising avenue for future development is the use of emulsions for targeted drug delivery, as demonstrated by the potential of cholesterol-rich emulsions to be taken up by LDL receptors of cancer cells (Azevedo et al., 2005). Monoclonal antibodies and other targeting moieties can also be explored. Targeting to folate receptors by a folate-linked microemulsion led to greater uptake of aclacinomycin A into tumors (Shiokawa et al., 2005). Further investigation of long-circulating emulsions derivatized by PEG (Liu and Liu, 1995) or sphingomyelin (Takino et al., 1994) is also warranted to extend the utility of emulsions for drug delivery.

Table of Registered Trademarks

Name	Company
Intralipid®; Vitalipid®	Kabi Vitrum, Stockholm, Sweden
Valium®	Roche Laboratories Inc., Nutley, New Jersey, USA
Diprivan®	Astra Zeneca, Wilmington Delaware, USA
Taxol®; Fungizone®	Bristol-Myers Squibb, Princeton, New Jersey, USA
Liposyn®	Hospira, Lake Forest, Illinois, USA
Gaulin®; Rannie®	Invensys APV, Denmark
Microfluidizer®	Microfluidics, Newton Massachusetts, USA
Five Star®	Five Star Technologies, Cleveland, Ohio, USA
Captex®	Abitec Corp, Columbus, Ohio, USA
Cremophor®; Solutol®; Pluronic®	BASF, Mount Olive, New Jersey, USA
Imwitor®; Miglyol®	Cremer Oleo GMBH, Hamburg Germany, USA
SPAN®; Tween®	Uniqema North America Inc., Chicago, Illinois, USA
Neobee®	Stepan Company, Northfield, Illinois, USA
Sandimmune®	Novartis Pharmaceuticals Corporation, East Hanover, New Jersey, USA
Phospholipon®	Lipoid GMBH, Ludwigshafen, Germany
Cleviprex®	The Medicines Company, Parsippany, New Jersey, USA
Ciclomulsion®	NeuroVive Pharmaceutical AB, Lund, Sweden

REFERENCES

Handbook of Pharmaceutical Excipients 1994. Wade, A., and P. J. Weller (Eds.), Pharmaceutical Press (London), pp. 352, 372, 377, 475.

Physicians Desk Reference 1995. Sifton, D. W. (Ed.), Medical Economics Co., Montvale, NJ, pp. 1019, 2436, 2618.

Physicians Desk Reference 1999. the PDR staff (Ed.), Medical Economics Co., Montvale, NJ, pp. 2063, 2079, 3411.

Abuja, P. M. and R. Albertini. 2001. Methods for monitoring oxidative stress, lipid peroxidation and oxidation resistance of lipoproteins. *Clin. Chim. Acta*, 306: 1–17.

Akkar, A., P. Namsolleck, M. Blaut, and R. H. Muller. 2004. Solubilizing poorly soluble antimycotic agents by emulsification via a solvent-free process. *AAPS Pharm Sci Tech.*, 5(1): 159–164.

Alford, K. M., M. A. Gales, B. J. Gales, and V. Ramgopal. 1994. Acute renal failure with amphotericin b in 20% lipid emulsion. *ASHP Midyear Clin. Meeting*, 29: 415.

Allen, T. M., C. Hansen, and J. Rutledge. 1989. Liposomes with prolonged circulation times: Factors affecting uptake by reticuloendothelial and other tissues. *Biochim. Biophys. Acta*, 981: 27–35.

Ames, M. M. and J. S. Kovach. 1982. Parenteral formulation of hexamethylmelamine potentially suitable for use in man. *Cancer Treat. Rep.*, 66: 1579–1581.

Antolovich, M., P. D. Prenzler, E. Patsalides, S. McDonald, and K. Robards. 2002. Methods for testing anti-oxidant activity. *Analyst*, 127: 183–198.

Arakane, K., K. Hayashi, N. Naito, T. Nagano, and M. Hirobe. 1995. pH lowering in liposomal dispersions induced by phospholipid peroxidation. *Chem. Pharm. Bull.*, 43: 1755–1758.

Attwood, D. and A. T. Florence. 1985. *Surfactant Systems*. Chapman & Hall, New York, pp. 469–568.

Azevedo, C. H. M., J. P. Carvalho, C. J. Valduga, and R. C. Maranhão. 2005. Plasma kinetics and uptake by the tumor of a cholesterol-rich microemulsion (LDE) associated to etoposide oleate in patient with ovarian carcinoma. *Gynecol. Oncol.*, 97: 178–182.

Behan, M., D. O'Connell, R. F. Mattrey, and D. N. Carney. 1993. Perfluorooctylbromide as a contrast agent for CT and sonography: Preliminary clinical results. *Am. J. Roentgenol.*, 160: 399–405.

Benita, S., D. Friedman, and M. Weinstock. 1986. Physostigmine emulsion: A new injectable controlled release delivery system. *Int. J. Pharm.*, 30: 47–55.

Biber, B., G. Johannesson, O. Lennander, J. Martner, H. Sonander, and O. Werner. 1984. Intravenous infusion of halothane dissolved in fat. Hemodynamic effects in dogs. *Acta Anesthesiol. Scand.*, 28: 385–389.

Caillot, D., P. Chavanet, O. Casasnovas, E. Solary, G. Zanetta, M. Buisson, O. Wagner, B. Cuisenier, A. Bonnin, P. Camerlynck, et al. 1992. Clinical evaluation of a new lipid-based delivery system for intravenous administration of amphotericin B. *Eur. J. Clin. Microbiol. Infect. Dis.*, 11: 722–725.

Cannon, J. B. 2007. Chemical and physical stability considerations for lipid-based drug formulations. *Amer. Pharm. Rev.*, 10: 132–138.

Carl, P., S. Hogskilde, J. W. Nielsen, M. B. Sorensen, M. Lindholm, B. Karlen, and T. Backstrom. 1990. Pregnanolone emulsion. A preliminary pharmacokinetic and pharmacodynamic study of a new intravenous anaesthetic agent. *Anaesthesia*, 45: 189–197.

Cave, G., M. Harvey, J. Willers, D. Uncles, T. Meek, J. Picard, and G. J. Weinberg. 2014. LIPAEMIC report: Results of clinical use of intravenous lipid emulsion in drug toxicity reported to an online lipid registry. *Med Toxicol.*, 10: 133–142.

Chansri, N., S. Kawakami, F. Yamashita, and M. Hashida. 2006. Inhibition of liver metastasis by all-trans retinoic acid incorporated into o/w emulsions in mice. *Int. J. Pharm.*, 321: 42–49.

Chavanet, P. Y., I. Garry, N. Charlier, D. Caillot, J. P. Kisterman, M. D'Athis, and H. Portier. 1992. Trial of glucose versus fat emulsion in preparation of amphotericin for use in HIV infected patients with candidiasis. *Brit. Med. J.*, 305: 921–925.

Chiang, C.-C., M. Longer, P. Tyle, D. Fessler, and B. Shetty. 1995. Formulation development of an oral dosage form for an HIV protease inhibitor, AG1284. *Int. J. Pharm.*, 117: 197–207.

Christie, W. W. and X. Han. 2010. *Lipid Analysis: Isolation, Separation, Identification and Lipidomic Analysis*, Fourth Edition (Oily Press Lipid Library Series). Woodhead Publishing, Cambridge, UK, p. 4.

Clark, LA., J. Beyer, and A. Graudins. 2014. An in vitro analysis of the effects of intravenous lipid emulsion on free and total local anaesthetic concentrations in human blood and plasma. *Crit. Care Res. Pract.*, 2014: 7.

Collins-Gold, L. C., R. T. Lyons, and L. C. Bartholow. 1990. Parenteral emulsions for drug delivery. *Adv. Drug Del. Rev.*, 5: 189–208.

Constantinides, P. P., A. Tustian, and D. R. Kessler, 2004. Tocol emulsion for drug solubilization and parenteral delivery. *Adv. Drug Del. Rev.*, 56: 1243–1255.

Cui, G., L. Wang, P. J. Davis, M. Kara, and H. Liu. 2006. Preparation and physical characterization of a novel marine oil emulsion as a potential new formulation vehicle for lipid soluble drugs. *Int. J. Pharm.*, 325: 180–185.

Davis, S. S. 1995. Drug delivery applications of multiphase systems. Multiphase systems for oral and parenteral drug delivery: Physical and biopharmaceutical aspects. *37th Annual International Industrial Pharmaceuticals R&D Conference*, Merrimac, WI, June 5–9.

Davis, S. S., C. Washington, P. West, L. Illum, G. Liversidge, L. Sternson, and R. Kirsch. 1987. Lipid emulsions as drug delivery systems. *Ann. NY Acad. Sci.*, 507: 75–88.

Derjaguin, B. V. and L. D. Landau. 1941. Theory of the stability of strongly lyophobic sols and of the adhesion of strongly charged particles in solutions of electrolytes. *Acta Physicochim.*, 14: 633–662.

Dietz, N. J., P. J. Cascella, J. E. Houglum, G. S. Chappell, and R. M. Sieve. 1988. Phenobarbital stability in different dosage forms: Alternatives for elixirs. *Pharm. Res.*, 5: 803–805.

Doenicke, A., A. Kugler, N. Vollmann, H. Suttmann, and K. Taeger, 1990. Etomidate using a new solubilizer. Experimental clinical studies on venous tolerance and bioavailability. *Anaesthesist*, 39: 475–480.

Dorlhiac-Llacer, P. E., M. V. Marquezini, O. Toffoletto, R. C. G. Carneiro, R. C. Maranhão, and D. A. F. Chamone. 2001. *In vitro* cytotoxicity of the LDE: Daunorubicin complex in acute myelogenous leukemia blast cells. *Braz. J. Med. Biol. Res.*, 34: 1257–1263.

Dundee, J. W. and R. S. J. Clarke. 1989. Propofol. *Eur. J. Anaesthesiol.*, 6: 5–22.

Ehinger, K. H., M. J. Hansson, F. Sjövall, and E. Elmér. 2013. Bioequivalence and tolerability assessment of a novel intravenous ciclosporin lipid emulsion compared to branded ciclosporin in Cremophor EL ®. *Clin Drug Investig.*, 33: 25–34.

El Sayed, A. A. A. and A. J. Repta. 1983. Solubilization and stabilization of an investigational antineoplastic drug (NSC-278214) in an intravenous formulation using an emulsion vehicle. *Int. J. Pharm.*, 13: 303–312.

Erickson, A. L., J. R. DeGrado, and J. R. Fanikos, 2010. Clevidipine: A short-acting intravenous dihydropyridine calcium channel blocker for the management of hypertension. *Pharmacotherapy*, 30: 515–528.

Fee, J. P. H., J. W. Dundee, P. S. Collier, and E. McClean. 1984. Bioavailability of intravenous diazepam. *Lancet*, 2: 813.

Floyd, A. G. 1999. Top ten considerations in the development of parenteral emulsions. *Pharm. Sci. Technol. Today*, 2: 134–143.

Forster, D., C. Washington, and S. S. Davis. 1988. Toxicity of solubilized and colloidal amphotericin B formulations to human erythrocytes. *J. Pharm. Pharmacol.*, 40: 325–328.

Fukushima, S., S. Kishimoto, Y. Takeuchi, and M. Fushima. 2000. Preparation and evaluation of o/w type emulsions containing antitumor prostaglandin. *Adv. Drug Del. Rev.*, 45: 65–75.

Gao, K., J. Sun, K. Liu, X. Liu, and Z. He, 2008. Preparation and characterization of a submicron lipid emulsion of docetaxel: Submicron lipid emulsion of docetaxel. *Drug Dev. Ind. Pharm.*, 34: 1227–1237.

Gasco, M. R., F. Pattarino, and F. Lattanzi. 1990. Long-acting delivery systems for peptides: Reduced plasma testosterone levels in male rats after a single injection. *Int. J. Pharm.*, 62: 119–123.

Gates, C. and R. J. Pinney, 1993. Amphotericin B and its delivery by liposomal and lipid formulations. *J. Clin. Pharm. Ther.*, 18: 147–153.

Gray, H. S. J., B. L. Holt, D. K. Whitaker, and P. Eadsforth, 1992. Preliminary study of a pregnanolone emulsion (KABI 2213) for i.v. induction of general anaesthesia. *Br. J. Anaesth.*, 68: 272–276.

Griffin, W. C. 1949. Classification of surface active agents by HLB. *J. Soc. Cosmetic Chem.*, 1: 311–326.

Halbaut, L., C. Barbe, M. Aroztegui, and C. de la Torre. 1997. Oxidative stability of semi-solid excipient mixtures with corn oil and its implication in the degradation of vitamin A. *Int. J. Pharm.*, 147: 31–40.

Hanauske, A. R., L. Goedhals, H. Gelderblom, Y. Lee, A. Awada, J. B. Vermorken, C. Bolling, A. Rui-Garcia, J. Pratt, and M. B. Stewart. 2005. Tocosol® paclitaxel and Cremophor EL® -paclitaxel: The pharmacokinetic comparison shows that a new paclitaxel formulation leads to increased drug exposure. *Eur. J. Cancer Suppl.*, 3: 427.

Handa, T., Y. Eguchi, and K. Miyajima. 1994. Effects of cholesterol and cholesteryl oleate on lipolysis and liver uptake of triglycerides/phosphatidylcholine emulsions in rats. *Pharm. Res.*, 11: 1283–1287.

Hanna, G., D. Saewert, J. Shorr, K. Flaim, P. Leese, M. Kopperman, and G. Wolf. 1994. Preclinical and clinical studies on lymph node imaging using perflubron emulsion. *Artif. Cells Blood Substit. Immobil. Biotechnol.*, 22: 1429–1439.

Hansrani, P. K., S. S. Davis, and M. J. Groves, 1983. The preparation and properties of sterile intravenous emulsions. *J. Parent. Sci. Technol.*, 37: 145–150.

Helson, L. A. 1984. Phase I study of vitamin E and neuroblastoma. In *Vitamins, Nutrition and Cancer*, Prasa, L., (Ed.), Krager, Basel, Switzerland, pp. 274–281.

Hering, W., R. Schlecht, G. Geisslinger, G. Biburger, M. Dinkel, K. Brune, and E. Ruegheimer. 1995. EEG analysis and pharmacodynamic modelling after intravenous bolus injection of eltanolone (pregnanolone). *Eur. J. Anaesthesiol.*, 12: 407–415.

Herman, C. J. and M. J. Groves. 1992. Hydrolysis kinetics of phospholipids in thermally stressed intravenous lipid emulsion formulations. *J. Pharm. Pharmacol.*, 44: 539–542.

Herman, C. J. and M. J. Groves, 1993. The influence of free fatty acid formation on the pH of phospholipid–Stabilized triglyceride emulsions. *Pharm. Res.*, 10: 774–776.

Hippalgaonkar, K., S. Majumdar, and V. Kansara. 2010. Injectable lipid emulsions—advancements, opportunities and challenges. *AAPS Pharm. Sci. Tech.*, 11: 1526–1540.

Hogskilde, S., J. W. Nielsen, P. Carl, and M. Sorenson, 1987a. Pregnanolone emulsion. *Anaesthesia*, 42: 586–590.

Hogskilde, S., J. Wagner, P. Carl, and M. Sorenson. 1987b. Anesthetic properties of pregnanolone emulsion. *Anaesthesia*, 42: 1045–1050.

Hwang, S. R., S. J. Lim, J. S. Park, and C. K. Kim. 2004. Phospholipid-based microemulsion formulation of all-trans-retinoic acid for parenteral administration. *Int. J. Pharm.*, 276: 175–183.

Ivancev, K., A. Lunderquist, A. Isaksson, P. Hochbergs, and A. Wretlind, 1989 Clinical trials with a new iodinated lipid emulsion for computed tomography of the liver. *Acta Radiol.*, 30: 449–457.

Jing, X., L. Deng, B. Gao, L. Xiao, Y. Zhang, X. Ke, J. Lian, Q. Zhao, L. Ma, J. Yao, and J. Chen. 2014. A novel polyethylene glycol mediated lipid nanoemulsion as drug delivery carrier for paclitaxel. *Nanomedicine*, 10: 371–380.

Johannesson, G., P. Alm, B. Biber, O. Lennander, and O. Werner. 1984. Halothane dissolved in fat as intravenous anesthetic to rats. *Acta Anesthesiol. Scand.*, 28: 381–384.

Jumaa, M. and B. W. Muller, 1998. The stabilization of parenteral fat emulsion using non-ionic ABA copolymer surfactant. *Int. J. Pharm.*, 174: 29–37.

Jumaa, M. and B. W. Müller, 2001. Development of a novel parenteral formulation for tetrazepam using a lipid emulsion. *Drug Dev. Ind. Pharm.*, 27: 1115–1121.

Junping, W., K. Takayama, T. Nagai, and Y. Maitani, 2003. Pharmacokinetics and antitumor effects of vincristine carried by microemulsions composed of PEG-lipid, oleic acid, vitamin E and cholesterol. *Int. J. Pharm.*, 251: 13–21.

Kam, E., M. S. Abdul-Latif, and A. McCluskey. 2004. Comparison of propofol-lipuro with propofol mixed with lidocaine 10 mg on propofol injection pain. *Anesthesia*, 59: 1167–1169.

Kawakami, S., F. Yamashita, and M. Hashida, 2000. Disposition characteristics of emulsions and incorporated drugs after systemic or local injection. *Adv. Drug Del. Rev.*, 45: 77–88.

Keipert, P. E. 1995. Use of Oxygent (R), a perfluorochemical-based oxygen carrier, as an alternative to intraoperative blood transfusion. *Artif. Cells, Blood Substit., Immobil. Biotechnol.*, 23: 381–394.

Kirsch, R. L. and L. J. Ravin. 1987. Polyene antibiotic emulsion formulation. *US Patent* 4,707,470.

Kulka, P. J., F. Bremer, and J. Schuttler. 1993. Anesthesia induction using etomidate in a lipid emulsion (Germany). *Anaesthesist*, 42: 205–209.

Kurihara, A., Y. Shibayama, A. Mizota, A. Yasuno, M. Ikeada, and M. Hisaoka. 1996. Pharmacokinetics of highly lipophilic autitumor agent palmitoyl Rhizoxin incorporated in lipid emulsion in rats. *Biol. Pharm. Bull.*, 19: 252–258.

Lamb, K. A., C. Washington, S. S. Davis. and S. P. Denyer. 1991. Toxicity of amphotericin B emulsion to cultured canine kidney cell monolayers. *J. Pharm. Pharmacol.*, 43: 522–524.

Lang, J. K. and A. Vigo-Pelfrey. 1993. Quality control of liposomal lipids with special emphasis on peroxidation of phospholipids and cholesterol. *Chem. Phys. Lipids*, 64: 19–29.

Laubli, M. W. and P. A. Bruttel. 1986. Determination of the oxidative stability of fats and oils comparison between the active oxygen method and the rancimat method. *J. Am. Oil Chem. Soc.*, 63: 792–795.

Lee, M. -J., M. -H. Lee, and C. -K. Shim, 1995. Inverse targeting of drugs to reticuloendothelial system-rich organs by lipid microemulsion emulsified with poloxamer 338. *Int. J. Pharm.*, 113: 175–187.

Levy, M. Y., L. Langerman, S. Gottschalk-Sabag, and S. Benita, 1989. Side effect evaluation of a new diazepam formulation venous sequalae reduction following i.v. injection of diazepam emulsion in rabbits. *Pharm. Res.*, 6: 510–516.

Levy, M. Y., I. Polacheck, Y. Barenholz, and S. Benita. 1995. Efficacy evaluation of a novel submicron miconazole emulsion in a murine Cryptococcosis model. *Pharm. Res.*, 12: 223.

Li, X., Y. Mao, K. Li, T. Shi, H. Yao, J. Yao, and S. Wang, 2015. Pharmacokinetics and tissue distribution study in mice of triptolide loaded lipid emulsion and accumulation effect on pancreas. *Drug Deliv.*, 20: 1–11.

Li, Y., W. Jin, H. Yan, H. Liu, and C. Wang. 2013. Development of intravenous lipid emulsion of vinorelbine based on drug-phospholipid complex technique. *Int. J. Pharm.*, 454: 472–477.

Lidgate, D. M., R. C. Fu, N. E. Byars, L. C. Foster, and J. S. Felitman. 1989. Formulation of vaccine adjuvant muramyldipeptides. 3. Processing optimization, characterization, and bioactivity of an emulsion vehicle. *Pharm. Res.*, 6: 748–752.

Lidgate, D. M., T. Trattner, R. M. Shultz, and R. Maskiewicz 1992. Sterile filtration of a parenteral emulsion. *Pharm. Res.*, 9: 860–863.

Liu, F. and D. Liu. 1995. Long-circulating emulsions (oil-in-water) as carriers for lipophilic drugs. *Pharm. Res.*, 12: 1060–1064.

Lopez-Berestein, G. 1988. Liposomal amphotericin b in antimicrobial therapy. In: *Liposomes as Drug Carriers*, Gregoriadis, G. (Ed.), John Wiley & Sons, New York, p. 345.

Lovell, M. W., H. W. Johnson, and P. K. Gupta, 1995. Stability of a less-painful intravenous emulsion of clarithromycin. *Int. J. Pharm.*, 118: 47–54.

Lovell, M. W., H. W. Johnson, H. -W. Hui, J. B. Cannon, P. K. Gupta, and C. C. Hsu. 1994. Less-painful emulsion formulations for intravenous administration of clarithromycin. *Int. J. Pharm.*, 109: 45–57.

Lundberg, B. 1994. The solubilization of lipophilic derivatives of podophyllotoxins in sub-micron sized lipid emulsions and their cytotoxic activity against cancer cells in culture. *Int. J. Pharm.*, 109: 73–81.

Lundberg, B. B., V. Risovic, M. Ramaswamy, and K. M. Wasan, 2003. A lipophilic paclitaxel derivative incorporated in a lipid emulsion for parenteral administration. *J Contr. Release.*, 86: 93–100.

Ma, W. C., Q. Zhang, H. Li, C. A. Larregieu, N. Zhang, T. Chu, H. Jin, and S. J. Mao. 2013. Development of intravenous lipid emulsion of α-asarone with significantly improved safety and enhanced efficacy. *Int. J. Pharm.*, 450: 21–30.

Malcolmson, C. and M. J. Lawrence, 1993. Comparison of the incorporation of model steroids into non-ionic micellar and microemulsion systems. *J. Pharm. Pharmacol.*, 45: 141–143.

Mao, C., J. Wan, H. Chen, H. Xu, and X. Yang, 2010. The composition of oil phase modulates venous irritation of lipid emulsion-loaded diallyl trisulfide. *Drug Dev. Ind. Pharm.*, 36: 698–704.

Marín-Quintero, D., F. Fernández-Campos, A. C. Calpena-Campmany, M. J. Montes-López, B. Clares-Naveros, and A. Del Pozo-Carrascosa. 2013. Formulation design and optimization for the improvement of nystatin loaded lipid intravenous emulsion. *J. Pharm. Sci.*, 102: 4015–4023.

Matsuo, H. 1998. Preliminary evaluation of AS-013 (prodrug of prostaglandin E1) administration for chronic peripheral arterial occlusive disease. *Int. J. Angiol.*, 7: 22–24.

Minagawa, T., Y. Kohno, T. Suwa, and A. Tsuji. 1994. Entrapping efficiency of an oil-in-water emulsion containing isocarbacyclin methyl ester (TEI-9090) in dog and human Sera. *Pharm. Res.*, 11: 1677–1679.

Muller, R. H., J. S. Lucks, J. Herbort, and P. Couvreur. 1991. Improved treatment of liver metastasis by titanocene dichloride using an emulsion carrier. *Arch. Pharma.*, 324: P37.

Muller, R. H., S. Schmidt, I. Buttle, A. Akkar, J. Schmitt, and S. Bromer. 2004. SolEmuls—novel technology for formulation of i.v. emulsions with poorly soluble drugs. *Int. J. Pharm.*, 269: 293–302.

Muller, S. H., J. H. Diaz, and A. D. Kaye. 2015. Clinical applications of intravenous lipid emulsion therapy. *J. Anesth.*, 29: 920–926.

Nakamoto, Y., M. Fujiwara, T. Naguchi, T. Kimura, S. Muranishi, and H. Sezaki, 1975. Studies on pharmaceutical modification of anticancer drugs. I. Enhancement of lymphatic transport of mitomycin C by parenteral emulsion. *Chem. Pharm. Bull.*, 23: 2232–2238.

Naylor, H. C. and A. N. Burlingham. 1985. Pharmacokinetics of diazepam emulsion. *Lancet*, 1: 518–519.

Oh, I., S. -C. Chi, B. R. Vishnuvajjala, and B. D. Anderson, 1991. Stability and solubilization of oxathiin carboxanilide a novel anti-HIV agent. *Int. J. Pharm.*, 73: 23–32.

Paborji, M., C. M. Riley, and V. J. Stella, 1988. A novel use of Intralipid for the parenteral delivery of perilla ketone (NSC-348407), an investigational cytotoxic drug with a high affinity for plastic. *Int. J. Pharm.*, 42: 243–249.

Park, K. M. and C. K. Kim, 1999. Preparation and evaluation of flurbiprofen-loaded microemulsion for parenteral delivery. *Int. J. Pharm.*, 181: 173–179.

Pathak, Y. V., A. Rubinstein, and S. Benita. 1990. Enhanced stability of physostigmine salicylate in submicron o/w emulsion. *Int. J. Pharm.*, 65: 169–175.

Porter, N. A. 1984. Chemistry of lipid peroxidation. *Meth. Enzymol.*, 105: 273.

Prankerd, R.J. and Stella, V.J. 1990. The use of oil-in-water emulsions as a vehicle for parenteral administration. *J. Parent. Sci. Technol.*, 44: 139–149.

Prankerd, R. J., S. Frank, and V. J. Stella, 1988. Preliminary development and evaluation of a parenteral formulation of penclomedine (NSC-338720); 3,5-dichloro-2,4-dimethoxy-6-trichloromethylpyridine): A novel, practically water insoluble cytotoxic agent. *J. Parent. Sci. Technol.*, 42: 76–81.

Ramreddy, S., P. Kandadi, and K. Veerabrahma, 2012. Formulation and pharmacokinetics of diclofenac lipid nanoemulsions for parenteral application. *PDA J. Pharm. Sci. Technol.*, 66: 28–37.

Reddy, P. R. and V. Venkateswarlu, 2005. Pharmacokinetics and tissue distribution of etoposide delivered in long circulating parenteral emulsion. *J. Drug Target*, 13: 543–553.

Rodriguez, D. G., D. A. Maria, D. C. Fernandes, J. V. Claudete, R. D. Couto, O. C. M. Ibanez, and R. C. Maranhão, 2005. Improvement of paclitaxel therapeutic index by derivatization and association to a cholesterol-rich microemulsion: *In vitro* and *in vivo* studies. *Cancer Chemother. Pharmacol.*, 55: 565–576.

Santos-Magalhaes, N. S., G. Cave, M. Seiller, and S. Benita. 1991. The stability and *in vitro* release kinetics of a clofibride emulsion. *Int. J. Pharm.*, 76: 225–237.

Sarker, D. K. 2005. Engineering of nanoemulsions for drug delivery. *Cancer Drug Deliv.*, 2: 297–310.

Sevanian, A. and F. Ursini. 2000. Lipid peroxidation in membranes and low-density lipoproteins: Similarities and differences. *Free Rad. Biol. Med.*, 29: 306–311.

Sherman, P. 1983. Rheological properties of emulsions. In *Encyclopedia of Emulsion Technology*, P. Becher, (Ed.), vol. II, Marcel Dekker, New York, p. 405.

Shi, S., H. Chen, Y. Cui, and X. Tang, 2009. Formulation, stability and degradation kinetics of intravenous cinnarizine lipid emulsion. *Int. J. Pharm.*, 373: 147–155.

Shi, S., H. Chen, X. Lin, and X. Tang. 2010. Pharmacokinetics., tissue distribution and safety of cinnarizine delivered in lipid emulsion. *Int. J. Pharm.*, 383: 264–270.

Shiokawa, T., Y. Hattori, K. Kawano, Y. Ohguchi, H. Kawakami, K. Toma, and Y. Maitani. 2005. Effect of polyethylene glycol linker chain length of folate-linked microemulsions loading aclacinomycin A on targeting ability and antitumor effect in vitro and in vivo. *Clin. Cancer Res.*, 11: 2018–2025.

Sila-on, W., N. Vardhanabhuti, B. Ongpipattanakul, and P. Kulvanich. 2008. Influence of incorporation methods on partitioning behavior of lipophilic drugs into various phases of a parenteral lipid emulsion. *AAPS Pharm. Sci. Tech.*, 9: 684–692.

Stella, V. J. 2013. Chemical drug stability in lipids, modified lipids, and polyethylene oxide-containing formulations. *Pharm. Res.*, 30: 3018–3028.

Stella, V. J., K. Umprayn, and W. Waugh. 1988. Development of parenteral formulations of experimental cytotoxic agents. I. Rhizoxin (NSC-332598). *Int. J. Pharm.*, 43: 191–199.

Strickley, R. G. and B. D. Anderson. 1993. Solubilization and stabilization of an anti-HIV thiocarbamate, NSC 629243, for parenteral delivery, using extemporaneous emulsions. *Pharm. Res.*, 10: 1076–1082.

Sundar S., J. Chakravarty, D. Agarwal, A. Shah, N. Agrawal, and M. Rai. 2008. Safety of a preformulated amphotericin B lipid emulsion for the treatment of Indian Kalaazar. *Trop. Med. Int. Health.*, 13: 1208–1212.

Sundar, S., K. Pandey, C. P. Thakur, T. K. Jha, V. N. Das, N. Verma, C. S. Lal, D. Verma, S. Alam, and P. Das, 2014. Efficacy and safety of amphotericin B emulsion versus liposomal formulation in Indian patients with visceral leishmaniasis: A randomized, open-label study. *PLoS Negl. Trop. Dis.*, 8: e3169.

Suzuki, Y., Y. Masumitsu, K. Okudaira, and M. Hayashi, 2004. The effects of emulsifying agents on disposition of lipid soluble drugs included in fat emulsion. *Drug Metab. Pharmacokinet.*, 19: 62–67.

Swern, D. 1995. Reactions of fats and fatty acids. In *Bailey's Industrial Oil and Fat Products*, Vol. 1, 4th Ed., John Wiley & Sons, New York, pp. 130–161.

Tadros, T., P. Izquierdo, J. Esquena, and C. Solans. 2004. Formation and stability of nano-emulsions. *Adv. Coll. Interface Sci.*, 108–109: 303–318.

Takino, T., K. Konishi, Y. Takadura, and M. Hashida. 1994. Long circulating emulsion carrier systems for highly lipophilic drugs. *Biol. Pharm. Bull.*, 17: 121–125.

Takino, T., E. Nagahama., T. Sakaeda, F. Yamashita, Y. Takakura, and M. Hashida, 1995. Pharmacokinetics disposition analysis of lipophlic drugs injected with various lipid carriers in the single-pass rat liver perfusion system. *Int. J. Pharm.*, 114: 43–54.

Tanigawa, N., T. Shimomatsuya, K. Takahashi, Y. Inomata, K. Tanaka, K. Satomura, Y. Hikasa, M. Hashida, S. Muranishi, and H. Sezaki. 1987. Treatment of cystic hygroma and lymphangioma with the use of bleomycin fat emulsion. *Cancer*, 60: 741–749.

Tarr, B. D., T. G. Sambandan, and S. H. Yalkowsky, 1987. A new parenteral emulsion for the administration of taxol. *Pharm. Res.*, 4: 162–165.

Teixeira, R. S., R. Curi, and R. C. Maranhão. 2004. Effects on Walker 256 tumour of Carmustine associated with a cholesterol-rich microemulsion (LDE). *J. Pharm. Pharmacol.*, 56: 909–914.

Tian, L., H. He, and X. Tang. 2007. Stability and degradation kinetics of etoposide loaded parenteral lipid emulsion. *J. Pharm. Sci.*, 96: 1719–1728.

Tibell, A., M. Larsson, and A. Alvestrand. 1993. Dissolving intravenous cyclosporin A in a fat emulsion carrier prevents acute renal side effects in the rat. *Transpl. Int.*, 6: 69–72.

Tibell, A., A. Linholm, J. Sawe, and B. Norrlind. 1995. Cyclosporin A in fat emulsion carriers: Experimental studies on pharmacokinetics and tissue distribution. *Pharmacol. Toxicol.*, 76: 115–121.

Toguchi, H., Y. Ogawa, and T. Shimamoto. 1990. Effects of the physicochemical properties of the emulsion formulation on the bioavailability of ethyl 2-chloro-3-[4-(2-methyl-2-phenylpropyloxy)phenyl] propionate in rats. *Chem. Pharm. Bull.*, 38: 2797–2800.

Ton, M. N., C. Chang, Y. A. Carpentier, and R. J. Deckelbaum. 2005. *In vivo* and *in vitro* properties of an intravenous lipid emulsion containing only medium chain and fish oil triglycerides. *Clin. Nutr.*, 24: 492–501.

Tyle, P. and S. M. Cady. 1990. Sustained release multiple emulsions for bovine somatotropin delivery. *Proc. Int. Sym. Cont. Rel. Bioact. Mater.*, 17: 49–50.

Valduga, C. J., D. C. Fernandes, A. C. Lo Prete, C. H. M. Azevedo, D. G. Rodrigues, R. C. Maranhão, 2003. Use of a cholesterol-rich microemulsion that binds to low-density lipoprotein as vehicle for etoposide. *J. Pharm. Pharmacol.*, 55: 1615–1622.

Van Berkel, T. J. C., J. Kar Kruijt, P. C. De Schmidt, and M. K. Bijsterbosch, 1991. Receptor-dependent targeting of lipoproteins to specific cell types of the liver. In *Lipoproteins as Carriers of Pharmacological Agents*, Shaw, J.M., (Ed.), Marcel Dekker, New York, p. 225–249.

Van Bloois, L., D. D. Dekker, and D. J. A. Crommelin. 1987. Solubilization of lipophilic drugs by amphiphiles improvement of the apparent solubility of almitrine bismesylate by liposomes mixed micelles and o–w emulsions. *Acta Pharm. Technol.*, 33: 136–139.

Velagaleti, R., and S. Ku. 2010. Solutol HS15 as a novel excipient. *Pharm. Tech.*, 34(11). Accessed on November 2, 2010, http://www.pharmtech.com/solutol-hs15-novel-excipient.

Venkatraman, S., W. M. Awni, K. Jordan, and Y. E. Rahman, 1990. Pharmacokinetics of two alternative dosage forms for cyclosporine liposomes and intralipid. *J. Pharm. Sci.*, 79: 216–219.

Verwey, E. J. W. and J. T. G. Overbeek. 1948. *Theory of the Stability of Lyophobic Colloids*. Elsevier, Amsterdam, The Netherlands.

Von Corswant, C., P. Thoren, and S. Engstrom. 1998. Triglyceride-based microemulsion for intravenous administration of sparingly soluble substances. *J. Pharm. Sci.*, 87: 200–208.

Von Dardel, O., C. Mebius, T. Mossberg, and B. Svensson. 1983. Fat emulsion as a vehicle for diazepam. A study of 9492 patients. *Br. J. Anesth.*, 55: 41–47.

Walstra, P. 1983. Formation of emulsions. In *Encyclopedia of Emulsion Technology*, Vol. I, P. Becher, (Ed.), Marcel Dekker, New York, p. 57.

Wang, J., Y. Maitani, and K. Takayama. 2002. Antitumor effects and pharmacokinetics of aclacinomycin A carried by injectable emulsions composed of vitamin E, cholesterol, and PEG-lipid. *J. Pharm. Sci.,* 91: 1128–1134.

Wang, J. J., K. C. Sung, O. Y. Hu, C. H. Yeh, and J. Y. Fang, 2006. Submicron lipid emulsion as a drug delivery system for nalbuphine and its prodrugs. *J Cont. Release.*, 115: 140–149.

Wang, Y., G. M. Mesfin, C. A. Rodríguez, J. G. Slatter, M. R. Schuette, A. L. Cory, and M. J. Higgins. 1999. Venous irritation., pharmacokinetics, and tissue distribution of tirilazad in rats following intravenous administration of a novel supersaturated submicron lipid emulsion. *Pharm Res.*, 16: 930–938.

Ward, D. S., R. J. Norton, P. -H. Guivarc'h, Litman, R. S. Bailey, P.L. 2002. Pharmacodynamics and pharmacokinetics of propofol in medium-chain triglyceride emulsion. *Anesthesiology*, 97: 140–1408.

Waring, W. S. (2012). Intravenous lipid administration for drug-induced toxicity: A critical review of the existing data. *Expert Rev. Clin. Pharmacol.*, 5: 437–444.

Washington, C., F. Koosha, and S. S. Davis. 1993. Physicochemical properties of parenteral fat emulsions containing 20% triglyceride; intralipid and Ivelip. *J. Clin. Pharm. Ther.*, 18: 123–131.

Wei, L., G. Li, Y. D. Yan, R. Pradhan, J. O. Kim, and Q. Quan. 2012b. Lipid emulsion as a drug delivery system for breviscapine: Formulation development and optimization. *Arch. Pharm. Res.*, 35: 1037–1043.

Wei, L., N. Marasini, G. Li, C. S. Yong, J. O. Kim, and Q. Quan, 2012a. Development of ligustrazine-loaded lipid emulsion: Formulation optimization, characterization and biodistribution. *Int. J. Pharm.*, 437: 203–212.

Williams, K. J. and A. R. Tall. 1988. Interactions of liposomes with lipoproteins. In *Liposomes as Drug Carriers,* Gregoriadis, G. (Ed.), John Wiley & Sons, New York, p. 93.

Woodle, M. C. and D. D. Lasic, 1992. Sterically stabilized liposomes. *Biochim. Biophys. Acta*, 113: 171–199.

Xiong, F., H. Wang, K. K. Geng, N. Gu, and J. B. Zhu, 2010. Optimized preparation, characterization and biodistribution in heart of breviscapine lipid emulsion. *Chem. Pharm. Bull.* (*Tokyo*)., 58: 1455–1460.

Yamaguchi, T. and Y. Mizushima, 1994. Lipid microspheres for drug delivery from the pharmaceutical viewpoint. *Crit. Rev. Drug Carrier Syst.*, 114: 215–229.

Yamaguchi, T., K. Nishizaki, S. Itai, H. Hayashi, and H. Oshima, 1995. Physicochemical characterization of parenteral lipid emulsion. *Pharm. Res.*, 12: 342–347.

You, J., J. Zhao, X. Wen, C. Wu, Q. Huang, F. Guan, R. Wu, D. Liang, and C. Li, 2015. Chemoradiation therapy using cyclopamine-loaded liquid-lipid nanoparticles and lutetium-177-labeled core-crosslinked polymeric micelles. *J. Cont. Release.*, 202: 40–48.

11 Emulsions, Microemulsions, and Lipid-Based Drug Delivery Systems for Drug Solubilization and Delivery—Part II: Oral Applications

John B. Cannon and Michelle A. Long

CONTENTS

INTRODUCTION

Owing to the large increase in the number of water-insoluble drugs in clinical development, lipids have come to the forefront as a formulation and drug delivery tool, particularly for drugs that exhibit dissolution rate-limited absorption. Most frequently lipid-based drug delivery systems (LBDDSs) for oral use are designed to present a poorly soluble drug in a solubilized form to eliminate dissolution of crystalline material as the rate-limiting step to absorption (Pouton, 2000). For poorly aqueous-soluble drugs, the dissolution rate can be extremely low under physiological conditions, leading to poor oral bioavailability and nonlinear exposure with increasing dose (Hörter and Dressman, 1997). Many of these lipophilic drugs will also exhibit a strong food effect where the bioavailability increases due to the solubilizing effects of ingested food and concomitant excretion of bile (Charman et al., 1997; Fleisher et al., 1999). By introducing the drug in solubilized form, lipid-based formulations have the potential to increase bioavailability and eliminate the food effect.

When considering oral formulations, the term *LBDDS* encompasses a broad array of formulations based on blends of acylglycerides, fatty acids, fatty acid derivatives, and emulsifiers. The unifying concept behind these formulations is that poor aqueous-soluble drugs that would normally exhibit dissolution rate-limited absorption are presented in a solubilized form *in vivo*. A number of reviews provide discussion of their design and performance (Armstrong and James, 1980; Humberstone and Charman, 1997; Pouton, 1997; Charman, 2000; Porter and Charman, 2001; Wasan, 2001; Porter et al., 2008; Porter et al., 2013; Williams et al., 2013a). While lipid-based parenteral formulations are typically administered as emulsions, oral LBDDSs are generally administered as a liquid or semisolid with high lipid and low or no aqueous content. These oral formulations form emulsions only after ingestion and mixing with gastric or intestinal contents. In this chapter, we will review approaches to develop LBDDSs for oral applications. We begin with basic definitions and functions of the main components, and build on that understanding to describe approaches to solubilization and characterization of performance. Additional information regarding special considerations for stability and manufacturing is provided. In addition to solubilization applications, there are examples where suspensions of poorly soluble drugs are presented in lipid matrices (e.g., for controlled release applications) (Hamdani et al., 2003; Bummer, 2004; Galal et al., 2004, Mengesha et al., 2013) and for taste masking (Robson et al., 2000), but these are not considered in the discussion here.

DEFINITIONS AND CONCEPTS

In addition to the concepts such as emulsions, submicron emulsions, and microemulsions introduced in Chapter 10 (Part I: Parenteral Applications), the following concepts and background information are important for oral formulations.

Lipids

The primary solvent in LBDDSs is the lipid component, which may be either a single material or blend of several types of lipids. As discussed in Part I, the operational definition of lipids is those components of biological material (either occurring naturally or easily derived from those that do occur naturally) that are water-insoluble but soluble in organic solvents such as methylene chloride. Alternatively, lipids are fatty acids and their derivatives, and substances related biosynthetically or functionally to these compounds. These definitions include materials such as cholesterol and other sterols in the category of lipids; however, it is the aliphatic chain lipids (fatty acids and fatty acid derivatives) that are most important for oral formulations. The physical form at room temperature can be solid or liquid depending on the degree of unsaturation of the fatty acid chains, chain length, and homogeneity of the fatty acid profile.

Aliphatic chain lipids can be classified into several groups according to their relative polarity; examples are shown in Table 11.1. The differences in polarity are an important guide in selecting solubilizing lipids for formulation. Among the most hydrophobic lipids are neutral fats (triglycerides), which are triesters of glycerol with fatty acids. The component fatty acids can be either saturated or unsaturated (e.g., palmitic or stearic acid versus oleic or linoleic acid), and chain lengths can vary,

TABLE 11.1

Lipids Used in Oral Lipid-Based Formulations

Class	Chemical Name	Trade or Common Name (Examples)
Long-chain triglycerides		Corn oil
		Soybean oil
		Safflower oil
		Olive oil
Medium-chain triglycerides	Glyceryl tricaprylate/caprate	Fractionated coconut oil
		Captex® 300
		Miglyol® 810
		Miglyol® 812
		Neobee® M-5
Propylene glycol esters	Propylene glycol monocaprylate	Capmul® PG-8
	Propylene glycol monolaurate	Capmul® PG-12; Lauroglycol
Fatty acids	cis-9 octadecenoic acid	Oleic acid
	hexadecanoic acid	Palmitic acid
	octadecanoic acid	Stearic acid
	Z,Z-9, 12 octadecadienoic acid	Linoleic acid
Monoglycerides/diglycerides	Glyceryl caprylate/caprate; glycerol monocaprylate	Capmul® MCM; Imwitor® 742
	Glycerol monooleate	Imwitor® 308
		Capmul® GMO
Lipid mixtures	Saturated C8-C18 triglycerides	Gelucire® 33/01
	Medium chain triglycerides + Phosphatidyl choline	Phosal® 53 MCT
	Phosphatidyl choline + safflower oil/ethanol	Phosal® 75 SA

with long chains having 14–20 carbons and medium chains consisting of 6–12 carbons. Common vegetable oils such as soybean, corn, sesame, olive, and peanut, contain blends of long-chain unsaturated triglycerides. Full or partial hydrogenation of vegetable oils will produce long-chain saturated triglycerides that will be solid or semisolid at room temperature. Medium-chain triglycerides (MCTs) are generally liquid at room temperature even when saturated and occur less commonly naturally, but can be prepared by fractionation of materials such as coconut oil. These materials are somewhat more polar than long-chain triglycerides (LCTs) and thus are generally better solvents.

Fatty acids, manufactured by hydrolysis of triglycerides, are somewhat more polar than the corresponding triglycerides. Oleic acid (cis-9 octadecenoic acid) is a particularly good solvent for a variety of drugs and is used in a number of commercial oral products (Strickley, 2004). Being ionizable, fatty acids can form ion pairs with basic drugs, which can confer solubility in triglyceride vehicles (Lovell et al., 1994).

Monoglycerides and diglycerides, also hydrolysis products of triglycerides, have similar polarity and solubilizing ability to fatty acids but are not ionizable. Glycerol monooleate (Capmul® GMO) and glycerol caprylate/caprate (Capmul MCM, Imwitor® 742) are among the more commonly used lipids in this class. As with all lipids, medium-chain derivatives will be more polar than the long-chain materials. As typically supplied, pharmaceutical grade medium-chain materials can be liquid at room temperature owing to the mixture of mono- and diglycerides and the presence of free glycerol.

Purified monoglycerides (e.g., glycerol monocaprylate, Imwitor 308) will be a waxy semisolid or solid at room temperature.

Substances related to the glycerides are the propylene glycol esters, chemically derived from propylene glycol and fatty acids. Important examples are propylene glycol monocaprylate (Capmul PG-8) and propylene glycol monolaurate (Capmul PG-12, Lauroglycol®). These are particularly good solvents and can be obtained in high purity.

A variety of less common lipids are available for formulation as well. Structured lipids are triglycerides composed of both long- and medium-chain fatty acids esterified to the same glycerol backbone. These lipids have been used in nutritional products where they take advantage of the faster hydrolysis of MCTs to deliver long-chain monoglycerides (Jandacek et al., 1987; Bell et al., 1997). These synthetic lipids are manufactured by transesterification of medium- and long-chain fatty acids with glycerol.

Additional naturally occurring lipids may be minor components of oral lipid-based formulations. Terpenes such as peppermint oil (>50% menthol) are fairly hydrophobic but can provide some solvent capacity. Steroids such as cholesterol, while important in topical and in parenteral liposomal products, are not important as oral pharmaceutical adjuvants. Phospholipids (e.g., egg or soybean phosphatidylcholine), an essential component of cell membranes, are considered polar lipids, and have surfactant properties.

Pharmacopeial specifications exist for many lipid materials. There are differences in criteria among the various pharmacopoeia. In general, the properties specified include the acid value (a measure of the free acids present in a sample, both organic and inorganic acids), hydroxyl value (a measure of the hydroxyl groups in a sample, related to mono- and diglyceride content), iodine number (a measure of unsaturation), peroxide value (a measure of the extent of oxidation—important to gelatin compatibility), saponification value (a measure of saponifiable matter, for example, esterified acids), and unsaponifiable matter (residual sterols, hydrocarbons, alcohols, etc.). Some additional properties that may be listed in the compendia that are useful to monitor include free fatty acid content, fatty acid distribution, alkaline impurities, solidification or congealing temperature, heavy metals, and water content. It is important to note that, owing to their natural origin, triglycerides and other lipids are heterogeneous in nature. For example, the fatty acid distribution of soybean oil consists of 50%–57% linoleic acid, 5%–10% linolenic acid, 17%–26% oleic acid, 9%–13% palmitic acid, and 3%–6% stearic acid (*Handbook of Pharmaceutical Excipients*, 1994). Similarly, the fatty acids found in fractionated coconut oil consist of caprylic (octanoic) and capric (decanoic) acid. As long as consistent sources and methods of manufacture are used and consistent specifications are employed, this generally will not impair their pharmaceutical function. If necessary, material of higher purity can be obtained from vendors at additional expense.

EMULSIFIERS

Often lipid-based oral formulations contain emulsifiers (surfactants) to facilitate dispersion of the drug and formulation components after ingestion. Surfactants can be classified according to their hydrophilic–lipophilic balance (HLB) number (Griffin, 1949); examples are shown in Table 11.2. Those with low HLB values (1–9) are more lipophilic, tend to be lipid soluble, and are useful in preparing water-in-oil emulsions; while those with high HLB values (>10) are more hydrophilic, often form transparent micellar solutions when added to water, and are useful in facilitating formation of oil-in-water (o/w) emulsions. Low HLB surfactants may also be an important component of oral lipid-based formulations by behaving as a coupling agent for the high HLB surfactant and lipophilic solvent components as well as contributing to solubilization by remaining associated with the lipophilic solvent post dispersion. Furthermore, using a blend of low and high HLB surfactants may also lead to more rapid dispersion and finer emulsion

TABLE 11.2
Surfactants Used in Oral Lipid-Based Formulations

Chemical or Common Name	Trade Name	HLB
Polyoxyethylene 20 sorbitan monolaurate	Polysorbate 20 (Tween 20)	16.7[a]
Polyoxyethylene 20 sorbitan monopalmitate	Polysorbate 40 (Tween 40)	15.6[a]
Polyoxyethylene 20 sorbitan monostearate	Polysorbate 60 (Tween 60)	14.9[a]
Polyoxyethylene 20 sorbitan monooleate	Polysorbate 80 (Tween 80)	15.0[a]
Polyoxyethylene 20 sorbitan trioleate	Polysorbate 85 (Tween 85)	11.0[a]
Sorbitan monooleate	SPAN 80	4.3[a]
Sorbitan trioleate	SPAN 85	1.8[a]
Sorbitan monostearate	SPAN 60	4.7[a]
Sorbitan monopalmitate	SPAN 40	6.7[a]
Sorbitan monolaurate	SPAN 20	8.6[a]
Polyoxyl 35 castor oil	Cremophor EL	12–14[a]
Polyoxyl 40 hydrogenated castor oil	Cremophor RH40	14–16[a]
Polyoxyethylene polyoxypropylene block copolymer	Poloxamer 188 (Pluronic F68); Poloxamer 407 (Pluronic 127)	29[b] 22[b]
Unsaturated polyglycolized glycerides	Labrafil M2125, M1944	4[b]
Saturated polyglycolized glycerides	Gelucire 44/14, 50/13	13–14[b]
PEG-8 Caprylic/capric glycerides	Labrasol	14[b]
PEG-8 Caprylic/capric glycerides	Labfac CM10	10[b]
Tocopherol PEG succinate	Vitamin E TPGS	13[b]
Polyoxyl 40 stearate	Myrj 52	16.9[a]
Phosphatidyl choline	Phospholipon	
Glyceryl caprylate/caprate	Capmul® MCM	5–6
Glycerol monooleate	Capmul® GMO	4–5
Propylene glycol monolaurate	Capmul® PG-12; Lauroglycol	4

[a] Handbook of Pharmaceutical ingredients.
[b] Vendor information (Abitec Corp.; BASF Corp.; Gattefosse SAS; Uniqema).

droplet size on addition to an aqueous phase, since in the initial stages of the dilution path, water will be taken up into the formulation, with intermediate formation of a water-in-oil emulsion before phase inversion. Monoglycerides and propylene glycol monoesters, lipids described earlier, also have surfactant properties as low HLB emulsifiers; thus these are also included in Table 11.2. Strickley (2004) has written a comprehensive review of commonly used lipids and emulsifiers with product examples.

Cosolvents

Hydrophilic cosolvents (e.g., ethanol, propylene glycol, polyethylene glycol 400 [PEG 400]) may be used in lipid-based oral formulations if needed to improve drug solubilization. These hydrophilic components may also aid dispersion by facilitating ingress of water into the formulation. An important advantage of lipid-based systems with a co-solvent over formulations consisting only of cosolvents is that after dissipation of the hydrophilic components, the lipids will remain to prevent drug precipitation, whereas in the absence of lipids, drug precipitation is likely. Figure 11.1 illustrates this point for a lipophilic drug RO-15-0778, for which a lipid-based self-emulsifying drug delivery systems (SEDDSs) exhibited a fourfold enhancement in

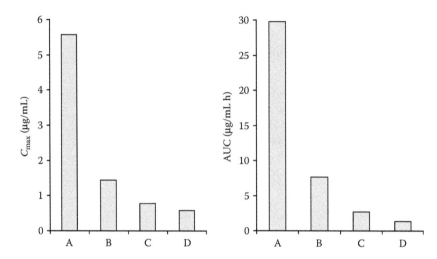

FIGURE 11.1 Comparison of the bioavailability for four formulations of a lipophilic drug, RO-15-0778, in dogs. (a) Lipid-based SEDDS; (b) PEG 400 solution; (c) capsule (powder); and (d) tablet. (Adapted from Gershanik, T. and Benita, S., *Eur. J. Pharm. Biopharm.*, 50, 179–188, 2000. With permission.)

bioavailability in dogs relative to a PEG 400 solution and over a 10-fold enhancement relative to a capsule or tablet (Gershanik and Benita, 2000). The amount of cosolvent used will be limited by the overall formulation compatibility with the encapsulation material. Certain cosolvents (e.g., propylene glycol) can migrate into gelatin capsule shells resulting in softening. Conversely, certain cosolvents may, by virtue of their hygroscopicity, induce water migration from the shell to the fill, resulting in brittle capsules. Compatibilities of various excipients with gelatin capsules have been summarized by Cole (1999).

Ideally, only excipients currently approved by the appropriate regulatory authorities should be used, in amounts established as safe, such as outlined in the approved inactive ingredients list of the US Food and Drug Administration (FDA) (http://www.accessdata.fda.gov/scripts/cder/iig/index. cfm). If novel excipients are required, regulatory hurdles will be encountered later in the development process, since safety of novel excipients is normally only evaluated in the context of a new drug application (NDA). However, pathways do exist for approval for novel excipients, requiring close cooperation between the pharmaceutical company and excipient manufacturers (Goldring, 2009). Tocopherol PEG succinate (tocophersolan) is a water-soluble (HLB ~13) Vitamin E derivative that can enhance solubilization and absorption of poorly water-soluble drugs (Wu and Hopkins, 1999). It was first used in the commercial formulation of the HIV protease inhibitor Amprenavir (Strickley, 2004).

SELF-EMULSIFYING DRUG DELIVERY SYSTEMS

Self-emulsifying drug delivery systems (SEDDSs) are oral dosage forms consisting of drug, oils, surfactants, and sometimes cosolvents (Constantinides, 1995; Pouton, 1997; Pouton, 2000). On addition to water (or on introduction to the gastrointestinal [GI] tract) and with gentle agitation, the system will easily form an emulsion or microemulsion (defined in the following). Self-emulsification may be driven by several mechanisms (López-Montilla et al., 2002). The mechanisms most likely involved in dispersion of pharmaceutical formulations are *diffusion and stranding*, those driven by osmotic pressure imbalances (Greiner and Evans, 1990), phase transformations, and changes owing to alteration of environmental conditions (e.g., pH). If the droplet size after dispersion is substantially less than 1 micron, the SEDDS is often designated as a self-nanoemulsifying drug delivery system (SNEDDS). Given the number of components found in pharmaceutical formulations, it is not unexpected for several mechanisms to operate in parallel. SEDDSs are more practical for oral applications than ready-to-use emulsions due to volume considerations and the ease of formulating them into a soft-gelatin capsule dosage form. Figure 11.1 shows the superior performance of a SEDDS formulation of a lipophilic drug compared to other formulations.

MICROEMULSION

The term *microemulsion* is often used to describe the state of certain LBDDSs after dispersion. Although the term would imply an emulsion of very fine particle size, microemulsions are not in fact emulsions. Microemulsions form spontaneously on mixing with little or no mechanical energy applied, in contrast to conventional emulsions, for which homogenization is critically important. The term was first introduced by Schulman in 1959, although they had actually been described as early as 1943 using terms such as "transparent water and oil dispersions," "hydrophilic oleomicelles" (for o/w), "oleophilic hydromicelles" (for water-in-oil [w/o]), or "swollen micellar solutions" (Friberg and Venable, 1983). Relative to emulsions, microemulsions have much smaller droplet diameter (6–80 nm), and thus are visually transparent or translucent. Unlike emulsions, which are thermodynamically metastable, a microemulsion is a single thermodynamically stable phase consisting of lipophilic domains separated from aqueous domains by an intervening surfactant layer (Strey, 1994). Structurally, a microemulsion can consist of oil droplets dispersed in an aqueous continuous medium, aqueous droplets dispersed in a lipophilic continuous medium, or maintain a bicontinuous structure best described as intertwining channels of each domain (Gelbart and Ben-Shaul, 1996; Hellweg, 2002). In addition to the aqueous phase, oily phase, and surfactant, they may include a *cosurfactant*, and the proportions of the components are chosen such that they are in a stable region of the respective phase diagram; oil content is generally 2%–20%. With pharmaceutically acceptable lipids, it is necessary to use high emulsifier content and cosurfactants to design a formulation capable of forming a microemulsion (Von Corswant et al., 1997; Malcolmson et al., 1998; Garti et al., 2001). As originally conceived, the cosurfactant was generally an alkanol of 4–8 carbons that are unsuitable for pharmaceutical use. More recently, there has been success in formulating alcohol-free microemulsions for oral use; frequently this can be achieved by using the appropriate ratios of lipophilic and hydrophilic surfactants, typically polyethoxylated nonionic surfactants (Constantinides, 1995; Lawrence, 1996). Self-microemulsifying drug delivery systems (SMEDDSs), as the name implies, are those self-emulsifying systems that form microemulsions on addition to water and gentle agitation.

MARKETED ORAL LIPID-BASED DRUG DELIVERY SYSTEM PRODUCTS

Table 11.3 shows marketed oral products that would be considered LBDDSs. None of them are emulsions in the marketed dosage form but yield an emulsion (e.g., Sandimmune®) or microemulsion (e.g., Neoral®) on dilution in the aqueous environment of the GI tract. Some of the liquids are mixed with water or juice, forming an emulsion, before ingestion. Not included in the table are products that are primarily surfactant based. These would include Gengraf® (cyclosporine) and Agenerase® (amprenavir), which are summarized in the review by Strickley (2004). Also not included are laxative products composed of emulsified castor or mineral oil. Some of the LBDDS products listed in Table 11.3 will be discussed in greater detail later.

TABLE 11.3

Marketed Products of Oral Lipid-Based Drug Delivery Systems

Drug	Product Name	Company	Drug Activity	Dosage Form	Components	References
Tipranavir	Aptivus	BI	AIDS	SGC	Ethanol, polyoxyl 35 castor oil, propylene glycol, mono/diglycerides of caprylic/capric acid	PDR[a]
Cyclosporine	Sandimmune oral	Novartis	Immunosuppressant	SGC	Corn oil, Labrafil, ethanol, glycerol	Strickley
Cyclosporine	Sandimmune oral	Novartis	Immunosuppressant	Liquid	Olive oil, Labrafil, ethanol, propylene glycol, α-tocopherol	Strickley
Cyclosporine	Neoral	Novartis	Immunosuppressant	SG, Liquid	Corn oil mono-diglycerides, Cremophor RH40, ethanol, propylene glycol, α-tocopherol	PDR
Ritonavir	Norvir	Abbott	AIDS	SGC	Butylated hydroxytoluene, ethanol, gelatin, iron oxide, oleic acid, polyoxyl 35 castor oil	PDR
Ritonavir/ Lopinavir	Kaletra	Abbott	AIDS	SGC	Oleic acid, Cremophor EL, propylene glycol	Strickley
Paricalcitol	Zemplar	Abbott	Calcium regulator	SGC	medium-chain triglycerides, alcohol, and butylated hydroxytoluene	PDR
Dutasteride	Avodart	GSK	BPH	SGC	mono-diglycerides of caprylic/capric acid and butylated hydroxytoluene	PDR
Isotretinoin	Accutane	Roche	Acne	SGC	Beeswax, butylated hydroxyanisole, hydrogenated soybean oil, hydrogenated vegetable oil, and soybean oil	PDR
Tretinoin	Vesanoid	Roche	Acne	SGC	Beeswax, butylated hydroxyanisole, hydrogenated soybean oil, hydrogenated vegetable oils, and soybean oil	PDR
Valproic acid	Depakene	Abbott	Epilepsy	SGC	Corn oil	PDR
Progesterone	Prometrium	Solvay	Endometrial hyperplasia	SGC	Peanut oil, glycerin, lecithin	PDR
Calcitriol	Rocaltrol	Roche	Calcium regulator	SG, Liquid	Medium-chain triglycerides	Strickley, 2004
Clofazimine	Lamprene	Geigy	Leprosy	SGC	Beeswax, Plant oils	Strickley, 2004
Doxercalciferol	Hectoral	Bone care	Calcium regulator	SGC	Medium-chain triglycerides	Strickley, 2004
Dronabinol	Marinol	Roxane	Anorexia	SGC	Sesame oil	Strickley, 2004
Saquinavir	Fortovase	Roche	AIDS	SGC	Medium-chain mono-diglycerides, povidone, α-tocopherol	Strickley, 2004
Sirolimus	Rapamune	WyethAyerst	Immunosuppression	Liquid	Phosal 50 PG	Strickley, 2004

(Continued)

TABLE 11.3 (*Continued*)
Marketed Products of Oral Lipid-Based Drug Delivery Systems

Drug	Product Name	Company	Drug Activity	Dosage Form	Components	References
Clomethiazole	Heminevrin	Astra-Zeneca	Sedation	SGC	Medium-chain triglycerides, gelatin, glycerin, sorbitol, manitol, oligosaccharides	Nanjwade et al., 2011
Alfacalcidol	Alfarol	Chugai	Vitamin D metabolic disorders	SGC	Medium-chain triglyceride, ethanol	Nanjwade et al., 2011
Menatetrenone	Glakay	Eisai	Osteoporosis	SGC	L-aspartic acid, carnauba wax, hydrogenated oil, D-sorbitol, glycerin, propylene glycol esters of fatty acid, glyceryl monooleate	Nanjwade et al., 2011
Tolterodine	Detrol® LA	Pharmacia Upjohn	Overactive bladder	HGC	Sucrose, starch, hypromellose, ethylcellulose, medium-chain triglycerides, oleic acid, gelatin	Nanjwade et al., 2011
Fenofibrate	Fenogal	Genus	Hyper-lipidemia	HGC	Lauryl macroglycerides, macrogol 20,000, hydroxypropylcellulose	Nanjwade et al., 2011
Testosterone undecanoate	Restandol	Organon	Hormone replacement therapy	SGC	Castor oil, propylene glycol laurate, medium-chain triglycerides, lecithin, glycerin	Kalepu et al., 2013
Tocopherol nicotinate	Juvela	Eisai	Hypertension	SGC	L-aspartic acid, carnauba wax, glycerol esters of fatty acids, titanium oxide, gelatin, D-sorbitol, medium chain fatty acid triglyceride, glycerin	Kalepu et al., 2013

[a] PDR: *Physicians Desk Reference*, PDR® Electronic Library, Thomson MICROMEDEX, 2007.

DESIGN AND CHARACTERIZATION OF LIPID-BASED DRUG DELIVERY SYSTEMS

Although there is an understanding in principle of the factors influencing bioavailability from LBDDSs, there are no definitive *in vitro* tests that reliably and accurately predict *in vivo* performance. What happens on ingestion of the formulation depends on the components selected. In a manner analogous to tablet disintegration and dissolution, the dispersion of the lipid-based formulation has been shown to affect the plasma profile of a given drug. Much emphasis in the literature has been placed on the use of self-emulsifying or self-microemulsifying formulations with the notable success of Novartis Neoral formulation of cyclosporine (Trull et al., 1993; Mueller et al., 1994a, 1994b; Ritschel, 1996). Self-emulsifying formulations are designed to disperse readily in the presence of an aqueous medium and thus lessen the inherent variability caused by reliance on gut motility and digestive mechanisms. Nevertheless, several marketed products, such as Depakene® and Accutane®, present the drug in a triglyceride without additional emulsifiers (Physicians Desk Reference). The natural process of digestion, which involves breakdown of the triglycerides to mono- and diglycerides and fatty acids, will facilitate emulsification of these types of formulations, and their simplicity may enhance their desirability as a commercial product.

Importantly, development of LBDDSs should not focus solely on the *in vivo* behavior of the lipid fill, but must consider additional factors such as compatibility with encapsulation material and the physical and chemical stability of the product. An LBDDS can be encapsulated in hard- or soft-gelatin capsule shells and in hydroxypropyl methylcellulose (HPMC) capsules. In the case of gelatin shells, special attention must be paid to the formation of aldehydes, which can occur with unsaturated lipids and induce gelatin cross-linking (Chafetz et al., 1984), and to migration of solvents between the shell and fill (Tahibi and Gupta, 2000, from R. Liu, 2000), which can induce softening or brittleness (Kuentz and Röthlisberger, 2002). Furthermore, as these LBDDSs are typically liquid solutions, degradation kinetics are accelerated relative to solid systems. Other minor components of oral lipid-based formulations may include antioxidants (probably required if unsaturated lipids are used), viscosity modifying agents, pH modifiers, and other excipients with specific functional purposes.

PROCESSING *IN VIVO* AND CLASSIFICATION OF LBDDS

Lipid-based drug delivery systems are typically presented as encapsulated liquid formulations, though as discussed later, examples of semisolid or solid formulations exist (Serajuddin et al., 1988; Khoo et al., 2000). Regardless of form, after ingestion, LBDDSs undergo GI processing. This processing includes emulsification to form lipid droplets, hydrolysis of di- and triglycerides, solubilization of these digestion products by bile acids and transport through mixed micelles to the intestinal wall (Patton et al., 1985; Thomson et al., 1993; Embleton and Pouton, 1997). Figure 11.2 summarizes these processes that occur for an LBDDS in the GI tract. As a result of the GI processing, the solvent environment provided by the LBDDS is constantly changing after ingestion, and the mechanism for release of the drug is not completely understood. The possibilities include simple partitioning from the emulsion oil droplets; partitioning from the bile salt mixed micelles; or micelle delivery to the intestinal wall, with absorption facilitated by breakdown of mixed micelles due to protonation of the bile salts or uptake of the fatty acids and monoglycerides (Charman et al., 1997). Although the exact mechanism for release of the drug is not known, certain properties of the formulation do enhance bioavailability from these vehicles. For example, release from emulsions can result in higher bioavailability than release from neat oil (Humberstone and Charman, 1997); self-emulsifying systems tend to provide more reproducible blood levels than emulsions that require more energy to form (Holt and Johnston, 1997); and formulations that form viscous liquid crystals have shown delayed or reduced release of drug (Alfons and Engstrom, 1998; Trotta, 1999).

The *in vivo* processing step that dominates the ultimate bioavailability of the drug is dictated by the composition of the formulation. If a formulation is simply drug dissolved in a triglyceride,

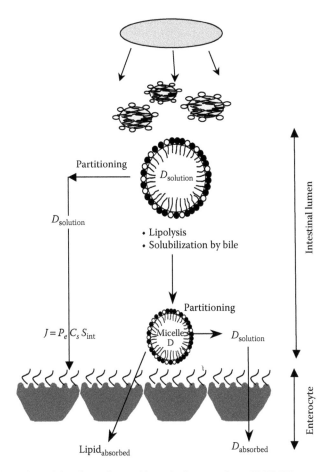

FIGURE 11.2   Illustration of the dispersion and intestinal processing of LBDDSs.

then the digestion process is responsible for the dispersion and breakdown of the formulation to extract the drug. In the 1970s, Carrigan and Bates assessed the absorption of griseofulvin in rats from a sesame oil suspension, an o/w emulsion, and an aqueous suspension (see Figure 11.3). While the emulsion was found to have the highest bioavailability, the oil suspension significantly increased absorption, apparently due to digestion of the oil and subsequent solubilization of the drug. Furthermore, the variability in C_{max} and AUC_{∞} decreased in the following order: aqueous suspension > oil suspension > emulsion. Hence, the emulsion formulation was found to enhance drug absorption in a reproducible and uniform manner (Carrigan and Bates, 1973). In contrast to formulations composed only of triglyceride, a self-emulsifying formulation may have very little dependence on digestive processes.

Pouton (2000) has proposed a classification system that balances the inherent dispersibility of the formulations and their reliance on digestion to facilitate breakdown (Table 11.4). Type I formulations are simple drugs in triglyceride or mixed glycerides. These are expected to form coarse emulsions and maintain their solubilizing capacity for the drug *in vivo*. Type II formulations have added surfactant to improve the dispersibility, but have used more lipophilic surfactants to reduce potential for partitioning of the surfactant into the aqueous phase and ensure continued solubilization of the drug. Type III formulations are self-emulsifying systems using hydrophilic surfactants and cosolvents that increase the driving force for formation of oil-in-water emulsions or, with the right composition, microemulsions. These formulations have a high potential to lose solubilizing

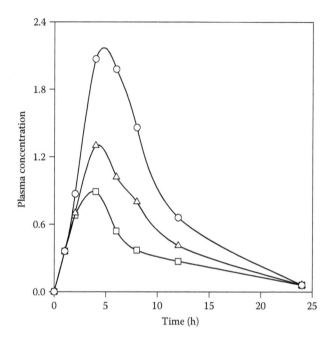

FIGURE 11.3 Mean plasma concentrations after oral administration of 50 mg/kg griseofulvin to rats. Key: (□) aqueous suspension, (△) oil suspension, and (o) o/w emulsion. (Adapted from Carrigan, P.J. and Bates, T.R., *J. Pharm. Sci.*, 62, 1476–1479, 1973. With permission.)

TABLE 11.4

Classification of Lipid-Based Delivery Systems Developed by C. Pouton

Typical Properties of Type I, II, IIIA, and IIIB Lipid Formulations

	Increasing Hydrophilic Content →			
	Type I	Type II	Type IIIA	Type IIIB
Typical composition (%)				
Triglycerides or mixed glycerides	100	40–80	40–80	<20
Surfactants	—	20–60 (HLB<12)	20–40 (HLB >11)	20–50 (HLB >11)
Hydrophilic cosolvents	—	—	0–40	20–50
Particle size of dispersion (nm)	Coarse	100–250	100–250	50–100
Significance of aqueous dilution	Limited importance	Solvent capacity unaffected	Some loss of solvent capacity	Significant phase changes and potential loss of solvent capacity
Significance of digestibility	Crucial requirement	Not crucial, but likely to occur	Not crucial, but may be inhibited	Not required and not likely to occur

Source: Pouton, C.W., *Eur. J. Pharm. Sci.*, 11, S93–S98, 2000.

capacity on dispersion due to partitioning of the components into the aqueous phase. This is especially true when hydrophilic cosolvents are used in the formulations to increase the initial loading capacity for the drug in the lipid formulation.

A fourth category, Type IV, that consists of surfactant/cosolvent mixtures without lipid was added in 2006 (Pouton, 2006; Porter et al., 2008). However, the lower oil content of Type IIIA and especially of Type IIIB and Type IV formulations increases the risk of drug precipitation upon mixing with the intestinal milieu, due to diffusion of the co-solvents and high HLB surfactant away from the emulsion droplet. Furthermore, surfactants in the formulation may also be digested by intestinal lipases and hence lose their solubilizing power, leading to drug precipitation. Thus, *in vitro* dissolution testing in biorelevant media (i.e., simulated intestinal fluids) such as those developed by Dressman (Jantratid et al., 2008) should be used to evaluate candidate formulations. Studies by Cuine et al. (2008) with a series of danazol lipid-based SMEDDS formulations showed that higher surfactant content led to smaller droplet size after *in vitro* dispersion, but under digestion conditions high surfactant content led to a greater occurrence of drug precipitation and lower bioavailability in dogs.

FEASIBILITY ASSESSMENT

Designing an LBDDS is daunting at first sight. An ideal oral lipid-based dosage form must meet a number of demands: It should solubilize therapeutic amounts of the drug in the dosage form; maintain adequate drug solubility over the entire shelf life of the drug product (generally 2 years) under all anticipated storage conditions; and provide adequate chemical and physical stability for the drug and formulation components. Additionally, it must be composed of approved excipients in safe amounts. When ingested, it should facilitate dispersion of the dosage form in the intestinal milieu and maintain drug solubilization in the dispersed form. It should adapt to the digestive processes of the GI tract such that digestion either maintains or enhances drug solubilization. Finally, it should present the drug to the intestinal mucosal cells such that absorption into the cells and into the systemic circulation is optimized. To meet these demands, the formulator is faced with a wide range of lipophilic solvents (e.g., fatty acids and fatty acid esters) available in various different chain lengths, and an even broader selection of emulsifiers. The formulation must balance the practical loading limitations for a unit dose dictated by the drug solubility in the available excipients, the stability of the drug in the formulation, and whether the formulation will rely on *in vivo* processing or self-emulsification. The development of the formulation will require a combination of *in vitro* laboratory-bench assessments and *in vivo* trials.

As a first step, it should be determined whether the bioavailability is in fact dissolution rate limited. Enhanced bioavailability when dosed with food is one indication that drug solubilization may be an important formulation design concept. A so-called food effect may also occur due to alterations of gastric pH (e.g., increased gastric pH results in higher solubility for acidic compounds) or slowing of gastric emptying and intestinal transit (influencing residence times for drugs exhibiting regional absorption windows) (Charman et al., 1997; Fleisher et al., 1999). The contributions of improved solubilization can be confirmed by appropriately designed *in vivo* studies such as rising dose in a simple hydrophilic cosolvent system (e.g., ethanol/PEG/water). If there is a nonlinear dose response in bioavailability from the cosolvent formulation, then a test using a simple formulation of drug solubilized in a triglyceride at one of the higher doses used in the cosolvent test would follow. A measurable improvement at the higher dose in the bioavailability from the lipid-based formulation suggests that the bioavailability is likely dissolution rate limited and it is worthwhile to pursue an LBDDS. A simple demonstration of this is provided by Burcham et al. (1997) who showed improved bioavailability of a lipophilic drug, DMP 565, in beagle dogs for a safflower oil formulation (F = 36.7% ± 10.7%) over PEG 300 (F = 13.1% ± 3.4%) or a suspension in an aqueous HPMC solution (F = 6.3% ± 0.7%). In another example, a water-insoluble steroid derivative, danazol, is known to lack dose-proportional absorption after oral administration. The oral administration of powder drug (i.e., capsule) demonstrated an almost threefold increase in bioavailability in fed versus the fasted state ($p = 0.0001$). A glycerol monooleate emulsion, where the drug was completely solubilized, provided good dose-proportional oral absorption in

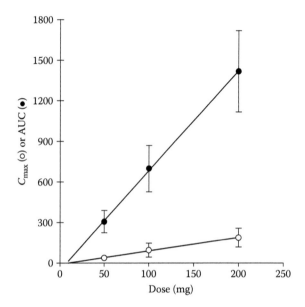

FIGURE 11.4 Correlation between the dose of danazol versus C_{max} (O; ng/mL, $r^2 = 0.999$) and dose versus AUC (●; ng h/mL, $r^2 = 0.999$) in humans. Bar represents SD of 12 humans per group. (Adapted from Charman W.N. et al., *J. Clin. Pharmacol.*, 33, 381–386, 1993. With permission.)

12 subjects (Figure 11.4). Furthermore, the bioavailability of the drug from the emulsion formulation was unaffected by food ($p = 0.47$) (Figure 11.5) (Charman et al., 1993). The change in the oral absorption profile of drug was attributed to the presence of triglycerides in the emulsion, which act as an intrinsic dissolution and emulsification aid for the drug. The study concluded that the factors that enhance drug solubilization also enhance its oral bioavailability.

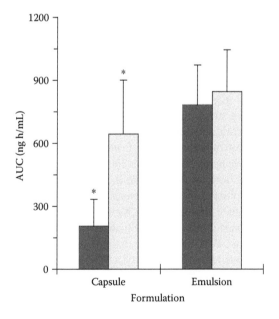

FIGURE 11.5 Effect of formulation type and food on AUC after oral administration of 100 mg danazol to group of eleven humans. Key: (■) AUC in fasting state and (□) AUC in fed state. (∗) represents significant difference. (Adapted from Charman, W.N. et al., *J. Clin. Pharmacol.*, 33, 381–386, 1993. With permission.)

The importance of drug solubilization by lipids is illustrated in a study by Abrams et al. (1978). The bioavailability of a lipophilic steroid was threefold higher for a solution of the drug in sesame oil relative to an aqueous suspension. As long as the solubility of the drug was not exceeded in the oil, absorption was dose proportional. However, above the solubility limit (i.e., when administered as a sesame oil suspension), absorption did not increase proportionately with dose. Alternative formulations designed to improve dissolution rate such as nanoparticles, solid dispersions or by modifying the solid form (through development of amorphous systems or salt selection) should also be considered when faced with the need to formulate poorly soluble drugs.

Once it is confirmed that a simple LBDDS provides measurable improvement in bioavailability, the next step is development and optimization of the formulation. Although considerable progress has been made, there are currently no definitive tests that will translate *in vitro* measures to *in vivo* performance. At the same time, this does not mean that development of such formulations should be conducted using a trial-and-error approach. Pouton's classification system points out that the factors to be considered in interpreting the *in vivo* behavior of the formulations are effects of lipolysis, dispersibility, and solubilization capacity on dilution. It is important to understand that the balance of each of these effects will depend on the drug being formulated, and that there is unlikely to be a universal formulation that works for all compounds.

In the next few sections, we will review the status of available techniques for evaluating each of these processes. While each area will be discussed separately, the optimization of the formulation cannot be approached in a linear fashion. As an example, Gao et al. (2004) describe the use of a statistical mixture experimental design as a rational strategy to identifying the balance of lipophilic solvent/surfactant/cosolvent to obtain a high loading, self-emulsifying formulation.

PHASE BEHAVIOR AND COMPLEX FLUID STRUCTURES

Before reviewing the steps for design of LBDDSs, it is necessary to have a brief review of the phase behavior of these systems and utility of phase diagrams. Mixtures of oil, water, and surfactant are known to create a variety of microstructures depending on the relative proportion of each component (Gelbart and Ben-Shaul, 1996). The various structures formed are the result of the amphiphilicity of the surfactant whose hydrophilic domain and lipophilic domain drive it to the interface of oil/water systems. These phases include the well-organized structure of lamellar, hexagonal and cubic liquid crystals, the water continuous L_1 phase, which includes micelles and o/w microemulsions, and the oil continuous L_2 phase, which includes inverse micelles and w/o microemulsions (Figure 11.6). The L_1 (micelle/microemulsion) and L_2 (water-in-oil microemulsion/isotropic oil continuous phase) phases are those most often encountered in developing LBDDSs. Pharmaceutical oral formulations that are blends of lipophilic solvent and emulsifier are typically L_2 phase systems. On dilution, the formulation may enter the L_1 phase, though this is not necessary, as many examples of formulations that form metastable emulsions on dilution exist with adequate bioavailability.

Ternary surfactant–oil–water phase diagrams are fundamental to understanding the relative role of each component in the system. The drug product will typically be a surfactant/oil blend with a composition represented by a point along the surfactant–oil axis. On ingestion, this formulation will necessarily be diluted by an aqueous phase and hence a line drawn from the original composition to the water apex will describe the equilibrium pathway and potential phase transitions that can occur. By constructing these diagrams, one can determine the potential for formation of viscous emulsions or liquid crystal phases that would inhibit dispersion. The realization that these phases are present allows for a rational approach to avoid them such as with the addition of cosolvents or substitution of surfactants or lipophilic solvents. These diagrams are also useful for exploring the solubilization capacity of formulations where cosolvents are added. The addition of cosolvents can influence the phase behavior and often has the effect of expanding the L_2 region, improving miscibility of lipophilic solvents and emulsifiers, and minimizing or reducing

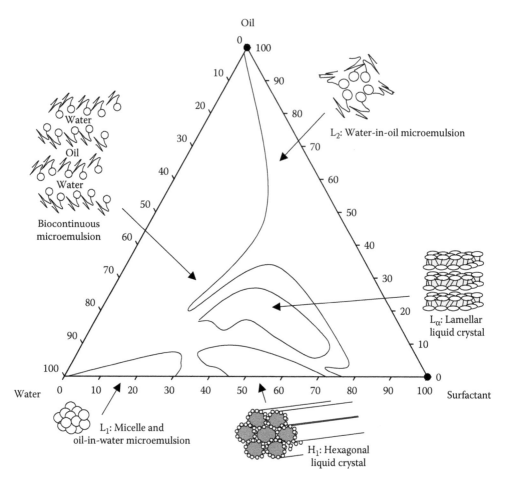

FIGURE 11.6 Example of a phase diagram for an oil–water-surfactant system. (Adapted from C12E10-water-oleic acid diagram Van Os et al., *Physio-Chemical Properties of Selected Anionic, Cationic and Nonionic Surfactants.* Elsevier Science Publishers, Amsterdam, The Netherlands, p. 301, 1993. With permission.)

the occurrence of liquid crystalline phases. These liquid crystalline phases are often viscous and can prevent dispersion of the lipid-based system if present along the dilution path.

Construction of phase diagrams can be tedious. They require preparation and equilibration of possibly hundreds of samples spanning all proportions of the components. These are thoroughly mixed and equilibrated under controlled temperatures, typically 37°C to mimic *in vivo* conditions. After equilibration, the samples are usually centrifuged to ensure separation of phases, and visual observations of the number and identity of phases are made. Single-phase regions are mapped on the phase diagram. Identification of lamellar and hexagonal liquid crystalline phases can be made using optical microscopy with polarized light (Laughlin, 1994). Additional characterization using light scattering or small angle X-ray scattering can provide particle sizes in L_1 and L_2 regions as well as repeat spacings in the case of liquid crystal phases. For blends of multiple components, sets of pseudo-ternary diagrams can be constructed using pseudo-components representing fixed ratios of components (e.g., a 9:1 ratio of MCT/ethanol as one component in ternary system including surfactant and water). While an understanding of the structures arising on a dilution path of a given formulation is important to assure formation of stable dispersed structures upon dilution, it is often unnecessary to construct the entire phase diagram.

SOLUBILIZATION

Drug candidates for lipid-based drug delivery are poorly aqueous- soluble and lipophilic (typically log $P > 3$). Being a poorly soluble drug alone is not sufficient, as solubility in the lipid components for LBDDSs is required. Initiating development of an LBDDS will begin with a solubility screening study in select lipid excipients, emulsifiers, and cosolvents (e.g., ethanol, propylene glycol, PEG 400). The primary solvent will typically be an alkylglyceride, and cosolvents are used to increase the solubility in the blend. The concentration of specific cosolvents (e.g., propylene glycol) must be restricted for two reasons: first, for formulations encapsulated in gelatin capsule shells, certain cosolvents (e.g., propylene glycol) will migrate into the capsule shell and cause softening. This will also cause a subsequent loss of solubilizing power for the encapsulated fill. Loss of solvency due to water migration from the shell into the fill has also been reported (Serajuddin et al., 1986). A second disadvantage is that excessive cosolvent will result in a loss of solubilizing power after dilution in an aqueous environment (namely, the GI tract), thus causing precipitation of solid drug and compromising the advantage of an LBDDS.

Addition of surfactants, which are used to improve dispersibility *in vivo*, may enhance or reduce solubility in the blend. To maintain a systematic approach to optimizing the solubility, the use of ternary phase diagrams are recommended. Ternary phase diagrams allow mapping of the blends to note regions of excipient immiscibility and record drug solubility to identify optimal compositions. These will also allow one to recognize systems where alternate excipients (e.g., exchanging surfactants) will provide systems of similar solubilization power. Compounds with ionizable groups present other alternatives. For example, amine-containing drugs may be soluble in oleic acid by formation of ion pairs, as exhibited by marketed formulations of ritonavir and ritonavir/lopinavir. Hydrophobic non-ionizable drugs (generally characterized by a Log $P_{octanol/water} > 3$) may be solubilized by long-chain triglycerides (LCT) or medium chain triglycerides (MCT) and/or by combination of a lipid with a low HLB surfactant such as phosphatidylcholine/medium chain triglyceride or oleoyl macrogolglycerides. Less hydrophobic drugs (viz., Log $P_{octanol/water} < 3$) may be solubilized by monoglycerides or propylene glycol monoesters, or by combinations of these lipids with high HLB surfactants or hydrophilic co-solvents. Often a combination of low HLB and high HLB surfactants give superior solubilization, which may also optimize the dispersion properties described later. Screening studies can be carried out by mixing the required drug amount in the formulation and monitoring the presence of drug crystals visually or microscopically, followed by more accurate determination of solubility values of drug in promising formulations by HPLC.

In parallel with optimizing the formulation for initial drug loading is an evaluation of the tendency for precipitation on dilution. This is still an exploratory area, and there are several studies describing evaluations in various media such as simulated gastric and intestinal fluids, water and media containing bile acids, and phospholipids at compositions to mimic fed and fasted conditions (Bravo González et al., 2002; Gao et al., 2003). Gao et al. (2003) used a conventional dissolution apparatus and simulated gastric fluid to test for precipitation over a period of 3 h from an LBDDS formulation of paclitaxel. In this case, addition of HPMC created a formulation capable of suppressing precipitation that translated into a 10-fold increase in bioavailability over the SEDDS formulation without HPMC.

At this time, systematic yet empirical approaches to identifying systems with sufficient drug solubility are necessary. High throughput screening systems have been employed to increase efficiency. For example, a robotic liquid dispenser was used to prepare a series of nilvadipine SMEDDS formulations with mixtures of oil, surfactant, and ethanol, followed by identification of the optimal low HLB/high HLB blend (Sakai et al., 2010). A rich area for research is the development of computational methods for predicting compound solubility in LBDDSs. Several models have potential application including linear free energy relationships, such as Abraham's model (Abraham and Le, 1999), and mobile order theory (Ruelle and Kesselring, 1994). An application of Abraham's model to solubilization in a MCT demonstrated the potential and complexity inherent in predicting solubility (Cao et al., 2004). The authors developed a model using six model solutes for which the Abraham descriptors had been established. They adjusted the solvency using mixtures of MCT with squalane. After demonstrating accurate prediction of partitioning in squalane, they developed a log-linear correction to partitioning with the added hydrogen-bond acidity, basicity, and polarizability contributions of the ester portions of the MCT. The study also attempted to model the effects of water typically resident in acylglycerides. The authors demonstrated experimentally that water modulated the solubility of the solutes studied (benzamide and N-methylbenzamide), but concluded that the current solute descriptors for water used in the modeling would require revision. More recently, Persson et al. (2013) measured the solubility of 30 structurally diverse lipophilic drug molecules in LCT, MCT, polysorbate, and PEG400. The experimental results were then used to develop a partial least squares model to predict drug solubility based on molecular descriptors such as melting point, octanol–water partition coefficient, polar surface area, and nitrogen content. The models could predict the solubility in LCT and MCT with r^2 values of 0.81 and 0.84, respectively. The use of computational models may be more appropriate for comparing partitioning of solutes into simple lipid solvents rather than actual solubility. This should be sufficient to use as a guide in selecting primary solvent systems versus modeling of more complex systems that include cosolvents and emulsifiers.

CHARACTERIZING DISPERSIBILITY AND DISSOLUTION/DISPERSION BEHAVIOR OF LBDDS

Much of the published literature on the design and performance of LBDDSs describes characterization of the dispersion properties. Attention has been focused on the resulting particle size, the concept being that smaller particle size increases the surface area for partitioning of drug or diffusion rate of the carrier droplets to the enterocyte. For particle size to be an important criterion there needs to be some assessment of the stability of the emulsion formed within the time period for measurement to allow the measurement to be meaningful. In addition, careful selection of the medium in which the measurement is carried out is required. Depending on the composition of the LBDDS, the medium pH, osmotic strength, and presence of bile can all affect the ultimate particle size formed after dispersion. In addition, the force of mechanical agitation can alter the particle size distribution.

While still sensitive to the medium environment, the ease of dispersion rather than particle size may be a better measure of the performance *in vivo*. Ease of dispersion refers to the facility for the formulation to mix with the aqueous phase and is typically represented by low interfacial tensions. It is this property that drives the process of self-emulsification. Mechanisms for promoting self-emulsification are a topic of current study (Pouton, 1997; Buchanan et al., 2000; Nishimi and Miller, 2000; Shahidzadeh et al., 2000; López-Montilla et al., 2002). The mechanisms most likely involved in dispersion of pharmaceutical formulations are *diffusion and stranding*, those driven by osmotic pressure imbalances (Greiner and Evans, 1990), phase transformations, and changes due to alteration of environmental conditions (e.g., pH). Given the number of components found in pharmaceutical formulations, it is not unexpected for several mechanisms to operate in parallel.

Diffusion and stranding is a mechanism of emulsion formation that relies on the presence of a solute in one phase that is in fact soluble in both phases and couples those phases within a limited composition range. Addition of a hydrophilic cosolvent can induce diffusion and stranding emulsification (Miller, 1988; Zourab and Miller, 1995; Pouton, 1997; Rang and Miller, 1999). The cosolvent may initially improve the miscibility of the lipid formulation with the aqueous medium, but as it continues to be diluted into the aqueous phase, the more lipophilic material is *stranded* as droplets. An osmotic mechanism is possible in the case of water-in-oil droplets where a solute is dissolved into the internal aqueous phase and the continuous oil phase presents a semipermeable barrier. The solute can be an additive such as a hydrophilic polymer or salt. Change in pH can trigger dispersion when ionizable components are used. For example, the ease of dispersion of fatty acids increases when the environmental pH is above the pK_a of the carboxylic acid (e.g., 4.89 for caprylic acid) (Lide, 1993).

Constructing phase diagrams of the LBDDS as a function of aqueous content and condition (e.g., change of pH or addition of bile components) can help identify factors influencing dispersion. Combinations of low HLB and high HLB surfactants often lead to smaller emulsion droplet size than single surfactants; these more complex systems can be examined by pseudo-ternary phase diagrams. Although *in vivo* processing of the formulations is dynamic, equilibrium-phase behavior studies can provide a guide to the driving forces behind the transitions that occur. For example, phase diagrams can be used to compare the equilibrium state of the formulation in the acidic environment of the stomach versus the more neutral conditions of the intestinal tract. Addition of bile components can address the ability to solubilize the formulation. Formulations that self-emulsify should avoid formation of viscous liquid crystals. Thus, compositional regions where these occur would be mapped on the phase diagram allowing the formulator to alter the composition of the LBDDS to avoid the region. These phase diagrams can then be used to compare the effect of excipient substitution (e.g., using the emulsifier Tween® 80 in place of Cremophor® EL). Lipid/emulsifier combinations with similar phase diagrams are likely to behave similarly *in vivo* assuming that the surface-active components of the intestinal milieu do not interact differently with these combinations.

Visual observations of ease of dispersion are useful for formulation screening. An example is provided by Khoo et al. (1998) who constructed a visual rating system that described the ultimate state of the formulation after diluting 1 into 200 mL of aqueous solution (either 0.1 N HCl or water in the publication). Extension of this approach using simulated fed and fasted fluids, such as those described by Nicolaides et al. (1999), would provide guidance on the solubilizing effects of bile. Dispersion behavior can also be assessed by measuring the droplet size after addition of the formulation to an aqueous medium using dynamic light scattering (DLS) techniques described in Chapter 10 (Part I: Parenteral Applications). Gao et al. (2004) used a custom-built DLS probe to optimize an SEDDS formulations using a statistical mixture experimental design. Assessment of a formulation's dispersion behavior can be coupled with quantitative analysis of solubilized drug concentration to assess the extent to which the formulation loses solubilizing power under these conditions. With respect to solubilizing capacity, it is important to consider that precipitation from solution may not occur immediately, and an evaluation of the kinetics may prove useful for comparison of formulations (Bravo González et al., 2002).

Shahba et al. (2012) examined the dispersion behavior and precipitation tendency of optimized SEDDS formulations of cinnarizine by measuring the drug solubility upon aqueous dilution, and measuring particle size after dilution. Type II formulations containing medium-chain mixed glycerides (e.g., Miglyol 810/Imwitor 308/Tween85 25/25/50) yielded droplet sizes of ≤50 nm and transparent appearance upon aqueous dilution, with ~90% of drug remaining in solution after dilution.

The effects of dispersion are highlighted by the differences in the properties of the marketed cyclosporine oral formulations and the resulting influence on pharmacokinetics. The Sandimmune capsule formulation is based on a blend of corn oil and the low HLB emulsifier Labrafil® M 2125 CS (polyoxyethylated glycerides, corn oil PEG 6 esters). On dilution, the formulation forms a coarse emulsion. Under similar dilution conditions, the Neoral formulation, which is based on corn oil mono- and diglycerides and the high HLB surfactant polyoxyl 40 hydrogenated castor oil, readily forms a microemulsion. The microemulsion is characterized by the formation of small and uniform particles. In nonfasting renal transplant patients, Neoral gave a shorter tmax (1.2 versus 2.6 h), a higher C_{max} (892 versus 528 µg/L), and a higher AUC (3028 versus 2432 µg h/L) relative to Sandimmune. A clinical study comparing cyclosporine bioavailability in transplant patients found increases of 39% in C_{max} and 15% in AUC for the Neoral soft-gelatin capsule formulation when compared to the Sandimmune soft-gelatin capsule formulation (Mueller et al., 1994a). Greater differences were found in a study of healthy volunteers given higher doses where it was shown that

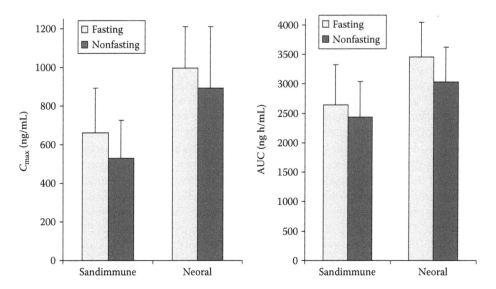

FIGURE 11.7 Comparison of marketed lipid-based cyclosporine formulations, Sandimmune (Olive oil SEDDS) and Neoral™ (Hydrolyzed Corn oil SMEDDS) in patients. (Adapted from Constantinides, P.P., *Pharm. Res.*, 12, 1561–1572, 1995. With permission.)

Neoral maintained dose linearity and improved relative bioavailability up to 239% when compared to Sandimmune (Mueller et al., 1994b). Fasting patients showed a similar trend, and the variability was lower for the Neoral dosage form (Holt et al., 1994). Bioavailability properties between Neoral and Sandimmune are compared graphically in Figure 11.7. While both formulations show a minimal food effect, Neoral shows somewhat higher C_{max} and area-under-the-curve (AUC) values for an equivalent dose in humans, which is attributed to its smaller droplet size after emulsification in the GI tract (Constantinides, 1995). Another example of the importance of particle size in oral lipid-based systems was demonstrated by a study by Myers and Stella (1992). Bioavailability of penclomedine in a 10% trioctanoin emulsion was 10-fold higher than from a solution of drug in the same amount of trioctanoin contained in the emulsion; this difference was attributed to the small particle size of the emulsion.

To gain insight into the phase behavior and dispersion at the atomic level, computational molecular dynamics modeling has been used to model drug dispersion from Type I lipid formulations. Combinations of several lipophilic drugs (acyclovir, danazol, hydrocortisone, ketoprofen, and progesterone) with mono- and dilauroyl glycerides with 0%–75% water were modeled. Phases present and location of the drugs at the interface were simulated; localization of the drugs is driven by the local polar/non-polar and hydrophobic/hydrophilic properties of the drug itself (Warren et al., 2013).

LIPOLYSIS AND LIPID ABSORPTION

In addition to the intrinsic dispersion properties created by choice of formulation components, *in vivo* processing of formulations facilitates dispersion. The digestive system has developed a very efficient mechanism for the breakdown and absorption of fats (Thomson et al., 1993; Embleton and Pouton, 1997; Norskog et al., 2001; Mu and Høy, 2004). Digestion begins in the stomach, initiated by gastric lipases. However, pancreatic lipase found in the small intestine is responsible for the majority of fat digestion. The activity of pancreatic lipase is low and is enhanced by colipase, which is in turn activated by bile acids. Triacylglycerides are hydrolyzed to monoglycerides and fatty acids, which are then rapidly absorbed. The process of triglyceride digestion generates crystalline, liquid crystalline, micellar, and vesicular phases consisting of mono- and diglycerides, fatty acids and calcium-fatty acid salts (Patton et al., 1985; Hernell et al., 1990; Staggers et al., 1990).

The efficiency of the lipases is dependent on the exposed surface area dictated by the number of droplets and their size in fat emulsions (Turnberg and Riley, 1985; Norkskog et al., 2001; Mu and Høy, 2004). This is one reason for the emphasis on dispersibility of lipid-based formulations as a measure of performance. Lipase activity is also a function of the acyl chain lengths, with LCTs hydrolyzed at a slower rate than MCTs (Mu and Høy, 2004). Furthermore, the lipases can be inhibited by surfactants in the formulations (MacGregor et al., 1997). Therefore, improving dispersibility by adding surfactant may not necessarily improve performance of the formulation. One avenue for minimizing the effects of digestion is to develop the LBDDS by formulating with the lipid digestion products, namely fatty acids and mono- and diglycerides.

After digestion, lipids are absorbed by the intestinal enterocyte and the majority are distributed into the portal blood (Mu and Høy, 2004). In addition, long-chain glycerides and fatty acids can contribute to chylomicron formation and enter the lymphatic system, bypassing hepatic first pass metabolism (Shen et al., 2001). Detailed reviews of this effect on improving drug bioavailability have been published (Charman and Stella, 1992; Porter and Charman, 1997). Improving the lymphatic uptake of drugs can affect the clearance of certain highly lipophilic drugs (i.e., those with Log $D > 5$). For example, up to 27% lymphatic uptake of the highly lipophilic antimalarial drug halofantrine from LCT vehicles has been demonstrated (Holm et al., 2003), as was lymphatic uptake of the leukotriene B4 inhibitor ontazolast (Log $D > 4$) dissolved in soybean oil (Hauss et al, 1998). However, the lymphatic route is normally a low capacity route of uptake, and therefore viability is limited to highly potent lipophilic drugs (Log $D > 5$). For this reason, discussions of formulation design and performance presented in this chapter are limited to the processes up to absorption by the enterocyte.

Formulators have recognized the importance of taking into account the role of digestive processes in the performance of LBDDSs, and of characterizing the products from digestion of candidate lipid formulations. *In vitro* assessments of the effects of lipolysis on the performance of lipid-based systems have been developed (Porter and Charman, 2001; Zangenberg et al., 2001a; Christensen et al., 2004; Kaukonen et al., 2004) and show promising correlations with *in vivo* performance (Kossena et al., 2005). While differences exist in digestion medium and specific techniques, the media generally consist of a buffered solution containing calcium salts, bile salt and phosphatidylcholine with digestion by pancreatic lipase (Zangenberg et al., 2001b; Christensen et al., 2004; Porter et al., 2004; Fatouros and Mullertz, 2008). Efforts are in progress by the Lipid Formulation Classification System (LFCS) Consortium to establish standardized *in vitro* tests for LBDDSs, especially in regard to digestion (Williams et al., 2012a,b, 2013, 2014). Recommended standard conditions are a pH 6.5 digestion buffer consisting of 2 mM tris maleate, 150 mM NaCl, 1.4 mM Ca^{2+}, 3 mM sodium taurodeoxycholate, and 0.75 mM phosphatidyl choline. The pancreatic lipase can be supplied as a crude mixture of digestive enzymes (e.g., porcine pancreatin) or, less commonly, in a purified form. The progress of digestion is monitored using a pH-stat titration to monitor fatty acid generation. The interest in monitoring the effects of digestion is to simulate the change in solubilization of the drug as the formulation undergoes chemical and physical (e.g., micelle, vesicle, and liquid crystal) transformation. To do this, the samples after digestion are centrifuged or undergo size exclusion chromatography to separate the various phases, and drug concentration is measured in each (Kossena et al., 2003). Dahan and Hoffman (2008) carried out *in vitro* lipolysis model studies and rat bioavailability studies of formulations of LCT, MCT, short chain triglycerides (SCT), and aqueous suspensions of griseofulvin. Both the *in vitro* and *in vivo* studies showed a rank ordering of drug solubilization of MCT > LCT > SCT > aqueous suspension, with a correlation $r^2 > 0.98$.

Sassene et al. (2014) investigated the effect of varying levels of porcine pancreatin and calcium in *in vitro* lipolysis models with danazol. Increasing pancreatin levels from 150 to 900 USPU increases the total extent of digestion by 51% and 59% for long-chain and medium-chain lipid formulations respectively. Varying calcium levels causes an indirect effect by interacting with digestion products (e.g., precipitating liberated fatty acids), which can lead to drug precipitation. Calcium levels of 1.4 mM are recommended to minimize precipitation, and a pancreatin level of 600 USPU/ml, both of which resemble *in vivo* activity under fasting conditions. While most studies are carried out at pH 6.5 and pancreatic lipase to focus on digestion in the small intestine, Bakala N'Goma et al. (2015) carried out lipolysis studies at lower pH (1.5–5.0) and with gastric lipase. Optimal pH for the gastric lipase was 4–5 and lipolysis was observed for 8 representative lipid formulations. The authors conclude, however, that carrying out standardized studies at pH 6.5 using pancreatic lipase is more practical and meaningful as a comparator for lipid formulations.

Other analytical methods have been successfully used to supplement the findings of *in vitro* digestion experiments and shed light on the mechanisms operating. Phan et al. (2013) removed samples at various points of time (0–60 min) from medium chain triglyceride (Captex® 355) undergoing digestion and examined them by synchrotron small-angle X-ray scattering and cryogenic transmission electron microscopy. The researchers were able to identify the types and structures of the vesicular phases formed upon digestion of the MCT; initially only micelles were present, but after 20–25 min, a lamellar phase was gradually formed. Stillhart et al. (2013) used in-line Raman spectroscopy to examine drug precipitation kinetics during digestion of a fenofibrate SMEDDS formulation composed of Miglyol 812/Imwitor 988/Cremophor RH40 (40/20/40). The Raman spectroscopy results were in good agreement with off-line nanofiltration measurements, and its higher sensitivity and time resolution allowed development of a mathematical model of precipitation kinetics and time-dependent drug solubility during digestion. Buyukozturk et al. (2013) used an electron paramagnetic resonance spin label probe (TEMPOL benzoate, $\log P_{o/w} = 2.46$) as a model of a water-insoluble drug to examine changes in a soybean oil/Tween 80 (1:1) SEDDS formulation. Drug solubility was 8 times higher in the presence of digested lipids, and drug release increased from 9% to 70% as a result of digestion. The method allowed development of a quantitative mechanistic model of drug solubility and partitioning during digestion, and rate constants of digestion, drug dissolution, and release were calculated. Computational models are becoming more important in understanding and optimization of LBDDSs; there were reviewed recently by Alskar and Bergstrom (2015).

Recently it has been appreciated that one of the factors involved in increased intestinal absorption of drugs from LBDDSs is a local supersaturation of drug near the enterocyte membrane, providing a high thermodynamic driving force for absorption. The supersaturation has been proposed to be induced at various stages after ingestion: from initial dispersion; from colloidal species generated after digestion; from structures generated from bile secretion and dilution; and from lipid absorption (Williams et al., 2013c). Drug precipitation due to supersaturation is possible, but studies with danazol, fenofibrate, and tolfenamic acid have indicated that local supersaturation ratios <3 (i.e., up to 3 times the aqueous equilibrium drug solubility) can be tolerated without drug precipitation (Williams et al., 2012b, 2013b), and formulations can be designed accordingly.

Porter et al. (2004) studied the correlation between *in vitro* digestion/solubilization and *in vivo* performance of lipid-based formulations of halofantrine consisting of LCT, MCT, or blends. Earlier studies had suggested that MCT formulations provided greater aqueous phase supersaturation than LCT formulations, and so the researchers anticipated greater absorption at early time-points from the MCT formulation. In fact, the LCT formulation showed enhanced absorption, and the authors demonstrated that the ability to support supersaturation depended on the amount of lipid in their *in vitro* lipolysis assay. Lowering the amount of MCT to 50 mg/10 mL of digest versus 250 mg/10 mL consequently reduced the fraction of vesicles that were better solubilizers for halofantrine than micelles. In comparison, the LCT formulation was able to sustain supersaturation even at the lower lipid levels used.

A final consideration in the absorption of drugs from lipid-based formulations is that many lipophilic compounds are substrates for *P*-glycoprotein (PgP) and for intestinal cytochrome P450 (CyP3A) enzymes (Kaminsky and Fasco, 1991; Seelig and Landwojtowicz, 2000; Wu and Benet, 2005). The former are membrane-bound efflux transporters that transport compounds from the enterocyte back out into the intestinal lumen, while the latter are hydroxylases that metabolize the drug to more polar and likely inactive species (Wacher et al., 1995; Wasan, 2001; Wang et al., 2003). The net effect of PgP is to decrease the absorption of drugs subject to efflux transport. Many of the surfactants listed in Table 11.2, including Cremophor EL, Cremophor RH40, polysorbate 80, and Vitamin E TPGS, are known to be PgP inhibitors in *in vitro* studies when used at high concentrations (Rege et al., 2002; Bogman et al., 2003). It is uncertain, however, whether these surfactants will have a net absorption enhancing effect *in vivo* due to PgP or CyP3A inhibition when used at normal levels. Nevertheless, during formulation development of a new drug candidate, it is important to gain understanding on the involvement of efflux transporters and CyP3A in the drug's absorption, and possibly consider the PgP and CyP3A inhibition properties of surfactants chosen in the formulation. *In vitro* and *in vivo* experiments with SNEDDS formulations of amiodarone and talimol indicate that along with increased solubilization, reduced PgP efflux and inhibition of CyP3A intraenterocyte metabolism contributed to the enhanced bioavailability (Elgart et al., 2013).

Absorption of drugs from LBDDSs can be examined in *ex vivo* models, allowing better *in vitro/in vivo* correlation. Yeap et al. (2013) used a single-pass rat jejunal perfusion model to examine the absorption of cinnarizine and ^{3}H-oleic acid from oleic acid–containing intestinal bile salt mixed micelles. Amiloride was used as an attenuator of the acidic microclimate, as it is a competitive inhibitor of the plasma membrane Na^+/H^+ exchanger. It was found that the acidic microclimate of the unstirred water layer promoted drug absorption from intestinal mixed micelles, and the results support that lipid absorption induces drug supersaturation and hence enhances drug absorption. Similarly, single pass *in situ* intestinal perfusion experiments in rats coupled with *in vitro* lipid digestion models allowed real-time analysis of absorption of fenofibrate from Type IIIA, IIIB, and IV formulations. While drug precipitation was observed *in vitro* resulting from supersaturation, the perfusion experiments showed that absorption still occurred, suggesting that if absorption is rapid enough, supersaturation can promote absorption without precipitation occurring. The authors conclude that the absence of an *absorptive sink* in *in vitro* digestion experiments can lead to under-estimation of *in vivo* performance (Crum et al., 2016).

The next step before clinical trials is testing in animals of candidate formulations to evaluate bioavailability of drugs in lipid-based systems and to assess *in vitro/in vivo* correlations. Rats and dogs have been the species most widely employed, but the pig has more recently been suggested as being more comparable in eating behavior and in GI physiology to humans (O'Driscoll and Griffin, 2008). In a series of soybean oil/long-chain triglyceride/Cremophor EL/ethanol formulations of danazol, it was found that increasing the surfactant/lipid ratio increased drug precipitation *in vitro* in digestion models. Accordingly, formulations with lower surfactant/lipid ratio had higher bioavailability, and a rank order *in vitro/in vivo* correlation was observed (Cuine et al., 2008). Pharmacokinetic aspects and *in vitro/in vivo* correlation trends of LBDDSs have been reviewed (Kollipara and Gandhi, 2014); a number of studies show fair or good correlation between *in vitro* dispersion and *in vivo* bioavailability (e.g. cyclosporin, ritonavir, lopinavir, arundic acid, and fenofibrate), and between correlation between *in vitro* lipolysis and *in vivo* bioavailability (e.g., halofantrine, griseofulvin, cinnarizine, dexamethasone, danazol, probucol, and vitamin D3).

Although this discussion has envisioned a stepwise development of LBDDSs to examine solubilization, dispersion, digestion, and absorption, these processes should not be examined in isolation, since each impacts the other. Furthermore, some surfactants are subject to digestion in the intestinal milieu (Cuine et al., 2008). For example, in studies with Labrasol (PEG-8 Caprylic/Capric glycerides), it was found that gastric lipase digested di-and triglycerides primarily to monoacylglycerols, while pancreatic lipase completed the digestion of PEG, fatty acids, and glycerol (Fernandez et al., 2013). Drug solubilization can either increase (e.g., for Type I formulations) or decrease after digestion. In a study of a Type IIIA cinnarizine SNEDDS formulations in sesame oil/oleic acid/Cremophor RH 40/Brij 97/ethanol (21:15:45:9:10), drug precipitation was observed for SNEDDSs with high loading (50 mg/g, corresponding to 85% saturation), but not at low (12.5 mg/g) loading (Larsen et al., 2013).

With regard to the interaction of solubilization, dispersion, digestion, and absorption, Porter et al. (2008) have outlined seven guidelines for design of lipid-based formulations:

1. It is critical to maintain drug solubility in the formulation after dispersion, and after digestion.
2. Properties of the colloidal species formed after digestive processing are probably more important than properties of the formulation itself in enhancing absorption. Higher proportions of lipid (>60%) and lower proportions of surfactant (<30%) and cosolvent (<10%) generally lead to more robust drug solubilization after dilution and digestion.
3. While MCT may afford greater drug solubility and stability in the formulation, LCT facilitate more efficient formation of bile salt-lipid colloidal species and therefore may yield higher bioavailability.
4. Type IIIB SMEDDS formulations give lower droplet sizes after dispersion. However, they are more dependent on the surfactant properties employed; non-digestible surfactants generally give higher bioavailability.
5. Dispersion of Type IV formulations containing two surfactants with cosolvent is likely to be more efficient than those with a single surfactant.
6. Type IV formulations may give higher drug solubility, but must be designed carefully to avoid drug precipitation after dispersion.

FINAL DOSAGE FORMS OF LIPID-BASED DRUG DELIVERY SYSTEMS

Lipid-based formulations can be (1) ready-to-use emulsions, (2) liquid systems that are either diluted with water or juice before administration, or (3) presented as liquid-filled capsules (Table 11.3). While capsules generally represent the most convenient dosage form, liquids are more acceptable to pediatric and geriatric patient populations. Furthermore, at early stages of drug development, liquid lipid-based formulations provide a relatively rapid means of entering First-in-Human studies due to the ease of manufacture of the formulation. The purpose of First-in-Human studies is generally for proof-of-concept of the drug's safety and efficacy, and the primary goal is usually to reach the clinic as fast as possible. In these studies, for greater patient or volunteer acceptance, it is desirable to dilute the formulation in juice, water, or other aqueous vehicle immediately before dosing; the administration of the resulting emulsion can also lead to more uniform dosing and absorption. If drug stability in the lipid vehicle is inadequate (<6 months) to support manufacture and storage of clinical supplies, it may be possible to extemporaneously prepare the dosage form from drug powder at the clinical site using a *powder-in-bottle* approach. During manufacture, weighed amounts of the drug powder, or a simple solid drug-excipient blend, are filled into the required number of suitable containers; a lipid/surfactant/co-solvent blend is prepared and weighed into other containers. At the clinical site, the drug powder and the lipid mixture are then combined as needed for use.

If time allows, use of liquid-filled capsule formulations in clinical trials provides a smoother transition to commercial dosage forms. Soft-gelatin capsules are most commonly used due to their applicability to a wide variety of liquid lipid vehicles (Jimerson, 1986). For most pharmaceutical companies, the manufacture of soft-gelatin capsule products requires the use of third party manufacturers due to the specialized manufacturing equipment. More recently, filling of liquids into hard gelatin capsules has been described, for example, using Capsugel's Li-Caps® system; this is particularly desirable for early drug development when batch sizes are relatively small (Cade et al., 1986). Compatibility of lipid vehicles with hard and soft-gelatin capsules differs, and must be considered (Cole, 1999). Recently, due to concerns with Bovine spongiform encephalopathy/transmissible spongiform encephalopathy (BSE/TSE) and the related trend to avoid animal-based products, there has been some interest in alternative shell materials such as HPMC, which was recently shown to exhibit *in vivo* disintegration times similar to gelatin capsules (Tuleu et al., 2007).

Lipid-based formulations can also be developed as semisolid formulations, which may be encapsulated in hard-gelatin capsules. Semisolid formulations can be defined as multiphase dispersions with a high proportion of solid mixed with a liquid phase. In general, they are prepared by combining a solid lipid with other liquid components and filling into capsules in the molten state (Walker et al., 1980). Banding or sealing of the capsules is usually necessary to prevent leakage. An additional option is a thixotropic gel semisolid formulation, wherein an agent such as colloidal silicon dioxide provides the matrix to prevent flow of the liquid vehicle. Special considerations and characterization methods for thixotropic formulations have been described (Lombardin et al., 2000). Advantages of semisolids over liquids are that they are more amenable to hard capsules, and may provide greater stability and compatibility between the capsule shells and fills.

Capsule softening, shell brittleness, and leakage of fill are all possible issues that must be monitored. Hydrophilic components (e.g., ethanol, propylene glycol, and glycerol) are particularly prone to lead to fill-shell incompatibilities. Glycerol can be an impurity in some mono- and diglyceride lipid excipients, and levels must be carefully controlled. While semi-solid fills can ameliorate some of the compatibility problems, they have potential physical stability problems, may require more time for development, and may be more difficult to characterize.

Several methods have been developed to transform lipid-based formulations into solid dosage forms that can be tabletted or filled into hard capsules (Cannon, 2005; Jannin et al., 2008; Tang et al., 2008; Tan et al., 2013; Dening et al., 2016). One alternative are solid dispersions, which can be defined as a solid matrix (e.g., polymers or lipids) containing dispersed or dissolved drug. Since there still may be some liquid component in a solid dispersion matrix (especially at temperatures above 37°C), there is a continuum between semisolids and solid dispersions, and there is often no clear distinction between the two types of systems in the literature. While polymers are the most common matrix for solid dispersion formulations (as reviewed by Breitenbach, 2002), solid lipids can also provide the matrix. Relatively high loading can be achieved with solid dispersions, but bioavailability will depend on whether dissolved or amorphous drug is required for absorption. A bio-study in humans for a vitamin E solid dispersion in Gelucire 44/14 melt filled into hard gelatin capsules showed improved bioavailability relative to the commercial product (Figure 11.8) (Barker et al., 2003). Unlike liquids and semisolids, solid dispersions with high melting points have potential to be compressed into tablets. Solid dispersions also can be designed for extended release formulations (Hamdani et al., 2003; Galal et al., 2004). Mixtures of Poloxamer 188 and PEG8000 with lipids (either glycerol or propylene glycol fatty acid monoesters) and drug (either fenofibrate or probucol)

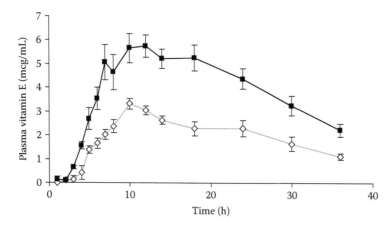

FIGURE 11.8 Plasma vitamin E concentration after oral administration of a vitamin E solid dispersion. Key: (■) PEG-32 glyceryl laurate (Gelucire® 44/14) solid dispersion and (◊) commercial product. (Adapted from Barker, S.A. et al., *J. Control. Rel.*, 91, 477–488, 2003. With permission.)

formed solid dispersions after melting at 75°C and cooling. The formulations showed no phase separation in the solid state and dispersed in water to form globules of 200–600 nm, or in some cases microemulsions, with drug remaining solubilized in the lipid phase. The poloxamer 188 served both as a solidifying agent as well as the emulsifying agent for the lipids (Shah and Serajuddin, 2012). A solid SEDDS formulation was prepared from mixtures of lauroyl polyoxyl glycerides (e.g., Acconon® C-44 and Gelucire® 44/14), medium-chain glycerides (e.g., Captex 355), and Cremophor EL by melting at 65°C and filling into hard gelatin capsules. DSC, powder XRD, and microscopic analysis showed that the drug (probucol) was dissolved in a liquid lipid phase interspersed between a solid phase and there was no crystallization of the drug. Dispersion in water gave emulsion particles that were <650 nm, and no precipitation of the drug from the solid formulations was evident (Patel et al., 2012).

Solid lipid nanoparticles (SLN) have size distributions in the submicron range and are similar in molecular structure to lipid solid dispersions. Manufacturing methods include hot melt homogenization, wherein a drug-lipid melt is emulsified and cooled; cold melt homogenization, wherein a drug-lipid melt is solidified, ground in a powder mill, dispersed, and emulsified; and solvent emulsification, wherein drug and lipid is dissolved in a lipophilic solvent, emulsified, and evaporated (Mehnert and Mader, 2001). A more recent variation are nanostructured lipid carriers (NLC); both SLN and NLC have been reviewed recently (Das and Chaudhury 2011). While the initial application of SLN formulations was parenteral, they have also used in oral administration, and can have a sustained release effect. Cyclosporine/stearic acid SLNs were prepared by hot melt homogenization. After oral administration to rats, the formulation showed a sustained release effect and had 80% of the bioavailability relative to the microemulsion (Zhang et al., 2000). SLNs containing torcetrapib were prepared from glyceryl palmitostearate by an anti-solvent precipitation method. The SLNs had an 11.6-fold increase in AUC in rats compared to torcetrapib powder, with a t_{max} of 1 h (Liu et al., 2015). SLNs with paclitaxel-loaded were prepared from stearylamine, soy lecithin, and poloxamer 188 by a modified solvent injection. A particle size of ~100 nm could be achieved; oral administration to mice gave a t_{max} of 6 h, compared to 2 h for paclitaxel solution, with a 6.4-fold improvement in AUC (Pandita et al., 2011).

There are several reports of solid SEDDS formulations formed from adsorption of lipid and surfactant on silicates. Liquid mixtures of medium chain glyceride (Capmul MCM and/or Captex 355) and surfactant (Cremophor EL) containing probucol were adsorbed onto Neusilin US2, a silicate that also contains other oxides such as magnesium, aluminum, and calcium oxide. At a ratio of 1:1 Neusilin/liquid, solid SEDDS powders could be prepared that had acceptable flow and compaction properties and could be compressed into tablets (Gumaste et al., 2013). A solid SEDDS of curcumin was prepared by spray-drying Aerosil 200 with drug dissolved in an oil phase of Lauroglycol/Labrasol/Transcutol. Administration of the solid SEDDS to rats gave a higher bioavailability compared to curcumin powder, with 4.6 and 7.6 times the C_{max} and AUC, respectively (Yan et al., 2011).

Other possible designs for solid dosage forms of oral lipid-based formulations include liquid–solid compacts and dry emulsions (Cannon, 2005; Tan et al., 2013). In the preparation of liquid–solid compacts, drug is dissolved in a non-aqueous solvent and adsorbed onto a solid carrier. Examples of solid carriers used include silica nanoparticles or microparticles, polysaccharide, polymers (Tan et al., 2013), and mesoporous inorganic materials (Dening et al., 2016). The resulting solid can be compressed into tablets or filled into capsules. An example is a Coenzyme Q10 self-emulsifying mixture containing lemon oil, Cremophor EL, and Capmul MCM adsorbed onto a maltodextrin/Avicel carrier (Nazzal et al., 2002). In the dry emulsion or solid-state emulsion approach, the drug is first dissolved in a lipophilic solvent, which is combined with an aqueous phase containing bulking agents (cryoprotectants) and homogenized to form an emulsion. Water is then removed by lyophilization, spray drying, or a similar drying method; the resulting dry powder can be filled into capsules or compressed into tablets. Examples of drugs formulated by this approach include hydrochlorthiazide

(Corvelyn and Remon, 1998), Vancomycin (Shively and Thompson, 1995), theophylline (Chambin et al., 2000), amlodipine (Jang et al., 2006), lovastatin (Ge et al., 2008), and indomethacin (Hamoudi et al., 2012; Wang et al., 2010). Both the liquid–solid compact and dry emulsion approaches have the disadvantage of low drug loading due to the requirement for the solid carrier, unless the drug itself is an oil (e.g., for vitamin E) (Takeuchi et al., 1991) and valproic acid (Cannon, 2005).

Use of these semisolid and solid approaches can potentially alleviate the chemical stability problems sometimes observed for liquid-filled formulations, and may eventually offer the possibility of development of a tablet dosage form using conventional equipment. Liquid lipid-based formulations, however, generally afford the greatest enhancement of bioavailability for water-insoluble drugs, as well as affording more rapid development for First-in-Human studies. Any decisions on the best formulation route would have to be evaluated on a case-by-case basis.

A commercial formulation must be robust, capable of reproducible and easily controlled manufacture, have minimal batch-to-batch variation in composition, characteristics, and performance. In earlier stages, characterization tests are primarily for functional performance, and assess drug solubility in the vehicle, dispersion characteristics, and bioavailability. Stability studies verify that there was minimal loss of drug potency and no significant change in these functional characteristics. These tests are still important at later stages, but must be complemented or replaced by those that best identify sources of batch-to-batch variability, monitor critical manufacturing parameters, and give meaningful specifications. Analytical tests and characterizations used at earlier stages of development will not necessarily be those tests that are suitable to set specifications.

Clinical studies of drugs with oral lipid-based formulations have been reviewed by Fatouros et al. (2007). Besides those listed in Table 11.3, drugs that have been examined using oral LBDDSs in clinical trials include atovaquone, clomethiazole, danazol, diazepam, dicumarol, flufenamic acid, griseofulvin, fenretinide, nitrofurantoin, paclitaxel, quingestrone, ubiquinone, retinyl palmitate, and tocotrienols.

CHALLENGES WITH LBDDS FORMULATIONS FOR DRUG SOLUBILIZATION AND DELIVERY

PHYSICAL STABILITY AND GELATIN COMPATIBILITY

Among the challenges often encountered when preparing lipid-based formulations is physical stability. With liquid formulations, a problem that is not uncommon includes interaction with and leakage from the capsule shell. Hydrophilic components such as glycerol (frequently a minor component found in lipid excipients), propylene glycol, ethanol, and water can migrate between the capsule shells and fills. The resulting change in shell composition can result in capsule brittleness or softening, impairing the capsule's physical integrity and potentially changing the dissolution profile of the product. Cole (1999) has compiled information on compatibility of excipients with hard gelatin capsules. In addition, the change in fill contents could alter the solubility of the drug in the fill, potentially leading to precipitation of drug and loss of bioavailability.

Additional challenges can arise with semisolid formulations, since they are dynamic systems containing both liquid and solid phases. Crystallinity of the matrix must be considered; this can be highly dependent on lipid purity and chain length distribution, as well as lipid polymorphism. For example, glycerides can exhibit a hexagonal (α) phase, an orthorhombic (β') phase, and a triclinic (β) phase (Mehnert and Mader, 2001). The latter is the most stable polymorph whereas the first two are metastable phases but nevertheless common. The manufacturing conditions (e.g., mixing, melting, and cooling rates) and storage conditions can affect the ratios of the polymorphs. Furthermore, crystallization of the matrix generally enhances drug crystallization, which can negatively affect *in vitro* and *in vivo* behavior. It is always important to monitor the crystalline nature of the drug and excipients by appropriate techniques during development [e.g., differential scanning calorimetry (DSC), powder X-ray diffraction (XRD), hot stage microscopy, Fourier transform infrared (FTIR), and FT-Raman]. Even when the formulation initially contains micronized solid drug and gives adequate bioavailability, the dynamic nature of semisolid formulations can eventually lead to an increase in drug particle size, with an adverse effect on bioavailability.

CHEMICAL STABILITY: TYPICAL MECHANISMS OF OXIDATION AND GELATIN CROSS-LINKING

As detailed in Part I, the two most important mechanisms that give rise to chemical instability of the components in lipid-based formulations are hydrolysis (for those components containing ester bonds) and oxidation (for unsaturated lipids and oxygen labile cosolvents and surfactants, for example, PEG 400 and Labrafil M2125 CS). The use of PEG-based surfactants and unsaturated lipids in lipid-based formulations make lipid peroxidation especially likely (Cannon 2005; Stella, 2013). While the products of lipid peroxidation can give rise to drug instability, a chief concern is that aldehyde products can react with the gelatin shell of both hard and soft-gel capsules; leading to cross-linking that can retard dissolution. Figure 11.9 shows the effect of various levels of aldehydes on gelatin cross-linking and the resultant change in dissolution profiles (Gold et al., 1997). Assay of aldehyde products and gelatin cross-linking should be considered for lipid-based formulations. In general, appropriate specifications for lipid and surfactant purity and source, and if necessary, use of antioxidants are critical for maintaining product stability.

As mentioned, hydrolysis is the other important mechanism by which some lipids (glycerides and phosphoglycerides) degrade and can lead to a reduction in pH due to liberation of free fatty acids; this was discussed in Chapter 10 (Part I: Parenteral Application). This phenomenon is less important for oral formulations when compared to parenteral products, since the former generally have low amounts of water in the formulation. Hydrolysis could occur on storage if water is absorbed from or through the gelatin shell.

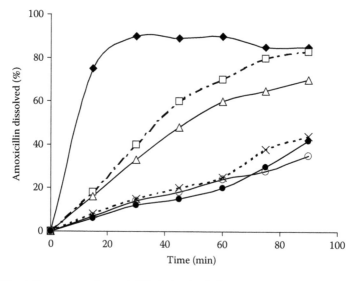

FIGURE 11.9 Dissolution curves of amoxicillin in hard gelatin capsules exposed to 150 ppb formaldehyde for various times. Key: (♦) control, (□) 2.25 h, (△) 4.60 h, (×) 9.42 h, (○) 16.0 h, and (●) 24.0 h. (From Gold, T.B. et al., *Pharm. Res.*, 14, 1046–1050, 1997.)

TOXICOLOGICAL CONSIDERATIONS FOR ORAL LIPID-BASED DRUG DELIVERY SYSTEMS

Compared to parenteral formulations, toxicity is rarely a concern for oral lipid-based formulations. Most lipids discussed here are considered generally recognized as safe (GRAS); indeed, long-chain tri-, di-, and monoglycerides are absorbed from foods in greater quantities than those administered in pharmaceutical dosage forms. Although there are reports that MCTs can accelerate small bowel transit time and induce diarrhea (Verkijk et al., 1997), dietary consumption of up to 1 g/kg of MCTs has been shown to be safe in human clinical trials (Traul et al., 2000). Toxicity of surfactants used in lipid-based formulations varies; levels should be kept within reported acceptable limits. In addition to toxicology, for lipid formulations administered orally as liquids, specialized efforts from the standpoint of taste, flavor and mouth feel must be considered.

CONCLUSIONS AND FUTURE PERSPECTIVES

While there has been much promise in the area of oral lipid-based formulations, there are several avenues of future research that will expand the utility of these systems. Although there are a number of excipients that can be used to prepare these formulations (Tables 11.1 and 11.2), novel lipids, and related substances for use in lipid formulations would be an important aid to future formulators. Desired attributes of new excipients would be enhanced solubilization of drug candidates across a wide range of drug properties; favorable toxicological profiles; stability; ease of manufacture; availability of adequate specifications and controls on purity; and compatibility with other lipids, surfactants, and capsule shells. It must be recognized that there are significant hurdles for approval of new excipients, and approval of a new excipient must generally be tied to that of a new drug product, which requires close cooperation between the pharmaceutical and excipient companies. A recent example of approval of a new excipient for lipid-based formulations is d-α-tocopheryl polyethylene glycol 1000 succinate (vitamin E TPGS, Eastman), first used in formulating the protease inhibitor Agenerase (amprenavir; GlaxoSmithKline). Vitamin E TPGS increased the solubility and permeability of amprenavir, and the resulting absorption enhancement by the excipient was regarded as essential to the development of the soft-gelatin capsule product for this HIV protease inhibitor (Yu et al., 1999).

An additional need is for improved methods of characterization of lipid-based formulations. In particular, although considerable progress has been made due to efforts of the LFCS consortium, there is still a need for improvements for *in vitro* characterization methods to provide *in vitro/in vivo* correlations. Owing to the need for sink conditions in dissolution methods required for regulatory submissions, surfactants must typically be added to the medium to achieve adequate drug solubility. This may alter the dispersion behavior of the formulation such that it is not predictive of the dispersion behavior *in vivo*. While traditional dissolution methods are probably adequate as quality control measures to assess batch-to-batch variability of an already developed formulation, other methods to measure dispersion behavior may be more suitable as a screening tool to compare a number of formulations. Possible methods include combination dissolution/Caco II models (Ginski and Polli, 1999; Kataoka et al., 2006) or dialysis methods such as the rotating dialysis cell (Takahashi et al., 1994). In addition, the extensive work underway to characterize the fate of drug on digestion of LBDDSs should provide new insight for development of simpler *in vitro* methods.

In conclusion, the recent increase in the number of water-insoluble drug candidates will doubtless enhance the importance of oral lipid-based formulations in the coming years. If a candidate has adequate solubility in the vehicles described in this chapter, lipid-based systems will usually provide an attractive approach for efficient in-house development of clinical and commercial formulations.

Table of Registered Trademarks

Name	Company
Accutane®	Roche Laboratories Inc., Nutley, New Jersey
Agenerase®	GlaxoSmithKline, Research Triangle Park, North Carolina
Capmul®; Captex®	Abitec Corp, Columbus,Ohio
Cremophor®; Pluronic®	BASF, Mount Olive, New Jersey
Depakene®	Abbott Laboratories, North Chicago, Illinois
Gelucire®; Labrafac®; Labrafil®; Labrasol®; Lauroglycol®	Gattefosse SAS, St. Priest Cedex, France
Imwitor®; Miglyol®	Cremer Oleo GMBH, Hamburg, Germany
Myrj®; SPAN®; Tween®	Uniqema North America Inc., Chicago, Illinois
Neobee®	Stepan Company, Northfield, Illinois
Neoral®; Sandimmune®	Novartis Pharmaceuticals Corporation, East Hanover, New Jersey
Phosal®; Phospholipon®	Lipoid GMBH, Steinhausen, Switzerland

REFERENCES

Abraham, M. H. and J. Le. (1999). The correlation and prediction of the solubility of compounds in water using an amended solvation energy relationship. *J. Pharm. Sci.*, 88: 868–880.

Abrams, L. S., H. S. Weintraub, J. E. Patrick, and J. L. McGuire. (1978). Comparative bioavailability of a lipophilic steroid. *J. Pharm. Sci.*, 67: 1287–1290.

Alfons, K. and S. Engstrom. (1998). Drug compatibility with the sponge phases formed in monoolein, water, and propylene glycol or poly(ethylene glycol). *J. Pharm. Sci.*, 87: 1527–1607.

Alskär, L. C. and C. A. S. Bergström. (2015). Models for predicting drug absorption from oral lipid-based formulations. *Curr. Mol. Bio. Rep.*, 1: 141–147.

Armstrong, N. A. and K. C. James. (1980). Drug release from lipid-based dosage forms. II. *Int. J. Pharm.*, 6: 195–204.

Bakala-N'Goma, J. C., H. D. Williams, P. J. Sassene, K. Kleberg, M. Calderone, V. Jannin, et al. (2015). Toward the establishment of standardized in vitro tests for lipid-based formulations. 5. Lipolysis of representative formulations by gastric lipase. *Pharm. Res.*, 32: 1279–1287.

Barker, S. A., S. P. Yap, K. H. Yuen, C. P. McCoy, J. R. Murphy, and D. Q. M. Craig. (2003). An investigation into the structure and bioavailability of alpha-tocopherol dispersions in Gelucire. *J. Control. Rel.*, 91: 477–488.

Bell, S. J. et al. (1997). The new dietary fats in health and disease. *J. Am. Dietetic Assoc.*, 97: 280–288.

Bogman, K., F. Erne-Brand, J. Alsenz, and J. Drewe. (2003). The role of surfactants in the reversal of active transport mediated by multidrug resistance proteins. *J. Pharm. Sci.*, 92: 1250–1261.

Bravo González, R. C., J. Huwyler, I. Walter, R. Mountfield, and B. Bittner. (2002). Improved oral bioavailability of cyclosporin A in male Wistar rats comparison of a Solutol HS 15 containing self-dispersing formulation and a microsuspension. *Int. J. Pharm.*, 245: 143–151.

Breitenbach, J. (2002). Melt extrusion: From process to drug delivery technology. *Eur. J. Pharm. Biopharm.*, 54: 107–117.

Buchanan, M. et al. (2000). Kinetic pathways of multiphase surfactant systems. *Phys. Rev. E: Stat. Phys., Plasm., Fluids, Relat. Interdisc. Topics*, 62: 6895–6905.

Bummer, P. M. (2004). Physical chemical considerations of lipid-based oral drug delivery—solid lipid nanoparticles. *Crit. Rev. Therap. Drug Carrier Syst.*, 21: 1–19.

Burcham, D. L. et al. (1997). Improved oral bioavailability of the hypocholesterolemic DMP 565 in dogs following oral dosing in oil and glycol solutions. *Biopharm. Drug Disp.*, 18: 737–742.

Buyukozturk, F., S. Di Maio, D. E. Budil, and R. L. Carrier. (2013). Effect of ingested lipids on drug dissolution and release with concurrent digestion: A modeling approach *Pharm. Res.*, 30: 3131–3144.

Cade, D., E. T. Cole, J. P. Mayer, and F. Wittwer. (1986). Liquid filled and sealed hard gelatin capsules. *Drug. Dev. Ind. Pharm.*, 12: 2289–2300.

Cannon, J. (2005). Oral solid dosage forms of lipid-based drug delivery systems. *Am. Pharm. Rev.*, 8: 108–113.

Cao, Y. et al. (2004). Predictive relationships for the effects of triglyceride ester concentration and water uptake on solubility and partitioning of small molecules into lipid vehicles. *J. Pharm. Sci.*, 93: 2768–2779.

Carrigan, P. J. and T. R. Bates. (1973). Biopharmaceutics of drugs administered in lipid containing dosage forms. I. GI absorption of griseofulvin from an oil-in-water emulsion in the rat. *J. Pharm. Sci.*, 62: 1476–1479.

Chafetz, L. et al. (1984). Decrease in the rate of capsule dissolution due to formaldehyde from Polysorbate 80 autoxidation. *J. Pharm. Sci.*, 73: 1186–1187.

Chambin, O., C. Bellone, D. Champion, M. H. Rochat-Gonthier, and Y. Poucelot. (2000). Dry adsorbed emulsion: I. characterization of an intricate physicochemical structure. *J. Pharm. Sci.*, 89: 991–999.

Charman, W. N. (2000). Lipids, lipophilic drugs, and oral drug delivery—some emerging concepts. *J. Pharm. Sci.*, 89: 967–978.

Charman, W. N. and V. J. Stella. (1992). *Lymphatic Transport of Drugs*, CRC Press, Boca Raton, FL.

Charman, W. N. et al. (1997). Physicochemical and physiological mechanisms for the effects of food on drug absorption: The role of lipids and pH. *J. Pharm. Sci.*, 86: 269–282.

Charman, W. N., M. C. Rogge, A. W. Boddy, and B. M. Berger. (1993). Effect of food and a monoglyceride emulsion formulation on danazol bioavailability. *J. Clin. Pharmacol.*, 33: 381–386.

Christensen, J. O. et al. (2004). Solubilisation of poorly water-soluble drugs during *in vitro* lipolysis of medium- and long-chain triacylglycerols. *Eur. J. Pharm. Sci.*, 23: 287–296.

Cole, E. (1999). Liquid filled and sealed hard gelatin capsules. Technical report, Capsugel, *Arlesheim, Switzerland*.

Constantinides, P. P. (1995). Lipid microemulsions for improving drug dissolution and oral absorption: Physical and biopharmaceutical aspects. *Pharm. Res.*, 12: 1561–1572.

Corvelyn, S. and J. P. Remon. (1998). Formulation of a lyophilized dry emulsion tablet for poorly soluble drugs. *Int. J. Pharm.*, 166: 65–74.

Crum, M. F., N. L. Trevaskis, H. D. Williams, C. W. Pouton, and C. J. Porter. (2016). A new in vitro lipid digestion in vivo absorption model to evaluate the mechanisms of drug absorption from lipid-based formulations. *Pharm. Res.*, 33: 970–982.

Cuiné, J. F., W. N. Charman, C. W. Pouton, G. A. Edwards, and C. J. Porter. (2007). Increasing the proportional content of surfactant (Cremophor EL) relative to lipid in self-emulsifying lipid-based formulations of danazol reduces oral bioavailability in beagle dogs. *Pharm. Res.*, 24: 748–757.

Cuine, J. F., C. L. McEvoy, W. N. Charman, C. W. Pouton, G. A. Edwards, H. Benameur, and C. J. Porter. (2008). Evaluation of the impact of surfactant digestion on the bioavailability of danazol after oral administration of lipidic self-emulsifying formulations to dogs. *J. Pharm. Sci.*, 97: 995–1012.

Dahan, A. and A. Hoffman, (2008). Rationalizing the selection of oral lipid based drug delivery systems by an in vitro dynamic lipolysis model for improved oral bioavailability of poorly water soluble drugs. *J. Control. Release*, 129: 1–10.

Das, S. and A. Chaudhury. (2011). Recent advances in lipid nanoparticle formulations with solid matrix for oral drug delivery. *AAPS Pharm. Sci. Tech.*, 12: 62–76.

Dening, T. J., S. Rao, N. Thomas, and C. A. Prestidge. (2016). Novel nanostructured solid materials for modulating oral drug delivery from solid state lipid based drug delivery systems. *AAPS J.*, 18: 23–40.

Elgart, A., I. Cherniakov, Y. Aldouby, A. J. Domb, and A. Hoffman. (2013). Improved oral bioavailability of BCS class 2 compounds by self nano-emulsifying drug delivery systems (SNEDDS): The underlying mechanisms for amiodarone and talinolol *Pharm. Res.*, 30: 3029–3044.

Embleton, J. K. and C. W. Pouton. (1997). Structure and function of gastro-intestinal lipases. *Adv. Drug Del. Rev.*, 25: 15–32.

Fatouros, D. G. and A. Mullertz. (2008). In vitro lipid digestion models in design of drug delivery systems for enhancing oral bioavailability. *Expert Opin. Drug Metab. Toxicol.*, 4: 65–76.

Fatouros, D. G., D. M. Karpf. F. S. Nielsen, and A. Mullertz. (2007). Clinical studies with oral lipid based formulations of poorly soluble compounds. *Ther. Clin. Risk Manag.*, 3: 591–604.

Fernandez, S., V. Jannin, S. Chevrier, Y. Chavant, F. Demarne, and F. Carrière. (2013). In vitro digestion of the self-emulsifying lipid excipient Labrasol® by gastrointestinal lipases and influence of its colloidal structure on lipolysis rate *Pharm. Res.*, 30: 3077–3087.

Fleisher, D. et al. (1999). Drug, meal and formulation interactions influencing drug absorption after oral administration. *Clin. Pharmacokinet.*, 36: 233–254.

Friberg, S. E. and R. L. Venable. (1983). Microemulsions. In *Encyclopedia of Emulsion Technology*, P. Becher, (Ed.), Vol. I, Marcel Dekker, New York, p. 287.

Galal, S., A. A. El Massik, O. Y. Abdallah, and N. A. Daabis. (2004). Study of *in vitro* release of carbamazepine extended release semi-solid matrix filled capsules based on Gelucires. *Drug Dev. Ind. Pharm.*, 30: 817–829.

Gao, P. et al. (2003). Development of a supersaturable SEDDS (S-SEDDS) formulation of paclitaxel with improved oral bioavailability. *J. Pharm. Sci.*, 92: 2386–2398.

Gao, P. et al. (2004). Application of a mixture experimental design in the optimization of a self-emulsifying formulation with a high drug load. *Pharm. Dev. Tech.*, 9: 301–309.

Garti, N. et al. (2001). Improved oil solubilization in oil/water food grade microemulsions in the presence of polyols and ethanol. *J. Agric. Food Chem.*, 49: 2552–2562.

Ge, Z., X. Zhang, L. Gan, and Y. Gan. (2008). Redispersible, dry emulsion of lovastatin protects against intestinal metabolism and improves bioavailability. *Acta Pharmacol. Sin.*, 29: 990–997.

Gelbart, W. M. and A. Ben-Shaul. (1996). The "new" science of "complex fluids." *J. Phys. Chem.*, 100: 13169–13189.

Gershanik, T. and S. Benita. (2000). Self-dispersing lipid formulations for improving oral absorption of lipophilic drugs. *Eur. J. Pharm. Biopharm.*, 50: 179–188.

Ginski, M. J. and J. E. Polli. (1999). Prediction of dissolution–absorption relationships from a dissolution/Caco-2 system. *Int. J. Pharm.*, 177: 117–125.

Gold, T. B., R. G. Bruice, R. A. Lodder, and G. A. Digenis. (1997). Determination of the extent of formaldehyde-induced cross-linking in hard gelatin capsules by near-infrared spectrophotometry. *Pharm. Res.*, 14: 1046–1050.

Goldring, J. (2009). Novel excipients: The next pharmaceutical frontier. *Amer. Pharm. Rev.*, 12: 56–59.

Greiner, R. W. and D. F. Evans. (1990). Spontaneous formation of a water-continuous emulsion from a w/o microemulsion. *Langmuir*, 6: 1793–1796.

Griffin, W. C. (1949). Classification of surface-active agents by "HLB." *J. Soc. Cos. Chem.*, 1: 311–326.

Gumaste, S.G., D. M. Dalrymple, and A. T. M. Serajuddin. (2013). Development of solid SEDDS, V: Compaction and drug release properties of tablets prepared by adsorbing lipid-based formulations onto Neusilin® US2. *Pharm. Res.*, 30: 3186–3199.

Hamdani, J., A. Moes, and K. Amighi. (2003). Physical and thermal characterization of Precirol and Compritol as lipophilic glycerides used for the preparation of controlled-release matrix pellets. *Int. J. Pharm.*, 260: 47–57.

Hamoudi, M. C., F. Bourasset, V. Domergue-Dupont, C. Gueutin, V. Nicolas, E. Fattal et al. (2012). Formulations based on alpha cyclodextrin and soybean oil: An approach to modulate the oral release of lipophilic drugs. *J. Cont. Release.*, 161: 861–867.

Handbook of Pharmaceutical Excipients. (1994). American Pharmaceutical Association. The Pharmaceutical Press, London. pp. 371, 375, 379, 473, 481.

Hauss, D. J., S. E. Fogal, J. V. Ficorilli, C. A. Price, T. Roy, A. A. Jayara, and J. J. Keirns. (1998). Lipid-based delivery systems for improving the bioavailability and lymphatic transport of a poorly water-soluble LTB4 inhibitor. *J. Pharm. Sci.*, 87: 164–169.

Hellweg, T. (2002). Phase structures of microemulsions. *Curr. Opin. Coll. Interf. Sci.*, 7: 50–56.

Hernell, O. et al. (1990). Physical–chemical behavior of dietary and biliary lipids during intestinal digestion and absorption. 2. Phase analysis and aggregation states of luminal lipids during duodenal fat digestion in healthy adult human beings. *Biochemistry*, 29: 2041–2056.

Holm, R., C. J. H. Porter, G. A. Edwards, A. Mullertz, H. G. Kristensen, and W. N. Charman. (2003). Examination of oral absorption and lymphatic transport of halofantrine in a triple-cannulated canine model after administration in self-microemulsifying drug delivery systems (SMEDDS) containing structured triglycerides. *Eur.J. Pharm. Sci.*, 20: 91–97.

Holt, D. W., E. A. Mueller, J. M. Kovarik, J. B. van Bree, and K. Kutz. (1994). The pharmacokinetics of Sandimmun Neoral: A new oral formulation of cyclosporine. *Transplant Proc.*, 26: 2935–2939.

Holt, D. W. and A. Johnston. (1997). Cyclosporin microemulsion. A guide to usage and monitoring. *BioDrugs*, 7: 175–197.

Hörter, D. and J. B. Dressman. (1997). Influence of physicochemical properties on dissolution of drugs in the gastrointestinal tract. *Adv. Drug Del. Rev.*, 25: 3–14.

Humberstone, A. J. and W. N. Charman. (1997). Lipid-based vehicles for the oral delivery of poorly water soluble drugs. *Adv. Drug Del. Rev.*, 25: 103–128.

Jandacek, R. J. et al. (1987). The rapid hydrolysis and efficient absorption of triglycerides with octanoic acid in the 1 and 3 positions and long-chain fatty acid in the 2 position. *Am J. Clin. Nutr.*, 45: 940–945.

Jang, D. J., E. J. Jeong, H. M. Lee, B. C. Kim, S. J. Lim, and C. K. Kim. (2006). Improvement of bioavailability and photostability of amlodipine using redispersible dry emulsion. *Eur. J. Pharm. Sci.*, 28(5): 405–411.

Jannin, V., J. Musakhanian, and D. Marchaud. (2008). Approaches for the development of solid and semi-solid lipid-based formulations. *Adv. Drug Deliv. Rev.*, 60: 734–746.

Jantratid, E., N. Janssen, H. Chokshi, K. Tang, and J. B. Dressman. (2008). Designing biorelevant dissolution tests for lipid formulations: Case example—lipid suspension of RZ-50. *Eur. J. Pharm. Biopharm.*, 69: 776–785.

Jimerson, R. F. (1986). Soft gelatin capsule update. *Drug. Dev. Ind. Pharm.*, 12: 1133–1144.

Kalepu, S., M. Manthina, and V. Padavala. (2013). Oral lipid-based drug delivery systems—An overview *Acta Pharm Sinica B*, 3: 361–372.

Kaminsky, L. S. and M. J. Fasco. (1991). Small intestinal cytochromes P450. *Crit. Rev. Toxicol.*, 21: 407–422.

Kataoka, M. et al. (2006). Effect of food intake on the oral absorption of poorly water-soluble drugs: *In vitro* assessment of drug dissolution and permeation assay system. *J. Pharm. Sci.*, 95: 2051–2061.

Kaukonen, A. M. et al. (2004). Drug solubilization behavior during *in vitro* digestion of simple triglyceride lipid solution formulations. *Pharm. Res.*, 21: 245–253.

Khoo, S.-M. et al. (1998). Formulation design and bioavailability assessment of lipidic self-emulsifying formulations of halofantrine. *Int. J. Pharm.*, 167: 155–164.

Khoo, S.-M. et al. (2000). The formulation of halofantrine as either non-solubilizing PEG 6000 or solubilizing lipid based solid dispersions: Physical stability and absolute bioavailability assessment. *Int. J. Pharm.*, 205: 65–78.

Kollipara, S. and R. K. Gandhi. (2014). Pharmacokinetic aspects and in vitro–in vivo correlation potential for lipid-based formulations. *Acta Pharm. Sin. B.*, 4: 333–349.

Kossena, G. A. et al. (2003). Separation and characterization of the colloidal phases produced on digestion of common formulation lipids and assessment of their impact on the apparent solubility of selected poorly water-soluble drugs. *J. Pharm. Sci.*, 92: 634–648.

Kossena, G. A. et al. (2005). Influence of the intermediate digestion phases of common formulation lipids on the absorption of a poorly water-soluble drug. *J. Pharm. Sci.*, 94: 481–492.

Kuentz, M. and D. Röthlisberger. (2002). Determination of the optimal amount of water in liquid-fill masses for hard gelatin capsules by means of texture analysis and experimental design. *Int. J. Pharm.*, 236: 145–152.

Larsen, A. T., P. Åkesson, A. Juréus. L. Saaby. R. Abu-Rmaileh. B. Abrahamsson, J. Østergaard, and A. Müllertz. (2013). Bioavailability of cinnarizine in dogs: Effect of SNEDDS loading level and correlation with cinnarizine solubilization during in vitro lipolysis. *Pharm. Res.*, 30: 3101–3113.

Laughlin, R. (1994). *The Aqueous Phase Behavior of Surfactants*. Academic Press, London.

Lawrence, M. J. (1996). Microemulsions as drug-delivery vehicles. *Curr. Opin. Coll. Interface Sci.*, 1: 826–832.

Lide, D. R. (Ed.). (1993). *CRC Handbook of Chemistry and Physics*, 74th edition. CRC Press, Boca Raton, FL, pp. 8–46.

Liu Y., G. M. Salituro, K. J. Lee, A. Bak, and D. H. Leung. (2015). Modulating drug release and enhancing the oral bioavailability of torcetrapib with solid lipid dispersion formulations. *AAPS PharmSciTech.*, 16: 1091–1100.

Lombardin, P., M. Seiller, E. Leverd, E. Goutay, J. Bougaret, and J. L. Grossiord. (2000). Study of thixotropic bases for the filling of hard capsules. *STP Pharm. Sci.*, 10: 429–437.

López-Montilla, J. C. et al., (2002). Spontaneous emulsification: Mechanisms, physicochemical aspects, modeling, and applications. *J. Disp. Sci. Tech.*, 23: 219–268.

Lovell, M. W., H. W. Johnson, H.-W. Hui, J. B. Cannon, P. K. Gupta, and C. C. Hsu. (1994). Less-painful emulsion formulations for intravenous administration of clarithromycin. *Int. J. Pharm.*, 109: 45–57.

MacGregor, K. J. et al. (1997). Influence of lipolysis on drug absorption from the gastro-intestinal tract. *Adv. Drug Del. Rev.*, 25: 33–46.

Malcolmson, C. et al. (1998). Effect of oil on the level of solubilization of testosterone propionate into nonionic oil-in-water microemulsions. *J. Pharm. Sci.*, 87: 109–116.

Mehnert, W. and K. Mader. (2001). Solid lipid nanoparticles: Production, characterization, and applications. *Adv. Drug Del. Rev.*, 47: 165–196.

Mengesha, A. E., R. J. Wydra, J. Z. Hilt, and P. M. Bummer. (2013). Binary blend of glyceryl monooleate and glyceryl monostearate for magnetically induced thermo-responsive local drug delivery system. *Pharm. Res.*, 30: 3214–3224.

Miller, C. A. (1988). Spontaneous emulsification produced by diffusion—a review. *Coll. Surf.*, 29: 89–102.

Mu, H. and C.-E. Høy. (2004). The digestion of dietary triacylglycerols. *Prog. Lipid Res.*, 43: 105–133.

Mueller, E. A. et al. (1994a). Improved dose linearity of cyclosporine pharmacokinetics from a microemulsion formulation. *Pharm. Res.*, 11: 301–304.

Mueller, E. A. et al. (1994b). Pharmacokinetics and tolerability of a microemulsion formulation of cyclosporine in renal allograft recipients—a concentration-controlled comparison with the commercial formulation. *Transplantation*, 57: 1178–1182.

Myers, R. A. and V. J. Stella. (1992). Factors affecting the lymphatic transport of penclomedine (NSC-338720), a lipophilic cytotoxic drug: Comparison to DDT and hexachlorobenzene. *Int. J. Pharm.*, 80: 51–62.

Nanjwade, B. K., D. J. Patel, R. A. Udhani, and F. V. Manvi. (2011). Functions of lipids for enhancement of oral bioavailability of poorly water-soluble drugs. *Sci Pharm.*, 79: 705–727.

Nazzal, S., M. Nutan, A. Palamakula, R. Shah, A. A. Zaghloul, and M. A. Khan. (2002). Optimization of a self-nanoemulsified tablet dosage form of Ubiquinone using response surface methodology: Effect of formulation ingredients. *Int. J. Pharm.*, 240: 103–114.

Nicolaides, E. et al. (1999). Forecasting the *in vivo* performance of four low solubility drugs from their *in vitro* dissolution data. *Pharm. Res.*, 16: 1877–1883.

Nishimi, T. and C. A. Miller. (2000). Spontaneous emulsification of oil in Aerosol-OT/water/hydrocarbon systems. *Langmuir*, 16: 9233–9241.

Norkskog, B. K. et al. (2001). An examination of the factors affecting intestinal lymphatic transport of dietary lipids. *Adv. Drug Del. Rev.*, 50: 21–44.

O'Driscoll, C. M. and B. T. Griffin. (2008). Biopharmaceutical challenges associated with drugs with low aqueous solubility—the potential impact of lipid-based formulations. *Adv Drug Deliv Rev.*, 60: 617–624.

Pandita, D., A. Ahuja, V. Lather, B. Benjamin, T. Dutta, T. Velpandian, and R. K. Khar. (2011). Development of lipid-based nanoparticles for enhancing the oral bioavailability of paclitaxel. *AAPS Pharm Sci Tech.*, 12: 712–722.

Patel, N., N. Hetal, H. N. Prajapati, D. D. Dalrymple, and A. T. M. Serajuddin. (2012). Development of Solid SEDDS, II: Application of Acconon® C-44 and Gelucire® 44/14 as solidifying agents for self-emulsifying drug delivery systems of medium chain triglyceride. *J. Excipients Food Chem.*, 3: 54–66.

Patton, J. S. et al. (1985). The light microscopy of triglyceride digestion. *Food Microstruct.*, 4: 29–41.

Persson, L. C., C. J. H. Porter, W. N. Charman, and C. A. S. Bergström, (2013). Computational prediction of drug solubility in lipid based formulation excipients. *Pharm. Res.*, 30: 3225–3237.

Phan, S., A. Hawley, X. Mulet, L. Waddington, C. A. Prestidge, and B. J. Boyd. (2013). Structural aspects of digestion of medium chain triglycerides studied in real time using sSAXS and Cryo-TEM. *Pharm. Res.*, 30: 3088–3100.

Physicians Desk Reference. (2007). Thompson PDR staff (eds.), PDR® Electronic Library, Thomson MICROMEDEX. Montvale, NJ, Physician's Desk Reference.

Porter, C. J., C. W. Pouton, J. F. Cuine, and W. N. Charman. (2008). Enhancing intestinal drug solubilisation using lipid-based delivery systems. *Adv. Drug Deliv. Rev.*, 60: 673–691.

Porter, C. J. H. and W. N. Charman. (1997). Uptake of drugs into the intestinal lymphatics after oral administration. *Adv. Drug Del. Rev.*, 25: 71–89.

Porter, C. J. H. and W. N. Charman. (2001). *In vitro* assessment of oral lipid based formulations. *Adv. Drug Del. Rev.*, 50: S127–S147.

Porter, C. J. H. et al. (2004). Use of *in vitro* lipid digestion data to explain the *in vivo* performance of triglyceride-based oral lipid formulations of poorly water-soluble drugs: Studies with halofantrine. *J. Pharm. Sci.*, 93: 1110–1121.

Porter, C. J. H., H. D. Williams, and N. L. Trevaskis. (2013). Recent advances in lipid-based formulation technology. *Pharm. Res.*, 30: 2971–2975.

Pouton, C. W. (2006). Formulation of poorly water-soluble drugs for oral administration: Physicochemical and physiological issues and the lipid formulation classification system. *Eur. J. Pharm. Sci.*, 29: 278–287.

Pouton, C. W. (1997). Formulation of self-emulsifying drug delivery systems. *Adv. Drug Del. Rev.*, 25: 47–58.

Pouton, C. W. (2000) Lipid formulations for oral administration of drugs: Non-emulsifying, self-emulsifying and "self-microemulsifying" drug delivery systems. *Eur. J. Pharm. Sci.*, 11 (Suppl. 2): S93–S98.

Rang, M-J. and C. A. Miller. (1999). Spontaneous emulsification of oils containing hydrocarbon, nonionic surfactant, and oleyl alcohol. *J. Coll. Interface Sci.*, 209: 179–192.

Rege, B. D., J. P. Kao, and J. E. Polli. (2002) Effects of nonionic surfactants on membrane transporters in Caco-2 cell monolayers. *Eur.J. Pharm. Sci.*, 16: 237–246.

Ritschel, W. A. (1996). Microemulsion technology in the reformulation of cyclosporine: The reason behind the pharmacokinetic properties of Neoral. *Clin. Transplant.*, 10: 364–373.

Robson, H., D. Q. M. Craig, and D. Deutsch. (2000). An investigation into the release of cefuroxime axetil from taste-masked stearic acid microspheres. II. The effects of buffer composition on drug release. *Int. J. Pharm.*, 195: 137–145.

Ruelle, P. and U. W. Kesselring. (1994). Solubility predictions for solid nitriles and tertiary amides based on the mobile order theory. *Pharm. Res.*, 11: 201–205.

Sakai, K., T. Yoshimori, K. Obata, and H. Maeda. (2010). Design of self-microemulsifying drug delivery systems using a high-throughput formulation screening system. *Drug Dev. Ind. Pharm.*, 36: 1245–1252.

Sassene, P., K. Kleberg, H. D. Williams, J. C. BakalaN'Goma, F. Carrière, M. Calderone et al. (2014). Toward the establishment of standardized in vitro tests for lipid-based formulations, part 6: Effects of varying pancreatin and calcium levels. *AAPS J.*, 16: 1344–1357.

Seelig, A. and E. Landwojtowicz. (2000). Structure–activity relationship of P-glycoprotein substrates and modifiers. *Eur. J. Pharm. Sci.*, 12: 31–40.

Serajuddin, A. T. M. et al. (1986). Water migration from soft gelatin capsule shell to fill material and its effect on drug solubility. *J. Pharm. Sci.*, 75: 62–64.

Serajuddin, A. T. M. et al. (1988). Effect of vehicle amphiphilicity on the dissolution and bioavailability of a poorly water-soluble drug from solid dispersions. *J. Pharm. Sci.*, 77: 414–417.

Shah, A. V. and A. T. Serajuddin. (2012). Development of solid self-emulsifying drug delivery system (SEDDS) I: Use of poloxamer 188 as both solidifying and emulsifying agent for lipids. *Pharm Res.*, 29: 2817–2832.

Shahba, A. A., K. Mohsin, and F. K. Alanazi. (2012). Novel self-nanoemulsifying drug delivery systems (SNEDDS) for oral delivery of cinnarizine: Design, optimization, and in-vitro assessment. *AAPS Pharm. Sci. Tech.*, 13: 967–977.

Shahidzadeh, N. et al. (2000). Dynamics of spontaneous emulsification for fabrication of oil in water emulsions. *Langmuir*, 16: 9703–9708.

Shen, H. et al. (2001). From interaction of lipidic vehicles with intestinal epithelial cell membranes to the formation and secretion of chylomicrons. *Adv. Drug Del. Rev.*, 50: S103–S125.

Shively, M. L. and D. C. Thompson. (1995). Oral bioavailability of vancomycin solid-state emulsions. *Int. J. Pharm.*, 117: 119–122.

Staggers, J. E. et al. (1990). Physical–chemical behavior of dietary and biliary lipids during intestinal digestion and absorption. 1. Phase behavior and aggregation states of model lipid systems patterned after aqueous duodenal contents of healthy adult human beings. *Biochemistry*, 29: 2028–2040.

Stella, V. J. (2013). Chemical drug stability in lipids, modified lipids, and polyethylene oxide-containing formulations. *Pharm. Res.*, 30: 3018–3028.

Stillhart, C., G. Imanidis, and M. Kuentz. (2013). Insights into drug precipitation kinetics during in vitro digestion of a lipid-based drug delivery system using in-line Raman Spectroscopy and mathematical modeling. *Pharm. Res.*, 30: 3114–3130.

Strey, R. (1994). Microemulsion microstructure and interfacial curvature. *Coll. Polym. Sci.*, 272: 1005–1019.

Strickley, R. G. (2004). Solubilizing excipients in oral and injectable formulations. *Pharm. Res.*, 21: 201–230.

Tahibi, S. E. and S. L. Gupta. (2000). Soft gelatin capsules development. In R. Liu, (Ed.) *Water Insoluble Drug Formulation*. Interpharm Press, Englewood, CO, pp. 609–633.

Takahashi, M., M. Mochizuki, K. Wada, T. Itoh, and M. Goto, (1994). Studies on dissolution tests of soft gelatin capsules. Part 5. Rotating dialysis cell method. *Chem. Pharm. Bull.*, 42: 1672–1675.

Takeuchi, H., H. Saski, T. Niwa, T. Hino, Y. Kawashima, K. Uesugi, M. Kayano, and Y. Miyake. (1991). Preparation of a powdered redispersible vitamin E acetate emulsion by spray-drying. *Chem. Pharm. Bull.*, 39: 1528–1531.

Tan, A., S. Rao, and C. A. Prestidge. (2013). Transforming lipid-based oral drug delivery systems into solid dosage forms: An overview of solid carriers, physicochemical properties, and biopharmaceutical performance. *Pharm. Res.*, 30: 2993–3017.

Tang, B., G. Cheng, J. C. Gu, and C. H. Xu. (2008). Development of solid self-emulsifying drug delivery systems: Preparation techniques and dosage forms. *Drug Discov. Today*, 13: 606–612.

Thomson, A. B. R. et al. (1993). Lipid absorption: Passing through the unstirred layers, brush-border membrane, and beyond. *Can. J. Physiol. Pharmacol.*, 71: 531–555.

Traul, K. A., A. Driedger, D. L. Ingle, and D. Nakhasf. (2000). Review of the toxicologic properties of medium-chain triglycerides. *Food Chem. Toxicol.*, 38: 79–98.

Trotta, M. (1999). Influence of phase transformation on indomethacin release from microemulsions. *J. Contr. Rel.*, 60: 399–405.

Trull, A. K. et al. (1993). Cyclosporine absorption from microemulsion formulation in liver transplant recipient. *Lancet*, 341: 433.

Tuleu, C., M. K. Khela, D. F. Evans, B. E. Jones, S. Nagata, and A. W. Basit. (2007). A scintigraphic investigation of the disintegration behavior of capsules in fasting subjects: A comparison of hypromellose capsules containing carrageenan as a gelling agent and standard gelatin capsules. *Eur. J. Pharm. Sci.*, 30: 251–255.

Turnberg, L. A. and S. A. Riley. (1985). Digestion and absorption of nutrients and vitamins. In *Handbook of Physiology*. Oxford Press, New York, pp. 977–1008.

Van Os, N. M. et al. (1993). *Physio-Chemical Properties of Selected Anionic, Cationic and Nonionic Surfactants*. Elsevier Science Publishers, Amsterdam, The Netherlands, p. 301.

Verkijk, M., J. Vecht, H. A. J. Gielkens, C. Lamers, and A. Masclee. (1997). Effects of medium-chain and long-chain triglycerides on antroduodenal motility and small bowel transit time in man. *Dig. Diseases Sci.*, 42: 1933–1939.

Von Corswant, C. et al. (1997). Microemulsions based on soybean phosphatidylcholine and triglycerides. Phase behavior and microstructure. *Langmuir*, 13: 5061–5070.

Wacher, V. J., C.-Y. Wu, and L. Z. Benet. (1995). Overlapping substrate specificities and tissue distribution of cytochrome P450 3A and P-glycoprotein: Implications for drug delivery and activity in cancer chemotherapy. *Mol. Carcinog.*, 13: 129–134.

Walker, S. E., J. A. Ganley, K. Bedford, and T. Eaves. (1980). The filling of molten and thixotropic formulations into hard gelatin capsules. *J. Pharm. Pharmacol.*, 32: 389–393.

Wang, J., Y. Hu, L. Li, T. Jiang, S. Wang, and F. Mo. (2010). Indomethacin-5-fluorouracil-methyl ester dry emulsion: A potential oral delivery system for 5-fluorouracil. *Drug Dev. Ind. Pharm.*, 36: 647–656.

Wang, R. B., C. L. Kuo, L. L. Lien, and E. J. Lien. (2003). Structure activity relationship: Analysis of P-glycoprotein substrates and inhibitors. *J. Clin. Pharm. Ther.*, 28: 203–228.

Warren, D. B., D. King, H. Benameur, C. W. Pouton, and D. K. Chalmers. (2013). Glyceride lipid formulations: Molecular dynamics modeling of phase behavior during dispersion and molecular interactions between drugs and excipients. *Pharm. Res.*, 30: 3238–3253.

Wasan, K. M. (2001). Formulation and physiological and biopharmaceutical issues in the development of oral lipid-based drug delivery systems. *Drug Dev. Ind. Pharm.*, 27: 267–276.

Williams, H. D., M. U. Anby, P. Sassene, K. Kleberg, J. C. BakalaN'Goma, M. Calderone, et al. (2012b). Toward the establishment of standardized in vitro tests for lipid-based formulations. 2. The effect of bile salt concentration and drug loading on the performance of type I, II, IIIA, IIIB, and IV formulations during in vitro digestion. *Mol. Pharm.*, 9: 3286–3300.

Williams, H. D., P. Sassene, K. Kleberg, J. C. BakalaN'Goma, M. Calderone, V. Jannin et al. (2012a). Toward the establishment of standardized in vitro tests for lipid-based formulations, part 1: Method parameterization and comparison of in vitro digestion profiles across a range of representative formulations. *Pharm. Sci.*, 101: 3360–3380.

Williams, H. D., P. Sassene, K. Kleberg, M. Calderone, A. Igonin, E. Jule, et al. (2014). Toward the establishment of standardized in vitro tests for lipid-based formulations, part 4: Proposing a new lipid formulation performance classification system. *J. Pharm. Sci.*, 103: 2441–2455.

Williams, H. D., P. Sassene, K. Kleberg, M. Calderone, A. Igonin, E. Jule. et al. (2013b). Toward the establishment of standardized in vitro tests for lipid-based formulations, Part 3: Understanding supersaturation versus precipitation potential during the in vitro digestion of Type I, II, IIIA, IIIB and IV lipid-based formulations. *Pharm. Res.*, 30: 3059–3076.

Williams, H. D., N. L. Trevaskis, S. A. Charman, R. M. Shanker, W. N. Charman, C. W. Pouton, and C. J. Porter, (2013a). Strategies to address low drug solubility in discovery and development. *Pharmacol. Rev.*, 65: 3154–3199.

Williams, H. D., N. L. Trevaskis, Y. Y. Yeap, M. U. Anby, C. W. Pouton, and C. J. H. Porter, (2013c). Lipid-based formulations and drug supersaturation: Harnessing the unique benefits of the lipid digestion/absorption pathway. *Pharm. Res.*, 30: 2976–2992.

Wu, C.-Y. and L. Z. Benet, (2005). Predicting drug disposition via application of BCS: Transport/absorption/elimination interplay and development of a biopharmaceutics drug disposition classification system. *Pharm. Res.*, 22: 11–23.

Wu, S. H. and W. K. Hopkins, (1999). Characteristics of D-alpha tocopheryl PEG 1000 succinate for applications as an absorption enhancer in drig delivery systems. *Pharm. Tech.*, 23: 52–58.

Yan, Y. D., J. A. Kim, M. K. Kwak, B. K. Yoo, C. S. Yong, H. G. Choi. (2011). Enhanced oral bioavailability of curcumin via a solid lipid-based self-emulsifying drug delivery system using a spray-drying technique. *Biol Pharm Bull.*, 34: 1179–1186.

Yeap, Y. Y., N. L. Trevaskis, and C. J. H. Porter, (2013). Lipid absorption triggers drug supersaturation at the intestinal unstirred water layer and promotes drug absorption from mixed micelles. *Pharm. Res.*, 30: 3045–3058.

Yu, L., A. Bridgers, J. Polli, A. Vickers, S. Long, A. Roy, R. Winnike, and M. Coffin. (1999). Vitamin E-TPGS increases absorption flux of an HIV protease inhibitor by enhancing its solubility and permeability. *Pharm. Res.*, 16: 1812–1817.

Zangenberg, N. H. et al. (2001a). A dynamic *in vitro* lipolysis model I. Controlling the rate of lipolysis by continuous addition of calcium. *Eur. J. Pharmaceut. Sci.*, 14: 115–122.

Zangenberg, N. H., A. Mullertz, H. G. Kristensen, and L. Hovgaard. (2001b). A dynamic in vitro lipolysis model. II: Evaluation of the model. *Eur. J. Pharm. Sci.*, 14: 237–244.

Zhang, Q., G. Yie, Y. Li, Q. Yang, and T. Nagai. (2000). Studies on the cyclosporin A loaded stearic acid nanoparticles. *Int. J. Pharm.*, 200: 153–159.

Zourab, S. M. and C. A. Miller. (1995). Equilibrium and dynamic behavior for systems containing nonionic surfactants, n-hexadecane, triolein and oleyl alcohol. *Coll. Surf.*, 95: 173–183.

12 Micellization and Drug Solubility Enhancement

*Rong (Ron) Liu, Rose-Marie Dannenfelser,
Shoufeng Li, and Zhanguo Yue*

CONTENTS

The ability of surfactants to enhance the solubility of poorly water-soluble compounds in an aqueous solution is widely known and used in many aspects of drug formulation development (Florence, 1981; Sweetana and Akers, 1996). For example, surfactants are used as wetting agents to improve tablet dissolution (Buckton et al., 1991; Efentakis et al., 1991; Chen and Zhang, 1993; Ruddy et al., 1999; Chen et al., 2015) and are commonly used in the media for dissolution testing to maintain sink conditions for the drug (Nagata et al., 1979; Crison et al., 1997; Rao et al., 1997; Desai et al., 2014; Deng et al., 2017). In addition, biologically relevant surfactants, bile salts as well as lecithin, can form mixed micelles that are responsible for solubilization and transport of fats and oils during digestion and likely facilitate dissolution and transport of poorly water-soluble drugs in the intestinal fluid (Humberstone et al., 1996; Kossena et al., 2003, 2004; Zhang et al., 2016).

Enhancement of the aqueous solubility by surfactants occurs as a result of the dual nature of the surfactant molecule. The term *surfactant* is derived from the concept of a surface-active agent. Surfactants typically contain discrete hydrophobic and hydrophilic regions, which allow them to orient at polar–nonpolar interfaces, such as water/air interfaces. Once the interface is saturated, the surfactants self-associate to form micelles and other aggregates, whereby their hydrophobic regions are minimized and shielded from aqueous contact by their hydrophilic regions. This creates a discrete hydrophobic environment suitable for solubilization of many hydrophobic compounds (Attwood and Florence, 1983; Li et al., 1999; Zhao et al., 1999).

Solubilization of drugs in micellar solutions has been investigated extensively. Excellent reviews on this topic can be found in the literature (Florence, 1981; Attwood and Florence, 1983; Ahmad et al., 2014). The benefits of micellar solutions as drug delivery vehicles arise mainly from the solubilization power of surfactants and thus the elimination of dissolution as a rate-limiting step in the process for absorption. They may also reduce toxicity caused by administering neat drug and improve stability of labile drugs. Nevertheless, there are disadvantages to formulating with surfactants, such as their own toxicity and low achievable drug load (Lawrence, 1994). Some of these deficiencies are being addressed by the development of amphiphilic block copolymers and other polymeric surfactants, which also form micellar aggregates consisting of a hydrophobic core surrounded by a hydrophilic corona (Kataoka et al., 1993, 1996; Kwon and Okano, 1996, 1999; Pasquali et al., 2005; Wei et al., 2013). In addition, less-toxic alternatives to the more common hydrocarbon surfactants have been developed (Meinert et al., 1992; Zuberi et al., 1997; Zuberi et al., 1999). The choice of a particular system for pharmaceutical development is largely dependent on the drug and the intended application (i.e., route of administration, solubilization, and/or absorption enhancement, stabilization of drug and toxicity buffering).

The scope of this chapter is to describe the use of surfactants to enhance aqueous solubility of water-insoluble drugs through micellar solubilization. In their book *Surfactant Systems*, Attwood and Florence (1983) provide a comprehensive reference for the use of surfactants in drug formulation development. The treatment by Florence (1981) of drug solubilization in surfactant systems is more focused on the question at hand and provides a clear description of surfactant behavior and solubilization in conventional hydrocarbon-based surfactants, especially nonionic surfactants. This chapter will discuss the conventional surfactant micelles in general as well as update the reader on recent practical/commercial solubilization applications utilizing surfactants. Other uses of surfactants as wetting agents, emulsifiers, and surface modifiers, and for other pharmaceutical applications are not emphasized. Readers can refer to other chapters in this book for details on these uses of surfactants. Polymeric surfactant micelles will be discussed in Chapter 13, "Micellization and Drug Solubility Enhancement Part II: Polymeric Micelles."

CLASSIFICATION OF TRADITIONAL SURFACTANTS

Traditional or conventional surfactants are made up of two discrete regions: a hydrophobic portion often referred to as the *tail* and a hydrophilic *head* group. The hydrophobic portion of these surfactants is commonly made up of straight- or branched-hydrocarbon chains, which may include cyclic or aromatic moieties. The hydrocarbon tails are normally flexible, and when aggregated, present a fluid hydrocarbon environment for the solubilization of hydrophobic materials (Tanford, 1980). Surfactant molecules with less than ten alkyl groups tend to be inefficient as solubilizing agents and those with more than eighteen alkyl groups are generally too insoluble to be effective. Tails consisting of fluorocarbons and hydrofluorocarbons are also available; however, their toxicity precludes them from use in pharmaceutical formulations (Kissa, 1994). Surfactant structures other than the traditional head/tail arrangement also exist. For instance, bile salts have a less common planar structure where the steroidal backbone presents a hydrophobic face and the reverse face is hydrophilic (Small et al., 1969). For traditional surfactants, the chemical nature of the hydrophilic portion (head group) provides the most useful way of characterizing or classifying surfactants. This allows the division of surfactants into four groups: nonionic, anionic, cationic, and zwitterionic.

NONIONIC SURFACTANTS

The head groups of these surfactant molecules contain no charged moieties, with their hydrophilic properties due to the presence of hydroxyl groups. Nonionic surfactants are most frequently used in pharmaceutical systems because of their compatibility with other formulation excipients, stability, and low toxicity. They can be divided into those that are water soluble and those that are water insoluble. Some examples of water-insoluble nonionic surfactants include long-chain fatty acid analogs such as fatty alcohols, glyceryl esters, and fatty acid esters. Fatty alcohols act as coemulsifiers in the presence of more hydrophilic amphiphiles, while glyceryl esters are mostly used in topical preparations. Fatty acid esters of, for example, cholesterol, sucrose, and sorbitan, find a wide range of applicability in pharmaceutical systems. These compounds may include unsaturated groups or aromatic moieties. To increase the water solubility of these compounds, polyoxyethylene (POE) groups are added through an ether linkage with one of the alcohol groups. Among the most widely used water-soluble surfactants are POE sorbitan fatty acid esters, which are commonly found in oral, parenteral, and topical pharmaceutical formulations.

ANIONIC SURFACTANTS

The head groups of these surfactant molecules are negatively charged. The most widely used anionic surfactants are those containing carboxylate groups, such as soaps, sulfonate, and sulfate ions. Soaps, which are salts of weak carboxylic acids, are formed by the hydrolysis of fats (triglycerides) by sodium hydroxide. Sulfonates, such as sodium docusate and decane sulfonate, have been widely used in pharmaceutical systems. The most popular alkyl sulfate is sodium lauryl sulfate, which is commonly used as an emulsifier and solubilizer in pharmaceutical systems. Unlike the sulfonates, sulfates are susceptible to hydrolysis, resulting in the formation of long-chain alcohols; thus pH control is essential for solutions containing sulfate surfactants. The degree of water solubility is greatly influenced by the length of the alkyl chain and the presence of double bonds. Multivalent ions, such as calcium and magnesium, can significantly decrease the water solubility of anionic surfactants, even those with a small alkyl chain length. In addition, mixed micelles of binary surfactant mixtures consisting of nonionic/nonionic and cationic/nonionic surfactants have been studied including chain length effect of the hydrophobic moiety on solubility (Chatterjee et al., 2006).

CATIONIC SURFACTANTS

Head groups of surfactants that ionize to yield a positive ion are classified as cationic. Some examples include amine, quaternary ammonium, and pyridiniumions. These surfactants are most commonly available as the halide salt form, for example, cetyltrimethylammonium bromide (CTAB), and are compatible with nonionic and amphotericin surfactants. Cationic surfactants cannot be used with anionic surfactants because they interact to form water-insoluble salts. Negatively charged substrates, such as skin, hair, glass, and many types of microorganisms strongly absorb positively charged surfactants. Quaternary amines retain their positive charge regardless of pH of solution. The use of cationic surfactants in pharmaceutical systems is generally limited to antimicrobial preservation. Their toxicity is due to the ability of cations to adsorb readily into cell membrane structures in a nonspecific manner, leading to cell lysis (including red blood cells), which destroy bacteria and fungi (Schott, 1995).

ZWITTERIONIC SURFACTANTS

Zwitterionic surfactants (such as amino acids, betaines, carnitines, and phosphatidylcholines) carry both a negatively and a positively charged moiety, and are pH-dependent. At high pH, they behave as anionic surfactants; at low pH, they behave as cationic surfactants; at intermediate pH values, they exhibit both anionic and cationic properties and have a neutral charge. Most of the molecules in this category are those containing carboxylate or phosphate groups as the anion and amino or quaternary ammonium groups as the cation. These long-chain amphoteric molecules are more surface active than ionic surfactants having the same hydrophobic groups, and are particularly useful as emulsifiers. Some examples include acrylic acid derivatives, such as alkylaminopropionic acids, substituted alkylamides, and phosphatides such as phospholipids. Phospholipids like lecithin are good emulsifiers for lipids and cholesterol. In the gastrointestinal tract, phospholipids combine with glycerides, fatty acids, and bile salts to form mixed micelles, which are effective solubilizers for cholesterol (Carey, 1983; Jin et at., 2014).

NONTRADITIONAL SURFACTANTS

BILE SALTS

Salts of cholic acid and its derivatives are known as bile salts. Bile salts are unlike traditional surfactants in that they are rigid and have multiple polar moieties on one side of the molecule thus exhibiting surface activity.

DRUGS

There are drug molecules themselves that resemble surfactant molecules with polar and nonpolar regions exhibiting surface-active properties. These drugs can thus self-associate and form small aggregates or micelles. Examples of drugs that are surface active include dexverapamil-HCl (Surakitbanharn et al., 1995), ibuprofen, and benzocaine.

THERMODYNAMICS

SURFACES AND INTERFACES

Concepts of surfaces and interfaces are described before the discussion of conventional surfactants to better understand surfactant behavior. A surface or an interface is a boundary between at least two immiscible phases, such as water and air. Geometrically, it is obvious that only a single surface can exist between two immiscible phases. If three phases are present, only a single line can be common among the various elements (Figure 12.1). Five basic types of interfaces exist. These include the solid–vapor (S/V), solid–liquid (S/L), solid–solid (S/S), liquid–vapor (L/V), and liquid–liquid (L/L) interfaces. The major impact of surface-active agents on the physical properties of a system will be found where at least one phase is liquid. Molecules at an interface have physical properties distinct from those of the bulk and, as a result, a definite free energy is associated with each unit of interfacial area. In particular, atoms and molecules located at an interface will experience significantly different force fields from those in the bulk because of different numbers and types of neighboring atoms and molecules. In a recent research study (Kalekar and Bhagwat, 2006), adsorption of various surfactants at the vapor liquid interface was studied with equilibrium and dynamic surface tension measurements; a new parameter is defined to quantify the dynamic behavior of adsorption, which gives the concentration of surfactant needed to reduce surface tension to half of its maximum reduction within a defined time available for adsorption.

One characteristic of phase boundaries, especially those involving an aqueous phase, is the probable existence of an electrical potential across the interface. Although such charge phenomena are not always present, when in existence, they have an enormous impact on system properties. Charge effects are usually most important in aqueous suspensions, emulsions, foams, aerosols, and other dispersions in which one phase is finely divided in another phase, creating a large interfacial area.

MODELING OF MICELLIZATION AND SOLUBILIZATION

The experimentally derived empirical expressions used in models such as the mass-action framework have contributed greatly to the logical selection of surfactants for efficient and effective solubilization of drugs. However, there is currently a need to develop more efficient, less toxic surfactants for use in drug delivery. A model that is able to provide quantitative prediction of the critical micelle concentration and micelle size without the need for extensive experimental measurements would greatly accelerate the development of novel surfactant chemistries for use in pharmaceutical applications.

Surfactant molecules, as illustrated in Figure 12.2a, are composed of a polar head that is compatible with water and a nonpolar or hydrophobic hydrocarbon tail that is compatible with oil. This dual

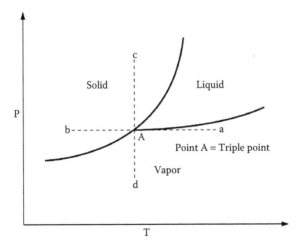

FIGURE 12.1 Illustration of a general temperature–pressure phase diagram.

nature endows the surfactants with their unique solution and interfacial characteristics. The most noteworthy characteristic is the behavior in dilute aqueous solutions, where the surfactant molecules self-assemble to form aggregates. This allows the segregation of the hydrophobic portions from water (Nagarajan and Ruckenstein, 1991). In dilute surfactant solutions, the polar head groups of the surfactant molecules are generally arranged in an outer spherical shell, while the hydrocarbon chains are oriented toward the center, forming a spherical core (Figure 12.2a). Various molecular architectures can result from this self-assembly. Depending on the type of surfactant and the solution conditions, the aggregates may be spherical, globular, or rodlike or have the structure of

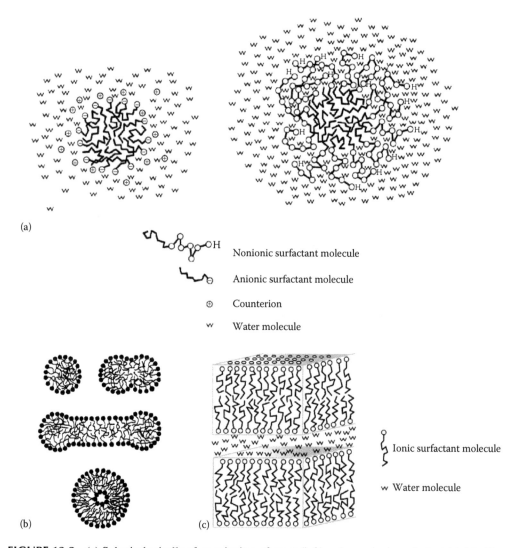

FIGURE 12.2 (a) Spherical micelle of an anionic surfactant (left) and a nonionic surfactant (right). (From Schott, H., Colloidal dispersions, in *Remington: The Science and Practice of Pharmacy*, ed. A. R. Gennaro, Vol. 1, Mack Publishing Co, Easton, PA, 1995. With permission.); (b) schematic representation of the structures of surfactant aggregates in dilute aqueous solutions. Shown are aggregates that are spherical, globular, and spherocylindrical micelles and spherical bilayer vesicles. (Reprinted with permission from Nagarajan, R. and Ruckenstein, E., *Langmuir,* 7, 2934–2969, 1991. Copyright 1991 American Chemical Society.); (c) lamellar mesophases of an ionic surfactant. (From Schott, H., Colloidal dispersions, in *Remington: The Science and Practice of Pharmacy*, A. R. Gennaro (Ed.), Vol. 1, Mack Publishing Co, Easton, PA, 1995. With permission.)   *(Continued)*

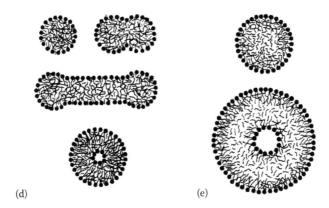

(d) (e)

FIGURE 12.2 (Continued) (d) schematic representation of solubilization of hydrophobic molecules in surfactants giving rise to type I aggregates, referred to as swollen aggregates. The solubilizates are present in the surfactant tail region which extends over the entire volume of the aggregate. The smaller dimension characterizing the aggregate is limited by the length of the surfactant tail. (Reprinted with permission from Nagarajan, R. and Ruckenstein, E., *Langmuir*, 7, 2934–2969, 1991. Copyright 1997 American Chemical Society.), and (e) structure of surfactant aggregates wherein the type II mode of solubilization occurs, also referred to as microemulsions. In these structures, the solubilizates are present both within surfactant tail region and in a domain made up of only the solubilizate. The solubilizate domain constitutes the core of the aggregate in the first structure shown and is a spherical shell region separating the two surfactant layers in the second structure shown. The dimensions of the aggregates are not limited by the extended length of the surfactant tail. (Reprinted with permission from Nagarajan, R. and Ruckenstein, E., *Langmuir*, 7, 2934–2969, 1991. Copyright 1997 American Chemical Society.)

spherical bilayers. The closed aggregates with hydrophobic interiors are known as micelles, whereas the spherical bilayers containing an encapsulated aqueous phase are called vesicles (Figure 12.2b).

In the spherical and spherocylindrical models represented by Figure 12.2a and b, the hydrocarbon chains that form the micellar interior are nonpolar and fluid. The representations of micelles in dilute solutions as perfect spheres or cylinders are *idealized* models (Lieberman et al., 1996). Examples of surfactants that form spherical micelles are sodium laureate ($C_{11}H_{23}COO^-Na^+$), sodium dodecyl sulfate ($C_{12}H_{25}SO_4^-Na^+$), and CTAB ($C_{16}H_{33}N^+(CH_3)_3Br^-$) (Mukerjee, 1979).

As micelles become larger, they have been shown to become more asymmetric, with their shape changing from spherical to cylindrical and lamellar. In lamellar mesophases (Figure 12.2c), the surfactant molecules are arranged in parallel sheets with the hydrocarbon tails forming the inner layers. The water is stratified between the sheets, hydrating the external polar head groups (Schott, 1995).

One of the distinguishable features of aqueous surfactant solutions is their ability to enhance the solubility of hydrophobic solutes that have otherwise very poor solubilities in water. This solubilization is a consequence of the presence of hydrophobic domains in the surfactant aggregates that act as compatible microenvironments for the location of hydrophobic solutes. The enhanced solubility of a hydrophobic solute has been found to be orders of magnitude larger than its aqueous solubility in the absence of surfactants (Nagarajan and Ruckenstein, 1991). The shape of the aggregates containing solutes may be similar to those in the absence of solubilization if the solute molecules are entirely located in the region of the surfactant tails. This mode of solubilization is designated as type I by Nagarajan and Ruckenstein (1991), and are referred to as swollen aggregates (Figure 12.2d). Alternately, the solute molecules may consist of a domain within the interior of the aggregates as well as being present among the surfactant tails. This mode of solubilization is designated as type II by the authors (Nagarajan and Ruckenstein, 1991), and are referred to as microemulsions (Figure 12.2e). Interested readers should refer to Nagarajan and Ruckenstein's article (1991) for more detailed theoretical modeling and prediction. More discussion on solubilization can be found in the related section in this chapter.

THERMODYNAMIC FUNCTIONS

Surfactants are compounds that exhibit surface activity, or more generally, interfacial activity, and migrate to the interface when placed in solution. This migration results in lowering the solution surface tension (interfacial tension) as compared to the surface tension of the pure solvent. Thermodynamically, adsorption of a surfactant is defined by the Gibbs adsorption equation:

$$\Gamma_2 = -\frac{a}{RT}\frac{d\gamma}{da} \qquad (12.1)$$

where Γ_2 is the excess surface concentration of a solute relative to the bulk solution, γ is the surface tension, a is the solute activity, R is the gas constant, and T is the temperature in degrees Kelvin (Lieberman et al., 1996). On the basis of this equation any material that reduces the free energy of the surface phase of a two-component system is a surfactant (Equation 12.4). The amphiphilic nature of surfactant molecules is responsible for their tendency to concentrate and align at interfaces and thereby reduce the free energy of the system in which they interact. Furthermore, their alignment at interfaces, with their hydrophobic tails in the air, and hydrophilic heads in the water, reflects the tendency of surfactant molecules to assume the most energetically favored orientation.

The primary mechanism for energy conservation is adsorption of surfactant molecules at various available interfaces. However, when, for instance, the water–air interface is saturated conservation may continue through other means (Figure 12.3). One such example is the crystallization or precipitation of the surfactant from solution, in other words, bulk phase separation. Another example is the formation of molecular aggregates or micelles that remain in solution as thermodynamically stable,

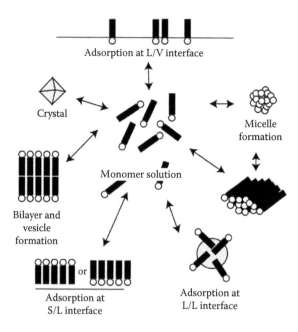

FIGURE 12.3 Modes of surfactant action for the reduction of surface and interfacial energies. (From Myers, D., Micellization and association, *Surfactant Science and Technology*, 2nd ed., D. Myers (Ed.), VCH Publishers, New York, 1992. With permission.)

dispersed species with properties distinct from those of an isotropic solution containing monomeric surfactant molecules (Myers, 1992).

Micelles are dynamic structures where a frequent exchange of monomers between micelles and the bulk solution occurs. Thermodynamics of the self-assembly of surfactants or aggregates is determined by the free energy of transfer of a surfactant monomer from water to the micelle.

Several models have been developed to interpret micellar behavior (Mukerjee, 1967; Lieberman et al., 1996). Two models, the mass-action and phase-separation models are described here in more detail. In the mass-action model, micelles are in equilibrium with the unassociated surfactant or monomer. For nonionic surfactants with an aggregation number of n, the mass-action model predicts that n molecules of monomeric nonionized surfactants, S, react to form a micelle, M:

$$nS \Leftrightarrow M \qquad (12.2)$$

with its equilibrium constant for micelle formation given as

$$K_m = \frac{[M]}{[S]^n} \qquad (12.3)$$

Values of K_m determine the extent of aggregation, in that as K_m increases, so does the amount of aggregation. The standard free energy of micellization at the critical micelle concentration (CMC) is

$$\Delta G_m^0 = RT \ln[S]_{CMC} \qquad (12.4)$$

The basis for the phase-separation model (Mukerjee, 1967) assumes that the occurrence of the phase change happens at the CMC. This model uses the chemical potentials of the free surfactant in the aqueous phase (μ_s) and the associated surfactant in the micellar phase (μ_m^0),

$$\mu_s = \mu_s^0 + RT \ln[S] \qquad (12.5)$$

where μ_s^0 refers to the standard state of the surfactant in the aqueous phase. The micellar material is in its standard state, and therefore $\mu_m = \mu_m^0$. The standard free energy of micellization is

$$\Delta G_m^0 = \mu_m^0 - \mu_s^0 = RT \ln X_S - \left(\frac{RT}{m} \right) \ln \left(\frac{X_m}{m} \right) \qquad (12.6)$$

where X_m and X_s are the mole fractions of monomer in the micellar and aqueous phase, respectively, and m is the number of monomers. For large micelles, m goes to infinity, and Equation 12.6 reduces to Equation 12.4. Micellization, in general, is exothermic and therefore negative values indicate spontaneous micelle formation. Equation 12.6 corresponds to a true phase separation, and according to the Gibbs Phase Rule, X_s is the single monomer concentration that can exist in equilibrium with the micelles (Marsh and King, 1986). However, this model is not very realistic because it predicts the change occurring at the CMC to be infinitely sharp, whereas in reality, the change is shown to be continuous (Mukerjee, 1967).

CRITICAL PARAMETERS

Critical Micellization Concentration

It has been well documented that surfactants self-associate in aqueous solution to minimize the area of contact between their hydrophobic tails and the aqueous solution (Mukerjee, 1979; Tanford, 1980). This phenomenon occurs at a critical concentration of surfactant, the critical

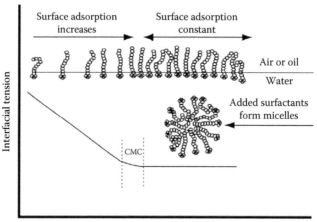

FIGURE 12.4 Schematic showing surfactant adsorption. Surfactants adsorb strongly to water–air interface or a water–oil interface owing to their amphiphilic nature (top). The accompanying reduction of interfacial tension (in accordance with the Gibbs adsorption equation, i.e., Equation 12.1) ceases in a narrow concentration range (the CMC). At concentrations above this range, added surfactant will aggregate to form micelles. (From Friberg and El-Nokaly (1985). With permission.)

micelle concentration or CMC (Figure 12.4) above where the surfactant molecules exist predominantly as monomeric units and above which micelles exist. The CMC can be measured by a variety of techniques, for example, surface tension, light scattering, and osmometry, each of which shows a characteristic break point in the plot of the operative property as a function of concentration. Knowing the CMC of the particular surfactant system and understanding the conditions that may raise or lower that critical concentration is important to the design of a formulation based on micellar solubilization.

In the literature, the change of the CMC with respect to a given parameter has provided insight through empirical expressions into the factors that control the onset of micellization. For example, CMC decreases as the hydrocarbon tail length increases, or as the molecular weight of a polyethylene oxide head group is reduced, or with the addition of salt to an ionic surfactant solution. In addition, the solvent environment also impacts the CMC values of the surfactant; it was reported that micelle formation occurred more easily in methanol than other higher alcohols (Andriamainty et al., 2007).

Mysels and Mukerjee (1979) define CMC as a small range of concentrations that separate the detection of micelles from monomers. CMC can also be defined as the maximum attainable chemical potential of the monomer, and is frequently the controlling factor in the transfer of lipid molecules between membranes. The CMC provides a convenient means of determining the properties of surfactants, many of which, if plotted against the concentration, appear to change at a different rate above and below this concentration range. By extrapolating the loci of such a property, the CMC value may be obtained.

The CMC values of surfactants are dependent on surfactant properties such as charge and hydrocarbon chain length. For example, ionic surfactants have higher CMC values than nonionic surfactants because the electrostatic repulsion of the charged head groups in the periphery of ionic micelles makes micellization more difficult. Anionic surfactants, however, such as long-chain fatty acid esters with Coenzyme A, have very low CMC values (5–250 μM depending on the assay conditions) owing to the presence of the charged and bulky hydrophilic head group (Constantinides and Steim, 1985). Attwood et al. (1994) investigated the surface properties of a series of nonionic surfactants in which a polar group was added into the hydrocarbon chain of octadecylpolyoxyethylene glycol monoether ($C_{18}E_{17}$). CMC values for these substituted surfactants were significantly higher than those for the unsubstituted octadecylpolyoxyethylene glycol monoether ($C_{18}E_{22}$). This behavior, according to the authors, was attributed to an increase in polarity of the hydrophobic group and its configuration in the micellar core. In general, the introduction of a polar group has been shown to increase the CMC. For example, the polyethylene oxide (PEO) chain repulsion on the external part of the micelles is much smaller than observed for ionic surfactants. Ionic charges can be localized on a defined external surface of the aggregate. In the case of nonionic surfactants, PEO polar chains have a typical size well above the alkyl chain dimension (Naylor et al., 1993). Addition of salts reduces the repulsive forces, resulting in lower CMC values for anionic and cationic surfactants. For example, increasing levels of sodium chloride lowers the CMC of alkyl sulfates. Length of the hydrocarbon surfactant chain is also a major factor in determining the CMC. Within any homologous series, the CMC decreases with increasing hydrocarbon chain length, as well as with increasing surface activity of the surfactant (Schott, 1995). CMC has been found to decrease logarithmically as the number of carbons in the chain of a homologous series increases. For straight-chain hydrocarbon surfactants of 16 carbon atoms or less, the CMC is usually reduced to half its value with the addition of each methylene group. In fact, these trends are independent of the nature and size of the polar head group. For ionic surfactants with highly charged and bulky head groups, such as C_{16}–C_{18} fatty acyl-CoA esters, the measured CMC values parallel the CMC order of the corresponding free fatty acids (Constantinides and Steim, 1985). For nonionic surfactants, the effect is much larger, with a decrease by a factor of 10 following the addition of carbons to the chain (Myers, 1992). In addition, Mysels and Mukerjee (1979) have shown that for compounds of the formula $C_mE_{1.25m}$, the CMC is related to m by:

$$\log_{10} CMC = 1.58 - 0.44\, m \quad \text{for } 4 \le m \le 16 \tag{12.7}$$

where m is the number of carbons in chain.

Various methods to measure CMC are all dependent on changes in an observable property on micellization, including surface tension, light scattering, dye solubilization, and surfactant ion electrodes (Carey, 1983). Different graphical procedures may also be used to evaluate the CMC. However, results of a single experiment may give more than one estimate of the CMC. Mysels and Mukerjee (1979) suggest that extrapolation of quasi-linear regions above and below the breakpoint be used to locate the CMC, particularly in cases where the overall plot of physical property versus concentration is nonlinear.

The micelle concentration in units of moles per liter can be calculated using the following formula:

$$[M] = \frac{\{[C_S] - CMC\}}{n} \tag{12.8}$$

where $[C_s]$ is the bulk molar concentration of surfactant, n is the mean aggregation number (refer to the following section), and CMC is the critical micellization concentration in moles per liter. For example, a solution containing octyl glucoside, with a CMC of 22 mM, at a bulk concentration of 100 mM mg/mL) in a phosphosaline buffer contains micelles at a concentration of approximately

$$\frac{(100 - 22\ \text{mM})}{27} \text{ or } 2.9\ \text{mM}$$

It is important to remember that an increase in the concentration of the surfactant beyond the CMC changes the number, size, and shape of the micelles, but does not increase the concentration of the monomeric species. In addition, care should be taken in interpreting the CMC values of some surfactants, for example, surfactants with bulky, rigid hydrophobic portions, such as bile salts that have a very broad concentration range of micellization. These surfactants also show variations in the monomer concentration above the CMC, and thus the CMC is not indicative of a critical phenomenon.

The following two items need to be considered from a practical perspective, especially for ionic surfactants, when measuring the CMC of surfactants (Constantinides and Steim, 1985): (a) surface-active impurities in commercial surfactants, such as SDS, give rise to a minimum in the surface tension–concentration plot, and unless a highly purified surfactant is used an approximate value of the CMC is obtained, and (b) in the dye solubilization method, it is important that the dye and the surfactant are of the same charge, to avoid premicellar association, that is, salt formation between the dye and the surfactant below the true CMC of the surfactant.

Micellar Size and Aggregation Number (n)

The second important characteristic of the micellar solution that relates to solubilization is the micelle size. Poor aqueous-soluble compounds are solubilized either within the hydrocarbon core of the micelle or, very commonly, within the head group layer at the surface of the micelle or in the palisade portion of the micelle. Predictions of the micelle size have relied on the use of empirical relationships employed within a thermodynamic model, for instance the law of mass action where micellization is in equilibrium with the associated and unassociated (monomer) surfactant molecules (Attwood and Florence, 1983).

The number of monomers that come together to form a micelle is called the aggregation number. Owing to the dynamic nature of micelles, this number represents a model of the micellar composition over a period of time. The aggregation number is calculated by dividing the micellar molecular weight by the molecular weight of the surfactant monomer. Micellar molecular weight may be determined by numerous methods, such as light scattering, sedimentation equilibrium, dynamic light scattering, and small-angle X-ray scattering. Micellar size is sensitive to the same experimental conditions as the CMC, including pH, temperature, ionic strength, and the presence of additives (Myers, 1992). The aggregation number for a particular surfactant may only be valid within a certain concentration range. Aggregation numbers for various surfactant types are given in Table 12.1. A few generalizations can be made about the aggregation number:

TABLE 12.1
Aggregation Numbers for Surfactants in Water

Surfactant	Temperature (°C)	Aggregation Number
$C_{10}H_{21}SO_3^-$	30	40
$C_{12}H_{25}SO_3^-Na^+$	40	54
$(C_{12}H_{25}SO_3^-)Mg^{2+}$	60	107
$C_{12}H_{25}SO_4^-Na^+$	23	71
$C_{14}H_{29}SO_3^-Na^+$	60	80
$C_{12}H_{25}N(CH_3)^+Br^-$	23	50
$C_8H_{17}O(CH_2CH_2O)_6H$	30	41
$C_{10}H_{21}O(CH_2CH_2O)_6H$	35	260
$C_{12}H_{25}O(CH_2CH_2O)_6H$	15	140
$C_{12}H_{25}O(CH_2CH_2O)_6H$	25	400
$C_{12}H_{25}O(CH_2CH_2O)_6H$	35	1400
$C_{14}H_{29}O(CH_2CH_2O)_6H$	35	7500

Source: Taken from Myers, D., Micellization and association, in *Surfactant Science and Technology.* 2nd ed., D. Myers (Ed.), VCH Publishers, New York, 1992.

---

1. In aqueous solutions, the greater the length of the hydrophobic chain of a homologous series of surfactants, the larger the aggregation number, n.
2. A similar increase in the aggregation number, n, is seen when there is a decrease in the hydrophilicity of the head group (i.e., a higher degree of ion binding, or shorter polyoxy-ethylene chain).
3. External factors that result in a reduction in the hydrophilicity of the head group, such as high neutral electrolyte concentrations, will cause an increase in the aggregation number, n.
4. For ionic surfactants, increasing the temperature results in a decrease in the aggregation number, n.
5. Addition of small amounts of nonsurfactant organic materials of low water solubility will produce an apparent increase in micelle size (Myers, 1992).

The Packing Parameter

The packing behavior of surfactant molecules in micelles is important because it directly relates to the structure of the micelles and other critical micellization parameters such as microviscosity (Berlepsch et al., 1998; Eads and Robosky, 1999; Zhang et al., 1999). A *packing parameter* concept was developed to relate the surfactant molecular structure to the expected aggregate shape (Nagarajan and Ruckenstein, 1991; Israelachvili, 1994). The volume-to-surface ratio of various aggregates normalized by the constrained dimension (V/Sr; sphere = 1/3, cylinder = 1/2, flat lamellar sheet = 1) is related to the volume-to-surface ratio of the surfactant molecule = v/al where v = surfactant tail volume, a = excluded area of the surfactant head group, and l = length of the surfactant tail (Israelachvili, 1994).

The packing parameter provides a simple semi quantitative model to interpret the influence of the dynamic surfactant structure on the size and shape of the resulting micelles (Israelachvili, 1994). An often cited example is micellization of sodium dodecyl sulfate. This molecule has a large excluded head group size of 60 Å^2, the tail length of 12 carbons leads to a volume of 350 Å^3 and a length of 18.4 Å. The resulting packing parameter is equal to 0.32, indicating spherical micelles should form. The large head group area of SDS is due to the electrostatic repulsion among the negatively charged head groups. The charge repulsion can be minimized by the addition of an electrolyte that would reduce the excluded head group area. By reducing the head group area, the calculated packing parameter increases changing the optimal micelle shape from spherical to cylindrical to eventually a lamellar structure. In a similar manner, the packing parameter can be used to interpret the effects of changing surfactant chain lengths that affect both the volume and length terms.

HYDROPHILIC–LIPOPHILIC BALANCE

Variations in the relative polarity or nonpolarity of surfactants (hydrophilic or hydrophobic) significantly influence its interfacial behavior. A measure of this parameter is useful to classify surfactants. An HLB number is a direct expression of the hydrophilic and hydrophobic character of surfactants and is a useful means for surfactant classification. HLB numbers for surfactants may be either calculated using the following empirical equation:

$$HLB = \sum (\# \text{ hydrophilic groups}) - \sum (\# \text{ hydrophobic groups}) + 7 \qquad (12.9)$$

or determined experimentally. These numbers range from 1 to 50, with larger HLB numbers indicating greater hydrophilicity. Surfactants with HLB numbers from 1 to 10 are considered lipophilic (Griffin, 1949). Table 12.2 lists some common surfactants and their HLB values. For example, on a molar basis,

TABLE 12.2
Approximate HLB Values for a Number of Surfactants

Generic or Chemical Name of Surfactant	HLB Value
Sorbitan trioleate	1.8
Propylene glycol monostearate	3.4
Glycerol monostearate	3.8
Propylene glycol monolaurate	4.5
Sorbitan monostearate	4.7
Glyceryl monostearate (self-emulsifying)	5.5
Sorbitan monolaurate	8.6
Polyoxyethylene-4-lauryl ether	9.5
Polyoxyethylene glycol 400 monostearate	11.6
Polyoxyethylene-4-sorbitan monolaurate	13.3
Polyoxyethylene-20-sorbitan monopalmitate	15.6
Polyoxyethylene-40-stearateb	16.9
Sodium stearate	17.6[a]
Sodium oleate	18.0
Sodium N-lauroyl sarcosinate	29[a]
Sodium lauryl sulfate	40.0

Source: Taken from Schott, H., Colloidal dispersions, in *Remington: The Science and Practice of Pharmacy*, A.R. Gennaro (Ed.), Vol. 1, Mack Publishing Co, Easton, PA, 1995; Treiner, C. et al., J. Coll. Interf. Sci., 125, 261–270, 1988.

[a] Data was obtained from Treiner, C. et al., *J. Coll. Interf. Sci.*, 125, 261–270, 1988.

a 100% hydrophilic molecule such as polyethylene glycol would have an HLB value of 20. Thus, an increase in the polyethylene oxide (PEO) chain length leads to an increase in the polarity and the HLB value. The advantage of such a system is that to a first approximation one can compare any chemical type of surfactant to another type when both polar and nonpolar groups are different (Schott, 1971). Values of HLB for nonionic surfactants are calculated based on the proportion of PEO chain present.

Temperature–Composition Phase Diagram

A temperature–composition phase diagram for a surfactant solution is a characteristic phase diagram that delineates the conditions under which crystalline surfactant, monomers, or micelles will exist. On the phase diagram shown in Figure 12.5 (Smirnova, 1995), L represents the liquid phase, S the solid phase, and X_1 the surfactant mole fraction. The critical micelle temperature, CMT, is defined as the line between the crystalline and micelle phases. Micelle formation occurs at temperatures greater than the CMT. The critical micelle concentration, CMC, line separates the micellar and monomeric phases. The Krafft point (point B) is defined as the triple point, or the CMT at the CMC, and at this point, the solubility curve intersects the CMC curve. At this temperature, the CMC is reached. Above it, a small increase in the solubility of the monomeric species involves a large increase in the concentration of the monomer and therefore, a large increase in the total concentration (Mukerjee, 1967). Point C (cloud point) occurs where a micellar solution is in equilibrium with both the solid (S) and the liquid crystalline (E) phases. Cloud point is a characteristic temperature at which solutions of surfactants undergo phase separation. Two lines going up from the points C and D are boundaries for the micellar solution (L) and liquid crystalline (E) phase equilibrium.

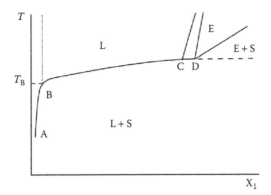

FIGURE 12.5 Fragment of the phase diagram for surfactant-water system. L, E, and S denotes liquid solution, liquid crystalline, and solid phases, respectively; the dotted line is the CMC curve. (Reprinted from Smirnova, N. A., *Fluid Phase Equilibria*, 110, 1–15, 1995. With permission.)

Experimental studies have shown a distinctive shape of the surfactant solubility curve that goes up steeply at the beginning, in the range of highly diluted solutions, and changes the slope near the Krafft point. The slope of the plateau is always positive, but varies for different surfactants. For zwitterionic and nonionic surfactants, the slope is very small, indicating that the surfactant solubility increases very rapidly with small temperature increases above the Krafft point. Smirnova (1995) used two models to interpret the temperature–composition dependencies for micellar solution–solid surfactant phase equilibrium: ideal monodispersed model and pseudo phase-separation model. The pseudo phase-separation model represents the micellar solution as a two-phase system consisting of aqueous and micellar phases. This model was found to be unrealistic because it states a zero temperature slope of the solubility curve. The ideal monodispersed micellar solution model applied to binary surfactant-water systems asserts a linear change of the temperature–composition phase diagram, with the Krafft boundary slope (line BC in Figure 12.5) being dependent on the aggregation number, temperature, and heat of surfactant dissolution. This model provided a good fit to the experimental data.

In the case of ionic surfactants, it is often observed that the solubility of the surfactant will undergo a sharp, discontinuous increase at some characteristic temperature, commonly referred to as the Krafft temperature, T_B (Figure 12.5). Below this temperature, the solubility of the surfactant is determined by the crystal lattice energy and the heat of hydration of the system. The concentration of the monomeric species in solution is limited to an equilibrium value determined by its properties. Above T_B, the solubility of the surfactant monomer increases to the point at which aggregate formation (micelles) begins, and the aggregated species becomes the thermodynamically favored form in solution. In the case of nonionic polyoxyethylene surfactants, at temperatures higher than the CMT, the physical state of the surfactants is affected. This is thought to be the result of dehydration of the oxyethylene head groups and consequent formation of *giant micelles*. This change in micellar size leads to a dependence of solubilization on temperature. The dependence of aqueous solubility on micellization temperature can also be found for anionic surfactants (Moroi et al., 1999).

MICELLAR SOLUBILIZATION

Solubilization Process

In simple terms, micellar solubilization can be defined as a process by which a water-insoluble substance (solute) is brought into solution by incorporation into micelles (solvent). The addition of solute may lead to changes in the packing of the micelle monomer unit. Compounds that are poorly soluble in water but soluble in hydrocarbon solvents can be dissolved in the interior of micelles, which consist of hydrocarbon tails surrounded by polar head groups (Florence, 1981; Saket, 1996, 1997). Thus, depending on its location and orientation in the micelles, a solute may be protected from the attack of solvent species that are insoluble in micelles (Mukerjee, 1979; Mall et al., 1996). Mukerjee presents a good overview of a number of fundamental issues in micellar solubilization. Micellar properties of nonionic surfactants in polar solvents depend mainly on the ability of the hydrocarbon core of the micelles to dissolve a nonpolar solute. Thus, the solubilization capacity for the solute is controlled mainly by the core volume. However, materials with some polarity, such as benzoic acid, are absorbed at the interface between the core and the hydrophilic layer of the micelle (Florence, 1981). Hence, the solubilization capacity is less controlled by the core and more dependent on the polar head group of the surfactant. For example, solubilizing efficiency decreases with increasing polyethylene oxide chain length when surfactants are compared on a weight basis, but the efficiency is reversed when compared on a molar basis (Florence, 1981; Saket, 1996; 1997).

The solubilization of drugs can be treated in terms of an association equilibrium between the solutes and the micelles in a micellar solution. Thus,

$$D_w + M \xleftrightarrow{\;\;K_m\;\;} D_m \qquad (12.10)$$

where D_w is the drug solubilized in the aqueous phase, M is the micellar concentration, K_m is the distribution coefficient between the micellar and aqueous phase, and D_m is the drug solubilized in the micellar phase. Then the solubility can be determined from

$$S_m = K_m S_o M \qquad (12.11)$$

where S_m and S_o are the nonionized solubilities in micellar and water phases, respectively (Fahelelbom et al., 1993). Every drug has a solubilization limit, which is dependent on the temperature, nature, and concentration of the surfactant. The solubilizing power or the solubilization capacity of the micelle is usually defined in terms of the ratio of the number of moles of solubilizate to the number of moles of micellized surfactant. Two categories of solubilizates have been determined by Hartley: (1) large, asymmetrical, rigid molecules forming crystalline solids that do not blend in with the tails making up the micellar core, and remain distinct as solute molecules, and (2) compounds that are liquid at room temperature and are made up of flexible molecules (McBain and Hutchinson, 1955). The second categories of solubilizates mix and blend in freely with the hydrocarbon portion of the surfactants in the core of the micelles and become indistinguishable from them. They are extensively solubilized and tend to swell the micelles, increasing both the volume of the hydrocarbon core and the number of surfactant molecules (McBain and Hutchinson, 1955). There are many drug molecules that are solid at room temperature but which nevertheless can be readily incorporated into micelles, suggesting that there is a third category.

Saket (1996, 1997) studied the micellar solubilization of meclozine hydrochloride (McHCl), which is slightly water soluble and mainly used as an antiemetic for nausea and vomiting. Improvement of its water solubility is desirable for formulating the drug in liquid dosage forms to facilitate absorption and bioavailability. The drug is solubilized at 30°C, 37°C, and 45°C in a series of different nonionic surfactant solutions, including polysorbates, Eumulgins, Brijs, and Myrjs. The solubility of the drug increased linearly with increasing surfactant concentrations, indicating that micellar solubilization obeys the partition model. Thus, the drug is distributed between the aqueous phase and the micellar pseudophase. The results showed that the longer the hydrocarbon chains in a homologous series, the more efficient the solubilizing power. Polysorbate 80 is thus more efficient as a solubilizer than polysorbate 20, and Brij 58 is more efficient than Brij 35, indicating that the drug is incorporated in the core more than the capsular region of the micelle. On the other hand, the shorter the polyoxyethylene chain in a homologous series, the more efficient the solubilizing power. Thus, Eumulgin C1000 is more efficient than Eumulgin C1500, and Myrj 53 is more efficient than Myrj 59.

Mall et al. (1996) applied a thermodynamic approach to study the solubilization of sulfonamides in a SDS micellar solution via the dissolution behavior of the drugs. From the surface energies of four sulfonamides assessed by contact angle data, the free energy of adhesion between the drugs and SDS head groups and tails was calculated. The most favored interaction was found to be for adhesion to the SDS tails, rather than the head groups. The thermodynamic parameters of activation were calculated from the dissolution rate data. A linear relationship exists between the enthalpy of transfer between water and SDS micelles and the free energy of adhesion between the drugs and both SDS head groups and tails. The interaction between the SDS head group and the drugs dominantly influences the solubilization when comparing the adhesion to the SDS head group and enthalpy of transfer data. The repulsion between the polar sulfanilamide and the SDS head group, as evidenced by the positive free energy of adhesion and positive enthalpy of transfer, may limit solubilization of this drug. The favorable free energy of adhesion and enthalpy of transfer can facilitate solubilization of the other three sulfonamides: sulfamerazine, sulfadiazine, and sulfamethazine. Therefore, the authors concluded that the highly nonpolar drugs had the most favored free energy of adhesion and the most favored enthalpy of transfer. The highly polar drug had a disfavored free energy of adhesion to the SDS head group and a disfavored enthalpy of transfer, thus demonstrating that the most important barrier to the passage from the aqueous media to the hydrophobic core of the micelle is the monopolar repulsion between the polar forces of the drug and head group surface energies. The authors claimed that this provided a new insight into a possible mechanism of solubilization and offered the prospect to better understand the complex partitioning behavior.

LOCATION OF SOLUTES IN MICELLAR SYSTEMS

The location of a solute within a micelle is largely dependent on the overall structure of the solute (Mukerjee, 1979). Thus, nonpolar solutes are primarily dissolved in the hydrocarbon core; whereas amphiphilic compounds containing both polar and nonpolar groups are oriented with the polar group at the surface, and the hydrophobic group is located inside the hydrophobic core of the micelle. Adsorption on the micellar surface has been postulated for some solutes, and suggested that certain solutes such as griseofulvin may be incorporated in the PEO exterior of nonionic surfactant micelles. Solutes that are located within the micelle core increase the size of the micelles and change the number of surfactant molecules per micelle. This means that the aggregation number increases in an effort to fill the swollen micelle core. In contrast, solutes that are located close to the surface of the micelle have little or no effect on the aggregation number, but do increase micelle size by the incorporation of solute molecules (Attwood and Florence, 1983).

Aliphatic hydrocarbon solutes are primarily solubilized within the hydrocarbon core region of the surfactant micelles. Solubilization isotherms (activity coefficient versus mole fraction, X) for these hydrophobic solutes exhibit curves that decrease from relatively large values at infinite dilution to lower values as X increases toward unity (Figure 12.6). The aromatic hydrocarbons are intermediate in behavior between highly polar solutes, which are anchored in the micelle surface region, and aliphatic hydrocarbons, which preferentially solubilize in the hydrocarbon core region (Kondo et al., 1993).

A two-state model of solubilization may be used to describe the location of solutes in micellar systems. This model involves a distribution between a dissolved state, which is associated with the core, and an adsorbed state, associated with the micellar water interface. The molecules in the dissolved state remain in the micelle because of the solvent properties of the core. Molecules in the adsorbed state are due to the surface activity of the dissolved species, similar to a surface excess (Mukerjee, 1979).

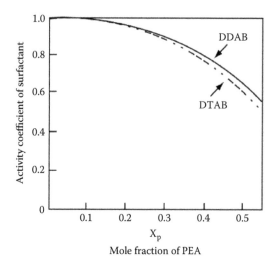

FIGURE 12.6 Dependence of the activity coefficients (γs) for DDAB and DTAB on the mole fraction of PEA. (From Kondo, Y. et al., *Langmuir*, 9, 899–902, 1993. With permission.)

SOLUTE PROPERTIES–MICELLAR SOLUBILIZATION RELATIONSHIPS

The properties of drugs (solutes) have been extensively studied to determine their relationship with micellar solubility and solubilization. In particular, Gadiraju et al. (1995) have characterized the solubility profile of amiodarone HCl as a function of pH, buffer concentration, and CMC. The solubility behavior of this amphoteric drug was found to be dependent on pH and the counter ions present in the buffer. Figure 12.7 demonstrates the increase in amiodarone HCl solubility with increasing buffer strength. This increase in solubility is expected for ionic surfactants owing to the denser packing of the micelles as the number of counter ions increases. More recently, Kondo et al. (1993) have determined the solubilization of 2-phenylethanol in dodecyl trimethyl ammonium bromide. They observed that small polar organic solutes such as acids and alcohols have their polar head groups anchored in the polar or ionic region of the aggregated ionic surfactants.

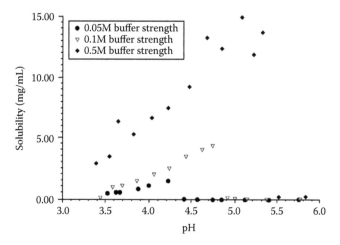

FIGURE 12.7 Solubility verse pH profiles at different acelate buffer strengths. (From Gadiraju, R. R. et al., The effect of buffer species, pH, and buffer strength on the CMC and solubility of amiodarone HCl, Poster presentation (AAPS annual meeting), 1995. With permission.)

The aliphatic or aromatic moieties of these polar solutes tend to be solubilized at least partly within the hydrocarbon core of the micelle.

The ability of nonionic surfactants to act as solubilizing agents for water-insoluble drugs has been extensively studied (Samaha and Naggar, 1988). The hydrophobic micellar moiety of both nonionic and anionic surfactants solubilizes nonionizable solutes with poor aqueous solubility. The polarity of the solute molecules is a major factor in determining the degree of solubilization. It has been observed that the solubilizing capacity of ionic and nonionic surfactants for solutes that are located in the micellar interior increases in the order of anionic < cationic < nonionic. This effect has been attributed to a corresponding increase in the area per head group of the series, leading to *looser* micelles with less dense hydrocarbon cores that can accommodate more solutes (Fahelelbom et al., 1993). The situation is different for solutes located at the interface. For example, the solubility of Furosemide, a diuretic, in a nonionic surfactant (polysorbate 80), an anionic surfactant (sodium lauryl sulfate), and a polymer (polyethylene glycol, PEG) has been studied as a function of polymer molecular weight and temperature by Shihab et al. (1979). They found that these solubilizers increase the solubility of the drug in water in the order of sodium lauryl sulfate > polysorbate 80 > PEG. The higher the molecular weight of PEG the greater the solubility of the drug. The linear increase of solubility with increasing surfactant concentration is typical of micellar solubilization (Figures 12.8 and 12.9).

Fahelelbom et al. (1993) have examined the influence of surfactant concentration on the solubility of clofazimine. They found that the pH of surfactant solutions, particularly sodium lauryl sulfate, increased solubility nonlinearly with an increase in surfactant concentration. The increase in solubility was believed to be due to the increased number of micelles in solution. Akbuga and Gursoy (1987) examined the effects of polysorbates and Myrj (polyoxyethylene fatty acid esters) on

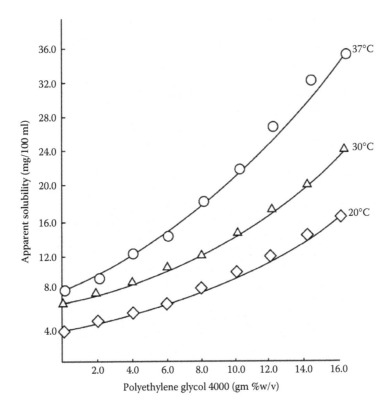

FIGURE 12.8 Solubility of furosemide in aqueous solutions of PEG 4000 at different temperatures. (From Shihab, F. A. et al., *Int. J. Pharm.*, 4, 13–20, 1979. With permission.)

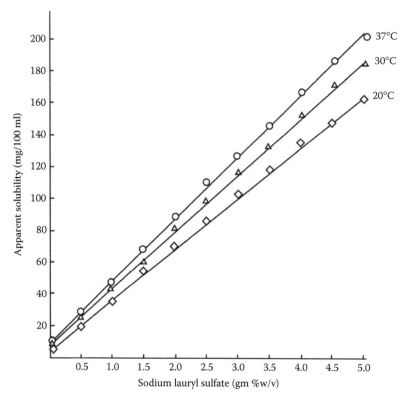

FIGURE 12.9 Solubility of furosemide in aqueous solutions of sodium lauryl sulfate at different temperatures. (From Shihab, F. A. et al., *Int. J. Pharm.*, 4, 13–20, 1979. With permission.)

the solubility of furosemide, and also determined the relationship between the solubility of this drug and the chemical structure of the surfactants. Table 12.3 shows the solubility capacities of the surfactants for furosemide. The solubilizing power of polysorbates was directly related to the alkyl chain lengths, with an increase in the chain length corresponding to an increase in the solubilizing capacity. Similar results were obtained by Hamza and Kata (1989) for allopurinol in a series of surfactants (Tween, Myrj, Brij, and Pluronic F Series). Extending the hydrocarbon core for a homologous series having the same polyoxyethylene chain length causes a decrease in the solubilized amount of the drug at various concentrations. On the other hand, for a series having the same hydrocarbon chain, extending the polyoxyethylene chains causes an increase in the solubilized amount of drug except at the highest concentration. (More detailed discussion of polymeric surfactants can be found in Chapter 13, "Micellization and Drug Solubility Enhancement Part II: Polymeric Micelles," of this book.) Interactions of solubilizers with other components in a particular formulation can influence their capacity to increase the solubility of drug substances (Florence, 1981). Polymers are frequently used as viscosity modifiers and suspension stabilizers. The interactions between a polymer and a surfactant can increase with increasing hydrophobicity of the macromolecule. It has been reported that the optimal interactions between a given polymer and a surfactant occur when the surfactant head group has a long, straight hydrocarbon chain, with the polar group terminal to the alkyl chain.

Chen et al. (1998) studied the rates of solubilization of triolein/fatty acid mixtures by nonionic surfactant solutions. Spontaneously generated convection and rapid initial solubilization were observed when oil drops containing mixtures of triolein and oleic acid were injected into aqueous solutions of nonionic surfactants including Tergitol 15-S-7. The latter is a mixture of species with the alcohol group located at various positions along a chain of 11–15 carbon atoms and with

TABLE 12.3
Effect of Surfactants on the Solubility of Furosemide

	Distilled Water		0.1 N Hydrochloric Acid	
Surfactant % (w/v)	Total Solubility (µg/mL)	Micellar Solubility (µg/mL)	Total Solubility (µg/mL)	Micellar Solubility (µg/mL)
0	41.2	—	15.0	—
Polysorbate 20 (C_{12})				
0.005	31.2	—	40.0	—
0.05	45.0	3.7	41.1	26.1
0.5	57.0	15.7	50.0	35.0
1.0	167.0	125.7	145.0	130.0
5.0	705.0	663.7	670.0	655.0
Polysorbate 40 (C_{16})				
0.005	32.5		25.0	
0.05	45.0	3.7	22.5	7.5
0.5	112.5	71.2	72.5	57.5
1.0	143.7	102.4	137.5	122.5
5.0	792.5	751.2	887.0	872.0
Polysorbate 80 (C_{18})				
0.005	43.7	2.4	15.9	0.9
0.05	43.7	2.4	18.7	3.7
0.5	141.2	100.0	74.0	59.0
1.0	205.0	163.7	160.0	145.0
5.0	980.0	938.7	808.0	793.0

Source: Taken from Akbuga, J. and Gursoy, A., *S.T.P. Pharma.*, 3, 395–399, 1987.

derivatized PEG having an average ethylene oxide number of 7, for example, $C_{12}E_6$ and $C_{12}E_8$, pure linear alcohol ethoxylates. For drops having oleic acid contents between 15% and 25% by weight, solubilization rates were at least an order of magnitude greater than those found for pure triolein. Drop volumes decreased by amounts ranging from 45% to 70% in less than 5 min. with no external stirring. It was assumed that the rapid solubilization occurred initially because most of the oleic acid had been solubilized. At later times, the solubilization rates were about the same as that for pure triolein with the same surfactant solutions. A similar effect was observed during the first minute or two after contact for a hydrocarbon/oleic acid mixture. The results indicate that solutes can significantly influence the rate of micellar solubilization.

FACTORS AFFECTING MICELLIZATION AND MICELLAR SOLUBILIZATION

Temperature

Temperature has a major impact on micellization and micellar solubilization. As discussed in the section of temperature–composition phase diagram, change in micellar size due to changes in temperature leads to a dependence of solubilization on temperature. As mentioned earlier, Saket (1996, 1997) studied the micellar solubilization of meclozine hydrochloride (McHCl). The drug was solubilized at 30°C, 37°C, and 45°C in series of different nonionic surfactant solutions, including polysorbates, Eumulgins, Brijs and Myrjs. It was found that raising the temperature from 30°C to 37°C to 45°C caused a positive effect on the solubilizing efficiencies of investigated solutions with McHCl and caused a decrease in the distribution coefficient (K_m) of the drug between micellar and aqueous phases. Other studies also showed similar results. For example, the effect of temperature on the solubilization of griseofulvin demonstrated about a 50% increase in solubility over a 30°C increase in temperature. However, there is a decrease in the apparent solubility of benzocaine in polyoxyethylene lauryl ether and in polysorbate solutions over the temperature range of 30°C–70°C (Hamid and Parrott, 1971).

In investigating temperature effects on drug solubilization in micellar systems, changes in the micellar properties as well as those in the aqueous solubility of the solute significantly affect the solubilization of the solute. For nonionic surfactants, the CMC values decrease with increasing temperature in line with an inverse temperature–surfactant solubility relationship. In the case of PEO surfactants, the aqueous solubility of the surfactants is attributed to hydrogen bonding between the ether oxygen of ethylene oxide chains and water molecules. When the temperature is increased, the hydrogen bonds break and the hydrophilicity of the polyethylene chain are reduced, rendering the surfactant less soluble so that micellization occurs at a lower concentration (Shahjahan and Enever, 1992). Thus, the solubilization for a solute occurs at lower surfactant concentrations. The solubilization capacity increases for the same amount of surfactant in the solution owing to the decrease of its CMC caused by an increase in temperature. Also, micelles of nonionic surfactants rapidly grow in size with increasing temperature, which may be in part due to greater hydrophobicity of the monomer and geometric considerations. Therefore, in general, the higher the temperature the larger the micellar solubilization capacity for a solute. As an example, increasing the temperature for PEO surfactants results in an increase in the aggregation number due to the progressive dehydration of the ethylene oxide chains. The change in micellar size leads to a dependence of solubilization on the temperature with an increase in solute uptake. The extent of increase in micelle size depends on the influence of temperature on the solution characteristics of the solubilizate molecules (Florence, 1981).

In the case of small ionic surfactants, such as sodium lauryl sulfate (SLS) and CTAB, the molecular movement in the surfactant solution is activated by an increase in temperature. It becomes more difficult for the ionic surfactant molecules to remain as micellar structures at a higher temperature than at a lower temperature. Since it is necessary to have a higher concentration of surfactant to maintain the aggregation state at higher temperatures, the CMC of ionic surfactants increases as temperature increases (Attwood and Florence, 1983).

Table 12.4 shows the effect of temperature on the solubilization of griseofulvin by bile salts. The data indicate that there is an approximate 50% increase in griseofulvin solubility over a 17°C temperature range.

Caution should be exercised when considering temperature effects on solubilization by micelles, since the aqueous solubility of the solute and thus its micelle/water partition coefficient can also change in response to temperature changes. For example, it has been reported that although the solubility of benzoic acid in a series of polyoxyethylene nonionic surfactants increases with temperature, the micelle/water partition coefficient, K_m, shows a minimum at 27°C, presumably due to

TABLE 12.4

The Effect of Temperature on the Maximum Additive Concentrations of Griseofulvin

Surfactant	MAC × 10³ (Moles of Drug per Mole of Surfactant)		
	27°C	37°C	45°C
None	4.59×10^{-4}	7.14×10^{-4}	10.2×10^{-4}
Sodium cholate	5.36	6.18	6.80
Sodium desoxycholate	4.68	6.18	6.54
Sodium taurocholate	3.77	4.90	6.15
Sodium glycocholate	3.85	5.13	5.29

the increase in the aqueous solubility of benzoic acid (Humphreys and Rhodes, 1968). The increase in K_m with increasing temperature was attributed to an increase in micellar size, as the cloud point temperature of the surfactant is approached (Humphreys and Rhodes, 1968).

pH

Many water-insoluble drugs are either weak bases or weak acids. There exists an equilibrium of ionized and unionized species for a weak base or a weak acid in an aqueous solution. The pH can affect the equilibrium between ionized and nonionized solute species, and consequently can have an effect on the capacity of micellar solubility. An example of this is the decreased uptake of 4-chlorobenzoic acid by polysorbate 80 micelles observed when the pH is changed from 3 to 4.4 (Collette and Koo, 1975). Another example regarding the effect of SDS micelles on the pK_a of atenolol, nadolol, midazolam, and nitrazepam is provided by Castro et al. (1998). Apparent acidity constants (pK_{app}) of the drugs were determined potentiometrically or spectrophotometrically in aqueous and SDS solutions at 25°C with 0.1 M NaCl. The concentration of SDS ranged from 5.0×10^{-4} to 2.0×10^{-2} M. The pK_{app} of a given compound is independent of the SDS concentration up to the CMC ($\sim 1.0 \times 10^{-3}$ M), but starts to decrease above this value. This behavior has been observed for many indicators, for which at least one form is cationic that interact with anionic micelles (Khaledi et al., 1990; Pal and Jana, 1996). In another case, for a pH-dependent drug cefpodoxime proxetil, a self-emulsifying system with <40% of surfactant was developed (Date and Nagarsenker, 2007), where the mean droplet size was not affected by the pH of the dilution medium. In general, stronger interactions with micelles cause larger shifts in the pK_a values (Khaledi et al., 1990). The pK_a of the β-blockers shifts approximately 0.5 log units and that of benzodiazepines changes approximately 1 log unit. As strong interactions of cationic species with anionic micelles drive the equilibrium from the protonated forms to the neutral forms of these substances, the values of pK_{app} thus increase. The results also suggest that the interactions of anionic micelles with protonated benzodiazepines are stronger than that with β-blockers.

An anionic surfactant is soluble only at a pH greater than the pK_a of its ionizable group, whereas a cationic surfactant (e.g., primary, secondary, or tertiary amines) is soluble only at a pH less than its pK_a. However, quaternary ammonium surfactants remain soluble at all pH values. Zwitterionic surfactants, for example, sulfobetaine surfactants, are neutral from pH 2 to 12, whereas some nonionic surfactants, for example, alkyldimethylamine oxides, are converted to cationic surfactants by protonation at acidic pH.

Shahjahan and Enever (1992) have determined the solubilization of nitrofurazone, uvinul D-50 (2,2′,4,4′-tetrahydroxy benzophenone), and uvinul N-35 (ethyl-2-cyano-3,3-diphenyl acrylate) in aqueous solutions of nonionic surfactants at various temperatures and pH values. They found that uvinul D-50 exhibits minimum solubility at pH 4, as shown by Figure 12.10, while nitrofurazone showed a decrease in solubility with increasing pH of the buffer solution (Figure 12.11). These results were interpreted in terms of a partition coefficient between the micellar and aqueous phases (K_m), which followed the order of uvinul N-35 > uvinul D-50 > nitrofurazone. In addition, K_m values increased with increasing oxyethylene chain length. The work by Ikeda et al. (1977) nicely illustrated the interactions between tetracycline antibiotics and anionic, cationic and nonionic surfactants as a function of pH. They studied the micellar interactions of drugs including tetracycline, oxytetracycline, chlortetracycline, and minocycline, and surfactants polyoxyethylene lauryl ether (PLE), sodium lauryl sulfate (SLS), and dodecyltrimethylammonium chloride (DTAC) at various pH values (2.1–5.6) using equilibrium dialysis. The tetracycline derivatives used in these studies existed in solution as zwitterions, positively charged and/or negatively charged species as a function of pH and therefore were expected to exhibit differences in their micellar interaction/binding in a given surfactant solution. The extent of these interactions was quantified by the corresponding partition coefficients (K_m) of the ionized and zwitterionic species. Table 12.5 shows the dependence of K_m on pH. K_m values for tetracycline, oxytetracycline, and chlortetracycline decreased as pH increased, while minocycline showed the opposite behavior. This indicates that

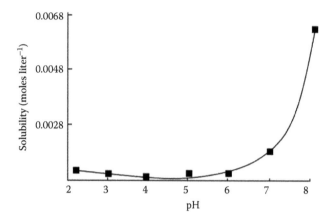

FIGURE 12.10   Effect of pH on the solubility of Uvinul D-50 at 25°C. (From Shahjahan, M. and Enever, R. P., *Int. J. Pharm.*, 82, 223–227, 1992. With permission.)

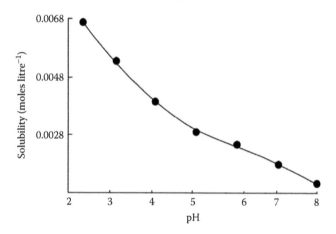

FIGURE 12.11   Effect of pH on the solubility of nitrofurazone at 25°C. (From Shahjahan, M. and Enever, R. P., *Int. J. Pharm.*, 82, 223–227, 1992. With permission.)

TABLE 12.5
Apparent Partition Coefficients in PLE Solution at Various pH Values (25°C)

Drug Substance	Apparent Partition Coefficient			
	pH 2.1	pH 3.0	pH 3.9	pH 5.6
Tetracycline	8.05	8.64	6.31	5.80
Oxytetracycline	8.01	7.61	6.54	5.68
Chlortetracycline	19.0	17.9	13.3	10.0
Minocycline	2.1	4.1	3.8	17.0

Source: Taken from Ikeda, K. et al., *Chem. Pharm. Bull.*, 25, 1067–1072, 1977.

all the cationic species were more soluble than the zwitterions. The micellar interactions with the antibiotics were determined not to be related either to the hydrogen bonding or to the lipophilicity of the species. Mechanistically, it appears that the cationic forms of these antibiotics were more solubilized by the orientation mechanism, whereas the zwitterionic species were solubilized by the intramolecular cancellation of charges (Ikeda et al., 1977). A useful conclusion from their studies was that the pH dependency of the tetracycline–PLE micelle interactions did not correlate with the octanol–water partition data. Octanol–water partition coefficients of a particular drug in model solvents/membranes are, in general, a useful predictor of mucosal absorption but cannot be used in a reliable manner to replace *in vivo* studies owing to other complex physicochemical and physiological factors that are involved during drug absorption (Nook et al., 1988; Alcorn et al., 1991, 1993).

Sheng et al. (2006) investigated the combined effect of pH and surfactant on the solubility and dissolution of ketoprofen. The solubility and dissolution rate enhancement were determined in buffers with pH range from 4.0 to 6.8 and sodium lauryl sulfate (SLS) concentration from 0% to 2.0%. It was found that the maximum solubility enhancement was approximately 232-fold whereas maximum dissolution amplification is only 54-fold because of the smaller diffusivity of micellar species. The authors further propose that the absorption of ketoprofen would be predominantly controlled by gastric emptying owing to the dramatic enhancement of solubility and rapid dissolution under *in vivo* condition similar to that of small intestine. This behavior is very similar to BCS I drugs, thus ketoprofen may be considered for possible waivers of bioequivalence. Similar results were reported in the literature (Granero et al., 2005; Joshi et al., 2006; Park et al., 2006).

Electrolytes and Ionic Strength

For ionic surfactant micelles, electrolyte addition results in an increase in micellar size (aggregation number) and a decrease in the CMC. Decrease in the CMC value is due to a decrease of the electrical double layer, reducing the charge interactions, which favors micellization. Therefore, the addition of electrolytes or increasing the ionic strength in a solution can increase the micellar solubilization capacity when using ionic surfactants as solubilizers. In the case of nonionic surfactants, it is important to consider the location of the solute within the micelle when determining the effect of electrolyte addition on the solubilization of a particular drug by surfactant micelles. Thus, for solutes that are located deep within the micelle core, solubilization may be increased owing to the increase in micellar volume following electrolyte addition. On the other hand, reduction in repulsion between head groups on electrolyte addition can lead to a closer packing of surfactant molecules and potentially result in a decrease in the solubilization of polar compounds that are located in this region. For example, several alkylparabens in the presence of increasing amounts of sodium chloride show a decrease in the partition coefficient between SDS micelles and water (Goto et al., 1980). The reduction in the alkylparabens solubility was also attributed to changes in the shape of the micelles from spherical to ellipsoid, leading to a concomitant decrease in surface area and thus limited penetration of the solute. Electrolyte addition also leads to an increase in aggregation number or micellar weight as well as an increase in the solubilization capacity for nonpolar compounds. This increase in solubilization parallels the depression in the cloud point temperature. Although the solubilization of polar compounds by nonionic surfactants in the presence of electrolytes follows no clear pattern, increase in the micelle/water partition coefficients has been reported in the case of sodium 2-naphthalene sulfonate and polysorbate 80 micelles.

Shihab et al. (1979) determined the effects of electrolytes on the solubility of furosemide in 5% polysorbate 80 solutions. It was found that the CMC of the surfactant decreased and the micellar volume increased in the presence of electrolytes (Table 12.6). All the electrolytes used increased the solubilizing power of the surfactant at the concentrations employed.

Some carboxylate surfactants, such as long-chain fatty acids or their anionic esters with Coenzyme A, are precipitated in the presence of Ca^{2+} and Mg^{2+} (Constantinides and Steim, 1986). Measurements of CMC in the presence of divalent ions should be avoided since the insoluble surfactant could introduce serious artifacts. Traces of transition-metal ions can catalyze autooxidation of some polyoxyethylene surfactants. In a recent article by Xiao (Xiao et al., 2006), interactions

TABLE 12.6

Effect of Electrolytes on the Solubility of Furosemide in 5% w/v Polysorbate 80

Concentration (M)	Solubility of Furosemide (mg/100 mL) in Electrolyte				
	NaCl	KCl	$MgCl_2$	Na_2SO_4	K_2SO_4
0.00	125.6	125.6	125.6	125.6	125.6
0.01	130.2	127.0	128.2	129.9	131.0
0.02	131.9	129.8	131.4	133.7	134.4
0.05	132.3	131.9	135.5	139.6	144.6
0.10	133.2	132.5	136.4	149.9	147.5
0.20	134.1	134.1	141.4	157.8	160.9

Source: Taken from Shihab, F. A. et al., *Int. J. Pharm.*, 4, 13–20, 1979.

between anionic surfactant (SDS) micellar solutions and several familiar metal salt solutions $(Al_2(SO_4)_3, FeCl_3, CaCl_2,$ and $MgCl_2)$ were investigated. Precipitates were formed in all systems except SDS-MgCl$_2$. The forming of these precipitates was attributed to adsorption-charge neutralization (Al^+), bridge connection (SDS-FeCl$_3$) and low solubility product of Ca(DS)$_2$ crystal respectively. SEM photographs of the precipitates can serve as additional vivid proofs of the above-mentioned conclusion.

Nature and Concentration of Surfactant and Solute

The effect of various surfactants—the cationics (cetyltrimethylammonium bromide [CTAB] and cetyl pyridinium chloride [CPC]), the anionic (sodium lauryl sulfate [SLS]), and the nonionic (polysorbate 80 [Tween 80]) —on the solubility and ionization constants of some sparingly soluble weak acids of pharmaceutical interest was studied (Gerakis et al., 1993). Benzoic acid (and its 3-methyl-, 3-nitro-, and 4-tert-butyl-derivatives), acetylsalicylic acid, naproxen, and iopanoic acid were chosen as model drugs. The cationics, CTAB and CPC, were found to considerably increase the ionization constant of the weak acids (ΔpK_a ranged from -0.21 to -3.57), while the anionic, SLS, showed a negligible effect and the nonionic, Tween 80, generally decreased the ionization constants. Solubility of the acids increased in aqueous micellar and in acidified micellar solutions.

Eda et al. (1996, 1997) studied the solubilization of isomeric alkanols in ionic surfactant micelles using a piezoelectric gas sensor method. The surfactants used included SLS and CTAB. The solutes were 1-, 2-, 3-, and 4-alkanol, as well as branched and cyclic alkanols. Free energy change of transfer of the alkanols from water to micelles was found to be in the order of 1- < 2- < 3- < 4-alkanol < branched alkanol < cyclic alkanol. The results seem to indicate that a bulkier alkanol was less favorably solubilized in the micelle. The results also agreed with the principle of hydrophobicity that a bulky alkyl group is less hydrophobic than a slender alkyl group with the same number of carbons, since the bulky one has a smaller surface area that is accessible to water. However, additional correlation work between the micelle/water and octanol/water partition coefficients showed a good correlation for the transfer free energy from water to micelle and from water to octanol ($r = 0.97-0.98$). This result indicates that the solubilization of alkanols in micelles depends only on the hydrophobicity of alkanols and that there is no effect of the molecular shape of alkanols on the solubilization in the micelles. Hence, a flexible micelle solubilization model for alkanols was proposed (Figure 12.12).

Some surfactant micelles exhibit concentration-dependent growth. That is, the micelles at concentrations much higher than the CMC are larger than those at concentrations smaller than the CMC. In the case where the solute is located within the hydrophobic core of the micelle, the micellar solubilization capacity increases with increasing alkyl chain length. Table 12.7 illustrates this

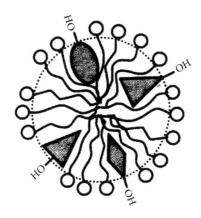

FIGURE 12.12 A possible model of a flexible micelle solubilizing alkanols. (Reprinted with permission from Eda, Y. et al., *Langmuir*, 12, 325–329, 1996. Copyright 1996 American Chemical Society.)

TABLE 12.7
Solubilizing Capacity of Surfactant Micelles and Distribution Coefficient of Timobesome Acetate in Aqueous Micellar Solutions at 25°C

Surfactant	Solubilizing Capacity (mmol/mol)	Distribution Coefficient
POE 20 sorbitan monolaurate (Polysorbate 20)	3.1 (0.1)[a]	5.19
POE 20 sorbitan monopalmitate (Polysorbate 40)	4.7 (0.1)	7.88
POE 20 sorbitan monostearate (Polysorbate 60)	5.2 (0.2)	8.58
POE 20 sorbitan monooleate (Polysorbate 80)	5.1 (0.4)	8.43
POE 23 lauryl ether (Brij 35)	4.7 (0.4)	7.82
POE 20 cetyl ether (Brij 58)	7.7 (1.3)	12.8
POE 20 stearyl ether (Brij 78)	8.4 (0.3)	14.1
POE 20 oleoyl ether (Brij 98)	7.5 (0.6)	12.6
POE 40 stearate (Myrj 52)	7.3 (0.3)	12.2
POE 100 stearate (Myrj 59)	6.9 (0.7)	11.6
Sucrose monolaurate (Crodesta SL40)	3.9 (0.1)	6.5

Source: Taken from Ong, J. T. and Manoukian, E., *Pharm. Res.*, 5, 704–708, 1988.
[a] ±95% confidence limit.

point and presents the solubilizing capacity of surfactant micelles and the distribution coefficient of timobesome acetate between the micellar and bulk aqueous phases (Ong and Manoukian, 1988). It is evident that for the polysorbate and Brij series, the solubilizing capacity and the distribution coefficient increase with increasing fatty acid chain length from laureate (C_{12}) to stearate (C_{18}). Since timobesome acetate is hydrophobic, it is expected to be solubilized in the hydrophobic core of the micelles. At a fixed fatty acid chain length, the nature of the hydrophilic group of the surfactant also affects the extent of solubilization. Thus, for surfactants containing laureate, the solubilizing capacity increased in the order of POE 20 sorbitan, < sucrose < POE 23 ether (Table 12.7). Similarly, for surfactants with palmitate or stearate, the ether-type surfactants (Brij) have a higher solubilizing capacity than the sorbitan (polysorbate) and ester-type (Myrj) surfactants. As shown by POE 40 stearate and POE 100 stearate, the length of the hydrophilic POE chain does not have any significant effect on the solubilizing capacity of the micelles. This further supports the fact that drug solubilization occurs in the hydrophobic core and not in the hydrophilic layer of the micelle. Finally, by comparing the solubilizing capacity of POE 20 oleoyl ether versus POE 20 stearyl ether, it can be concluded that surfactants containing an unsaturated fatty acid chain exhibit lower solubilizing capacity than surfactants containing saturated fatty acid chains. This is possibly due to the cis configuration of oleic acid, which causes packing constraints and leads to less effective hydrophobic interactions (Ong and Manoukian, 1988). However, depending on the size of the hydrophilic group, it is possible to accommodate the cis configuration of oleic acid without imposing structural constraints on the micelles. This point is clearly illustrated in the comparison of the solubilizing capacities of polysorbate 80 and polysorbate 60, as shown in Table 12.7, where no differences between the two surfactants were found. This is most likely attributed to the presence of the bulky sorbitan group.

Although it is possible to correlate solute solubility to different physical properties, such as molar volume, polarity, polarizability, and chain length, the most frequently used property is the solute octanol/water partition coefficient ($P_{o/w}$). Rank order correlations between the $P_{o/w}$ values of a series of substituted barbituric acids and the amount solubilized by polyoxyethylene stearates have been reported (Ismail et al., 1970). Similarly, linear relationships have been established between the octanol/water partition coefficients of a series of substituted benzoic acids and micelles of polysorbate 20 and water coefficient (Tomida et al., 1978).

Other Ingredients

Addition of nonelectrolytes can also have a profound effect on the solubilizing capacity of surfactant solutions. Such additives can either increase the solubilization potential of a surfactant (synergistic effect) or decrease it (antagonistic effect). For example, the addition of mono- and polyhydroxy alcohols was found to have a synergistic effect on the solubility of several compounds by different surfactants and this effect was shown to increase with the alcohol chain length. Surfactants may precipitate in the presence of some organic additives. Micellization may not occur if high enough concentrations of, for example, alcohols are present. Excipients such as phospholipids also affect CMC. When hydroxylated additives are added or incorporated into nonionic surfactant solutions, they increase the solubilizing efficiencies and reduce the concentration of solubilizers needed to attain a therapeutic dose.

Abdel-Rahman et al. (1991) have studied the effects of surfactant structure, pH, temperature, and organic additives on the solubilization of chlordiazepoxide. They found that the volume of various hydrocarbons solubilized by potassium laureate (i.e., the solubilizing capacity) was inversely related to the molar volume of the hydrocarbons. This relationship is to be expected if solubilization is a consequence of drug incorporation in the micelles. In addition to volume, polarity and shape are contributory factors. Solubility increased with increasing surfactant concentration. Polysorbate 80, with a longer hydrocarbon chain, was shown to be more efficient as a solubilizer than polysorbate 20. Extending the POE chain length in a homologous series of surfactants led to a decrease in the amount of drug solubilized. Rao et al. (2006) investigated the combined effect of micellization and complexation on solubilization of poorly soluble drugs. The authors developed a mathematical model to provide the quantitative basis for this approach, the model shows good agreement with two literature cases, where the combined solubility is less than the sum of the individual solubility values in cyclodextrins and surfactants.

Mixed Micelles

Solubilization in Mixed Micelles

Surfactant mixtures are commonly used in many practical surfactant applications. Mixtures are advantageous because purification of a single compound may be too costly or difficult and because surfactant mixtures often perform better than a single surfactant (Shiloach and Blankschtein, 1998a–c). For example, in skin care applications, synergism in a surfactant mixture can minimize the total surfactant monomer concentration (Garcia et al., 1992), which in turn has been shown to reduce skin irritation. The synergistic behavior of surfactant mixtures may also be exploited to reduce the total amount of surfactant used in a particular application, thus reducing both cost and environmental impact. In addition, as environmental regulations on producing and releasing new materials become more restrictive, it may be preferable from a regulatory perspective to combine existing surfactants rather than introducing new ones (Shiloach and Blankschtein, 1998a).

Surfactant mixtures are also often employed in drug solubilization since such mixtures exhibit high solubilization potential for lipophilic drugs and also are physiologically relevant (Humberstone et al., 1996; Krishnadas et al., 2003; Rhee, 2007). Christensen et al. (2004) applies solubilization in mixed micelles to *in vitro* lipid digestion models to simulate drug in an *in vivo* setting. Mixtures of surfactants can lead to changes in the size and shapes of micelles, as well as to increases in the amount of oil solubilized in some surfactant solutions (Florence, 1981; Hammad and Muller, 1998; Sugioka and Moroi, 1998). Mixed micelles act as solubilizing vehicles for nonswelling amphiphilic such as long-chain fatty acids and cholesterol. As early as 1969, Small et al. (1969) have studied simple and mixed bile salt micelles using NMR. They found that the hydrophobic side of the bile salt molecule containing methyl groups is hindered in its molecular form by the addition of lecithin. Furthermore, by assuming a disk-shaped micelle model in which the outer perimeter of bile salt molecules encloses a small disc of lecithin molecules, they found that as the molar ratio of lecithin increases, the diameter of the micellar disc would increase. This leads to a decrease in the fraction of lecithin molecules in contact with bile salts.

Naylor et al. (1993) studied the ability of lecithin to modify the rate and mechanism of dissolution of hydrocortisone in the presence of sodium taurocholate (NaTC) solutions. They found that in the presence of lecithin, the CMC of NaTC dropped owing to the *more effective solubilization capacity of the mixed micelle*. Furthermore, the CMC value dropped more on saturation with hydrocortisone, implying some interaction between hydrocortisone and the NaTC/lecithin micelles. These results indicated that in the NaTC-only system, wetting effects predominated dissolution, whereas in the NaTC/lecithin system, the dissolution rate of hydrocortisone was enhanced mainly through solubilization.

Humberstone et al. (1996) investigated the solubilization and intrinsic dissolution of halofantrine hydrochloride (Hf·HCl), a highly lipophilic phenanthrenemethanol antimalarial with poor and erratic absorption of Hf after oral administration, using micellar composition (NaTC alone) and mixed micellar composition (NaTC and lecithin). Studies were initiated based on the fact that food increases the oral bioavailability of Hf in humans approximately three- to fivefold. The solubility and intrinsic dissolution rate of Hf·HCl were investigated as a function of bile salt concentration (NaTC, 0–30 mM) and micellar composition (4:1 NaTC:lecithin). At premicellar (fasted) concentrations of NaTC (<5 mM), the solubility and intrinsic dissolution rate were very low (<15 μg/mL; <0.01 μg s^{-1} cm^{-2}). At NaTC concentrations typical of the postprandial state, the solubility and dissolution rate improved dramatically. For example, solubility in 30 mM NaTC increased approximately 1000-fold relative to buffer control, with even greater enhancement (3000-fold) associated with mixed micellar systems. These data suggest that the improved absorption of Hf·HCl in the fed state is most likely due to the increased solubilization and dissolution of the drug in the presence of mixed micelles containing bile salts.

Comparison of Solubilizing Capacity Among Different Types of Micelles

Hammad and Muller (1998) investigated the solubility of clonazepam in bile salt/soya phosphatidylcholine-mixed micelles (BS/SPC-MM). The solubility of clonazepam in different micellar systems was studied as a function of the concentration. The linear increase in clonazepam solubility is attributed to the parallel increase in the number of micellar species available to solubilize clonazepam (Alkan-Onyuksel et al., 1994). Hammad and Muller (1998) also compared the solubilization capacity of BS/SPC-MM with other surfactant systems such as pluronic F68, sugar ether, and BS. It was found that BS/SPC-MM was proven superior in enhancing the solubility of clonazepam. At a concentration of 10%, 3.5-, 30-, 40-, and 50-fold increases in clonazepam solubility were observed in pluronic F68, BS, sugar ether, and BS/SPC-MM, respectively. The results showed that BS/SPC-MM systems displayed the highest solubilizing capacity, while pluronic F68 showed the lowest. The authors believed that lower solubilizing capacity of pluronic F68 could be explained by the fact that it has a semipolar micelle core that is not suitable for the accommodation of the lipophilic side of clonazepam molecules that would be responsible for interaction and orientation of the drug in the micelle. Moreover, water may penetrate into the oxypropylene region of the micelle. This effect would render this region too polar for solubilizate molecules (Elworthy and Patel, 1983). In addition, incomplete micellization is expected from the structural features of pluronic surfactants which could be another reason for the decreased solubilizing capacity of these surfactants for this drug. On the other hand, higher solubility could be achieved in MM probably owing to the simultaneous presence of both the charged palisade layer (the charges of PC and BS) and lipophilic core (PC fatty acids residue and the lipophilic side of BS) in the MM, which result in enhanced interaction with polar and nonpolar regions, respectively, of the clonazepam molecule. Lower solubility in sodium glycocholate (SGC) micelles compared with that in BS/SPC-MM was thought to be due to its smaller micelle size and higher hydrophilicity. Balzer (1996) showed that sugar ether or glucoside 81s forms anisometric *worm-like* micelles with high aggregation numbers favoring higher solubilization. However, it has a lower solubilizing capacity compared with that of BS/SPC-MM. This can be explained by lower lipophilicity of the micelle core (C8–10) compared with that of BS/SPC-MM. In addition, the bulky hydrophilic palisade layer of the glucose units is expected to hinder interaction of clonazepam molecules with the micelles.

However, only slight differences in solubilizing capacity were observed among MM prepared from different bile salts, sodium cholate (SC) and SGC. The slight difference between SC/SPC-MM and SGC/SPC-MM is accounted for by the small difference in micellar size, as these two BS are trihydroxy bile salts and expected to form more or less similar micelles.

Moreover, increasing SPC ratio in MM led to a parallel increase in solubility due to the parallel increase of both size and lipophilicity of the formed BS/SPC-MM. This effect has also been noted during the solubility study of diazepam in MM from SC and egg phosphatidylcholine (Rosoff and Serajuddin, 1980).

Additive Effect on Solubilization of Mixed Micelles

Hammad and Muller (1998) studied the effect of addition of alcohols with different hydrophilicity, such as ethanol, propanol, butanol, pentanol, cyclohexanol, and benzyl alcohol, as well as 2-phenylethanol, on clonazepam solubility in MM. Addition of alcohols with ascending lipophilicity, beginning with ethanol, propanol, and up to butanol, insignificantly affected clonazepam solubility in MM. Addition of pentanol cyclohexanol, benzyl alcohol, or 2-phenylethanol increased the solubility to different degrees. The increase in the lipophilicity of alcohol increased its affinity to the micellar phase and hence a higher concentration of the alcohol in the micellar phase is expected.

It has been reported that water-soluble alcohols (methanol to butanol) are predominantly dissolved in the water phase and may decrease or increase the micellar aggregation number, n, depending on the alcohol concentration. Moderately soluble alcohols (pentanol and hexanol) are distributed between the aqueous and micellar phases and may increase the association number (Backland et al., 1981). Moreover, more hydrophilic alcohols were found to increase the CMC, while more lipophilic alcohols were found to decrease the CMC (Green, 1972). Although the decrease in CMC could partially contribute to the increase in the solubilizing capacity, it could also be considered as an indication of the formation of micellar species with larger size. These results furnish a basis that agrees with the explanations of Hammad and Muller (1998). In addition, Roe and Barry (1982) reported that addition of 2-phenylethanol at concentrations in the same range used in this study to different bile salt solutions showed an increase in the micellar size. The increase in the size of bile salt micelles as a function of 2-phenylethanol concentration occurred in a more or less similar fashion to the increase of clonazepam solubility in MM.

Incorporation of alcohol into MM could result in the swelling of MM, and this in turn increases its solubilizing capacity. This increase in size does not appear to be the only factor that is responsible for the higher solubility. Comparing the chemical structures alcohols that have aromatic rings showed the highest potential to increase the solubility of clonazepam in MM. The saturation solubility of clonazepam in these alcohols was considerably higher compared to its solubility in the other alcohols. This leads to the assumption that the solubilization capacity of MM is influenced by the nature of the incorporated alcohol. Accordingly, it could explain why benzyl alcohol is more effective than pentanol in increasing the solubility of clonazepam, even though the latter is more lipophilic.

On the other hand, 2-phenylethanol has a similar chemical structure to benzyl alcohol and hence a similar solubilizing capacity after incorporation in MM. The saturation solubility of 2-phenylethanol in the aqueous 5% MM phase is about 4%, while this is about 5% for benzyl alcohol. From the pharmaceutical point of view, the increase in clonazepam solubility in MM by addition of either benzyl alcohol or 2-phenylethanol makes their usual use as preservatives more advantageous owing to the possibility of decreasing the concentration of MM.

Marszall (1988) studied the effect of electrolytes on the cloud point of mixed ionic–nonionic surfactant solutions such as SDS and Triton X-100. It was found that the cloud point of the mixed micellar solutions is drastically lowered by a variety of electrolytes at considerably lower concentrations than those affecting the cloud point of nonionic surfactants used alone. The results indicate that the factors affecting the cloud point phenomena of mixed surfactants at very low concentrations of ionic surfactants and electrolytes are primarily electrostatic in nature. The change in the original charge distribution of mixed micelles at a fixed SDS-Triton X-100 ratio (one molecule per micelle), as indicated by the cloud point measurements as a function of electrolyte concentration, depends mostly on the valency number of the cations (counterions) and to some extent on the kind of the anion (co-ion) and is independent of the type of monovalent cation.

Mixed Micelles in Physiological Conditions

In vivo, bile salts enhance secretion of cholesterol into bile and its subsequent solubilization with phosphatidylcholine in mixed micelles. Sphingomyelin, a major structural lipid of the hepatocyte canalicular membrane, and disaturated phosphatidylcholines are known to impede nucleation of solid cholesterol crystals in supersaturated model systems. To understand these physicochemical effects, Erpecum and Carey (1997) compared the influence of bile salts on interactions of cholesterol with natural sphingomyelins, as well as with dipalmitoyl and egg yolk phosphatidylcholines using various *in vitro* systems. Submicellar bile salts significantly enhanced the bidirectional transfer of dehydroergosterol (a fluorescent cholesterol analog) between sphingomyelin and egg yolk phosphatidylcholine vesicles in the rank order taurocholate < tauroursodeoxycholate < taurodeoxycholate. Quasielastic light scattering of serially diluted sphingomyelin-taurocholate mixtures (1:1 molar ratio, 3 g/dL) revealed metastable temperature-dependent transitions between globular rod-shaped micelles and vesicles, suggesting that phase transitions under these experimental conditions were metastable only at temperatures below 37°C. Ternary phase diagrams vof all sphingomyelins and dipalmitoyl phosphatidylcholine with cholesterol and taurocholate (37°C, 3 g/dL, 0.15 M NaCl) were identical. Compared to systems containing egg yolk phosphatidylcholine, the one-phase micellar zone and two- and three-phase solid cholesterol crystal-containing zones were markedly reduced, whereas the three-phase zone with stable cholesterol-sphingomyelin liquid crystals was greatly expanded. Their results suggest that the high affinity of cholesterol for sphingomyelin is lost in the presence of bile salts. These findings may be relevant to secretion of cholesterol into bile and to its inability to crystallize in the hepatocyte canalicular lumen or its surrounding membranes.

Modeling of Mixed Micelles

In spite of their widespread use, surfactant mixtures are fundamentally not well understood at a molecular level. For specific applications, such mixtures are often chosen based on experience, empirical evidence, or trial and error research. A comprehensive, predictive, molecular theory would thus advance our understanding of surfactant mixture behavior. Such a theory would also facilitate the design and optimization of new surfactant mixtures by reducing the experimentation necessary to identify suitable mixtures and optimize their performance (Shiloach and Blankschtein, 1998a).

Binary surfactant mixtures have traditionally been modeled using the pseudophase-separation approach, in which the micelles are treated as a separate, infinite phase in equilibrium with the monomer phase. Because the micelles are considered to be infinitely large, this approach cannot provide information on micelle shape or size (Shiloach and Blankschtein, 1998a). According to the development history, two models one based on a regular solution theory and another based on a molecular-thermodynamic theory exists and, are discussed in the following.

Model Based on Regular Solution Theory

Regular solution theory can be applied to understand the thermodynamics of micellization in binary micelle mixtures and to determine critical mixed micelle concentrations, as well as aggregation numbers. Treiner et al. (1988) used this analysis to study the micellar solubilization of 1-pentanol in mixed surfactant systems. For anionic–cationic surfactant mixtures, and the sign and amplitude of the micellar solubilization was found to change when a second surfactant was added to the micellar solution. This behavior was governed by the interaction forces between two surfactants in the mixed micelle. Regular solution theory developed for the solubility of a gas in binary liquid systems was applied. The solubility decreased for 1-pentanol in the case of strongly interacting micellar systems (anionic + cationic mixtures), and increased over the additivity rule (a positive synergistic effect) when repulsive interactions occurred. The micellar solubilization of mixed surfactant systems was further investigated by studying the micellar solubilization of barbituric acids for two binary surfactant systems. Variation of partition coefficients (K_m) between micelle and water as a function of micellar composition was represented by a relationship similar to that obtained from regular solution theory with a single empirical coefficient (β). This parameter was found to be negative for all systems studied. Moreover, the sign and amplitude of β, and therefore the variation of K_m with surfactant composition, were determined to be governed by the interaction between unlike surfactants in the micelles. In most cases, the K_m values of polar hydrophobic molecules should be less in mixed surfactant systems than that calculated from the ideal additivity rule.

$$K_m = \frac{(C_m/C_w)}{(V_w/V_m)} \qquad (12.12)$$

where m refers to the micellar phase, w, the water phase, and V, an estimate of the partial molar volume. For mixed systems, the apparent partition coefficient may be written as

$$P = \frac{(C_m - C_w)}{[C_w(C_S - C_m)]} \qquad (12.13)$$

where C_s is the total surfactant concentration and C_m is the total monomer concentration. C_m has to be calculated for each surfactant by

$$C_m = Xf_1\,CMC \qquad (12.14)$$

where X is the micellar mole fraction of the binary surfactant, and f_1 is the activity coefficient. The simplest way to estimate f values is through regular solution theory where

$$f = \exp(\beta x^2) \qquad (12.15)$$

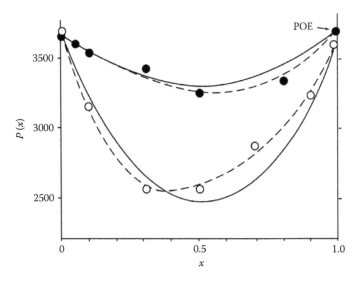

FIGURE 12.13 Variation of $P(x)$ with micellar composition for pentobarbital: (o) SDS + POE; solid line: Equation 12.15 with $\beta = -1.4$; (•) TTAB + POE; solid line; Equation 12.15 with $\beta = -0.4$. (From Treiner C. et al., *J. Coll. Interf. Sci.*, 125, 261–270, 1988. With permission.)

and β is the interaction coefficient, which for mixed surfactant solution is determined from CMC measurements. Therefore, a plot of K_m versus X will give β values, as shown in Figure 12.13.

More recently, Treiner et al. (1990) examined the effect of surfactant–surfactant interaction energy on solubilization in strong interacting micellar systems. Their approach, based on regular solution theory as outlined earlier is purely thermodynamic and does not take into account any structural changes on surfactant mixing, which might influence the solubilization phenomena. The hypothesis was that if the interaction energy between two surfactants forming a mixed micelle is attractive, then the solubilization of a solute should be less in the mixed micelle than in either pure surfactant. They found that the variation of the distribution constant of complex molecules between mixed micelles and water as a function of micellar composition can be represented with an equation having a single adjustable parameter (β). This parameter is closely related to the binary interaction coefficient of the regular solution approximation. The more negative the β value, the lower the decrease of micellar solubilization of polar solutes on surfactant mixing. Micellization of a number of solutes was examined using cationic, anionic, and nonionic surfactants with alkyl chain lengths ranging from C_{10} to C_{14}. Micellar solubilization of babituric acids involves the hydrophobic moieties of these molecules, such that the polar group plays no part in the interaction with mixed micelles. Their results, shown in Table 12.8, demonstrate that the large increase of micellar size for anionic–cationic surfactant systems does not lead to an increase in the partition coefficient. In this table, ΔN refers to the change in the aggregation number and ΔK_m, the change in the partition coefficient. A plus sign for these values indicates a positive deviation from the additivity rule, while a minus sign indicates a negative deviation. For these mixtures, the solubilization shows the largest negative deviations from ideality. The rate of change of K_m (ΔK_m) with micellar composition is a function of intramicellar interaction energies between unlike surfactants. Furthermore, they found that solubilization of nonpolar solutes (hydrocarbons) increased in mixed micelles over that of single micellar results. This is expected, since the enthalpy of mixing for the mixed hydrocarbon core in which the nonpolar solute will be located should be close to zero, and thus, the solubilization should follow the ideal mixing rule. For nonpolar compounds, the increase in the aggregation number on surfactant mixing with the change in structure from spherical to cylindrical symmetry favors solubilization of those solutes that penetrate the hydrocarbon core. The effect of polar solutes is more difficult to analyze. With polar

TABLE 12.8

Micellar Solubilization and Other Physicochemical Parameters for Binary Mixed Surfactant Systems

Solute	Mixed Surfactant	β	ΘN	ΘK_m
Benzene	NaPFO + NaDEC	1.8	+	+
1-Pentanol	NaPFO + NaDEC	1.8	+	−
1-Octanol	DMLL + C_{12}Na	−15	+	+
1-Octanol	DMLL + C_{14}Br	−1	−	−
1-Hexanol	C_{16}PyCl + NPE$_{15}$	−1.3	NA	−
1-Hexanol	C_{12}Cl + C_{12}Na	−25	+	−
1-Pentanol	C_{10}Na + C_{10}Br	−13.2	+	−
1-Pentanol	C_{12}E$_{23}$ + C_{12}Na	−2.6	0	−
1-Pentanol	LiPFO + C_{12}Li	2.2	+	+
1-Decane	C_{12}Cl + C_{12}Na	−25	+	+
1-Hexane	NPE$_{10}$ + C_{16}PyCl	−1.3	NA	+
1-Hexane	NPE$_{10}$ + C_{12}Na	−4.8	NA	+
1-Hexane	C_{16}PyCl + C_{12}Na	−25	NA	+

NaPFO, sodium perfluorooctanoate; NaDEC, sodium decanoate; DMLL, N^{α}, N^{α}-dimethyl-N^{ε}-lauroyl lysine; LiPFO, lithium perfluorooctanesulfonate; NPE$_{10}$, nonylphenolpoly(oxyethylate); C_{16}PyCl, hexadecylpyridinium chloride; NA, not available.

Additional values of β have been tabulated for many binary surfactant mixtures (Rosen, M. J., *Surfactants and Interfacial Phenomena*, 2nd ed., Wiley, New York, 1978).

Source: Taken from Treiner, C. et al. *Langmuir*, 6, 1211–1216, 1990.

solutes, there was an increase in the micellar aggregation number on surfactant mixing for anionic/nonionic mixtures. However, this increase is not responsible for micellar solubilization changes of polar solutes. Furthermore, the structural changes should have little effect on the micellar solubilization of polar solutes that interact with the micelle by surface adsorption.

Others have studied the volumetric changes occurring in mixed micelles of anionic–anionic and nonionic–nonionic surfactants as a determinant of intermolecular interactions and a measure of the thermodynamic ideality of mixing. In particular, Funasaki et al. (1986) have studied the volumetric behavior of mixed micelles of ionic and nonionic surfactants and analyzed their results in terms of regular solution theory. They found that in water, anionic surfactants such as SDS bind to PEG, but cationic surfactants (such as DTAB) do not, likely due to differences observed in ΔV_m. For two surfactants, the micelle has a smaller volume than the liquid. Even highly charged anionic surfactant mixtures such as esters of coenzyme A (CoA) with fatty acids (palmitic, stearic, and oleic) can be described using regular solution theory (Constantinides and Steim, 1988). The behavior of the palmitoyl-CoA/stearoyl-CoA mixture is ideal, while the palmitoyl-CoA/oleoyl-CoA mixture, although not exhibiting ideal behavior, can be fitted reasonably well by nonideal theory. In both mixtures, selective micellization takes place and, unlike the case of pure fatty acyl-CoAs, above the CMC of the mixtures the concentration of free molecules in solution is strongly dependent on total concentration (Constantinides and Steim, 1988). The regular solution theory approach has also been extended to multicomponent surfactant mixtures, by decomposing the interactions into pair-wise interactions between every possible surfactant pair.

In spite of the wide use and convenience of regular solution theory, the theoretical validity of using it to describe nonideal mixing in mixed surfactant micelles has been questioned (Hoffmann and Poessnecker, 1994). Regular solution theory assumes that the excess entropy of mixing is zero; calorimetric measurements or calculations of the enthalpy of mixing combined with mixture CMC measurements (Osborne-Lee and Schechter, 1986; Foerster et al., 1990) have shown that the excess mixing entropy in some mixed surfactant systems is nonzero. In addition, if the theory accurately models the nonideal mixing, the parameter should be strictly constant as a function of composition. However, calculations of the β parameter based on CMC measurements for many types of binary surfactant mixtures, including cationic/nonionic (Desai and Dixit, 1996), anionic/nonionic (Carrion Fite, 1985), anionic/anionic (Bharadwaj and Ahluwalia, 1996), anionic/zwitterionic (Bakshi et al., 1993), and mixtures containing bile salts (Haque et al., 1996), demonstrate that β can vary widely with solution composition. Although some variability in β may be due to experimental error in measurements of the mixture CMC (Hoffmann and Poessnecker, 1994), a large variability of β with solution composition indicates that regular solution theory may not appropriately describe the nonideal micellar mixing behavior.

Regardless of these limitations, the pseudophase separation/regular solution theory approach remains a very widely used and convenient method for analyzing experimental CMC measurements of mixed micellar systems. The approach is conceptually simple and straightforward to apply given experimental CMC data. The β parameter quantitatively captures the extent of nonideality in a single number that can be easily compared among different pairs of surfactants (Shiloach and Blankschtein, 1998).

Model Based on Molecular-Thermodynamic Theory

In an effort to go beyond regular solution theory and better understand the molecular basis of mixed surfactant system behavior, several molecular-thermodynamic theories for surfactant mixtures have been developed. The molecular-thermodynamic theory will be briefly introduced and discussed in the following. Readers are referred to a recent summary (Shiloach and Blankschtein, 1998) or can obtain more detailed description and discussion in literature (Nagarajan, 1985, 1986; Puvvada and Blankschtein, 1990, 1992a; Nagarajan and Ruckenstein, 1991; Bergstroem and Eriksson, 1992; Sarmoria et al., 1992; Zoeller and Blankschtein, 1995, 1998; Almgren et al., 1996; Barzykin and Almgren, 1996; Bergstroem, 1996; Zoeller et al., 1996; Blankschtein et al., 1997; Shiloach and Blankschtein, 1997, 1998; Thomas et al., 1997; Shiloach et al., 1998).

The theory is based on calculating the size and composition distribution of the mixed micelles, which in turn depends on the free energy of forming a mixed micelle, g_{mic}. The free energy of mixed micellization is modeled as the sum of several free-energy contributions and an ideal entropy of mixing (Puvvada and Blankschtein, 1992; Shiloach and Blankschtein, 1998), as illustrated conceptually in Figure 12.14. For each free-energy contribution, the authors have highlighted schematically only the relevant characteristics of the surfactant tails or the surfactant heads. g_{mic} is a function of the shape, sh, the micelle core minor radius, I_c, and the composition of the mixed micelles, α, and expressed as

$$g_{mic} \cdot (sh, I_c, \alpha) = g_{tr} + g_{int} + g_{pack} + g_{st} + g_{elec} + kT[\alpha \ln \alpha + (1-\alpha)\ln(1-\alpha)] \qquad (12.16)$$

where k is the Boltzmann constant and T is the absolute temperature. Other free-energy terms are discussed.

The first three free-energy contributions involve only the surfactant tails. The transfer contribution, g_{tr}, accounts for transferring the surfactant tails of both surfactant types, drawn as long black tails and shorter grey tails (Figure 12.14), from the aqueous solution to the core of the mixed micelle, which is modeled at this stage as a binary oil mixture composed of the two tail types. The transfer free energy can be calculated as a function of temperature and of the number of carbon atoms in the corresponding hydrocarbon tail, using experimental solubility data for hydrocarbons in water (Puvvada and Blankschtein, 1992).

The interfacial contribution, g_{int}, accounts for forming the interface, which is drawn in Figure 12.14 as a heavy dashed line, between the oil mixture representing the micellar core and

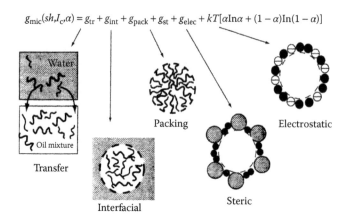

$$g_{mic}(sh,I_c,\alpha) = g_{tr} + g_{int} + g_{pack} + g_{st} + g_{elec} + kT[\alpha\ln\alpha + (1-\alpha)\ln(1-\alpha)]$$

Water

Oil mixture

Transfer

Interfacial

Packing

Steric

Electrostatic

FIGURE 12.14 Schematic conceptual representation of the various free-energy contributions involved in the free energy of the mixed micellization (see text for details). The schematic highlights only the surfactant characteristics relevant to each free-energy contribution. The free-energy contributions include transferring the tails of both surfactant types from the aqueous solution to the core of the mixed micelle, which is modeled as an oil mixture composed of the longer black tails and the shorter grey tails (g_n); forming the interface, drawn as a heavy dashed line, between the oil mixture representing the micellar core and the aqueous solution (g_{int}); anchoring the surfactant tails at the micellar core/water interface and packing them in the micellar core (g_{pack}); accounting for steric interactions among the large grey surfactant heads and the small black surfactant heads (g_{st}); and accounting for electrostatic interactions among the negatively charged surfactant heads and the black uncharged surfactant heads (g_{elec}). (Reprinted with permission from Shiloach, A., and Blankschtein, D., *Langmuir,* 14, 7166–7182, 1998. American Chemical Society.)

the aqueous solution. In other words, it represents the free-energy change per surfactant molecule associated with forming an interface between the hydrocarbon micellar core and the surrounding aqueous solution. The interfacial free energy is a function of interfacial area, interfacial tension of hydrocarbons, and composition.

The packing contribution, g_{pack}, accounts for anchoring one end of the tails of both surfactant types at the micellar core/water interface and packing the surfactant tails in the micellar core. If, as illustrated in Figure 12.14, the two-surfactant types have tails of different lengths, they may pack better in the micellar core than tails that are all of the same length and, thus, contribute to synergism in mixed micelle formation. This contribution is evaluated using a single-chain mean-field model in which the effect of neighboring chains on a single chain is calculated (Szleifer et al., 1987). In mixed micelles, the mean-field approach implies that two different tails mix homogeneously in the micellar core, and g_{pack} is function of α. In general, g_{pack} is a nonlinear function of α and therefore, it can contribute to nonideality in mixed micelle formation.

The last two free-energy contributions involve only the surfactant heads. The steric contribution, g_{st}, accounts for steric interactions between the surfactant heads at the micellar interface. This contribution can be responsible for synergism in mixed micelle formation if the heads of the two-surfactant types have different sizes, as illustrated by the large grey heads and small black heads in Figure 12.14. The steric contribution depends only on the size of the surfactant heads.

The surfactant heads are treated as a monolayer adsorbed at the micellar interface, and their interactions are a function of the head cross-sectional areas of both surfactants as well as the composition. The larger the surfactant heads, the higher the g_{st}. A smaller area per surfactant molecule, as in cylindrical micelles, leads to a higher g_{st}, while a larger area per surfactant molecule, as in spherical micelles, leads to a lower g_{st} (Shiloach and Blankschtein, 1998).

Finally, the electrostatic contribution, g_{elec}, accounts for electrostatic interactions between the surfactant heads. If, for example, negatively charged surfactant heads are mixed with uncharged surfactant heads (shown in grey in Figure 12.14), the uncharged heads reduce the electrostatic repulsion between the charged heads and thus facilitate mixed micelle formation. The electrostatic contribution depends only on the electrostatic characteristics of the surfactant head, such as the valence of the charge and its location in the surfactant head.

The electrostatic free energy, g_{elec}, is calculated as the reversible work of charging the mixed micelle to its final surface charge density. For ionic/nonionic mixed micelles, in general, the higher the ionic mixed micelle composition, the higher g_{elec}. Also, the higher the surface charge density, the higher g_{elec}. If the charged surfactant heads are closer together, as in cylindrical micelles, where the area per surfactant molecule is smaller, gelec is higher. If the charged heads are farther apart, as in spherical micelles, g_{elec} is lower.

The last term in Equation 12.16 accounts for an ideal entropy of mixing. This ideal mixing entropy reflects the random mixing of the hydrocarbon tails in the bulk hydrocarbon phase.

In the molecular-thermodynamic theory of mixed micellization, the size and shape of the mixed micelles can also be predicted by calculating the size and composition distribution. This distribution can be expressed as a function of two fundamental parameters that control the size of the mixed micelles. The first parameter, K, is defined as (Puvvada and Blankschtein, 1992a, b) to be

$$K = e^{\Delta\mu/kT} \tag{12.17}$$

where:

$$\Delta\mu = n_{sph}[g_m^{sph} - g_m^{cyl}] + kT \tag{12.18}$$

and n_{sph} is the aggregation number of a spherical mixed micelle, and g_m^{sph} and g_m^{cyl} are modified free energies of mixed micellization of the optimum spherical and infinite cylindrical mixed micelles, respectively. The parameter determines whether the mixed micelles form spheres or cylinders. If $\Delta\mu < 0$ (and thus $K < 1$), spheres are free-energetically more favorable, while if $\Delta\mu > 0$ ($K > 1$), cylinders are more favorable, and the mixed micelles grow. The second parameter, X_{cyl}, is defined as (Puvvada and Blankschtein, 1992)

$$X_{cyl} = e^{g_m^{cyl}/kT} \tag{12.19}$$

$$g_m^{cyl}/kT = g_{mic}^{cyl}/kT - 1 - \alpha \ln\alpha_1 - (1-\alpha)\ln(1-\alpha_1) \tag{12.20}$$

and g_{mic}^{cyl} is the free energy of mixed micellization of an infinite cylindrical mixed micelle, α is them mixed micelle composition, and α_1 is the monomer composition. Since g_m^{cyl} is a measure of the free-energy cost of adding a surfactant molecule to the cylindrical portion of the mixed micelle, then X_{cyl} can be viewed as the CMC for forming an infinitely large cylindrical mixed micelle. The lower the value of g_m^{cyl}, the more favorable it is to add a surfactant molecule to the cylindrical portion of the mixed micelle, and the easier it is for the mixed micelle to grow. A detailed discussion of the parameters K and X_{cyl} can be found in the works of Puvvada and Blankschtein (1992a, b).

Prediction of the aggregation number of mixed micelles and calculation of other molecular parameters are discussed thoroughly in Blankschtein's articles listed in the reference section. Interested readers can read these articles for details.

OTHER MICELLES

Solid Micelle Dispersion and Solution

Solid micelle dispersions may be defined as a solid dispersion containing surfactants that can dissolve water-insoluble drugs rapidly and prevent the precipitation of drugs by forming micelles in aqueous medium (Sjoekvist et al., 1991; Alden et al., 1992; Sjoekvist et al., 1992; Alden et al., 1993; Hwang et al., 1996; Kim et al., 1996; Shin et al., 1996; Joshi et al., 2004). They can also be referred to as solid solutions containing surfactants (Sjoekvist et al., 1991; Alden et al., 1992; Sjoekvist et al., 1992; Alden et al., 1993; Smirnova, 1996; D'Antona et al., 2000) and there are those that are microemulsions or self-microemulsifying (Kim and Ku, 2000; Kim et al., 2001; Itoh et al., 2002a,b; Li et al., 2002; Kang et al., 2004; Li et al., 2005).

Griseofulvin solid dispersion of PEG 3000 containing surfactant aggregates (micelles) were studied for solubilization and enhancement of dissolution of this water-insoluble drug (Sjoekvist et al., 1991; Alden et al., 1992; Sjoekvist et al., 1992; Alden et al., 1993). SDS, DTAB, Brij 35, and polysorbate 80 were used. A melting (fusion) method was employed to manufacture these solid dispersion/solution containing surfactants. An almost instant and complete dissolution was obtained for dispersions with 1% and 2% (by weight) SDS. X-ray diffraction revealed that a complete molecular dispersion or solution of griseofulvin in PEG/SDS was obtained when 2% SDS was incorporated. A relationship between the solubilizing efficiency of the surfactant in aqueous solutions and its ability to increase the solid solubility of a drug in PEG, and subsequently the dissolution rate was obtained.

In another example of a polyethylene glycol/surfactant, solid dispersion is presented by Dannenfelser et al. (2004) with a poorly water-insoluble drug exhibiting only a 0.17 µg/mL aqueous solubility. At 40 mg/mL, the PEG 3350/polysorbate 80 solid dispersion exhibited similar exposure as that of a cosolvent-surfactant solution and a 10-fold increase over a dry blend formulation, thus enabling a solid oral dosage form for clinical trials.

Other methods to prepare solid micelle dispersion, such as spray drying of a drug containing micelle solution onto solid core materials or solvent emulsification technique to prepare solid lipid nanoparticles, can be found in literature (Karmazina, 1997; Burruano et al., 1999; Luo et al., 2006; Radomska-Soukharev et al., 2006).

El Haskouri et al. (1999) studied the formation of hexagonal mesostructured mixed-valence oxovanadium phosphates ($[CTA]xVOPO_4 \cdot zH_2O$), in ICMUV-2 solids, through a S^+I^- cooperative mechanism using cationic surfactant (CTAB) rodlike micelles as a template. On the lines of the hypothesis that the driving force leading to the formation of mesostructured solid is the charge density matching at the interface between the supramolecular-organic and supramolecular-inorganic4 moieties, the self-assembling process between CTA^+ micelles and $VOPO_4^{q-}$ planar anions can be thought of as a consequence of the adequate adjustment of the metal mean oxidation state. The S^+I^- cooperative mechanism is illustrated in Figure 12.15. The interesting mesostructured laminar solids could be useful implications in water-insoluble drug delivery.

Although additional discussion on this topic can be found in the section of case studies, solid micelle dispersion/solution is not the primary scope of this chapter. Readers interested in this topic can refer to a corresponding chapter in this book or literature elsewhere (for characterization and thermodynamic modeling of solid micelles: Smirnova, 1995, 1996; Berret, 1997; Fujiwara et al., 1997; Marques, 1997; Markina et al., 1998; El Haskouri et al., 1999; for pharmaceutical applications and methods to prepare solid micelle dispersions: Fontan et al., 1991; Sjoekvist et al., 1991; Alden et al., 1992; Sjoekvist et al., 1992; Alden et al., 1993; Hwang et al., 1996; Kim et al., 1996; Shin et al., 1996; Karmazina, 1997; Burruano et al., 1999).

Micellization in Nonaqueous Systems

Some surfactants undergo an aggregation process in hydrocarbon and other nonpolar solvents. The forces involved in surfactant aggregation with nonaqueous solvents must differ considerably from

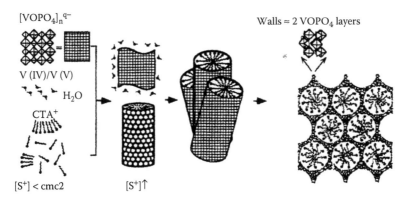

$[VOPO_4]_n^{q-}$

V (IV)/V (V)

H_2O

CTA^+

$[S^+] < cmc2$

$[S^+]\uparrow$

Walls ≈ 2 $VOPO_4$ layers

FIGURE 12.15 Schematic representation of the S^+I^- cooperative formation mechanism for ICMUV-2 mesostructured oxovanadium phosphates. (Reprinted with permission from El Haskouri J. et al., *Chem. Mater.*, 11, 1446–1454, 1999. Copyright 1999 American Chemical Society.)

those already discussed for water-based systems. The orientation of the surfactant relative to the bulk solvent will be opposite to that in water; therefore, these systems are referred to as reverse micelles. These micelles will not have any significant electrical properties relative to the bulk solvent (Luisi et al., 1988).

In nonaqueous solvents, the significant energetic source of micelle formation is the reduction of unfavorable interactions between the ionic head group of the surfactant and the nonpolar solvent molecules. In these systems, small spherical micelles appear to be the most favored, especially when the reduction of solvent/polar group interactions is important (Luisi et al., 1988; Huruguen et al., 1991).

Reversed micelles are usually used for the solubilization of oil-insoluble substances such as proteins, peptides (Brown and Slusser, 1994; Shapiro et al., 1994; Ichikawa et al., 1998), fatty acid esters, phospholipids, and tocopherols (Nielsen, 1998). Usefulness of reversed micelles can also be found in the development of delivery systems for antitumor drugs such as daunomycin, doxorubicin, verapamil (multidrug resistance), and genistein (multidrug resistance) (Frazier and Karukstis, 1997; Thompson and Karukstis, 1997; Karukstis et al., 1998). Sodium *bis*(2-ethylhexyl) sulfosuccinate (AOT) was employed as the anionic surfactant in these reversed micelles. Other reversed micelles using AOT as the surfactant include the studies of piroxicam (Andrade and Costa, 1996) and water-soluble vitamins (Ihara et al., 1995). Reversed micelles can also be used in aerosol formulations to deliver proteins and peptides (Evans et al., 1991; Evans and Farr, 1992, 1993; Brown and Slusser, 1994). Because it is not the scope of this chapter, for more information of micellization in nonaqueous systems, the readers can find related literature cited in this section or elsewhere.

DRUG DELIVERY APPLICATIONS

Solubilization of water-insoluble drugs by surfactant micelles has long been considered to enhance drug solubility, particularly for parenteral and oral administrations. Additional protection of labile drugs from the environment through solubilization within the micelles has also been proposed. To date, several reports have appeared in the literature on the incorporation of a wide variety of drugs into surfactant micelles, focusing on nonionic surfactants in particular (Lawrence, 1994). Drug products in micellar systems, however, are limited because the solubilization capacity is usually too low to be of practical use. For an average dose of a drug in the order of tens of milligrams and the concentration of the micellar solution not exceeding 20 wt% surfactant, only highly potent lipophilic drugs, such as testosterone, can be developed in such systems. Even if it is possible to increase solubilization to a sufficient degree, preferably to about 100 mg/g of surfactant, there are a number of other issues that need to be addressed. One issue is potential drug precipitation with subsequent local irritation due to a large dilution of the micellar solution, particularly on intravenous and oral administration. However, high drug concentration can be achieved by solubilizing the drug in binary surfactant–cosolvent mixtures to form a drug concentrate, such as Sandimmune® Injection (cyclosporine concentrate for injection). The concentrate can be diluted with an IV diluent to a desired concentration just before the intravenous dosing takes place. The micelles are formed during dilution on mixing. For topical applications, controlled release of drugs such as estradiol can be achieved with polymer/surfactant formulations (Barreiro-Iglesias et al., 2003).

Surfactants are employed in nanoparticle suspensions. Chen et al. (2002) evaluated the preparation of amorphous nanoparticle suspensions containing cyclosporine A, using the evaporative precipitation into aqueous solution (EPAS) system. The effect of particle size was studied varying the drug: surfactant ratios, type of surfactants, temperature, drug load, and solvent. Acceptable particle sizes suitable for both oral and parenteral administration were also studied. Additional articles in the nanoparticle delivery of poorly water-soluble drugs include Kipp (2004), Perkins et al. (2000), Young et al. (2000), and Tyner et al. (2004).

Quite often micellar solutions can solubilize other formulation additives in addition to the active, such as preservatives and sweetening agents. Such cosolubilization can lead either to a decrease or to an increase in drug solubilization (Attwood et al., 1994). The effect of one solute on the solubilization of another will depend on the mechanisms of solubilization. Competition between the drug and additive for uptake sites within the micellar interior can result in a decrease of drug solubilization. One solute might induce a reorganization of the micellar structure and thus increase solubility. For example, it has been found that benzoic acid increases the solubility of methylparaben in cetomacrogol solutions, but dichlorophenol decreases its solubilization (Crooks and Brown, 1973). Chloroxylenol reduces the solubility of methylparaben, and methylparaben reduces the solubility of chloroxylenol in cetomacrogol, there being no effect on mutual solubilities in the absence of surfactant. Althesin (Glaxo), a marketed preparation of intravenous anesthetics, contains a mixture of steroids. The more active anesthetic is alphadalone (present at 9 mg/mL) and the less active alphadalone acetate has been added (at 3 mg/mL) to improve the solubility of the alphaxolone in the Cremophor® EL vehicle (20%). From a similar study, it was assumed that this effect follows from an increase in micellar volume.

GENERAL DEVELOPMENT PROCEDURE FOR A MICELLAR DRUG SOLUBILIZATION SYSTEM

Preformulation data such as pH-partition coefficient, pH-solubility, pK_a, and pH-stability profiles can provide very useful information for the development of a micellar solubilization system for a water-insoluble drug. Therefore, before the initiation of formulation development, it is desirable to have the preformulation data of the water-insoluble drug. Readers can refer to the Chapter 9, "Solubilization Using Cosolvent Approach," for details. Following are several selection criteria and general methodologies that may be helpful for the development of a micellar solubilization system for a water-insoluble drug.

Surfactant Selection Based on Toxicology Profiles

Surfactant selection for drug solubilization and formulation development should be first based on the toxicology profile of the surfactant. A pharmaceutically acceptable surfactant is preferred, especially one that is already present in marketed drugs. Surfactants approved as food additives can also be considered. Surfactants are known permeation enhancers and therefore the route of administration must also be considered. Owing to this property, a surfactant given parenterally has hemolytic potential and therefore should be cautiously used in parenteral formulations (Ross et al., 2004).

Additional toxicology studies may be required. For example, acute oral toxicity in rats and mice, mutagenicity evaluation, 28-day oral toxicity in rodents and possibly nonrodents may be required for a food grade surfactant that is intended for oral dosage form development. Surfactants that have not been approved as either pharmaceutical or food grade should be used with caution since required toxicological studies may be extensive.

Surfactant Selection Based on Drug Solubility in Surfactants

For liquid surfactants, drug solubility can be approximated using a simple method, in which the drug is added to a fixed amount of a liquid surfactant while stirring at room temperature until the solid drug cannot further dissolve. For more accurate data, the drug solubility should be determined using an equilibrium solubility method.

For semisolid surfactants, the surfactant can be heated to a temperature higher than its melting point until it completely melts. A drug can then be added to a fixed amount of surfactant while stirring at that temperature until the solid drug cannot further dissolve. However, the drug should be stable at that temperature within the experimental period. Alternatively, the experiment can be done in an aqueous surfactant solution. The solid drug in excess can be equilibrated at a desirable temperature by constantly mixing for 24–48 h. The solubility of the drug in the surfactant solution can be determined using a suitable analytical method. This equilibrium solubility method can be also used to determine the solubility of a water-insoluble drug in an aqueous solution containing a solid surfactant.

In many cases, the solubility of a water-insoluble drug can be enhanced by adding a cosurfactant to a surfactant solution. Such solubility enhancement is useful for mixed micelle and emulsion formulation development.

Dilution tests should be performed for a drug-surfactant solution to determine whether precipitation of the drug occurs on dilution. Readers can refer to the Chapter 9, "Solubilization Using Cosolvent Approach," for the dilution test methods.

Surfactant Selection Based on Drug-Surfactant Compatibility Study

Physical and chemical compatibility of the water-insoluble drug with surfactants should be used in the surfactant selection procedure. Physical compatibility may include precipitation/crystallization, phase separation, and color change in the drug-surfactant solution during the course of the study. Chemical compatibility is primarily regarded as the chemical stability of the drug in a surfactant solution. A surfactant is then considered for further development only if it is physically and chemically compatible with the drug.

Prototype Formulations

Several good surfactants in terms of solubility, compatibility, and toxicity can be selected for prototype formulation development. In general, one surfactant can be used as the primary solubilizer in a prototype formulation. Functional excipients, such as antioxidants, tonicity agents for parenteral products and sweeteners, and taste-masking agents for oral products, may be added to the prototype formulation.

General Preparation Procedure of a Micellar Solution

For the preparation of a micellar solution, the water-insoluble drug and lipophilic excipients can be dissolved in a liquid surfactant by mixing at a relatively high temperature (45°C–60°C) until a clear solution is obtained. If necessary, a cosolvent can be added to aid solubility in the surfactant. Then a water or buffer solution containing hydrophilic excipients is added to the desired volume while mixing. In some cases, the aqueous solution needs to be heated to the same temperature as that of the surfactant to obtain desirable results.

SURFACTANT TOXICITY CONSIDERATIONS

Surfactants act as solubilizers, stabilizers, emulsifiers, and wetting agents. They can also cause toxicity and disrupt normal membrane structure. Surfactant toxicity is directly related to its concentration. This should be considered by the pharmaceutical formulator so levels below the toxic concentration will be used for a particular application. Many of the toxic effects of the surfactants are related to their physicochemical properties and their interaction with biological membranes and other macromolecular assemblies. The observed protein binding and lipid solubilization is directly related to the surface activity and structure of these surfactants. In general, the oral toxicity of surfactants is in the order of nonionic < anionic < cationic with nonionics and anionics reported as having low oral toxicity, whereas the cationics are considered moderately toxic (Lieberman et al., 1996). A recent research article (Soederlind and Karlsson, 2006) reported the hemolytic activity of a number of maltopyranoside surfactants. The study included octyl, nonyl, decyl, dodecyl, tetradecyl, cyclohexyl-propyl, cyclohexyl-hexyl, and dimethyl-heptyl maltopyranoside. It was found that alkyl maltopyranosides become more haemolytic the longer the alkyl chain. Branching or presence of cyclic groups clearly decreases haemolytic activity, but it also increases the critical micelle concentration. The most useful surfactant, for pharmaceutical applications, appears to be tetradecyl maltopyranoside, which is the least haemolytic surfactant relative to its critical micelle concentration. The influence of vitamin E TPGS poly(ethylene glycol) chain length on apical efflux transporters in Caco-2 cell monolayers was investigated by Collnot (2006).

Biological markers such as DNA, mucus, phospholipid, protein, lysosomal, and cytoplasmic enzymes have been used as toxicity indicators. In particular, Oberle et al. (1995) have studied the toxic effects of the nonionic surfactants, polysorbate 80, and Triton X-100, perfused in rat jejunum and colon using lactate dehydrogenase and mucus as markers of intestinal damage. In addition, morphological changes were assessed using light microscopy and scanning electron microscopy. Authors found that the release rate of lactate dehydrogenase (LDH) increased in the order of saline < 1% polysorbate 80 < 1% Triton X-100 in both the jejunum and colon. Significant changes were noted with Triton X-100 exposure, indicating that although the nonionic surfactant polysorbate 80 would be a nonirritating putative enhancer, Triton X-100 would not be recommended. Furthermore, the authors concluded that the single-pass *in situ* perfusion model allows for early evaluation of intestinal damage due to both excipients and active ingredients and simultaneous measurement of drug absorption.

Reviews of surfactant toxicity as related to a specific pharmaceutical application can be found elsewhere (Gloxbuber, 1974). When surfactants are used as dispersants or as emulsifiers for parenteral (IV) administration, the toxicity issue is further complicated by the physical properties of the surfactant vehicle/emulsion. For example, emulsions with a small droplet size have been shown to be less toxic than those with a larger droplet size (Doris et al., 1985). Another complicating factor is the purity of the surfactants. Most commercially available surfactants are generally of low purity, so toxicity may arise from the presence of surface-active impurities. The use of highly pure surfactants, however, is not always desirable since in addition to cost considerations, elimination of some surface-active impurities may impact the emulsion stabilization properties of surfactants. For example, lecithin from either plant or animal sources is a complex mixture of phospholipids. Phosphatidylcholine, the major component in lecithin, is a poor emulsifier, and the stability of an emulsion incorporating lecithin is largely dependent on the nature of lecithin. Particularly, the presence of some ionic phospholipids such as phosphatidic acid or phosphatidylserine will help stabilize the emulsion.

SPECIFIC APPLICATIONS AND CASE STUDIES

Surfactants are becoming increasingly important in the field of pharmaceuticals. They are commonly used excipients in all major routes of drug administration. The level of surfactant in a particular dosage form will vary depending on its role in the formulation. In a solid dosage form it may be added at levels <0.1% to aid wetting of the drug substance and thus increase the dissolution rate. In liquid and semisolid dosage forms, the surfactant levels in self-emulsifying drug delivery systems or microemulsions can vary from 10% to 40%, and in addition to its role as a solvent for the drug, the surfactant also serves as absorption enhancer. Thus, both drug dissolution and oral absorption can be improved using surfactant(s) in liquid and semisolid dosage forms. In parenterals, the surfactant in a dosing solution may be an emulsion stabilizer (1%–2%) or a dispersant (<1%). In some cases, its role is to solubilize the drug (5%–20%). Finally, in topicals the surfactant is present usually at levels between 2% and 10% to help in the formation of the microstructure (gel, cream, emulsion) and improve transmucosal absorption. In many cases, the role of a surfactant is in fact multifunctional.

Strickley (2004) has compiled a comprehensive review of solubilizing excipients, including surfactants, in various oral and injectable formulations.

SOLID DOSAGE FORMS

Several marketed products of lipophilic drugs incorporate various surfactants to aid drug dissolution and oral absorption. An interesting method has been reported on the preparation of solid dosage forms of lipophilic drugs, primarily in a powder form using solid micelle dispersion (Hwang et al., 1996; Kim et al., 1996). According to this method, the drug is first solubilized in solvent-surfactant(s) mixtures. Subsequently the resulting mixture is adsorbed onto porous dextrin while the solvent is removed to generate a drug powder that subsequently can be filled into hard gelatin capsules for oral administration. Improved oral absorption of cyclosporine from a solid micelle dispersion incorporating a nonionic hydrophilic surfactant and a porous carrier was obtained when compared to that obtained with the commercial Sandimmune formulation. The solid micelle dispersion had less intersubject variation compared with Sandimmune (Kim et al., 1996; Shin et al., 1996). Applicability of this method to other lipophilic drugs needs to be determined.

SEMISOLID ORAL DOSAGE FORMS

There is increasing interest in the use of semisolid formulations to solubilize lipophilic drugs for oral administration in a hard gelatin capsule. These formulations incorporate solvents (ethanol, propylene glycol, PEGs) along with surfactants and glyceride bases. On dilution with aqueous media or biological fluids, they form micellar solutions/dispersions or microemulsions (oil-in-water). It has been shown that absorption of cyclosporine from these formulations is fast with more consistent pharmacokinetic profiles than the reference formulation (Sandimmune). This improvement in drug absorption has been attributed to improved dissolution and thus instantaneous absorption (Ritschell, 1996).

LIQUID/PARENTERAL FORMULATIONS

For parenteral uses, drug products can be formulated as parenteral solutions or concentrates. Before administration, the parenteral concentrates, such as intravenous infusion, micelles are formed on dilution with diluents. Examples of these drug formulations can be found in several marketed products, such as Taxol® (paclitaxel) Injection, Sandimmune Injection (cyclosporin for injection concentrate), and Vumon (teniposide) for Injection Concentrate. Taxol is used here as a case study to illustrate the use of micellar solubilization in a liquid/parenteral dosage form (PDR® 1997).

Taxol Injection, a product by Bristol-Myers Squibb, consists of 6 mg paclitaxel, 527 mg of Cremophor EL (polyoxyethylated castor oil) and 49.7% (v/v) dehydrated alcohol, USP in 1 mL parenteral concentrate. Paclitaxel is highly lipophilic and insoluble in water with a melting point of 216°C–217°C and a molecular weight of 854. It has to be in a soluble form to prepare an intravenous formulation. Cremophor EL is a nonionic surfactant and its main component is glycerol polyethyl-eneglycol ricinoleate, in which fatty acid esters of glycerol represent the hydrophobic portion, and polyethylene glycols represent the hydrophilic portion of the surfactant. Cremophor EL is a pale yellow, oily, and viscous liquid with an HLB value lying between 12 and 14. In the commercial paclitaxel formulation, Cremophor EL is used as the solubilizer and alcohol as the thinning agent and cosolvent for the drug.

Taxol is commercially available in 30 mg (5 mL) and 100 mg (16.7 mL) multidose vials. This parenteral concentrate is intended for dilution with a suitable parenteral dilution media before intra-venous infusion. Taxol should be diluted with 0.9% sodium chloride injection, USP, 5% Dextrose injection, USP (or combinations thereof), or 5% Dextrose in Ringer's Injection to a final concentra-tion of 0.3–1.2 mg/mL. This dilution covers a range from 5- to 20-fold dilution of the drug concen-trate. The final dosing preparation is a micellar dispersion.

It is known, however, that Cremophor EL can cause hypersensitivity (Gelderblom et al., 2001).

Thus, patients with history of severe hypersensitivity reactions to products containing Cremophor EL should not be treated with Taxol. To avoid the occurrence of severe hypersensitivity reactions, all patients treated with Taxol should be premedicated with corticosteroids (such as dexamethasone), diphenhydramine, and H2 antagonists (such as cimetidine or ranitidine). It is evident that adverse reaction and surfactant toxicity should be taken into account when using a particular surfactant as the solubilizer for a water-insoluble drug.

As alternatives to Taxol Injection, several formulations are being developed (Terwogt et al., 1997). Among these formulations, a filter sterilizable o/w emulsion of paclitaxel at high drug load (8–10 mg/mL) using surfactants other than Cremophor EL has been developed (Constantinides et al., 2000, 2004). In preclinical studies, this injectable emulsion of paclitaxel showed good physi-cal and chemical stability, low toxicity, and efficacy at least as good as that of Taxol.

ACKNOWLEDGMENTS

The authors would like thank Dr. Negar Sadrazadeh and Dr. Panayiotis P. Constantinides for their contributions to the first edition of this book.

REFERENCES

Abdel-Rahman, A. A., A. E. Aboutaleb, and E. M. Samy. 1991. Factors affecting chloideazepoxide solubiliza-tion by nonionic surfactants. *Bull. Pharm. Sci. Assiut University.* 14: 35–45.

Ahmad, Z., A. Shah, M. Siddiq, and H. B. Kraatz. 2014. Polymeric micelles as drug delivery vehicles. *Rsc. Adv. 4*(33): 17028–17038.

Akbuga, J. and A. Gursoy. 1987. The effect of surfactants on the solubility and tablet dissolution of furose-mide. *S.T.P. Pharma.* 3: 395–399.

Alcorn, C. J., R. J. Simpson, D. Leahy, and T. J. Peters. 1991. *In vitro* studies of intestinal drug absorption. Determination of partition and distribution coefficients with brush border membrane vesicles. *Biochem. Pharmacol.* 42: 2259–2264.

Alcorn, C. J., R. J. Simpson, D. Leahy, and T. J. Peters. 1993. Partition and distribution coefficients of solutes and drugs in brush border membrane vesicles. *Biochem. Pharmacol.* 45: 1775–1782.

Alden, M., J. Tegenfeldt, and E. S. Evan. 1993. Structures formed by interactions in solid dispersions of the system polyethylene gycol-griseofulvin with charged and noncharged surfactants added. *Int. J. Pharm.* 94: 31–38.

Alden, M., J. Tegenfeldt, and E. Sjoekvist. 1992. Structures of solid dispersions in the system polyethylene gycol-griseofulvin with additions of sodium dodecyl sulfate. *Int. J. Pharm.* 83: 47–52.

Alkan-Onyuksel, H., S. Ramakrishnan, H. Chai, and M. J. Pezzuto. 1994. A mixed micellar formulation suit-able for the parenteral administration of taxol. *Pharm. Res.* 11: 206–212.

Almgren, M., P. Hansson, and K. Wang. 1996. Distribution of surfactants in a nonideal mixed micellar sys-tem. Effect of a surfactant quencher on the fluorescence decay of solubilized pyrene. *Langmuir.* 12: 3855–3858.

Andrade, S. M. and S. M. B. Costa. 1996. Fluorescence studies of the drug piroxicam in reverse micelles of AOT and microemulsions of Triton X-100. *Prog. Colloid Polym. Sci.* 100: 195–200.

Andriamainty, F., J. Cizmarik, Z. Zudorova, I. Malik, and E. Sedlarova. 2007. Influence of alcohols on the critical micelle concentration of heptacainiurn chloride. Study of local anesthetics, part 171. *Pharmazie.* 62: 77–78.

Attwood, D. and A. T. Florence. 1983. *Surfactant Systems: Their Chemistry, Pharmacy and Biology.* New York: Chapman and Hall.

Attwood, D., P. H. Elworthy, and M. J. Lawrence. 1994. Effect of structural variations of non-ionic surfactants on surface properties: Surfactants with semi-polar hydrophobes. *J. Pharm. Pharmacol.* 42: 581–583.

Backland, S., K. Rundt, K. S. Birdi, and S. Dalsager. 1981. Aggregation behavior of ionic surfactant micelles in aqueous alcoholic solutions at different temperatures. *J. Coll. Interface Sci.* 79: 578–580.

Bakshi, M. S., R. Crisantino, R. De Lisi, and S. Milioto. 1993. Volume and heat capacity of sodium dodecyl sulfate-dodecyldimethylamine oxide mixed micelles. *J. Phys. Chem.* 97: 6914–6919.

Balzer, D. 1996. Zum eigenschaftsbild der alkylpolyglucoside. *Tenside Surf. Det.* 33: 102–110.

Barreiro-Iglesias, R., C. Alvarez-Lorenzo, and A. Concheiro. 2003. Controlled release of estradiol solubilized in carbopol/surfactant aggregates. *J. Cont. Rel.* 93: 319–330.

Barzykin, A. V. and M. Almgren. 1996. On the distribution of surfactants among mixed micelles. *Langmuir.* 12: 4672–4680.

Bergstroem, M. 1996. Derivation of size distributions of surfactant micelles taking into account shape, composition, and chain packing density fluctuations. *J. Coll. Interface Sci.* 181: 208–219.

Bergstroem, M. and J. C. Eriksson. 1992. Composition fluctuations promoting the formation of long rod-shaped micelles. *Langmuir.* 8: 36–42.

Berlepsch, H. V., U. Keiderling, and H. Schnablegger. 1998. Characterization of sodium sulfopropyl octadecyl maleate micelles by small-angle neutron scattering. *Langmuir.* 14: 7403–7409.

Berret, J.-F. 1997. Transient rheology of wormlike micelles. *Langmuir.* 13: 2227–2234.

Bharadwaj, S. and J. C. Ahluwalia. 1996. Mixed-surfactant system of dodecylbenzene sulfonate and alpha olefin sulfonate: Micellar and volumetric studies. *J. Am. Oil Chem. Soc.* 73: 39–45.

Blankschtein, D., A. Shiloach, and N. Zoeller. 1997. Thermodynamic theories of micellar and vesicular systems. *Curr. Opin. Coll. Interface Sci.* 2: 294–300.

Brown, A. R. and J. G. Slusser. 1994. Propellant-driven aerosols of functional proteins as potential therapeutic agents in the respiratory tract. *Immunopharmacology.* 28: 241–257.

Buckton, G., M. Efentakis, H. Al-Hmoud, and Z. Rajan. 1991. The influence of surfactants on drug release from acrylic matrixes. *Int. J. Pharm.* 74: 169–174.

Burruano, B., M. R. Hoy, R. D. Bruce, and J. D. Higgins. 1999. Method for producing water dispersible sterol formulations. US Patent 6,110,502.

Carey, M. C. 1983. Measurement of the physical–chemical properties of bile salt solutions. In *Bile Acids in Gastroenterology*, Barbara, L., et al. (Ed.), 19 Boston, MA: MTP Press.

Carrion Fite, F. J. 1985. The formation of micelles in mixtures of sodium dodecylsulfate and ethoxylated non-ylphenol with different degrees of ethoxylation. *Tenside Deterg.* 22: 225–229.

Castro, B. D., P. Gameiro, C. Guimaraes, J. L. F. C. Lima, and S. Reis. 1998. Acid/base properties of β-blockers and benzodiazepines in sodium dodecyl sulfate micelles. A spectrophotometric and potentiometric study. *J. Pharm. Sci.* 87: 356–359.

Chatterjee, S., P. K. Sen, K. Das, S. C. Bhattacharya, and R. Palepu. 2006. Mixed micellization of ionic and nonionic surfactants in aqueous solution. *J. Dispers. Sci. Technol.* 27: 751–759.

Chen, B. H., C. A. Miller, and P. R. Garrett. 1998. Rates of solubilization of triolein/fatty acid mixtures by nonionic surfactant solutions. *Langmuir.* 14: 31–41.

Chen, D. and R. Zhang. 1993. Effects of surfactants on the dissolution rate of aspirin from tablets in water. *Shenyang Yaoxueyuan Xuebao.* 10: 240–246, 292.

Chen, J., J. D. Ormes, J. D. Higgins, and L. S. Taylor, 2015. Impact of surfactants on the crystallization of aqueous suspensions of celecoxib amorphous solid dispersion spray dried particles. *Mol. Pharm.,* 12(2): 533–541.

Chen, X., T. J. Young, M. Sarkari, R. O. Williams III, and K. P. Johnston. 2002. Preparation of cyclosporine A nanoparticles by evaporative precipitation into aqueous solution. *Int. J. Pharm.* 242: 3–14.

Christensen, J. O., K. Schultz, B. Mollgaard, H. G. Kristensen, and A. Mullertz. 2004. Solubilisation of poorly water-soluble drugs during *in vitro* lipolysis of medium- and long-chain triacylglycerols. *Eur. J. Pharm. Sci.* 23: 287–296.

Collette, J. H. and L. Koo. 1975. Interaction of substituted benzoic acids with polysorbate 20 micelles. *J. Pharm. Sci.* 64: 1253–1255.

Collnot, E. M., C. Baldes, M. F. Wempe, J. Hyatt, C. M. Lehr, et al. 2006. Influence of vitamin E TPGS poly(ethylene glycol) chain length on apical efflux transporters in Caco-2 cell monolayers. *J. Control. Rel.* 111: 35–40.

Constantinides, P. P., A. Tustian, and D. R. Kessler. 2004. Tocol emulsions for drug solubilization and parenteral delivery. *Adv. Drug Del. Rev.* 56: 1243–1255.

Constantinides, P. P. and J. M. Steim. 1985. Physical properties of fatty-acyl CoA: Critical micelle concentrations and micellar size and shape. *J. Biol. Chem.* 260: 7573–7580.

Constantinides, P. P., and J. M. Steim. 1986. Solubility of palmitoyl-coenzyme A in acyltransferase assay buffers containing magnesium ions. *Arch. Biochem. Biophys.* 250: 267–270.

Constantinides, P. P. and J. M. Steim. 1988. Micellization of fatty acyl-CoA mixtures and its relevance to the fatty acyl selectivity of acyltransferases. *Arch. Biochem. Biophys.* 261: 430–436.

Constantinides, P. P., K. Lambert, A. Tustian, S. Lalji, B. Schneider, W. Ma, B. Wentzel, D. Kessler, D. Worah, and S. Q. Quay. 2000. Formulation development and antitumor activity of a filter-sterilizable emulsion of paclitaxel. *Pharm. Res.* 17: 175–182.

Crison, J. R., N. D. Weiner, and G. L. Amidon. 1997. Dissolution media for *in vitro* testing of water-insoluble drugs: Effect of surfactant purity and electrolyte on *in vitro* dissolution of carbamazepine in aqueous solutions of sodium lauryl sulfate. *J. Pharm. Sci.* 86: 384–388.

Crooks, M. J. and K. F. Brown. 1973. A note on the solubilization of preservative mixtures by cetomacrogol. *J. Pharm. Pharmacol.* 25: 281–284.

D'Antona, P., W. O. Parker, M. C. Zanirato, E. Esposito, and C. Nastruzzi. 2000. Rheologic and NMR characterization of monoglyceride-based formulations. *Biomed. Mater. Res.* 52: 40–52.

Dannenfelser, R.-M., H. He, Y. Joshi, S. Bateman, and A. T. M. Serajuddin. 2004. Development of clinical dosage forms for a poorly water soluble drug I: Application of polyethylene glycol-polysorbate 80 solid dispersion carrier system. *J. Pharm. Sci.* 93: 1165–1175.

Date, A. A. and M. S. Nagarsenker. 2007. Design and evaluation of self-nanoemulsifying drug delivery systems (SNEDDS) for cefpodoxime proxetil. *Int. J. Pharm.* 329: 166–172.

Deng, J., S. Staufenbiel, S. Hao, B. Wang, A. Dashevskiy, and R. Bodmeier. 2017. Development of a discriminative biphasic in vitro dissolution test and correlation with in vivo pharmacokinetic studies for differently formulated racecadotril granules. *J. Contr. Rel.*, 255: 202–209.

Desai, D., B. Wong, Y. Huang, Q. Ye, D. Tang, H. Guo, M. Huang, and P. Timmins. 2014. Surfactant-mediated dissolution of metformin hydrochloride tablets: Wetting effects versus ion pairs diffusivity. *J. Pharm. Sci.* 103(3): 920–926.

Desai, T. R. and S. G. Dixit. 1996. Interaction and viscous properties of aqueous solutions of mixed cationic and nonionic surfactants. *J. Coll. Interface Sci.* 177: 471–477.

Doris, S. S., J. Handgratt, and K.J. Palin. 1985. Medical and pharmaceutical applications of emulsions. In *Encyclopedia of Emulsion Technology*. Vol. 2, pp. 159–237. New York: Marcel Dekker.

Eads, C. D. and L. C. Robosky. 1999. NMR studies of binary surfactant mixture thermodynamics: Molecular size model for asymmetric activity coefficients. *Langmuir.* 15: 2661–2668.

Eda, Y., N. Takisawa, and K. Shirahama. 1996. Solubilization of 1-alkanols in ionic micelles measured by piezoeletric gas sensors. *Langmuir.* 12: 325–329.

Eda, Y., N. Takisawa, and K. Shirahama. 1997. Solubilization of isomeric alkanols in ionic micelles. *Langmuir.* 13: 2432–2435.

Efentakis, M., H. Al-Hmoud, G. Buckton, and Z. Rajan. 1991. The influence of surfactants on drug release from a hydrophobic matrix. *Int. J. Pharm.* 70: 153–158.

El Haskouri, J., M. Roca, S. Cabrera, J. Alamo, A. Beltran-Porter, D. Beltran-Porter, M. D. Marcos, and P. Amoros. 1999. Interface charge density matching as driving force for new mesostructured oxovanadium phosphates with hexagonal structure, [CTA]xVOPO4×zH$_2$O. *Chem. Mater.* 11: 1446–1454.

Elworthy, P. H. and M. S. Patel. 1983. Solubilizing capacity of a polyoxybutylene–polyoxypropylene surfactant. *J. Pharm. Pharmacol.* 35: 55–68.

Erpecum, K. J. V. and M. C. Carey. 1997. Influence of bile salts on molecular interactions between sphingomyelin and cholesterol: Relevance to bile formation and stability. *Biochem. Biophys. Acta.* 1345: 269–282.

Evans, R. M. and S. J. Farr. 1992. The development of novel, pressurized aerosols formulated as solutions. *J. Biopharm. Sci.* 3: 33–40.

Evans, R. M. and S. J. Farr. 1993. Aerosol formulations including proteins and peptides solubilized in reverse micelles and process for making the aerosol formulations. US Patent 5,230,884.

Evans, R. M., S. J. Farr, N. A. Armstrong, and S. M. Chatham. 1991. Formulation and *in vitro* evaluation of pressurized inhalation aerosols containing isotropic systems of lecithin and water. *Pharm. Res.* 8: 629–635.

Fahelelbom, K. M., R. F. Timoney, and O. I. Corrigan. 1993. Micellar solubilization of clofazimine analogues in aqueous solutions of ionic and nonionic surfactants. *Pharm. Res.* 10: 631–634.

Florence, A. T. 1981. Drug solubilization in surfactant systems. In *Techniques of Solubilization of Drugs*, S. H. Yalkowsky (Ed.). New York: Marcel Dekker.

Foerster, T., W. Von Rybinski, and M. J. Schwuger. 1990. Mixed micelle formation. *Tenside. Surf. Deterg.* 27: 254–256.

Fontan, J. E., P. Arnaud, and J. C. Chaumeil. 1991. Enhancing properties of surfactants on the release of carbamazepine from suppositories. *Int. J. Pharm.* 73: 17–21.

Frazier, A. A. and K. K. Karukstis. 1997. Investigation of competitive binding between daunomycin and verapamil or genistein in AOT reverse micelles. *Abstracts of 213th ACS National Meeting*, p. 262. Washington, DC: Amer Chemical Soc.

Friberg, S. E. and M. A. El–Nokaly. 1985. Surfactant association structures of relevance to cosmetic preparations. RIEGER, MM Surfactants in cosmetics. New York: M. Dekker, p. 488.

Fujiwara, M., T. Okano, H. Amano, H. Asano, and K. Ohbu. 1997. Phase diagram of a-sulfonated palmitic acid methyl ester sodium salt-water system. *Langmuir.* 13: 3345–3348.

Funasaki, N., S. Hada, and S. Neya. 1986. Volumetric study of intermolecular interactions in mixed micelles. *J. Phys. Chem.* 90: 5469–5473.

Gadiraju, R. R., R. I. Poust, and H. S. Huang. 1995. The effect of buffer species, pH and buffer strength on the CMC and solubility of amiodarone HCl, Poster presentation (AAPS annual meeting). Miami Beach, Florida.

Garcia, M. T., I. Ribosa, and J. Sanchez Leal. 1992. Diffusion of anionic surfactant/amphoteric surfactant mixtures through collagen. *Invest. Inf. Text. Tensioactivos.* 35: 21–27.

Gelderblom, H., J. Verweij, K. Nooter, and A. Sparreboom. 2001. Cremophor EL: The drawbacks and advantages of vehicle selection for drug formulation. *Eur. J. Cancer.* 37: 1590–1598.

Gerakis, A. M., M. A. Koupparis, and C. E. Efstathiou. 1993. Micellar acid–base potentiometric titrations of weak acidic and/or insoluble drugs. *J. Pharm. Biomed. Anal.* 11: 33–41.

Gloxbuber, C. 1974. Toxicological properties of surfactants. *Arch. Toxicol.* 32: 245–270.

Goto, A., R. Sakura, and F. Endo. 1980. Gel filtration of solubilized systems. V. Effects of sodium chloride on micellar sodium lauryl sulfate solutions solubilizing alkylparabens. *Chem. Pharm. Bull.* 28: 14–22.

Granero, G. E., C. Ramachandran, and G. L. Amidon. 2005. Dissolution and solubility behavior of fenofibrate in sodium lauryl sulfate solutions. *Drug Dev. Ind. Pharm.* 31: 917–922.

Green, F. A. 1972. Interactions of a nonionic detergent. III. Further observations on hydrophobic interactions. *J. Coll. Interface Sci.* 41: 124–129.

Griffin, W. C. 1949. Classification of surface-active agents by "HLB." *J. Soc. Cosmet. Chem.* 1: 311–326.

Hamid, I. A. and E. L. Parrott. 1971. Effect of temperature on solubilization and hydrolytic degradation of solubilized benzocaine and hematropine. *J. Pharm. Sci.* 60: 901–906.

Hammad, M. A. and B. W. Muller. 1998. Solubility and stability of clonazepam in mixed micelles. *Int. J. Pharm.* 169: 55–64.

Hamza, Y. E. and M. Kata. 1989. Influence of certain non-ionic surfactants on solubilization and *in-vitro* availability of allopurinol. *Pharm. Ind.* 51: 1441–1444.

Haque, M. E., A. R. Das, A. K. Rakshit, and S. P. Moulik. 1996. Properties of mixed micelles of binary surfactant combinations. *Langmuir.* 12: 4084–4089.

Hoffmann, H. and G. Poessnecker. 1994. The mixing behavior of surfactants. *Langmuir.* 10: 381–389.

Humberstone, A. J., C. J. H. Porter, and W. N. Charman. 1996. A physicochemical basis for the effect of food on the absolute oral bioavailability of halofantrine. *J. Pharm. Sci.* 85: 525–529.

Humphreys, K. J. and C. T. Rhodes. 1968. Effect of temperature upon solubilization by a series of nonionic surfactants. *J. Pharm. Sci.* 57: 79–83.

Huruguen, J. P., M. Authier, J. L. Greffe, and M. P. Pileni. 1991. Percolation process induced by solubilizing cytochrome c in reverse micelles. *Langmuir.* 7: 243–249.

Hwang, S.-J., S. H. Park, and E. J. Jeong. 1996. Solid formulations for oral administration of cyclosporin A. *PCT Int. Appl.* 30. PCT/KR1996/000008.

Ichikawa, S., M. Nakajima, S. Sugiura, H. Sano, H. Nabetani, M. Seki, and S. Kosaki. 1998. *Jpn. Kokai Tokkyo Koho.* 4.

Ihara, T., N. Suzuki, T. Maeda, K. Sagara, and T. Hobo. 1995. Extraction of water-soluble vitamins from pharmaceutical preparations using AOT (sodium di-2-ethylhexylsulfosuccinate)/pentane reversed micelles. *Chem. Pharm. Bull.* 43: 626–630.

Ikeda, K., H. Tomida, and T. Yotsuyanagi. 1977. Micellar interaction of tetracycline antibiotics. *Chem. Pharm. Bull.* 25: 1067–1072.

Ismail, A. A., M. W. Gouda, and M. M. Motawi. 1970. Micellar solubilization of barbiturates. I. Solubilities of certain barbiturates in polysorbates of varying hydrophobic chain length. *J. Pharm. Sci.* 59: 220–224.

Israelachvili, J. 1994. Self-assembly in two dimensions: Surface micelles and domain formation in monolayers. *Langmuir.* 10: 3774–3781.

Itoh, K., S. Matsui, Y. Tozuka, T. Oguchi, and K. Yamamoto. 2002a. Improvement of physicochemical properties of N-4472 part I: Formulation design by using self-microemulsifying system. *Int. J. Pharm.* 238: 153–160.

Itoh, K., S. Matsui, Y. Tozuka, T. Oguchi, and K. Yamamoto. 2002b. Improvement of physicochemical properties of N-4472 part II: Characterization of N-4472 microemulsion and the enhanced oral absorption. *Int. J. Pharm.* 246: 75–83.

Jin, Q., Y. Chen, Y. Wang, and J. Ji. 2014. Zwitterionic drug nanocarriers: A biomimetic strategy for drug delivery. *Colloids Surf. B: Biointerfaces.* 124: 80–86.

Joshi, H. N., R. W. Tejwani, M. Davidovich, V. P. Sahasrabudhe, M. Jemal, M. S. Bathala, S. A. Varia, and A. T. M. Serajuddin. 2004. Bioavailability enhancement of a poorly water-soluble drug by solid dispersion in polyethylene glycol-polysorbate 80 mixture. *Int. J. Pharm.* 269: 251–258.

Joshi, V. Y. and M.R. Sawant. 2006. Study on dissolution rate enhancement of poorly water soluble drug: Contributions of solubility enhancement and relatively low micelle diffusivity. *J. Dispers. Sci. Technol.* 27: 1141–1150.

Kalekar, M. S. and S. S. Bhagwat. 2006. Dynamic behavior of surfactants in solution. *J. Dispers. Sci. Technol.* 27: 1027–1034.

Kang, B. K., J. S. Lee, S. K. Chon, S. Y. Jeong, S. H. Yuk, G. Khang, H. B. Lee, and S. H. Cho. 2004. Development of self-microemulsyfying drug delivery systems (SMEDDS) for oral bioavailability enhancement of simvastatin in beagle dogs. *Int. J. Pharm.* 274: 65–73.

Karmazina, T. V. 1997. Neutron spectroscopy for study of micelle-forming surfactants adsorbed on solid surfaces from aqueous solutions. *Khim. Tekhnol. Vody.* 19: 350–364.

Karukstis, K. K., E. H. Z. Thompson, J. A. Whiles, and R. J. Rosenfeld. 1998. Partitioning of daunomycin and doxorubicin in AOT reverse micelles. *Abstracts of 215th ACS National Meeting*, p. 173.

Kataoka, K., G. S. Kwon, M. Yokoyama, T. Okano, and Y. Sakurai. 1993. Block copolymer micelles as vehicles for drug delivery. *J. Cont. Rel.* 24: 119–132.

Kataoka, K., H. Togawa, A. Hareda, K. Yasugi, T. Matsumoto, and S. Katayose. 1996. Spontaneous formation of polyion complex micelles with narrow distribution from antisense oligonucleotide and cationic block copolymer in physiological saline. *Macromolecules* 29: 8556–8557.

Khaledi, M. G., J. K. Strasters, A. H. Rodgers, and E. D. Breyer. 1990. Simultaneous enhancement of separation selectivity and solvent strength in reversed-phase liquid chromatography using micelles in hydro-organic solvents. *Anal. Chem.* 62: 130–136.

Kim, C.-K., Y.-J. Cho, and Z-G. Gao. 2001. Preparation and evaluation of biphenyl dimethyl dicarboxylate microemulsions for oral delivery. *J. Cont. Rel.* 70: 149–155.

Kim, J. W., H. J. Shin, J. K. Park, and K. B. Min. 1996. Cyclosporin containing powder composition. US Patent 5,543,393.

Kim, J. Y. and Y. S. Ku. 2000. Enhanced absorption of indomethacin after oral or rectal administration of a self-emulsifying system containing indomethacin to rats. *Int. J. Pharm.* 194: 81–89.

Kipp, J. E. 2004. The role of solid nanoparticle technology in the parenteral delivery of poorly water-soluble drugs. *Int. J. Pharm.* 284: 109–122.

Kissa, E. 1994. *Fluorinated Surfactant: Synthesis, Properties and Applications.* Surfactant Science Series, Vol. 50, New York: Marcel Dekker.

Kondo, Y., M. Abe, K. Ogino, H. Uchiyama, J. F. Scamehorn, E. E. Tucker, and S. D. Christian. 1993. Solubilization of 2-phenylethanol in surfactant vesicles and micelles. *Langmuir.* 9: 899–902.

Kossena, G. A., B. J. Boyd, C. J. H. Porter, and W. N. Charman. 2003. Separation and characterization of the colloidal phases produced on digestion of common formulation lipids and assessment of their impact on the apparent solubility of selected poorly water-soluble drugs. *J. Pharm. Sci.* 92: 634–648.

Kossena, G. A., W. N. Charman, B. J. Boyd, D. E. Dunstan, and C. J. H. Porter. 2004. Probing drug solubilization patterns in the gastrointestinal tract after administration of lipid-based delivery systems: A phase diagram approach. *J. Pharm. Sci.* 93: 332–348.

Krishnadas, A., I. Rubinstein, and H. Onyuksel. 2003. Sterically stabilized phospholipid mixed micelles: *In vitro* evaluation as a novel carrier for water-insoluble drugs. *Pharm. Res.* 20: 297–302.

Kwon, G. S. and T. Okano. 1996. Polymeric micelles as new drug carriers. *Adv. Drug Del. Rev.* 16: 107–116.

Kwon, G. S. and T. Okano. 1999. Soluble self-assembled block copolymers for drug delivery. *Pharm. Res.* 16: 597–600.

Lawrence, M. J. 1994. Surfactant systems: Their use in drug delivery. *Chem. Soc. Rev.* 417–424.

Li, L., I. Nandi, and K. H. Kim. 2002. Development of an ethyl laureate-based microemulsion for rapid-onset intranasal delivery of diazepam. *Int. J. Pharm.* 237: 77–85.

Li, P., A. Ghosh, R. F. Wagner, S. Krill, Y. M. Joshi, and A. T. M. Serajuddin. 2005. Effect of combined use of nonionic surfactant on formation of oil-in-water microemulsions. *Int. J. Pharm.* 288: 27–34.

Li, P., S. E. Tabibi, and S. H. Yalkowsky. 1999. Solubilization of ionized and un-ionized Flavopiridol by ethanol and polysorbate 20. *J. Pharm. Sci.* 88: 507–509.

Lieberman, H. A., M. M. Rieger, and G. S. Banker. 1996. *Pharmaceutical Dosage Forms: Disperse Systems*, Vol. 1. New York: Marcel Dekker.

Luisi, P. L., M. Giomini, M. P. Pileni, and B. H. Robinson. 1988. Reverse micelles as hosts of proteins and small molecules. *Biochim. Biophys. Acta* 947: 209–246.

Luo, Y., D. W. Chen, L. X. Ren, X. L. Zhao, and J. Qin. 2006. Solid lipid nanoparticles for enhancing vinpocetine's oral bioavailability. *J. Control. Rel.* 114: 53–59.

Mall, S., G. Buckton, and D. A. Rawlines. 1996. Dissolution behavior of sulphonamides into sodium dodecyl sulfate micelles: A thermodynamic approach. *J. Pharm. Sci.* 85: 75–78.

Markina, Z. N., G. A. Chirova, and N. M. Zadymova. 1998. Structure-related mechanical properties of hydrogels of micelle-forming surfactants. *Coll. J.* 60: 568–572.

Marques, C. M. 1997. Bunchy Micelles. *Langmuir.* 13: 1430–1433.

Marsh, D. and M. D. King. 1986. Prediction of the critical micelle concentrations of mono- and di-acyl phospholipids. *Chem. Phys. Lipids.* 42: 271–277.

Marszall, L. 1988. Cloud point of mixed ionic-nonionic surfactant solutions in the presence of electrolytes. *Langmuir.* 4: 90–93.

McBain, M. E. L. and E. Hutchinson. 1955. *Solubilization and Related Phenomena.* New York: Academic Press.

Meinert, H., P. Reuter, J. Mader, L. Haidmann, and H. Northoff. 1992. Syntheses, interfacial active properties and toxicity of new perfluoroalkylated surfactants. *Biomater., Artif. Cells, Immobilization Biotechnol.* 20: 115–124.

Moroi, Y., A. Otonishi, and N. Yoshida. 1999. Micelle formation of sodium 1-decanesulfonate and change of micellization temperature by excess counterion. *J. Phys. Chem. B.* 103: 8960–8964.

Mukerjee, P. 1967. Association equilibria and hydrophobic bonding. *Advan. Coll. Interface Sci.* 1: 241–275.

Mukerjee, P. 1979. Solubilization in aqueous micellar systems. In *Solution Chemistry of Surfactants.* Vol. 1, K. Mittal (Ed.), pp. 153–174. New York: Plenum Publishing Corp.

Myers, D. 1992. Micellization and association. In *Surfactant Science and Technology.* 2nd edn., D. Myers (Ed.). New York: VCH Publishers.

Mysels, K. J. and P. Mukerjee. 1979. Reporting experimental data dealing with critical micellization concentrations (CMCs) of aqueous surfactant systems. *Pure Appl. Chem.* 51: 1083–1089.

Nagarajan, R. 1985. Molecular theory for mixed micelles. *Langmuir.* 1: 331–341.

Nagarajan, R. 1986. Micellization, mixed micellization and solubilization: The role of interfacial interactions. *Adv. Coll. Interf. Sci.* 26: 205–264.

Nagarajan, R. and E. Ruckenstein. 1991. Theory of surfactant self-assembly: A predictive molecular thermodynamic approach. *Langmuir.* 7: 2934–2969.

Nagata, M., K. Matsuba, S. Hasegawa, T. Okuda, M. Harata, K. Hisada, M. Ishijima, and J. Watanabe. 1979. Pharmaceutical studies on commercial phytonadion tablets and effect of polysorbate 80 on the dissolution test. *Yakugaku Zasshi.* 99: 965–970.

Naylor, L. J., V. Bakatselou, and J. B. Dressman. 1993. Comparison of the mechanism of dissolution of hydrocortisone in simple and mixed micelle systems. *Pharm. Res.* 10: 865–870.

Nielsen, L. S. 1998. A bioadhesive drug delivery system based on liquid crystals. *PCT Int. Appl.* 176.

Nook, T., E. Doelker, and I. Bori 1988. The role of bile and biliary salts in drug absorption. *Int. J. Pharm.* 43: 119–129.

Oberle, R. L., T. J. Moore, and D. A. P. Krummel. 1995. Evaluation of mucosal damage of surfactants in rat jejunum and colon. *J. Pharm. Toxicol. Methods.* 33: 75–81.

Ong, J. T. and E. Manoukian. 1988. Micellar solubilization of timobesome acetate in aqueous and aqueous propylene glycol solutions of nonionic surfactants. *Pharm. Res.* 5: 704–708.

Osborne-Lee, I. W. and R. S. Schechter. 1986. Nonideal mixed micelles. Thermodynamic models and experimental comparisons. *ACS Symp. Ser.* (*Phenom. Mixed Surfactant Syst.*). 311: 30–43.

Pal, T. and N. R. Jana. 1996. Polarity dependent positional shift of probe in a micellar environment. *Langmuir.* 13: 3114–3121.

Park, S. H. and H. K. Choi. 2006. The effects of surfactants on the dissolution profiles of poorly water-soluble acidic drugs. *Int. J. Pharm.* 321: 35–41.

Pasquali, R. C., D. A. Chiappeta, and C. Bregni. 2005. Amphiphilic block copolymers and their pharmaceutical applications. *Acta Farmaceutica Bonaerense.* 24: 610–618.

Perkins, W. R., I. Ahmad, X. Li, D. J. Hirsh, G. R. Masters, C. J. Fecko, J. Lee et al. 2000. Novel therapeutic nano-particles (lipocores): Trapping poorly water soluble compounds. *Int. J. Pharm.* 200: 27–39.

Puvvada, S. and D. Blankschtein. 1990. Molecular-thermodynamic approach to predict micellization, phase behavior and phase separation of micellar solutions. I. Application to nonionic surfactants. *The Journal of chemical physics*, 92(6), pp. 3710–3724.

Puvvada, S. and D. Blankschtein. 1992a. Thermodynamic description of micellization, phase behavior, and phase separation of aqueous solutions of surfactant mixtures. *J. Phys. Chem.* 96: 5567–5579.

Puvvada, S. and D. Blankschtein. 1992b. Theoretical and experimental investigations of micellar properties of aqueous solutions containing binary mixtures of nonionic surfactants. *J. Phys. Chem.* 96: 5579–5592.

Radomska-Soukharev, A. and R. H. Mueller. 2006. Chemical stability of lipid excipients in SLN-production of test formulations, characterization and short-term stability. *Pharmazie* 61: 425–430.

Rao, V. M., M. Lin, C. K. Larive, and M. Z. Southard. 1997. A mechanistic study of griseofulvin dissolution into surfactant solutions under laminar flow conditions. *J. Pharm. Sci.* 86: 1132–1137.

Rao, V. M., M. Nerurkar, S. Pinnamaneni, F. Rinaldi, and K. Raghavan. 2006. Co-solubilization of poorly soluble drugs by micellization and complexation. *Int. J. Pharm.* 319: 98–106.

Rhee, Y. S., C. W. Park, T. Y. Nam, Y. S. Shin, E. S. Park et al. 2007. Formulation of parenteral microemulsion containing itraconazole. *Arch. Pharm. Res.* 30: 114–123.

Ritschell, W. A. 1996. Microemulsion technology in the reformulation of cyclosporine: The reason behind the pharmacokinetic properties of neoral clinical transplantation. *Clin. Transplant.* 10: 364–373.

Roe, J. M. and B. W. Barry. 1982. Micellar properties of sodium salts of ursodeoxycholic chenodeoxycholic, deoxycholic and cholic acids. *J. Pharm. Pharmacol.* 34 (Suppl.): 24–25.

Rosen, M. J. 1978. *Surfactants and Interfacial Phenomena*, 2nd ed. New York: Wiley.

Rosoff, M. and A. T. M. Serajuddin. 1980. Solubilization of diazepam in bile salts and in sodium cholate-lecithin-water phases. *Int. J. Pharm.* 6: 137–146.

Ross, B. P., A. C. Braddy, R. P. McGeary, J. T. Blanchfield, L. Prokai, and I. Toth. 2004. Micellar aggregation and membrane partitioning of bile salts, fatty acids, sodium dodecyl sulfate, and sugar-conjugated fatty acids: Correlation with hemolytic potency and implications for drug delivery. *Mol. Pharm.* 1: 233–245.

Ruddy, S. B., B. K. Matuszewska, Y. A. Grim, D. Ostovic, and D. E. Storey. 1999. Design and characterization of a surfactant-enriched tablet formulation for oral delivery of a poorly water-soluble immunosuppressive agent. *Int. J. Pharm.* 182: 173–186.

Saket, M. 1996. Comparative evaluation of micellar solubilization and cyclodextrin inclusion complexation for meclozine hydrochloride. *Alexandria J. Pharm. Sci.* 10: 13–18.

Saket, M. 1997. Improvement of solubility and dissolution rate of meclozine hydrochloride utilizing cyclodextrins and non-ionic surfactant solutions containing cosolvents and additives. *Acta Technol. Legis Med.* 8: 33–48.

Samaha, M. W. and V. F. Naggar. 1988. Micellar properties of non-ionic surfactants in relation to their solubility parameters. *Int. J. Pharm.* 42: 1–9.

Sarmoria, C., S. Puvvada, and D. Blankschtein. 1992. Prediction of critical micelle concentrations of nonideal binary surfactant mixtures. *Langmuir.* 8: 2690–2697.

Schott, H. 1971. Hydrophilic–lipophilic balance and distribution coefficients of nonionic surfactants. *J. Pharm. Sci.* 60: 648–649.

Schott, H. 1995. Colloidal dispersions. In *Remington: The Science and Practice of Pharmacy*, Vol. 1, A. R. Gennaro (Ed.). Easton, PA: Mack Publishing Co.

Shahjahan, M. and R. P. Enever. 1992. Some parameters for the solubilization of nitrofurazone and ultraviolet light absorbers by nonionic surfactants. *Int. J. Pharm.* 82: 223–227.

Shapiro, Y., V. Gorbatyuk, A. A. Mazurov, and S. A. Andronati. 1994. Stabilization of the peptide conformation on the micellar surface. *A. V. Bogatsky Physico-Chem. Inst.* 119: 647–652.

Sheng, J. J., N. A. Kasim, R. Chandrasekharan, and G. L. Amidon. 2006. Solubilization and dissolution of insoluble weak acid, ketoprofen: Effects of pH combined with surfactant. *Eur. J. Pharm. Sci.* 29: 306–314.

Shihab, F. A., A. R. Ebian, and R. M. Mustafa. 1979. Effect of polyethyleneglycol, sodium laurylsulfate and polysorbate-80 on the solubility of furosemide. *Int. J. Pharm.* 4: 13–20.

Shiloach, A. and D. Blankschtein. 1997. Prediction of critical micelle concentrations and synergism of binary surfactant mixtures containing zwitterionic surfactants. *Langmuir.* 13: 3968–3981.

Shiloach, A. and D. Blankschtein. 1998a. Predicting micellar solution properties of binary surfactant mixtures. *Langmuir.* 14: 1618–1636.

Shiloach, A. and D. Blankschtein. 1998b. Measurement and prediction of ionic/nonionic mixed micelle formation and growth. *Langmuir.* 14: 7166–7182.

Shiloach, A. and D. Blankschtein. 1998c. Prediction of critical micelle concentrations of nonideal ternary surfactant mixtures. *Langmuir.* 14: 4105–4114.

Shiloach, A., N. Zoeller, and D. Blankschtein. 1998. Predicting surfactant solution behavior. Speeding the process with new computer programs. *Cosmet. Toiletries* 113: 75–76, 78–79.

Shin, H.-J., J.-K. Park, J.-W. Kim, E.-J. Lee, and C.-K. Kim. 1996. Preparation and bioequivalence test of new oral solid dosage form of cyclosporin A. *Proc. Int. Symp. Controlled Release Bioact. Mater.* 23: 519–520.

Sjoekvist, E., C. Nystroem, and M. Alden. 1991. Physicochemical aspects of drug release. XIII. The effects of sodium dodecyl sulfate additions on the structure and dissolution of a drug in solid dispersions. *Int. J. Pharm.* 69: 53–62.

Sjoekvist, E., C. Nystroem, M. Alden, and N. Caram-Lelham. 1992. Physicochemical aspects of drug release. XIV. The effects of some ionic and nonionic surfactants on properties of a sparingly soluble drug in solid dispersions. *Int. J. Pharm.* 79: 123–133.

Small, D. M., S. A. Penkett, and D. Chapman. 1969. Studies on simple and mixed bile salt micelles by nuclear magnetic resonance spectroscopy. *Biochim. Biophy. Acta.* 176: 178–189.

Smirnova, N. A. 1995. Thermodynamic study of micellar solution—solid surfactant equilibrium. *Fluid Phase Equilibria.* 110: 1–15.

Smirnova, N. A. 1996. Modeling of the micellar solution—solid surfactant equilibrium. *Fluid Phase Equilibria.* 117: 320–333.

Soederlind, E. and L. Karlsson. 2006. Haemolytic activity of maltopyranoside surfactants. *Eur. J. Pharm. Biopharm.* 62: 254–259.

Strickley, R. G. 2004. Solubilizing excipients in oral and injectable formulations. *Pharm. Res.* 21: 201–230.

Sugioka, H. and Y. Moroi. 1998. Micelle formation of sodium cholate and solubilization into the micelle. *Biochim. Biophy. Acta.* 1394: 99–110.

Surakitbanharn, Y., R. McCandless, J. F. Kryzyzaniak, R.-M. Dannenfelser, and S. H. Yalkowsky. 1995. Self-association of dexverapamil in aqueous solution. *J. Pharm. Sci.* 84: 720–723.

Sweetana, S. and M. J. Akers. 1996. Solubility principles and practices for parenteral drug dosage from development. *PDA J. Pharm. Sci. Technol.* 50: 330–342.

Szleifer, I., A. Ben-Shaul, and W. M. Gelbart. 1987. Statistical thermodynamics of molecular organization in mixed micelles and bilayers. *J. Chem. Phys.* 86: 7094–7109.

Tanford, C. 1980. *The Hydrophobic Effect.* New York: Wiley.

Terwogt, J. M. M., B. Nuijen, W. W. Ten Bokkel Huinink, and J. H. Beijnen. 1997. Alternative formulations of paclitaxel. *Cancer Treat. Rev.* 23: 87–95.

Thomas, H. G., A. Lomakin, D. Blankschtein, and G. B. Benedek. 1997. Growth of mixed nonionic micelles. *Langmuir.* 13: 209–218.

Thompson, E. H. Z. and K. K. Karukstis. 1997. Fluorescence studies of doxorubicin in corporation in AOT reversed micelles. *Abstracts of 213th ACS National Meeting,* San Francisco, CA, p. 261.

Tomida, H., T. Yotsuyanagi, and K. Ikeda. 1978. Solubilization of benzoic acid derivatives by polyoxyethylene lauryl ether. *Chem. Pharm. Bull.* 26: 2824–2831.

Treiner, C., M. Nortz, and C. Vaution. 1990. Micellar solubilization in strongly interacting binary surfactant systems. *Langmuir.* 6: 1211–1216.

Treiner, C., M. Nortz, C. Vaution, and F. Puisieux. 1988. Micellar solubilization in aqueous binary surfactant systems: Barbituric acids in mixed anionic + nonionic or cationic + nonionic mixtures. *J. Coll. Interf. Sci.* 125: 261–270.

Tyner, K. M., S. R. Schiffman, and E. P. Giannelis. 2004. Nanobiohybrids as delivery vehicles for camptothecin. *J. Cont. Rel.* 95: 501–514.

Wei, H., Zhuo, R. X., and Zhang, X. Z., 2013. Design and development of polymeric micelles with cleavable links for intracellular drug delivery. *Progr. Poly. Sci.* 38(3): 503–535.

Xiao, J.-L. V., W. Dong, and J. T. Zhou. 2006. Interaction mechanisms between anionic surfactant micelles and different metal ions in aqueous solutions. *J. Dispers. Sci. Technol.* 27: 1073–1077.

Young, T. J., S. Mawson, K. P. Johnston, I. B. Henriksen, G. W. Pace, and A. K. Mishra. 2000. Rapid expansion from supercritical to aqueous solution to produce submicron suspensions of water-insoluble drugs. *Biotechnol. Prog.* 16: 402–407.

Zhang, R., P. A. Marone, P. Thiyagarajan, and D. M. Tiede. 1999. Structure and molecular fluctuations of *n*-alkyl-β-d-glucopyranoside micelles determined by x-ray and neutron scattering. Langmuir. 15: 7510–7519.

Zhang, Y., Song, W., Geng, J., Chitgupi, U., Unsal, H., Federizon, J., Rzayev, J., Sukumaran, D.K., Alexandridis, P., and Lovell, J.F., 2016. Therapeutic surfactant-stripped frozen micelles. *Nat. Comm.*, 7: 11649. Doi:10.1038/ncomms11649.

Zhao, L., P. Li, and S. H. Yalkowsky. 1999. Solubilization of fluasterone. *J. Pharm. Sci.* 88: 967–969.

Zoeller, N. J., A. Shiloach, and D. Blankschtein. 1996. Predicting surfactant solution behavior. *Chemtech.* 26: 24–31.

Zoeller, N. J. and D. Blankschtein. 1995. Development of user-friendly computer programs to predict solution properties of single and mixed surfactant systems. *Ind. Eng. Chem. Res.* 34: 4150–4160.

Zoeller, N. J. and D. Blankschtein. 1998. Experimental determination of micelle shape and size in aqueous solutions of dodecyl ethoxy sulfates. *Langmuir.* 14: 7155–7165.

Zuberi, S., T. Zuberi, S. Sultana, and J. Lawrence. 1999. Characterization of a new generation of surfactants with the potential to act as drug delivery vehicles. *Abstracts of 218th ACS National Meeting,* New Orleans, LA, p. 119.

Zuberi, T., S. Sultana, and J. Lawrence. 1997. Synthesis and physico-characterization of some novel surfactants. *Abstracts of 214th ACS National Meeting,* Las Vegas, NV, p. 47.

Polymeric Micelles in
Water-Insoluble Drug Delivery

Rong (Ron) Liu, M. Laird Forrest, Glen S. Kwon,
Xiaobing Xiong, and Zhihong (John) Zhang

CONTENTS

OVERVIEW

Polymeric surfactants are finding increasing use in pharmaceutical applications. Although polymeric micelles have mostly been studied as delivery systems for anticancer drugs, they could be used to transport plasmid DNA (Katayose and Kataoka, 1997, 1998), antisense oligonucleotides (Kataoka et al., 1996), or for the delivery of diagnostic agents to a specific organ in the body (Park et al., 2002; Torchilin, 2002). The structures of the copolymers vary widely and include random copolymers, grafted copolymers, and the most commonly used block copolymers (Kataoda et al., 1993; Kwon and Okano, 1996, 1999; Alakahov and Kabanov, 1998; Kwon, 1998, 2003; Seymour et al., 1998). Novel polymer chemistries, including drugs covalently bound to the hydrophobic blocks of micelle-forming block copolymer conjugates Kwon and Okano, 1996, 1999) have shown success in clinical trials. In all cases, the relative hydrophilic/lipophilic balance is achieved by using a combination of hydrophilic and hydrophobic monomers. In a solvent compatible with one monomer but incompatible with the other, micelles form with the poorly soluble monomers forming the core and the easily soluble monomers forming the corona (Xing and Mattice, 1998).

The advantages of polymers over conventional surfactants include their lower toxicity, ability to prevent the adsorption of proteins such as immunoglobuins (Abuchowski et al., 1977), and ability to prevent adhesion of the drug vehicle onto the surfaces of phagocytes. The latter phenomena would otherwise lead to the clearance of drug vehicles. Therefore, polymeric micelles possess great potential for extending the circulation time of a drug (Kwon and Kataoka, 1995; Kwon, 2003; Aliabadi and Lavasanifar, 2006). To date, several polymeric micellar formulations have reached preclinical and clinical trials, and one of paclitaxel micellar formulation has been approved for clinical use.

CLASSIFICATION OF COPOLYMERS

Copolymers are defined as polymers composed of several different monomer units and are classified into four types by monomer organization: random copolymers, alternating copolymers, graft copolymers, star copolymers, and block copolymers (Nagarajan and Ganesh, 1989a,b; Yokoyama, 1992). If A is defined as a monomer unit soluble in the solvent and B as a solvent-phobic monomer unit, the five types of copolymers can be pictured as in Figure 13.1. For the purposes of this chapter, monomer A will always be a water-soluble monomer, and B will refer to water-insoluble monomers.

Random copolymers are characterized by the statistical placement of comonomer repeating units along the backbone chain. Alternating copolymers, as the name suggests, are characterized by the alternate placement of monomers. Graft copolymers are made of chemically linked pairs of homopolymers and resemble a comb. Block copolymers are composed of terminally connected structures.

(1) Random copolymer

AABAAABBABAAABBA

(2) Alternative copolymer

ABABABABABABABAB

(3) Graft copolymer

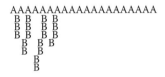

(4) Star copolymers

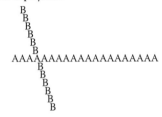

(5) Block copolymers

Diblock copolymer (AB-type)

AAAAAAAAAABBBBBBBBBB

Triblock copolymer (ABA-type)

AAAAAAAAAABBBBBBBBBBAAAAAAAAAA

Triblock copolymer (BAB-type)

BBBBBBBBBBAAAAAAAAAABBBBBBBBBB

(AB)n block copolymers ((AB)n multi-segment type)

$\{$AAAAAAABBBBBBBBBB$\}_n$

FIGURE 13.1   Classification of copolymers.

Pharmaceutical research on polymeric micelles has mainly focused on two kinds of block copolymers, namely, AB block copolymers or diblock copolymers and ABA or BAB block copolymers known as triblock copolymers (Bader et al., 1984; Yokoyama et al., 1990, 1991; Kwon and Okano, 1996, 1999; Alakahov and Kabanov, 1998; Kwon, 1998, 2003). The most common hydrophilic block (A) of the block copolymers is polyethylene oxide (PEO). This polymer is highly hydrated through hydrogen bonding and sterically stabilizes surfaces of the polymeric micelles in aqueous systems.

Of the triblock copolymers, the Pluronic series are the most popular. According to the product information by BASF, the nomenclature of Pluronic surfactants can be described based on the molecular weight ranges of the hydrophobe propylene oxide (PO) against the weight-percent of the hydrophile ethylene oxide (EO) present in each molecule. The letter-number combinations can be used to identify the various products of the Pluronic series. The alphabetical designation explains the physical form of the product: "L" for liquids, "P" for pastes, "F" for solid forms. The first digit (two digits in a three-digit number) in the numerical designation, multiplied by 300, indicates the approximate molecular weight of the hydrophobe. The last digit, when multiplied by 10, indicates the approximate EO content in the molecule. For example, Pluronic F-68 is a solid material. The molecular weight of the hydrophobe is approximately 1800 (6 × 300). The hydrophile represents approximately 80% of the molecule, by weight (8 × 10).

The Pluronic R surfactant shows the relationship between the hydrophobe and hydrophile of each product. The letter "R" found in the middle of each designation signifies that this product has a *reverse* structure compared with the Pluronic products, that is, the EO hydrophile is sandwiched between the PO blocks. The numeric designation preceding the "R," when multiplied by 100, indicates the approximate molecular weight of the PO block. The number following the "R," when multiplied by 10, indicates the approximate weight percent EO in that product. For example, Pluronic 25R4 contains 40% EO (4 × 10) and the approximate molecular weight of the combined PO blocks is 2500 (25 × 100).

As with normal hydrocarbon-based surfactants, polymeric micelles have a core-shell structure in aqueous systems (Jones and Leroux, 1999). The shell is responsible for micelle stabilization and interactions with plasma proteins and cell membranes. It usually consists of chains of hydrophilic nonbiodegradable, biocompatible polymers such as PEO. The biodistribution of the carrier is mainly dictated by the nature of the hydrophilic shell (Yokoyama, 1998). PEO forms a dense brush around the micelle core, preventing interaction between the micelle and proteins, for example, opsonins, which promote rapid circulatory clearance by the mononuclear phagocyte system (MPS) (Papisov, 1995). Other polymers such as poly(*N*-isopropylacrylamide) (PNIPA) (Cammas et al., 1997; Chung et al., 1999) and poly(alkylacrylic acid) (Chen et al., 1995; Kwon and Kataoka, 1995; Kohori et al., 1998) can impart additional temperature or pH-sensitivity to the micelles, and may eventually be used to confer bioadhesive properties (Inoue et al., 1998).

The hydrophobic B block forms the core of the micelle that serves as a reservoir for an insoluble drug, thus protecting it from contact with the aqueous environment. Four major classes of core-forming blocks have been widely investigated for drug delivery, including polypropyleneoxide (i.e., Pluronics), poly(l-amino acids), and poly(esters), and phospholipids. Poly(l-amino acids), such as poly(β-benzyl-l-aspartate) (PBLA) (La et al., 1996) offer the ability to tailor extensively core properties, both by design of the amino acid sequence in the repeating block and by adding substituent groups to the functionized amino acids, for example, poly(l-aspartamide)-*graph* fatty acid esters) (Lavasanifar et al., 2001). Although the biodegradablility of artificial poly(l-amino) acids is unknown, phase I trials of a PEO-*b*-P(Asp)-DOX micelle encapsulating doxorubicin have demonstrated the clinical potential of poly(l-amino acid) micelles (Matsumura et al., 2004). Ester hydrolysis and ubiquitous esterases ensure the biodegradability of poly(esters), hence micelles of PEO-*b*-poly(esters) have been investigated extensively as drug carriers, for example, poly(dl-lactic acid) (PDLLA), poly(lactic-*co*-glycolic acid) (PLGA), and poly(ε-caprolactone) (PCL) (Connor et al., 1986; Shin et al., 1998; Jones and Leroux, 1999). The hydrophobic inner core can also consist of a highly hydrophobic small chain such as an alkyl chain (Ringsdorf et al., 1991, 1992; Yoshioka et al., 1995) or a diacyllipid (e.g., distearoyl phosphatidyl ethanolamine [DSPE]) (Trubestkoy et al., 1995). The hydrophobic chain can be either attached to one end of a polymer (Winnik et al., 1995) or randomly distributed within the polymeric structure (Schild and Tirrell, 1991; Ringsdorf et al., 1992) (Figure 13.2, right part).

The B block may consist of a water-soluble polymer, for example, poly(aspartic acid) P(Asp), that is rendered hydrophobic by the chemical conjugation of a hydrophobic drug (Yokoyama et al., 1992, 1993, 1996; Nakanishi et al., 2001), or is formed through the association of two oppositely charged polyions (polyion complex micelles) (Hatada et al., 1995, 1998; Kataoka et al., 1996). Drugs used to couple the B block include cyclophosphamide, doxorubicin, cisplatin, pyrene, and iodine derivative of benzoic acid (Kwon and Kataoka, 1995; Trubetskoy et al., 1997; Yu et al., 1998).

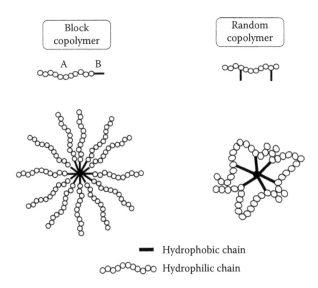

FIGURE 13.2 Schematic representation of block and random copolymer micelles. (Reprinted from *Eur. J. Pharm. Biopharm.*, 48, Jones, M.C. and Leroux, J.C., Polymeric micelles—A new generation of colloidal drug carries, 101–111, Copyright 1999, with permission from Elsevier.)

As summarized in Jones and Leroux's review article (1999), the use of non- or poorly biodegradable polymers such as polystyrene (PST) (Zhao et al., 1990; Zhang et al., 1995) or poly(methyl methacrylate) (PMMA) (Inoue et al., 1998) as constituents of the B block offer interesting properties such as a glassy state that confers remarkable stability to the micelle core. Though it must be pointed out that, to be considered clinically relevant drug carriers, nonbiodegradable polymers must be nontoxic and have a molecular weight sufficiently low to be excreted through the renal route (ca. less than 50,000 Da) (Seymour et al., 1987).

THERMODYNAMICS MICELLIZATION AND SOLUBILIZATION

Polymeric micelle formation occurs as a result of two forces. One is an attractive force that leads to the association of molecules, while the other one is a repulsive force, preventing unlimited growth of the micelles to a distinct macroscopic phase (Price, 1983; Astafieva et al., 1993; Jones and Leroux, 1999). Amphiphilic copolymers form micellar structures through self-association of the insoluble segments when placed in a solvent that is selective for the other monomer (Kataoka et al., 1993; Jones and Leroux, 1999). The process of micellization for amphiphilic copolymers is similar to the process described for conventional hydrocarbon chain-based surfactants as described in the first part of this chapter.

At very low concentrations, the polymers exist only as single chains. As the concentration increases to reach a critical value, called the critical micelle concentration (CMC), polymer chains start to associate to form micelles in such a way that the hydrophobic segment of the copolymer will avoid contact with the aqueous media in that the polymer is diluted. At the CMC, a significant amount of solvent may still be found inside the micellar core, and micelles are described as loose aggregates that exhibit larger size than micelles formed at higher concentrations (Gao and Eisenberg, 1993). At those higher concentrations, the equilibrium will favor tighter micelle formation; micelles will adopt their low-energy state configuration and the remaining solvent will gradually be released from the hydrophobic core resulting in a decrease in micellar size (Jones and Leroux, 1999). Two techniques for the formation of micelles, flash nanoprecipitation (Johnson and Prud'homme, 2003a, b) and azeotropic dialysis (Jette et al., 2004), replace a miscible organic solvent with water to derive micellization of amphiphilic block copolymers.

The micellization of amphiphilic copolymers can result in two different types of micelles, depending on whether the hydrophobic portion is randomly bound to the hydrophilic polymer or grafted to one end of the hydrophilic portion. When terminal hydrophobic groups associate to form micelles, the water clusters immobilized around the hydrophobic segments are excluded from the core and no direct interaction exists between the core and the hydrophilic shell that remains as mobile linear chains in the micellar structure (Winnik et al., 1992; Chung et al., 1999). Randomly modified polymers, however, associate in such a manner that hydrophobic and hydrophilic segments of the polymer are entangled, allowing possible contact between the core and the aqueous media. In this case, the hydrophilic chains forming the shells are less mobile (Chung et al., 1999). This is an important issue, since exposed hydrophobic cores may result in secondary aggregation of polymeric micelles (Gao and Eisenberg, 1993; Yokoyama et al., 1994; La et al., 1996).

Gadelle et al. (1995) investigated the solubilization of various aromatic solutes in PEO-b-PPO-b-PEO (ABA)/PPO-b-PEO-b-PPO (BAB) triblock copolymers. According to the experimental results, they indicated two different solubilization processes. To understand better the mechanism for solubilization in the polymeric surfactant solutions, it was postulated that (1) the addition of apolar solutes promotes micellization of the polymeric surfactant molecules, (2) the central core of the polymeric micelles contains some water molecules, and (3) solubilization is initially a replacement process in which water molecules are displaced from the micellar core by the solubilizate. A detailed discussion of the solubilization process can be found in the next section and the pharmaceutical application section of this chapter.

MODELING OF MICELLIZATION AND SOLUBILIZATION

Diblock Copolymeric Micelles

In an early diblock copolymeric micellar model, an isolated chain in solution was described as having a tadpole configuration with a short collapsed head-block connected to a solvent swollen tail. Each solvent-phobic head is assumed to be a molten liquid globule that merges with other heads in order to minimize exposure to the poor solvent. The resulting micellar aggregate is thus a molten spherical core surrounded by the swollen tails (Daoud and Cotton, 1982; Kwon and Kataoda, 1995; Marques, 1997) (Figure 13.3). The liquid nature of the core allows for mixing the chains and enables the assembly to reach a thermodynamic equilibrium state where the balance between core-solvent interfacial tension and stretching of the chains can be achieved. Under these equilibrium conditions, the micelle aggregation number has been theoretically predicted (Halperin, 1987; Marques et al., 1988) with reasonable agreement in experimental data.

There is evidence to suggest that the hypothesized liquid nature of the core does not generally hold (Antonietti et al., 1994; Marques, 1997). If the core is not a molten globule but is instead in a glass-like state, Marques (1997) indicated that two possible core structures can be considered, and the structure formed depends on the preparation method. First, for micelles prepared in an equilibrium solution (usually at high temperature) and then quenched, the molten core will undergo a glassy transition leading to a final structure that carries the signature of the micellization temperature and of the quenching process. The central glassy region is then likely to have a uniform monomer density of entangled glassy chains. The initial aggregation number is defined by the micellization that occurs at the equilibrium solution state before quenching. Faster quenching rates produce micelles closer to the initial state.

The second possible geometry will arise if the micellization proceeds by aggregation of copolymer chains that already have a glassy head. Although little is known about the structure of individual glassy chains in solution, the characteristic relaxation time of the chain is likely to depend on the amount of solvent actually present in the collapsed globule. In the extreme case of zero solvent content (zero plasticizing effect) and infinite relaxation time, the core will have a porous structure (Figure 13.4), and the pores are filled with solvent and copolymer tails. This bunchy aspect leads to a new distribution of monomers in the micelles and provides simple geometric rules determining

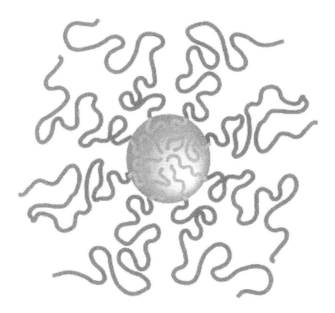

FIGURE 13.3 Sketch for the structure of a diblock copolymer micelle with a molten liquid core. The core is free of solvent or tail monomers. (Reprinted with permission from Marques, C.M., *Langmuir*, 13, 1430–1433, 1997. Copyright 1997 American Chemical Society.)

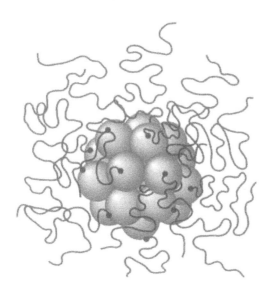

FIGURE 13.4 Core structure of a bunchy micelle, which allows for a significant penetration of solvent and tails in the core region. The tails are assumed to be repelled by the beads and therefore to protrude toward the solvent in order to escape confinement. (Reprinted with permission from Marques, C.M., *Langmuir*, 13, 1430–1433, 1997. Copyright 1997 American Chemical Society.)

the micellar aggregation number. As is being discussed, this picture leads to a different micellization scenario and to new predictions for the properties of the micelles.

The process of constructing a bunchy micellar core is represented by Marques (1997) as a process by which individual beads are added until saturation or some equilibrium aggregation number is reached. It is assumed that the solid, spherical heads behave like impenetrable, repulsive walls with respect to the monomers from the soluble block. The amount of space filled by the solvent and by the tails will depend on the exact packing geometry of the solid heads and on how deformable the solid is. For an infinitely rigid head, the porosity may vary from a minimum of 26%, when spherical heads close pack in a crystal hexagonal close packed or face centered cubic structure, to the most likely case, corresponding to an amorphous structure of approximately 45% porosity. A particular feature of these micelles is that the exchange of a bead from the central core region to the bulk is practically forbidden. At a given moment, only the surface beads may be easily exchanged. This contradicts with the classical micelles where all the micelle chains are *surface chains* and may then be directly exchanged with the bulk. Marques (1997) has shown that the calculated scaling form for the aggregation number in diblock copolymers with a glassy head is in close agreement with results by Antonietti et al. (1994). This suggests that bunchy micelles are good candidates for modeling micellization in that system. However, care should be exerted when extracting information from a single set of data, because alternative explanations could be invoked.

The configuration of the polymers in the micelle has also been studied within the framework of the Daoud-Cotton model (Daoud and Cotton, 1982) for star polymers. However, this model assumes that all the chain ends lie at the outer surface of the corona, therefore overlooking the possibility of a chain-end distribution Marques (1997).

Solubilization by block copolymers has been investigated by Nagarajan and Ganesh (1989) who developed a theory of solubilization of low molecular weight compounds in micelles of AB diblock copolymers in a selective solvent. The theory predicts that the solubilization behavior of the micelles and their geometrical characteristics are significantly influenced by the interactions between the solubilizate and the solvent-compatible block of the copolymer as well as by the solubilizate-solvent interfacial tension. The scaling relationship obtained was compared with previous experimental data where the micellar core was composed of poly(propylene oxide)/PST. This polymer core showed substantial solubilization of aromatic hydrocarbon solubilizates in contrast to negligible solubilization of aliphatics. The conclusion was made that the solubilizate that is more compatible with the polymer block that constitutes the core of the micelle is solubilized to a greater extent.

Triblock Copolymeric Micelles

Hydrophilic terminal blockmicelles: Water-soluble poly(EO)-poly(PO)-poly(EO) (PEO-*b*-PPO-*b*-PEO) triblock copolymers can aggregate to form micelles with a core presumably dominated by PPO and a corona dominated by hydrated PEO blocks. Hurterr et al. (1993a) developed a self-consistent mean field lattice theory to predict the aggregation behavior of PEO-*b*-PPO-*b*-PEO block copolymers and the solubilization of naphthalene in these micelles as a function of polymer composition and molecular weight. The predictions compared favorably with experimental results. It was found that the dependence of the micelle-water partition coefficient on polymer composition is not simply related to the proportion of the hydrophobic constituent but depends on the details of the micelle structure. A strong effect of the molecular weight and PPO content of the polymer on the amount of naphthalene solubilized was observed. A more detailed discussion of Pluronics and other ABA triblock polymers can be found in the next section and the pharmaceutical application section in this chapter.

Hydrophobic terminal blockmicelles: Xing and Mattice (1998) applied Monte Carlo simulation techniques to study the models of BAB triblock copolymeric micelles with solubilizates in a selected solvent. They focused on a microscopic picture regarding the locus of solubilizates in BAB triblock copolymer micelles when the solubilizate molecules are energetically equivalent to a segment of the insoluble block. This situation is of practical interest since monomer or homopolymer impurities are hard to eliminate from block copolymer synthesis.

Two models for micelle structure were identified in their studies (Xing and Mattice, 1998). In analogy with the structural models for systems involving low molecular weight surfactants, two kinds of aggregates of spherical shape can be pictured, depending on how the solubilizates are located inside the block copolymer micelles. Solubilization takes places in two steps in the Xing and Mattice's simulations (1998).

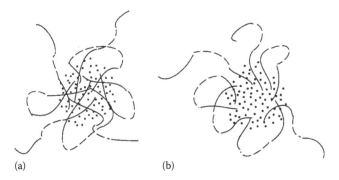

FIGURE 13.5   Two models for the structure of micelles. (a) Uniform dissolution of I in B. (b) Stabilization of a microdroplet of I by putting A on the interface. (Reprinted with permission from Xing, L. and Mattice, W.L., *Langmuir*, 14, 4074–4080, 1998. Copyright 1998 American Chemical Society.)

Solubilization initially takes place by displacing the solvent molecules from the micellar core. Unlike with conventional surfactant micelles, a substantial amount of solvent is present in the micellar core of the small BAB triblock copolymers. This is supported by Hurterr et al. (1993b) and Linse and Malmsten (1992). At this stage, the micellar structure complies with the model drawn in Figure 13.5a, which is the uniform dissolution of solute in B.

Subsequent solubilization takes place by further displacing the solvent molecules and by excluding the insoluble blocks away from the center of the core. If the B blocks cannot stretch into the centers of the cores of the swollen micelles, solute will accumulate in the centers. The corresponding micellar structure is as shown in Figure 13.5b. The distinct characteristic of this structure is that there is a region where only pure solute molecules are present. This can be described as stabilization of a microdroplet of solute by putting B at the interface. The structure gradually changes from part a to part b of Figure 13.5 as more solute is added to the system. Besides the addition of solute, a higher incompatibility between solvent and solute also promotes switching from the first model to the second.

Other copolymers that may show micellization similar to that of BAB triblock copolymers include random copolymers if the hydrophobic units are located near both ends of the polymeric structure (Schild and Tirrell, 1991; Ringsdorf et al., 1992; Chung et al., 1999; Jones and Leroux, 1999), and graft copolymers if the hydrophobic blocks are grafted near both ends of a hydrophilic backbone.

Flory–Huggins Modeling of Solubilization

Flory–Huggins analysis was developed to predict the compatibility of polymers and solvents (Flory, 1941) but has found application in pharmaceutics for predicting water absorption of pharmaceutical solids (Hancock and Zografi, 1993) and interactions of polymers and excipients with small drug molecules (Lacoulonche et al., 1998; Nair et al., 2001). Interactions between the hydrophobic core of block copolymer micelles and the drug molecule strongly influence solubilization (Nagarajan et al., 1986), and it has been found that Flory–Huggins may be applied to micellar drug systems to predict solubility (Liu et al., 2003).

For two components of a mixture (i.e., drug molecules and the hydrophobic block of the copolymer) to be mutually miscible, the Gibbs free energy of mixing, ΔG_{mix}, must be negative.

$$\Delta G_{\text{mix}} = \Delta H_{\text{mix}} - T\Delta S_{\text{mix}}$$

$$\Delta H_{\text{mix}} = \chi\varphi(1-\varphi)RT$$

Therefore, the enthalpy of mixing, ΔH_{mix}, must be minimized for the drug to be soluble in the micelle core, as the mixing entropy, ΔS_{mix} is dependent on the volume fraction drug in the core, φ, and not the dispersion and adhesion energy interactions between components. The Flory–Huggins solubility parameter, χ, can be calculated using the Hildebrand solubility parameters:

$$\chi = \frac{V_{drug}(\delta_{drug} - \delta_{poly})^2}{RT}$$

where the Hildebrand solubility parameters, δ_{poly} and δ_{poly}, are square roots of the cohesive energy densities of the drug molecule and hydrophobic repeating group of the copolymer, respectively; V_{drug} is the molar volume of the drug molecule; R is the ideal gas constant; and T is the temperature. The Hildebrand solubility parameters may be calculated using group contribution methods, wherein the overall solubility parameter is the sum of contributions from Van der Waals dispersion forces, δ_d; dipole–dipole interactions, δ_p; and hydrogen bonding, δ_h.

$$\delta_{total} = [\delta_d^2 + \delta_p^2 + \delta_h^2]^{1/2}$$

$$\delta_d = \frac{\sum F_{di}}{V} \quad \delta_p = \frac{\sqrt{\sum F_{pi}^2}}{V} \quad \delta_h = \frac{\sqrt{\sum E_{hi}}}{V}$$

The molar attraction constants of dispersion, F_{di}; dipole–dipole interactions, F_{pi}; hydrogen bonding, E_{hi}; and the molar volume, V; for the drug and the hydrophobic block may be determined from group contribution tables provided by Hoftyzer-Van Krevelen and Fedor (Krevelen, 1990).

Liu et al. (2003) recently applied classic Flory–Huggins solution theory to predict the solubility of the hydrophobic drug ellipticine in several block copolymers (Table 13.1). Solution theory predicted the solubility of ellipticine in block copolymers to be PBLA > PCL > PDLA > PGA. Liu et al. found PEO-*b*-PCL to encapsulate up to 21% w/w ellipticine, whereas PDLA encapsulated a maximum of 0.1% w/w.

FACTORS AFFECTING MICELLIZATION AND SOLUBILIZATION

Temperature and Concentration Effects on Micellization

Before discussing the temperature and concentration effects, some terms need to be defined. First, a solvent is considered a *selective solvent* if it is a thermodynamically good solvent for one type of block but a nonsolvent for the other type of block. Next, the CMC of copolymers can be defined as the concentration below which only single chains are present but above which both single chains and micellar aggregates coexist. Then *critical micelle temperature* (CMT) is the temperature below which only single chains are present, while above the CMT both single chains and micelles coexist. Therefore, by monitoring an appropriate property of the system of interest, an inflection point, which corresponds to the CMC or CMT, can usually be found on the concentration or temperature curve.

TABLE 13.1
Solubility Parameters and Heat of Mixing of Ellipticine in Various Polymers

Polymer	δ_{total} (MPa$^{1/2}$)	$\delta_{ellipticine} - \delta_{polymer}$	ΔH_{mix}(MJ/m^3)
Poly(benzyl l-aspartate) (PBLA)	25	0.8	2.2
Poly(ε-caprolactone) (PCL)	20.2	5.9	10.8
Poly(dl-lactic acid) (PDLA)	23.3	2.8	14.3
Poly(glycolic acid) (PGA)	28	−1.9	21.7
Ellipticine	26.1	–	–

Source: Liu, J. et al., *J. Pharm. Sci.*, 93, 132–143, 2003.

The values of the CMC or CMT collected as a function of temperature or concentration can be used to extract the enthalpic and entropic contributions to the association process. For a closed association mechanism with relatively large aggregation number and a narrow distribution, the standard free energy and standard enthalpy of micelle formation ($\Delta G°$ and $\Delta H°$, per mole of the solute in the micelle) are related to the CMC and its temperature dependence in the form (Lindman and Wennerstrom, 1980; Zhou and Chu, 1994).

$$\Delta G° = RT \ \ln \ (\text{CMC}) \tag{13.1}$$

$$\Delta H° = R[\text{d} \ \ln \ (\text{CMC})/\text{d}(1/T)] \tag{13.2}$$

where the CMC is in molar concentration, the two standard states are the polymer molecules and micelles in ideally dilute solution at unit molarity. Equation 13.2 can be integrated to yield

$$\ln \ (\text{CMC}) \approx \Delta H°/RT + \text{constant} \tag{13.3}$$

provided that $\Delta H°$ is approximately a constant in the temperature interval involved.

At a given temperature, micellization of copolymers in aqueous solutions depends on their concentration. Therefore, the application of micelles as drug carriers raises the fundamental question about their stability during dissolution by body fluids. The multimolecular micelles are formed at copolymer concentrations equal to or exceeding the CMC, which may serve as a thermodynamic parameter characterizing the micelle stability during dissolution. Temperature can affect the CMC as well as other thermodynamic parameters such as aggregation number and micelle size. Linse and Malmsten (1992) used gel permeation chromatography (GPC) and data obtained from the literature to study the temperature-dependent micellization in aqueous block copolymer solutions. Pluronic 127 was used as the model copolymer in their study. They concluded that temperature has a great effect on micellization of the Pluronic copolymer: with increasing temperature, the CMC decreases, the fraction of polymer molecules in micellar form increases, the average aggregation number increases, and the micelle hydrodynamic radius (size) increases.

Almgren et al. (1992) examined aqueous solutions of Pluronic L-64 with static and dynamic light scattering (DLS), pulsed-gradient spin-echo (PGSE) NMR and fluorescence spectroscopy over a range of concentrations from 0.2% to 25% and temperature from 15°C to 60°C. Relaxation time distributions from DLS show L-64 to be molecularly dissolved at 21°C and to form micelles at higher temperatures. The aggregation numbers at the temperatures 21.0°C, 25.9°C, 40.0°C, and 60.0°C were calculated to be 2, 4, 19, and 85, respectively, indicating a smooth increase with temperature. The data are in agreement with earlier reported results (McDonald and Wang, 1974; Al-Saden et al., 1982). These micelles persist at high concentrations (25%) without the formation of gel or liquid crystalline phases. The temperature where micelle formation starts is strongly concentration dependent, in contrast to the cloud point (CP) that remains fairly constant at 60°C. Similar results were obtained by Pandya using static light scattering (Pandya et al., 1993).

The data from PSGE NMR indicate that the exchange between monomers and micelles is fast and the large aggregates involve only a small fraction of L-64 (Almgren et al., 1992). At low concentrations, the observed diffusion coefficient (D) grows initially with the temperature to a maximum, and decreases steeply thereafter. The decrease in D is due to micelle formation, which starts at a lower temperature when the concentration is high. The steep decrease on approaching the CP is probably due to micelle-micelle interactions.

The pronounced sensitivity of the CMC to temperature, or the CMT to concentration, is commonly found for poloxamers (Zhou and Chu, 1987, 1988), but not for the normal alkyl polyethylene glycol ethers, $C_x EO_y$ (35). The decrease of the hydrophilicity of the PEO blocks with increasing temperature has comparatively little effect on the CMC for $C_x EO_y$. For $C_{12} EO_8$ the CMC is reported as 9.7×10^{-5} M at 15°C and 5.8×10^{-5} M at 40°C (Megufo et al., 1987). In addition, the number of

EO units has little effect on CMC. CMC is given as 6.5×10^{-5} M for $C_{12}EO_5$ and 7.2×10^{-5} M for $C_{12}EO_8$ (Megufo et al., 1987). The main determinant of the CMC for C_xEO_y is the length of the alkyl chain; for the poloxamers an increasing hydrophobicity of the PO block with increasing temperature, in combination with the size polydispersity of the PO blocks, could explain the temperature dependence of the CMC.

Bohorquez et al. (1999) also studied the temperature-dependent micellization of the pharmaceutically important Pluronic F-127 using static light scattering and various aspects of the pyrene fluorescence spectrum (monomer intensity, excimer formation, and the I_1/I_3 ratio). All techniques gave essentially the same values for the CMT of various F-127 solutions and agreed with those in the literature. CMT values decrease with increasing F-127 concentrations. Significant solubilization of pyrene in F-127 solutions below the CMT was observed, indicating that hydrophobic molecules such as water-insoluble drugs may be substantially solubilized in F-127 before micelle formation. For pyrene, this solubilization was observed at approximately 1°C–2°C below the CMT. Although this temperature difference appears small, it indicates that changes in body temperature (which are usually of the order of 1°F–5°F) may have an effect on the behavior of F-127 systems.

The thermodynamics of the micellization process were studied and gave different results at low and high F127 concentrations. In the low F-127 concentration range (up to ~50 mg/mL), $\Delta H = 312$ kJ/mol and $\Delta S = 1.14$ kJ/mol·K were obtained, while above 50 mg/mL, $\Delta H = 136$ kJ/mol and $\Delta S = 0.54$ kJ/mol·K were found. This discontinuity in thermodynamic behavior can be due to a change in aggregation number with temperature and/or a change in the micellization process at higher concentrations such as progressive entanglements between PEO chains.

The thermodynamic parameters were also calculated for Pluronic L-64 in water. Zhou and Chu (1994) took the CMT data obtained by scattered light intensity measurements from Pandya et al. (1993) and the CMC data by surface tension measurements from Reddy et al. (1990). The CMT values of L-64 were 28°C, 30°C, and 33°C for the concentrations of 20, 10, and 5 mg/mL, respectively. The CMC values of L-64 were 7.1, 2.8, and 0.9 mg/mL at 27.0°C, 34.5°C, and 40.0°C, respectively. It appears that for aqueous L-64 solutions, these two sets of micellization data from different sources with different experimental methods are basically consistent with each other except for the CMC data at 27.0°C. From these they calculated the standard enthalpy of micellization, $\Delta H° = 210 \pm 11$ kJ/mol. At 40.0°C, $\Delta G°$, and $\Delta S°$ were estimated to be -21 kJ/mol and 1.74 kJ/K/mol, respectively.

A broader study of the dilute solution behavior of ABA copolymers was reported by Beezer et al. (1994) who analyzed scanning microcalorimetric transition data for 27 members of Pluronic ABA block copolymer family. These data were used to correlate the thermodynamic parameters of the observed transitions to poly(propylene oxide) content. The observed phase transition is an event related to hydrophobic aggregation, but independent of the polymer CP. They hypothesized that a coiled colloidal poly(propylene oxide) core was surrounded by the solvated poly(EO) portion of the molecule. On temperature-induced phase transition at these concentrations, the central poly(propylene oxide) core must associate to produce larger aggregates.

However, some contradictory data on Pluronic CMC can be found in the literature (Schmolka, 1977; Alexandris et al., 1994a, b). The reported CMC values differ by a factor of 1 or 2 for the same Pluronic polymers (Kabanov et al., 1995). Kabanov et al. (1995) employed several independent methods to study micellization of Pluronic polymers F-68, P-85, and F-108 in aqueous solutions, and determined the CMC for these Pluronics. These methods included surface tension measurements and fluorescent probes (pyrene, 1,6-diphenyl-1,3,5-hexatriene). The temperature ranged from 25°C to 50°C in these experiments and the CMC decreased with increasing temperature for all three Pluronics. The CMC values are in reasonable agreement with the values reported by Schmolka and Raymond (Schmolka and Raymond, 1965) for F68, P85, and F108, and also consistent with the data obtained by Zhou and Chu (1987, 1988,) and Nakashima et al. (1994) for F68. However, some CMC values are not in agreement with those by Alexandris et al. (1994a, b). These CMC values by Alexandris et al. were affected by the relaxation process in the measurement (Kabanov et al., 1995).

Zhou and Chu (1994) studied the phase behavior and association properties of Pluronic R17R4, a PPO-*b*-PEO-*b*-PPO (BAB) triblock copolymer in aqueous solutions. At room temperature, 17R4 $[(PO)_{14}(EO)_{24}(PO)_{14}]$ exists in the form of single coils with a radius of approximately 1 nm even at fairly high concentrations (0.2 g/mL). However, at 40°C, the light-scattering measurements taken as a function of concentration show an inflection at a concentration of 0.091 g/mL. This inflection was interpreted as the CMC. Thus, BAB triblock polymers do form micelles in aqueous solution at elevated temperatures, and they exhibit a temperature induced micellization behavior similar to that of ABA triblock copolymers. At 25°C, remarkable solute-solvent interactions exist owing to the hydrogen bond formation between ether oxygen atoms and water molecules. In addition, the strong repulsive interactions between the segments can explain why no micelles are formed at room temperature even for concentrated solutions of 17R4 in water. However, at 40°C, a profound enhancement of solute–solute interactions was found with increasing temperature. In the dilute region, such attractive interactions are, most likely, of intrachain nature, and consequently, collapsed unimers are observed at 40°C. At high concentrations, the interchain attractive interactions become important, leading to the self-assembly phenomenon observed at 40°C when a certain concentration threshold is exceeded. Although 17R4 forms associated structures only at high copolymer concentrations within a narrow temperature region, the temperature dependent micellization of BAB triblock copolymers could be interesting for pharmaceutical applications. For example, this property can be utilized to make thermosensitive drug carriers.

17R4 and L-64 are very similar in chemical composition and have only a small difference of about 9% in the total molar mass. Therefore, they constitute a good pair of subjects to compare the effect of chain architecture on phase behavior and association properties.

By comparing the thermodynamic quantities of micellization of both 17R4 and L-64, Zhou and Chu (1994) concluded, that micellization of both surfactants is an endothermic process that accounts for the fact that the CMC decreases as the temperature increases. In both cases, the entropically driven hydrophobic interactions of the poly(propylene oxide) blocks in an aqueous environment are mainly responsible for micelle formation.

For 17R4 in water, the entropy loss arising from the looping geometry of the middle poly(EO) block may largely reduce the driving force for micellization. As a result, the free energy of micellization becomes much less negative, being about −9 kJ/mol at 40.0°C as compared with $\Delta G° = -21$ kJ/mol for L-64. Correspondingly, the critical micelle concentration of 17R4 at this temperature, the reciprocal of which may serve as a measure of micellization ability, is significantly greater than that of L-64, that is, by a factor of about 100.

These differences also appear in the phase diagrams of the two surfactants (Figure 13.6a, b). In Figure 13.6a, the CPs of 17R4 solutions are denoted by open circles. As reported in a BASF brochure (BASF, 1989), the CPs of 1% and 10% aqueous 17R4 solutions are 46°C and 31°C (shown by filled circle in Figure 13.6a). Figure 13.6a also shows the relevant CMT data (open triangles) and CMC data (filled triangle). The solid line represents a fit to the data and the slope is interpreted using Equation 13.3 to provide $\Delta H° = 115$ kJ/mol (Zhou and Chu, 1994). The dotted line represents an extension of the solid line to the dilute solution region where the two physical quantities in Equation 13.3 ($\Delta H°$ and constant) are assumed to have the same values as those determined in concentrated 17R4 solutions.

There exist three regions of interest in these diagrams, namely, the one-phase unimer region (I), the one-phase micelle region (II), and the two-phase region where two immiscible (isotropic) solutions are observed (III). The phase behavior of L-64 in water is relatively simple. Below the cloud-point curve, as illustrated by the extensive region II, L-64 forms micelles over a large temperature range as well as a large concentration range. Unimers exist only in a small-restricted area, mainly, at low temperatures and in dilute solutions. As reported elsewhere (Zhou and Chu, 1988a,b; Reddy et al., 1990; Almgren et al., 1991a,b; Pandya et al., 1993a,b), the aggregation number and L-64 micellar size increase with increasing temperature in region II.

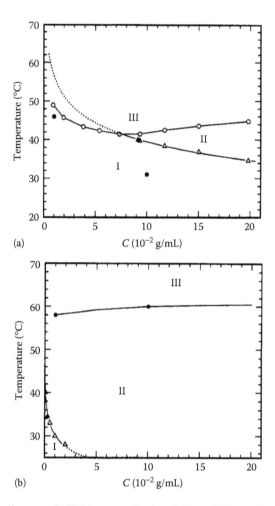

FIGURE 13.6 (a) Phase diagram of 17R4 in water. Regions I, II, and III are the one-phase unimer region, one-phase micelle region, and two-phase region of two immiscible isotropic solutions, respectively. (b) Phase diagram of L-64 in water. Also, three-phase regions are shown. See text for an explanation of the symbols and curves. (Reprinted with permission from Zhou, Z. and Chu, B., *Macromolecules*, 27, 2025–2033, 1994. Copyright 1994 American Chemical Society.)

The phase behavior of 17R4 in water and its tendency toward self-assembly differ dramatically from those of L-64, meaning that for triblock copolymers, the construction sequence of blocks has a significant influence on their solution properties. In strong contrast to L-64, the 17R4 unimer region extends over a broad concentration range and a large temperature range. However, 17R4 forms micelles only at high concentrations ($C > 7.5 \times 10^{-2}$ g/mL) within a narrow, wedged-shape temperature range, the width of which expands moderately with increasing concentration. Moreover, the location of the cloud-point curve in the neighborhood of an intermediate temperature (~42°C) largely restricts the effective temperature range of the micelle region. For instance, even at the highest concentration ($C = 20\%$ (w/v)), a temperature interval of only 10°C is in effect. In the dilute region (e.g., $C < 7.5 \times 10^{-2}$ g/mL), when raising the temperature, the cloud-point curve was met rather than the CMT curve, and therefore, the formation of micelles becomes completely impossible, no matter what temperature has been selected.

Table 13.2 summarizes the effect of the chain architecture, and provides a detailed comparison of micellar parameters between 17R4 and L-64 micelles, including the thermodynamic quantities of the micellization process.

TABLE 13.2

Comparison in Micellar Parameters between 17R4 and L-64 Micelles in Water

	Pluronic L-64	Pluronic 17R4
Composition	$(EO)_{13}(PO)_{30}(EO)_{13}$	$(PO)_{14}(EO)_{24}(PO)_{14}$
HLB value	15	7–12
CMC at 40°C, g/mL	9.0×10^{-14a}	9.1×10^{-2}
Mw, g/mol	2.8×10^{5a}	2.65×104 (40.0°C)
Aggregation number	88 (42.5°C)[b]	10 (40.0°C)
A_2, cm³mol g⁻²	$\sim 6.0 \times 10^{-4}$ (42.5°C)[b]	$\sim 6.0 \times 10^{-5}$
R_h, nm	10.2 (42.5°C)[b]	4.0 (40.0°C)
$\Delta H°$, kJ/mol	210	115
$\Delta G°$, at 40.0°C, kJ/mol	−21	−9
$\Delta S°$, at 40.0°C, kJ/(mol K)	0.74	0.40

Source: Zhou, Z. and Chu, B., *Macromolecules*, 27, 2025–2033, 1994.

Note: Mw is the weight-average molecular weight, A_2 the second virial coefficient, R_h, hydrodynamic radius.

[a] Reddy, N.K. et al., *J. Chem. Soc., Faraday Trans.*, 86, 1569–1572, 1990.

[b] Zhou, Z. and Chu, B., *Macromolecules*, 21, 2548–2554, 1988a.

Linse (1993) compared the micellization behavior of an ABA triblock copolymer (PEO-*b*-PPO-*b*-PEO) with a BAB triblock copolymer (PPO-*b*-PEO-*b*-PPO) with the same composition as that of Pluronic P-105 (i.e., $(EO)_{74}(PO)_{56}$). He concluded that PPO-*b*-PEO-*b*-PPO forms micelles only within a narrow temperature range and only at high concentrations. However, the CMC value of Pluronic P105 is a factor of two lower than that of the PPO-*b*-PEO-*b*-PPO copolymer. It was predicted that the PPO-*b*-PEO-*b*-PPO forms larger micelles than P105. Additional studies of other BAB triblock copolymers can be found elsewhere (Mortensen et al., 1994; Yekta et al., 1995; Yang et al., 1996; Zhou et al., 1996).

Temperature and Concentration Effects on Solubilization

In investigating temperature effects on drug solubilization in micellar systems, changes in the micellar properties as well as those in the aqueous solubility of the solute significantly affect the solubilization of the solute. As discussed in the "Temperature and Concentration Effects on Micellization" section, the CMC values decrease with increasing temperature in line with an inverse temperature-surfactant solubility relationship. In the case of PEO surfactants, the aqueous solubility of the surfactants is attributed to hydrogen bonding between the ether oxygens of EO chains and water molecules. When the temperature is increased, these hydrogen bonds break and the hydrophilicity of the PEO chain is reduced, rendering the surfactant less soluble so that micellization occurs at a lower concentration (Almgren et al., 1995). This suggests that the solubilization of a solute will occur at lower surfactant concentrations, and the solubilization capacity increases per gram of surfactant in solution, owing to the decrease of CMC caused by an increase in the temperature. In addition, micelles of polymeric surfactants rapidly grow in size with increasing temperature, which may be in part due to greater hydrophobicity of the monomer and geometric considerations. Therefore, in general, the higher the temperature, the larger the micellar solubilization capacity for a solute.

Lin and Yang (1987) found that the diazepam solubilizing capacities of Pluronics increased with increasing temperature and rank in the order: F-68 < F-88 < F-108. These results, along with partition coefficient (K_m) values, are shown below in Table 13.3. The higher the K_m, the greater the amount of diazepam entrapped within the micelles. The difference in K_m values at different temperatures is because micellar solubility increases more rapidly with temperature than does the solubility in water. The rise in solubility of diazepam in the presence of Pluronic

TABLE 13.3

Solubilizing Capacities and Partition Coefficients of Diazepam as a Function of Temperature

Pluronics	Solubilizing Capacity[a]			Partition Coefficient (K_m)		
	25°C	37°C	50°C	25°C	37°C	50°C
F-68	0.0253	0.0522	0.1811	272.32	460.37	1292.76
F-88	0.0334	0.1206	0.3167	358.77	1059.43	2464.44
F-108	0.0342	0.3751	0.6771	367.38	3326.63	4294.74

Source: Lin, S.Y. and Yang, J.C., *Acta Pharm. Technol.*, 33, 222–224, 1987.
[a] Units: mol diazepam/mol Pluronic.

TABLE 13.4

Thermodynamic Parameters for the Solubilization of Diazepam by Pluronic Surfactants

Temperature	F-68			F-88			F-108		
	ΔG	ΔH	ΔS	ΔG	ΔH	ΔS	ΔG	ΔH	ΔS
25°C	−3.32	−11.61	−27.83	−3.48	−14.53	−37.07	−3.50	−2.74	6.71
37°C	−3.78	—	—	−4.29	—	−33.03	−4.99	—	7.28
50°C	−4.59	—	−21.69	−5.01	—	−29.47	−5.37	—	8.14

Source: Lin, S.Y. and Yang, J.C., *Acta Pharm. Technol.*, 33, 222–224, 1987.
Note: Units of ΔG and ΔH are kcal/mol, and ΔS is cal/K/mol.

surfactants with increasing temperature is believed to be the result of an increase in the micellar aggregation number at higher temperatures, leading to the formation of a larger micelle, capable of entrapping more diazepam.

Lin and Yang (1987) also calculated the thermodynamic parameters of diazepam for micellar solubilization in Pluronic surfactant solutions at different temperatures (Table 13.4). For all systems, ΔG was negative, indicating micellar solubilization was spontaneous. The sign of entropy has been associated with the location of solubilized molecules within the micelles. Positive values have been observed for molecules embedded in the micelle center and negative values for adsorption of the molecules on the micelle surface. The results in this paper indicate that in the F-108 and F-88 Pluronics, diazepam molecules can penetrate into the micelle interior, whereas for F-68 and lower concentrations of F-88, diazepam is adsorbed on the micelle surface without penetration into the micellar core.

Croy and Kwon (2004) found increasing temperature from 25°C to 37°C increased the partitioning coefficient and decreased the critical aggregation concentration (CAC) of the polyene antimycotic nystatin in micelles of F-98, P-105, and F-127 (Figure 13.7; Table 13.5). The trend in increased partitioning followed decreased CMC, enlarged core size, and increased aggregate number; hence, the solubility of nystatin improved with the presence of greater available micellar core surface area, indicating amphiphilic nystatin was solubilized at the core-shell interface of these micelles. Croy and Kwon further investigated the effect of temperature on the core polarity of Pluronic micelles, finding the polarity decreased with increasing temperature. Although nystatin partitioning increased at 37°C in the Pluronics, partitioning was much lower in the less numerous F-98 micelles although its core polarity was similar to P-105 and F-127, indicating solubility of nystatin was dependent on total micellar core surface area.

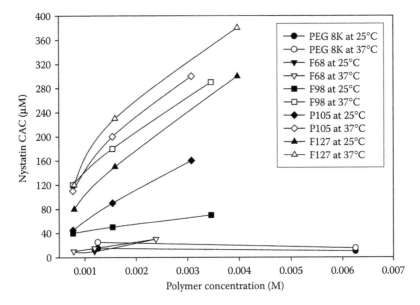

FIGURE 13.7   Effect of polymer concentration and temperature on the critical aggregation concentration of nystatin, as interpreted from dynamic light scattering data. (Reprinted from *J. Control. Rel.*, 95, Croy, S. R. and Kwon, G. S., The effects of Pluronic block copolymers on the aggregation state of nystatin, 161–171, Copyright 2004, with permission from Elsevier.)

TABLE 13.5

Nystatin Micelle-Water Partition Coefficients and Pluronic Micelle Core Polarities as a Function of Pluronic and Temperature

Pluronic	Nystatin Partition Coefficient		Core Polarity[a]	
	25°C	37°C	25°C	37°C
F-127	17 ± 1	79 ± 8	1.204 ± 0.001	1.179 ± 0.003
P-105	16 ± 5	73 ± 6	1.214 ± 0.003	1.180 ± 0.004
F-98	N/A	21 ± 5	1.221 ± 0.001	1.193 ± 0.002
F-68	N/A	15 ± 5	1.405 ± 0.003	1.332 ± 0.001

Source: Croy, S. R. and Kwon, G. S., *J. Control. Rel.*, 95, 161–171, 2004.

[a]   Determined by ratio of pyrene I and III fluorescence peaks.

Effect of Copolymeric Architecture on Micellization

It has been demonstrated for several copolymers that the onset of micellization is mainly dependent upon the length of the hydrophobic polymer chains, while the effect of the hydrophilic chain length on the CMC is less pronounced (Astafieva et al., 1993; Gao and Eisenberg, 1993; Kataoka et al., 1993). Astafieva et al. (1993) measured the CMC of a range of block copolyelectrolytes based on styrene (the insoluble block) and sodium acrylate. The lengths of the styrene blocks ranged from ca. 300 to ca. 1400. The pyrene fluorescent probe technique was utilized, and the data were treated by five different methods. CMC results were interpolated for a constant polyelectrolyte block length of 1000 units. It was found that changing the insoluble block length from 6 to 110 lowered the CMC from 1.6×10^{-5} to 5×10^{-8} M. In contrast, changing the soluble block length from 300 to 1400 typically changed the CMC values by less than a factor of two. For very short PST blocks, the CMC decreased very rapidly with increasing length of the insoluble block. For longer lengths (above 12) the drop in the CMC was much more gradual.

Guo et al. (1999) studied the temperature-dependent micellization of PEO-*b*-PPO-*b*-PEO block copolymers with different lengths of EO and PO segments by FT-Raman spectroscopy in the range of 5°C–50°C. Four triblock copolymers of Pluronic P103, P104, P105, and F88 along with homopolymers of PPO and PEO in aqueous solution were used in the study. The frequencies and relative intensities of C–H stretching bands in FT-Raman spectra are sensitive to the local polarity and conformation of block copolymer chains, and the variations with temperature are indicators of micellization.

Transitions corresponding to the CMT are observed in wavenumber shifts. The CMT values of various block copolymers are obtained from the first break in the wavenumber versus temperature curves. The results indicate that the values of CMT for 10% Pluronic copolymer solutions are 29.0°C, 16.5°C, 16.0°C, and 15.0°C for F88, P105, P104, and P103, respectively. Guo et al. (1999) found that the CMT values for the Pluronic copolymer solutions (at a given copolymer concentration) decrease with an increase of the number of PO segments. These results indicate that copolymers with larger hydrophobic domains form micelles at lower temperatures. Micelle formation of the block copolymer with a smaller PPO segment (such as Pluronic F88) is more difficult, but micelle formation is much easier for the Pluronics P103, P104, and P105 with larger PPO segments. These results are in reasonable agreement with the temperature-dependent micellization of aqueous copolymers investigated with other techniques (Zhou and Chu, 1988; Tontisakis et al., 1990; Almgren et al., 1991a,b; Bahadur et al., 1992a,b).

Chung et al. (1998) studied the micellar solutions of terminally modified PIPAAms, such as PIPAAm-$C_{18}H_{35}$ and PIPAAm-PST. These show nearly the same lower critical solution temperature (LCST) as that of pure PIPAAm. The LCST is the temperature above which the polymer solution phase separates (Heskins and Guillet, 1968) and is related to how the hydrophobic–hydrophilic balance of the polymer changes. In contrast, randomly modified PIPAAm [P(IPAAm-*g*-MASE)] (MASE, i.e., methacrylic acid stearyl ester) exhibited an LCST shift to a lower temperature that was proportional to the hydrophobic mole fraction, even above its CMC. These observations suggest that the supramolecular assemblies are quite different in nature. When terminally hydrophobic groups self-aggregate by hydrophobic interactions, water clusters immobilized around the hydrophobic segments are excluded from the hydrophobically aggregated inner core, and the isolated hydrophobic micellar core does not directly interfere with PIPAAm chain dynamics in aqueous media. The PIPAAm chains of the micellar outer shell remain as mobile linear chains in this core-shell micellar structure. As a result, the thermoresponsive properties of PIPAAm in the outer PIPAAm chains of this structure are unaltered (Winnik et al., 1992; Chung et al., 1998). In contrast, aggregation of the hydrophobic domains of randomly modified P(IPAAm-MASE)s entangles parts of the PIPAAm main chain in the inside of the core. Simultaneously, hydrophobic aggregates remain partially exposed to water. Moreover, PIPAAm chains surrounding hydrophobic aggregates are immobile hydrated loops without a freely mobile end (Figure 13.8). Such a structure slows down the phase transition rate of PIPAAm (Takei et al., 1994; Matsukata et al., 1996). Terminal-modification of PIPAAm appears to be an essential key for a design strategy to fabricate polymeric micelles as stable carriers maintaining thermoresponses of pure linear PIPAAm in their outer shells.

Adams and Kwon (2003) investigated the effect of substituted acyl chain length on the properties of PEO-*b*-poly(*N*-hexyl-l-aspartamide) P(6-HHA) micelles. The CMC and the core polarity of P(6-HA-acyl) micelles decreased with increasing acyl chain length (Table 13.6) while the micelle hydrodynamic diameters and relative core viscosities increased. Therefore, the packing of hydrophobic chains in long acyl cores was much tighter with less freedom of movement, substantially increasing the core viscosity. Further studies (2003) found that the modified P(6-HHA) cores were able to entrap substantially more amphotericin B, and time-course hemolysis studies indicated the more viscous cores resulted in more graduate release of the hemolytic drug into saline medium. Yokoyama et al. (1998) substantially increased the capacity of PEO-*b*-PBLA micelles for

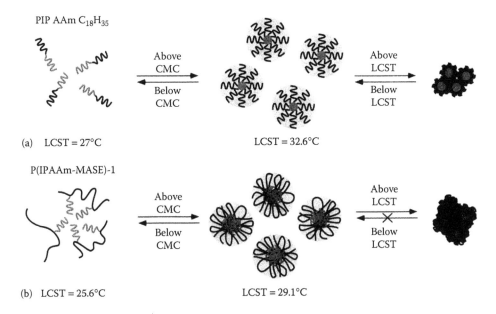

PIP AAm C$_{18}$H$_{35}$

(a) LCST = 27°C   LCST = 32.6°C

P(IPAAm-MASE)-1

(b) LCST = 25.6°C   LCST = 29.1°C

FIGURE 13.8 Schematic of micellar structure and thermoresponsive reversibility of (a) PIPAAm-C18H35 and (b) P(IPAAm-MASE). (Reprinted from *J. Control. Rel.*, 53, Chung, J.E. et al., Effect of molecular architecture of hydrophobically modified poly(*N*-isopropylacrylamide) on the formation of thermo-responsive core-shell micellar drug carriers, 119–130, Copyright 1998, with permission from Elsevier.)

TABLE 13.6
Effect of Micelle Core Structure on Core Properties and Drug Encapsulation in Micelles Derived from PEO-*b*-P(6-HHA)

Polymer	CMC (µg/mL)	Core Polarity	Core Viscosity[a]	Size (nm)	Amphotericin B-Polymer (mol:mol)
PEO-*b*-PBLA, 12:25	18.3 ± 0.5	1.55 ± 0.01	0.05 ± 0.01	46	N/A
PEO-*b*-P(6-HHA)	454.6 ± 7.2	1.76 ± 0.09	0.24 ± 0.01	80	0.08 ± 0.01
PEO-*b*-P(6-HA-2-acyl)	27.2 ± 0.9	1.72 ± 0.01	0.02 ± 0.01	39	1.94 ± 0.08
PEO-*b*-P(6-HA-6-acyl)	23.3 ± 0.6	1.41 ± 0.01	0.06 ± 0.01	47	1.43 ± 0.03
PEO-*b*-P(6-HA-12-acyl)	20.6 ± 0.8	1.35 ± 0.01	0.04 ± 0.01	56	2.25 ± 0.03
PEO-*b*-P(6-HA-18-acyl)	17.5 ± 0.4	1.33 ± 0.01	0.04 ± 0.01	68	1.96 ± 0.01

Source: Adams, M.L. and Kwon, G.S., *J. Biomater. Sci. Polym. Edn.*, 13, 991–1006, 2002; Adams, M.L. and Kwon, G.S., *J. Control. Rel.*, 81, 23–32, 2003.

[a] Relative core viscosity based on dipyrene excimer/monomer ratio; SDS micelles were 0.64 ± 0.01.

doxorubicin by substitution of doxorubicin side chains to the PBLA core, which allowed high levels of drug to be physically entrapped in the micelle. It appears the capacity and release behavior of micelle drug delivery systems may be manipulated by modification of the core properties.

Covalently cross-linking of the micelle core or shell can substantially increase the drug capacity of micelles and decrease the CMC (Shuai et al., 2004; Joralemon et al., 2005); however, it is doubtful if such cross-linked carriers would be acceptable clinically as it is unknown if resulting micelles could be renally cleared. In addition, the cross-linking agents may react nonspecifically with the encapsulated drug. An interesting approach to cross-linking investigated by Xu et al. (2004) involved

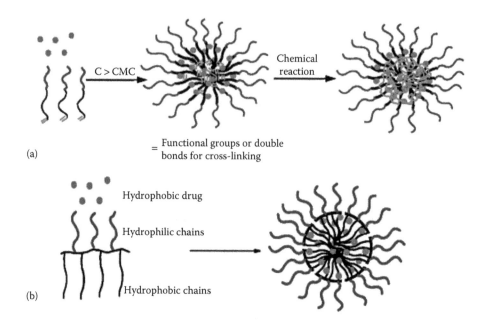

forming short series of unimers linked at the junction of the amphiphilic blocks (Figure 13.9). The unimers were sufficiently short to be excluded renally, yet the CMC of the micelles decreased 10-fold over the unlinked micelles. This approach may avoid long-term accumulation of carrier and prevent the use of cross-linking agents in the presence of drug, reducing the likelihood of cross-linking agents and side products in the final formulation.

Effects of Solubilizates and Additives on Solubilization

As with traditional surfactants, additives may influence the onset of micellization of polymeric surfactants and thus affect solubilization. These additives can include inorganic salts and sugars used to adjust isotonicity and even the solubilizate drug itself. In addition to micellization, these additives can influence the LCST or CP and even the structure of micelles formed.

Several factors affecting solubilization of aromatic solutes in triblock oxyalkylene copolymers (PEOn-*b*-PPOm-*b*-PEOn or PPOm-*b*-PEOn-*b*-PPOm) known to form micelles have been investigated (Gadelle et al., 1995). Solubilization isotherms of toluene, benzene, chlorobenzene, and p-xylene in various aqueous polymeric solutions were determined using headspace gas chromatography. The solute partition coefficient in the polymer was shown to have a strong dependence on the solute concentration for all polymers. The amount solubilized was at its highest for the high molecular weight hydrophobic polymers. For the less hydrophobic or lower molecular weight polymers, it was determined that solubilization capacity was a function of the polymer concentration. Comparisons between the different solute solubilization isotherms indicate that PPO-PEO, polymer–water, and polymer–solute interactions have a strong influence on aggregation and solubilization.

The effect of the medium composition or the loaded drug on the CMC may be difficult to predict. Zhang et al. (1996a) found that the incorporation of 10% paclitaxel into MePEO-*b*-PDLLA micelles did not cause the CMC to change significantly. Those authors also showed that the CMC of methoxy (Me) PEO-*b*-PDLLA (poly[dl-lactic acid]) micelles remained the same in water, 0.9% saline solution, and 5% dextrose solutions. This is not surprising considering the nonionic nature of the polymer.

At first glance, additives would be expected to alter the behavior of charged polymers. According to the theory of Marko and Rabin (1992), micelle formation in block polyelectrolytes is determined by a balance of the core-solvent interfacial energy and Coulombic repulsions of the charged polyelectrolyte chains. In block polyelectrolyte micelles, electrostatic effects play a major role in micelle formation and dominate at low salt concentrations. According to this theory, micelle formation will not occur for highly charged diblock polyelectrolytes because of the strong electrostatic repulsive forces along the chain. At low salt concentrations, electrostatic correlations dominate the chain configurations, and thus also the aggregation behavior (Dan and Tirrell, 1993). As the salt concentration increases from very low concentrations, the electrostatic repulsions decrease and the aggregation number increases. At moderate salt concentrations, the aggregation numbers do not vary significantly with the addition of salt and the micellar properties are dominated by the core block properties. Therefore, N, the CMC, and the chemical potential of the micelles are identical to those calculated for micelles of neutral diblock copolymers. This was observed PNIPA copolymerized with octadecylacrylate and methacrylic acid that had the same CMC in water and phosphate buffered saline (PBS) (Jones and Leroux, 1999). In another study, Khougaz et al. (1995) studied the influence of a broad range of NaCl salt concentrations on the micellar properties of a series of poly(styrene-b-sodium acrylate) (PS-b-PANa), block polyelectrolytes. At low salt concentrations, the aggregation numbers (N) were found to increase with increasing salt concentration. For instance, the N values for PS(6)-b-PANa(160) in 0.050 and 2.5 M NaCl increased from 11 to 26, respectively. Similarly, for PS(23)-b-PANa(300), the N values in 0.050 and 2.5 M NaCl increased from 90 to 150, respectively. At higher salt concentrations (>ca. 0.10 M), the aggregation numbers were found to remain essentially constant. The N values for PS(6)-b-PANa(89) and PS(6)-b-PANa(400) were essentially the same in 0.10 and 2.5 M NaCl. Similar results for the dependence of N on salt concentration have been obtained by Solb and Gallot (1980) in a mixed solvent system of water-methanol-LiBr.

The clouding behavior of nonionic block copolymeric surfactants in water is an interesting feature influencing their practical usefulness. The clouding phenomenon results from the attractive interactions between PEO chains at elevated temperature in water. In other words, water becomes a less good solvent for PEO with increasing temperature. The molecular mechanism behind this has been disputed. A reasonable explanation is found in the conformational equilibrium of the PEO chains as suggested by Karlstrom (1985).

As the CP of a nonionic surfactant is a unique characteristic that helps in deciding its function and practical utility under various conditions, Pandya et al. (1993) extensively investigated the effect of additives on the clouding behavior of Pluronic L-64 (MW = 2900, % PEO = 40) in aqueous solution.

First, they studied the effect of inorganic salts on the CP of L-64 (Figure 13.10). These salts increase or decrease the CP depending on their nature; a CP decrease is generally due to dehydration of the EO chain by the salt (salting out), whereas an increase reflects enhanced solubility of the EO chain in water (salting in). The influence of salts on the CP of L-64 is similar to what has been observed for PEO and follows the Hofmeister or lyotropic series. Anions with a low lyotropic number, high hydration, or a strong water-structure-making tendency decrease the CP. Usually, the higher the valency of the anion, the more the CP decreases. Multivalent cations, due to their interaction with the ether oxygens of PEO, show a CP increase. Similarly, the ions CNS^- and I^- show an increase in the CP due to the enhanced solubility of L-64 in water. The net effect of salt on the CP of L-64 is reflected by the combined influences of both the anion and cation.

The effect of salts on the CP may be explained in terms of the polarity of the solute and the solvent. Ions prefer a water environment, and thus they increase the polarity of the solvent, which decreases the solubility of L-64. CNS^- and I^- ions have a slight preference to associate with the L-64 molecule and increase its polarity, and thus they increase the solubility, resulting in an increase in the CP.

Apart from the effect of pure inorganic salts, Pandya et al. (1993) studied two series of electrolytes, one with increasing anion size (carboxylates: formate, acetate, propionate, butyrate, valerate,

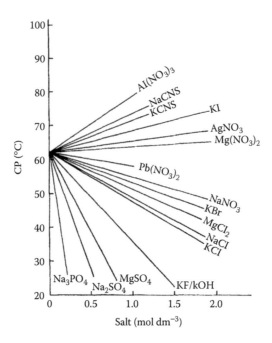

FIGURE 13.10 Cloud point of L-64 in aqueous salt solutions. (With kind permission from Taylor & Francis: *J.M.S. Pure Appl. Chem. A*, Effect of additives on the clouding behavior of an ethylene oxide-propylene oxide block copolymer in aqueous solution 30, 1993a, 1–18, Pandya, K. et al.)

caproate, caprylate) and the other with increasing cation size (tetraalkylammonium ions: methyl, ethyl, propyl, butyl, amyl) (Figures 13.11 and 13.12). Figure 13.11 shows that smaller carboxylate ions show a CP decrease, similar to that of inorganic anions with the *salting out* effect. With an increasing chain length of carboxylate ion, the effect on CP diminishes. On the other hand, larger carboxylate ions induce a remarkable increase in the CP. This CP increase can be interpreted in the same manner as the presence of a very small amount of an ionic surfactant that comicellizes with L-64 to form a mixed micelle. Valerate, caproate, and caprylate ions possess fairly long chains, and they behave like ionic surfactants. In the case of tetraalkylammonium ions, an increase in the CP was observed (which attains a constant value after a certain concentration) for all cations except tetraamylammonium ion, which at low concentration first shows an increase in the CP, then the CP rapidly decreases at higher concentrations (Figure 13.12). The increase in the CP by tetraalkylammonium ions at lower concentrations can generally be considered to be due to the more favorable interaction between water and the PEO chain. The tetraamylammonium ion at higher concentrations, owing to its longer amyl chain, increases the hydrophobicity of the solvent (water) and makes the hydrophilic PEO chain less soluble, and thus the CP decreases. Figure 13.12 also shows the effect of a cationic surfactant, trimethylammonium bromide, for comparison.

The effect of sodium dodecyl sulfate (SDS) on the CP of L-64 in water is shown in Figure 13.13. A drastic increase in the CP of nonionic surfactants in the presence of a small amount of ionic surfactant was observed, which is in agreement with previous studies on ionic + nonionic surfactant systems (Vaiaulikar and Manohar, 1985; Marshall, 1988). The incorporation of an ionic surfactant into nonionic micelles creates an electric charge on the micellar surface and thus causes repulsion between the micelles and increases the CP of L-64. Incorporation of SDS into L-64 micelles has been experimentally determined (Almgren et al., 1991a,b). The influence of the SDS on the L-64 CP can be neutralized with added salt. The CP of aqueous solutions of L-64 in NaCl in the presence of SDS is shown in Figure 13.14. As observed earlier, without salt addition, the CP increases steeply in the presence of SDS. A high SDS concentration is required to increase the CP in the presence of salt. However,

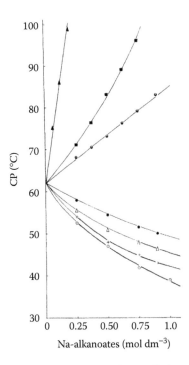

FIGURE 13.11 Cloud point of L-64 in the presence of tetraalkylammonium bromides: (•) NH₄Br, (+) (CH₃)₄NBr, (Δ) (C₂H₅)₄NBr, (half-filled ○) (C₅H₁₁)₄NBr, (filled Δ) C₁₀H₂₃N(CH₃)₃Br. (With kind permission from Taylor & Francis: *J.M.S. Pure Appl. Chem. A*, Effect of additives on the clouding behavior of an ethylene oxide-propylene oxide block copolymer in aqueous solution 30, 1993a, 1–18, Pandya, K. et al.)

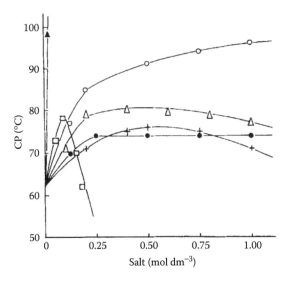

FIGURE 13.12 Cloud point of L-64 in water in the presence of sodium alkanoates: (+) Na-formate, (○) Na-acetate, (Δ) Na-propionate, (•) Na-butyrate, (half-filled ○) Navalerate, (filled Δ) Na-caproate, (filled Δ) Na-caprylate. (With kind permission from Taylor & Francis: *J.M.S. Pure Appl. Chem. A*, Effect of additives on the clouding behavior of an ethylene oxide-propylene oxide block copolymer in aqueous solution 30, 1993a, 1–18, Pandya, K. et al.)

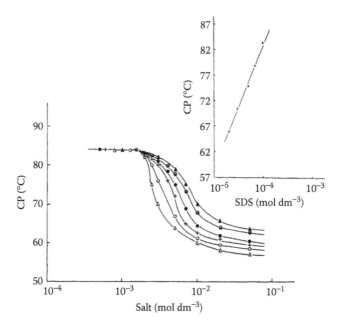

FIGURE 13.13 Cloud point of L-64 in the presence of SDS (0.1 mM) as a function of molar concentration of added salts: (filled Δ) KCNS, (half-filled ○) KI, (•) KBr, (+) KCl, (○) KF, (Δ) K$_2$SO$_4$. The inset figure shows the cloud point of L-64 in the presence of SDS. (With kind permission from Taylor & Francis: *J.M.S. Pure Appl. Chem. A*, Effect of additives on the clouding behavior of an ethylene oxide-propylene oxide block copolymer in aqueous solution 30, 1993a, 1–18, Pandya, K. et al.)

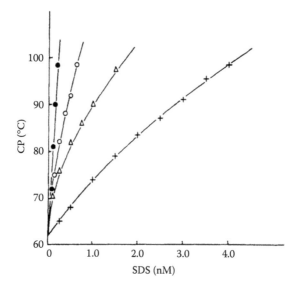

FIGURE 13.14 Cloud point of L-64 in the presence of NaCl as a function of the molar concentrations of added SDS: (•) 5 mM, (○) 10 mM, (Δ) 25 mM, (+) 50 mM. (With kind permission from Taylor & Francis: *J.M.S. Pure Appl. Chem. A*, Effect of additives on the clouding behavior of an ethylene oxide-propylene oxide block copolymer in aqueous solution 30, 1993a, 1–18, Pandya, K. et al.)

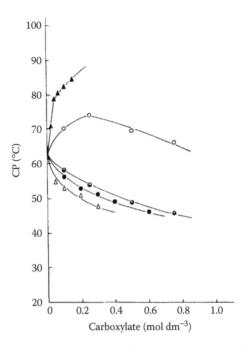

FIGURE 13.15   Cloud point of L-64 in water-containing carboxylates: (O) Na-oxalate, (half-filled O) Na-malonate, (•) Na-succinate, (Δ) Na-adipate, (filled Δ) Na-salicylate. (With kind permission from Taylor & Francis: *J.M.S. Pure Appl. Chem. A*, Effect of additives on the clouding behavior of an ethylene oxide-propylene oxide block copolymer in aqueous solution 30, 1993a, 1–18, Pandya, K. et al.)

no minimum in CP was observed, as noted earlier by Carlsson et al. (1986). Similar observations of the effects on CP of a nonionic surfactant, Triton X-100, in the presence of SDS and salt were made by Marshall (1988).

Figure 13.15 shows the effect of sodium dicarboxylates with an increasing number of methylene groups (Pandya et al., 1993). Their effect on the CP is opposite to that shown by monocarboxylates. The two-carboxylate groups at the ends of methylene chains perhaps put constraints on the incorporation of the ion into the micelle. The dicarboxylate ions thus lower the CP. A remarkably steep rise in CP was observed for sodium salicylate.

Different kinds of nonelectrolytes were also examined for their effect on the CP (Pandya et al., 1993). The effect of different amides on the CP is first considered. Amides such as urea, thiourea, acetamide, and formamide were used; each showed an increase in CP (Figure 13.16). The increasing CP effect of ureas and other amides on solutions of nonionic surfactants has been examined before (Han et al., 1989; Briganti et al., 1991). These amides decrease the water structure and thus favor hydration of PEO chain, resulting in an increase in the CP.

The effect of various hydroxy compounds on the CP of L-64 was studied in detail (Pandya et al., 1993). The effect of monohydric alcohols on the CP is shown in Figure 13.17. While lower alcohols (C_1–C_3) have a slight increasing effect on the CP, higher alcohols decrease the CP; the longer the carbon chain in the alcohol, the stronger is the CP decrease. Furthermore, this effect weakens with branching in the chain or a shift of the -OH group from the end of the chain. The effect of added alcohols on the CP can be interpreted by assuming that short-chain alcohols prefer a water environment while long-chain alcohols are effectively attracted to the L-64 molecules to an extent that depends on the chain length of the alcohol. Therefore, short-chain alcohols will decrease the polarity of the solvent, thereby increasing the solubility of L-64 and also the CP. Long-chain alcohols, on the other hand, will tend to associate with the L-64 molecules, making the polymer more hydrophobic and therefore also less water soluble.

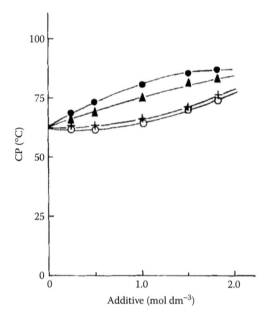

FIGURE 13.16   Cloud point of L-64 in the presence of amides: (•) Urea, (filled Δ), (+) acetamide, (O) thiaourea. (With kind permission from Taylor & Francis: *J.M.S. Pure Appl. Chem. A*, Effect of additives on the clouding behavior of an ethylene oxide-propylene oxide block copolymer in aqueous solution 30, 1993a, 1–18, Pandya, K. et al.)

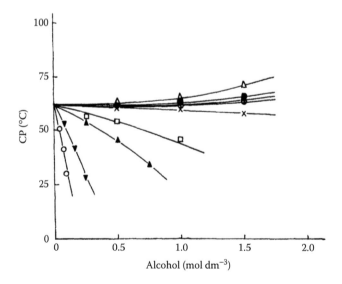

FIGURE 13.17   Cloud point of L-64 in the presence of alcohols: (half-filled O) Methanol, (•) ethanol, (+) propanol-1, (Δ) propanol-2, (X) 2 methyl propanol-2, (▲) butanol-1, (□) butanol-2, (▼) pentranol-1, (o) phenol. (With kind permission from Taylor & Francis: *J.M.S. Pure Appl. Chem. A*, Effect of additives on the clouding behavior of an ethylene oxide-propylene oxide block copolymer in aqueous solution 30, 1993a, 1–18, Pandya, K. et al.)

A very small amount of phenol decreases the CP of L-64 significantly to room temperature (Figure 13.17). A similar behavior was observed by Donbrow and Azaz (1976) for cetomacrogel in the presence of various phenols. It is thought that the sharp fall in the CP of L-64 in the presence of phenols at specific solute concentrations might be due to saturation of the micelles. The influence of phenols on the CP of L-64 may be due to a combination of hydrogen bonding, favoring retention of these molecules in the EO region of the micelles, and water structuring exercised by solubilizate molecules in this environment.

The effect of ethylene glycol (EG), its oligomers, and its polymers on the CP of L-64 is shown in Figure 13.18a. A slight increase in CP by EG and DEG (diethylene glycol) is due to preferential solvation of the surfactant molecules. Micelle formation of a nonionic surfactant in water-EG mixtures has been examined by Ray and Nemethy (1971). These authors observed an increase in CMC and have accounted for this effect as owing to partial changes in the solvent environment of the EO chain of the surfactant. Polyethylene glycols (PEGs) (polyethylene oxides), on the other hand, decrease the CP of nonionic surfactants. The effect of PEGs on the clouding behavior of polyoxyethylene nonyl phenol ethers has been studied by Marshall (1988). Depending on the chain length of the surfactant, the CP decreases or increases in the presence of PEGs. A decrease in the CP of L-64 upon the addition of PEGs (which are themselves very hydrophilic and have CP > 100°C) reveals some interaction between L-64 and PEG, although such an interaction may be very weak.

The effect of EG and its monoalkylether substitutes is shown in Figure 13.18b. A linear increase in the CP in the following order was always seen: MBEEG > MEEEG > MMEEG (butyl, ethyl, and methyl, respectively). The increase in the CP of L-64 by glycol and its ethers is mainly because of the weakening of hydrophobic interaction, although the interaction of the PEO moiety of L-64 with these additives and the self-aggregating behavior of glycol ethers, particularly for monobutyl ether, may also affect the clouding phenomena. A detailed study on the effect of glycol ethers on CMC and the CP of nonionic surfactants has been conducted by Marshall (1988). The trend in the results of Pandya et al. (1993) resembles that observed by Marshall for polyoxyethylene nonyl phenols.

Figure 13.18 shows the effect of sorbitol. A gradual decrease in the CP with an increase in sorbitol concentration was observed. Some other polyhydric alcohols (including saccharides, viz. mannitol, glucose, sucrose, fructose, etc.) induced a similar decrease. A decrease in CP with

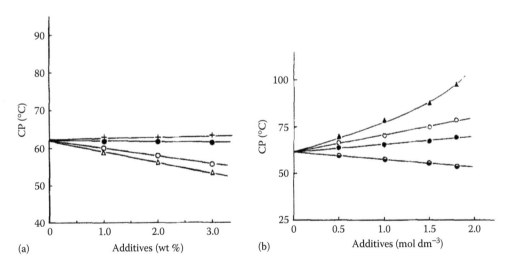

FIGURE 13.18 (a) Cloud point of L-64 in the presence of additives: (+) Ethylene glycol, (•) diethylene glycol, (○) PEG-400, (Δ) PEG-6000. (b) Cloud point of L-64 in the presence of monoalkylethers of ethylene glycol: (•) methyl, (○) ethyl, (▲) butyl, (◓) sorbitol. (With kind permission from Taylor & Francis: *J.M.S. Pure Appl. Chem. A*, Effect of additives on the clouding behavior of an ethylene oxide-propylene oxide block copolymer in aqueous solution 30, 1993a, 1–18, Pandya, K. et al.)

saccharides has been observed for polyethylene glycol (PEG) and for sorbitol on polysorbate, a nonionic surfactant (Zatz and Lue, 1987; Attwood et al., 1989). Sjoberg et al. (1989) showed that all saccharides decrease the CP of PEG, which is well described by mean field theory. Also, an explanation was given for the difference between the saccharides in their ability to decrease the CP in aqueous PEG solutions.

Comparison of Polymeric Micelles with Other Colloidal Drug Carriers

As compared with other types of carrier systems, the polymeric micelle systems possess several benefits (Yokoyama, 1992, 1994) including the wide applicability of polymeric micelle systems to drugs, through either chemical conjugation or physical entrapment; and the small size of polymeric micelles. In the case of physical entrapment, utilizing hydrophobic interactions can be applied to many kinds of drugs (Kwon et al., 1994a,b) because most drugs contain hydrophobic moiety(ies) in their chemical structures.

The size of polymeric micelles, with an approximate diameter range of 20–60 nm, is smaller than achievable by liposomes and micro(nano)spheres. The smaller carrier systems are expected to show higher vascular permeability at target sites by a diffusion mechanism. Furthermore, the diameter range of the polymeric micelle systems is considered to be appropriate to evade renal excretion and nonspecific capture by the reticuloendothelial systems (RES).

In comparing the advantages of micelle-forming lipid-polymer conjugates with liposomes used as diagnostic agent carriers, Trubetskoy and Torchilin (1995) pointed out the main feature that makes PEO-lipid micelles attractive for diagnostic imaging applications is their size. Owing to the lipid bilayer curvature limitations, it is not possible to prepare liposomes smaller than a certain minimal diameter (usually 70–100 nm) (Enoch and Strittmatter, 1979). For some diagnostic applications, the administration of diagnostic particulates of significantly smaller size is required. One such situation arises during percutaneous lymphography. It was shown that uptake of PST nanospheres in the primary lymph node after subcutaneous injection is drastically increased with decreasing particle size especially for nanospheres with a diameter below 100 nm (Davis et al., 1993).

Another benefit of polymeric surfactants over traditional surfactants is the potential for much lower CMCs. Amphiphiles with a high CMC may not be suitable as drug-targeting devices since they are unstable in an aqueous environment and easily dissociate upon dilution (Jones and Leroux, 1999). It must be noted that while some polymers exhibit very low CMCs—for instance, the CMC of poly(β-benzyl-l-aspartate) (PEO-b-PBLA), poly(N-isopropylacrylamide-polystyrene (PNIPA-PST), and poly(ε-caprolactone) (PEO-b-PCL) are between 0.00005% and 0.002% (La et al., 1996; Cammas et al., 1997; Aliabadi et al., 2005a)—other copolymers may have much higher CMCs, reaching values, for example, of up to 0.01%–10% in the case of poloxamers (Prasad et al., 1979; Torro and Chung, 1984; Kabanov et al., 1992).

In terms of solubilization ability, Gadelle et al. (1995) showed that there were distinct differences between conventional surfactant micelles and polymeric surfactant micelles. Solubilization in block copolymer micelles is a strong function of the solute concentration and may also be dependent on the polymer concentration. However, in a solubilization study of some aromatic compounds using low molecular weight surfactants such as SDS, cetyl pyridinium chloride (CPC), and polyoxyethylene dodecylphenyl ether (RC630), the partition coefficient is a weak function of the solute and surfactant concentration (Gadelle et al., 1995). The partition coefficients for the two conventional surfactants (CPC and RC630) are essentially constant for the entire range of solute concentration, and the partition coefficient of polymeric surfactants (Pluronic P184 and P103) depends strongly on the aromatic solute concentration. Another difference is that, for a given PPO unit number, solubilization in the copolymers is a strong function of the PEO content; this is somewhat different for solubilization in low molecular weight nonionic surfactants, where it was observed that increasing the EO number had only a moderate effect when the solute concentration was close to the aqueous saturation. It was assumed that the hydrophobic core of the polymeric micelles contains substantial quantities of water and, initially, solubilization is a replacement process in which water is displaced from the core by the solubilizates. In addition, the formation of the polymeric micelles is directed by polymer-polymer and water-polymer interactions (Gadelle et al., 1995). In contrast, the hydrophobic core of a conventional surfactant micelle is essentially void of water, and the aggregation process is mostly dependent on interfacial tension.

To compare the solubilization capacity of the copolymers and the conventional surfactants, a different representation of the solubilization capability can be found (Gadelle et al., 1995). It was shown that the block copolymer (P103) yields a higher solubilization capacity than the conventional surfactants (CPC and RC630) for high toluene concentrations. On the other hand, the extent of solubilization in P103 is comparable to that in CPC for lower solute concentrations. The results indicate that some polymeric surfactants could advantageously replace conventional low molecular weight surfactants in processes where solubilization is involved (Gadelle et al., 1995).

In terms of biodistribution, Zhang et al. (1997) were not able to demonstrate any difference between the biodistribution of paclitaxel loaded into MePEO-b-PDLLA micelles versus paclitaxel solubilized in Cremophor EL (a conventional surfactant). These two formulations also showed similar *in vitro* distribution between the lipoprotein and lipoprotein-deficient fraction of plasma (Ramaswamy et al., 1997). As for other drug carriers, plasma half-life and uptake of polymeric micelles by the MPS depend on the molecular weight (Kwon et al., 1994a,b) and density of the hydrophilic shell (Hagan et al., 1996).

Weissig et al. (1998a,b) compared liposomes with similar surface characteristics to polymeric micelles. Liposomes seem to have a longer circulation time than polymeric micelles, possibly because extravasation of liposomes from the vasculature is more difficult due to their larger size. The capacity of polymeric micelles to reach regions of the body that are poorly accessible to liposomes has been exemplified by Trubetskoy and Torchilin (1996). They showed that after subcutaneous injection in the dorsum of rabbit hindpaw, polymeric micelles exhibited higher accumulation in the primary lymph node than liposomes and reached the systemic circulation after massage of the lymph node. A more detailed discussion of this work can be found in the case study of micelle-forming diacyllipid-polymer conjugates in the Pharmaceutical Application section of this chapter.

Aliabadi and Lavasanifar (2006) recently compiled a comprehensive review of the solubilities and loading levels of many hydrophobic drugs in block copolymer micelle systems. The diversity of drugs that may be incorporated in block copolymers testifies to the vesitility of these systems owing to the wide structural diversity possible in the core forming block (Table 13.7).

TABLE 13.7
Drug Loading in Block Copolymer Micelles

Drug	Solubility of Free Drug	Block Copolymer	Loading (% w/w)
Cisplatin	1.2 mg/mL	PEO-b-P(glutamic acid)	31–39
		PEO-b-P(aspartic acid)	49
		PEO-b-P(lysine)-succinate	5.5
Doxorubicin	≤50 µg/mL	PEO-b-P(benzyl-l-aspartate)	10–20
		PEO-b-P(aspartic acid)-DOX	18–53
		Pluronic P-85	13
Indomethacin	35 µg/mL	PEO-b-P(benzyl-l-aspartate)	20–22
		PEO-b-P(ε-caprolactone)	42
		PEO-b-P(dl-lactic acid)	22
Paclitaxel	1 µg/mL	PEO-b-P(dl-lactic acid)	25
		PEO-b-P(ε-caprolactone)	5–21
		PEO-b-P(N-[2-hydroxypropyl] methacrylamide lactate)	22

Source: Aliabadi, H.M. and Lavasanifar, A., *Expert Opin. Drug Deliv.*, 3, 139–162, 2006.

PREPARATION OF POLYMERIC MICELLES

Aliabadi and Lavasanifar (2006) recently reviewed some pharmaceutical examples of drugs loaded into polymeric micelles as well as the corresponding drug loading procedures. Polymeric micelle formation and insoluble drugs incorporation in micelles can be achieved by chemical conjugation or by physical entrapment through dialysis and emulsification techniques (Figure 13.19), cosolvent evaporation (Figure 13.20), flash nanoprecipitation, and mechanical dispersion methods. Each of these techniques are described as follows.

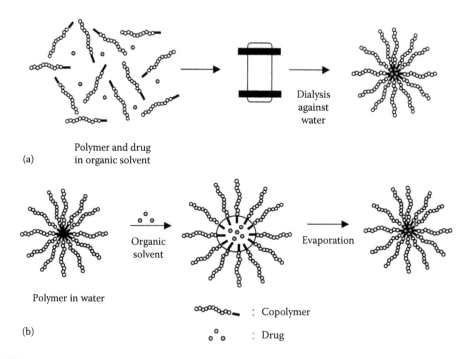

FIGURE 13.19 Drug loading of polymeric micelles by the dialysis (a) and the oil-in-water emulsion methods (b). (Reprinted from *Eur. J. Pharm. Biopharm.*, 48, Jones, M. C. and Leroux., J. C., Polymeric micelles—A new generation of colloidal drug carries, 101–111, Copyright 1999, with permission from Elsevier.)

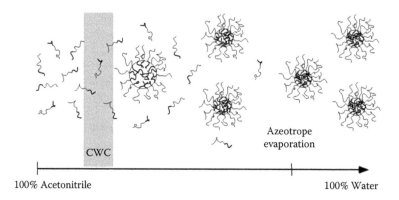

FIGURE 13.20 Drug loading by cosolvent evaporation. (With kind permission from Springer Science+Business Media: *Pharm. Res.*, Preparation and drug loading of poly(ethylene glycol)-block-poly(ε-caprolactone) micelles through the evaporation of a cosolvent azeotrope, 21, 2004, 1184–1191, Jette, K.K. et al.)

PHYSICAL ENTRAPMENT

Mechanical Dispersion Methods

In the mechanical dispersion methods, insoluble drugs and the copolymers can be dissolved in an organic solvent or a blend of solvents followed by evaporation of the solvent through a rotary evaporator for small-scale preparation, that is, thin-film method, or an explosion-proof spray dryer for larger-scale production. After drying, hydration, and micelle formation, the drug-copolymer complex can be carried out by addition of an aqueous solution with agitation. This method is most successful with block copolymers that have a relatively large hydrophilic fraction, and ultrasonification may assist formation of the micelles.

This process was used to prepare diblock copolymer micelle carriers of paclitaxel (Zhang, 1996b). In this case, the drug and the copolymer were dissolved in acetonitrile (ACN) followed by evaporation of the solvent under a stream of nitrogen at 60°C for about 2 h to obtain a solid paclitaxel/PDLLA-b-MePEG matrix. Residual ACN remaining in the taxol/copolymer matrix was determined by gas chromatographic analysis using flame ionization detection. Dissolution of the solid paclitaxel/copolymer matrix was carried out by preheating the matrix in a warm water bath (about 60°C) to obtain a transparent gel-like sample. This was followed by the addition of water at about 60°C and stirring by a vortex mixer or a glass rod to obtain a clear micellar solution.

Dialysis Method

The dialysis method consists of replacing a water-miscible solvent in which the drug and copolymer are both soluble (e.g., ethanol, N, N-dimethylformamide (DMF), ACN) with a solvent that is selective only for the hydrophilic part of the polymer (e.g., water). As the good solvent is replaced by the selective one, the hydrophobic portion of the polymer associates to form the micellar core incorporating the insoluble drug in the process. Extending the dialysis over several days helps ensure the complete removal of the organic solvent (Jones and Leroux, 1999).

The initial solvent used to prepare micelles by dialysis in water drastically affects the stability of the polymeric micelles. For example, PEO-b-PBLA micelles prepared by dialysis using DMF have a relatively large average diameter with a considerable amount of secondary aggregation (Kataoka et al., 1993). La et al. (1996) used the dialysis method to prepare PEO-b-PBLA micelles from several solvents. In their experiment, 100 mg of PEO-b-PBLA block copolymer was dissolved in 20 mL each of DMF, ACN, tetrahydrofuran (THF), dimethyl sulfoxide (DMSO), N, N-dimethylacetamide (DMAc), and ethyl alcohol, respectively, and stirred overnight at room temperature. Then, the block copolymer solution was dialyzed against distilled water using molecular porous dialysis tubing (molecular weight cutoff (MWCO) 12,000–14,000), followed by lyophilization. The yield of PEO-b-PBLA micelles from dialysis against water using the DMAc solution was 87% w/w. The average particle size, based on the number distribution of the micelles, was estimated to be ca. 19 nm. The secondary aggregates were less than 0.01% of the total amount and have a diameter of 115 nm. In addition, the PEO-b-PBLA micelles generated by using DMAc as an initial solvent had a narrow size distribution compared with other samples.

Cosolvent Evaporation Method

The cosolvent evaporation method consists of dissolving the drug and block copolymer in a volatile water-miscible organic solvent, for example, ACN, THF, acetone, or methanol. Water is added gradually pushing the self-assembly of the hydrophobic blocks into micelles (Figure 13.20). The organic cosolvent is then removed by evaporation (Jette et al., 2004; Shuai et al., 2004; Aliabadi et al., 2005b).

Jette et al. (2004) investigated the assembly of PEG-b-PCL micelles formed by addition of water to an ACN unimer solution, using DLS and ^{1}H-NMR. At the critical water content (CWC) between 10% and 30% water, depending on the PCL block size, micelle assembly was observed by DLS. Initial micelle structures were swollen having a diameter ranging from 200 to 800 nm, but when

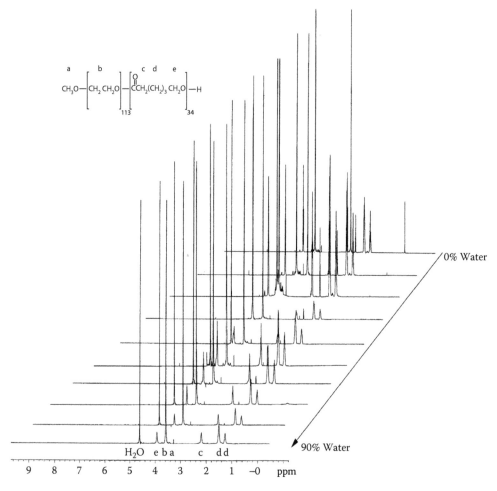

FIGURE 13.21 1H-NMR spectra of PEG-*b*-PCL (5000:4000 MW) in ACN-*d₃* with gradual addition of D₂O to 10% D₂O (v/v). (With kind permission from Springer Science+Business Media: *Pharm. Res.*, Preparation and drug loading of poly(ethylene glycol)-block-poly(ε-caprolactone) micelles through the evaporation of a cosolvent azeotrope, 21, 2004, 1184–1191, Jette, K.K. et al.)

the water fraction increased to ca. 40%, there was sharp collapse into 20–60 nm monodisperse micelles. At the CWC, the ^{1}H-NMR (D$_2$O/ACN-d_3) resonances of the PCL block groups broadened and diminished in intensity, whereas the PEG ethylene resonance was unchanged (Figure 13.21).

Flash Nanoprecipitation

The flash nanoprecipitation technique is a variation of cosolvent extraction, wherein the micelle unimers and drug are dissolved in a volatile water-miscible organic solvent and then added to an agitated aqueous nonsolvent, that is, water or buffer solution. On addition to the aqueous nonsolvent, the unimers and drug are in a supersaturated state and spontaneously nucleate into nanoaggregates on the ms time scale (ca. 10 ms). The aggregates fuse until steric hindrance of the brush, that is, the hydrated PEO block, prevents rapid uniner exchange, kinetically freezing the micelle (Johnson and Prud'homme, 2003a). Johnson and Prud'homme (2003b) have provided a detailed study on the scale-up of flash nanoprecipitation to large production levels.

Ge et al. (2002) prepared triblock copolymer micelles of PCL-*b*-PEO-*b*-PCL encapsulating nimodipine by flash nanoprecipitation. The PCL-*b*-PEO-*b*-PCL copolymer, 100 mg, and nimodipine,

10 mg, were dissolved in 20 mL of acetone, and then the organic phase was dropped into 50 mL of water under moderate stirring. The acetone was removed under reduced pressure and the aqueous suspension was concentrated to 20 mL and filtered, 15 μm, to remove aggregates and unincorporated drug. The resulting micelles were 89 to 144 nm in diameter, incorporating 3% to 5% w/w nimodipine. Forrest et al. (2006) formed PEO-*b*-PCL micelles encapsulating rapamycin using a similar technique. The resulting micelles were 46 to 76 nm in diameter and encapsulated 6% to 11% w/w rapamycin.

Oil-in-Water Emulsion Method

The oil-in-water (o/w) emulsion method consists first of preparing an aqueous solution of the copolymer. To this a solution of the drug in a water-insoluble volatile solvent (e.g., chloroform) is added to form an o/w emulsion (Jones and Leroux, 1999). The micelle-drug complex forms as the solvent evaporates. The main advantage of the dialysis procedure over this method is that potentially toxic solvents can be avoided. Both dialysis and o/w emulsion methods were compared for the incorporation of doxorubicin (DOX) in PEO-*b*-PBLA micelles (Kwon et al., 1997). The emulsification method was more efficient with a doxorubicin (DOX) loading of 12% (w/w) (Kwon et al., 1997) compared with 8% (w/w) for the dialysis technique (Kwon et al., 1995).

La et al. (1996) used the o/w emulsion method to prepare IMC-incorporated micelles. Sixty mg of PEO-PBLA without drug was dissolved in 120 mL of distilled water and homogenized by sonication for 30 s. To the solution of PEO-*b*-PBLA micelle in distilled water, a chloroform solution of IMC (6 mg in 1.8 mL) was added drop-wise under vigorous stirring at room temperature. The chloroform was removed by evaporation from the open system. The solution was then filtered, using an Amicon YM-30 ultrafiltration membrane (MWCO 50,000) to remove unbound IMC and low molecular weight contaminants, and lyophilized.

CHEMICAL CONJUGATION

Poly(ethylene glycol)-b-poly(L-amino acid) and poly(ethylene glycol)-b-polyester are most commonly used block copolymers for drug conjugation. Yokoyama et al. (1998) reported the procedures for chemical conjugation of adriamycin (ADR) into polymeric micelles that was based on a reference (Yokoyama et al., 1994) with some modifications. The copolymer used by Yokoyama et al. (1998) was poly(ethylene glycol)-b-poly(aspartic acid) block copolymer (PEG-P(Asp)). Molecular weight of the PEG chain and the (P(Asp)) chain was 12,000 and 2,100, respectively. PEG-b-P(Asp) was dissolved in DMF, and adriamycin hydrochloride (ADR·HCl) and triethylamine (TEA) (1.3 mol. equivalents to ADR) were consecutively added to the block copolymer solution. The mixture was cooled to 0°C, and the conjugation reaction initiated by addition of 1-ethyl-3-(3-dimethylaminopropyl) carbodiimide hydrochloride (EDC·HCl). Four hours after initiation of the reaction at 0°C, EDC·HCl was again added. Twenty hours after the second addition of EDC·HCl, the reaction mixture was dialyzed with a Spectrapor 2 dialysis membrane, followed by ultrafiltration using an Amicon ultrafiltration membrane PM 30 (MWCO = 30,000) in distilled water. Content of the chemically conjugated ADR in PEG-b-P(Asp-g-ADR) with respect to the aspartic acid residues was determined by measuring an amount of unreacted ADR in the reaction mixture by reversed-phase chromatography. By subtracting this amount from that of the added ADR as a substrate, an amount of the conjugated ADR was obtained.

Conjugation of drugs to PEO-*b*-poly(ester)s has usually been accomplished by functionalization of the terminal poly(ester) end which is followed by reaction with drugs. Zhang et al has attached the water-insoluble anticancer drug, paclitaxel, to the PLA section of the PEO-*b*-PLA to increase its solubility (Figure 13.22a) (Zhang et al., 2005). Toward this goal, hydroxyl-terminated diblock copolymer of monomethoxy-poly(ethylene oxide)-*b*-poly(lactide) (MPEO-*b*-PLA) was first synthesized by ring-opening polymerization of L-lactide, using MPEO as a macroinitiator. The terminal hydroxyl group of the PLA block was then converted to carboxyl group by reacting PEO-*b*-PLA with mono-t-butyl ester of diglycolic acid and subsequent deprotection of the t-butyl group with trifluoroacetic

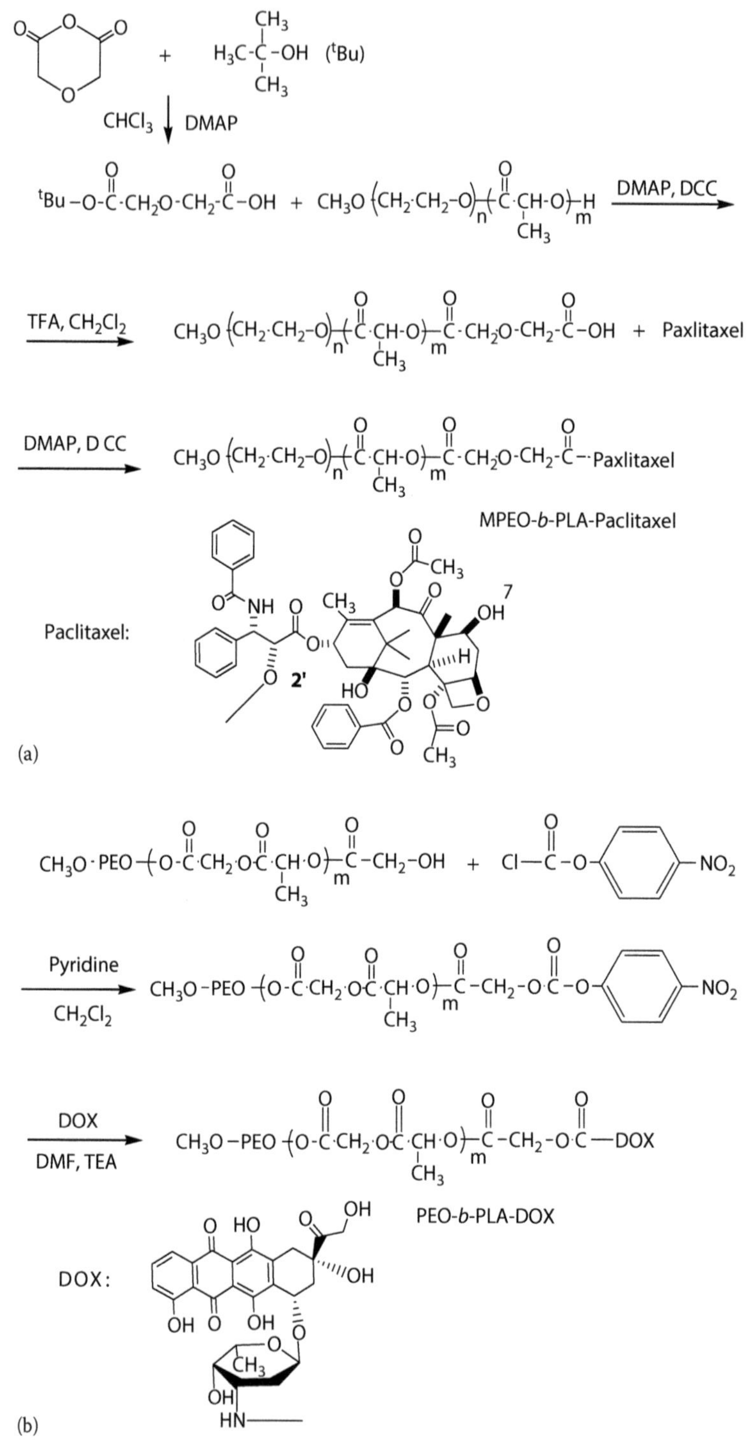

FIGURE 13.22 Synthesis of polymer-drug conjugates: (a) PEO-*b*-PLA-Paclitaxel; (b) PEO-*b*-PLA-DOX.

(Continued)

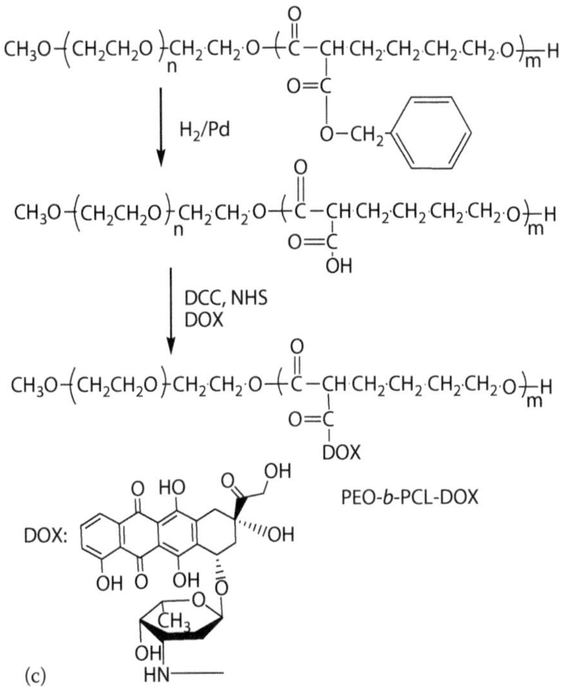

(c)

FIGURE 13.22 (Continued) Synthesis of polymer-drug conjugates: (c) PEO-*b*-PCL-DOX.

acid (TFA). Paclitaxel was then conjugated to the copolymer through formation of ester bonds between the terminal carboxylic groups of the copolymer and the hydroxyl group of paclitaxel in the presence of dicyclohexylcarbodiimide (DCC) and dimethylaminopyridine (DMAP). Because of the spatial hindrance in paclitaxel, 2'-hydroxyl is more active than the 7-hydroxyl for esterification and preferentially used for paclitaxel conjugation. Paclitaxel was released from the conjugate upon hydrolysis without loss of cytotoxicity.

Conjugation of DOX to the PEO-*b*-PLGA after activation of the PLGA terminus by *p*-nitrophenyl chloroformate has also been reported (Yoo et al., 2001) (Figure 13.22b). The micelles containing chemically conjugated DOX exhibited a more sustained release profile than PEG–*b*-PLGA micelles containing physically entrapped DOX. Interestingly, the cellular uptake of the DOX-conjugated micelles was more efficient than free DOX against HepG2 cells, leading to higher cytotoxic activity than free DOX.

By the introduction of one functional group to the end of the poly(ester) chain in each copolymer molecule, the chemical drug loading efficiency can achieve only a 1:1 molar ratio at most. In our group, DOX was conjugated to the PCL section of the PEO-*b*-PCL copolymers by the reaction between the –COOH side group on the PCL (in PEO-b-PCCL block copolymer) and amine group of DOX (Figure 13.22c). The degree of DOX conjugation reached 1.5:1 molar ratio in our preliminary study (Mahmud et al., 2008).

CHARACTERIZATION

Critical Micelle Concentration and Critical Micelle Temperature

There are many techniques available for the determination of critical micelle concentrations. Theoretically, one can use any physical property, which depends on the particle size or the number of particles. Frequently, discontinuities or sudden changes at or near the CMC, in which plots of such properties as the surface tension, electrical conductivity, osmotic pressure, interfacial tension, or light scattering as a function of concentration, have been used for this purpose (Kakamura et al., 1976; Astafieva et al., 1993; Lieberman et al., 1996). However, for polymeric micelles, the CMC is generally too low to be determined by such methods. Light scattering is widely used for the determination of the molecular weight, size, shape, and aggregation number of micelles. However, the onset of micellization can be detected only if the CMC falls within the sensitivity of the scattering method that is rarely the case for polymers in water (Astafieva et al., 1993; Jones and Leroux, 1999). GPC under aqueous conditions can be employed since single chains and micellar chain fractions of copolymers exhibit different elution volumes (Weissig et al., 1998a,b).

CMC can also be determined from the change in the spectral characteristics of some dye probes added to the surfactant solution. A preferred method to determine the CMC involves the use of fluorescent probes (Turro and Chung, 1984; Wilhelm et al., 1991; Astafieva et al., 1993), among which pyrene is the most widely used. Pyrene is a condensed aromatic hydrocarbon that is highly hydrophobic and sensitive to the polarity of the surrounding environment (Kalyanasundaram and Thomas, 1977). Below the CMC, pyrene is solubilized in water, a medium of high polarity. When micelles are formed, pyrene partitions preferentially toward the hydrophobic domain afforded by the micellar core and thus, experiences a nonpolar environment (Kalyanasundaram and Thomas, 1977). Consequently, numerous changes such as an increase in the fluorescence intensity, a change in the vibrational fine structure of the emission spectra and a red shift of the (0,0) band in the excitation spectra, are observed. The apparent CMC can be obtained from a plot of the fluorescence of pyrene, the I1/I3 ratio from the emission spectra or the I333/I338 ratio from the excitation spectra, against concentration. A major change in the slope indicates the onset of micellization (Kalyanasundaram and Thomas, 1977) (Figure 13.23). The I1/I3 ratio is the intensity ratio between the first and third highest energy emission peaks and is measured at a constant excitation wavelength and variable emission wavelengths corresponding to I1 and I3. Some claim that I1/I3 ratio should be reserved for evaluation of polarity since it is affected by the wavelength of excitation and may result in an erroneous CMC (Astafieva et al., 1993). Thus, CMC may be better ascertained by the I333/I338 ratio (Astafieva et al., 1993; Shin et al., 1998). The CMC determined with fluorescence techniques

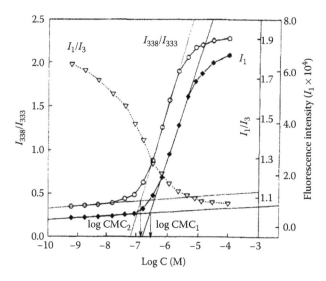

FIGURE 13.23 Plots of the fluorescence intensity I_1 and intensity ratios I_1/I_3 (from pyrene emission spectra) and I_{333}/I_{338} as a function of PST-b-poly(sodium acrylate) concentration. Values of CMC_{app} are indicated by arrows. (Reprinted with permission from Astafieva, I. et al., *Macromolecules*, 26, 7339–7352, 1993. Copyright 1993 American Chemical Society.)

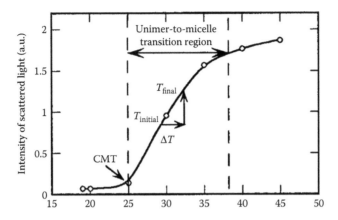

FIGURE 13.24 Scattered light intensity as a function of temperature showing the unimer-to-micelle transition region and a typical temperature jump experiment. (Reprinted with permission from Goldmints, I. et al., *Langmuir*, 13, 6130–6134, 1997. Copyright 1997 American Chemical Society.)

needs to be carefully interpreted for two reasons. First, the concentration of pyrene should be kept extremely low (10^{-7} M) so that a change in slope can be precisely detected as micellization occurs. Second, a gradual change in the fluorescence spectrum can sometimes be attributed to the presence of hydrophobic impurities or association of the probe with individual polymer chains or premicellar aggregates (Chen et al., 1995). Changes in anisotropy of fluorescent probes have also been associated with the onset of micellization (Zhang et al., 1996a, b).

Similar to the measurement of CMC, CMT can be determined using light scattering indicated by a temperature/intensity jump. Temperature jump experiments can be carried out using the iodine laser temperature jump apparatus described by Holzwarth et al. (1977) and Goldmints et al. (1997). Besides CMT, relaxation times of the polymeric solutions can also be obtained from temperature jump measurements. Experiments are conducted in the unimer-to-micelle transition region as shown in Figure 13.24, which shows the intensity of scattered light for an equilibrated system as a function of temperature. Following rapid heating, the solution will relax to a new equilibrium state at T_{final} for which the final value of scattered light intensity is higher than that in the initial equilibrium state at $T_{initial}$.

Aggregation Number and Micelle Molecular Mass

The aggregation number of the polymeric micelles is a parameter of great interest. The aggregation number can be obtained by static light scattering or fluorescence quenching measurements. Although the light scattering of block copolymers is generally quite complex, the optical similarity between PEO and PPO allows a straightforward evaluation of the average molecular weight, and hence of the aggregation number. Fluorescence quenching, on the other hand, relies on the determination of the number of micelles, which, in conjunction with the total amount of material, gives the aggregation number (Linse and Malmsten, 1992).

It is also possible to determine simultaneously by GPC the micelle molecular weight and aggregation number. It is important to ensure that the integrity of polymeric micelles during their elution through the size exclusion column is maintained. Adsorption of the polymer on the column may prove to be a problem (Yokoyama et al., 1993), especially at concentrations close to the CMC, where micelles consist of large loose aggregates (Jones and Leroux, 1999).

Ultracentrifugation techniques (Kabanov et al., 1995) may also provide the molecular mass (M) of the polymeric micelles through the Svedberg equation:

$$M = \frac{s^{\circ}RT}{D^{\circ}(1-v\rho)} \tag{13.4}$$

where $s°$ and $D°$ are the sedimentation and translational diffusion coefficients at infinite dilutions, ν is the partial specific volume of the micelle, T is the temperature, R is the universal gas constant, and ρ is the solvent density.

In order to obtain $s°$ and $D°$ experimentally, both sedimentation coefficients and translational diffusion coefficients of the micellar solutions need to be measured. Sedimentation coefficients of the micellar solutions can be measured either by scanning using an analytical ultracentrifuge such as Beckman E equipped with a photoelectrical scanning device with monocromator and multiplexor or using a schliren mode available on the same equipment with a schliren-optic registration system. The (z-average) translational diffusion coefficients can be determined by quasielastic light-scattering method using an Autosizer 2c (Malvern) small-angle laser photometer. The $s°$ and $D°$ values are then determined using the extrapolation of the sedimentation and translational diffusion coefficients to infinite dilutions. The ν value can be determined using a pycnometer. Dynamic light-scattering measurements for estimation of unimer diffusion coefficients can be made using the Brookhaven Model BI-200SM laser light-scattering system (Brookhaven Instrument Corporation) at a scattering angle of 90° (Goldmints et al., 1997).

Micelle Size and Size Distribution

Small size (10–100 nm) is one of the most interesting features of polymeric micelles. Besides allowing the extravasation of the carriers, it permits the sterilization of the preparation to be done simply by filtration and minimizes the risks of embolism in capillaries, contrary to larger drug carriers (Kwon and Okano, 1996). Micellar size seldom exceeds 100 nm, but depends on several factors, including copolymer molecular weight, relative proportion of hydrophilic and hydrophobic chains, and aggregation number (Yokoyama et al., 1990; Trubetskoy and Torchilin, 1996; Shin et al., 1998).

Micellar diameter and size polydispersity can be obtained directly in water or in an isotonic buffer by DLS. DLS can also provide some information on the sphericity of polymeric micelles (Kataoka et al., 1996; Nagasaki et al., 1998). Ultracentrifugation velocity studies are sometimes performed to assess the polydispersity of polymeric micelles (Yokoyama et al., 1994; Hagan et al., 1996).

Microscopic methods such as atomic force microscopy (AFM) (Cammas et al., 1997; Kohori et al., 1998), transmission electron microscopy (TEM) (Yu et al., 1998), and scanning electron microscopy (SEM) (Kim et al., 1998) have been applied. These methods allow the characterization of the micelle shape and size dispersity. Conventional SEM is widely used in the field of colloidal carriers since it has high resolution and the sample preparation is relatively easy. However, it is analyzed, the samples must withstand high vacuum. Furthermore, the visualization of the particles requires them to be conductive, which is achieved by coating their surface with gold. The thickness of the coating, which can reach several nanometers, has to be taken into account in the size determination. New imaging tools such as AFM enable the visualization of polymeric micelles at atmospheric pressure without gold coating (Allemann et al., 1998). By AFM, Cammas et al. (1997) showed that micelles of poly(N-isopropylamide)-block-polystyrene (PNIPA-b-PST) had a discus shape with a 5 nm height and a 20 nm diameter, which was close to the 24 nm size measured by DLS.

Size measurements can be done to study the interaction of polymeric micelles with biological media (Jones and Leroux, 1999). For instance, PEO-b-PPO-b-PEO micelles were found to maintain their initial size in the presence of antibodies and bovine serum albumin, suggesting the apparent absence of interaction with plasma proteins (Kabanov et al., 1992).

Lower Critical Solution Temperature and Cloud Point

As is being discussed, polymers used to prepare micelles exhibit a LCST that can be defined as the temperature at which the polymer phase separates (Heskins and Guillet, 1968). Below the LCST, the polymer/micelle is soluble, but it precipitates at temperatures above the LCST. The diameter of these micelles rapidly rises at temperatures above the LCST, due to hydrophobic interactions that result in the aggregation of the micelles (Kohori et al., 1998). This effect of temperature on size was shown to be reversible, since the micellar architecture was maintained after lowering the temperature below the LCST (Chung et al., 1999).

Copolymers such as poly(N-isopropylacrylamide) (PIPAAm) in aqueous solution are well known to exhibit a thermoresponsive phase transition (32°C for PIPAAm) (Heskins and Guillet, 1968). The copolymers, water soluble and hydrophilic, usually show an extended chain conformation below their LCSTs, undergoing a phase transition to an insoluble and hydrophobic aggregate above the LCSTs. This phase transition for PIPAAm remarkably occurs with narrow temperature changes through the LCST and is reversible corresponding to temperature changes (Chung et al., 1999).

CPs of copolymers can be determined using the optical transmittance method (Chung et al., 1999), and even using a visual observation method (Pandya et al., 1993). Optical transmittance of aqueous polymer solutions at various temperatures can be measured using a UV/visible spectrometer. Sample and reference cells are thermostated with a circular water jacket, and the sample is monitored for the onset of turbidity. For the visual observation method, copolymer solutions at different concentrations are measured by heating them in glass tubes immersed in a well-stirred heating bath. The temperature of first appearance of turbidity is taken as the CP. For both methods, the samples must be well stirred.

Core Viscosity

The viscosity of the micellar core may influence the physical stability of the micelles as well as drug release (Jones and Leroux, 1999). The intrinsic viscosity of the hydrophobic core, or microviscosity, can be determined by using fluorescent probes such as bis(1-pyrenyl-methyl) ether (dipyme) (Winnik et al., 1992), 1,2-(1,1°-dipyrenyl)propane (Kwon et al., 1993a,b), or 1,6-diphenyl-1,3,5-hexatriene (DPH) (Ringsdorf, 1991). Dipyme is sensitive to both polarity and viscosity changes in its local environment. The extent of intramolecular excimer emission depends upon the rate of conformational change of the chain linking the two pyrenyl groups. The local friction in the environment causes resistance to motion (Winnik et al., 1992). As a consequence, the excimer to monomer intensity ratio (*IE/IM*) provides information on the microviscosity of the dipyme local environment. A small ratio correlates with a low mobility and a solid-like core. Winnik et al. (1992) showed with dipyme that the microviscosity of the inner core of poly(N-isopropylacrylamide) (PNIPA) micelles was dependent on the position of the hydrophobic moiety (random versus end-grafted chain).

Internal viscosity can also be obtained from the depolarization of DPH (Ringsdorf, 1991; Zhang et al., 1996b). Anisotropy values are directly related to the rotational freedom of DPH: the higher the local viscosity of the associated DPH region, the higher the anisotropy values will be (Ringsdorf, 1991).

Chung et al. (1999) used 1,3-bis(1-pyrenyl) propane (PC$_3$P) as a sensitive probe for local viscosity measurements (Almeida et al., 1982; Zachariasse et al., 1982) by forming an intramolecular excimer. In the emission spectra for PC$_3$P in PIPAAm and PIPAAm-b-PBMA solutions above their CMC as a function of temperature, PIPAAm solutions showed a continuous reduction in *IE/IM* as the temperature increased below the LCST, since hydrophobic polymer-rich phases solubilizing PC$_3$P probes were getting rigid as the polymer chain dehydrated. However, the value of *IE/IM* discontinuously decreased by a temperature increase through the LCST, implying the phase transition of PIPAAm chains. Above the LCST, it remains essentially unaffected by further temperature increase. It implied that the motion of PC$_3$P is suppressed by the microviscosity created by hydrophobic contracted polymer chain aggregation. On the other hand, the ratios (*IE/IM*) of PC$_3$P dissolved in PIPAAm-b-PBMA micelle solutions were markedly lower than those of PIPAAm solutions over the entire temperature region, owing to highly compact cores of aggregated PBMA chains.

[1]H-nuclear magnetic resonance (NMR) also provides some information on the viscosity of the micellar core (Jones and Leroux, 1999). The copolymers are usually dissolved in D2O and in a solvent where micelle formation is not expected and where all the peaks proper to the hydrophilic and hydrophobic part of the polymer can be detected (e.g., CDC$_{13}$). In D$_2$O, the presence of micelles

with a highly inner viscous state result in a restricted motion of the protons within the micellar core, as demonstrated by the weak signals associated with the hydrophobic part of the copolymer (Nakamura et al., 1977; Bahadur et al., 1988).

Solution Viscosity

Intrinsic viscosity serves as a measure of the hydrodynamic volume of a single particle in the solution under study. Viscosity of micellar solutions can be measured using an Ubbelohde viscometer at a given temperature (Astafieva et al., 1993; Pandya et al., 1993; Zhou and Chu, 1994). The temperature of the thermostatted bath is usually controlled within 0.02°C to obtain an accurate measurement. After a desired temperature is set, each solution should be temperature-equilibrated for at least 20 min before viscosity measurement. An average flow time is taken for several consecutive measurements on the same copolymer solution to calculate the viscosity value.

Pandya et al. (1993) determined the viscosity of L-64 solutions in the presence of electrolytes at different temperatures. The reduced viscosities of L-64 solutions at different concentrations in water and sodium acetate (0.1–0.65 M) showed linear plots from which extrapolation yielded the intrinsic viscosity.

Stability of Polymeric Micelles and Drug Release

The rate of dissociation of the polymeric micelles into single chains and their interaction with plasma components is as important as the CMC and the micellar size in drug delivery. Once injected, polymeric micelles should maintain their integrity for a sufficient period of time to deliver the drug to its site of action (Jones and Leroux, 1999). High *in vitro* stability of DOX-loaded polymeric micelles was correlated with efficient *in vivo* antitumor activity against murine colon adenocarcinoma 26 (Yokoyama et al., 1994). Conversely, unstable conjugates were not effectively delivered to the tumor.

Physical stability is often assessed by GPC. Yokoyama et al. (1993) showed that PEO-*b*-P(Asp/DOX) micelles had a very slow rate of dissociation in water and PBS. Dissociation was accelerated in a 1:1 mixture of serum rabbit and PBS but was still below 30% after 6 h. In this case, the stability could be modulated by varying the amount of DOX and the length of the P(Asp) and PEO chains. Polymers containing long hydrophobic chains of P(Asp/DOX) were less stable, while longer hydrophilic chains of PEO yielded higher *in vitro* stability (Yokoyama et al., 1993, 1994). Lipid moieties can impart good stability to polymeric micelles, since the presence of two fatty acid acyls increases the hydrophobic interactions between polymeric chains in the micelle core. Indeed, no dissociation into individual polymeric chain was observed upon the chromatography of serial dilutions of diacyllipid-PEO conjugates (Trubetskoy and Torchilin, 1995).

Chung et al. (1999) studied the micellar stability of the thermoresponsive polymeric micelles. The hydrophobic microenvironment of PIPAAm-*b*-PBMA micelle aqueous solutions was characterized by fluorescence spectroscopy using pyrene and 1,3-bis(1-pyrenyl) propane (PC_3P) as fluorescent probes. The fluorescence spectrum of pyrene at the low concentration possesses a vibrational band structure, which exhibits a strong sensitivity to polarity of the pyrene environment (Dong and Winnik, 1984). The ratio (I_1/I_3) of intensity of the first band (I_1) to that of the third band (I_3) was monitored as a function of each PIPAAm-PBMA micelle concentration (Kalyanasundaram and Thomas, 1977). The ratio (I_1/I_3) of intensity or micropolarity ratio was plotted against polymer concentration to study the relationship of polymer concentration and micellar micropolarity. As concentrations of PIPAAm-*b*-PBMA increased, a large decrease in I_1/I_3 was observed. This indicates partitioning of the hydrophobic probe into a hydrophobic environment. From these plots, it is possible to estimate a concentration corresponding to the onset of hydrophobic aggregation of PBMA segments. The value determined from the midpoints of the plots for I_1/I_3 changes was a low concentration of 20 mg/L, providing evidence for an apparent stability of the polymeric micelles and allowed their use in very dilute aqueous milieu such as body fluids.

La et al. (1996) studied *in vitro* release pattern of indomethacin (IMC) from IMC/ poly(ethylene oxide)-poly(β-benzyl l-aspartate) (PEO-PBLA) micelles. Five milligrams of IMC/PEO-*b*-PBLA micelles was put in 5 mL of various test solutions and introduced into Spectra/por 4 dialysis membrane (MWCO 12,000–14,000) bags. The bags were placed in 900 mL of the release media, and the media was stirred at 100 rpm at 37°C. At predetermined time, intervals up to 6 h, 1 mL samples of the solution were withdrawn from the release media and replaced with an equal volume of the fresh solution. The samples were assayed by using a UV derivative method (Nabeshima et al., 1987). La et al. found IMC to release slowly in acid medium, 0.58 μg/L/h at pH 1.2, and to increase with alkalinity to 11.29 μg/L/h at pH 6.8. The carboxylic acid of IMC ionized partially at more alkaline conditions, causing IMC to partition near the hydrophobic-hydrophilic interface of the micelles core-shell; hence, pH affected the micelle-water partition coefficient.

Soo et al. (2002) studied the *in vitro* release of hydrophobic fluorescent probes from PEO-*b*-PCL micelles. Micelle solutions were placed in dialysis bags (MWCO 50,000) in a stirred water bath with a constant overflow of distilled water. This maintained the release environment at near perfect sink conditions, so the limited solubility of the probes in the medium did not affect release kinetics. Release was determined by removing aliquots of the dialysis bag contents and measuring fluorescently. Soo et al. found an initial burst release of probe followed by slow diffusional release. For the probes studies, benzo-[*a*]-pyrene and Cell-Tracker-CM-Dil, diffusion constants were of the order 10^{-15} cm^2/s.

Chung et al. (1999) measured ADR release from thermo-responsive micelles at various temperatures through the micelle LCST using LTV absorbance at 485 nm in a time-course. The results of the ADR release from the thermo-responsive micelles can be referred to the discussion of thermo-responsive polymeric micelles by Chung et al. (1999) in the section titled Pharmaceutical Applications.

Savić et al. (2006) report a method to evaluate micelle integrity both *in vitro* and *in vivo*. PEO-*b*-PCL micelles were synthesized with a fluorogenic dye, fluorescein-5-carbonyl azide diacetate, covalently attached to the PCL block. In the hydrophobic core of intact micelles, the dye remained essentially nonfluorescent, but on exposure to the aqueous mileu, the probe was hydrolyzed to a highly fluorescent derivative. Using whole-body fluorescent imaging, Savić et al. quantified micelle integrity in live mice after subcutaneous and intramuscular injections. The results are discussed in the Biopharmaceuts Aspects section.

Entrapment Efficiency

The drug entrapment efficiency in polymeric micelles can be measured simply by HPLC or spectrophotometric methods by dissolving the lyophilized micelle powder without free drug in a solvent suitable for both the drug and the copolymer. La et al. (1996) used the spectophotometric method to measure the entrapment efficiency of PEO-*b*-PBLA micelles for IMC. The amount of drug entrapped was determined by measuring the absorbance at 319 nm after the disruption of the micelle by addition of DMAc. For this analysis, a calibration curve of standard solutions containing 0–100 g/mL of IMC by UV absorbance at 319 nm was obtained. Using a calibration curve of IMC, the amount of IMC entrapped in the PBLA portion of the micelles was determined.

Kwon et al. (1997) applied reversed-phase HPLC to determine DOX loading in PEO-*b*-PBLA micelles. Samples of 20 mL diluted to 10 μg/mL DOX with 0.10 M sodium phosphate buffer, pH 7.4, were separated at 40°C at a flow rate of 1.0 mL/min. The mobile phase was a linear gradient mixture of an aqueous solution of 1% acetic acid and ACN (15% v/v to 85% v/v). Detection of DOX was done by measuring its UV absorbance at 485 nm.

Evidence of drug incorporation can also be obtained by GPC or DLS, since both methods can detect a change in micellar size that usually increases in the presence of drugs (Kwon et al., 1997; Yu et al., 1998). The location of a drug inside the micelle core is sometimes demonstrated by quenching experiments (Kwon et al., 1995, 1997). For instance, iodide (I$^-$) that is a water-soluble quencher of DOX, does not affect the fluorescence of the micelle-incorporated drug, but quenches the fluorescence of the free drug. Such experiments showed that DOX was retained in PEO-*b*-PBLA after freeze-drying and reconstitution in water (Kwon et al., 1997). In the case of DOX, the self-association of the drug in the micelle core also results in a decrease in the fluorescence intensity of the drug (Kwon et al., 1995).

Recently, the retention and slow release of amphotericin B from polymeric micelles was indirectly ascertained by measuring the decrease of its hemolytic activity after incorporation into PEO-*b*-PBLA micelles (Yu et al., 1998).

BIOPHARMACEUTIC ASPECTS

Polymeric micelles serve mainly for the transport of water insoluble drugs and can increase drug efficiency by targeting specific cells or organs, therefore lowering accumulation of the drug in healthy tissues, and minimizing its toxicity, sometimes allowing higher doses to be administered. Theoretically, following intravenous administration, polymeric micelles should have a prolonged systemic circulation time due to their small size and hydrophilic shell, which minimize uptake by the MPS, and their high molecular weight prevents renal excretion (Jones and Leroux, 1999) (Figure 13.25). Indeed, intact polymeric micelles have been recovered from plasma several hours after intravenous injection (Rolland et al., 1992; Kwon et al., 1994a,b).

Polymeric micelle-incorporated drugs may accumulate to a greater extent than free drug into tumors and show a reduced distribution in nontargeted areas such as the heart (Kwon et al., 1994a,b). Accumulation of polymeric micelles in malignant or inflamed tissues may be due to an increased vascular permeability and impaired lymphatic drainage enhanced permeability and retention (EPR) effect (Maeda et al., 1992; Jain, 1997). Tumor vessels are leakier and less permselective than normal vessels (Figure 13.25). Large pores exist and may account for the perivascular accumulation of macromolecules and colloidal drug carriers (Yuan et al., 1994, 1995). However, differences in the biodistribution pattern cannot be always evidenced. Therefore, understanding of biopharmaceutics, pharmacokinetics, and toxicity of a specific pharmaceutical application of polymeric micelles will certainly help the drug development process.

To study the absorption characteristic of copolymers, Batrakova et al. (1998) investigated the effects of Pluronic copolymers on the transport of a P-gp-dependent probe, rhodamine 123 (R123) and a P-gp-independent probe rhodamine 110 (R110) in Caco-2 cell monolayers. The solutions of the Pluronic P-85 and L-81 were prepared at concentrations below the CMC to study the effect of the unimers and above the CMC to investigate the effects of the polymeric micelles. At concentrations below the CMC Pluronic block copolymers enhanced accumulation and inhibited efflux of R123 in Caco-2 monolayers. The block copolymer unimers did not alter the transport of the P-gp-independent probe, R110 under these conditions. This suggests that the unimers are blocking P-gp efflux system rather than altering the membrane permeability in a nonspecific way. Furthermore, inhibition of R123 efflux with P-85 unimers supports their effects on P-gp efflux pump in Caco-2

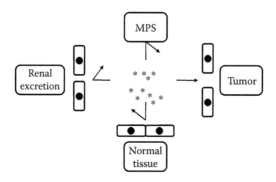

FIGURE 13.25   Accumulation of polymeric micelles in tumors. (Reproduced from Kataoka, K., *J. Macromol. Sci.—Pure Appl. Chem. A*, 31, 1759–1769, 1994. With permission.)

monolayers. Batrakova et al. (1998) also compared the effects of Pluronics on R123 accumulation in Caco-2 monolayers with the effects of Cremophor EL and Tween 60. The results suggest that the most effective Pluronic P-85 and L-81 induce significantly higher levels of cellular R123 than these detergents. Therefore, Pluronic copolymers can be useful in increasing oral absorption of P-gp substrates (Batrakova et al., 1998).

The effects of the Pluronics on R123 transport in Caco-2 monolayers vary, depending on the segment length of the polymers. The activity of unimers increases with elevation of hydrophobic copolymers. Longer PO segments or shorter EO segments, that is, more hydrophobic copolymers, cause higher R123 accumulations at lower concentrations, that is, are more *potent* P-gp inhibitors. However, copolymers with intermediate hydrophobicity cause higher R123 accumulations and are more efficient at intermediate concentrations.

At concentrations above the CMC, the effects of the micelles on R123 accumulation in cells were very different from those of the P-85 unimers (Batrakova et al., 1998). In the case of the micelles there was an initial rapid increase in R123 accumulation during the first 15 min, with cellular R123 leveling off at incubation times more than 15 min. Conversely, the free R123 or R123 and P-85 unimer mixtures revealed steady increase in R123 levels during the entire incubation period. Furthermore, in contrast to P-85 unimers, the P-85 micelles increased the efflux of R123 in Caco-2 monolayers, rather than inhibited it.

At physiological conditions, P-85 micelles represent aggregates of ca. 15 nm (Kabanov et al., 1995). The hydrophilic shell of these micelles is made of EO chain segments and their core consists of tightly packed hydrophobic PO chain segments. Above the CMC, the hydrophobic and amphiphilic probes such as R123 incorporate into the micelle core, thus becoming masked from the external medium. The fraction of the micellar R123 increases and the fraction of the free R123 decreases with elevating the micelle concentration. At 11 mM P85 (5% w/v), about 95% of R123 is incorporated into the P-85 micelles and only 5% of the probe is still in the free form (Miller et al., 1997). Under these conditions, interactions of the micellar form of R123 with cells become very significant. Indeed, the effects of the P-85 micelles have been previously shown to involve vesicular transport of the micelle-incorporated probe, which is different from the free probe entering the cell through transmembrane diffusion (Miller et al., 1997). Miller et al. (1997) studied the interactions of Pluronic block copolymers with brain microvessel endothelial cells. The effects of the Pluronics on the absorptions were similar to those in the Caco-2 cells.

To evaluate polymeric micelles as a drug carrier, Zhang et al. (1997) used poly(dl-lactide)-*b*-methoxy polyethylene glycol (PDLLA-*b*-MePEG) micellar paclitaxel to investigate the cytotoxicity, antitumor activity, and biodistribution of the drug. Hs578T breast, SKMES nonsmall cell lung, and HT-29 colon human tumor cells were exposed for 1 h or continuously, either to conventionally formulated paclitaxel (Cremophor paclitaxel, Cremophor is a low molecular weight surfactant) or polymeric micellar paclitaxel. In the *in vivo* antitumor study, B6D2F1 mice, bearing P388 leukemia tumor intraperitoneally (i.p.), were treated with polymeric micellar paclitaxel or Cremophor paclitaxel by i.p. injection. In the biodistribution study, CD-1 mice were given micellar paclitaxel i.p. at a dose of 100 mg/kg. The copolymer concentrations in the *in vitro* cytotoxicity studies were all less than 30 μM, which is below the CMC (Zhang et al., 1996b). Since the single copolymer chain can form a core-shell structure itself (Evans and Wennerstrom, 1994), the paclitaxel might be considered to be associated with the polymer molecule. The polymeric micellar paclitaxel showed similar *in vitro* cytotoxicity to Cremophor paclitaxel against the tumor cell lines, which indicate that paclitaxel is readily available to the cells under these conditions or that the polymer molecule-*bound* paclitaxel is itself cytotoxic. The polymeric micellar formulation of paclitaxel produced a fivefold increase in the maximum tolerated dose (MTD) as compared with Cremophor paclitaxel. The higher MTD with polymeric micellar paclitaxel is probably attributable to the following circumstances. First, the dissociation rate of paclitaxel from the polymeric micelles is probably slower than the Cremophor micelles. Second, the PDLLA-*b*-MePEG copolymers may not possess the toxicity associated with the Cremophor/ethanol vehicle and the amount of vehicle used in the polymer formulation is about 18 times lower than that required for the Cremophor formulation (Zhang et al., 1997a,b). In the *in vivo* experiment, polymeric micellar paclitaxel produced greater efficacy in terms of extending the survival time of tumor-bearing mice and produced animals that were long-term survivors (20%), compared with Cremophor/ethanol, when both were administered i.p. at their MTDs. Paclitaxel peak concentrations in blood, liver, kidney, heart, lung, and spleen represented 11%, 9%, 6%, 4%, 2%, and 2% of the dose/g tissue, respectively. The AUC_{0-12} h value in blood was 968 μg h/mL. In one study (Zhang et al., 1997a,b), the bioavailability of i.p. injected Cremophor paclitaxel in CD2F1 mice was found to be approximately 10% and $AUC_{0-\infty}$ value in the plasma was about 6 μg h/mL (dose 22.5 mg/kg). In another study (Innocenti et al., 1995), AUC_{1-30} h in plasma was found to be 113.2 μg h/mL (dose 18 mg/kg) or 141.9 μg h/mL (dose 36 mg/kg) after i.p. injection of Cremophor paclitaxel into Swiss female mice.

Kwon and Kataoka (1995) summarized earlier studies of the pharmacokinetics and disposition poly(ethylene oxide-*b*-aspartate)-doxorubicin conjugates (PEO-*b*-PAsp-DOX) (Yokoyama et al., 1991) and poly(ethylene oxide-*b*-isoprene-*b*-ethylene oxide) (PEO-*b*-PI-*b*-PEO) micelles (Rolland et al., 1992). The pharmacokinetics and disposition of PEO-*b*-PAsp-DOX conjugates were studied in female, ddy mice (6 weeks old) after intravenous injection following radioiodination of the conjugate through the aglycone moiety (Yokoyama et al., 1991). The PEO-*b*-PAsp-DOX conjugate circulated for prolonged periods ($t_{1/2} \approx 70$ min) in the mice relative to free DOX and did so in the form of micelles as evidenced by size exclusion chromatography (SEC) analysis of blood samples taken at 1 h. For PEO-*b*-PAsp-DOX, the volume of distribution was 3.6 mL, whereas for free DOX it was 2000 mL, suggesting that the PEO-*b*-PAsp-DOX conjugate was somewhat confined to the blood pool. The disposition of PEO-*b*-PAsp-DOX conjugate in the mice at 1 h after intravenous injection is shown in Table 13.8. Compared with free DOX, lower levels of PEO-*b*-PAsp-DOX conjugate at the heart, lung, and liver were revealed (2.9%, 4.0%, and 7.1% dose/g organ versus 3.7%, 7.5%, and 13.4% dose/g organ for flee DOX). Such drastic alterations in the pharmacokinetics and disposition of PEO-*b*-PAsp-DOX relative to free DOX were believed due to core/shell polymeric micellar structure (Kwon and Kataoka, 1995). PEO located in the shell prohibits adsorption of proteins, which occurs quickly after intravenous injection, and prohibits adhesion of cells, which precedes endocytosis of the drug vehicles. In addition, the increased size of the micelle in comparison to the monomeric conjugate precludes renal clearance. It is pointed out that the covalent binding of hydrophobic molecules such as drugs to soluble polymers promotes the uptake of the polymeric conjugates at sites of RES such as the liver (Ambler et al., 1992). But in the case of the PEO-*b*-PAsp-DOX

TABLE 13.8

Disposition of PEO-*b*-PAsp-DOX Conjugates 1 h After Intravenous Injection

Organ	% Dose/g Organ	DOX Equiv. (μg/g Organ)	% Dose/Organ
Blood	17 ± 2.3[a]	75.5 ± 7.8[b]	32.7 ± 3.3
Liver	7.1 ± 1.0	31.0 ± 7.4	7.9 ± 0.8
Kidney	9.6 ± 2.2	41.9 ± 9.6	2.7 ± 0.8
Spleen	11.6 ± 1.8	50.6 ± 7.8	1.0 ± 0
Heart	2.9 ± 0.5	12.6 ± 2.2	0.3 ± 0
Lung	4.0 ± 1.2	17.4 ± 5.2	0.6 ± 0.2
Stomach	5.3 ± 1.4	23.1 ± 6.1	1.3 ± 0.4
Small intestine	5.8 ± 2.1	25.3 ± 9.2	Not determined

Source: Kwon, G. S. and Kataoda, K., *Adv. Drug Delivery Rev.*, 16, 295–309, 1995.

[a] % dose/mL blood.

[b] % μg/mL for blood.

conjugates, DOX is masked in the core of the micelles by PEO, resulting in relatively low uptake at the liver (7.1% ± 1.0% dose/g organ) and at the spleen (11.6% ± 1.8% dose/g organ).

In another study (Kwon et al., 1993a,b), the effect of PEO-*b*-PAsp-DOX composition on its pharmacokinetics and disposition was investigated. Several compositions of PEO-*b*-PAsp-DOX conjugates were synthesized and their micellization was determined by SEC. Overall, PEO-*b*-PAsp-DOX conjugates with high molecular weight PEO blocks (5,000–12,000 g/mol) and low molecular weight PAsp blocks (2000 g/mol) formed the most stable micelles, whereas PEO-*b*-PAsp-DOX conjugates with low molecular weight PEO blocks (1000 g/mol) and high molecular weight PAsp blocks (5000 g/mol) formed unstable micelles. In fact, a significant fraction of PEO-*b*-PAsp-DOX in the latter case eluted as monomeric conjugate in the SEC study. Accordingly, this PEO-*b*-PAsp-DOX conjugate readily dissociates and is cleared quickly renally with low accumulation in the RES. In contrast, the other compositions of PEO-*b*-PAsp-DOX conjugate circulated for prolonged periods, with longer circulation times for those with high molecular weight PEO blocks and low molecular weight PAsp-DOX blocks. Approximately 68%–10% of the injected dose of PEO-*b*-PAsp-DOX conjugate were in the blood at 4–24 h, respectively, when it had a PEO molecular weight of 12,000 g/mol and a PAsp molecular weight of 2,100 g/mol. The circulation time of PEO-*b*-PAsp-DOX decreases as the molecular weight of the PAsp block increases, and there is a concurrent increase in the uptake at the sites of the RES (liver, spleen). The PAsp-DOX block, therefore, is less effectively shielded from biological components by PEO as its size increases.

PEO-*b*-PAsp-DOX conjugates that circulated for prolonged periods were also evaluated in tumor-bearing mice after intravenous injection (Kwon et al., 1994a,b). PEO-*b*-PAsp-DOX conjugates had similar plasma profiles and disposition characteristics that were noted earlier (Kwon and Kataoka, 1995). The levels of PEO-*b*-PAsp-DOX conjugates at the solid tumors were found to be elevated in comparison with free DOX. The selectivity of PEO-*b*-PAsp-DOX conjugates for tumors relative to the heart was also improved significantly from 0.90 for DOX to 12 for the PEO-*b*-PAsp-*g*-DOX conjugate, which consists of a PEO molecular weight of 12,000 g/mol and a PAsp molecular weight of 2,100 g/mol. This composition of PEO-*b*-PAsp-DOX conjugate circulates for prolonged periods in blood with 7.0% of the injected dose in the blood after 24 h.

The finding that the long-circulating PEO-*b*-PAsp-DOX conjugates accumulate at solid tumors had been earlier borne out in the case of long-circulating liposomes in animals and recently in humans (Yuan et al., 1994). There is evidence that suggests that solid tumors have leaky vessels that allow extravasation of molecules and vehicles (Maeda and Matsushima, 1989; Wu et al., 1993; Yuan et al., 1994), including those of colloidal dimensions, in contrast to the continuous endothelium. For long-circulating liposomes, their retention at solid tumors after extravasation was revealed. Thus, vehicles that slowly release drug, such as poly(ethylene oxide) block copolymer micelles, may act as drug depots after extravasation at solid tumors. Finally, the high accumulations of the PEO-*b*-PAsp-DOX conjugates are consistent with their high antitumor activity as judged by decreases in tumor volumes and in some cases, complete disappearance of tumors (Kataoka et al., 1993). Aliabadi and Lavasanifar (2006) recently compiled a comprehensive review of the pharmacokinetic parameters and biodistribution of reported doxorubicin micelle formulations.

For the case of PEO-b -PI-b -PEO micelles, the pharmacokinetics and disposition of PEO-PI-PEO in mice was studied after intravenous injection (Rolland et al., 1992). In this study, the cores of the PEO-PI-PEO micelles were cross linked by reaction of isoprene double bonds using UV irradiation along with a photoinitiator. By the addition of [$_{14}$C] styrene within the micellar cores, the radiolabeling of the micelles took place along with the cross linking reaction. PEO-*b*-PI-*b*-PEO micelles cross linked in this manner were stable with regard to dissociation to monomeric PEO-*b*-PI-*b*-PEO. Notably, PEO-*b*-PI-*b*-PEO micelles had sizes ranging from 14.1 to 206 nm, depending on the method of PEO-*b*-PI-*b*-PEO solubilization in water and depending on the method used to size the micelles (the larger sizes of micelles may reflect secondary association of PEO-*b*-PI-*b*-PEO micelles or incomplete solubilization of PEO-*b*-PI-*b*-PEO). The levels of PEO-*b*-PI-*b*-PEO, as expressed as percentage of *in vivo* label, at 2–24 h are shown, along with data of long-circulating

TABLE 13.9

Murine Pharmocokinetics and Biodistribution of Cyclosporine A in a PEO-*b*-PCL Micelle Formulation and the Cremophor Preparation (Sandimmune©, Novartis Pharmaceuticals)

Parameter	Cremophor EL	PEO-*b*-PCL Micelles
AUC_{0-24} h (μg h/mL)	25.3 ± 7.64	167 ± 18.8
$AUC_{0-\infty}$ (μg h/mL)	32.7 ± 13.8	199 ± 20.9
$t_{1/2}$ (h)	11.5 ± 4.58	9.40 ± 1.20
MRT (h)	14.4 ± 6.62	9.24 ± 2.06
CL (L/kg/h)	0.195 ± 0.131	0.0255 ± 0.00319
V_d (L/kg)	2.33 ± 0.785	0.232 ± 0.0425
Organ	Cremophor EL (μg·h/g)	PEO-*b*-PCL (μg·h/g)
Blood	31.8 ± 1.59	118 ± 8.07
Plasma	29.5 ± 3.23	143 ± 5.61
Kidney	128 ± 7.12	91.4 ± 6.12
Liver	176 ± 27.5	119 ± 8.52
Spleen	188 ± 32.1	90.0 ± 10.1
Heart	107 ± 13.8	155 ± 13.4

Source: Aliabadi, H. M. et al., *J. Control. Rel.*, 104, 301–311, 2005a.

liposomes of (Allen et al., 1989). PEO-*b*-PI-*b*-PEO micelles circulate for prolonged periods with low uptake at the liver and spleen. Again, the data are comparable to long-circulating liposomes. It is noteworthy that the PEO-*b*-PI-*b*-PEO micelles used in the study had diameters of 100 nm so it is not clear that forms of PEO-*b*-PI-*b*-PEO other than micelles did not exist. However, the results indicate that as long as the micelles dissociated slowly or not at all, they may circulate for prolonged periods with low uptake by the RES.

Although prolonged circulation is expected to be an essential criteria for micellar carriers; however, micellar carriers with limited stability *in vivo* have been shown to still alter the biodistribution and pharmacokinetics of incorporated drugs. Savić et al. (2006) investigated the integrity of PEO-*b*-PCL micelles both *in vitro* and *in vivo*. In animal serum, PEO-*b*-PCL micelles lost 37% integrity after 1 h and 74% integrity after 24 h. In murine studies, Saviæ et al. found a significant loss of local micelle integrity after intramuscular and subcutaneous injections. However, studies by Aliabadi et al. (2005a) found PEO-*b*-PCL micelles dramatically altered the murine pharmocokinetics and biodistribution of cyclosporine A as compared with a commercial Cremophor EL preparation (Table 13.9). Although the $t_{1/2}$ was unchanged, the $AUC_{0-\infty}$ increased 6-fold and the V_d decreased 10-fold between the Cremophor EL and PEO-*b*-PCL preparations, respectively.

PHARMACEUTICAL APPLICATIONS

Theoretically, polymeric micelles may find practical applications in a variety of pharmaceutical fields, from oral delivery to sustained release and site-specific drug targeting. However, until now polymeric micelles have been almost exclusively evaluated for the parenteral administration of anticancer drugs and serve primarily for the transport of water-insoluble drugs (Jones and Leroux, 1999). Several *in vivo* studies showed that polymeric micelles were able to improve the efficiency of anticancer drugs against leukemia (Yokoyama et al., 1990; Zhang et al., 1997a,b) and solid tumors (Yokoyama et al., 1991; Zhang et al., 1997a,b). Specific pharmaceutical applications are discussed subsequently.

DIBLOCK POLYMERIC MICELLES

Yu et al. (1998) used amphotericin B (AmB), an antifungal drug, as a model to study the release profile of poly(ethylene oxide)-block-poly(benzyl-aspartate) (PEO-*b*-PBLA) block copolymer micelles. AmB is a poorly water-soluble drug that is currently formulated with the bile salt deoxycholate (Fungizone®). This formulation induces hemolysis and slowed release of AmB is shown to prevent this toxic side effect. In addition, Yu et al. investigated the effect of freeze-drying and reconstitution on the micelles.

The drug-loaded PEO-*b*-PBLA micelles were prepared as follows. The PEO-*b*-PBLA was first dissolved in dimethylfomamide and the AmB added to this solution. The polymer/drug solution was then dialyzed against distilled water to remove the DMF and unencapsulated AmB. The pH of the dialysis medium was maintained at pH 11.3 to ensure ionization of the unencapsulated AmB that facilitates its removal. The dialysis medium was neutralized to pH 5.6 upon completion. The isotonicity of the micellar solution in the dialysis bag was adjusted with dextrose. Adjustment of the isotonicity was not made for the micelles that were freeze-dried. The loading of AmB was measured by UV-vis spectroscopy after dilution with DMF that breaks down the PEO-PBLA micelles to release the AmB. The loading efficiency was approximately 30%, and the molar ratio of AmB to polymer ranged from 0.40 to 1.0.

TEM can resolve nanoscopic colloids such as polymeric micelles. TEM pictures revealed spherical PEO-*b*-PBLA micelles, confirming earlier dynamic light-scattering measurements on the polymeric micelles. The mean diameters of the unloaded PEO-*b*-PBLA micelles and AmB-loaded PEO-*b*-PBLA micelles were 20.0 ± 3.9 and 25.8 ± 4.2 nm, respectively, indicating a slight increase in size upon drug loading. The size distributions of the PEO-*b*-PBLA micelles are very narrow, characteristic of polymeric micelles.

Intravenous solutions of AmB were administered at levels of 50–100 mg/mL. The loading of AmB into PEO-*b*-PBLA micelles drastically lowers the hemolytic activity of AmB, even at an AmB level of 10 µg/mL. When deoxycholate solubilizes AmB (Fungizone), AmB is very hemolytic, reaching a 100% hemolysis at a level of ca. 3.0 µg/mL. Without deoxycholate, which exhibits its own hemolytic activity, micelles of AmB itself formed by dialysis are slightly less hemolytic. In contrast, AmB-loaded PEO-*b*-PBLA micelles caused no hemolysis at 3.0 µg/mL for a period of up to 5.5 h versus 30 min. This indicates that the release of AmB from PEO-*b*-PBLA micelles is slow. The lack of hemolytic activity may also reflect the release of monomeric AmB from PEO-*b*-PBLA micelles as opposed to Fungizone, which releases both aggregated and monomeric forms of the drug.

The nonhemolytic effect of AmB-loaded PEO-*b*-PBLA micelles was supported by another study on the *in vitro* dissociation of antifungal efficacy and toxicity for these diblock copolymeric micelles (Yu et al., 1998). Since the aggregation state of AmB is a determinant factor for toxicity, AmB has been loaded into PEO-block-PBLA micelles in a monomeric state, resulting in a formulation that has uncoupled efficacy from toxicity for concentrations up to 15 µg/mL as measured by hemolytic activity and minimal inhibitory concentration (MIC). The antifungal efficacy of AmB-loaded PEO-*b*-PBLA micelles in terms of MIC is greater than Fungizone, perhaps owing to a stabilizing role of the polymeric micelles and/or enhanced interaction of AmB at a membrane level. The results support findings on the selective activity of monomeric AmB against fungal cells over mammalian cells.

It was found that unloaded PEO-*b*-PBLA micelles cause no hemolysis, even at a level of 0.70 mg/mL. PEO-*b*-PBLA has an extremely low critical micelle concentration (Kwon et al., 1993a,b), and thus, there is little monomeric PEO-*b*-PBLA for the lysis of lipid bilayer membranes. In addition, PEO-*b*-PBLA micelles may break apart slowly to monomers. The lack of hemolytic activity of PEO-*b*-PBLA contrasts strongly with other amphiphiles used for drug solubilization and intravenous drug administration. Sodium deoxycholate causes 100% hemolysis at a level of 0.32 mg/mL. This is due to disruption of lipid bilayer membranes of red blood cells.

The high structural integrity of PEO-PBLA micelles, along with slow release of AmB, may be due to the solid-like cores of PEO-*b*-PBLA micelles (Kwon et al., 1993a,b). Strong secondary interactions along with the bulky benzyl side chains in the cores of PEO-*b*-PBLA micelles lead to high core viscosity (Kwon et al., 1993a,b), which may deter micelle breakup and AmB release. For polymeric micelles with core-forming poly(styrene) blocks (phenyl side chains), there is no inter-micellar exchange of diblock copolymers at 25°C (Wang et al., 1992). On the other hand, detergent micelles have liquid-like cores, and in this case intermicellar exchange happens in the order of μs (Yu et al., 1998).

Finally, freeze-dried, AmB-loaded PEO-*b*-PBLA micelles easily dissolved within a few seconds in aqueous solutions. This contrasts with the behavior of PEO-*b*-PBLA and AmB, both of which are insoluble when directly placed in water. TEM reveals that the PEO-*b*-PBLA micelles remain intact, and the size distribution confirms the absence of any secondary aggregation that may have resulted from the freeze-drying and reconstitution processes. Further, the resultant AmB-loaded PEO-*b*-PBLA micelles cause no hemolysis at 10 μg/mL, indicating that AmB is still present inside the polymeric micelles. An AmB level of 5.0 mg/mL was obtained; this is 10,000 times the solubility of AmB. Thus, reconstitution of freeze-dried micelles allows high AmB levels in solution. It is the same with doxorubicin-loaded PEO-*b*-PBLA micelles (Kwon et al., 1997).

Yu et al. (1998) were able to increase the *in vitro* antifungal efficiency of amphotericin B while at the same time decreasing its hemolytic activity by loading the drug into polymeric micelles. It was suggested that polymeric micelles could stabilize amphotericin B against autooxidation and/or enhance membrane perturbation of fungal cells.

TRIBLOCK POLYMERIC MICELLES

Solubilization of insoluble drugs using poloxamers (Pluronics), PEO-*b*-PPO-*b*-PEO triblock copolymers, has been extensively studied. Kabanov et al. (1992) designed and formulated targeted drug delivery systems for the hydrophobic neuroleptic haloperidol. Other drugs studied include tropicamide, a poorly water-soluble mydriatic/cycloplegic drug (Saettone et al., 1988); allopurinol (Hamza and Kata, 1989); diazepam (Lin, 1987); and naproxen (Suh and Jun, 1996). A brief summary of the highlights of each of these studies is given subsequently.

Micelles for drug targeting were prepared using polymeric surfactant PEO-*b*-PPO-*b*-PEO block copolymers such as Pluronic P-85, F-64, L-68, and L-101 (Kabanov et al., 1992). Holoperidol was dissolved in Pluronic micelle solutions at pH 6, and the solutions were incubated at 37°C for 1 h. The drug was incorporated into the inner hydrophobic core formed by PPO blocks. The polymeric micellar solubilization of low molecular weight compounds, such as fluorescein isothiocyanate (FITC) and haloperidol, was characterized using various techniques including fluorescence, ultra-centrifugation, and quasielastic light scattering. In a majority of cases, the diameter of Pluronic micelles including those containing solubilized compounds ranged from 12 to 36 nm.

To target these microcontainers to a certain cell, the Pluronic molecules were conjugated with antibodies against a target-specific antigen or with protein ligands selectively interacting with target cell receptors. These conjugates were then incorporated into the drug-containing micelles by simple mixing of the corresponding components. Solubilization of FITC in Pluronic micelles shows its distribution in animal (mouse) tissues. Unconjugated micelles concentrate in the lung. Conjugation of FITC-containing micelles with insulin vector results in increase of FITC penetration in all tissues including the brain. Specific targeting of the brain occurred when the Pluronic was conjugated with antibodies to the antigen of brain glial cells (α2-glycoprotein). When haloperidol was solubilized in these conjugated micelles, there was a drastic increase of drug effect. This result indicates that vector-containing Pluronic micelles provide an effective transport of solubilized neuroleptics across blood-brain barrier.

Solubilization of tropicamide, a poorly water-soluble mydriatic/cycloplegic drug, by poloxamers or Pluronics was studied (Saettone et al., 1988). The polymers evaluated as solubilizers for the drug included L-64, P-65, F-68, P-75, F-77, P-84, P-85, F-87, F-88, and F-127. The authors measured a range of physicochemical properties, such as solubility of tropicamide in polymer solutions, partition coefficient of the drug between isopropyl myristate and copolymer solutions, critical micelle concentration of the copolymers, and viscosity of the copolymeric solutions containing tropicamide.

The solubility isotherms at 25°C showed that the solubility of the drug increased linearly with increasing surfactant concentration in the 4.0%–20.0% w/v. concentration range. In the presence of 20% wt./vol. Pluronics, the drug solubility increased substantially, ranging from 1.9-fold (F-88) to approximately 3.0-fold (P-85). The solubility of tropicamide increased as the ethylene oxide (EO) content of the surfactants increased. However, the amount of drug solubilized per EO unit decreased with increasing hydrophilicity (increasing PEO chain length) of surfactants. Calculation of the relative amount of drug bound to the PEO and to the PPO portions of the surfactant molecules indicated that binding occurs in part of the hydrophilic (PEO) outer mantle, and in part to the hydrophobic (PPO) inner core of the micellar aggregates, with PEO/PPO binding ratios varying from 1.17 to 3.13, depending on the polymer type.

Mydriatic activity on rabbits and humans, and cycloplegic activity on humans were tested. It was found that tropicamide bioavailability, both in rabbits and in humans, was not decreased by micellar solubilization. The conclusion was that some poloxamers perform satisfactorily as solubilizing vehicles for tropicamide, producing neutral 1.0%–1.5% drug solutions that are better tolerated and more effective than the standard aqueous eyedrops.

The effect of block structure on solubilization was also observed for other drugs. Hamza and Kata (1989) studied solubilization of allopurinol in a series of surfactants, including the Pluronic F series. Extending the hydrophobic core of a homologous series having the same polyoxyethylene chain length causes a decrease in the solubilized amount of the drug at various concentrations. On the other hand, for a series having the same hydrophobic block, extending the polyoxyethylene chains causes an increase in the solubilized amount of drug except at the highest concentration. Such results were obtained for the solubility of diazepam in three types of Pluronic surfactant aqueous solutions (F-108 $\gg$ F-88 > F-68) (Lin, 1987). The solubility and release of naproxen from Pluronic PF-127 micelles were studied as a function of temperature and pH by Suh and Jun (1996). The solubility of the drug at pH 2 was significantly increased as a linear function of PF-127 concentrations for three temperatures. Naproxen was highly entrapped by the micelles as indicated by large partition coefficient. The micellar solubilization was a spontaneous ($\Delta G < 0$) and exothermic ($\Delta H < 0$) process that resulted in a less ordered state ($\Delta S > 0$). In the presence of PF-127, the release of naproxen was sustained at pH 2 and inversely proportional to the surfactant concentration. In contrast, at pH 7, PF-127 had little effect on the membrane transport of naproxen. The release of naproxen from the PF-127 gel into isopropanol myristate was also found to be dependent on the medium pH with the highest release observed at pH 6.3.

Thermo-Responsive Polymeric Micelles

For the purpose of evading the RES (Matsumura and Maeda, 1986; Maeda et al., 1992), thermo-responsive micelles are able not only to utilize spatial specificity in a passive manner owing to their sizes but also to increase the spatial specificity in combination with a physical targeting mechanism, which is achieved by the introduction of a thermo-responsive polymer segment such as PIPAAm. The thermo-response is expected to accomplish multiple functions for a double targeting system in both passive and stimuliresponsive manners enhancing vascular transport and drug release, and/or embolization induced by local temperature change. Selective accumulation of micelles at a malignant tissue site could be increased as a result of micelle adsorption enhancement to cells mediated by hydrophobic interactions between polymeric micelles and cells. Simultaneously, this strategy can achieve temporal drug delivery control: drug expresses its activity only for a time period defined by local heating and cooling (Chung et al., 1999).

Poly(N-isopropylacrylamide) (PIPAAm) in aqueous solution is well known to exhibit a thermo-responsive phase transition at 32°C (Heskins and Guillet, 1968). PIPAAm surfaces can be grafted with a hydrophobic segment such as polystyrene, creating hydrophilic/hydrophobic switchable surfaces (Yamada et al., 1990; Okano et al., 1993, 1995). This AB-type block copolymer of PIPAAm and a hydrophobic segment shows thermo-responsive water solubility and can form heterogeneous microstructures, that is, micellar structures composed of hydrophilic microdomains of soluble PIPAAm segments together with hydrophobic aggregated microdomains of incorporated hydrophobic segments in aqueous solution below the LCST. The hydrophobic inner core of the micelle contains water-insoluble drugs, while the PIPAAm outer shell plays a role of stabilization and temperature-response. The outer shell hydrophilicity that prevents inner core interaction with biocomponents and other micelles can be suddenly switched to hydrophobicity at a specific site by a temperature increase above the LCST (Chung et al., 1999).

In order to design and facilitate a reversibly temperature-responsive micelle for a drug delivery system, Chung et al. (1997, 1999) and Cammas et al. (1997) conducted extensive research on the micelle formation mechanism, the structural stability and the temperature-response relating to intra- or intermolecular hydrophilic/hydrophobic interactions and molecular architectures.

In general, incorporation of hydrophilic or hydrophobic groups into PIPAAm chains changes the LCST (Taylor and Cerankowski, 1975; Dong and Hoffman, 1991; Takei et al., 1993; Chen and Hoffman, 1995). PIPAAms with hydrophilic groups raised the LCST to higher temperatures than that of the corresponding pure PIPAAm and slowed down phase transition phenomena by stabilizing polymer dissolution through strengthened interactions between polymer chains and water (Dong and Hoffman, 1991; Chen and Hoffman, 1995). The hydrophilic contribution to the LCST transition is especially great for terminal-located hydrophilic groups (Chung et al., 1997). In the same way that the hydrophilic contribution alters the PIPAAm LCST, the hydrophobic contribution also depends on the locations of the hydrophobic group. Hydrophobic groups alter the hydrophilic/hydrophobic balance in PIPAAm and promoted a PIPAAm phase transition at lower solution temperatures than the LCST of the corresponding pure PIPAAm (Taylor and Cerankowski, 1975; Takei et al., 1993).

However, supramolecular structures comprising hydrophobically modified PIPAAm at terminal positions showed the same LCST and same phase transition kinetics as freely mobile, linear PIPAAm chains (Chung et al., 1997). When terminal hydrophobic groups self-aggregate by hydrophobic interactions, water clusters immobilized around the hydrophobic segments are excluded from the hydrophobically aggregated inner core, and the isolated hydrophobic micellar core does not directly interfere with PIPAAm chain dynamics in aqueous media. The PIPAAm chains of the micellar outer shell remain as mobile linear chains in this core-shell micellar structure. As a result, the thermo-responsive properties of PIPAAm in the outer PIPAAm chains of this structure are unaltered (Winnik et al., 1992; Chung et al., 1997). It has been shown earlier that strongly hydrophobic terminally modified PIPAAm formed clearly phase-separated micellar structures and preserved the stable structures during thermo-responsive structural changes when responding to thermal stimuli (Cammas et al., 1997; Chung et al., 1997, 1998).

Chung et al. (1999) constructed a plot of micropolarity of PIPAAm-b-PBMA against temperature (Figure 13.26). The solution showed increased polarity of the pyrene environment with increasing temperature through the LCST, while the solution showed a constant micropolarity and was less polar below the LCST. Pure PIPAAm solutions showed an abrupt decrease in polarity when the temperature was raised through its LCST, indicating the transfer of pyrene into the precipitated polymer-rich phase (Chung et al., 1997). On the other hand, a micelle solution showed lower polarity than that of pure PIPAAm solution for the entire temperature region owing to a presence of hydrophobic PBMA cores of the micelles. Aggregation of collapsed PIPAAm outer shells could have induced micelle structural deformation that increased the polarity of the pyrene microenvironment above the LCST. The structural deformation that allowed the change in pyrene partitioning was reversed upon rehydration of the PIPAAm chains below the LCST. A small hysteresis around the LCST was observed to be caused by the delayed hydration of the PIPAAm chains on cooling

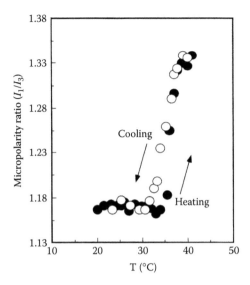

FIGURE 13.26 Plot of the ratio of intensities (I_1/I_3) of the vibrational bands in the pyrene fluorescence spectrum as a function of temperature for PIPAAm-*b*-PBMA, $\lambda_{ex} = 340$ nm, [pyrene] $= 1.6 \times 10^{-7}$ M, 1°C/min, [polymer] = 5000 mg/L. (Reprinted from *J. Control. Rel.*, 62, Chung, J. E. et al., Thermo-responsive drug delivery from polymeric micelles constructed using block copolymers of poly(*N*-isopropylacrylamide) and poly(butylmethacrylate), 115–127, Copyright 1999, with permission from Elsevier.)

(Chung et al., 1997). These results suggest potential for the polymeric micelle structural changes selectively to modulate drug release from the inner cores on heating.

PIPAAm-*b*-PBMA micelle formation and drug loading resulting from solvent exchange during dialysis was significantly affected by interaction of the solvents with both polymers and drugs, solvent exchange speed, and solution temperature. In the gradual decrease of organic solvent composition during dialysis, spontaneous hydrophobic association of PBMA segments both with themselves and with hydrophobic drugs is a driving force for micelle formation and drug loading into micelle cores. Therefore, drug choice and drug loading are defined by interactions of drugs with both the hydrophobic segments and solvents. Control of the optimum conditions should provide important information to generalize optimum drug loading conditions in polymeric micelles. Optimum hydrophobic interactions to form PIPAAm-*b*-PBMA micelles containing ADR was regulated by modulating variables such as hydrophilic/hydrophobic block lengths of the polymer, concentration of both the polymer and ADR in the dialysis bag, TEA amounts and dialysis temperature. PIPAAm(6100)-*b*-PBMA(8900) was most successful for both micelle formation and drug (ADR) load (14.6 wt.%) by choosing *N*-ethylacetamide as a good solvent for both the polymers and the ADR and other selected conditions. The polymer-ADR solution of *N*, *N*-dimethylformamide or DMSO precipitated during dialysis against water. A dialysis membrane (Spectra/Por) with a pore size of MWCO = 12,000–14,000 provided optimum solvent exchange rates for micelle formation of this PIPAAm-*b*-PBMA/ADR combination. The micelle-ADR solution was obtained as a transparent red solution at ca. 20°C (dialysis temperature) relating to polymer solubility, especially for PIPAAm segments in water. Other higher or lower dialysis temperatures than 20°C led to precipitates.

Chung et al. (1999) monitored the drug release from micelles using a UV spectrophotometer. ADR release profile from polymeric micelles showed drastic changes with temperature alterations through the LCST (Figure 13.27). ADR release was selectively accelerated upon heating through the LCST, while ADR release was well suppressed below the LCST. Temperature-accelerated ADR release was consistent with temperature-induced structural change of the polymeric micelle (Figure 13.26). Figure 13.28 shows that ADR release from polymer micelles is thermo-responsively

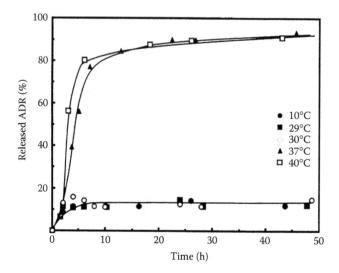

FIGURE 13.27 Drug (ADR) release from thermo-responsive PIPAAm-*b*-PBMA micelles containing ADR. (Reprinted from *J. Control. Rel.*, 62, Chung, J.E. et al., Thermo-responsive drug delivery from polymeric micelles constructed using block copolymers of poly(*N*-isopropylacrylamide) and poly(butylmethacrylate), 115–127, Copyright 1999, with permission from Elsevier.)

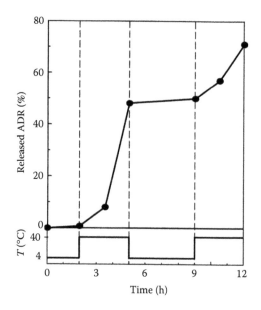

FIGURE 13.28 On/off switched drug (ADR) release from PIPAAm-*b*-PBMA micelles containing ADR responding temperature changes. (Reprinted from *J. Control. Rel.*, 62, Chung, J.E. et al., Thermo-responsive drug delivery from polymeric micelles constructed using block copolymers of poly(*N*-isopropylacrylamide) and poly(butylmethacrylate), 115–127, Copyright 1999, with permission from Elsevier.)

on/off-switched corresponding to reversible structural changes of micelles by temperature changes through the LCST. The ADR release initiated on heating above the LCST was accelerated as increasing ADR concentration surrounding the micelles. Moreover, it was by just cooling below the LCST and accelerated again upon another heating.

In the thermo-responsive *in vitro* cytotoxicity studies for PIPAAm-*b*-PBMA micelles containing ADR at 29°C and 37°C compared with that of free ADR, Chung et al. (1999) found that polymeric micelles showed higher cytotoxic activity than that of free ADR at 37°C (above the LCST), while it showed lower cytotoxic activity than that of free ADR at 29°C (below the LCST). Cytotoxicity was remarkably well enhanced corresponding to both the micelle structural change (Figure 13.26) and ADR release (Figure 13.27) was selectively initiated by heating through the LCST.

MICELLE-FORMING COPOLYMER-DRUG CONJUGATES

Micelle-forming copolymer-drug conjugates may provide prolonged circulating time, higher efficacy, and low toxicity compared with the free drug. Kwon and Okano (1999) summarized the recent advance of micelle-forming copolymer-drug conjugates. A poly(ethylene oxide-*b*-poly(aspartic acid)-doxorubicin (PEO-*b*-PAA-DOX) conjugate can self-assemble into a spherical micelle-like structure in water (Yokoyama et al., 1990, 1992). It has a nonpolar core composed of a PAA block with attached DOX, and a hydrophilic shell composed of PEO. Its diameter is ca. 30 nm, based on DLS measurements, corresponding to the size of lipoproteins and viruses (Yokoyama et al., 1990). The attachment of DOX onto PEO-*b*-PAA occurs at high levels without a loss of water solubility. A loss of water solubility often limits the degree of drug substitution of soluble synthetic polymers. The micelle-like structure of a PEO-*b*-PAA-DOX conjugate is held tightly together by self-association of DOX in the core region, as evidenced by quenching of drug fluorescence (Yokoyama et al., 1992). Even in blood, the micelle-like structure of a PEO-*b*-PAA-DOX conjugate breaks apart gradually (hours). This unique stability toward break-up enables PEO-*b*-PAA-DOX conjugate micelles to have a prolonged blood half-life, versus the rapid renal clearance of unimer (Yokoyama et al., 1991). PEO plays a recognized role in blood, preventing protein adsorption and cellular adhesion steps that precede phagocytosis by cells of the MPS. An inordinately dense layer of PEO (polymer brush) masks the nonpolar core of drug. PEO-*b*-PAA-DOX conjugate micelles, therefore, passively accumulate at solid tumors by the EPR effect (Kwon et al., 1994a,b). Conjugated DOX on PAA plays on direct role in antitumor activity expressed in murine tumor models (Yokoyama et al., 1998). It was found instead that unconjugated DOX is held tightly in cores of PEO-*b*-PAA-DOX conjugate micelles and carried to tumors where it exerts antitumor effects.

However, Yokoyama et al. (1994) reported that a ratio between the chemically conjugated and physically entrapped ADR (i.e., DOX) was not determined, and considerable amounts of adriamycin derivatives formed and were incorporated in the micelles. Yokoyama et al. (1998) quantitatively measured the ADR incorporated in the inner core using the improved synthetic method, and analyzed the effects of the ADR contents (both by chemical conjugation and physical entrapment) on micelle stability and *in vivo* antitumor activity. The copolymer used by Yokoyama et al. (1998) was poly(ethylene glycol)-*b*-poly(aspartic acid) block copolymer (PEG-*b*-P(Asp)). The chemical conjugation and physical entrapment methods can be referred to in the earlier section of preparation of polymeric micelles.

Large enhancement of antitumor activity of ADR was successfully achieved by its incorporation into polymeric micelles with the controlled amounts of the chemically conjugated and physically entrapped ADR. The high *in vivo* antitumor activity is considered to result from selective delivery of the physically entrapped ADR to solid tumor sites, since the block copolymer-drug conjugate along without physically entrapped ADR did not show any *in vivo* activity. However, *in vivo* antitumor activity was found to depend on contents of both the physically entrapped and chemically conjugated ADR. Gel-filtration analyses revealed differences in micelle structural stability. The polymeric micelle with high structural stability shown by a small elution volume expressed high *in vivo* antitumor activity. These results indicate that stable physical entrapment of ADR was essential for *in vivo* antitumor activity in this polymeric micelle drug carrier system.

Kwon et al. (1994) reported that polymeric micelles were found to selectively accumulate at C26 tumors by radioisotope label on block copolymers. This selectivity was considered to be based on hyperpermeability of the vascular endothelia at tumor sites (Dvorak et al., 1979, 1995). This unique phenomenon was clearly defined as EPR effect for a drug targeting strategy to solid tumors (Matsumura and Maeda, 1986, Maeda et al., 1992). Although this EPR effect was originally reported for proteins such as albumin, Yokoyama et al. (1998) believed that it might be applied also to polymeric micelles that have much larger diameters than those of the proteins. In order to utilize the EPR effect for drug targeting to solid tumors, interactions (e.g., hydrophobic interactions) of drug carrier systems with the vascular endothelial cells should be avoided, since these hydrophobic interactions may considerably reduce contribution of diffusive and convectional transport (through intracellular channels or intercellular junctions of endothelia) on which the EPR effect is based. The polymeric micelles with the PEG (i.e., PEO) outer shells are considered to inherently possess selective targeting ability to tumors by the EPR effect, since PEG is known to be an inert polymer with very small interactions with cells and proteins, as demonstrated by prolongation of plasma half-lives of several proteins by PEG modification (Abuchowski et al., 1977; Katre et al., 1987). Stability of the polymeric micelles measured by gel-filtration chromatography is considered to show how completely the hydrophobic inner cores were shielded by the PEG outer shells. Consequently, the stable polymeric micelles could more effectively utilize the EPR effect by more efficiently inhibiting the hydrophobic interactions. To obtain the stable entrapment, large amounts of the chemically conjugated and physically entrapped ADR were required probably for tight packing of the hydrophobic inner cores (Yokoyama et al., 1998).

Yokoyama et al. (1998) considered that the chemically conjugated ADR did not play a major role in antitumor activity, since polymeric micelle consisting chemically conjugated ADR alone did not show any *in vivo* activity, and did show no or low *in vitro* cytotoxic activity. Such no or low activities are considered to result from no or slow (if any) release of free ADR from the block copolymer owing to the absence of cleavable spacer groups such as tetrapeptide of Kopecek's study (Patnum and Kopecek, 1995). However, it still remains unknown whether the chemically conjugated ADR could express any pharmacological effects or not. According to Tritton's study (Wingard et al., 1985), the conjugated ADR can express cytotoxic activities without any release of free ADR. On the other hand, the chemically conjugated ADR was shown to contribute to physically entrap free (unconjugated) ADR in a stable manner inside the inner core, since no physical entrapment of ADR was attained by mixing ADR and poly(ethylene glycol)-*b*-poly(aspartic acid) block copolymer (Yokoyama et al., 1998). Martin (1980) reported self-association of daunomycin (an adriamycin analogue). Therefore, the conjugated ADR is considered to work as a very good carrier of the physically entrapped ADR by providing specific interactions between the two ADR molecules as well as nonspecific hydrophobic interactions (Yokoyama et al., 1998).

Kwon and Okano (1999) added that synthetic micelle-like structures of block copolymers might pose as functional analogues of biological transport systems, such as low-density lipoprotein. A major function of plasma lipoproteins is the solubilization of lipids, and synthetic micelle-like structures of block copolymers may play an analogous role for water-insoluble drugs. Synthetic micelle-like structures of block copolymers may deliver unconjugated drug to solid tumors without an excessive loss of drug. Lastly, synthetic micelle-like structures of block copolymers may be more easily scaled-up and less costly than lipoproteins for drug delivery.

MICELLE-FORMING DIACYLLIPID-POLYMER CONJUGATES

Trubetskoy and Torchilin (1995) studied diacyllipid-PEO conjugates as micelle-forming polymers to deliver therapeutic and diagnostic agents. They based on the theory that the stability of amphiphilic micelles in its major part depends on the strength of Van der Waals interactions between hydrophobic blocks forming the core of the particle and the molecular size of the hydrophilic block counterbalancing the non-water-soluble part of the macromolecule. Use of lipid moieties as hydrophobic blocks capping PEO chains can provide additional advantages for particle stability when compared with conventional amphiphilic polymer micelles, since the existence of two fatty acid acyls might contribute considerably to the increase of the hydrophobic interactions between the polymeric chains in the micelle's core. More hydrophobic membranes anchor result in a stronger interaction of the amphiphilic polymer with the lipid membrane (Trubetskoy and Torchilin, 1995). Upon incorporation into the liposome membrane, the hydrophilic polymer capped with palmityl (C_{16}) fatty acid acyls served as a better steric protector than decyl (C10) derivatives.

Diacyllipid-polyethyleneoxide conjugates have been introduced into the controlled drug delivery area as polymeric surface modifiers for liposomes (Klibanov et al., 1990). Being incorporated into the liposome membrane by insertion of their lipidic anchor into the bilayer, such molecules can sterically stabilize the liposome against interaction with certain plasma proteins in the blood, which results in significant prolongation of the vesicle circulation time. The diacyllipid-PEO molecule itself represents a characteristic amphiphilic polymer with a bulky hydrophilic (PEO) portion and a very short but extremely hydrophobic diacyllipid part. Typically, for other PEO-containing amphiphilic block copolymers, diacyllipid-PEO conjugates were found to form micelles in an aqueous environment (Lasie et al., 1991). It seems that the use of PEO-diacyllipid conjugates that represent micelle-forming amphiphilic copolymers with larger hydrophilic blocks and more lipophilic hydrophobic blocks might result in colloid particles that are more stable at physiologic conditions.

Owing to their size and macrophage avoiding properties, the use of PEO-lipid conjugates can be especially advantageous for some specific routes of drug delivery. For example, it is known from experiments with [198]Au gold colloids that the optimal size for a particulate lymphatic adsorption from the interstitial space after subcutaneous administration is rather small (~5 nm) (Strand and Petsson, 1979). The structure of the particulate's surface is another factor that can regulate its disappearance from the injection site as well as uptake by the lymph node. The importance of PEO-coated particulates in percutaneous administration and lymph node delivery has already been demonstrated with poloxamer-coated polystyrene latex particles (Moghimi et al., 1994). However, as others pointed out (Tan et al., 1993), the potential of polystyrene nanospheres as vehicles for delivery of practical bioactive agents remains to be established. At the same time, polymeric micelles already proved themselves effective carriers for a variety of hydrophobic substances. Proper size, surface coating, and ability to be loaded with sufficient quantities of drug or diagnostic agent make PEO-lipid micelles a perfect choice for percutaneous lymphatic delivery.

The supramolecular structure of PEO-diacyllipid micelles is somewhat similar to that of PEO-lipid-containing liposomes: both particulates possess a lipidic portion and its outer surrounded by a hydrophilic PEO shell facing the aqueous phase. As a consequence, one may expect similar *in vivo* properties including half-life in the blood. Macrophage-evading properties might be an important issue not only for intravenous drug carriers but also for other administration routes. Trubetskoy and Torchilin (1995) presented the results of some of their experiments on the delivery of micelle-loaded amphiphilic diagnostic agents to the elements of local lymphatics. A series of PEO-phosphatidylethanolamine (PEO-PE) conjugates were synthesized using egg PE (transphosphotidylated) and *N*-hydroxysuccinimide esters of methoxy-PEO succinates (molecular weights of 2, 5, and 12 kDa) (Klibanov et al., 1990). HPLC-based GPC showed that these polymers formed micelles of different sizes in an aqueous environment. The stability of the polymeric micelles was confirmed using the same method: no dissociation into individual polymeric chains was found upon chromatography of the serially diluted samples of PEO (5 kDa)-PE. PEO-PE micelles can efficiently incorporate some sparingly soluble and amphiphilic substances. For example, spectral analysis of the micellar HPLC peak shows that polymeric micelles can incorporate the topoisomerase II inhibitor ellipticine, a substance with water solubility of 1.5 μg/mL. Nevertheless, the most successful examples of hydrophobic substance incorporation into PEO-lipid micelles were different amphiphilic lipid derivatives. Unlike ellipticine that can be successfully incorporated into PEO(5 kDa)-PE micelles only at the drug: PEO-PE molar ratio 1:25, the fluorescent lipid probe rhodamine-PE incorporates into the same micelles up to 2:1 drug: PEO-PE molar ratio. One can suggest that the most successful therapeutic applications of PEO-lipid polymeric micelles as drug carriers would require the use of the appropriate hydrophobized prodrugs. The hydrophobized prodrug approach in the area of drug delivery systems has been successfully used for increased permeation of peptides across the intestinal membrane (Yodoya et al., 1994) and for increased loading of anticancer drug derivatives into reconstituted low-density lipoproteins, owing to the covalent coupling of lipophilic anchor directly to the drug (Samadi-Boboli et al., 1993).

During biodistribution experiments *in vivo* ^{111}In-labeled PEO-PE micelles demonstrated that half-life was up to 2.5 h in mice. This value is long enough compared with the majority of nonsurface-modified particulates, but somewhat shorter than for PEO-containing liposomes. Several circumstances might explain this difference. First, particles might extravasate from the vasculature, owing to a considerably smaller size compared with liposomes. Another possibility is an exchange of the amphiphilic label with the plasma proteins possessing affinity to lipidic moieties (such as albumin).

Macrophage-evading properties of polymeric micelles are important not only for intravenous applications but also for another route of drug carrier administration. A good example for the practical application of these properties of PEO-lipid polymeric micelles can be found in the delivery of diagnostically important heavy metal ions *in vivo*. Apart from the practical value for diagnosis itself, this area has significant importance for the delivery of drugs, as it allows to visualize the exact sites of the drug carrier deposition within the body with extraordinary anatomical resolution. Chelated paramagnetic metal moieties (Gd, Mn, or Dy aqueous ions) represent the major interest for the design of MR positive (T_1) contrast agents. Chelated metal ions possess a definitely hydrophilic character: the complex of diethylenetriamine pentaacetic acid (DTPA) with Gd^{3+} for example, has a water molecule bound directly to the metal coordination sphere. In order to be incorporated into micelles, such structures should acquire an amphiphilic nature. Several chelating probes of this type have been developed earlier for liposome membrane incorporation studies (DTPA-PE [Grant et al., 1989], DTPA-stearylamine, DTPA-SA [Kabalka et al., 1989], and amphiphilic acylated paramagnetic complexes of Mn and Gd [Unger et al., 1994]). In these agents, the hydrophilic chelating residue is covalently linked to a hydrophobic (lipid) chain. The lipid part of the molecule can be anchored in the liposome bilayer or the hydrophobic core of the micelle, while the more hydrophilic chelate is localized on the liposome surface or hydrophilic polymer shell of the micelle. Incorporation of radioactive ion chelate allows one to follow the pharmacokinetic parameters *in vivo*, including blood half-life and biodistribution. The amphiphilic chelating probes (paramagnetic Gd-DTPA-PE and radioactive ^{111}In-DTPA-SA) were incorporated into PEO(5 kDa)-PE micelles and used *in vivo* for MR and scintigraphy imaging.

In Trubetskoy and Torchilin's (1995) experiments, they incorporated amphiphilic chelating probes Gd(^{111}In)-DTPA-PE and ^{111}In-DTPA-SA into PEO(5 kDa)-PE micelles (20 nm in diameter) and surface-modified liposomes (200 nm in diameter), and tried to compare these particulate agents in experimental percutaneous lymphography using γ-scintigraphy and MR imaging in rabbits. It was demonstrated that the localization of ^{111}In-labeled DTPA-SA/ PEO(5 kDa)-PE micelles in local lymphatics follows subcutaneous administration of a 20 μCi dose into the dorsum of the hind paws of a rabbit. The popliteal lymph node can be visualized within seconds after injection. Gentle massage of the injection site can increase the nodal accumulation and push the labeled material further down the lymphatic pathway to the thoracic duct. Direct massage of the popliteal node can *squeeze*. ^{111}In-labeled micelles to the systemic circulation. However, it is evident that the micelles as smaller particles exhibit higher accumulation in the primary lymph node without massage. Interestingly, injection site massage leveled up the difference in lymph node accumulation between these two particulates (micelle and liposome). On the contrary, popliteal lymph node massage removes smaller particles more readily than liposomes. The micellar particulates due to their size and surface properties can be moved with ease from the injection site along the lymphatics to the systemic circulation evidently with the lymph flow. Taking into account the ease and rapidity of the primary lymph node visualization, one can suggest that unlike the other lymphotropic contrast media, polymeric micelles are lymphangiogsaphic in nature. Their action is based on the visualization of lymph flowing through different elements of the lymphatics. The action of other lymphotropic contrast media is based primarily on their active uptake by the nodal macrophages (i.e., lymph nodes become visible only after the concentration of the medium in the lymph node has achieved a certain threshold value that usually requires prolonged periods of time).

As can be seen, lipid-PEO conjugates can be successfully used as drug and diagnostics carriers in experimental systems *in vivo*. Using copolymers with different sizes of PEO block, it is possible to control the diameter of polymeric micelles. Different sparingly soluble or amphiphilic drugs and diagnostic agents can be incorporated into their hydrophobic core. But the future of this perspective type of drug carriers probably lies in their use together with hydrophobized prodrugs where an active drug is attached to the hydrophobic anchor through some sort of cleavable spacer (Trubetskoy and Torchilin, 1995).

CLINICAL TRIALS

Block copolymer micelle formulations of doxorubicin and paclitaxel are both in Phase I/II trials for the treatment of advanced cancers. To date, seven polymeric micellar formulations have reached preclinical and clinical trials (Table 13.10). Among them, Genexol-PM® has been approved for clinical use as the first-line treatment for breast cancer, lung cancer, and ovarian cancer.

TABLE 13.10
Polymeric Micellar Delivery Systems in Clinical Trials

Trade Name	Polymer Category	Incorporated Drug	Progress	Most Significant Outcome	References
NK911	PEO-b-PLAA	DOX/chemically conjugated and physically loaded	Phase II	Significant pharmacokinetic improvement and tumor accumulation	Matsumura (2008)
NK105	PEO-b-PLAA	Paclitaxel/ physically loaded	Phase I	Improved tumor accumulation and anti-tumor activity in mice	Danson (2004)
NC-6004	PEO-b-PLAA	Cisplatine/to form complex	Phase I	Reduced nephrotoxicity and neurotoxicity in rats (preclinical)	Hamaguchi (2005)
SP1049C	Pluronic	DOX/physically loaded	Phase II	Partial response in some patients	Kim (2004)
PAXCEED®	PEO-b-poly(ester)	Paclitaxel/ physically loaded	Phase I/II	Lower toxicity (mice) and increase in solubility (no pharmacokinetic improvement)	Angiotech Pharmaceuticals (2006)
Genexol®-PM	PEO-b-poly(ester)	Paclitaxel/ physically loaded	Clinical use	Increased MTD (no pharmacokinetic improvement)	Zhang (2005)
NK012	PEO-b-(Glu)	7-ethyl-10-hydroxy camptothecin/ chemically conjugated	Phase I	Enhanced and prolonged distribution of free SN-38 in the tumor, improved anti-tumor activity in mice (preclinical)	Yoo (2001)

DOXORUBICIN

NK-911

NK-911 was the first polymeric micelle system to enter human clinical trials successfully in Japan. NK-911 is a PEO-*b*-poly(asptaric acid) with covalently linked doxorubicin side groups in the hydrophobic block (PEO-*b*-P(Asp)-DOX). The modified core block copolymer is used to physically entrap large quantities of DOX. Studies revealed that it is the physically entrapped DOX, and not the chemically conjugated DOX, that plays a significant role in the anti-tumor activity of PEO-*b*-P(Asp)-DOX micelles (Yokoyama et al., 1994). Preclinical studies of NK-911 revealed up to a 28.9-fold increase in the plasmal AUC compared with the commercial formulation, and a 3.4- to 7.4-fold increase in tumor AUC and activity in C26-bearing mice (Yokoyama et al., 1998; Nakanishi et al., 2001). Phase I studies of NK-911 against several advanced tumors determined the micelle formulation to be well tolerated, with major side effects being moderate nausea and vomiting. Currently, phase II studies are underway for patients with metastatic pancreatic cancer at an MTD of 50 mg/m^2 (Matsumura, 2004).

SP-1049C

SP-1049C is a Pluronic formulation of doxorubicin, which uses a mixture of two Pluronics that is, L-61 and F-127, to form a mixed micelle physically entrapping DOX. Preclinical studies of SP-1049C showed a 1.2-fold increase in plasma AUC, a 1.2-fold decrease in CL, and a 1.4-fold decrease in V$_d$ in Lewis lung carcinoma–bearing mice, as compared to free DOX. The toxicity profiles were similar for the micelle formulation and the free drug, but biodistribution experiments indicated a 1.6-fold increase in the brain AUC and 1.7-fold increase in the tumor AUC for SP-1049C (Alakahov, 1999). Phase I clinical trials in Canada of SP-1049C found a slower terminal clearance compared with free conventional DOX, but otherwise phamacokinetics were similar. Dose excalation studies determined that the recommended phase II MTD of SP-1049C be 70 mg/m^2, with dose-limiting myelosuppression at 90 mg/m^2. Evidence of activity was observed in some patients with refractory solid tumors (Danson et al., 2004). A phase II study in inoperable esophagus carcinoma observed partial responses at 75 mg/m^2, and the major side effects were haematological, neutropenia, leucopenia, nausea, anorexia, lethargy, neutropaenia, weight loss, vomiting, mucositis, and alopecia. Half of the recipients had to be reduced to 55 mg/m^2 after the first cycle, and there was a significant fall in cardiac function in some patients, measured as left ventricular ejection fraction (Valle et al., 2004).

PACLITAXEL

NK-105

NK-105 is the only micellar formulation of paclitaxel (PAX) so far to show improved pharmacokinetics in preclinical trials compared with the commercial Cremophor EL paclitaxel formulation, Taxol. NK-105 is a PEO-*b*-PBLA formulation physically encapsulating PAX. Preclinical trials found the plasma AUC was 90-fold higher for NK-105 compared with free PAX, owing to lower leakage from normal blood vessels and reduced uptake by the RES. The tumor AUC in a colorectal xenograph was 25-fold higher for NK-105. Furthermore, neurotoxicity was significantly less for NK-105 compared with free PAX (Hamaguchi et al., 2005). Phase I trials of NK-105 began in April 2004, and results are pending.

PAXCEED

The PEO-*b*-P(d, l-lactic acid) (PEO-*b*-PDDLA) formulation of PAX, PAXCEED, was reported by Zhang et al. (1996a) to increase the solubility of PAX 5000-fold, encapsulating 25% w/w PAX. However, preclinical studies found PEO-*b*-PDLLA decreased the AUC of PAX 5.5-fold, and PAX was found to rapidly disassociate from the micelle after intravenous administration to rats

(Zhang et al., 1997a,b). Leung et al. (2000) found in a LNCaP prostate tumor xenograph that PAXCEED reduced the tumor size 91% after three treatment cycles and caused no significant side effects or mortality, whereas the conventional Taxol formulation killed all the rodents within 1 day. In a phase II pilot trial of PAXCEED for severe psoriasis, all patients ($n = 5$) showed a significant response (60% reduction in Psoriasis Area and Severity Index [PASI]), and PAXCEED was well tolerated (Ehrlich et al., 2004). A phase II trial of PAXCEED for multiple sclerosis failed to improve patient outcome, but a phase II trial of PAXCEED for rheumatoid arthritis is ongoing (Angiotech Pharmaceuticals, 2006).

Genexol-PM

Genexol-PM is another PEO-*b*-PDDLA micellar formulation of PAX, similar to PAXCEED. It has been approved for clinical use in Korea. It is also the first micellar formulation in clinical use. Similarly, the reduced toxicity of Genexol-PM over Taxol allowed much higher dosing levels to be used in preclinical studies (MTD > 100 mg/kg) than Taxol (MTD 20 mg/kg), although resulting plasma maximum concentrations and AUCs were lower (Kim et al., 2001). Genexol-PM showed better tumor response in murine models of both ovarian and breast cancer (2001). A phase I trial of Genexol-PM showed partial response in 3 of 21 patients, 2 of which were refractory to Taxol. Although the plasma AUC and half-life of Genexol-PM were low ever than Taxol, they were higher than the recently approved Abraxan, an albumin nanoparticle formulation of PAX (Kim et al., 2004). Testing to date has demonstrated significant pharmaceutical and biological advantages for polymeric micelle formulations as compared to standard preparations. The technology enables development of pharmaceutically acceptable formulations with enhanced stability and improved bioavailability of highly water-insoluble drugs. Additional potential of the technology may be realized for manipulating pharmacokinetic parameters and distribution of drug in tissues.

ACKNOWLEDGMENT

The authors would like sincerely to thank Dr. Michelle Long from Abbott Laboratories for her helpful discussion and valuable inputs during the writing of this chapter.

REFERENCES

Abuchowski, A., J. R. McCoy, N. C. Palezuk, J. V. E. Es, and F. F. Davis. 1977. Effect of covalent attachment of polyethylene glycol on immunogenicity and circulating life of bovine liver catalase. *J. Biol. Chem.* 252: 3582–3586.

Adams, M. L. and G. S. Kwon. 2002. The effects of acyl chain length on the micelle properties of poly(ethylene oxide)-block-poly(*N*-hexyl-l-aspartamide)-acyl conjugates. *J. Biomater. Sci. Polym. Edn.* 13: 991–1006.

Adams, M. L. and G. S. Kwon. 2003. Relative aggregation state and hemolytic activity of amphotericin B encapsulated by poly(ethylene oxide)-block-poly(*N*-hexyl-l-aspartamide)-acyl conjugate micelles: Effects of acyl chain length. *J. Control. Rel.* 81: 23–32.

Alakahov, V., E. Klinski, S. Li, G. Pietrzynski, A. Venne, E. Batrakova, T. Bronitch, and A. Kabanov. 1999. Block copolymer-based formulation of doxorubicin. From cell screen to clinical trials. *Coll. Surf. B. Biointerf.* 16: 113–134.

Alakahov, V. Y. and A. V. Kabanov. 1998. Block copolymeric biotransport carriers as versatile vehicles for drug delivery. *Expert Opin. Investig. Drugs.* 7: 1453–1473.

Alexandris, P., V. Athanassiou, S. Fukuda, and T. A. Hatton. 1994a. Surface activity of poly(ethylene oxide-block-poly(propylene oxide)-block-poly(ethylene oxide) copolymers. *Langmuir* 10: 2604–2612.

Alexandris, P., J. F. Holzwarth, and T. A. Hatton. 1994b. Micellization of poly(ethylene oxide)-poly(propylene oxide)-poly(ethylene oxide) triblock copolymers in aqueous solutions: Thermodynamics of copolymer association. *Macromolecules* 27: 2414–2425.

Aliabadi, H. M., D. R. Brocks, and A. Lavasanifar. 2005b. Polymeric micelles for the solubilization and delivery of cyclosporine A: Pharmacokinetics and biodistribution. *Biomaterials* 26: 7251–7259.

Aliabadi, H. M. and A. Lavasanifar. 2006. Polymeric micelles for drug delivery. *Expert Opin. Drug Deliv.* 3: 139–162.

Aliabadi, H. M., A. Mahmud, A. D. Sharifabadi, and A. Lavasanifar. 2005a. Micelles of methoxy poly(ethylene oxide)-*b*-poly(ε-caprolactone) as vehicles for the solubilization and controlled delivery of cyclosporine A. *J. Control. Rel.* 104: 301–311.

Allemann, E., J. C. Leroux, and R. Gurny. 1998. Biodegradable nanoparticles of poly(lactic acid) and poly(lactic-*c*-glycolic acid) for parenteral administration. In *Pharmaceutical Dosage Forms: Disperse Systems*, Lieberman, H., Rieger, M., Banker, G. (Eds.), Vol. 3, New York, Marcel Dekker, pp. 163–193.

Allen, T. M., C. Hansen, and J. Rutledge. 1989. Liposomes with prolonged circulation times: Factors affecting uptake by reticuloendothelial and other tissues. *Biochim. Biophys. Acta.* 981: 27–35.

Almeida, L. M., W. L. C. Vaz, K. A. Zachariasse, and X. C. Madeta. 1982. Fluidity of satcoplasmic reticulum membranes investigated with dipyrenylpropane, an intramolecular excimer probe. *Biochemistry* 21: 5972–5977.

Almgren, M., J. Alsins, and P. Bahadur. 1991a. Fluorescence quenching and excimer formation to probe the micellization of a poly(ethylene oxide)-poly(propylene oxde)-poly(ethylene oxide) block copolymer, as modulated by potassium fluoride in aqueous solution. *Langmuir* 7: 446–450.

Almgren, M., P. Bahadur, M. Jansson, P. Li, W. Brown, and A. Bahadur. 1992. Static and dynamic properties of a (PEO-PPO-PEO) block copolymer in aqueous solution. *J. Coll. Interf. Sci.* 151: 157–165.

Almgren, M., W. Brown, and S. Hvidt. 1995. Self-aggregation and phase behavior of poly(ethylene oxide)-poly(propylene oxide)-poly(ethylene oxide) block copolymers in aqueous solution. *Coll. Polym. Sci.* 273: 2–15.

Almgren, M., J. Van Stam, C. Lindblad, P. Stilbs, and P. Bahadur. 1991b. Aggregation of poly(ethylene oxide)-poly(propylene oxide)-poly(ethylene oxide) triblock copolymers in the presence of sodium dodecyl sulfate in aqueous solution. *J. Phys. Chem.* 95: 5677–5684.

Al-Saden, A. A., A. T. Florence, T. K. Whatley, F. Puisieux, and C. Vautuion. 1982. Characterization of mixed nonionic surfactant micelles by photon correlation spectroscopy and viscosity. *J. Coll. Interf. Sci.* 86: 51–56.

Ambler, L. E., L. Brookman, J. Brown, P. Goddard, and K. Petrak. 1992. Soluble polymeric carriers for drug delivery. 5. Solution properties and biodistribution behavior of n-(2-hydroxypropyl)methacryl-amide-co-*n*-(2-[4-hydroxy phenyl]ethyl)-acrylamidecopolymers substituted with cholesterol. *J. Bioact. Compat. Polym.* 7: 223–241.

Angiotech Pharmaceuticals, specialize in the design and manufacturing of high performance surgical knives and wound closure products. 2006. http://www.angiotech.com/.

Antonietti, M., S. Heinz, M. Schmidt, and C. Rosenauer. 1994. Determination of the micelle architecture of polystyrene/poly(4-vinylpyridine) block copolymers in dilute solution. *Macromolecules* 27: 3276–3281.

Astafieva, I., X. Zhong, and F. A. Eisenberg. 1993. Critical micellization phenomena in block polyelectrolyte solutions. *Macromolecules* 26: 7339–7352.

Attwood, D., G. Ktistic, Y. McCormick, and M. J. Story. 1989. Solubilization of indomethacin by polysorbate 80 in mixed water-sorbitol solvents. *J. Pharm. Pharmacol.* 41: 83–86.

Bader, H., H. Ringsdorf, and B. Schmidt. 1984. Water soluble polymers in medicine. *Angew. Chem.* 123/124: 457–463.

Bahadur, P., M. Almgren, M. Jansson, P. Li, W. Brown, and A. Bahadur. 1992a. Static and dynamic properties of a (PEO-PPO-PEO) block copolymer in aqueous solution. *J. Coll. Interf. Sci.* 151: 157–165.

Bahadur, P., P. Li, P. M. Almgren, and W. Brown. 1992b. Effect of potassium fluoride on the micellar behavior of Pluronic F-68 in aqueous solution. *Langmuir* 8: 1903–1907.

Bahadur, P., N. V. Sastry, and Y. K. Rao. 1988. Interaction studies of styrene-ethylene oxide block copolymers with ionic surfactants in aqueous solution. *Colloids Surf.* 29: 343–358.

BASF. 1989. Corporation brochure on pluronic and tetronic surfactants.

Batrakova, E., H. Han, V. Y. Alakhov, D. W. Miller, and A. V. Kabanov. 1998. Effects of pluronic block copolymers on drug absorption in Caco-2 cell monolayers. *Pharm. Res.* 15: 850–855.

Beezer, A. E., W. Loh, J. C. Mitchell, P. G. Royall, D. O. Smith, M. S. Tute, J. K. Armstrong. et al. 1994. An investigation of dilute aqueous solution behavior of poly(oxyethylene)+poly(oxypropylene)+poly(oxyethylene) block copolymers. *Langmuir* 10: 4001–4005.

Bohorquez, M., C. Koch, T. Trygstad, and N. Pandit. 1999. A study of the temperature-dependent micellization of Pluronic F127. *J. Coll. Interf. Sci.* 216: 34–40.

Briganti, G., S. Puvvada, and D. Blankschtein. 1991. Effect of urea on micellar properties of aqueous solutions of nonionic surfactants. *J. Phys. Chem.* 95: 8989–8995.

Cammas, S., K. Suzuki, Y. Sone, Y. Sakurai, K. Kataoka, and T. Okano. 1997. Thermoresponsive polymer nanoparticles with a core-shell micelle structure as site specific drug carriers. *J. Control. Rel.* 48: 157–164.

Carlsson, A., G. Karlstrom, and B. Lindman. 1986. Synergistic surfactant-electrolyte effect in polymer solutions. *Langmuir* 2: 536–537.

Chen, G. and A. S. Hoffman. 1995. Grafted copolymers that exhibit temperature-induced phased transitions over a wide range of pH. *Nature* 373: 49–52.

Chen, W. Y., P. Alexandridis, C. K. Su, C. S. Patrickios, W. R. Hertler, and T. A. Hatton. 1995. Effect of block size and sequence on the micellization of ABC triblock methacrylic acid polyampholytes. *Macromolecules* 28: 8604–8611.

Chung, J. E., M. Yokoyama, T. Aoyagi, Y Sakurai, and T. Okano. 1998. Effect of molecular architecture of hydrophobically modified poly(*N*-isopropylacrylamide) on the formation of thermo-responsive core-shell micellar drug carriers. *J. Control. Rel.* 53: 119–130.

Chung, J. E., M. Yokoyama, K. Suzuki, T. Aoyagi, Y. Sakurai, and T. Okano. 1997. Reversibly thermoresponsive alkyl-terminated poly(*N*-isopropylacrylamide) core-shell micellar structures. *Coll. Surf. (B. Biointerf.)* 9: 37–48.

Chung, J. E., M. Yokoyama, M. Yamato, T. Aoyagi, Y. Sakurai, and T. Okano. 1999. Thermo-responsive drug delivery from polymeric micelles constructed using block copolymers of poly(*N*-isopropylacrylamide) and poly(butylmethacrylate). *J. Control. Rel.* 62: 115–127.

Connor, J., N. Noriey, and L. Huang. 1986. Biodistribution of immunoliposomes. *Biochem. Biophys. Acta* 884: 474–481.

Croy, S. R. and G. S. Kwon. 2004. The effects of Pluronic block copolymers on the aggregation state of nystatin. *J. Control. Rel.* 95: 161–171.

Dan, N. and M. Tirrell. 1993. Self-assembly of block copolymers with strongly charged and a hydrophobic block in a selective, polar solvent. Micelles and adsorbed layers. *Macromolecules* 26: 4310–4315.

Danson, S., D. Ferry, V. Alakhov, J. Margison, D. Kerr, D. Jowle, M. Brampton, G. Halbert, and M. Ranson. 2004. Phase I dose escalation and pharmacokinetic study of pluronic polymer-bound doxorubicin (SP1049C) in patients with advanced cancer. *Br. J. Cancer* 90(11): 2085–2091.

Daoud, M. and J. P. Cotton. 1982. Star shaped polymers: A model for the conformation and its concentration dependence. *J. Phys.* 43: 531–538.

Davis, S. S., L. Ilium, S. M. Moghimi, M. C. Davies, C. J. H. Porter, L. S. Miur, A. Brindley. et al. 1993. Microspheres for targeting drugs to specific body sites. *J. Control. Rel.* 24: 157–163.

Donbrow, M. and E. Azaz. 1976. Solubilization of phenolic compounds in nonionic surface-active agents. II. Cloud point and phase changes in solubilization of phenol cresols, xylenols, and benzoic acid. *J. Coll. Interf. Sci.* 57: 20–27.

Dong, D. C. and M. A. Wittalk. 1984. The Py scale of solvent polarities. *Can. J. Chem.* 62: 2560–2568.

Dong, L.-C. and A. S. Hoffman. 1991. A novel approach for preparation of pH-sensitive hydrogels for enteric drug delivery. *J. Control. Rel.* 15: 141–152.

Dvorak, F., B. Lawrence, M. Detmar, and A. M. Dvorak. 1995. Vascular permeability factor/vascular endothelial growth factor, microvascular hyperpermeability, and angiogenesis. *Am. J. Pathol.* 146: 1029–1039.

Dvorak, H. F., N. S. Orenstein, A. C. Carvalho, W. H. Churchill, A. M. Dvorak, S. J. Galli, J. Feder, A. M. Bitzer, J. Rypysc, and P. Giovinco. 1979. Induction of a fibrin-gel investment: An early event in line 10 hepatocarcinoma growth mediated by tumor-secreted products. *J. Immunol.* 122: 166–174.

Enoch, H. G. and P. Strittmatter. 1979. Formation and properties of 1000-A-diameter, single bilayer phospholipid vesicles. *Proc. Natl. Acad. Sci. USA* 76: 145–148.

Ehrlich, A., S. Booher, Y. Becerra, D. L. Borris, W. D. Figg, M. L. Turner, and A. Blauvelt. 2004. Micellar paclitaxel improves severe psoriasis in a prospective phase II pilot study. *J. Am. Acad. Dermatol.* 50: 533–540.

Evans D. F. and H. Wenerstrom. 1994. *The Colloidal Domain, Where Physics, Chemistry, Biology, and Technology Meet*, New York, VCH.

Flory, P. J. 1941. Thermodynamics of high polymer solutions. *J. Chem. Phys.* 9: 660.

Forrest, M. L., C.-W. Won, A. W. Malick, and G. S. Kwon. 2006. *In vitro* release of the mTOR inhibitor rapamycin from poly(ethylene glycol)-*b*-poly(ε-caprolactone) micelles. *J. Control. Rel.* 110: 370–377.

Gadelle, F., W. J. Koros, and R. S. Schechter, 1995. Solubilization of aromatic solutes in block copolymers. *Macromolecules* 28: 4883–4892.

Gao, Z. and A. Eisenberg. 1993. A model of micellization for block copolymers in solutions. *Macromolecules* 26: 7353–7360.

Ge, H., Y. Hu, X. Jiang, D. Cheng, Y. Yuan, H. Bi, and C. Yang. 2002. Preparation, characterization, and drug release behaviors of drug nimodipine-loaded poly(ε-caprolactone)-poly(ethyleneoxide)-poly(ε-caprolactone) amphiphilic triblock copolymer micelles. *J. Pharm. Sci.* 91: 1463–1473.

Goldmints, I., J. F. Holzwarth, K. A. Smith, and T. A. Hatton. 1997. Micellar dynamics in aqueous solutions of PEO-PPO-PEO block copolymers. *Langmuir* 13: 6130–6134.

Grant, C. W. M., S. Karlik, and E. Florio. 1989. A liposomal MRI contrast agent: Phosphatidyl ethanolamine. *Magn. Res. Med.* 11: 236–243.

Guo, C., J. Wang, H. Z. Liu, and J. Y. Chen. 1999. Hydration and conformation of temperature-dependent micellization of PEO-PPO-PEO block copolymers in aqueous solutions by FT-Raman. *Langmuir* 15: 2703–2708.

Hagan, S. A., G. A. Coombes, M. C. Garnett, S. E. Dunn, M. C. Davies, L. Illum, S. S. Davis, S. E. Harding, S. Parkiss, and P. R. Gellert. 1996. Polylactide-poly(ethylene glycol) copolymers as drug delivery systems. 1. Characterization of water dispersible micelle-forming systems. *Langmuir* 12: 2153–2161.

Halperin, A. 1987. Polymeric micelles: A star model. *Macromolecules* 20: 2943–2946.

Hamaguchi, T., Y. Matsumura, M. Suzuki, K. Shimizu, R. Goda, I. Nakamura, I. Nakatomi, M. Yokoyama, K. Kataoka, and T. Kakizoe. 2005. NK105, a paclitaxel-incorporating micellar nanoparticle formulation, can extend *in vivo* antitumour activity and reduce the neurotoxicity of paclitaxel. *Br. J. Cancer.* 92: 1240–1246.

Hamza, Y. E. and M. Kata. 1989. Influence of certain hydrotropic and complexing agents on solubilization of allopurinol. *Pharm. Ind.* 51: 1159–1162.

Han, S. K., S. M. Lee, M. Kim, and H. Schott. 1989. Effect of protein denaturants on cloud point and Krafft point of nonionic surfactants. *J. Coll. Interf. Sci.* 132: 444–450.

Hancock, B. C. and G. Zografi. 1993. The use of solution theories for predicting water vapor absorption by amorphous pharmaceutical solids: A test of the Flory-Huggins and Vrentas models. *Pharm. Res.* 10: 1262–1267.

Hatada, A. and A. Kataoka. 1995. Formation of polyion complex micelles in an aqueous milieu from a pair of oppositely-charged block copolymers with poly(ethylene glycol) segments. *Macromolecules* 28: 5294–5299.

Hatada, A. and K. Kataoka. 1998. Novel polyion complex micelles entrapping enzyme molecules in the core: Preparation of narrowly-distributed micelles from lysozyme and poly(ethylene glycol)-poly(aspartic acid) block copolymer in aqueous medium. *Macromolecules* 31: 288–294.

Heskins, M. and J. E. Guillet. 1968. Solution properties of poly(*N*-isopropylacrylamide). *J. Macromol. Sci. Chem. A* 2: 1441–1455.

Holzwarth, J. F., A. Schmidt, H. Wolff, and R. Volk. 1977. Nanosecond temperature-jump technique with an iodine laser. *J. Phys. Chem.* 81: 2300–2301.

Hurterr, P. N., J. M. H. M. Scheutjens, T. A. Hatton, and T. Alan. 1993a. Molecular modeling of micelle formation and solubilization in block copolymer micelles. 1. A self-consistent mean-field lattice theory. *Macromolecules* 26: 5592–5601.

Hurterr, P. N., J. M. H. M. Scheutjens, T. A. Hatton, and T. Alan. 1993b. Molecular modeling of micelle formation and solubilization in block copolymer micelles. 2. Lattice theory for monomers with internal degrees of freedom. *Macromolecules* 26: 5030–5040.

Innocenti, F., R. Danesi, A. D. Paolo, C. Agen, D. Nardini, G. Bocci, and M. D. Tacca. 1995. Plasma and tissue disposition of paclitaxel after intraperitoneal administration in mice. *Drug Metab. Dispos.* 23: 713–717.

Inoue, T., G. Chen, K. Nakamae, and A. S. Hoffman. 1998. An AB block copolymer of oligo(methyl methacrylate) and poly(acrylic acid) for micellar delivery of hydrophobic drugs. *J. Control. Rel.* 51: 221–229.

Jain, R. K. 1997. Delivery of molecular and cellular medicine to solid tumors. *Adv. Drug Deliv. Rev.* 26: 71–90.

Jette, K. K., D. Law, E. A. Schmitt, and G. S. Kwon. 2004. Preparation and drug loading of poly(ethylene glycol)-block-poly(ε-caprolactone) micelles through the evaporation of a cosolvent azeotrope. *Pharm. Res.* 21: 1184–1191.

Johnson, B. K. and R. K. Prud'homme. 2003a. Mechanism for rapid self-assembly of block copolymer nanoparticles. *Phys. Rev. Lett.* 91: 118302.1–118302.4.

Johnson, B. K. and R. K. Prud'homme. 2003b. Chemical processing and micromixing in confined impinging jets. *AIChE J.* 49: 2264–2282.

Jones, M. C. and J. C. Leroux. 1999. Polymeric micelles—A new generation of colloidal drug carries. *Eur. J. Pharm. Biopharm.* 48: 101–111.

Joralemon, M. J., R. K. O'Reilly, C. J. Hawker, and K. L. Wooley. 2005. Shell click-crosslinked (SCC) nanoparticles: A new methodology for synthesis and orthogonal functionalization. *J. Am. Chem. Soc.* 127: 16892–16899.

Kabalka, G., E. Buonocore, K. Hubner, M. Davis, and L. Huang. 1989. Gadolinium-labeled liposomes containing paramagnetic amphipatic agents: Targeted MRI contrast agent for the liver. *Magn. Res. Med.* 8: 89–95.

Kabanov, A. V., E. V. Batrakova, N. S. Melik-Nubarov, N. A. Fedoseev, T. Y. Dorodnich, V. Y. Alakhov, V. P. Chekhonin, I. R. Nazarova, and V. A. Kabanov. 1992. A new class of drug carriers: Micelles of poly(oxyethylene)-poly(oxypropylene) block copolymers as microcontainers for drug targeting from blood in brain. *J. Control. Rel.* 22: 141–158.

Kabanov, A. V., I. R. Nazarrova, I. V. Astafieva, E. V. Batrakova, V. Y. Alakhov, A. A. Yaroslavov, and V. A. Kabanov. 1995. Micelle formation and solubilization of luorescent probes in poly(oxyethylene-*b-o*ypropylene-*b*-oxyethylene) solutions. *Macromolecules* 28: 2303–2314.

Kalyanasundaram, K. and J. K. Thomas. 1977. Environmental effects on vibronic band intensities in pyrene monomer fluorescence and their application in studies of micellar systems. *J. Am. Chem. Soc.* 99: 2039–2044.

Karlstrom, G. 1985. A new model for upper and lower critical solution temperatures in poly(ethylene oxide) solutions. *J. Phys. Chem.* 89: 4962–4964.

Kataoda, K., G. S. Kwon, M. Yokoyama, T. Okano, and Y. Sakurai. 1993. Block copolymer micelles as vehicles for drug delivery. *J. Control. Rel.* 24: 119–132.

Kataoka, K. 1994. Design of nanoscopic vehicles for drug targeting based on micellization of amphiphilic block copolymers. *J. Macromol. Sci.—Pure Appl. Chem. A* 31: 1759–1769.

Kataoka, K., H. Togawa, A. Hareda, K. Yasugi, T. Matsumoto, and S. Katayose. 1996. Spontaneous formation of polyion complex micelles with narrow distribution from antisense oligonucleotide and cationic block copolymer in physiological saline. *Macromolecules* 29: 8556–8557.

Katayose, S. and K. Kataoka. 1997. Water-soluble polyion complex associates of DNA and poly(ethylene glycol)-poly(l-lysine) black copolymer. *Bioconj. Chem.* 8: 702–707.

Katayose, S. and K. Kataoka. 1998. Remarkable increase in nuclease resistance of plasmid DNA through supramolecular assembly with poly(ethylene glycol)-poly(l-lysine) block copolymer. *J. Pharm. Sci.* 87: 160–163.

Katre, N. V., M. J. Knauf, and W. J. Lair. 1987. Chemical modification of recombinant interleukin 2 by polyethylene glycol increases its potency in the murine Meth A sarcoma model. *Proc. Natl. Acad. Sci. USA* 84: 1487–1491.

Khougaz, K., I. Astafieva, and A. Eisenberg. 1995. Micellization in block polyelectrolyte solutions. 3. Static light scattering characterization. *Macromolecules* 28: 7135–7147.

Kim, S. C., D. W. Kim, Y. H. Shim, J. S. Bang, H. S. Oh, S. W. Kim, and M. H. Seo. 2001. *In vivo* evaluation of polymeric micellar paclitaxel formulation: Toxicity and efficacy. *J. Control. Rel.* 53: 131136.

Kim, S. Y., I. G. Shin, Y. M. Lee, C. S. Cho, and Y. K. Sung. 1998. Methoxy poly(ethylene glycol) and ε-caprolactone amphiphilic block copolymeric micelle containing indomethacin. II. Micelle formation and drug release behaviors. *J. Control. Rel.* 51: 13–22.

Kim, T.-Y., D.-W. Kim, J.-Y. Chung, S. G. Shin, S.-C. Kim, D. S. Heo, N. K. Kim, and Y.-J. Bang. 2004. Phase I and pharmacokinetic study of Genexol-P, a Cremophor-free polymeric micelle-formulation paclitaxel with advanced malignancies. *Clin. Cancer Res.* 10: 3708–3716.

Klibanov, A. L., K. Maruyama, V. P. Torchtlin, and L. Huang. 1990. Amphipathic polyethyleneglycols effectively prolong the circulation time of liposomes. *FEBS Lett.* 268: 235–238.

Kohori, F., K. Sakai, T. Aoyagi, M. Yokoyama, Y. Sakurai, and T. Okano. 1998. Preparation and characterization of thermally responsive block copolymer micelles comprising poly(*N*-isopropylacrylamide-*b*-dl-lactide). *J. Control. Rel.* 55: 87–98.

Krevelen, D. V. 1990. Cohesive properties and solubility, In *Properties of Polym: Their Correlation with Chemical Structure*, Krevelen, D. V. (Ed.), New York, Elsevier Scientific Publication Co, pp. 189–224.

Kwon, G., M. Naito, M. Yokoyama, T. Okano, Y. Sakurai, and K. Kataoka. 1993a. Micelles based on ab block copolymers of poly(ethylene oxide) and poly(-benzyl-aspartate). *Langmuir* 9: 945–949.

Kwon, G. S. 1998. Diblock copolymer nanoparticles for drug delivery. *CRC Crit. Rev. Ther. Drug Carrier Syst.* 20: 357–512.

Kwon, G. S. 2003. Polymeric micelles for delivery of poorly water-soluble compounds. *Crit. Rev. Ther. Drug Carrier Syst.* 25: 357–403.

Kwon, G. S. and K. Kataoda. 1995. Block copolymer micelles as long-circulating drug vehicles. *Adv. Drug Delivery Rev.* 16: 295–309.

Kwon, G. S., M. Naito, K. Kataoka, M. Yokoyama, Y. Sakurai, and T. Okano. 1994a. Block copolymer micelles as vehicles for hydrophobic drugs. *Coll. Surf. B: Bioint.* 2: 429–434.

Kwon, G. S., M. Naito, M. Yokoyama, T. Okano, Y. Sakurai, and K. Kataoka. 1995. Physical entrapment of adriamycin in AB block copolymer micelles. *Pharm. Res.* 12: 192–195.

Kwon, G., M. Naito, M. Yokoyama, T. Okano, Y. Sakurai, and K. Karaoka. 1997. Block copolymer micelles for drug delivery: Loading and release of doxorubicin. *J. Control. Rel.* 48: 195–201.

Kwon, G. S. and T. Okano. 1996. Polymeric micelles as new drug carriers. *Adv. Drug Del. Rev.* 16: 107–116.

Kwon, G. S. and T. Okano. 1999. Soluble self-assembled block copolymers for drug delivery. *Pharm. Res.* 16: 597–600.

Kwon, G. S., S. Suwa, M. Yokoyama, T. Okano, Y. Sakurai, and K. Kataoka. 1994b. Enhanced tumor accumulation and prolonged circulation times of micelle-forming poly(ethylene oxide-aspartate) block copolymers-adriamycin conjugates. *J. Control. Rel.* 29: 17–23.

Kwon, G. S., M. Yokoyama, T. Okano, Y. Sakurai, and K. Kataoka. 1993b. Biodistribution of micelle-forming polymer-drug conjugates. *Pharm. Res.* 10: 970–974.

La, S. B., T. Okano, and K. Kataoka. 1996. Preparation and characterization of the micelle-forming polymeric drug indomethacin-incorporated poly(ethylene oxide)-poly(-benzyl l-aspartate) block copolymer micelles. *J. Pharm. Sci.* 85: 85–90.

Lacoulonche, F., A. Chauvet, J. Masse, M. A. Egea, and M. L. Garcia. 1998. An investigation of FB interactions with poly(ethylene glycol) 6000, poly(ethylene glycol) 4000, and poly-ε-caprolactone by thermoanalytical and spectroscopic methods and modeling. *J. Pharm. Sci.* 87: 543–551.

Lasie, D. D., M. C. Woodie, F. J. Martin, and T. Valentincic. 1991. Phase behavior of "stealth-lipid" decithin mixtures. *Period. Biol.* 93: 9287–9290.

Lavasanifar A., J. Samuel, and G. S. Kwon. 2001. The effect of alkyl core structure on micellar properties of poly(ethylene oxide)-block-poly(l-aspartamide) derivatives. *Coll. Surf. B: Bioint.* 22: 115–126.

Leung, S. Y. L., J. Jackson, H. Miyake, H. Burt, and M. E. Gleave. 2000. Polymeric micellar paclitaxel phosphorylates Bcl-2 and induces apoptotic regression of androgen-independent LNCaP prostate tumors. *Prostate* 44: 156–163.

Lieberman, H. A., M. M. Rieger, and G. S. Banker. 1996. *Pharmaceutical Dosage Forms: Disperse Systems*, Vol. 1, New York, Marcel Dekker Inc.

Lin, S. Y. 1987. Pluronic surfactants affecting diazepam solubility, compatibility, and absorption from i.v. admixture solutions. *J. Parenteral Sci. Technol.* 41: 83–87.

Lin, S. Y. and J. C. Yang. 1987. Solubility and thermodynamic parameters of diazepam in Pluronic surfactant solutions. *Acta Pharm. Technol.* 33: 222–224.

Lindman, B. and H. Wennerstrom. 1980. Micelles. Amphiphile aggregation in aqueous solution. *Top. Curr. Chem.* 87: 1–83.

Linse, P. 1993. Micellization of poly(ethylene oxide)-poly(propylene oxide) block copolymers in aqueous solution. *Macromolecules* 26: 4437–4449.

Linse, P. and M. Malmsten. 1992. Temperature-dependent micellization in aqueous block copolymer solutions. *Macromolecules* 25: 5434–5439.

Liu, J., Y. Xiao, and C. Allen. 2003. Polymer-drug compatibility: A guide to the development of delivery systems for the anticancer agent, ellipticine. *J. Pharm. Sci.* 93: 132–143.

Maeda, H. and Y. Matsushima. 1989. Tumoritropic and lymphotropic principles of macromolecular drugs. *CRC Crit. Rev. Ther. Drug Carrier Syst.* 6: 193–210.

Maeda, H., L. W. Seymour, and Y. Miyamoto. 1992. Conjugates of anticancer agents and polymers: Advantages of macromolecular therapeutics *in vivo*. *Bioconj. Chem.* 3: 351–361.

Mahmud, A., X. B. Xiong, and A. Lavasanifar. 2008. Development of novel polymeric micellar drug conjugates and nano-containers with hydrolyzable core structure for doxorubicin delivery. *Eur. J. Pharm. Biopharm.* 69(3): 923–934.

Marko, J. F. and Y. Rabin. 1992. Microphase separation of charged diblock copolymers: Melts and solutions. *Macromolecules* 25: 1503–1509.

Marques, C. M. 1997. Bunchy micelles. *Langmuir* 13: 1430–1433.

Marques, C. M., J. F. Joanny, and L. Leibler. 1988. Adsorption of block copolymers in selective solvents. *Macromolecules* 21: 1051–1059.

Marshall, L. 1988. Cloud point of mixed ionic-nonionic surfactant solutions in the presence of electrolytes. *Langmuir* 4: 90–93.

Martin, S. R. 1980. Absorption and circular dichroic spectral studies in the self-association of daunomycin. *Biopolymers* 19: 713–721.

Matsukata, M., T. Aoki, K. Sanui, N. Ogata, A. Kikuchi, Y. Sakurai, and T. Okano. 1996. Effect of molecular architecture of poly(N-isopropylacrylamide)-trypsin conjugates on their solution and enzymatic properties. *Bioconj. Chem.* 7: 96–101.

Matsumura, Y. 2008. Poly (amino acid) micelle nanocarriers in preclinical and clinical studies. *Adv. Drug Deliv. Rev.* 60(8): 899–914.

Matsumura, Y. and H. Maeda. 1986. A new concept for macromolecular therapeutics in cancer chemotherapy: Mechanism of tumoritropic accumulation of proteins and the antitumor agent sroaries. *Cancer Res.* 46: 6387–6392.

Matsumura, Y., T. Hamaguchi, T. Ura, K. Muro, Y. Yamada, Y. Shimada, K. Shirao. et al. 2004. Phase I clinical trial and pharmacokinetic evaluation of NK911, a micelle-encapsulated doxorubicin. *Br. J. Cancer.* 91: 1775–1781.

McDonald, C. and C. K. Wong. 1974. The effect of temperature on the micellar properties of a polyoxypropylene-polyoxyethylene polymer in water. *J. Pharm. Pharmalol.* 26: 556–557.

Megufo, K., M. Ueno, and K. Esumi. 1987. Nonionic surfactants: Physical chemistry. In *Nonionic Surfactants*: *Physical Chemistry*, Schick, M. J. (Ed.), Surfactant Science Series, Vol. 23, New York, Marcel Dekker, p. 109.

Miller, D. W., E. V. Batrakova, T. O. Waltner, V. Y. Alakhov, and A. V. Kabanov. 1997. Interactions of Pluronic block copolymers with brain microvessel endothelial cells: Evidence of two potential pathways for drug. *Bioconj. Chem.* 8: 649–657.

Moghimi, S. M., A. E. Hawley, N. M. Christy, T. Gray, L. Ilium, and S. S. Davis. 1994. Surface engineered nanospheres with enhanced drainage into lymphatics and uptake by macrophages of the regional lymph node. *FEBS Lett.* 344: 25–30.

Mortensen, K., W. Brown, and E. Jorgensen. 1994. Phase behavior of poly(propylene oxide)-poly(ethylene oxide)-poly(propylene oxide) triblock copolymer melt and aqueous solutions. *Macromolecules* 27: 5654–5666.

Nabeshima, Y., A. Maruyama, T. Tsuruta, and K. Kataoka. 1987. A polyamine macromonomer having controlled molecular weight—Synthesis and mechanism. *Polym. J.* 19: 593–601.

Nagarajan, R., M. Barry, and E. Ruckenstein. 1986. Unusual selectivity in solubilization by block copolymer micelles. *Langmuir* 2: 210–215.

Nagarajan, R. and K. Ganesh. 1989a. Block copolymer self-assembly in selective solvents: Theory of solubilization in spherical micelles. *Macromolecules* 22: 4312–4325.

Nagarajan, R. and K. Ganesh. 1989b. Block copolymer self-assembly in selective solvents: Spherical micelles with segregated cores. *J. Chem. Phys.* 90: 5843–5856.

Nagasaki, Y., T. Okada, C. Scholz, M. Iijima, M. Kato, and Kataoka. 1998. The reactive polymeric micelle based on an aldehyde-ended poly(-ethylene glycol)/poly(lactide) block copolymer. *Macromolecules* 31: 1473–1479.

Nair, R., N. Nyamweya, S. Gonen, L. J. Martinez-Miranda, and S. W. Hoag. 2001. Influence of various drugs on the glass transition temperature of poly(vinylpyrolidone): A thermodynamic and spectroscopic investigation. *Int. J. Pharm.* 225: 83–96.

Nakamura, K., R. Eodo, and M. Takeda. 1977. Study of molecular motion of block copolymers in solution by high-resolution proton magnetic resonance. *J. Polym. Sci. Polym. Phys. Ed.* 15: 2095–2101.

Nakanishi, T., S. Fukushima, K. Okamoto, M. Suzuki, Y. Matsumura, M. Yokoyama, T. Okano, Y. Sakurai, and K. Kataoka. 2001. Development of the polymer micelle carrier system for doxorubicin. *J. Control. Rel.* 74: 295–302.

Nakashima, K., T. Anzai, and Y. Fujimoto. 1994. Fluorescence studies on the properties of a Pluronic F68 micelles. *Langmuir* 10: 658–661.

Okano, T., N. Yamada, M. Okuhara, H. Sakai, and Y. Sakurai. 1995. Mechanism of cell detachment from temperature-modulated hydrophilie-hydrophobie polymer surfaces. *Biomaterials* 16: 297–303.

Okano, T., N. Yarnada, H. Sakai, and Y. Sakural. 1993. A novel recovery system for cultured cells using plasma-treated polystyrene dishes graphed with poly(N-isopropylacrylamida). *J. Biomed. Mater. Res.* 27: 1243–1251.

Pandya, K., P. Bahadur, T. N. Nagar, and A. Bahadur. 1993b. Micellar and solubilizing behavior of Pluronic L64 in water. *Coll. Surf. A: Phys. Eng.* 70: 219–227.

Pandya, K., K. Lad, and P. Bahadur. 1993a. Effect of additives on the clouding behavior of an ethylene oxide-propylene oxide block copolymer in aqueous solution. *J.M.S. Pure Appl. Chem. A* 30: 1–18.

Papisov, M. L. 1995. Modeling *in vivo* transfer of long-circulating polymers (two clases of long circulating polymers and factors affecting their transfer *in vivo*). *Adv. Drug Deliv. Rev.* 16: 127–139.

Park, J. P., J. Y. Lee, Y. S. Chang, J. M. Jeong, J. K. Chung, M. C. Lee, K. B. Park, and S. J. Lee. 2002. Radioisotope carrying polyethylene oxide-polycaprolactone copolymer micelles for targetable bone imaging. *Biomaterials* 22: 873–879.

Patnum, D. and J. Kopecek. 1995. Polymer conjugates with anticancer activity. *Adv. Polym. Sci.* 122: 55–123.

Prasad, K. N., T. T. Luong, A. T. Florence, J. Paris, C. Vaution, M. Seiller, and F. Puisieux. 1979. Surface activity and association of ABA polyoxyethylene-polyoxypropylene block copolymers in aqueous solution. *J. Coll. Interf. Sci.* 69: 225–232.

Price, C. 1983. Micelle formation by block copolymer in organic solvents. *Pure Appl. Chem.* 55: 1563–1572.

Ramaswamy, M., X. Zhang, H. M. Burt, and K. M. Wasan. 1997. Human plasma distribution of free paclitaxel and paclitaxel associated with diblock copolymers. *J. Pharm. Sci.* 86: 460–464.

Ray, A. and G. Nemethy. 1971. Micelle formation by nonionic detergents in water-ethylene glycol mixtures. *J. Phys. Chem.* 75: 809–815.

Reddy, N. K., P. J. Fordham, D. Attwood, and C. Booth. 1990. Association and surface properties of block-copoly(oxyethylene/oxypropylene) L64. *J. Chem. Soc., Faraday Trans.* 86: 1569–1572.

Ringsdorf, H., I. Simon, and F. M. Winnik. 1992. Hydrophobically-modified poly(N-isopropylacrylamides) in water: Probing of the microdomain composition by nonradiative energy transfer. *Macromolecules* 25: 5353–5361.

Ringsdorf, H., J. Venzmer, and F. M. Winnik. 1991. Fluorescence studies of hydrophohically modified poly (N- isopropylacrylamides). *Macromolecules* 24: 1678–1686.

Rolland, A., I. E. O'Mullane, P. Goddard, L. Brookman, and K. Pettrak. 1992. New macromolecular carriers for drugs, I. Preparation and characterization of poly(oxyethylene-b-isoprene-b-oxyethylene) block copolymer aggregates. *J. Appl. Polym. Sci.* 44: 1195–1203.

Saettone, M. F., B. Giannaccini, G. Delmonte, V. Campigli, G. Tota, and F. La Marca. 1988. Solubilization of tropicamide by poloxamers: Physicochemical data and activity data in rabbits and humans. *Int. J. Pharm.* 43: 67–76.

Samadi-Boboli, M., G. Favre, P. Canal, and G. Soula. 1993. Low density lipoprotein for cytotoxic drug targeting: Improved activity of elliptinium derivative against B16 melanoma in mice. *Br. J. Cancer* 68: 319–326.

Savić, R., T. Azzam, A. Eisenberg, and D. Maysinger. 2006. Assessment of the integrity of poly(caprolactone)-b-poly(ethylene oxide) micelles under biological conditions: A fluorogenic-based approach. *Langmuir* 22: 3570–3578.

Schild, H. G. and D. A. Tirrell. 1991. Microheterogenous solutions of amphiphilic copolymers of N-isopropylacrylamide, an investigation via fluorescence methods. *Lungmuir* 7: 1319–1324.

Schmolka, I. R. 1977. A review of block polymer surfactants. *J. Am. Oil Chem. Soc.* 54: 110–116.

Schmolka, I. R. and A. J. Raymond. 1965. Micelle formation of polyoxyethylene-polyoxypropylene surfactants. *J. Am. Oil Chem. Soc.* 42: 1088–1091.

Seymour, L. W., R. Duncan, J. Strohalm, and I. Kopecek. 1987. Effect of molecular weight (Mw) of N-(2-hydroxypropyl)methacrylamide copolymers on body distribution and rate of excretion after subcutaneous, intraperitoneal, and intravenous administration to rats. *J. Biomed. Mater. Res.* 21: 1341–1358.

Seymour, L. W., K. Kataoka, and A. V. Kabanov. 1998. Cationic block copolymers as self-assembling vectors for gene delivery. In *Self-Assembling Complexes for Gene Delivery from Laboratory to Clinical Trial*, Kabanov, A. V., Seymour, L. W., and Felgner, P. (Eds.), Chichester, UK, John Wiley & Sons, 219–239.

Shin, I. L., S. Y. Kim, Y. M Lee, C. S. Cho, and Y. K. Sung. 1998. Methoxy poly(ethylene glycol) ∈-caprolactone amphiphilic block copolymeric micelle containing indomethacin. I. Preparation and characterization, *J. Control. Rel.* 51: 1–11.

Shuai, X., T. Merdan, A. K. Schaper, F. Xi, and T. Kissel. 2004. Core-cross-linked polymeric micelles as paclitaxel carriers. *Bioconj. Chem.* 15: 441–448.

Sjoberg, A., G. Karlstrom, and F. Tjerneld. 1989. Effects on the cloud point of aqueous poly(ethylene glycol) solutions upon addition of low molecular weight saccharides. *Macromolecules* 22: 4512–4516.

Solb, J. and Y. Gallot. 1980. In *Polymeric Amines and Ammonium Salts*, Goethals, E. J. (Ed.), New York, Pergamon Press, pp. 205–218.

Soo, P. L., L. Luo, D. Maysinger, and A. Eisenberg. 2002. Incorporation and release of hydrophobic probes in biocompatible polycaprolactone-block-poly(ethylene oxide) micelles: Implications for drug delivery. *Langmuir* 18: 996–1004.

Strand, S.-E. and B. R. R. Petsson. 1979. Quantitative lymphoscintigraphy I: Basic concepts for optimal uptake of radiocolloids in the parasternal lymph nodes of rabbits. *J. Nucl. Med.* 20: 1038–1046.

Suh, H. and H. W. Jun. 1996. Physicochemical and release studies of naproxen in poloxamer gels. *Int. J. Pharm.* 129: 13–20.

Takei, Y. G., T. Aoki, K. Sanui, N. Ogata, T. Okano, and Y. Sakurai. 1993. Temperature-responsive bioconjugates. 2. Molecular design for temperature-modulated bioseparations. *Bioconj. Chem.* 4: 341–346.

Takei, Y. G., T. Aoki, K. Sanui, N. Ogata, Y. Sakurai, and T. Okano. 1994. Dynamic contact angle measurement of temperature-responsive surface properties for poly(*N*-isopropylacrylamide) grafted surfaces. *Macromolecules* 27: 6163–6166.

Tan, J. S., D. E. Butterfield, C. L. Voycheck, K. D. Caidwell, and J. T. Li. 1993. Surface modification of nanoparticles by PEO/PPO block copolymers to minimize interactions with blood components and prolong blood circulation in rats. *Biomaterials* 14: 823–833.

Taylor, L. D. and L. D. Cerankowski. 1975. Preparation of films exhibiting a balanced temperature dependence to permeation by aqueous solutions. *J. Polym. Sci. Poly. Chem.* 13: 2551–2570.

Tontisakis, A., R. Hilfiker, and B. Chu. 1990. Effect of xylene on micellar solutions of block-copoly(oxyethylene/oxypropylene/oxyethylene) in water. *J. Coll. Interf. Sci.* 135: 427–434.

Torchilin, V. P. 2002. PEG-based micelles as carriers of contrast agents for imaging modalities. *Adv. Drug Del. Rev.* 54: 235–252.

Trubetskoy, V. S., G. S. Gazelle, G. L. Wolf, and P. Torchilin. 1997. Block-copolymer of polyethylene glycol and polylysine as a carrier of organic iodine: Design of a long circulating particulate contrast medium for x-ray computed tomography. *J. Drug Targeting* 4: 381–388.

Trubetskoy, V. S. and V. P. Torchilin. 1995. Use of polyoxyethylene-lipid conjugates as long-circulating carriers for delivery of therapeutic and diagnostic agents. *Adv. Drug Del. Rev.* 16: 311–320.

Trubetskoy, V. S. and V. P. Torchilin. 1996. Polyethyleneglycol based micelles as carriers of therapeutic and diagnostic agents. *S.T.P. Pharma Sci.* 6: 79–86.

Turro, N. J. and C. J. Chung. 1984. Photoluminescent probes for water-water soluble polymers, pressure and temperature effect on a polyol surfactant. *Macromolecules* 17: 2123–2126.

Unger, E., T. Fritz, G. Wu, D. Shen, B. Kulik, T. New, M. Crowell, and N. Wilke. 1994. Liposomal MR contrast agents. *J. Liposome Res.* 4: 811–834.

Vaiaulikar, B. S. and C. Manohar. 1985. The mechanism of clouding in triton X-100: The effect of additives. *J. Coll. Interf. Sci.* 108: 403–406.

Valle, J. W., J. Lawrance, J. Brewer, A. Clayton, P. Corrie, V. Alakhov, and M. Ranson. 2004. A phase II, window study of SP1049C as first-line therapy in inoperable metastatic adenocarcinoma of the oesophagus. *J. Clin. Oncol.* 22: 4195.

Wang, Y., R. Ballaji, P. Quirk, W. L. Mattice. 1992. Detection of the rate of exchange between micelles formed by diblock copolymers in aqueous solution. *Polym. Bull.* 28: 333–338.

Weissig, V., C. Lizano, and V. P, Torchilin. 1998a. Micellar delivery system for dequalinium. *Proceed. Intern. Symp. Control. Rel. Bioact. Mater.* 25: 415–416.

Weissig, V., K. R. Whiteman, and V. P. Torchilin. 1998b. Accumulation of protein-loaded long-circulating micelles and liposomes in subcutaneous Lewis lung carcinoma in mice. *Pharm. Res.* 15: 1552–1556.

Wilhelm, M., C. L. Zhao, Y. Wang, R. Xu, M. A. Winnik, J. L. Mura, G. Riess, and M. D. Croucher. 1991. Poly(styrene-ethylene oxide) block copolymer micelle formation in water: A fluorescence probe study. *Macromolecules* 24: 1033–1040.

Wingard, Jr., L. B., T. R. Tritton, and K. A. Egler. 1985. Cell surface effect of adriamycin and carminomycin immobilized on cross-linked polyvinyl alcohol. *Cancer Res.* 45: 3529–3536.

Winnik, F. M., A. Adronov, and H. Kitann. 1995. Pyrene-labeled amphiphilic poly-(*N*-isopropylacrylamides) prepared by using a lipophilic radical initiator: Synthesis, solution properties in water, and interactions with liposomes. *Can. J. Chem.* 73: 2030–2040.

Winnik, F. M, A. R. Davidson, G. K. Hamer, and H. Kitano. 1992. Amphiphilic poly(*N*-isopropylacrylamide) prepared by using a lipophilic radical initiator: Synthesis and solution properties in water. *Macromolecules* 25: 1876–1880.

Wu, N. M., D. Da, T. L. Rudoll, D. Needham, A. R. Whorton, and M. W. Dehirst. 1993. Increased microvascular permeability contributes to preferential accumulation of stealth liposomes in tumor tissue. *Cancer Res.* 53: 3765–3770.

Xing, L. and W. L. Mattice. 1998. Large internal structures of micelles of triblock copolymers with small insoluble molecules in their cores. *Langmuir* 14: 4074–4080.

Xu, P., H. Tang, S. Li, J. Ren, E. V. Kirk, W. J. Murdoch, M. Radosz, and Y. Shen. 2004. Enhanced stability of core-surface cross-linked micelles fabricated from amphiphilic brush copolymers. *Biomacromolecules* 5: 1736–1744.

Yamada, N., T. Okano, H. Sakai, F, Karikusa, Y. Sawasaki, and Y. Sakurai. 1990. Thermoresponsive poly-meric surfaces; Control of attachment and detachment of cultured cells. *Makromol. Chem., Rapid Cornmun.* 11: 571–576.

Yang, Y. W., Z. Yang, Z. K. Zhou, D. Attwood, and C. Booth. 1996. Association of triblock copolymers of ethyl-ene oxide and butylene oxide in aqueous solution. A study of B*n*EmB*n* copolymers. *Macromolecules* 29: 670–680.

Yekta, A., B. Xu, J. Duhamel, H. Adiwidjaja, and M. A. Winnik. 1995. Fluorescence studies of associating polymers in water: Determination of the chain end aggregation number and a model for the association process. *Macromolecules* 28: 956–966.

Yodoya, E., K. Uemura, T. Tenma, T. Fujita, M. Murakami, A. Yamamoto, and S. Muranishi. 1994. Enhanced permeability of tetragastrin across the rat intestinal membrane and its reduced degradation by acylation with various fatty acids. *J. Pharmacol. Exp. Ther.* 271: 1509–1513.

Yokoyama, M. 1992. Block copolymers as drug carriers. *Crit. Rev. Ther. Drug Carrier Syst.* 9: 213–248.

Yokoyama, M. 1994. Site specific drug delivery using polymeric carriers. In *Advances in Polymeric Systems for Drug Delivery*, M. Yokoyama (ed.). Yverdon, Switzerland, Gordon & Breach Science Publishers, pp. 24–66.

Yokoyama, M. 1998. Novel passive targetable drug delivery with polymeric micelles. In *Biorelated Polymers and Gels*, Okano, T. (Ed.), San Diego, CA, Academic Press, pp. 193–229.

Yokoyama M., S. Fukushima, R. Uehara, K. Okamoto, K. Kataoka, Y. Sakurai, and T. Okano. 1998a. Characterization of physical entrapment and chemical conjugation of adriamycin in polymeric micelles and their design for *in vivo* delivery to a solid tumor. *J. Control. Rel.* 50: 79–92.

Yokoyama, M., G. S. Kwon, T. Okano, Y. Sakurai, M. Naito, and K. Kataoka. 1994a. Influencing factors on *in vitro* micelle stability of adriamycin-block copolymer conjugates. *J. Control. Rel.* 28: 59–65.

Yokoyama, M., G. S. Kwon, T. Okano, Y. Sakurai, T. Sero, and K. Kataoka. 1992. Preparation of micelle-forming polymer-drug conjugate. *Bioconj. Chem.* 3: 295–301.

Yokoyama, M., M. Miyauchi, N. Yamada, T. Okano, Y. Sakurai, K. Kataoda, and S. Inoue. 1990a. Characterization and anticancer activity of the micelle-forming polymeric anticancer drug adriamycin-conjugated poly(ethylene glycol)-poly(aspartic acid) block copolymer. *Cancer Res.* 50: 1693–1700.

Yokoyama, M., M. Miyauchi, N. Yamada, T. Okano, Y. Sakurai, K. Kataoka, and S. Inoue. 1990b. Characterization and anticancer activity of the micelle-forming polymeric anticancer drug adryamicin-conjugated poly(ethylene glycol)-poly(aspartic acid) block copolymer. *Cancer Res.* 50: 1700–1993.

Yokoyama, M., M. Miyauchi, N. Yamada, T. Okano, Y. Sakurai, K. Kataoda, and S. Inoue. 1990c. Polymer micelles as novel carrier: Adriamycin-conjugated poly(ethylene glycol)-poly(aspartic acid) block copo-lymer. *J. Control. Rel.* 11: 269–278.

Yokoyama, M., T. Okano, Y. Sakurai, H. Ekimoto, C. Shibazaki, and K. Kataoda. 1991. Toxicity and antitu-mor activity against solid tumors of micelle-forming polymeric anticancer drug and its extremely long circulation in blood. *Cancer Res.* 51: 3229–3236.

Yokoyama, M., T. Okano, Y. Sakurai, and K. Kataoka. 1994b. Improved synthesis of adriamycin-conjugated poly(ethylene oxide)-poly(aspartic acid) block copolymer and formation of unimodal micellar structure with controlled amount of physically entrapped adriamycin. *J. Control. Rel.* 32: 269–277.

Yokoyama, M., T. Okano, Y. Sakurai, S. Suwa, and K. Kataoka. 1996. Introduction of cisplatin into polymeric micelles. *J. Control. Rel.* 39: 351–356.

Yokoyama, M., A. Satoh, Y. Sakurai, T. Okano, Y. Matsumara, T. Kakizoe, and K. Kataoka. 1998b. Incorporation of water-insoluble anticancer drug into polymeric micelles and control of their particle size. *J. Control. Rel.* 55: 219–229.

Yokoyama, M., T. Sugiyama, T. Okano, Y. Sakurai, M. Naito, and K. Kataoka. 1993. Analysis of micelle for-mation of an adriamycin-conjugated poly(ethylene glycol)-poly(aspartic acid) block copolymer by gel permeation chromatography. *Pharm. Res.* 10: 895–899.

Yoo, H. S. and T. G. Park. 2001. Biodegradable polymeric micelles composed of doxorubicin conjugated PLGA-PEG block copolymer. *J. Control. Rel.* 70(1–2): 63–70.

Yoshioka, H., K. Nonaka, K. Fukuda, and S. Kazama. 1995. Chitosan-derived polymer-surfactants and their micellar properties. *Biosci. Biotechnol. Biochem.* 59: 1901–1904.

Yu, B. G., T. Okano, K. Kataoka, and G. Kwon. 1998a. Polymeric micelles for drug delivery: Solubilization and hemolytic activity of amphotericin B. *J. Control. Rel.* 53: 131–136.

Yu, B. G., T. Okano, K. Kataoka, S. Sardari, and G. S. Kwon. 1998b. *In vitro* dissociation and antifungal efficacy and toxicity of amphotericin B-loaded poly(ethylene oxide)-block-poly(β-benzyl l-aspartate) micelles. *J. Control. Rel.* 56: 285–291.

Yuan, F., M. Dellian, D. Fukumura, M. Leunig, D. A. Berk, V. P. Torchilin, and R. K. Jain. 1995. Vascular permeability in a human tumor xenograft: Molecular size dependence and cutoff size. *Cancer Res.* 55: 3752–3756.

Yuan, F., M. Leuning, S. K. Huang, D. A. Berk, D. Papahadjopoulos, and R. K. Jain. 1994. Microvascular permeability and interstitial penetration of sterically-stabilized (stealth) liposomes in human tumor xenograft. *Cancer Res.* 54: 3352–3356.

Zachariasse, K. A., W. L. C. Vaz, C. Sotomayor, and W. Kuhnle 1982. Investigation of human erythrccyte ghost membrane with intramolecular excimer probes. *Biochim. Biophys. Acta* 688: 323–332.

Zatz, J. L. and R-Y. Lue. 1987. Flocculation of suspensions containing nonionic surfactants by sorbitol. *J. Pharm. Sci.,* 76: 157–160.

Zhang, L. and A. Eisenberg. 1995. Multiple morphologies of "crew-cut" aggregates of polystyrene-*b*-poly(acrylic acid) block copolymers. *Science* 268: 1728–1731.

Zhang, X., H. M. Burt, D. Von Hoff, D. Dexter, G. Mangold, D. Degen, A. M. Oktaba, and W. L. Hunter. 1997a. An investigation of the antitumour activity and biodistribution of polymeric micellar paclitaxel. *Cancer Chemother. Pharmacol.* 40: 81–86.

Zhang, X., H. M. Butt, G. Mangold, D. Dexter, D. Von Hoff, L. Mayer, and W. L. Hunter. 1997b. Antitumor efficacy and biodistribution of intravenous polymeric micellar paclitaxel. *Anti-Cancer Drugs* 8: 686–701.

Zhang, X., J. K. Jackson, and H. M. Burt. 1996a. Development of amphiphilic diblock copolymers as micellar carriers of paclitaxel. *Int. J. Pharm.* 132: 195–206.

Zhang, X., J. K. Jackson, and H. M. Burt. 1996b. Determination of surfactant micelle concentration by a novel fluorescence depolarization technique. *J. Biochem. Biophys. Methods* 31: 145–150.

Zhang X, and Y. Li, 2005. Synthesis and characterization of the paclitaxel/MPEG-PLA block copolymer conjugate. *Biomaterials* 26(14): 2121–2128.

Zhao, C. L., M. A. Winnik, G. Riess, and M. D. Croucher. 1990. Fluorescence probe techniques used to study micelle formation in water-soluble block copolymers. *Langmuir* 6: 514–516.

Zhou, Z. and B. Chu. 1987. Anomalous association behavior of an ethylene oxide/propylene oxide ABA block copolymer in water. *Macromolecules* 20: 3089–3091.

Zhou, Z. and B. Chu. 1988a. Anomalous micellization behavior and composition heterogeneity of a triblock ABA copolymer of (a) ethylene oxide and (b) propylene oxide in aqueous solution. *Macromolecules* 21: 2548–2554.

Zhou, Z. and B. Chu. 1988b. Light-scattering study on the association behavior of triblock polymers of ethylene oxide and propylene oxide in aqueous solution. *J. Coll. Interf. Sci.* 126: 171–180.

Zhou, Z. and B. Chu. 1994. Phase behavior and association properties of poly(oxypropylene)-poly(oxyethylene)-poly(oxypropylene) triblock copolymer in aqueous solution. *Macromolecules* 27: 2025–2033.

Zhou, Z., B. Chu, V. M. Nace, Y. W. Yang, and C. Booth. 1996. Self-assembly characteristics of BEB-type triblock copolymers. *Macromolecules* 29: 3663–3664.

14 Liposomes in Solubilization

Rong (Ron) Liu, John B. Cannon, and Sophia Y. L. Paspal

CONTENTS

INTRODUCTION

HISTORY OF LIPOSOMES

Over 40 years ago, Alec D. Bangham, a British physician, investigated the relation of cell membranes to phospholipid molecules and discovered phospholipid vesicles, which he initially called smectic mesophases or *tiny fat bubbles*, and later named liposomes. He demonstrated that in water these phospholipid molecules arrange themselves spontaneously into bilayer structures, so that the hydrophobic tails are shielded from the water by hydrophilic heads (Bangham et al., 1965, 1992). Since then, liposomes have been extensively investigated by scientists from many disciplines. The enthusiasm for liposome research had by 1989 resulted in the publication of more than 20,000 scientific articles on liposomes in fields as diverse as gene transfer and nutrition (Ostro and Cullis, 1989); since that time, this number has more than doubled. In addition, more than 1000 patents have been issued or were filed dealing with specific aspects of liposomes (Crommelin and Schreier, 1994). However, early research interests in liposomes were limited primarily to physiologists and biophysicists. The physiologists used liposomes as models to investigate ionic flow across cell membranes, and the biophysicists used them to study the phase behavior of lipids under precisely controlled conditions (Ostro and Cullis, 1989). Later on, biopharmaceutical scientists started to utilize liposomes as delivery or targeting systems for many drug substances (Ostro, 1992; Sharma and Sharma, 1997). More recently, pharmaceutical formulation scientists found that liposomal delivery is an exciting technique and particularly useful to deliver water-insoluble compounds (Chen et al., 1986; Lidgate et al., 1988; Tasset et al., 1992). Many drugs such as anticancer and anti-HIV compounds are water insoluble, and the proportion of new drug candidates that are water insoluble has increased dramatically. The lipophilic phase of the lipid bilayer membrane affords a useful environment to dissolve lipid-soluble compounds. Hence, liposomal delivery offers the possibility of formulating highly promising but water-insoluble compounds that otherwise could not be developed for medical uses because of solubility problems in aqueous solution (Vries et al., 1996; Sharma and Sharma, 1997).

IN VIVO BEHAVIOR OF LIPOSOMES

A variety of routes, including intravenous (IV), intramuscular (IM), and subcutaneous (SC) are used to introduce liposomes into a human body; however, IV injection is the most common and effective means. On injection, liposomes interact with at least two groups of plasma proteins (namely, lipoproteins, and opsonins), and cells in blood. Depending on the liposome composition, lipoproteins can attack and degrade liposomes by removing phospholipid molecules from the lipid bilayer structure. This leads to the destabilization of the bilayers of vesicles, leading to release of the entrapped drug molecules into the blood circulation. Opsonins adsorb onto the surface of the vesicles; the resulting opsonin–liposome complexes, along with the entrapped drug, fall prey to the phagocyte cells of the reticuloendothelial system (RES) (Gregoriadis, 1990).

Of the postulated mechanisms by which liposomes can interact with cells of the RES, adsorption, endocytosis, lipid exchange, and fusion are believed to be the most important (Figure 14.1) (Ostro, 1987).

In the mechanism of adsorption, liposomes can be adsorbed onto the membrane of any cell under suitable conditions, for example, by electrostatic attraction. During liposome–cell adsorption, the

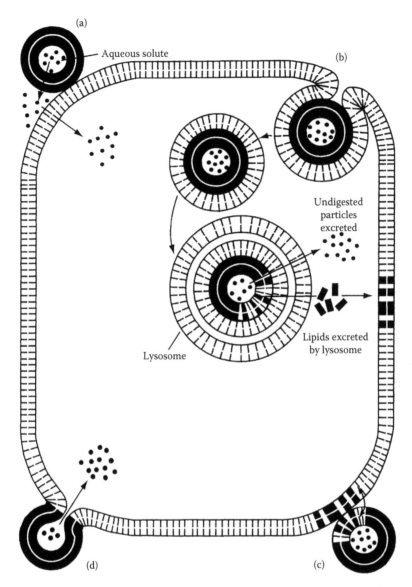

(a)

Aqueous solute

(b)

Undigested
particles
excreted

Lysosome

Lipids excreted
by lysosome

(d)

(c)

FIGURE 14.1 Scheme of the proposed interaction mechanisms of liposomes with cells: (a) adsorption, (b) endocytosis, (c) lipid exchange, and (d) fusion. (From Ostro, M. J., *Sci. Am.*, 257, 102–111, 1987. With permission.)

encapsulated drug molecules are slowly released into the extracellular fluid, and some of the drug molecules may penetrate through the cell membrane into the cell. Endocytosis is one of the most important among all the proposed mechanisms (Weiner, 1990), but only a few types of cells can efficiently endocytose liposomes. Cells derived from the bone marrow, such as the monocytes, macrophages, and other white blood cells, are adept in the endocytotic process of liposomes. In the case of binding of liposomes to cells such as macrophages, they are first engulfed in vesicles called phagosomes. These phagosomes fuse with lysosomes, whose degradative enzymes (e.g., phospholipases) degrade the engulfed liposomes. The lipid components of the liposomes are reused by the cells as membrane constituents. Any entrapped drug molecules in the liposomes are then released into cytoplasm if they survive the lysosomal environment. The third type of liposome–cell interaction is lipid exchange that involves the transfer of individual lipid molecules from the liposomes to the plasma membrane of the cell. Since lipophilic drug molecules are entrapped in lipid bilayers of the liposomes, during the process of lipid exchange the drug molecules may penetrate into the cell. Lipid exchange can also occur between liposomes and circulating lipoproteins. The lipophilic drug molecules may transfer from liposomes to lipoproteins. The last type of interaction is fusion, which can be regarded as the intercalation of outer membrane of the liposome into the cell membrane. However, liposome fusion is thought to occur rarely *in vivo*, being a low-level process at best (Betageri et al., 1993). The incidence of liposome fusion may be augmented by the incorporation of fusogenic substances (e.g., peptides) into the lipid bilayer.

Local administration of liposomes can be achieved through IM injection or SC injection. Liposomes can remain at the site of injection, maximizing local drug concentration while minimizing systemic levels, and may also prolong the release of the drug (Juliano, 1981). After local injection, the larger liposomes are disintegrated locally, and as a result, they disappear very slowly from the site of injection. The small vesicles may eventually enter the circulation through the lymphatic system and interact with lipoproteins and cells in RES. Some of them end up in the lymph nodes near the injection site and circulate through the lymphatic system. In general, only a small percentage of liposomes are adsorbed into the blood since the majority are taken up by cells in the lymph and degraded to release their contents (Gregoriadis, 1990).

Oral administration of liposomally encapsulated drugs such as insulin, glucose oxidase, turbocurarine, clotting factor VIII, and heparin have been reported. Although liposomes are readily digested by phospholipases and bile salts in the gastrointestinal (GI) tract, it was reported that entrapped drugs, especially water-insoluble drugs, can be adsorbed through phospholipid-bile salt–drug complexes (Gregoriadis, 1990). In this case, mechanisms of absorption are probably similar to other oral lipid-based drug delivery systems, which are discussed in another chapter. In an oral liquid formulation of the immunosuppressant sirolimus (Rapamune®), the drug is solubilized by Phosal PG50, which contains phosphatidylcholine and propylene glycol (Strickley, 2004). Thus, it is likely that liposomes are formed transiently to solubilize the drug when the dosage form is dispersed in water.

Liposomally formulated drugs distribute differently in the body than conventional pharmaceuticals since liposomes have distinct pharmacokinetic pathways of distribution and elimination (Hwang, 1987). When administered intravenously, liposome formulations act as a drug reservoir and offer sustained release in the blood stream. Liposomes are selectively taken up by the RES (such as the liver, spleen, lungs, lymph node, and to a lesser degree, bone marrow), being ingested like other foreign particles by phagocytic cells such as macrophages. This indicates that liposomes can also act as a carrier for intracellular drug delivery, making them well suited to the treatment of diseases of the mononuclear phagocyte system, including systemic fungal infections in immunocompromised patients undergoing treatment for cancer or those with immunodeficiency disorders.

Water insoluble drugs will be incorporated into the liposome bilayer, and it is possible that the drug will be removed from the carrier by blood components fairly soon after injection. In this case, distribution of the drug will be different from that of the liposome. For example, propofol was rapidly released from the carrier in a liposomal propofol formulation such that distribution was indistinguishable from that of emulsion formulations (Jensen et al, 2008).

ADVANTAGES OF USING LIPOSOMES AS A DRUG CARRIER

Liposomes are unique as drug carriers in that they can encapsulate drugs with widely varying polarities. Hydrophilic drugs can be entrapped in the aqueous spaces while lipophilic drugs can be incorporated into the lipid membranes. Using a liposomal formulation can dramatically increase the apparent aqueous solubility of a lipophilic drug, making possible delivery of a dose much higher than the water solubility. Therefore, a stable formulation with a water-insoluble drug is often achievable with no precipitation on dilution. Liposomal drugs can target the sites of inflammation, infection, and neoplasm. This may be because at those sites, the disease states lead to increased spaces between the endothelial cells lining the local capillaries (Bangham, 1992; Ostro, 1992). Encapsulation of drugs in liposomes thus results in an increase of drug levels at the targeted sites when compared with the conventional formulations. This site-specific action reduces the toxicity of drugs without loss of their efficacies, and has been used to improve the therapeutic indices of several classes of drugs. For example, the liposome formulation of Amphotericin B, an antifungal agent with serious toxicity, has been proven to be as much as 70 times less toxic in mice than the conventional formulation. Similarly, the serious irreversible cardiomyopathy side effect of doxorubicin, a widely used anticancer drug, can be reduced using liposome technology.

MARKETED PRODUCTS AND CLINICAL TRIAL PROJECTS

With the development of the liposome technology, more and more marketed products and clinical trial projects have been developed. Table 14.1 summarizes marketed liposomal products, and Table 14.2 give a representative list of products that are in clinical trials as liposomal formulations.

AmBisome®, a liposomal formulation of Amphotericin B developed by Nexstar (now Gilead Sciences), has been approved for use in more than 40 countries since 1990 and was approved for the U.S. market by the Food and Drug Administration (FDA) in 1997. Several other forms of liposomal

TABLE 14.1
Marketed Liposomal Products

Drug	Product Name	Company*	Route	Drug Activity	Status	References
Doxorubicin	Doxil	Alza/Janssen	IV	Cancer	Marketed	PDR (2006)
	Myocet	Cephalon	IV	Cancer	Marketed (EU)	Allen and Cullis (2013)
Amphotericin B	Ambisome	Gilead/Astellas	IV	Antifungal	Marketed	PDR (2006)
	Abelcet	Liposome Co./Sigma-Tau	IV	Antifungal	Marketed	PDR (2006)
	Amphotec	Alza/Three Rivers	IV	Antifungal	Marketed	Dupont (2002)
Daunorubicin	DaunoXome	Gilead/Galen US	IV	Cancer, Kaposi's Sarcoma	Marketed	Allen and Cullis (2013)
Cytarabine	DepoCyt	SkyePharma/ Sigma-Tau	Intrathecal	Lymphomatous meningitis	Marketed	PDR (2006); Dupont (2002)
Morphine sulfate	Depodur	SkyePharma/ Pacira	Epidural	Pain	Marketed	PDR (2006); Dupont (2002)
Verteporfin	Visudyne	QLT/Valeant	IV	Age related macular degeneration	Marketed	PDR (2006); Dupont (2002)
Vincristine	Marquibo	Talon	IV	Leukemia	Marketed	PDR (2006); Dupont (2002)
Bupivacaine	Exparel	Pacira	Surgical site	Anesthesia	Marketed	Allen and Cullis (2013) Viscusi et al. (2014); PDR (2006); Dupont (2002)
Muramyl tripeptide PE	Mepact; Junovan	IDM pharma	IV	Osteosarcoma	Marketed (EU) NDA (US)	Nardin et al. (2006)
Irinotecan hydrochloride	Onivyde	Merrimack pharmaceuticals	IV	Cancer	Marketed	PDR (2006)
Paclitaxel	Lipusu	Luye pharma	IV	Cancer	Marketed (China)	PDR (2006)

PDR: Physician's Desk Reference.

TABLE 14.2

A Representative List of Liposomal Products in Clinical Trials

Drug	Product Name	Company	Route	Drug Activity	Status	References
Paclitaxel	EndoTag	Medigene/SynCor	IV	Cancer	Phase III	Schuch (2005)
Factor VIII	Kogenate	Zilip	IV	Hemophilia	Phase III	Yoshioka et al. (2006)
Cis-platin	Lipoplatin	Regulon	IV	Lung cancer	Phase III	Allen (2013)
Vincristine	Onco TCS	Inex	IV	Non-Hodgkins Lymphoma	Phase III	Drugs in R&D (2004)
Thermally responsive liposomal doxorubicin	Thermodox	Celsion	IV	Primary liver cancer	Phase III	Miller (2013)
Anti-MUC-1 Cancer Vaccine	Stimuvax (L–BLP25)	Merck/Oncothyreon	IV	Non-small lung cancer	Phase III	Allen (2013); Wu et al. (2011)
Alprostadil	Liprostin	Endovasc	IV	Ischemia	Phase III	–
Amikacin	Arikayce	Insmed	Inhalation	cystic fibrosis	Phase III	–
Annamycin	L-Annamycin	Callisto	IV	Leukemia	Phase II	Wetzler et al. (2013)
Amikacin	MiKasome	Gilead	IV	Drug-resistant tuberculosis	Phase II	–
Lurtotecan	OSI-211 (NX 211)	OSI Pharma/Gilead	IV	ovarian and lung cancer	Phase II	Dark et al. (2005)
Thymidylate synthase inhibitor	OSI-7904L (GS7904L)	OSI Pharma/Gilead	IV	Gastric Cancer	Phase II	Sen and Mandal (2013)
Paclitaxel	LEP-ETU	Neopharm/Insys	IV	Metastatic breast cancer	Phase II	Sen and Mandal (2013)
Cytarabine:daunorubicin	CPX-351	Celator pharmaceuticals	IV	Acute myeloid leukemia	Phase II	Lancet et al. (2014); Allen (2013)
Irinotecan:floxuridine	CPX-1	Celator pharmaceuticals	IV	Colorectal cancer	Phase II	Allen (2013)
Alendronate	LABR-312	Biorest	IV	Restenosis	Phase II	Banai et al. (2013)
Transferrin targeted oxaliplatin	MBP-426	Mebiopharm	IV	Gastric cancer	Phase II	Allen (2013)
Irinotecan (CPT-11)	MM-398	Merrimack	IV	Gastric and pancreatic cancer	Phase II	Allen (2013)
Topotecan	Brakiva	Talon	IV	Relapsed solid tumors	Phase I	Allen (2013)
Vinorelbine	Alocrest	Talon	IV	Relapsed solid tumors	Phase I	Allen (2013)
Anti-transferrin targeted p53 cDNA	SGT-53	SynerGene	IV	Advanced solid tumors	Phase I	Senzer et al. (2013)
Docetaxol	LEP-DT	Neopharm/Insys	IV	Metastatic solid cancer	Phase I	Sen and Mandal (2013); Deeken et al. (2013)
Antisense oligonucleotide	LEP-rafAON	Neopharm/Insys	IV	Pancreatic cancer	Phase I	Dritschilo et al. (2006)
Immunoliposomal doxorubicin	MM-302	Merrimack	IV	HER-2 over-expressing cancers	Phase I	Allen (2013)
Prostaglandin E1	TLC C-53	The liposome company (Elan)	IV	Acute inflammatory and veso-occlusive conditions	Phase II (discontinued)	Vincent et al. (2001)

Amphotericin B or Amphotericin–phospholipid complex have already been approved. Plaux® (Lipo-alprostadil), a cardiovascular and an anti-diabetic drug incorporated in liposome formulation, was launched in Japan in 1988. The use of liposomes as drug carriers for chemotherapeutic agents or biologic response modifiers has been actively pursued by several companies. DOXIL®, a liposomal formulation of doxorubicin developed by Sequus Pharmaceuticals (now Alza, part of Johnson and Johnson) was approved by the United States in 1995. DOXIL, one of the most successful liposome products, uses polyethylene glycol to increase circulation time, as discussed later. Myocet® is a non-pegylated liposomal doxorubicin product marketed in Europe. A liposomal formulation of muramyl tripeptide phosphatidylethanolamine, an immunomodulator, is marketed in Europe and has been submitted for a new drug application (NDA) in the United States. Other formulations, such as a topical formulation of minoxidil, a dermatological agent from Taisho developed by Upjohn, were launched worldwide in 1986. Iodinated liposome, a diagnostics from Sequus Pharmaceuticals (now Alza) is currently in use. Verteporfin is a photodynamic therapy agent developed by QLT Phototherapeutics. It was originally tested as an anticancer agent and is now marketed as Visudyne®, a treatment for age-related macular degeneration. Daunorubicin, cytarabine, morphine sulfate, and vincristine are other drugs that have come to the market as liposomal formulations (Table 14.1). Liposomal delivery of paclitaxel has been studied in a number of clinical trials for cancer, as have the chemotherapeutic agents docataxol, irinotecan, lurtotecan, topotecan, and cis-platin, with promising results. Besides those listed in Table 14.2, liposomal drugs that have been examined in clinical trials include mitoxantrone (Yang et al., 2014), lactoferrin (Ishikado et al., 2004), and tretinoin (Bernstein et al., 2002). Antisense oligonucleotides such as LEP-rafAON (Dritschilo et al., 2006), and siRNA (Schultheis et al., 2014) have been studied clinically. Liposomal combination therapies (Combiplex®) such as irinotecan:floxuridine and cytarabine:daunorubicin have been explored by Celator Pharmaceuticals. Besides injectables, nebulized liposomal formulations have shown some advantages in drug delivery to the lungs. For example, Amphotericin B (Monforte et al., 2009), cis-platin (Wittgen et al., 2007), and camptothecin (Verschraegen et al., 2004) have been examined clinically in nebulized liposomal formulations. Similarly, since there is evidence that liposomes and/ or their components enhance penetration of drugs into the skin (Cevc, 2004), topical liposomal formulations of dithranol (Saraswat et al., 2007), superoxide dismutase (Riedl et al., 2005), idoxuridine (Seth et al., 2004), tretinoin (Patel et al., 2001), and heparin (Górski et al., 2005) have been tested in the clinic. Since 1990, there have been more than a dozen liposome projects in phase III/New Drug Application (NDA) stages, and numerous in phase I and phase II clinical studies. As of 2014, there were at least 107 active clinical trials containing the terms *liposome* listed by the Food and Drug Administration (FDA) (Kraft et al., 2014).

LIPIDS AND LIPID BILAYERS CLASSIFICATION OF LIPIDS

Phospholipids are found in all living cells and typically constitute about half the mass of animal cell plasma membranes (Cevc, 1992). The reason for the variety of membrane lipids might simply be that these amphiphilic structures have in common the ability to arrange as bilayers in an aqueous environment (Paltauf and Hermetter, 1990). Thus, the use of endogenous phospholipids to form vesicles as drug carriers may have much less adverse effects in patients compared to synthetic drug carrier molecules.

Almost all naturally occurring phospholipids are constructed from the combination of a polar headgroup and a glycerol backbone moiety substituted with either one or two acyl or alkyl chains or an *N*-acylated sphingoid base (i.e., a ceramide). Therefore, the phospholipids from natural sources can be classified into phosphodiglycerides and sphingolipids, together with their corresponding hydrolysis products. The basic structures of these two classes are illustrated in Figure 14.2.

Phosphatidylcholines (PC) are the major phosphodiglycerides that can be obtained from natural and synthetic sources. When extracted from plant and animal sources (primarily egg yolk and soybean), PCs, known in the unpurified form as *lecithins*, are composed of a mixture of PCs varying in chain length and degree of unsaturation. Unless highly purified, these naturally derived

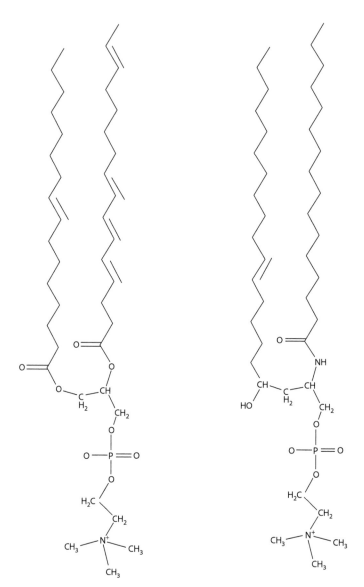

FIGURE 14.2 Chemical structures of two representative classes of phospholipids.

materials also contain small amounts of phosphatidyl ethanolamine (PE), phosphatidyl inositol (PI), and sphingomyelin. Lecithin obtained from animal sources contains a higher portion of saturation in the acyl or alkylated chains, while that derived from plant sources has a high degree of unsaturation in the fatty chains. Owing to relatively low cost, neutral charge, and chemical inertness, PCs are usually used as the principal phospholipids in liposomal formulations. Other phospholipids are often incorporated into liposomes to impart a charge; these include phosphatidyl serine (PS), phosphatidyl glycerol (PG), phosphatidic acid (PA), and PI. PI is a major component of soybean-derived phospholipids; however, there are some pharmacological effects associated with PI, because it may serve as a precursor for certain messenger molecules (Bleasdale et al., 1985). Thus, PI-containing liposomes may not be acceptable for parenteral use. An exception might be made for cancer chemotherapeutic agents, in which cytotoxicity of PI has been shown to be selective for tumor cells (Jett and Alving, 1988). More rarely used are *ether-linked* PCs, in which an ether linkage replaces the ester between the choline group and the glycerol backbone, and accordingly have greater resistance to hydrolysis and enzymatic degradation. However, these synthetic lipids may present a toxicity associated with the inability to metabolize ether linkages.

STRUCTURE AND PROPERTIES OF LIPID BILAYER

Mechanism of Formation of Lipid Bilayers

Phospholipids, by virtue of their hydrophobic acyl hydrocarbon chains and the hydrophilic polar headgroup are amphipathic molecules, with a hydrophilic–lipophilic balance (HLB) number generally around 4–6. As such, molecules of PC are not soluble in water in the accepted sense, and in aqueous media, they align themselves closely into planar bilayer sheets to minimize the unfavorable interactions between the bulk aqueous phase and the long hydrocarbon fatty acid chains. Such interactions are completely eliminated when the sheets fold on themselves to form closed sealed vesicles. Their geometry dictates that phospholipids form lamellar bilayers, owing to the double tails, in contrast to most other surfactants, whose geometry (single tails) leads to micelles. Under certain conditions, an alternate form, the inverse hexagonal phase (H_{II}), can exist, wherein water is entrapped as cylinders surrounded by the polar headgroups of the lipid while the tail groups fill the interstitial regions of the hexagonal lattice. This can be prominent at high lipid/water ratios (>20% lipid), particularly for PE with unsaturated fatty acyl chains (due to its small headgroup). The kinetics of the lamellar (L_α) to H_{II} phase transition has been studied by time resolved X-ray diffraction techniques (Tate et al., 1992). The H_{II} and other phases could be transient intermediates on hydration of phospholipids.

Temperature Effect and Phase Transitions

At different temperatures, phospholipid bilayer membranes can exist in different phases and states of fluidity. This aspect of the order/disorder properties of membranes can be complex. For example, fully hydrated distearoyl phosphatidyl choline (DSPC) undergoes as many as three transitions. Two transitions, a pretransition at 51°C ($\Delta H = 1.3$ kcal/mol) and the main transition at 55°C ($\Delta H = 10.8$ kcal/mol), are well known. An additional non-reversible subtransition around 30°C can also be observed upon prolonged refrigerated storage (Mattai et al., 1987). The pretransition involves a *rippling* or undulation of the lipid bilayer (Cevc, 1991). The main phase transition is the most relevant and general phenomenon, and reflects the passage of the membrane from a tightly ordered *gel* or *solid* phase, to a fluid phase. The fluid phase retains some order and is hence termed a liquid crystalline phase, but the freedom of movement of individual molecules (in terms of translational movement and acyl chain conformational changes) is higher than in the gel phase. As the temperature increases, the fatty acid chains tend to adopt conformations other than the all-trans straight chain configuration, such as the gauche conformation state. This has the effect of expanding the area occupied by the chains, reducing the overall length of the hydrocarbon chains, and decreasing the bilayer thickness on transition from a gel to a liquid crystalline phase. For single-component systems, especially for saturated diacyl phospholipids of chain length C_{12}–C_{20}, the transition occurs over a narrow temperature range above room temperature, with the melting temperature (T_m) increasing with increasing chain length. A theoretical expression of the dependence of T_m on chain length has been devised by Marsh (1991), wherein the incremental effects of methylene groups on changes in transition entropy and enthalpy are accounted for. Detailed analysis of the transition region reveals strong density fluctuations, and it has been suggested from computer simulations that transient domains form on a nanoscale, that is, domains of fluid lipid form within the gel phase, or domains of gel-phase lipid form within the fluid phase, just before or after the crystallization temperature (T_c), respectively (Mouritsen and Jorgensen, 1993). An increase in volume is associated with the gel to liquid crystalline phase, with $\Delta V = 15.2, 22.5, 30.0$, and 27.4 mL/mol for dimyristoyl phosphatidyl ethanolamine (DMPE), dipalmitoyl phosphatidyl ethanolamine (DPPE), distearoyl phosphatidyl ethanolamine (DSPE), and dipalmitoyl phosphatidyl choline (DPPC), respectively (Mason and O'Leary, 1990). T_m can be most easily determined by differential scanning calorimetry and other microcalorimetric methods. However, a variety of other techniques, such as X-ray diffraction, NMR spectroscopy, and fluorescence, have been used to study the transition.

If unsaturation is present in the phospholipid acyl chains, T_m is generally below room temperature, and the transition is somewhat broader. For multicomponent systems, the main phase transition is considerably broadened or essentially abolished. Cholesterol is the most important molecule that moderates lipid bilayer fluidity (both in physiological membranes and in synthetic vesicles) owing to its ability to interact with the phospholipid headgroup and tailgroups by hydrogen-bonding and hydrophobic attractions, respectively. Above 20 mol% cholesterol, a unique and stable phase termed the *liquid-ordered phase* arises, characterized by a high-lateral (translational) diffusion but high conformational order (Mouritsen and Jorgensen, 1993). At higher concentrations, however, cholesterol may perturb the tight packing of the bilayer.

An understanding of phase transitions and fluidity of phospholipid membranes is important in both the manufacture and application of liposomes. The phase behavior of a liposome membrane determines such properties as permeability, fusion, aggregation, and protein binding, all of which can markedly affect the stability of liposomes as well as their behavior in biological systems. In addition, drugs can change the transition temperature. For example, cationic amphiphilic compounds were shown to depress the transition temperatures of dipalmitoyl phosphatidic acid (DPPA) liposomes, apparently because of both headgroup and tailgroup interactions (Haupft and Mohr, 1985; Borchardt et al., 1991). A neutral hydrophobic anticancer drug, teniposide, has been shown to decrease and broaden the main T_m of dimyristoyl phosphatidyl choline (DMPC) and DPPC liposomes in a linear fashion from 1 to 5 mol%. The pretransition was decreased by teniposide concentrations as low as 0.1 mol% and abolished by 1 mol% drug (Wright and White, 1986).

Conformation of Lipid Chain

In the gel phase, the bulky headgroup of PC occupies a 42 Å^2 area of the membrane, while the two straight chain fatty acids occupy a smaller area (~39 Å^2). Accordingly, the hydrocarbon chains are thought to tilt relative to the plane of the membrane at an angle of 58°, thereby filling up the extra space created by the headgroups. Chain fluidization and transition to the liquid crystalline phase eliminates some degree of the chain tilt, with the result that there is looser chain packing; consequently fluid bilayers will be thinner than the corresponding ordered ones (Cevc and Seddon, 1993).

Phase Separation

Normally, lipid bilayer components will be randomly and uniformly distributed, even when non-phospholipid compounds such as cholesterol are introduced into the bilayer to confer desirable properties. Under some conditions, however, the unwanted phenomenon of phase separation will occur, wherein like components will segregate into zones or domains within the bilayer. This can result in bilayer leakage, aggregation of vesicles, and membrane fusion. Thus, care should be taken in devising liposome compositions and keeping the number of components widely divergent in structure at a minimum (Cevc, 1992). Like-charged lipids will generally be electrostatically repelled from one another, yielding a uniform distribution, but the presence of high concentrations of divalent salts may cause clustering of charged lipids and phase separation. Mixtures of shortand long-chain PC liposomes were shown to undergo phase separation in the gel state (Bian and Roberts, 1990).

Membrane Permeability and Partitioning

Liposome membranes, like biological membranes, are semipermeable. They serve as a very tenuous barrier to molecules with a high solubility in both organic and aqueous media. In contrast, polar solutes (such as glucose) and higher molecular weight compounds generally pass very slowly across intact phospholipid bilayers. Diffusion across the bilayer is quite rapid for smaller molecules of neutral charge (e.g., water and urea), and somewhat slower for protons and hydroxyl ions. Sodium and potassium ions traverse the membrane very slowly. Gel-phase bilayers are less permeable than the corresponding fluid bilayers, that is, increasing the temperature above T_m will increase the permeability.

Phospholipid packing can also affect bilayer permeability. At the membrane boundary, where the lipid compartment interfaces with the bulk aqueous phase, the limited rotational and translational freedom normally manifests itself in alignment of lipids in a regular two-dimensional array with molecules all adopting a set distance and orientation with respect to each other. However, packing abnormalities (point defects, line defects, and grain boundaries) can occur as a result of impurities resulting from an altered configuration or change in conformation of the acyl chain carbons from trans to gauche. Packing abnormalities thus lead to small exposed areas of the membrane, which facilitate the passage of small molecules through that area of the bilayer, increasing the permeability.

When considering hydrophobic drugs that are localized primarily in the lipid tail-group region of the bilayer, the more important parameter is the partition coefficient of drug between lipid bilayer and aqueous phase. One of the main goals of formulation development would be to maximize this number. Partition coefficient is a static parameter, whereas rate of efflux from the bilayer would be the corresponding kinetic parameter, analogous to the permeability parameter of water-soluble molecules.

Properties of Negatively Charged Phospholipids

In negatively charged phospholipids, three possible forces, namely, steric hindrance, hydrogen-bonding, and electrostatic charge, regulate headgroup interactions of the bilayer. For example, dipalmitoyl phosphatidyl glycerol (DPPG), with its bulky glycerol group and electrostatic repulsion of the deprotonated phosphate at pH 7, has a phase transition temperature about 10°C below that of DPPC. In contrast, DPPA, with a small headgroup and negative charge at neutral pH (leading to hydrogen-bonding), has a higher relative main transition temperature. Another factor is a pH effect: at high and low pH, the T_m is brought down, particularly at high pH, where electrostatic repulsion can push the headgroup apart. Similarly, acidic phospholipids can bind strongly to divalent cations (Ca^{2+}, Mg^{2+}), which will decrease the electrostatic charge of the headgroups, condense the bilayer (i.e., increase the packing density in the gel phase), and thus increase the T_m. Therefore, at the appropriate ambient temperature, the addition of cations can induce a phase change from liquid crystalline to gel phase.

Properties of Cholesterol-Containing Lipid Bilayers

Sterols are important components of most natural membranes, with cholesterol and its derivatives being the most important and predominant sterol in animal tissues. Incorporation of sterols into liposome bilayers can bring about major changes in the properties of these membranes. Cholesterol does not form bilayer structures by itself, but having some degree of amphipathic nature, it can be incorporated into phospholipid membranes at very high concentrations (up to 2:1 molar ratios of cholesterol to PC). While it will generally have little effect on the actual phase transition temperature, it can broaden the transition of the bilayer considerably, and in some cases can completely abolish the heat of transition. In the presence of cholesterol, the freedom of molecular motion of the bilayer above the phase transition is decreased, but below the phase transition, mobility is increased. Thus, the overall effect of cholesterol is to moderate the differences between gel and liquid crystalline phases. A corollary to this is that cholesterol will not only fluidize bilayers containing saturated phospholipids, but also will increase the fluidity of bilayers containing unsaturated phospholipids. Some of the benefits that may result from use of cholesterol in a liposomal formulation are decreased permeability of the bilayer, smaller and more uniform size distribution, and prevention of phase separation. The influence of cholesterol on a particular liposomal-drug formulation would have to be evaluated on an individual basis and often involve empirical trial and error.

TYPES AND STRUCTURES OF LIPOSOMES

Liposomes can be characterized by their size (related to number of lamellae, that is, bilayers) and shape. Classification of liposomes according to size is the most common index, as given in the following.

MULTILAMELLAR VESICLES

Multilamellar vesicles (MLVs) usually consist of a population of vesicles covering a wide range of sizes (100–1000 nm), each vesicle generally consisting of five or more concentric lamellae (Figure 14.3). Vesicles composed of just a few concentric lamellae are sometimes called oligolamellar liposomes, or paucilamellar vesicles. In general, oligolamellar liposomes are considered to be 2–5 bilayers, and range in size from 50 to 250 nm. Multivesicular structures can also occur, wherein two or more liposomes are enclosed together in a nonconcentric manner within another larger one. Multivesicular liposomes have been shown to entrap a greater proportion of aqueous space than multilamellar liposomes with only concentric bilayers (Jain et al., 2005). A multivesicular liposomal bupivacaine formulation (Exparel) is marketed for treatment of pain at the surgical site (Chahar and Cummings, 2012). Preparation of a multivesicular hydroxycamptothecin liposomal demonstrated that this type of structure could be used for sustained release of water insoluble drugs (Zhao et al., 2010).

SMALL UNILAMELLAR VESICLES

Small unilamellar vesicles (SUVs) are defined here as those unilamellar (i.e., single-bilayer) liposomes at the lowest limit of size possible for phospholipid vesicles. This limit varies slightly according to the ionic strength of the aqueous medium and the lipid composition of the membrane, but is about 15 nm for pure egg lecithin in normal saline, and 25 nm for DPPC liposomes. Since, according to definition, these liposomes are at or close to the lower size limit, they will be a relatively homogeneous population in terms of size (Figure 14.4).

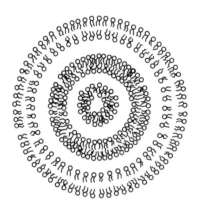 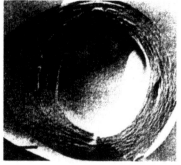

FIGURE 14.3 Diagram and freeze-fracture electron micrograph of a MLVs. (From Ostro, M.J. and Cullis, P.R., *Am. J. Hosp. Pharm.*, 46, 1576–1587, 1989. With permission.)

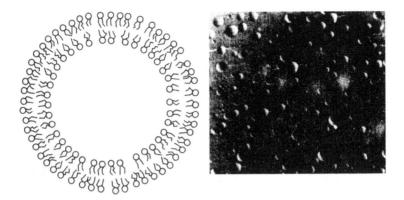

FIGURE 14.4 Diagram of a single unilamellar vesicle and freeze-fracture electron micrograph of many unilamellar vesicles. (From Ostro, M.J. and Cullis, P.R., *Am. J. Hosp. Pharm.*, 46, 1576–1587, 1989. With permission.)

INTERMEDIATE-SIZED UNILAMELLAR VESICLES

Intermediate-sized unilamellar vesicles (IUVs) have diameters of the order of magnitude of 100 nm, and are called *large unilamellar vesicles* (LUVs) if the size is more than 100 nm and they consist of a single bilayer. For unilamellar vesicles, the phospholipid content is related to the surface area of the vesicles, which is proportional to the square of the radius, while the entrapped volume varies with the cube of the radius. In addition, because of the finite thickness of the membrane (ca. 4 nm), as the vesicles become smaller, their aqueous volume is further reduced since the phospholipids occupy more of the internal space. Consequently, for a given quantity of lipid, large unilamellar liposomes entrap a far greater aqueous volume than do small liposomes. These relationships are illustrated in Figure 14.5. Note that this concern is related only to encapsulation of water-soluble compounds.

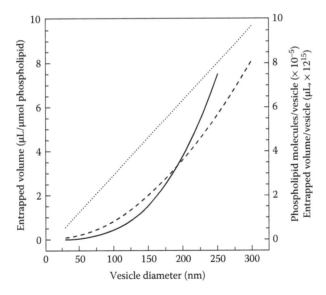

FIGURE 14.5 Entrapped volume and number of phospholipid molecules per liposome as a function of diameter of unilamellar egg PC vesicles. Theoretical curves were calculated assuming a bilayer thickness of 3.7 nm and a phospholipid specific volume of 1.253 nm^3/molecule. (········) Entrapped volume, μL/μmol phospholipid; (— — —) entrapped volume/vesicle, μL × 10^{15}; (- - - - -)/phospholipid molecules per vesicle, μL × 10^{-5}. (Adapted from Enoch, H.G. and Strittmatter, P., *Proc. Nat. Acad. Sci. USA*, 76, 145–149, 1979. With permission.)

POLYMERIZED AND FLUORINATED LIPOSOMES

Early in the development of liposomes, it was recognized that their plasma instability could be a serious detriment in certain applications. Consequently, there were efforts to first incorporate polymerizable lipids into the liposomal bilayers, and then initiate polymerization by, for example, photolysis, to form interchain crosslinks to stabilize the bilayer. The most commonly used polymerizable lipids have been PCs-containing diacetylene or butadiene moieties in the tailgroups (Hupfer et al., 1983; Freeman et al., 1987). The permeability of polymeric liposomes to the water-soluble marker 6-carboxy flourescein was substantially decreased and resistance to organic solvents and detergents was increased relative to nonpolymeric liposomes (Hupfer et al., 1983). Recently, pH-sensitive polymeric liposomes containing ampicillin were prepared using polydiacetylene lipids at neutral pH 7; under acidic conditions, drug is released rapidly (Won et al., 2013) Polymerized liposomes have not been used clinically, perhaps owing to concern for the potential toxicity of the polymerizable lipids. Use of polymeric liposomes in solubilization of water-insoluble drugs would probably have limited value, since in this case partitioning from the bilayer is of greater importance than *trans*bilayer permeability. Stability of drugs located in the lipid bilayer under the polymerization conditions would also be of serious concern.

A related technology is the use of fluorinated vesicles, composed of an amphiphile with a fluorocarbon rather than hydrocarbon tail group. Fluorocarbon chains tend to be more hydrophobic and more rigid than the hydrocarbon chains, providing a driving force for fluorinated amphiphiles to self-organize into lamellar systems that are better organized and more stable than the corresponding hydrocarbon systems (Riess, 1994). This results in a significant decrease in permeability for fluorinated vesicles, both in buffer and in human serum. For example, there was a 100-fold reduction of 6-carboxyfluorescein permeability coefficient at 75°C for DMPC liposomes when the myristoyl groups were replaced with $C_6F_{13}C_6H_{12}CO-$ groups, or a 2000-fold reduction when replaced with $C_8F_{17}C_4H_8CO-$ groups (Riess, 1994). For DSPC liposomes, there was a 10-fold reduction in 6-carboxyfluorescein permeability coefficient in buffer at 75°C when stearoyl groups were replaced with $C_6F_{13}C_{10}H_{20}CO-$ groups. This change resulted in improved serum stability at 37°C, with the DSPC and fluorinated vesicles showing 40% versus 15% loss of entrapped marker after 28 h, respectively, as well as up to a 13-fold increase in circulating half-life (Riess, 1994). Similarly, fluorinated liposomes were shown to be more resistant to the lytic action of detergents compared to conventional DSPC liposomes (Gadras et al., 1999). Fluorinated vesicles have the advantage over polymerized liposomes in that conventional methods for preparation can be used, without use of photoactivation. The fluorinated bilayer does not prevent the use of remote-loading techniques for vesicle preparation, as has been shown for encapsulation of doxorubicin into fluorinated vesicles (Frezard et al., 1994). Fluorinated vesicles have not been used clinically, perhaps owing to unknown toxicity.

LONG-CIRCULATING STERICALLY STABILIZED LIPOSOMES

Recently there has been a great deal of interest in liposomes whose surfaces have been derivatized or modified to prolong their circulating lifetime. There have been several approaches to this modification: the earliest utilized incorporation of sialic acids (e.g., ganglioside GM1) into the bilayer (Allen and Chonn, 1987; Gabizon and Papahadjopoulos, 1988; Allen et al., 1989). More recently, polyethylene glycol (PEG)-derivatized liposomes, normally prepared by incorporating 10–20 mol% of PE to which PEG has been covalently attached at the amino group of PE, have become the method of choice for preparing long-circulating (*Stealth*) liposomes (Woodle, 1993). The surface modification can increase the circulating half-life from 2 to 3 h for conventional liposomes to over 24 h for sterically stabilized liposomes (SSL) owing to reduced RES uptake. For example, an 18-fold increase in half-life was observed when PEG lipid was included in small

DSPC liposomes (Allen et al., 1995). IV injection of partially hydrogenated egg PC/cholesterol (2:1) liposomes containing entrapped marker 67Ga desferoxamine mesylate into rats led to only 1% of the marker found in blood after 24 h, with 31% found in liver and spleen. In contrast, the same liposomes containing 0.15 mol 5000PEG-DSPE showed 21% of the marker in the blood and 10% in the liver and spleen after 24 h (Woodle et al., 1994). A sterically stabilized formulation of doxorubicin is marketed as DOXIL (Table 14.1). This IV formulation showed a circulating half-life of 40–60 h in humans (Woodle, 1995). In general, clearance of sterically stabilized liposomes follows first-order log-linear elimination kinetics, whereas conventional liposomes follow saturation-type Michaelis-Menton kinetics, with a biphasic elimination profile at low doses (Allen et al., 1995); that is, steric stabilization avoids the saturation of RES uptake seen by conventional liposomes. The marked reduction in RES uptake of sterically stabilized liposomes leads to increased uptake in other target areas (e.g., tumors).

The mechanism by which the surface modification alters the pharmacokinetics is not yet fully understood. The primary effect seems to be that the PEG or sialic acid *masks* the surface charge of the phospholipids. This masking, which has been described as a steric barrier, reduces the recognition and binding of the opsinizing agents (plasma proteins) to the liposomes, which leads to lack of RES uptake (Woodle, 1995). The surface charge masking is shown by zeta potential measurements: incorporation of PEG of more than 2000 MW onto the surface of PC liposomes altered the apparent surface zeta potential from −65 to −10 mV; the corresponding thickness of the PEG polymer coat was estimated to be 5 nm (Woodle et al., 1994). Other factors have also been proposed as contributing to the mechanism of prolonging circulation, for example, PEG's role in imparting a greater degree of hydrophilicity to the liposome surface (Woodle, 1993) and the flexibility of the polymer chain (Torchilin and Papisov, 1994). Possible mechanisms have been reviewed; it appears that pegylated liposomes may still be prone to opsonization, and factors leading to their prolonged circulation are complex (Moghimi and Szebeni, 2003; Immordino et al., 2006).

The value of using SSL for delivery of a water-insoluble drug would have to be evaluated on a case-by-case basis. Factors to consider would include the target organ or tissue, desired half-life, and removal of drug from liposomes by albumin and other plasma proteins. For example, if liver and spleen are the primary sites of action of the drug, then SSL would have little or no value. Also, if albumin, lipoproteins, and other plasma proteins remove drug from conventional liposomes before the latter's uptake by the RES and drug is subsequently available for binding to its receptor, SSL would also have questionable value. On the other hand, if a prolonged drug circulating half-life is a formulation goal and/or RES uptake is a problem, delivery by means of SSL might be a viable option. Decisions whether to use SSL versus conventional liposomes should be driven by the specific application and knowledge of tissue targets. Some of these decisions should be based on available data and on direct comparisons in animal or clinical studies with regard to drug pharmacokinetics, tissue distribution, efficacy, and toxicity.

Targeted Liposomes

Early in the development of liposomes, it was recognized that by binding selectively to a certain cell type or releasing the contents in a specific organ, liposomes could potentially afford targeting of their contents to desired locations. This approach would be especially attractive for delivery of cancer drugs with relatively small therapeutic indices. One type of targeted liposome that has been extensively examined is immunoliposomes, wherein a monoclonal antibody is linked to the surface of the liposome (Allen et al., 2002). Clinical development of immunoliposomes has only recently begun, perhaps due to the complexity of manufacture of large quantities of this type of formulation. In a phase I clinical trial, doxorubicin encapsulated in a pegylated immunoliposome was well tolerated in 23 patients in Japan with metastatic stomach cancer, although no objective tumor response was observed (Matsumura et al., 2004). An immunoliposomal delivery system for doxorubicin

(MM-302; Table 14.2) is being developed clinically by Merrimack Pharmaceuticals. This is a doxorubicin liposome conjugated to an anti-HER2 scFv antibody targeting cancer cells that express HER2, and is in Phase II clinical trials in patients with locally advanced/metastatic breast cancer. Another immunoliposomal delivery system in clinical development is SGT-53 (Table 14.2), which uses an anti-transferrin receptor single-chain antibody fragment to target liposomes encapsulating a p53 DNA plasmid to cancer cells *via* the transferrin glycoprotein receptor (Senzer et al., 2013).

Another targeting approach involves coupling a molecule such as folate or transferrin to the liposome surface; folate and transferrin receptors are expressed to a higher extent in cancer cells, and thus such receptor-targeted liposomes would be expected to have increased uptake in cancer cells (Sapra and Allen, 2003; Felnerova et al., 2004). MBP-426 (Table 14.2) is a pegylated liposome encapsulating oxaliplatin targeted with transferrin to cancer cells expressing transferrin receptors; it is currently in Phase II trials (Suzuki et al., 2008).

Another method to enhance the release of liposomal drugs at specific locations is by use of pH- and thermosensitive liposomes. These are destabilized by an acidic environment or by an elevated temperature, respectively, and release their contents at specific tissues meeting the criteria (Simoes et al., 2004; Andresen et al., 2005). Thermodox (Table 14.2) is a thermally responsive liposomal doxorubicin that releases drug at induced temperatures above 37°C in Phase III trials for liver cancer (Miller, 2013).

OTHER STRUCTURES

Although not strictly within the scope of this chapter, a few other delivery systems are worth mentioning by virtue of their similarity to liposomes. Bilayer vesicle structures are not limited to phospholipids. For example, cholesterol hemisuccinate vesicles have been proposed as a delivery system for poorly soluble substances (Janoff et al., 1988). Similarly, an Amphotericin B/cholesterol sulfate (1:1) complex, Amphotericin B Colloidal Dispersion, was originally developed by Sequus Pharmaceuticals and now marketed by Three Rivers Pharmaceuticals as Amphotec® (Hiemenz and Walsh, 1996; Noskin et al., 1998; AHFS Drug Information, 2006) (Table 14.1). Niosomes are lamellar structures composed of certain nonionic surfactants, and also have the potential for formulation of water-insoluble drugs.

A related consideration is that incorporation of a hydrophobic drug into a phospholipid bilayer may lead to formation of nonbilayer structures, if high drug/lipid ratios destabilize the lipid bilayer. In general, in situations in which bilayers are destabilized by drug, there will be a threshold lipid/drug ratio below which alternate structures (e.g., micelles, mixed micelles), will be formed. Size exclusion chromatography is probably the best method to measure the relative amounts of liposomes and alternate structures, and to determine the optimum lipid/drug ratio for liposome formation. For example, the metalloporphyrins heme and tin mesoporphyrin form micellar structures at lipid/porphyrin ratios of less than 5 (Cannon et al., 1984; Cannon et al., 1993). Formation of such nonliposomal structures does not preclude their clinical use and commercial development, provided that the structures are well characterized. For example, Amphotericin B destabilizes the liposome bilayer structure when present at a lipid/drug ratio of less than 5:1, giving rise to unusual ribbonlike lipid complexes. A DMPC/DPMP/Amphotericin B (7:3:1) formulation, called Amphotericin B Lipid Complex (ABLC®), is currently marketed as Abelcet® (Table 14.1) (Hiemenz and Walsh, 1996; Physicians Desk Reference (PDR), 2006).

PREPARATION OF LIPOSOMES

The driving force behind the formation of liposomes is the interaction between water and phospholipids, which have an amphiphilic nature. On one hand, the hydrophilic headgroup prefers the water phase through the hydrophilic interaction. For example, the zwitterionic headgroup of phosphatidylcholine has approximately 15 water molecules weakly bound to it. On the other hand, the hydrophobic hydrocarbon tails of the lipid prefer one another's company to that of water through hydrophobic interaction. This hydrophobic interaction leads to the fact that the chemical potential of the lipids is lowered substantially in going from an aqueous to an oil-like environment. Tanford (1980) estimated the chemical potential loss was 3.7 kJ/mol per methylene group. The large free-energy change between the lipids and water owing to these interactions explains the overwhelming preference of typical phospholipids to form the bilayer structure.

Since phospholipids are the principal raw material for forming liposomes, it is worthwhile to list some of the precautions in the handling process for them. Storage conditions are very important for the chemical stability of phospholipids. In general, there are two possible pathways for the degradation of phospholipids. First, phospholipids are susceptible to hydrolysis, and second, phospholipids containing unsaturated acyl chains are vulnerable to oxidative degradation. These degradation products are considered to be impurities and can significantly affect the physical and chemical properties of liposomes. For these reasons, lipids are usually stored either as solids in bottles filled with an inert gas such as argon or nitrogen in the head space, or in organic solvents at subzero temperatures, to minimize the possibility of hydrolysis and oxidation reactions.

A large variety of techniques for generating liposome systems exist. The methods that will be discussed in the following sections are mechanical dispersion, organic solvent dilution, dialysis, freezing-drying, pH-gradient, and gas-bubbling. In addition, two steps that are involved in the preparation of liposome for parenteral formulation, namely aseptic filtration and lyophilization of the liposome, will be briefly discussed.

MECHANICAL DISPERSION METHODS

Mechanical dispersion methods are the most frequently used methods in the production of the laboratory scale liposomes. Usually two steps are included in these methods: the film preparation and hydration step, and the particle size reduction step. Some liposomes can be prepared by employing just the first step. The hand-shaken method and proliposome method are the two commonly used methods in the first step. Sonication, high-pressure homogenization, or high-pressure membrane extrusion, are usually involved in the particle size reduction step.

The general and common feature of the mechanical dispersion methods is as follows: first, lipids and lipophilic drugs are dissolved in organic solvent(s). The solvents can be chloroform, methylene chloride, methanol, ethanol, ether, or mixtures of these solvents. Many water-insoluble compounds can dissolve in chloroform and methylene chloride. Compounds that are sparingly soluble in either chloroform or methanol alone will often dissolve readily in 2:1 mixture of these two solvents. Second, the solution of lipid with or without drug is dried down onto a solid support (which can be the sides of the flask) by slowly evaporating the organic solvent(s). Third, the dried film is hydrated by addition of an aqueous medium followed by agitation until the lipid film has been completely dispersed. At this point, lipid bilayers are formed. A particle size reduction or homogenization step can be used to reduce the particle size to the desired range.

The lipid bilayer structure is readily formed using the above-mentioned method. Even before exposure to the aqueous medium, the lipids in the dried film are thought to be oriented in such a way as to separate hydrophilic and hydrophobic regions from each other in a manner resembling their conformation in the finished membrane preparation. On hydration, the lipids are said to swell and peel off the support in sheets, generally to form MLVs. The aqueous volume enclosed within the lipid membrane is usually only a small proportion of the total volume used for swelling (about 5%–10%). This method is, therefore very wasteful of water-soluble compounds to be entrapped. Lipid-soluble compounds, on the other hand, can be incorporated with great efficiency (up to 100% encapsulation) if they are not present in quantities that alter the integrity of the membrane.

Although the evaporation step removes the organic solvents, traces may remain in the final formulation, which would be concern for a clinical product. The use of safer alternative solvent mixtures such as ethanol/ethyl acetate to prepare liposomes has been demonstrated (Cortesi et al., 1999). More recently, supercritical fluid technology has been explored as a means of decreasing or avoiding the use of organic solvents and facilitating scale-up of liposomal formulations (Bridson et al., 2002; Imura et al., 2003). This could have significant advantages in liposome manufacture and be an important factor in expanding the commercial applications of liposomal-drug formulations.

Hand-Shaken Multilamellar Vesicles

The classical method of mechanical dispersion is commonly known as *hand-shaking*, since the lipids are suspended from the walls of a glass vessel into the aqueous medium by gentle manual agitation. The main equipments are a rotary evaporator, a water bath, and a round-bottomed flask. A drug-lipid film is formed using the general procedure discussed earlier. The hydration step is carried out by gently shaking the flask until a homogeneous milky white suspension free of visible particles is formed. The suspension is then allowed to stand for several hours for the swelling process to be completed.

The liposomes prepared by this method are usually MLVs, but the structure inside the vesicles can be highly formulation dependent. MLVs composed entirely of neutral lipids tend to be very tightly packed multilayer assemblies with the adjacent bilayers stacked closely on one another, with very little aqueous space between them. The presence of negatively charged lipids in the membrane tends to push the bilayers apart from each other and increase the aqueous volume of entrapment significantly for water-soluble compounds.

The hand-shaken method is the most practical method of making liposomes for water-insoluble compounds, particularly in preclinical studies. Batch size can be made as small as the 5 mL and as large as up to 20 L when using rotary evaporators with different sizes. The advantages of the *hand-shaken* method are that it provides an easy and quick way of preparing liposomes, and the vesicles prepared are relatively stable on storage. However, there are several disadvantages associated with this method, the first being that the liposome entrapment volume is low. Hence, this is not a good method for water-soluble compounds, although it may be an advantage in entrapping water-insoluble compounds in the lipophilic lipid bilayers. A second disadvantage is that the solute distribution may be uneven in the liposome, raising a major concern when preparing liposomes for pharmaceutical use. The third disadvantage is that the liposome size distribution is heterogeneous; particles as large as 30 μm and as small as 0.050 μm can exist in the system (Lichtenberg and Barenholz, 1988). A final disadvantage is that this method is difficult to scale-up. For example, in the filmmaking step, the thickness and the final batch size is determined by the size of the round-bottomed flask. The thickness of the film will affect the efficiency of the hydration process. For a large batch, it is not feasible to build a large flask to make the film with a proper thickness.

Proliposomes

To increase the deposition surface for phospholipids or to make much thinner films, a method has been developed in which the lipids are dried down onto a finely divided particulate support such as powdered sodium chloride, sorbitol, lactose, or polysaccharide, giving a product known as *proliposomes*. When hydrating the dry powder while mixing with a whirl mixer, the phospholipids swell whereas the support rapidly dissolves to give a liposomal suspension of MLVs in an aqueous solution.

The equipment used to prepare small-scale proliposomes are the same as the hand-shaken method, except that some modifications have been made to the rotary evaporator, as follows: the end of the glass solvent inlet tube of the evaporator is drawn out to a fine point so that the lipid solution is introduced into the flask as a fine spray, and a thermocouple is introduced into the evaporator through a vacuum line. An organic solution of phospholipids and drug is sprayed onto the core material while under vacuum. The thermocouple monitors the temperature; once it has dropped below a certain value (due to evaporation), the spraying is stopped by closure of a valve, and drying under vacuum continues. When the temperature rises, spraying is resumed, and the cycle is repeated until all the solution is sprayed onto the core materials. From this process, one can conclude that an effective monitoring and controlling of the temperature during the process of drying the lipids onto the support is important to assure that the components remain in a finely dried form and are evenly dispersed.

For supporting of core materials, sorbitol has received much attention, both because of its acceptability for clinical use and because the solutions formed from it have lower osmolarity than do those of lower molecular weight compounds. The sorbitol granules consist of a microporous matrix, so that the actual area available for deposition is considerably greater than that calculated on the basis of the outer surface of the granule alone, and is equal to approximately 33.1 m²/g. At a loading of about 1 g of lipid for 5 g of sorbitol, a coverage of 6 mg/m² is obtained, which is equivalent to a continuous lipid coating of just a few bilayers over the whole surface. Because water has much greater access to lipids in the form of proliposomes than when they are dried onto a glass wall (where the coating ratio may be 10 g/m²), liposomes are formed much more rapidly by this method, and a higher proportion of smaller vesicles is obtained. For example, MLVs composed of DMPC and dimyristoyl phosphatidyl glycerol (DMPG) with a 7:3 molar ratio made by the hand-shaking method have a mean diameter of 1.8 μm, compared with proliposomes of the same composition that have a mean diameter of 0.13 μm. The mean size of liposomes produced by hydration of the proliposome powder also increases with increasing loading, and decreases with decreasing negatively charged lipid components.

Essentially any combination of lipids can be used in this method. When working with lipids with a low melting temperature such as PC, care must be taken not to allow the temperature to rise too high, or agglomeration of powder particles will result. Any solvent that will dissolve the lipids can be used, but with ethanol or methanol, very precise regulation of evaporation conditions is required to ensure that dissolution of the sorbitol does not occur as the temperature rises. In these situations, it is important to maintain a high vacuum, so that the solvent may be removed rapidly. If one is depositing high-melting lipids onto sorbitol in chloroform or methylene chloride, it may be possible to conduct the operation without temperature control by the thermocouple, considerably reducing the complexity of the setup.

Even though the proliposome method has some of the same disadvantages as the hand-shaken method (such as the low entrapment efficiency for the hydrophilic compounds and the possible existence of an uneven distribution of the solutes), the proliposome method has unique advantages. It provides a novel solution to product stability problems associated with the storage of aqueous liposome dispersions, in that it produces a dry product that can be stored for long periods and hydrated immediately before use. Moreover, the liposome sizes prepared by this method can be controlled by careful consideration of carrier type, surface area, and relative lipid loading.

On the basis of the proliposome concept, large-scale production of lipid powder can be made using a fluid-bed method and a spray-drying method, similar to particle coating technology. Sorbitol, lactose, and other polysaccharides can be used as the core materials. When using a fluid-bed method, the organic lipid solution that contains water-insoluble drug can be sprayed onto the floating powder through a nozzle. At the same time, the organic solvent is removed by applying vacuum to the fluid bed. To remove the trace amount of residual solvent the finished lipid-coated powder needs to be dried under vacuum overnight. A unit Glatt fluid-bed and a Strea-1 fluid-bed (Niro-Airomatic) can be used to produce a relatively small batch (0.5–1 kg of core materials). Fluid-bed coating was used to manufacture beclometasone dipropionate liposomes; after high-pressure homogenization and freeze-drying, liposomes <150 nm were produced (Gala et al., 2015). Similarly, a spray-drying device can be used for the large-scale manufacture of dried lipid-coated powders.

Particle Size Reduction

For parenteral uses, the sizes of MLVs prepared by the above-mentioned methods need to be small enough to pass through the aseptic filter. Three methods that are used in reducing the particles sizes will be discussed as follows: sonication, high-pressure homogenization, and extrusion.

Size Reduction Using Sonication

Sonication is an effective method for reducing the liposome particle size for small batches. On the basis of the sonicator type, probe sonication and bath sonication have been developed. Difficulty in uniformly sonicating large batches of material, generation of personal hazard, risk of causing the degradation of the components by elevated temperatures, and production of the *limiting size* vesicles are shortcomings of the sonication method.

> Probe sonication: This type of sonication is conducted by immersing a metal probe below the liquid surface. Because of the high input of energy in this method, there are high risks of lipid degradation resulting from the high temperatures and increased gas exchange associated with operation of the probe. It is essential, therefore, that the sonicator vessel be cooled efficiently at all times. However, it is also desirable that the lipids are sonicated above their transition temperature T_c since breaking and resealing of vesicles does not occur efficiently below this temperature. While this can be achieved very easily for egg lecithin (which has a T_c around $-15°C$ with an ice bath), saturated lipids such as DMPC need to be maintained at room temperature or above. In these cases, a circulating water bath with a high rate of flow is essential. Owing to the high energy input of this method, the particle size of the MLV can be reduced rapidly and reproducibly. Small and homogeneously distributed SUV liposomes can be produced by this method. However, this method may introduce contamination due to metal leaching from the sonicator probes.
>
> Bath sonication: Traditional laboratory bath sonicators normally do not impart enough energy to liposomes to reduce vesicle sizes; only *cup-horn* type sonicators (e.g., of Branson) are powerful enough for liposome preparation. This setup has the advantage of avoiding direct contact of the formulation with the probe, but is limited to small quantities (<100 mL) of material.

Size Reduction Using High-Pressure Homogenization

There are several homogenizers capable of generating sufficient high-shear forces to produce both unilamellar and MLVs with defined size distributions (Mayhew et al., 1984; Vidal-Naquet et al., 1989). For example, the Microfluidizer® (Microfluidics, Inc.) is a machine that pumps fluid at a very high pressure (up to 18,000 psi) through a membrane filter, after which it is forced along defined microchannels that direct the two streams of fluid to collide at right-angles with very high velocities in an interaction chamber, thus providing a very efficient transfer of energy (Figure 14.6). The lipids can be introduced into the fluidizer either as a suspension of large MLVs, or as slurry of lipid in an aqueous medium. In the latter case, use of organic solvents may sometimes be unnecessary. The fluid collected can be recycled through the pump and the interaction chamber until vesicles of the required dimensions are obtained.

The homogenization method of the Microfluidizer is very efficient. After a single pass, the size of nondrug loaded vesicles can be reduced to between 0.1 and 0.2 μm in diameter, the exact size distribution depending on the nature of the components of lipids and of the hydration medium. In general, the presence of negatively charged lipids tends to decrease the vesicle size, while increasing the amount of cholesterol in the formulation gives larger liposomes. The nature of the drug can also affect the final size distribution of a liposomal-drug formulation. Continuing the cycling time generally brings the size to a narrow size distribution of low value. However, in some cases (e.g., liposome-containing doxorubicin) the diameter can increase after prolonged recycling, demonstrating that the nature of the drug is very important for reduction of particle size.

Large-scale Microfluidizer homogenizers capable of producing liposomes at high rate, such as 3.8–5.7 L/min for the Microfluidizer Model 210EH, are available, meaning that relatively large volumes of liposomes can be prepared easily. A larger size unit (Microfluidizer Model 610) with a much higher rate is also available; however, the efficiency of its interaction chamber is not as high as the smaller model. The liposomes produced at low lipid concentrations usually contain very high

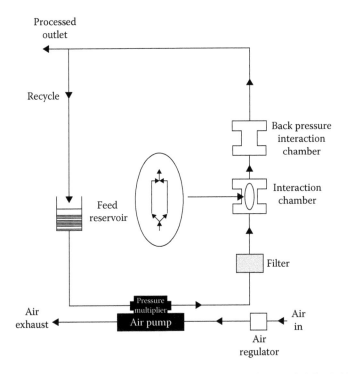

FIGURE 14.6 Schematic presentation of a Microfluidizer. (From Vuillemard, J.C., *J. Microencapsul.*, 8, 547–562, 1991. With permission.)

bulk aqueous proportions inside the liposomes, thereby resulting in high efficiency in encapsulation of water-soluble compounds. At higher lipid concentration, homogenization is also efficient in entrapping water-insoluble drugs and has the ability to process samples with a very high proportion of lipid (>20%), which is difficult to achieve with other methods of making MLVs. Liposomes prepared using a microfluidizer are generally homogeneous in size and reproducible. The drawbacks of microfluidization method are the cost of maintenance of the apparatus and an additional step of hydration of the phospholipids required in most circumstances.

Another advantage of using the Microfluidizer for manufacture is that liposomes can often be produced without the step of formation of a dry lipid film (i.e., instead starting from dry lipid powders); thus organic solvents can be eliminated from the process. If a drug is a water-insoluble weak base or a weak acid, there are at least two ways to produce a liposomal formulation with this drug without using organic solvents. Because the solubility of the drug is pH dependent, one method is to solubilize the drug in an aqueous solution with an appropriate pH in which the drug is more soluble. Then, phospholipids can be hydrated in this drug containing solution. Once the phospholipids are hydrated, the liposomal suspension can be passed through a microfluidizer to produce liposomes. Finally, the drug can be entrapped into the lipid bilayers by adjusting the pH of the aqueous phase to one at which the drug is less soluble. Another method is to solubilize drug in placebo liposomes by adjusting the bulk pH to a value at which the drug has a high solubility. As soon as the drug dissolves, the drug molecules can be entrapped into the lipid bilayers by adjusting the pH to a value at which the drug is less soluble in the aqueous phase. Because the process involves changing the bulk pH, the effect of pH on the stability of both drug and phospholipid must be taken into account.

A related technology for small scale production of liposomes is microfluidics, using a device such as the NanoAssemblr™. For example, this method was used for incorporation of water-insoluble drugs into liposomes, and for manufacture of cationic liposomes for DNA transfection (Kastner et al., 2014; Kastner et al., 2015).

There are a number of commercial homogenizers (e.g., Five-Star, Manton-Gaulin, Avestin Emulsiflex, and Rannie homogenizers) that operate on similar principles (namely, high shear forces and high liquid pressures). These are commonly used for manufacturing emulsions and are adaptable for particle size reduction of liposomes in large scale.

Size Reduction Using the Membrane Extrusion Method

The membrane extrusion method is another homogenization method for the reduction of the particle size of liposomes (Olson et al., 1979). This process can be accomplished by employing an extruder, which is a machine equipped with a pump that pushes fluids through membranes (Figure 14.7). The membranes used in the extrusion method are called *nucleation track* membranes that consist of a thin continuous sheet of polymer (usually polycarbonate) in which straight-sided pores of exact diameter have been created by, for example, laser and chemical etching. As a result, the pore size distribution is narrow and precise. Because the pores go straight though from one side to the other, they offer low resistance to material passing through the membrane. The inherent flexibility of phospholipid lamellae enables liposomes to change their conformations so that they can be squeezed though the pores, and thus may pass through even if the sizes are larger than the pore diameter. However, liposomes that are much larger than the pore size are broken up in the process. After several passes through the membrane, a population of liposomes will be reduced in size to an average diameter somewhat smaller than the membrane pore diameter, but with a small proportion still slightly larger than the pores. The advantages of the membrane extrusion method are as follows:

1. It produces liposomes with relatively homogeneous size distribution.
2. The method is fast and reproducible.
3. Liposomes with high lipid concentrations can be processed by this method.

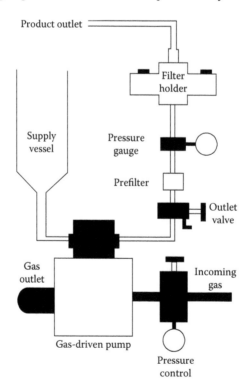

FIGURE 14.7 Schematic presentation of the high-pressure extrusion apparatus. (From Schneider, T. et al., *Int. J. Pharm.*, 117, 1–12, 1995. With permission.)

4. The liposomes produced can have high entrapment efficiency.
5. The method is relatively gentle and nondestructive compared with other methods.
6. The method has a certain flexibility in size reduction, which can produce liposomes of different sizes by changing the membranes with different pore sizes.

The disadvantages of this method are as follows:

1. The procedure is discontinuous.
2. The size of the batch is relatively small compare to the high-pressure homogenization method.
3. Preliminary preparation of MLV is necessary.

OTHER PREPARATION METHODS

Organic Solvent Dilution Method

The organic solvent dilution method has been developed for large-scale production of liposomes containing water-insoluble compounds. This method is based on the ether infusion method, introduced by Deamer and Bangham (1976), and the ethanol injection method, introduced by Batzi and Korn (1973). The basic procedures are first, the lipids and the water-insoluble compounds are dissolved into water miscible organic solvents (usually ethanol). Then the organic solution is mixed with the aqueous phase with defined tonicity. Finally, the organic phase is then dialyzed out by cross-flow filtration.

The instruments involved in this method are dynamic mixing devices with two pumps, and a cross-flow filtration device with proper membranes (Figure 14.8). One pump is used to push the organic phase with a slow rate and the other is used to pump the aqueous phase with a fast rate. Liposomes can be prepared by continuously pumping the organic phase and the aqueous phase together and then flow through the dialysis devices. The method can be used for scale-up and good manufacturing practice (GMP) manufacture of drug-containing liposomes (Wagner et al., 2006).

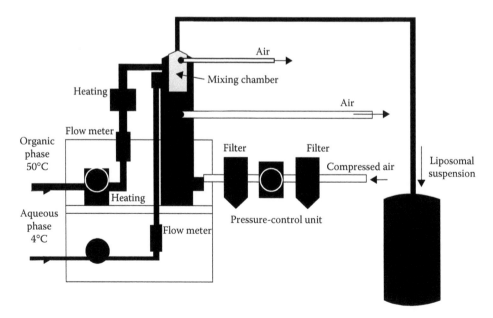

FIGURE 14.8 Schematic presentation of a dynamic mixing device. (From Isele, U. et al., *J. Pharm. Sci.*, 83, 1608–1616, 1994. With permission.)

The advantages of this method are (1) this method is a fast and simple procedure, (2) the method can be used to produce LUVs, and (3) the production can be easily scaled up. The drawbacks of this method are (1) liposomes that are heterogeneous in size may be produced; (2) removing the organic solvent from the mixture is necessary; and (3) due to the large dilution in the dynamic mixing process, the product produced is very dilute, perhaps necessitating concentration procedures.

Dialysis Method

Following its introduction in the early 1970s, the dialysis method has since developed into a useful method of preparing relatively large batches of liposomes for clinical use (Schwendener, 1986). The general procedures of this method are first, the mixture of lipids, drug, and detergent is dissolved in an organic phase and the organic solvent(s) is evaporated to form a film; next, the film is hydrated to form mixed micelles; and finally the unilamellar vesicles are produced by removing the detergent using dialysis systems. The commonly used detergents are sodium cholate, sodium deoxycholate, and some synthetic detergents such as octylglucoside. These all have reasonably high critical micelle concentrations (5–20 mM) to facilitate their removal.

The dialysis system is low cost and includes valves, pumps, capillary dialysis cartridges, and reservoirs. The number and the types of the dialysis cartridges can be varied, for example, two or more cartridges can be connected in a consecutive mode. Several types of disposable cartridges are available that differ in the total surface area available, void volume, and ultrafiltration rate.

In the dialysis method, the parameters that can be adjusted to control the size and homogeneity of the liposomes produced are (1) lipid and drug concentrations, (2) number and type of cartridges used, (3) the flow rates of the mixed micelles and of the dialysis buffer, and (4) the physicochemical properties of the detergent used. These parameters influence the kinetics of the detergent removal from the mixed micelles systems. For example, increasing lipid concentrations usually cause slower detergent removal and less homogeneous liposomes. With an increase of both the membrane surface of the dialysis cartridge and the flow rate of the dialysis buffer, the size of the liposomes can be kept small. The type of the detergent used has a more profound effect on the liposome sizes than the other factors.

The dialysis method is well suited for the encapsulation of lipophilic drugs. The liposomes prepared by this method are usually homogeneous in size with good reproducibility, and the encapsulation condition is mild compared with other methods. The drawbacks include (1) low entrapment efficiency for hydrophilic molecules, (2) the complete removal of residual detergent is impossible, (3) the procedure is lengthy, and (4) scale-up is difficult.

Freeze-Drying Method

The freeze-drying (or dehydration–rehydration) method was developed by Ohsawa et al. (1984) and Kirby and Gregoriadis (1984). This method is used to prepare MLVs with high entrapment efficiency. In this method, small *empty* unilamellar vesicles are first prepared, which are then mixed with the aqueous phase containing the molecules to be encapsulated. The mixture is freeze dried by conventional means. The liposome will be generated by adding an aqueous phase, followed by shaking, usually resulting in large MLVs as products. Alternatively, if the drug has a stability problem during the freeze-drying process, an aqueous solution containing the drug can be mixed with a prefabricated freeze-dried lipid product to produce liposomal drug.

The advantages of this method are as follows:

1. It produces liposomes with high entrapment efficiency.
2. The procedure's flexibility may aid product stability, as noted earlier.
3. Scale-up is possible.
4. The lyophile can be stored and rehydration can be done immediately before use.

The drawbacks of the method are possible particle size instability of the liposome during the freeze-drying process and the high cost of the freeze-drying process.

pH-Gradient Method ("Remote Loading")

The pH-gradient method has been designed to improve the encapsulation efficiency of ionizable amphoteric compounds (Mayer et al., 1993; Cullis et al., 1997). In this method, liposomes with or without the drug are first prepared by the techniques described earlier. The transmembrane pH-gradient of the liposomes is then generated either by adding an alkalinizing agent to increase the pH of the external medium to a desired level or by exchanging the extravesicular media with a buffer using gel exclusion chromatography or dialysis techniques. The drugs will be redistributed across the lipid bilayers in response to the pH-gradient, and can potentially achieve entrapment efficiencies of almost 100%. One advantage of this method is its high efficiency to encapsulate lipophilic amines such as doxorubicin and dopamine. DOXIL (Table 14.1) is prepared by this method. Another advantage is that this technique allows the drug to be encapsulated just before use, which eliminates the stability problems associated with the postencapsulation processing and long-term storage. Any lipids or mixture of lipids can be used as long as they form liposomes capable of maintaining a stable transmembrane pH-gradient. However, this technique is not applicable to nonionizable drugs.

Gas-Bubbling Method

The gas-bubbling method is a simple method developed by Talsma et al. (1994). In this method, a stream of gas is introduced into the bottom of a bottle that contains an aqueous dispersion of lipid particles. After bubbling for a sufficient time, liposomes are formed in the reservoir. To reduce the processing time, the size of the lipid particles is usually decreased (e.g., by micronization), and the temperature of the bubbling process is controlled above the gel/liquid phase transition temperature of the lipids. This method is a simple and inexpensive single-step process using no organic solvents or strong mechanical forces; the bubbling gas can be recycled and reused in the production. The drawbacks of this method are (1) the production time is long; (2) the particle size tends to be large and heterogeneous; (3) heating the system above the gel/liquid transition could induce the degradation of the drugs; (4) scale-up is difficult; and (5) encapsulation of water-insoluble drugs is inefficient, as they must be solubilized in the system before liposome formulation. If liposome preparation by the gas-bubbling method is followed by one of the size reduction methods discussed earlier, the size heterogeneity will be diminished.

ASEPTIC FILTRATION FOR PARENTERAL FORMULATIONS

Aseptic filtration is necessary for parenteral formulations. Because both lipids and the structure of liposomes are unstable at high temperatures, conventional terminal steam sterilization is not suitable for liposome formulations. Thus, the membrane aseptic filtration is the most reliable method for sterilizing liposome formulations. Since the possibility exists for the membrane being defective, it is advisable to test the integrity of the assembled unit by carrying out a *bubble-point* test. This test relies on the fact that after a membrane has been wetted, the surface tension between water and air is such that air cannot be passed through the membrane until sufficient pressure has been reached to overcome that surface tension. The critical pressure at which air will pass (i.e., the point at which a bubble will appear) is directly related to the size of the pores. For a filtration unit to be effective, the size of the pore should be within the limit.

Membrane filters used for sterile filtration are usually the *tortuous pore* type membrane, which consists of fibers crisscrossed over each other to give a matrix in which channels are formed from the random spaces winding in and out between the fibers, tracing a tortuous path from one side of the membrane to the other. The average diameter of these channels is controlled by the density of the fibers in the matrix. Because of the convoluted nature of the channels, microorganisms and liposomes that are larger than the channel diameter (usually 0.22 μm) are retained when passing through such a membrane, and thus the filter clogs up easily.

Freeze Drying of Liposomes

After aseptic filtration, the liposomes are usually freeze dried to prolong their shelf lives. Freeze drying (lyophilization) involves the removal of water from the liposomal formulation in the frozen state at low pressure. In the freezing step, the aqueous liposomal formulation is filled into vials and then the vials are loaded onto temperature-controlled shelves in a large chamber. The shelf temperature is lowered to about –40°C. The drying step starts after the product is completely frozen at this temperature. This step can be further divided into two steps, primary drying and secondary drying. During primary drying, the shelf temperature is increased to a designated temperature and the ice in the frozen system is evaporated. In the secondary drying process, the shelf temperature is further increased and the residual adsorbed water is removed by high vacuum. To preserve the liposome structures during the freeze-drying process, lyoprotectants such as lactose, sucrose, or trehalose are added in the liposomal formulation.

There are several characteristics of the freeze-drying process that make it desirable for liposomal formulations. First, since the drying takes place at low temperatures, chemical decomposition of labile drugs and aggregation of liposomes are minimized. Second, the resulting product has a very high specific surface area, which makes the product be easily rehydrated before use. Third, freeze drying is more compatible with sterile operations compared with other drying methods; the liposomal solution can be sterile-filtered immediately before the vial filling process.

MECHANISMS AND STRATEGIES FOR SOLUBILIZATION OF LIPID-SOLUBLE COMPOUNDS

One advantage of liposome is their singular ability to take up material of all shapes and sizes regardless of their individual chemical peculiarities. The most relevant to this discussion is for lipid-soluble compounds, which are incorporated into the lipid bilayer of the liposome. Thus, the maximum amount taken up into liposomes is directly proportional to the quantity of membrane components, but is independent of the size of the liposomes used, except in a few cases where the structure of the encapsulated compound may restrict the final size of the liposome. Theoretically, any type of liposome is suitable for the incorporation of lipid-soluble substances, but practical considerations make some choices more preferable over others. MLVs are the best choice for sustained release, whereas SUVs are particularly suitable for rapid intermembrane transfer.

For optimal loading of lipid-soluble drugs, the most desirable formulations would be those having the highest lipid/aqueous distribution ratio. Thus, MLV and SUV will be suitable, although the higher curvature of the SUV bilayer may reduce its capacity for drug molecules. LUVs prepared by the reverse-phase evaporation or solvent-injection methods, while optimal for water-soluble drugs, will generally have a lower capacity for lipid-soluble drugs owing to the lower lipid/aqueous distribution ratio.

The preferred preparation methods for incorporation of water-insoluble drugs are generally those that involve organic solvents. Thus, drug will be dissolved in the appropriate solvent and preparation will proceed as normal, as in the film forming/rehydration (MLV, SUV) methods, organic dilution methods, spray-dried proliposomes, and others. During processing, as the lipid bilayer forms, drug molecules will naturally become incorporated into the bilayer.

Incorporation of water-insoluble drugs into previously formed liposomes is possible but may be problematic. Preparation by stirring solid drug with liposomes would require an initial dissolution of drug into the bulk aqueous phase before partitioning into the lipid bilayer. While the equilibrium may favor this resulting incorporation into liposomes, the overall rate will be limited by the intrinsic dissolution rate and the aqueous solubility of the compound, and thus may not be rapid enough to be practical. On the other hand, if the drug is ionizable and has appreciable solubility at any pH, it may be possible to utilize the pH-gradient methods described earlier, whereby changing the pH to render the drug unionized and water insoluble will load drug into the liposome bilayer.

Care must be taken that the pH change is gradual enough such that partitioning of the drug into the liposome bilayer will occur rather than drug precipitation.

Another important factor is the actual location and orientation of the drug molecule within the lipid bilayer. These would be determined by the molecular size, lipophilicity, and geometry of the drug molecule. Relatively flat, amphiphilic molecules that are roughly the same size and shape as phospholipid molecules would be most favorably incorporated and oriented in parallel with the tail chains of phospholipids, analogously to cholesterol. Hydrogen-bonding and/or electrostatic attractions of the polar portions of drug with the phospholipid headgroups would render this orientation especially favorable. Flat molecules with no polar regions (e.g., aromatic compounds) can be envisioned as being sandwiched between the two tail groups of the liposomal membrane. An example of the former orientation is heme (Tipping et al., 1979; Ginsburg and Demel, 1983; Cannon et al., 1984), while tetraphenyl porphyrin and its analogs exhibit the latter orientation (Tsuschida et al., 1983; Yuasa et al., 1986).

CHARACTERIZATION OF LIPOSOMES

To ensure reproducibility of the performance of drug-loaded liposomes in vivo, one must assess the appropriate physicochemical parameters of the formulation. Some of the key parameters, along with the most commonly used techniques, are listed in Table 14.3.

Liposome size is probably the parameter that has the largest influence on the physical properties and appearance of the formulation. Dynamic and quasielastic light-scattering techniques (e.g., Malvern and Coulter Counter apparatus), including laser light scattering (e.g., Nicomp, Sympatec-Helos), are probably the most commonly used method for measuring size. It has the advantage of quickly giving quantitative results on size distribution. A related technique, forward laser light scatter by flow cytometry (fluorescence activated cell sorter), was used to characterize liposomes prepared using the Microfluidizer. The results correlated well with those of electron microscopy (Childers et al., 1989). Size exclusion chromatography such as molecular sieve chromatography,

---

TABLE 14.3
List of Parameters and Common Techniques for Characterizing Liposomes

Parameter	Technique
Size	Light-scattering
	Size exclusion/molecular sieve chromatography
	Electron microscopy
	Ultracentrifugation
	Ultrafiltration
Number of lamellae	NMR spectroscopy
	Small-angle X-ray scattering
Encapsulation volume	Encapsulation of water-soluble markers
Encapsulation efficiency	Size exclusion/molecular sieve chromatography
	Ultrafiltration/dialysis
	Ultracentrifugation
Bilayer fluidity	Fluorescent probes
	Spin label EPR
	NMR probes
	Calorimetry
Charge	Microelectrophoresis
	Zeta potential

gel permeation chromatography, is also convenient and capable of giving quantitative size distribution results. A variety of size exclusion high-performance liquid chromatography (HPLC) columns are now commercially available, and thus the technique is adaptable to an industrial laboratory setting that requires high throughput. One must be careful in choice of column to ensure that the molecular size range of the column encompasses all expected size ranges of the formulation. If a significant fraction of the product elutes in the void volume of the column, the technique is probably not sensitive enough for quality control purposes. Electron microscopy will yield size as well as structural information (lamellarity, shape, etc.), but is limited to semiquantitative information about a small sampling of the formulation. In addition, care must be taken that sample preparation (e.g., freeze etching, fixation) does not introduce any change in the physical properties of the liposomes. Ultra-centrifugation will also yield semiquantitative information on size distribution, but is not commonly used at present due to low throughput, expense, and other confounding factors.

Number of lamellae is another important parameter that is important to monitor, since it can influence the amount of water-insoluble drug that can be incorporated into the liposome bilayers. Knowledge of the size distribution and method of preparation can give some clue to the number of lamellae, but it is preferable to utilize a technique that gives a direct measure of the parameter. The most routinely used is electron-scanning microscopy, subject to the same precautions mentioned earlier. More sophisticated techniques include nuclear magnetic resonance (NMR) spectroscopy and small-angle X-ray scattering (Hauser, 1993) can be used.

If one knows the average size and the number of lamellae, one can theoretically estimate the average encapsulation volume for water-soluble drugs, which is the total volume of the enclosed aqueous space within the core and between the lipid bilayers. This can be measured directly by encapsulation of water-soluble markers. Knowledge of this parameter is more critical for water-soluble compounds than for water-insoluble ones.

Encapsulation efficiency is an expression of the amount of drug incorporated into the liposome, and is normally defined as the percentage of drug bound to liposome relative to total amount of drug. It can also be expressed as absolute encapsulation efficiency, which is a ratio of moles of bound drug/mole lipid. For example, if a liposomal preparation contains 4 mM total drug, 3 mM bound drug, 1 mM free drug, and 30 mM lipid, the percentage encapsulation efficiency would be 75%, corresponding to an absolute encapsulation efficiency of 0.1 mole bound drug/mole lipid. Determination of the parameter generally requires separation of free drug from liposomes. Analysis of drug in both the free and liposomal-drug fractions allows calculation of encapsulation efficiency. For the latter, it may be necessary to first disrupt the liposomes by treatment with detergent (e.g., Triton X100) or other suitable means to obtain accurate determinations of drug concentration. Separation of free and liposomal drug is usually accomplished by size exclusion chromatography using a column that elutes the liposomes in the void volume and retains free drug. Other techniques include dialysis, ultrafiltration, and ultracentrifugation. In the dialysis and ultrafiltration method, membranes with a molecular weight cutoff between those of the drug and the lowest expected liposome fraction are selected. Control experiments must be performed to ensure that no free drug is adsorbed onto the membrane and that no liposomal material comes through the membrane into the ultrafiltrate or dialysate. This is also applied to ultracentrifugation method, wherein liposomal drug is pelleted, leaving free drug in the supernatant. Care must be taken that no liposomal material (namely, small liposomes) remains in the supernatant to give inaccurate results. One study compared several methods for separation of LUV liposomal from nonencapsulated drug. The conclusions from these studies were that (1) ultrafiltration appeared to be the fastest method; (2) dialysis was unsuitable owing to equilibration of encapsulated drug as dialysis of free drug proceeded; (3) size-exclusion chromatography led to dilution of liposomes, unless a minicolumn was used; (4) precipitation of liposomes by protamine aggregation was an inexpensive and efficient method for separation and measurement of free drug; and (5) a density-gradient method was judged to be the best method for separation (Dipali et al., 1996).

Encapsulation efficiencies for water-insoluble drugs will normally be quite high, since the amount of drug in the external aqueous phase will be limited by the solubility. In this case, the encapsulation efficiency will be related to the partition coefficient of drug between the aqueous phase and the lipid bilayers, or actually the distribution coefficient if working with an ionizable drug at a particular pH. If there is any appreciable water solubility, the partition or distribution coefficient will actually reflect a lower limit for the encapsulation efficiency, since there could be drug dissolved in the aqueous regions within the liposome. Partition coefficient is usually expressed in terms of ratio of drugs in respective volumes of lipid bilayer and buffer, in which case the former must be estimated on the basis of lipid weight and density. Austin et al. (1995) measured the distribution coefficients of four ionizable molecules into DMPC SUV liposomes as a function of pH, using an ultrafiltration method to separate free drug from liposomes. Results were consistent with the known pK_a values of the compounds, and the partition coefficient of the unionized species was generally within an order of magnitude to those from octanol/buffer partition coefficients. However, for the charged species of some compounds (especially protonated amines), the partitioning profiles in the lipid/buffer did not agree with octanol/water distribution coefficient data, in that they partitioned into the lipid bilayer while not into the octanol. This is not surprising, since charged moieties would be expected to interact favorably with the headgroups of phospholipids. Similarly, membrane partition coefficients for a series of steroids in egg PC liposomes were measured by determining the solubility in buffer and liposomes by a dialysis technique; the partition coefficient was then determined by calculating the ratio of the two solubility values times the calculated volume ratio of lipid to buffer (Heap et al., 1970). Other factors affect the distribution coefficient as well. For example, lipid/buffer distribution coefficients for a 5-lipoxygenase inhibitor in liposomes, determined by ultrafiltration, were found to be dependent on lipid composition and concentration, with 50% cholesterol increasing in the formulation; the distribution coefficient increased almost twofold (Gupta et al., 1996).

Bilayer fluidity is an important parameter that affects liposome stability, liposome behavior in vivo, and other properties. As discussed earlier, calorimetric methods (e.g., DSC and mDSC) are useful to determine actual phase transition temperatures for the gel to liquid crystalline transition. Alternatively, one can incorporate fluorescent probes into the bilayer that have different fluorescent properties depending on the molecular motion of their environment, and thus are sensitive to whether the bilayer is in the gel or liquid crystalline state. Examples of these probes are dipyrenyl PC (Vaukonen et al., 1990), diphenyl hexatriene (Diederichs et al., 1992), indolyl-labeled PC, and carbazole-labeled PC (Gardam and Silvius, 1990). Motion in the headgroup region can be monitored by dansyl PE (Diederichs et al., 1992). Similarly, NMR probes such as deuterated PC (Davis, 1983), spin label electron paramagnetic resonance (EPR) probes such as nitroxide tagged lipids (Cevc and Seddon, 1993), or FT-IR of 13C-DPPS liposomes (Huber et al., 1994) can be used to obtain the same information. The EPR method is not widely used because of the expense of the equipment, and has been supplanted by the other techniques. The experiments with probes need to be done at several temperatures spanning storage and physiologic temperatures, and the probe concentration must be kept low enough to ensure that the probe itself does not alter the fluidity.

The charge on the liposomal surface is a property that has major effects on the stability, biodistribution, and cellular uptake of liposomes, and is governed by lipid headgroup composition and by pH. It can be monitored by micro electrophoresis (i.e., capillary zone electrophoresis), or by measurement of the zeta potential (Egorova, 1994).

STABILITY OF LIPOSOMES

When evaluating the stability of liposomal formulations, there are a number of factors to consider. The physical characteristics of the liposomes (parameters listed in Table 14.3) can be altered on storage and should be monitored by the appropriate technique as a function of time of storage. In addition, chemical stability of the phospholipid and other components is also an important parameter to assess. Chemical degradation of the lipid can in turn alter the physical properties of the liposome. Accelerated stability studies may be misleading, since storage above the transition temperature of the phospholipids used would give results not indicative of those at room temperature. Thus real-time studies may be necessary (Betageri et al., 1993). Both physical and chemical stability are addressed in the following.

PHYSICAL STABILITY

Changing in the size distribution of the liposomal dispersion is probably the parameter most likely to affect efficacy and biodistribution of the formulation, and thus is most important to measure. In common with emulsions, small unilamellar liposomes can be considered to be in a thermodynamically unstable state. Processes such as fusion and invagination will eventually cause SUV preparations to increase in size and lamellarity to become MLV liposomes. The process could take years, but it is nevertheless necessary to monitor the size distribution using appropriate techniques, as shown in Table 14.3, as part of the stability evaluation of a liposomal formulation. In general, liposomes with a neutral surface charge (e.g., those containing only PC) will have the highest tendency to aggregate, hence the desirability of incorporating small amounts of charged lipids. Crommelin (1984) found that negatively charged liposomes composed of PC/Chol/PS (10:4:1) were stable with respect to size over a 7-day period regardless of ionic strength. However, positively charged liposomes [PC/Chol/SA (10:4:1)] were stable for the same period only at low ionic strength, suggesting that factors other than electrical repulsion control stability. Changes in size due to aggregation will also alter the number of lamellae and the encapsulation volume. Bilayer fluidity also has an effect on stability of liposome size (Saez et al., 1985).

Monitoring encapsulation efficiency is another high priority for inclusion in a stability protocol for liposomal formulations. Inclusion of cholesterol increases the bilayer fluidity of phospholipids containing saturated tailgroups that decreases the permeability and stabilizes the encapsulation efficiency. For example, leakage of fluorescent marker (6-carboxyl fluorescein) from PC/chol (1:1) liposomes was 250 times slower than from liposomes containing only PC (Noda et al. 1993). Leakage of drug out of liposomes can arise from changes in liposome fluidity, bilayer permeability, pore formation, and other phenomena. Liposome surface charge will be affected by chemical changes in the phospholipid headgroups and should be monitored to assess stability. The other parameters outlined in Table 14.3 should also be monitored as a function of time to assess physical stability.

CHEMICAL STABILITY

Hydrolysis and oxidation are the two primary degradation routes to which liposomal phospholipids are susceptible. Hydrolytic attack at the fatty acyl carbonyl will produce free fatty acids and lysophosphatides (e.g., lyso-phosphatidyl choline [LPC]). Hydrolysis generally follows first-order kinetics, with a strong dependence on pH; the pH for optimum stability is around 6.5 (Martin, 1990). The fatty acids produced will lead to a decrease in pH, hence the need to monitor pH-stability. The production of lysophosphatides will generally lead to an increase in bilayer fluidity and permeability, and hence decrease encapsulation efficiency. For example, Hernandez-Caselles et al. (1990) found that LPC formation led to release of fluorescent marker (carboxy fluorescein) from the liposomes. Hydrolysis can also occur to a lesser extent in the headgroup region (e.g., PC will yield PA and choline). This will result in changes in pH and liposome surface charge.

The oxidative route involves peroxidation of unsaturated tailgroups, particularly linoleic and linolenic acids. The resulting products (free radicals, aldehydes, etc.) can have a serious adverse effect on drug stability. The mechanism of lipid peroxidation is complex (see the Chemical Stability section in Chapter 10, "Emulsions and Microemulsions for Drug Solubilization and Delivery"), and is usually characterized by a lag phase. The reaction can be initiated by trace amounts of heavy metals (e.g., iron or copper), and propagated by peroxides and free radicals. Thus, the rate of oxidative degradation for a given liposome preparation would be dependent on a variety of factors and difficult to predict. Preparation method has some effect: sonication (Almog et al., 1991) and other high shear processes (Lang and Vigo-Pelfrey, 1993) have been shown to increase the rate of lipid peroxidation. Contact of formulations with the metal parts of certain size reducing equipment (e.g., the Microfluidizer) may also render them more susceptible to degradation (Lang and Vigo-Pelfrey, 1993). Liposome peroxidation can lead to changes in bilayer fluidity, permeability, and encapsulation efficiency in the same way as hydrolysis; thus, it is necessary to monitor and reduce this problem.

Lipid peroxidation can be monitored by several methods. These include determination of thiobarbituric acid reactive species (i.e., malondialdehyde and other aldehyde products), changes in UV absorbance at 234 nm (arising from formation of conjugated dienes from radical catalyzed rearrangement of, for example, linoleic and linolenic acid), and other methods. Since the various methods monitor the extent of oxidation at different points in the mechanism and may actually monitor transient species, care must be taken to choose the method most indicative of stability of the formulations of interest, and if necessary, two different methods. Lang and Vigo-Pelfrey, (1993) compared several different methods for monitoring peroxidation as a quality control procedure for liposomes, and found that conjugated diene measurement at 234 nm increased continuously and correlated well with changes in fatty acid composition, whereas neither malondialdehyde formation nor lipid hydroperoxide formation (measured by an iodometric assay) showed any such correlation. In any case, such procedures should be considered as screening methods, and final conclusions on excipient stability should be based on assays of individual phospholipids by HPLC or gas chromatography methods. Cholesterol has also been shown to be susceptible to peroxidation (Lang and Vigo-Pelfrey, 1993); thus, formulations containing it should also be assayed for cholesterol as part of a stability protocol. If the formulation is found to be susceptible to peroxidation, antioxidants such as BHA, BHT, or tocopherols can be added to improve stability, or phospholipids containing only saturated phospholipids can be used. Tris buffer has been shown to retard oxidation of PC liposomes due to its ability to scavenge hydroxyl free radicals (Almog et al., 1991).

There is some evidence that the processes of hydrolysis and peroxidation are interrelated. Since the latter process generally has a lag phase, hydrolysis usually begins first. The resulting increase in bilayer fluidity and permeability due to hydrolysis may render the phospholipid tailgroups more exposed to initiators and propagators of lipid peroxidation. Thus, incorporation of 3 mol% LPC into diarachidonyl PC liposomes increased malodialdehyde production by about 25% (Montfort et al., 1987). Similarly, LPC formation has been found to be retarded in liposomes stored under nitrogen, suggesting that peroxidation renders the bilayer more susceptible to hydrolysis (Hernandez-Caselles et al., 1990). SUV liposomes have been found to undergo both hydrolysis and peroxidation more rapidly than MLV structures due to the greater curvature (Lang and Vigo-Pelfrey, 1993). This is in line with the findings that phospholipids in mixed micelles undergo peroxidation faster compared with those in bilayers (Maiorino et al., 1995). Compounds that decrease bilayer fluidity (e.g., cholesterol and to an even greater extent, ergosterol and estradiol) have been found to retard lipid peroxidation (Wiseman et al., 1990). Tocopherol appears to have a dual role in stabilizing liposomes: it serves primarily not only as an antioxidant but also stabilizes the bilayer by specific binding to phospholipid molecules (Hernandez-Caselles et al., 1990). This interaction appears to be between the hydroxyl groups of alpha-tocopherol and the fatty acyl carbonyl of phospholipids (Urano et al., 1990).

In general, liposomes cannot be frozen and thawed to overcome chemical stability problems, since this leads to increases in liposome size and decreases in encapsulation efficiency. A better approach to extend the shelf life of liposomes has been lyophilization, with reconstitution just before use. Early attempts to do this generally led to an unacceptable increase in particle size of liposomes and decrease in encapsulation efficiency, but it has been found that inclusion of a disaccharide (e.g., lactose, sucrose, or, especially, trehalose) in the formulation prevents this (Crommelin and Van Bommel, 1984; Crowe et al., 1987; Crowe and Crowe, 1992). It has been proposed that the mechanism for the stabilization is that the disaccharide can substitute for water in binding to the headgroup region of the phospholipid and retain the bilayer in a liquid crystalline phase in the dry state (Crowe and Crowe, 1992). If one decides to use lyophilization and storage in the dry state to extend the shelf life of a liposomal formulation, one should monitor liposome size, lamellarity, encapsulation efficiency, drug potency, and other parameters both before and after lyophilization and reconstitution. Such a protocol was followed for a liposomal hemoglobin formulation containing trehalose, proposed as a blood substitute (Cliff et al., 1992).

PHARMACEUTICAL APPLICATIONS

The delivery of water-insoluble drugs into the target sites in the human body has always been a challenge, because these compounds have low solubilities and will precipitate out in an aqueous environment. Liposomes, as one of the latest new drug delivery systems, efficiently meet this challenge. Compared with other solubilization techniques for water-insoluble drugs, liposome technology is a superior choice in many cases. In a study conducted by van Bloois et al. (1987), the improvement of the apparent solubility of almitrine bismesylate, a poorly water-soluble lipophilic compound was compared among three techniques: liposomes, mixed micelles, and oil-in-water (o/w) emulsions. Liposomes possessed superior properties with respect to almitrine solubilization and stability compared with the other two types of formulations. A 100-fold increase in apparent almitrine solubility relative to the aqueous buffer could be achieved. In addition to their function of solubilizing the water-insoluble drugs, liposomes as drug delivery systems can change the biodistribution of a drug and thereby alter its therapeutic index. Hence, liposome technology has been successfully used to formulate water-insoluble pharmaceutical agents. Examples of water-insoluble drugs that have been examined in liposomal formulations include annamycin, vincristine, mitoxantrone, and ciprofloxacin. The cancer therapeutic agent camptothecin and its analogs are also particularly challenging to formulate due to their poor water solubility and toxic effects. Hence, liposomal formulations have been evaluated for a number of camptothecin analogs, for example, topotecan, lurtotecan, 9-nitrocamptothecin, irinotecan, gimatecan (Pantazis et al., 2003; Stano et al., 2004; Castor 2005; Glaberman et al., 2005; Zamboni 2005). Four other examples are discussed more fully in the following section.

Amphotericin B

Amphotericin B, a polyene macrolide antibiotic, is a broad-spectrum antifungal agent for the treatment of systematic fungal infections (Gold et al., 1955; Gallis et al., 1990; Lyman and Walsh, 1992). It has remained the drug of choice for life-threatening invasive fungal infections over the past 30 years. Amphotericin B is practically water insoluble at pH 6–7, while at pH 2 or 11 in water it is very slightly soluble (ca. 0.1 mg/mL). The mechanism of pharmacological effect of amphotericin B is well established. This macrolide primarily binds with ergosterol, a common sterol in fungal membrane. Reaction with ergosterol produces pores in the cell membrane, allowing salts and other small molecules to escape the fungal cell. This action is fungicidal, a significant advantage in antifungal chemotherapy (Palacios and Serrano, 1978; Kerridge, 1986). However, amphotericin B also has toxic effects due to the binding with other sterols, including cholesterol, a common sterol in mammalian membranes (Medoff and Kobayashi, 1980). This leads to a range of serious side effects such as chills, fever, headache, nausea, azotemia, hypolalemia, hypomagnesemia, nephrotoxicity, and thrombophlebitis at the infusion site with associated local tissue damage. As a result, the usefulness of amphotericin B has been limited by its narrow therapeutic index. To increase its therapeutic index and reduce its toxic effects, liposomal formulations of amphotericin B have been investigated since 1981 (Adler-Moore, 1994). This polyene antibiotic can be incorporated into the lipid bilayer owing to its high lipophilicity (Hiemenz and Walsh, 1996).

Three lipid formulations of amphotericin B are now either marketed for clinical use or undergoing further study before they can be approved in various countries worldwide (Hiemenz and Walsh, 1996).

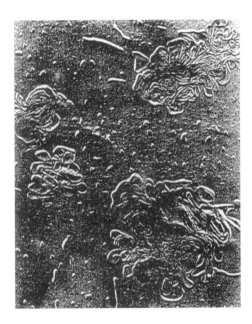

FIGURE 14.9 Freeze-fracture electron micrograph of the ribbon-like amphotericin B lipid complexes. (From Bangham, A. D., *Hosp. Pract.*, 27, 51–62, 1992. With permission.)

Amphotericin B lipid complex (Abelcet®, Enzon Pharmaceuticals, Inc., Bridgewater, New Jersey) is a suspension of ribbonlike structures of a bilayered membrane formed by combining a 7:3 molar ratio of DMPC and DMPG with amphotericin B (Figure 14.9). Amphotericin B colloidal dispersion (Amphotec®, developed by Sequus and now marketed by Three Rivers Pharmaceuticals) is composed of disk-like structures of cholesteryl sulfate complex with amphotericin B in a ratio of 1:1. Ambisome® (developed by Gilead Sciences and now marketed by Astellas Pharma US, Deerfield, Illinois) is the only true liposomal preparation among the three lipid formulations of amphotericin B. In this formulation, the drug is incorporated into the bilayer of small unilamellar liposome within a size range of 45–80 nm. The lipid bilayer is made up of hydrogenated soy phosphatidylcholine (HSPC), distearoyl phosphatidylglycerol (DSPG), cholesterol, and amphotericin B in a 2:0.8:1:0.4 molar ratios (Adler-Moore and Proffitt, 1993). In the development of this formulation, unilamellar liposomes with a range of different chemical compositions were tested. Although both HSPC and hydrogenated egg phosphatidylcholine performed comparably as the primary phospholipid, HSPC was chosen for the final formulation since there was less variation in the length of its hydrocarbon chains. Hydrogenated rather than nonhydrogenated phospholipids were used because of the chemical stability provided by the saturated phospholipids. Formulations that contained no cholesterol or low molar ratios of cholesterol exhibited more toxicity in mice than formulations with a cholesterol content greater than 25 mol% of total lipid component. The reduced toxicity associated with the presence of cholesterol in AmBisome may be due to increased bilayer stability that is imparted by the sterol, and possibly to the affinity of Amphotericin B for the cholesterol in the membrane (Papahadjopoulos et al., 1973a, b; Medoff et al., 1983). Increased toxicity was also observed in mice either when the molar ratio of DSPG: amphotericin B was less than 2:1 or when shorter chain phospholipids, such as dilauryl phosphatidylglycerol, were substituted for DSPG (Adler-Moore and Proffitt, 1993).

In the manufacturing process for the marketed products, the lipids, cholesterol, and amphotericin B were first dissolved in an organic solvent, and a dry film was obtained using a rotary evaporator. The film was dehydrated and a microemulsification technique (Gamble, 1988) was used in the preparation of small unilamellar liposomes. In the microemulsification process, a modified Gaulin

Homogenizer, Model 15M was used. The modification consists of two heat exchange reservoirs that maintain the lipid solution at a selected temperature. In the operation, the solution is subjected to very high shearing forces in the homogenizing valve area while maintaining the solution at a selected temperature. A certain period of time is selected to allow multiple circulations of the entire lipid solution through the homogenizer. The final product can be readily sterilized by aseptic filtration. The microemulsification procedure produced small liposomes with less toxicity and a more consistently homogeneous size distribution than sonicated liposomes (Adler-Moore and Proffitt, 1993). Electron microscopic examination of the AmBisome by negative staining and freeze fracture confirmed the small, unilamellar, and spherical morphology of the liposomes (Adler-Moore and Proffitt, 1993).

AmBisome is a sterile, lyophilized powder with a shelf life of up to 4 years when stored at or below 25°C. This form can be easily reconstituted by adding sterile water and shaking by hand. The physicochemical and biological properties of the rehydrated products do not change during this time. The amount of drug association with the liposomes was confirmed by applying AmBisome to a Sephadex G25M chromatographic column. All the amphotericin B was recovered from the liposomal fraction of the column (Adler-Moore and Proffitt, 1993).

AmBisome has proven its efficacy in both controlled and randomized clinical trials. There are more than 150 publications on the safety and efficacy of AmBisome in the treatment of life-threatening fungal infections. The incidence of adverse effects for AmBisome is low, namely, 5%–10%, compared with 80% of the conventional amphotericin B formulation. The effective dose for AmBisome ranges from 1 to 3 mg/kg and achieves peak liposomal amphotericin B level of 29 μg/mL at 1 mg/kg dose, compared to 3.6 μg/mL for the conventional amphotericin B at the same dose. AmBisome is well tolerated when used with Cyclosporin A, an important consideration when treating organ transplant patients. AmBisome can be administrated rapidly, usually within 30–60 min, and without need for administering a test dose or pretreating patient with antihistamines or fever-reducing agents. To date, AmBisome has been used to treat more than 100,000 patients worldwide.

Doxorubicin

Doxorubicin is a cytotoxic anthracylcine chemotherapeutic agent isolated from cultures of *Streptomyces peucetius*. The cytotoxic effect is thought to be related to its ability to intercalate between nucleotide bases of DNA and RNA of target cells, thereby inhibiting nucleotide replication and action of DNA and RNA polymerases. It has been used for a variety of malignancies and cancers such as disseminated neoplastic conditions such as acute lymphoblastic leukemia, acute myeloblastic leukemia, neuroblastoma, soft tissue and bone sarcomas, breast cancer, ovarian cancer, Hodgkin's disease, malignant lymphoma, AIDS-related Kaposi's sarcoma, and multiple myeloma. However, it has several adverse side effects, most notably cardiotoxicity, that significantly limit its dosage. The cardiotoxic effects include cumulative dose-related congestive heart failure, left ventricular ejection fraction, and histological changes (Rahman et al., 2007). Hence, liposomes have been successfully investigated to ameliorate the cardiotoxic effects of doxorubicin, to enhance preferential uptake by tumor cells rather than cardiac tissue. Whereas blood vessels in cardiac tissues have tight capillary junctions, those in tumors allow more extravasation of species such as liposomes into the tumor, which enhances uptake of a liposome-encapsulated chemotherapeutic agent into the tumor (Green and Rose, 2006). Doxorubicin liposomes were first examined clinically as early as the 1980s (Rahman et al., 1990). Doxil (US; Caelyx® in the EU) a long-circulating (pegylated) doxorubicin liposomal formulation, was approved in 1995 for Karposi's sarcoma, and in 1999 for ovarian cancer. A non-pegylated lipsomal formulation, Myocet, was approved in Europe in 2000 (Barenholz, 2012; Allen and Cullis, 2013). For Doxil, Phase III trials showed similar efficacy compared to conventional doxorubicin, but had a superior safety profile, with lower incidence of alopecia, myelosuppression, nausea and vomiting, and a significantly lower incidence ($p < 0.001$) of cardiotoxicity even at higher cumulative doses (Rivera, 2003). Liposomal encapsulation has a large effect on the pharmacokinetic properties of doxorubicin, which contributes to its increased therapeutic index. The half-lives are 30, 16, and 74 hours, while the volumes of distribution are 900 L/m^2, 34 L/m^2, and 1.9 L/m^2 for free doxorubicin, non-pegylated liposomal doxorubicin, and pegylated liposomal doxorubicin, respectively, (Macpherson and Evans, 2009).

Doxil is manufactured by the remote loading technique discussed earlier, which allows high loading of the drug in the liposomes. The drug actually precipitates inside the liposome, which increases loading and retention within the liposome (Allen and Cullis, 2013). Doxil has become one of the most widely used agents for treatment of ovarian cancer, AIDS-related Kaposi's sarcoma, multiple myeloma, and breast cancer. Due to manufacturing issues, there was a drug supply shortage in 2011; the FDA allowed temporary use of an alternate form (Berger et al., 2014), and eventually an alternate manufacturing site for Doxil was approved to alleviate the shortage.

PACLITAXEL

Paclitaxel, a natural diterpene product isolated from the bark of *Taxus brevifolia*, is clinically active against advanced ovarian and breast cancer. Its use in treating other malignancies such as head, lung, and neck cancers is being explored. Paclitaxel is the first of a new class of antineoplastic drugs (Rowinsky et al., 1990; Huizing et al., 1995). The unique mechanism of action of paclitaxel includes stabilization of abnormal microtubules (Schiff et al., 1979), thus interfering with tumor cellular progress through mitosis, and arresting cell replication (DeBrabander et al., 1981). In spite of its powerful antitumor activity, the drug has presented a considerable challenge to formulation scientists owing to its poor water solubility. It does not contain any functional ionizable groups (Wani et al., 1971). For this reason, the solubility problem cannot be improved by alteration of pH, salt formation, or addition of charged complexing agents. The current clinical dosage form, Taxol® consists of concentrations of 0.3–1.2 mg/mL of paclitaxel dispersed in an equal parts mixture of ethanol and polyethoxylated castor oil (Cremophor EL®) (Meerum et al., 1997). This formulation is associated with a number of concerns, including stability, filtering requirements, and use of nonplasticized solution containers, and administration sets. Moreover, some of the side effects, such as severe hypersensitivity reactions, are considered to be formulation related. The adverse effects of the formulation are considered to be related to the use of Cremophor EL as the vehicle (Lorenz et al., 1977; Liebmann et al., 1994).

To eliminate the side effects caused by the excipients and possibly increase the antitumor activity of paclitaxel, liposome formulations have been investigated (Sharma et al., 1993; Straubinger et al., 1993; Sharma and Straubinger, 1994). The rationale of using liposomes as a carrier for the water-insoluble paclitaxel is similar to that for amphotericin B. More than 300 liposome formulations were evaluated. Preliminary results suggested that using PC as the principal lipid can incorporate higher concentrations of paclitaxel than any other lipids. However, the formulation containing only PC was highly aggregated, and incorporation of a negatively charged lipid, PG, reduced the aggregation. A molar ratio of PC:PG 9:1 was selected based on the stability results, as indicated by the crystallization of paclitaxel from the aqueous liposomal formulations (Sharma and Straubinger, 1994).

The production process of paclitaxel liposome formulation was similar to that of amphotericin B. However, owing to the very low solubility of paclitaxel, several different procedures were involved. First, solvation of the lipid-drug film was done using tert-butanol. Second, the solution was then lyophilized for 24 h. The lyophilized powder was hydrated with buffer (NaCl/Tes/EDTA:14 mM/10 mM/0.1 mM). Third, in the size-reduction process, a sonication method was used, wherein the suspension of MLVs was sonicated under argon in a bath sonicator for 30 min at 20°C. On the basis of the method, SUVs can be obtained with the size range of 25–50 nm. Paclitaxel was stable in the liposome for more than 3 months at both 4°C and 20°C, as indicated by a reverse-phase HPLC method. The liposomal formulations have been demonstrated to be able to increase the therapeutic index of paclitaxel in human ovarian tumor models (Sharma et al., 1997). A commercial liposomal formulation of paclitaxel, EndoTAG® (MediGene), is currently in Phase III clinical trials, while another, LEP-ETU (Neopharm/Insys) is in Phase II trials (Table 14.2).

Verteporfin (BPDMA)

Porphyrin compounds have been known as photosensitizers for the treatment and diagnosis of malignant cells (Kessel, 1983). The porphyrins have a natural tendency to localize in malignant tissue, where they absorb light at certain wavelengths when irradiated, thus providing a means to detect the tumor by the location of fluorescence. Verteporfin is a porphyrin that belongs to benzo-porphyrin derivatives. It is a water-insoluble compound at physiological pH, requiring an expensive and complicated synthetic procedure to produce. On the basis of the preliminary studies, this compound is also insoluble in pharmaceutically acceptable aqueous-organic cosolvent mixtures, aqueous polymeric solutions, and surfactant/micelle solutions. However, this photosensitizer can still be solubilized in a form suitable for parenteral administration using liposomes (Liu, 1998).

A stable verteporfin liposome formulation has been developed that includes DMPC as the principal neutral lipid, egg PG as the negatively charged lipid, and the drug (Liu, 1998). The molar ratio of the phospholipid to the photosensitizer should be greater than or equal to 7:1 to make a stable liposomal formulation with particle size of 150–300 nm and nearly 100% encapsulation of the verteporfin. The manufacturing process of the liposome (which includes dissolving the lipids and verteporfin in an organic solvent, formation of film by rotary evaporator, hydration of the film, and homogenizing the particle size) is similar to the method developed in making AmBisome. However, several features are unique to manufacturing of the liposomal formulation of verteporfin. First, the media used to hydrate the drug-lipid film is a solution of a disaccharide such as lactose, which serves as a cryoprotectant and facilitates the hydration process. Second, the hydration step should be done at a temperature lower than 30°C and preferably below the glass transition temperature of the photosensitizer–phospholipid complex formed, since at higher temperatures, phase separation and the portion of membrane defects increases, resulting in leakage of the photosensitizer from the liposome. On the basis of the method developed, the designed formulation generally gives liposomes smaller than 300 nm, which has a high filterability. Large batches can be produced using this method. In vitro studies have shown that verteporfin is rapidly transferred from the liposomal formulation to serum proteins, thereby providing a mechanism for delivery to cells (Chowdhary 2003). Currently, this verteporfin liposomal formulation is in clinical trials for cancer, and is already marketed as Visudyne for treatment of age-related macular degeneration. After IV injection, a laser is used to treat the affected area of the retina and arrest the degeneration process.

CONCLUSIONS AND FUTURE PROSPECTS

With the inception of liposome research in the drug delivery field over five decades ago, there was high optimism that liposomes would provide a delivery system that could be applied successfully to a large variety of pharmaceutical problems. In retrospect, it is now clear that liposomes will not provide the panacea for all delivery problems as had originally been hoped. However, the introduction of liposomal formulations for amphotericin B, doxorubicin, daunorubicin, and verteporfin into the marketplace within the past three decades, as well as the multiple products that have recently entered advanced clinical trials for cancer (Table 14.2), have demonstrated that the technology can potentially fill an important niche to solve delivery problems for selected drug molecules. In particular, when formulating poorly water-soluble substances, especially for parenteral administration, one should always consider liposomes as a possible approach. When compared to other vehicles used for water-insoluble drugs such as cosolvents, micelles, and emulsions, liposomes stand out as an attractive alternative owing to the low toxicity of phospholipids. Water insolubility is increasingly becoming a dominant characteristic of new drug candidates developed in pharmaceutical discovery areas. Thus, it is likely that use of liposomes in pharmaceutical products will be an increasingly important tool to the pharmaceutical formulator, and that more products using liposomal technology will reach the marketplace in the years to come.

ABBREVIATIONS

CMC	critical micelle concentration
DLPC	dilauroyl phosphatidyl choline
DMPC	dimyristoyl phosphatidyl choline
DMPE	dimyristoyl phosphatidyl ethanolamine
DMPG	dimyristoyl phosphatidyl glycerol
DOPC	dioleyl phosphatidyl choline
DPPA	dipalmitoyl phosphatidic acid
DPPC	dipalmitoyl phosphatidyl choline
DPPG	dipalmitoyl phosphatidyl glycerol
DPPE	dipalmitoyl phosphatidyl ethanolamine
DSPC	distearoyl phosphatidyl choline
DSC	differential scanning calorimetry
mDSC	modulated differential scanning calorimetry
DSPE	distearoyl phosphatidyl ethanolamine
DSPG	distearoyl phosphatidyl glycerol
EPR	electron paramagnetic resonance
HLB	hydrophilic-lipophilic balance
HPLC	high-performance liquid chromatography
HSPC	hydrogenated soy phosphatidyl choline
IUV	intermediate-sized unilamellar vesicle
LPC	lyso-phosphatidyl choline
LUV	large unilamellar vesicle
MLV	multi-lamellar vesicle
NMR	nuclear magnetic resonance
PA	phosphatidic acid
PC	phosphatidyl choline
PE	phosphatidyl ethanolamine
PEG	polyethylene glycol
PG	phosphatidyl glycerol
PI	phosphatidyl inositol
PS	phosphatidyl serine
RES	reticulo-endothelial system
REV	reverse-phase evaporation vesicle
SPLV	stable plurilamellar vesicle
SSL	sterically stabilized liposomes
SUV	small unilamellar vesicle

REFERENCES

Adler-Moore, J. (1994). AmBisome targeting to fungal infections. *Bone Marrow Transplant.*, 14 (Suppl.): 3–7.

Adler-Moore, J. P. and R. T. Proffitt. (1993). Development, characterization, efficacy, and mode of action of AmBiSome, a unilamellar liposomal formulation of Amphotericin B. *J. Liposome Res.*, 3: 429–450.

AHFS Drug Information (2006). American Society of Health-System Pharmacist, Bethesda, MD.

Allen, T. M. and A. Chonn. (1987). Large unilamellar liposomes with low uptake into the reticuloendothelial system. *FEBS Lett.*, 223: 42–46.

Allen T. M. and P. R. Cullis. (2013). Liposomal drug delivery systems: From concept to clinical applications. *Advan. Drug Deliv. Rev.*, 65: 36–48.

Allen, T. M., C. Hansen, and J. Rutledge. (1989). Liposomes with prolonged circulation times: Factors affecting uptake by reticuloendothelial and other tissues. *Biochim. Biophys. Acta*, 981: 27–35.

Allen, T. M., C. B. Hansen, and D. E. Lopes de Menezes. (1995). Pharmacokinetics of long-circulating liposomes. *Adv. Drug Deliv. Rev.*, 16: 267–284.

Allen, T. M., P. Sapra, E. Moase, J. Moreira, and D. Iden. (2002). Adventures in targeting. *J. Liposome Res.* 12: 5–12.

Almog, R., R. Forward, and C. Samsonoff. (1991). Stability of sonicated aqueous suspensions of phospholipids under air. *Chem. Phys. Lipid.*, 60: 93–99.

Andresen, T. L., L. Thomas, S. S. Jensen, and K. Jørgensen. (2005). Advanced strategies in liposomal cancer therapy: Problems and prospects of active and tumor specific drug release. *Prog. Lipid. Res.*, 44: 68–97.

Austin, R. P., A. M. Davis, and C. N. Manners. (1995). Partitioning of ionizing molecules between aqueous buffers and phospholipid vesicles. *J. Pharm. Sci.*, 84: 1180–1183.

Banai, S., A. Finkelstein, Y. Almagor, A. Assali, Y. Hasin, U. Rosenschein, P. Apruzzese et al. (2013). Targeted anti-inflammatory systemic therapy for restenosis: The Biorest Liposomal Alendronate with Stenting Study (BLAST) - A double blind, randomized clinical trial. *Am. Heart. J.*, 165: 234–240.

Bangham, A. D. (1992). Liposomes: Realizing their promise. *Hosp. Pract.*, 27: 51–62.

Bangham, A. D., M. M. Standish, and J. C. Watkins. (1965). Diffusion of univalent ions across the lamellae of swollen phospholipids. *J. Mol. Biol.*, 13: 238–252.

Barenholz, Y. (2012). Doxil® - The first FDA-approved nanodrug: Lessons learned. *J Control. Rel.*, 160: 117–134.

Batzi, S. and E. D. Korn. (1973). Single bilayer liposomes prepared without sonication. *Biochim. Biophys. Acta*, 298: 1015–1019.

Berger, J. L., A. Smith, K. K. Zorn, P. Sukumvanich, A. B. Olawaiye, J. Kelley, and T. C. Krivak. (2014). Outcomes analysis of an alternative formulation of PEGylated liposomal doxorubicin in recurrent epithelial ovarian carcinoma during the drug shortage era. *Onco. Targets Ther.*, 7: 1409–1413.

Bernstein, Z. P., A. Khan, K. C. Miller, D. W. Northfelt, G. Lopez-Berestein, and P. S. Gill. (2002). A multicenter phase II study of the intravenous administration of liposomal tretinoin in patients with acquired immunodeficiency syndrome-associated Kaposi's sarcoma. *Cancer*, 95: 2555–2561.

Betageri, G. V., S. A. Jenkins, and D. L. Parsons. (1993). *Liposome Drug Delivery Systems*, Technomic Publishing Company, Lancaster, UK, pp. 65–88.

Bian, J. and M. F. Roberts. (1990). Phase separation in short-chain lecithin/gel state long-chain lecithin aggregates. *Biochemistry*, 29: 7928–7935.

Bleasdale, J. E., J. Eichberg, and H. Hauser (1985). *Inositol and Phosphoinositides Metabolism and Regulation*, Human Press Inc., Clifton, NJ.

Borchardt, K., D. Heber, M. Klingmuller, K. Mohr, and B. Muller. (1991). The ability of cationic amphiphilic compounds to depress the transition temperature of DPPA liposomes depends on the spatial arrangement of the lipophilic moiety. *Biochem. Pharmacol.*, 42: S61–S65.

Bridson, R. H., B. Al-Duri, R. C. D. Santos, S. M. McAllister, J. Robertson, and H. O. Alpar. (2002). The preparation of liposomes using supercritical fluid technology. *J. Pharm. Pharmacol.*, 54 (Suppl.): S51.

Cannon, J. B., F. S. Kuo, R. F. Pasternack, N. M. Wong, and U. Muller-Eberhard. (1984). Kinetics of the interaction of hemin liposomes with heme binding proteins. *Biochemistry*, 23: 3715–3721.

Cannon, J. B., C. Martin, G. S. Drummond, and A. Kappas. (1993). Targeted delivery of a heme oxygenase inhibitor with a lyophilized liposomal tin mesoporphyrin formulation. *Pharm. Res.*, 10: 715–721.

Castor, T. P. (2005). Phospholipid nanosomes. *Curr. Drug Deliv.*, 2: 329–340.

Cevc, G. (1991). Polymorphism of the bilayer membranes in the ordered phase and the molecular origin of the lipid pretransition and rippled lamellae. *Biochimica et Biophysica Acta*, 1062: 59–69.

Cevc, G. (1992). Lipid properties as a basis for membrane modeling and rational liposome design. In *Liposome Technology*, Gregoriadis, G. (Ed.), Vol. I, CRC Press, Boca Raton, FL, pp. 1–36.

Cevc, G. (2004). Lipid vesicles and other colloids as drug carriers on the skin. *Adv. Drug Deliv. Rev.*, 56: 675–711.

Cevc, G. and J. M. Seddon. (1993). Physical characterization. In *Phospholipids Handbook*, Cevc, G. (Ed.), Marcel Dekker, New York, pp. 351–401.

Chahar, P. and K. C. Cummings. (2012). Liposomal bupivacaine: A review of a new bupivacaine formulation. *J. Pain Res.*, 5: 257–264.

Chen, T., J. M. Lausier, and C. T. Rhodes. (1986). Possible strategies for the formulation of antineoplastic drugs. *Drug Dev. Ind. Pharm.*, 12: 1041–1106.

Childers, N. K., S. M. Michalek, J. H. Eldridge, F. R. Denys, A. K. Berry, and J. R. McGhee. (1989). Characterization of liposome suspensions by flow cytometry *J. Immunol. Methods*, 119: 135–143.

Chowdhary, R. K., I. Shariff, and D. Dolphin. (2003). Drug release characteristics of lipid based benzoporphyrin derivative. *J. Pharm. Pharm. Sci.*, 6: 13–19.

Cliff, R. O., F. Ligler, B. Goins, P. M. Hoffmann, H. Spielberg, and A. S. Rudolph. (1992). Liposome encapsulated hemoglobin: Long-term storage stability and in vivo characterization. *Biomat. Artif. Cells Immob. Biotechnol.*, 20: 619–626.

Cortesi, B., E. Esposito, S. Gambarin, P. Telloli, E. Menegatti, and C. Nastruzzi. (1999). Preparation of lipo-somes by reverse-phase evaporation using alternative organic solvents. *J. Microencapsul.*, 16: 251–256.

Crommelin, D. J. A. (1984). Influence of lipid composition and ionic strength on the physical stability of lipo-somes. *J. Pharm. Sci.*, 73: 1559–1563.

Crommelin, D. J. A. and H. Schreier. (1994). Liposomes. In *Colloidal Drug Delivery Systems*, Kreuter, J. (Ed.), Marcel Dekker, New York, pp. 73–190.

Crommelin, D. J. A. and E. M. G. Van Bommel. (1984). Stability of liposomes on storage: Freeze-dried, frozen or as an aqueous dispersion. *Pharm. Res.*, 1: 159–163.

Crowe, J. H., L. M. Crowe, J. F., Carpenter, and A. Wistrom. (1987). Stabilization of dry phospholipid bilayers and proteins by sugars. *Biochem. J.*, 242: 1–10.

Crowe, L. M. and J. H. Crowe, (1992). Stabilization of dry liposomes by carbohydrates. *Dev. Biol. Stand.*, 74: 285–294.

Cullis, P. R., M. J. Hope, M. B. Bally, T. D. Madden, L. D. Mayer, and D. B. Fenske. (1997). Influence of pH gradients on the transbilayer transport of drugs, lipids, peptides and metal ions into large unilamellar vesicles. *Biochim. Biophys. Acta*, 1331: 187–211.

Dark, G. G., A. H. Calvert, R. Grimshaw, C. Poole, K. Swenerton, S. Kaye, R. Coleman et al. (2005). Randomized trial of two intravenous schedules of the topoisomerase I inhibitor liposomal lurtotecan in women with relapsed epithelial ovarian cancer: A trial of the national cancer institute of Canada clinical trials group. *J. Clin. Oncol.*, 23: 1859–1866.

Davis, J. H. (1983). The description of membrane lipid conformation, order and dynamics by 2H-NMR. *Biochim. Biophys. Acta*, 737: 117–171.

Deamer, D. and A. D. Bangham. (1976). Large volume liposomes by an ether vaporization method. *Biochim. Biophys. Acta*, 443: 629–634.

DeBrabander, M. G., R. Nuydens, R. Willebrods, and J. Demay. (1981). Taxol induces the assembly of free microtubules in living cells and blocks the organizing capacity of centrosomes and kinetochores. *Proc. Natl. Acad. Sci.*, 78: 5608–5612.

Deeken, J. F., R. Slack, G. J. Weiss, R. K. Ramanathan, M. J. Pishvaian, J. Hwang, and K. Lewandowski et al. (2013). A phase I study of liposomal-encapsulated docetaxel (LEDT) in patients with advanced solid tumor malignancies. *Cancer Chemother. Pharmacol.*, 71: 627–633.

Diederichs, J. E., W. Mehnert, J. S. Lucks, and R. H. Muller. (1992). Microviscosity measurements for the optimization of liposome and emulsion formulations. *Congr. Int. Technol. Pharm. USA*, 5: 138–147.

Dipali, S. R., S. B. Kulkari, and G. V. Betageri. (1996). Comparative study of separation of non-encapsulated drug from unilamellar liposomes by various methods. *J. Pharm. Pharmacol.*, 48: 1112–1115.

Dritschilo, A., C. H. Huang, C. M. Rudin, J. Marshall, B. Collins, J. L. Dul, and C. Zhang et al. (2006). Phase I study of liposome encapsulated craf antisense oligodeoxyribonucleotide infusion in combination with radiation therapy in patients with advanced malignancies. *Clin. Cancer Res.*, 12: 1251–1259.

Drugs, R. D. (2004). Vincristine liposomal—INEX: Lipid-encapsulated vincristine, Onco TCS, transmembrane carrier system—vincristine, vincacine, vincristine sulfate liposomes for injection, *VSLI.* 5(2): 119–123.

Dupont, B. (2002). Overview of the lipid formulations of amphotericin B. *J. Antimicrob. Chemother.* 49 (Suppl 1): 31–36.

Egorova, E. M. (1994). The validity of the Smoluchowski equation in electrophoretic studies of lipid mem-branes. *Electrophoresis*, 15: 1125–1131.

Enoch, H. G. and P. Strittmatter. (1979). Formation and properties of 1000 Angstrom-diameter, single-bilayer phospholipid vesicles. *Proc. Nat. Acad. Sci. USA*, 76: 145–149.

Felnerova, D., J. F. Viret, R. Glück, and C. Moser. (2004). Liposomes and virosomes as delivery systems for antigens, nucleic acids and drugs. *Curr. Opin. Biotechnol.*, 15: 518–529.

Freeman, F. J., J. A. Hayward, and D. Chapman. (1987). Permeability studies on liposomes formed from polymerizable diactylenic phospholipids and their potential applications as drug delivery systems. *Biochim. Biophys. Acta*, 924: 341–451.

Frezard, F., C. Santella, M. J. Montisci, P. Vierling, and J. G. Riess. (1994). Fluorinated PC-based liposomes: H^+/Na^+ permeability, active doxorubicin encapsulation and stability in human serum. *Biochim. Biophys. Acta*, 1194: 61–68.

Gabizon, A. and D. Papahadjopoulos. (1988). Liposome formulations with prolonged circulation time in blood and enhanced uptake by tumors. *Proc. Natl. Acad. Sci. USA*, 85: 6949–6953.

Gadras, C., C. Santaella, and P. Vierling. (1999). Improved stability of highly fluorinated phospholipid-based vesicles in the presence of bile salts. *J. Control. Rel.*, 57: 29–34.

Gala, R. P., I. Khan, A. M. Elhissi, and M. A. Alhnan. (2015). A comprehensive production method of self-cryoprotected nanoliposome powders. *Int. J. Pharm.*, 486: 153–158.

Gallis, H. A., R. H. Drew, and W. W. Pickard. (1990). Amphotericin B: 30 years of clinical experience. *Rev. Infect. Dis.*, 12: 308–329.

Gamble, R. C. (1988). Method for preparing small vesicles using microemulsification, US Patent 4,753,788.

Gardam, M. A. and J. R. Silvius. (1990). Interactions of different lipid species in multicomponent membranes. *Biochem. Soc. Trans.*, 18: 831–835.

Ginsburg, H. and R. A. Demel. (1983). The effect of ferriprotoporphyrin IX and chloroquine on phospholipid monolayers and the possible implications to antimalarial activity. *Biochim. Biophys. Acta*, 732: 316–319.

Glaberman, U., I. Rabinowitz, and C. F. Verschraegen. (2005). Alternative administration of camptothecin analogues. *Expert Opin. Drug Deliv.*, 2: 323–333.

Gold, W., H. A. Stout, J. F. Pagona, and R. Donovick. (1955). Amphotericins A and B, antifungal antibiotics produced by a streptomycete. I. In vitro studies. *Antibiot. Ann.*, 3: 579–586.

Górski, G., P. Szopiński, J. Michalak, A. Marianowska, M. Borkowski, M. Geremek, and M. Trochimczuk et al. (2005). Liposomal heparin spray: A new formula in adjunctive treatment of superficial venous thrombosis. *Angiology*, 56: 9–17.

Green, A. E. and P. G. Rose. (2006). Pegylated liposomal doxorubicin in ovarian cancer. *Int. J. Nanomedicine.*, 1: 229–239.

Gregoriadis, G. (1990). Biological behavior of liposomes. In *Phospholipids*, Hanin, I., and Papeu, G. (Eds.), Plenum Press, New York, pp. 123–132.

Gupta, P., J. Cannon, and A. Adjei. (1996). Liposomal formulations of ABT-077: In vitro characterization studies. *Int. J. Pharm.*, 140: 119–129.

Haupft, R. and K. Mohr. (1985). Influence of cationic amphiphilic drugs on the phase transition temperature of phospholipids with different polar headgroups. *Biochim. Biophys. Acta*, 814: 156–162.

Hauser, H. (1993). Phospholipid vesicles. In *Phospholipids Handbook*, Cevc, G. (Ed.), Marcel Dekker, New York, pp. 603–637.

Heap, R. B., A. M. Symons, and J. C. Watkins. (1970). Steroids and their interactions with phospholipids: Solubility distribution coefficient and effect on potassium permeability of liposomes. *Biochim. Biophys. Acta*, 218: 482–495.

Hernandez-Caselles, T., J. Villalain, and J. C. Gomez-Fernadez. (1990). Stability of liposomes on long term storage. *J. Pharm. Pharmacol.*, 42: 397–400.

Hiemenz, J. W. and T. J. Walsh. (1996). Lipid formulations of amphotericin B: Recent progress and future directions. *Clin. Infect. Dis.*, 22 (Suppl 2): S133–144.

Huber, W., H. H. Mantsch, F. Paltauf, and H. Hauser. (1994). Conformation of phosphatidyl serine in bilayers as studied by FT-IR spectroscopy. *Biochemistry*, 33: 320–326.

Huizing, M. T., V. H. Sewberath Misser, and R. C. Pieters. (1995). Taxanes: A new class of antitumor agents. *Cancer Invest.*, 13: 381–404.

Hupfer, B., H. Rinsdorf, and H. Schupp. (1983). Liposomes form polymerizable lipids. *Chem. Phys. Lipid.*, 33: 355–374.

Hwang, K. J. (1987). Liposome pharmacokinetics. In *Liposome: From Biophysics to Therapeutics*, Ostro, M. J. (Ed.), Marcel Dekker, New York, pp. 109–156.

Immordino, M. L., F. Dosio, and L. Cattel. (2006). Stealth liposomes: Review of the basic science, rationale, and clinical applications, existing and potential. *Inter. J. Nanomed.*, 1: 297–315.

Imura, T., K. Otake, S. Hashimoto, T. Gotoh, M. Yuasa, S. Yokoyama, H. Sakai, J. F. Rathman, and M. Abe. (2003). Preparation and physicochemical properties of various soybean lecithin liposomes using supercritical reverse phase evaporation method. *Coll. Surf. B—Biointerf.*, 27: 133–140.

Isele, U., P. van Hoogevest, R. Hilfiker, H. Capraro, K. Schieweck, and H. Leuenberger. (1994). Large-scale production of liposomes containing monomeric zinc phthalocyanine by controlled dilution of organic solvents. *J. Pharm. Sci.*, 83: 1608–1616.

Ishikado, A., H. Imanaka, M. Kotani, A. Fujita, Y. Mitsuishi, T. Kanemitsu, Y. Tamura, and T. Makino. (2004). Liposomal lactoferrin induced significant increase of the interferon-alpha (IFNalpha) producibility in healthy volunteers. *Biofactors*, 21: 69–72.

Jain, S. K., R. K. Jain, M. K. Chourasia, A. K. Jain, K. B. Chalasani, V. Soni, and A. Jain. (2005). Design and development of multivesicular liposomal depot delivery system for controlled systemic delivery of acyclovir sodium. *AAPS Pharm. Sci. Tech.*, 6: E35–E40.

Janoff, A. S., C. L. Kurtz, R. L. Jablonski, S. R. Minchey, L. T. Boni, S. M. Gruner, P. R. Cullis, L. D. Mayer, and M. J. Hope. (1988). Characterization of cholesterol hemisuccinate and alpha-tocopherol hemisuccinate vesicles. *Biochim. Biophys. Acta*, 941: 165–175.

Jensen, G. M., C. S. Ashvar, S. W. Bunte, C. D. Barzak, T. H. Bunch, R. L. Fahrner, and N. Hu et al. (2008). A liposomal dispersion formulation of propofol: Formulation, pharmacokinetics, stability, and identification of an oxidative degradant. *Theor. Chem. Acc.*, 119: 291–296.

Jett, M. and C. R. Alving. (1988). Phospholipase A2 substrates: A novel approach to cancer chemotherapy. In *Liposomes as Drug Carriers*, Gregoriadis, G. (Ed.), Wiley, Chichester, UK, pp. 419–429.

Juliano, R. L. (1981). Pharmacokinetics of liposome-encapsulated drugs. In *Liposomes: From Physical Structure to Therapeutic Applications*, Knight, C. G. (Ed.), Elsevier, Amsterdam, the Netherlands, pp. 391–407.

Kastner, E., R. Kaur, D. Lowry, B. Moghaddam, A. Wilkinson, and Y. Perrie. (2014). High throughput manufacturing of size-tuned liposomes by a new microfluidics method using enhanced statistical tools for characterization. *Int. J. Pharm.*, 477: 361–368.

Kastner, E., V. Verma, D. Lowry, and Y. Perrie. (2015). Microfluidic controlled manufacture of liposomes for the solubilisation of a poorly water soluble drug. *Int. J. Pharm.*, 485: 122–130.

Kerridge, D. (1986). Mode of action of clinically important antifungal drugs. *Adv. Microb. Physiol.*, 27: 1–72.

Kessel, D. (1983). *Porphyrin Photosensitization*, Plenum Press, New York.

Kirby, C. J. and G. Gredgoriadis. (1984). A simple procedure for preparing liposomes capable of high encapsulation efficiency under mild conditions. In *Liposome Technology*, Gregoriadis, G. (Ed.), Vol. I, CRC Press, Boca Raton, FL.

Kraft, J. C., J. P. Freeling, Z. Wang, and R. J. Y. Ho. (2014). Emerging research and clinical development trends of liposome and lipid nanoparticle drug delivery systems. *J. Pharm. Sci.*, 103: 29–52.

Lancet, J. E., J. E. Cortes, D. E. Hogge, M. S. Tallman, T. J. Kovacsovics, L. E. Damon, and R. Komrokji et al. (2014). Phase 2 trial of CPX351, a fixed 5:1 molar ratio of cytarabine/daunorubicin, vs cytarabine/daunorubicin in older adults with untreated AML. *Blood.*, 123: 3239–3246.

Lang, J. K. and C. Vigo-Pelfrey, (1993). Quality control of liposome lipids with special emphasis on peroxidation of phospholipids and cholesterol. *Chem. Phys. Lipid.*, 64: 19–29.

Lichtenberg, D. and Y. Barenholz, (1988). Liposome preparation, characterization, and preservation. *Methods Biochem. Anal.*, 33: 337–462.

Lidgate, D. M., P. L. Felgner, J. S. Fleitman, J. Whatley, and R. C. Fu. (1988). In vitro and in vivo studies evaluating a liposome system for drug solubilization. *Pharm. Res.*, 5: 759–764.

Liebmann, J., J. Cook, and C. Lipschultz. (1994). The influence of Cremophor EL on the cell cycle effects of paclitaxel (Taxol.) in human tumor cell lines. *Cancer Chemother. Pharmacol.*, 33: 331–339.

Liu, R. (1998). Methods of making liposomes containing hydro-monobenzoporphyrin photosensitizer. QLT photo therapeutics, US Patent 5,707,608.

Lorenz, W., H. J. Reimann, and A. Schmal. (1977). Histamine release in dogs by Cremophor EL and its derivatives. *Agents Act.*, 7: 63–67.

Lyman, C. A. and T. J. Walsh, (1992). Systemically administered antifungal agents. A review of their clinical pharmacology and therapeutic applications. *Drugs*, 44: 9–35.

Macpherson, I. R. and T. J. Evans, (2009). New approaches in the management of advanced breast cancer role of combination treatment with liposomal doxorubicin. *Breast Cancer*, 1: 1–18.

Maiorino, M., A. Zamburlini, A. Roveri, and F. Ursini. (1995). Copper-induced lipid peroxidation in liposomes, micelles, and LDL: Which is the role of Vitamin E.? *Free Radic. Biol. Med.*, 18: 67–74.

Marsh, D. (1991). Analysis of the chain length dependence of lipid phase transition temperatures. *Biochim. Biophys. Acta*, 1062: 1–6.

Martin, F. J. (1990). Pharmaceutical manufacturing of liposomes. In *Specialized Drug Delivery Systems: Manufacturing and Production Technology*, Tyle, P. (Ed.), Marcel Dekker, New York, pp. 267–316.

Mason, J. T. and T. J. O'Leary, (1990). Effects of head group methylation and acyl chain length on the volume of melting of phosphatidyl ethanolamines. *Biophys. J.*, 58: 277–281.

Matsumura, Y., M. Gotoh, K. Muro, Y. Yamada, K. Shirao, Y. Shimada, and M. Okuwa et al. (2004). Phase I and pharmacokinetic study of MCC-465, a doxorubicin (DXR) encapsulated in PEG immunoliposome, in patients with metastatic stomach cancer. *Annal. Oncol.*, 15: 517–525.

Mattai, J., P. K. Sripada, and G. G. Shipley. (1987). Mixed-chain PC bilayers: Structure and properties. *Biochemistry*, 26: 3287–3297.

Mayer, L. D., T. D. Madden, M. B. Bally, and P. R. Cullis. (1993). pH-gradient-mediated drug entrapment in liposomes. In *Liposome Technology*, Gregoriadis, G. (Ed.), Vol. II, CRC Press, Boca Raton, FL, pp. 27–44.

Mayhew, E., R. Lazo, W. J. Vail, J. King, and A. M. Green. (1984). Characterization of liposomes prepared using a microemulsifier. *Biochim. Biophys. Acta*, 775: 169–174.

Medoff, G., J. Brajtburg, G. S. Kobayashi, and J. Bolard. (1983). Antifungal agents useful in therapy of systemic fungal infections. *Ann. Rev. Pharmacol. Toxicol.*, 23: 303.

Medoff, G. and G. S. Kobayashi. (1980). Strategies in the treatment of systemic fungal infections. *N. Engl. J. Med.*, 302: 145–155.

Meerum, T. J. M., B. Nuijen, B. H. W. W. Ten, and J. H. Beijnen. (1997). Alternative formulations of paclitaxel. *Cancer Treat. Rev.*, 23: 87–95.

Miller, A. D. (2013). Lipid-based nanoparticles in cancer diagnosis and therapy. *J. Drug Deliv.*, 2013. Article ID 165981: http://dx.doi.org/10.1155/2013/16598.

Moghimi, S. M. and J. Szebeni. (2003). Stealth liposomes and long circulating nanoparticles: Critical issues in pharmacokinetics, opsonization and protein-binding properties. *Prog. Lipid Res.*, 42: 463–478.

Monforte, V., P. Ussetti, J. Gavaldà, C. Bravo, R. Laporta, O. Len, C. L. García-Gallo et al. (2009). Feasibility, tolerability, and outcomes of nebulized liposomal amphotericin B for Aspergillus infection prevention in lung transplantation. *J. Heart Lung Transplant.*, 29: 523–530.

Montfort, A., K. Bezstartosi, M. M. J. Groh, and T. J. A. Metsa-Ketala. (1987). The influence of the lipid composition on the degree of lipid peroxidation of liposomes. *Biochem. Int.*, 15: 525–543.

Mouritsen, O. G. and K. Jorgensen. (1993). Dynamical order and disorder in lipid bilayers. *Chem. Phys. Lipid.*, 73: 3–25.

Nardin, A., M. L. Lefebvre, K. Labroquère, O. Faure, and J. P. Abastado. (2006). Liposomal muramyl tripeptide phosphatidylethanolamine: Targeting and activating macrophages for adjuvant treatment of osteosarcoma. *Curr. Canc. Drug Targ.*, 6: 123–133.

Noda, H., M. Hurono, N. Ohishi, and K. Yagi. (1993). Stabilization of egg PC liposomes by the insertion of sulfatide. *Biochim. Biophys. Acta*, 1153: 127–131.

Noskin, G. A., L. Pietrelli, G. Coffey, M. Gurwith, and L. J. Liang. (1998). Amphotericin B colloidal dispersion for treatment of candidemia in immunocompromised patients. *Clin. Infect. Dis.*, 26: 461–467.

Ohsawa, T., H. Miura, and K. Harada. (1984). A novel method for preparing liposome with a high capacity to encapsulate proteinous drugs: Freeze-drying method. *Chem. Parm. Bull.*, 32: 2442–2445.

Olson, F., C. A. Hunt, F. C. Szoka, W. J. Vial, and D. Papahadjopoulos. (1979). Preparation of liposomes of defined size distribution by extrusion through polycarbonate membranes. *Biochim. Biophys. Acta*, 557: 9–23.

Ostro, M. J. (1987). Liposomes. *Sci. Am.*, 257: 102–111.

Ostro, M. J. (1992). Drug delivery via liposomes. *Drug Ther.*, 10: 61–65.

Ostro, M. J. and P. R. Cullis. (1989). Use of liposomes as injectable drug delivery systems. *Am. J. Hosp. Pharm.*, 46: 1576–1587.

Palacios, J. and R. Serrano. (1978). Proton permeability induced by polyene antibiotics. A plausible mechanism for their inhibition of maltose fermentation in yeast. *FEBS Lett.*, 91: 198–201.

Paltauf, F. and A. Hermetter. (1990). Phospholipids-natural, semisynthetic, and synthetic. In *Phospholipids*, Hanin, I. and Pepeu, G. (Eds.), Plenum Press, New York, pp. 1–12.

Pantazis, P., Z. Han, K. Balan, Y. Wang, and J. H. Wyche. (2003). Camptothecin and 9-nitrocamptothecin (9NC) as anti-cancer, anti-HIV and cell-differentiation agents. *Anticancer Res.*, 23: 3623–3638.

Papahadjopoulos, D., M. Cowden, and H. Kimelberg. (1973a). Role of cholesterol in membranes. Effects of phospholipid-protein interactions, membrane permeability and enzymatic activity. *Biochim. Biophys. Acta*, 330: 8.

Papahadjopoulos, D., K. Jacobson, S. Nir, and T. Isac. (1973b). Phase transitions in phospholipid vesicles. Fluorescence polarization and permeability measurements concerning the effect of temperature and cholesterol. *Biochimica et Biophysica Acta*, 311: 330.

Patel, V. B., A. Misra, and Y. S. Marfatia. (2001). Clinical assessment of the combination therapy with liposomal gels of tretinoin and benzoyl peroxide in acne. *AAPS Pharm. Sci. Tech.*, 2(3): 1–5.

Physician's Desk Reference (PDR) (2006). PDR staff (eds.). Thomson PDR, Montvale, NJ, http://www.pdr.net/.

Rahman, A., J. Treat, J. K. Roh, L. A. Potkul, W. G. Alvord, D. Forst, and P. V. Woolley. (1990). A phase I clinical trial and pharmacokinetic evaluation of liposome-encapsulated doxorubicin. *J. Clin. Oncol.*, 8: 1093–1100.

Rahman, A. M., S. W. Yusuf, and M. S. Ewer. (2007). Anthracycline-induced cardiotoxicity and the cardiac-sparing effect of liposomal formulation. *Int. J. Nanomed.*, 2: 567–583.

Riedl, C. R., P. Sternig, G. Gallé, F. Langmann, B. Vcelar, K. Vorauer, and A. Wagner et al. (2005). Liposomal recombinant human superoxide dismutase for the treatment of Peyronie's disease: A randomized placebo controlled double blind prospective clinical study. *Eur. Urol.*, 48: 656–661.

Riess, J. G. (1994). Fluorinated vesicles. *J. Drug Target*, 2: 455–468.

Rivera, E. (2003). Liposomal anthracyclines in metastatic breast cancer: Clinical update. *Oncologist*, 8 (Suppl 2): 3–9.

Rowinsky, E. K., L. A. Cazenave, and R. C. Donehower. (1990). Taxol—a novel investigational antimicrotubule agent. *J. Natl. Cancer Inst.*, 82: 1247–1259.

Saez, R., F. Goni, and A. Alonso. (1985). The effect of bilayer order and fluidity on detergent-induced liposome fusion. *FEBS Lett.*, 179: 311–315.

Sapra, P. and T. M. Allen. (2003). Ligand-targeted liposomal anticancer drugs. *Prog. Lipid Res.*, 42: 439–462.

Saraswat, A., l. R. Agarwa, O. P. Katare, I. Kaur, and B. Kumar. (2007). A randomized, double-blind, vehicle-controlled study of a novel liposomal dithranol formulation in psoriasis. *J. Dermatolog. Treat.*, 18: 40–45.

Schiff, P. B., J. Fant, and S. B. Horwitz. (1979). Promotion of microtubule assembly in vitro by taxol. *Nature*, 277: 665–667.

Schneider, T., A. Sachse, G. Bossling, and M. Brandl. (1995). Generation of contrast-carrying liposomes of defined size with a new continuous high pressure extrusion method. *Int. J. Pharm.*, 117: 1–12.

Schuch, G. (2005). EndoTAG-1 MediGene. *Curr. Opin. Investig. Drugs*, 6: 1259–1265.

Schultheis, B., D. Strumberg, A. Santel, C. Vank, F. Gebhardt, O. Keil, and C. Lange et al. (2014). First-in-human phase I study of the liposomal RNA interference therapeutic Atu027 in patients with advanced solid tumors. *J. Clin. Oncol.*, 32: 4141–4148.

Schwendener, R. A. (1986). The preparation of large volumes of homogeneous, sterile liposomes containing various lipophilic cytostatic drugs by the use of a capillary dialyzer. *Cancer Drug Deliv.*, 3: 123–129.

Sen, K. and M. Mandal. (2013). Second generation liposomal cancer therapeutics: Transition from laboratory to clinic. *Int. J. Pharm.*, 448: 28–43.

Senzer, N., J. Nemunaitis, D. Nemunaitis, C. Bedell, G. Edelman, M. Barve, and R. Nunan et al. (2013). Phase I study of a systemically delivered p53 nanoparticle in advanced solid tumors. *Mol. Ther.*, 21: 1096–1103.

Seth, A. K., A. Misra, and D. Umrigar. (2004). Topical liposomal gel of idoxuridine for the treatment of herpes simplex: Pharmaceutical and clinical implications. *Pharm. Dev. Technol.*, 9: 277–289.

Sharma, A., E. Mayhew, L. Bolcsak, and C. Cavanaugh. (1997). Activity of paclitaxel liposome formulation against human ovarian tumor xenografts. *Int. J. Cancer*, 71: 103–107.

Sharma, A., E. Mayhew, and R. M. Straubinger. (1993). Antitumor effect of taxol-containing liposomes in a taxol-resistant murine tumor model. *Cancer Res.*, 53: 5877–5881.

Sharma, A. and U. S. Sharma. (1997). Liposome in drug delivery—progress and limitations. *Int. J. Pharm.*, 154: 123–140.

Sharma, A. and R. M. Straubinger. (1994). Novel taxol formulations: Preparations and characterization of taxol-containing liposomes. *Pharm. Res.*, 11: 889–896.

Simoes, S., J. N. Moreira, C. Fonseca, N. Düzgünes, and M. C. P. de Lima. (2004). On the formulation of pH-sensitive liposomes with long circulation times. *Adv. Drug. Deliv. Rev.*, 56: 947–965.

Stano, P., S. Bufali, C. Pisano, F. Bucci, M. Barbarino, M. Santaniello, P. Carminati, and L. Luisi-Pier. (2004). Novel camptothecin analogue (gimatecan)-containing liposomes prepared by the ethanol injection method. *J. Liposome Res.*, 14: 87–109.

Straubinger, R. M., A. Sharma, and M. Murray. (1993). Novel taxol formulations: Taxol-containing liposomes. *J. Natl. Cancer Inst. Monogr.*, 15: 69–78.

Strickley, R. G. (2004). Solubilizing excipients in oral and injectable formulations. *Pharm. Res.*, 21: 201–230.

Suzuki, R., T. Takizawa, Y. Kuwata, M. Mutoh, N. Ishiguro, N. Utoguchi, and A. Shinohara et al. (2008). Effective anti-tumor activity of oxaliplatin encapsulated in transferrin-PEG-liposome. *Int. J. Pharm.*, 346: 143–150.

Talsma, H., M. J. Vansteenbergen, J. C. H. Borchert, and D. J .A. Crommelin. (1994). A novel technique for the one-step preparation of liposomes and nonionic surfactant vesicles without the use of organic solvents. *J. Pharm. Sci.*, 83: 276–280.

Tanford, C. (1980). *The Hydrophobic Effect: Formation of Micelles and Biological Membranes*, John Wiley & Sons, New York.

Tasset, C., V. Preat, and M. Roland. (1992). Galenical formulations of amphotericin B. *J. Pharm. Belg.*, 47: 523–536.

Tate, M. W., E. Shyamsunder, S. M. Gruner, and K. L. D'Amico. (1992). Kinetics of the lamellar-inverse hexagonal phase transition determined by time resolved X-ray diffraction. *Biochemistry*, 31: 1081–1092.

Tipping, E., B. Ketterer, and L. Christodoulides. (1979). Interactions of small molecules with phospholipid bilayers. Binding to egg phosphatidylcholine of some organic anions (bromosulphophthalein, oestrone sulphate, haem and bilirubin) that bind to ligandin and aminoazo-dye-binding protein A. *Biochem. J.*, 180: 327–337.

Torchilin, V. P. and M. I. Papisov. (1994). Why do polyethylene glycol-coated liposomes circulate so long? *J. Liposome Res.*, 4: 725–739.

Tsuschida, E., H. Nishide, M. Sekine, and A. Yamagishi. (1983). Liposomal heme as oxygen carrier under semi-physiological conditions. Orientation study of heme embedded in a phospholipid bilayer by an electrooptical method. *Biochim. Biophys. Acta*, 734: 274–278.

Urano, S., M. Kitahara, Y. Kato, Y. Hasegawa, and M. Matsuo. (1990). Membrane stabilizing effect of Vitamin E: Existence of a hydrogen bond between alpha-tocopherol and phospholipids in bilayer membranes. *J. Nutr. Sci. Vitaminol.*, 36: 513–519.

Van Bloois, L., D. D. Dekker, and D. J. A. Crommelin. (1987). Solubilization of lipophilic drugs by amphiphiles: Improvement of the apparent solubility of almitrine bismesylate by liposomes, mixed micelles and O/W emulsions. *Acta Pharm. Technol.*, 33: 136–139.

Vaukonen, M., M. Sassaroli, P. Somerhraju, and J. Eisinger. (1990). Dipyrenylphosphatidyl cholines as membrane fluidity probes *Biophys. J.*, 57: 291–300.

Verschraegen, C. F., B. E. Gilbert, E. Loyer, A. Huaringa, G. Walsh, R. A. Newman, and V. Knight. (2004). Clinical evaluation of the delivery and safety of aerosolized liposomal 9-nitro-20(s) camptothecin in patients with advanced pulmonary malignancies. *Clin. Cancer Res.*, 10: 2319–2326.

Vidal-Naquet, A., J. L. Goosage, T. P. Sullivan, J. W. Haynes, B. H. Giruth, R. L. Beissinger, L. R. Seghal, and A. L. Rosen. (1989). Liposome-encapsulated hemoglobin as an artificial red blood cell: Characterization and scale-up. *Biomat. Artif. Cells Artif. Organs*, 17: 531–552.

Vincent, J. L., R. Brase, F. Santman, P. M. Suter, A. McLuckie, J. F. Dhainaut, Y. Park, and J. Karmel. (2001). A multicentre, double-blind, placebo-controlled study of liposomal prostaglandin E1 (TLC C53) in patients with acute respiratory distress syndrome. *Inten. Care Med.*, 27: 1578–1583.

Viscusi, E. R., R. Sinatra, E. Onel, and S. L. Ramamoorthy. (2014). The safety of liposome bupivacaine, a novel local analgesic formulation. *Clin. J. Pain.*, 30: 102–110.

Vries, J. D. J., K. P. Flora, A. Bult, and J. H. Beijnen. (1996). Pharmaceutical development of investigational anticancer agents for parenteral use—a review. *Drug Dev. Indust. Pharm.*, 22: 475–494.

Vuillemard, J. C. (1991). Recent advances in the large-scale production of lipid vesicles for use in food products: Microfluidization. *J. Microencapsul.*, 8: 547–562.

Wagner, A., M. Platzgummer, G. Kreismayr, H. Quendler, G. Stiegler, B. Ferko, and G. Vecera et al. (2006). GMP production of liposomes: A new industrial approach. *J. Liposome Res.*, 16: 311–319.

Wani, M. C., H. L. Taylor, and M. E. Wall. (1971). Plant antitumor agents. VI. The isolation and structure of taxol, a novel antileukemic and antitumor agent from *Taxus brevifolia*. *J. Am. Chem. Soc.*, 93: 2325–2327.

Weiner, A. (1990). Chemistry and biology of immunotargeted liposomes. In *Targeted Therapeutic Systems*, Tyle, P. and Ram, B. (Eds.), Marcel Decker, New York, pp. 305–336.

Wetzler, M., D. A. Thomas, E. S. Wang, R. Shepard, L. A. Ford, T. L. Heffner, and S. Parekh et al. (2013). Phase I/II trial of nanomolecular liposomal annamycin in adult patients with relapsed/refractory acute lymphoblastic leukemia. *Clin. Lymphoma Myeloma Leukemia*, 13: 430–434.

Wiseman, H., M. Cannon, R. V. Arnstein, and B. Halliwell. (1990). Mechanism of inhibition of lipid peroxidation by tamoxifen and 4-hydroxytamoxifen introduced into liposomes. *FEBS Lett.*, 274: 107–110.

Wittgen, B. P., P. W. Kunst, K. van der Born, A. W. van Wijk, W. Perkins, F. G. Pilkiewicz, and R. Perez-Soler et al. (2007). Phase I study of aerosolized SLIT cisplatin in the treatment of patients with carcinoma of the lung. *Clin. Cancer Res.*, 13: 2414–2421.

Won, S. H., J. U. Lee, and S. J. Sim. (2013). Fluorogenic pH-sensitive polydiacetylene (PDA) liposomes as a drug carrier. *J. Nanosci. Nanotechnol.*, 13: 3792–3800.

Woodle, M. C. (1993). Surface-modified liposomes: Assessment and characterization for decreased stability and prolonged blood circulation. *Chem. Phys. Lipid.*, 64: 249–262.

Woodle, M. C. (1995). Sterically stabilized liposome therapeutics. *Adv. Drug Deliv. Rev.*, 16: 249–265.

Woodle, M. C., M. S. Newman, and J. A. Cohn. (1994). Sterically stabilized liposomes: Physical and biological properties. *J. Drug Target*, 2: 397–403.

Wright, S. E. and J. C. White. (1986). Teniposide-induced changes in the physical properties of phosphatidyl choline liposomes. *Biochem. Pharmacol.*, 16: 2731–2735.

Wu, Y. L. K. Park, R. A. Soo, Y. Sun, K. Tyroller, D. Wages, and G. Ely et al. (2011). Inspire: A phase III study of the BLP25 liposome vaccine (L-BLP25) in Asian patients with unresectable stage III non-small cell lung cancer. *BMC Cancer*, 11: 430.

Yang, J., Y. Shi, C. Li, L. Gui, X. Zhao, P. Liu, and X. Han et al. (2014). Phase I clinical trial of pegylated liposomal mitoxantrone plm60s: Pharmacokinetics, toxicity and preliminary efficacy. *Cancer Chemother. Pharmacol.*, 74: 637–646.

Yoshioka, A., K. Fukutake, J. Takamatsu, and A. Shirahata. (2006). Clinical evaluation of recombinant factor VIII preparation (Kogenate) in previously treated patients with hemophilia A: Descriptive meta-analysis of post-marketing study data. *Int. J. Hematol.*, 84: 158–165.

Yuasa, M., K. Aiba, Y. Ogata, H. Nishide, and E. Tsuchida. (1986). Structure of the liposome composed of lipid-heme and phospholipids. *Biochim. Biophys. Acta*, 860: 558–565.

Zamboni, W. C. (2005). Liposomal, nanoparticle, and conjugated formulations of anticancer agents. *Clin. Cancer Res.*, 11: 8230–8234.

Zhao, Y., J. Liu, X. Sun, Z. R. Zhang, and T. Gong. (2010). Sustained release of hydroxycamptothecin after subcutaneous administration using a novel phospholipid complex-DepoFoam technology. *Drug Dev. Ind. Pharm.*, 36: 823–831.

15 Pharmaceutical Salts

Steven H. Neau and Nikhil C. Loka

CONTENTS

INTRODUCTION

In formulation development or in the *in vivo* performance of a dosage form, the occasion may arise when the inherently low aqueous solubility of a drug does not meet the solution concentration required. If the solubility of a drug is less than 10 mg/mL, bioavailability or absorption problems are likely to exist (Greene, 1979). If the drug to be formulated as a liquid product possesses an ionizable group, adjustment of the pH in which the drug is to be dissolved might be sufficient to enhance the solubility. This is understandable since there are strong interactions between the solute ion and the ions and dipoles of water, likely overcoming the drawback of a large hydrophobic portion of the drug molecule. However, to become ionized, acidic or basic drugs might require extremes in pH that are outside acceptable physiological limits, or at which stability problems arise (Anderson, 1985; Ansel et al., 1995). In general, aqueous solubility is limited by polarizability, lipophilicity, and the electron arrangement of the drug (Bergström et al., 2007), and salts represent the class of drugs that are most likely to attain the desired extent of solubility in water owing to their increased polarizability (Motola and Agharkar, 1984). A pharmaceutical salt is an ionizable drug presented in a neutral complex with a counterion (Patel et al., 2009). By producing a salt form of a drug, its chemical stability, manufacture into drug products, handling, and administration might be improved, but it is expected that its pharmacokinetics profile is likewise altered (Patel et al., 2009). Furthermore, solid state properties might halt pursuit of certain salt forms mostly due to the influence of these properties on solubility and stability (Ravin and Radebaugh, 1990; Ando and Radebaugh, 2000; Huang and Tong, 2004).

Approximately half of drugs approved for use in the United States are salts (Patel et al., 2009; Thackaberry, 2012). This is not surprising since an ionizable functional group on a drug molecule provides an opportunity for it to engage in an electrostatic, or Coulombic, force of attraction with an oppositely charged ion, with its counterion in a salt form, or with the dipole of water. If that force of attraction can be retained through the crystallization process, a salt product will be obtained (Bhattachar et al., 2006). The salt form of a drug is usually substantially more soluble than the non-ionized form in an aqueous medium, although it should be noted that not all salts have an improved solubility in water when compared to the uncharged form of the drug. Procaine penicillin is often cited as an example of a poorly soluble salt (Amidon, 1981). Nevertheless, salt formation is a simple, cost-effective means to improve solubility and thus enhance the oral bioavailability of ionizable drugs (Berge et al., 1977; Gould, 1986; Serajuddin, 2007; Elder et al., 2013). The crystalline nature of the salt form can also improve processability and dosage form development, but solid state properties such as crystallinity, crystal habit, particle size, flowability, melting point, enthalpy of fusion, hygroscopicity, and the potential for solvate formation or polymorphic changes must be considered when choosing a salt form for a drug (Berge et al., 1977; Gould, 1986; Huang and Tong, 2004; Serajuddin, 2007; Guerrieri et al., 2010; Elder et al., 2013).

The physical form of the salt must be taken into account, and several issues must be considered (Serajuddin and Pudipeddi, 2002). For example, a salt form might prove to be amorphous material. Even if crystalline, the salt form might prove to be polymorphic. David et al. (2012) reported that benzylamine salts are likely to be polymorphic, whereas cyclohexylamine and t-butylamine produced salts with good physicochemical properties that are unlikely to undergo polymorphic transitions, presumably due to the lack of the ability to stack by π–π interactions. Aakeröy et al. (2007) reported that about 45% of N-heterocyclic salts of carboxylic acids have some tendency toward solvate formation. Formation of a hydrate or a solvate might occur on crystallization or recrystallization, and the effect of temperature and humidity on this should be investigated. In general, hydrates and solvates are more stable, but less soluble in the respective solvent, than the anhydrous or non-solvated form (Khankari and Grant, 1995), although they will be more soluble in a solvent that is not involved in the solid form (Davies, 2001). A particular counterion for a drug salt will affect the melting point, solubility, dissolution rate, and hygroscopicity (Huang and Tong, 2004). Both the physical and chemical stability of the different candidate salts in the solid state will ultimately determine the optimal form of the drug.

Miller and Heller (1975) pointed out that different salts of the same drug rarely differ in their pharmacological effect. Differences are usually limited to the physical and chemical properties exhibited by the salts that ultimately affect absorption and bioavailability. Typically, a low bioavailability of less than 20% leads to dose-to-dose differences that result in variable drug levels, pharmacological effects, and side effects (Schoenwald, 2002). Wagner (1961) stated that, although the biological response elicited by salts of the same drug might not differ qualitatively, the intensity of the response may differ markedly in relation to the time after administration. Nelson (1957) pointed out that the dissolution rate of the drug from a particular dosage form largely determines the rate of drug appearance in the blood, as well as the timing and magnitude of the maximum concentration attained. Since salt formation can increase the solubility by several orders of magnitude, this approach to improving drug solubility can have a profound effect on the dissolution rate (Serajuddin, 2007) as described by the Nernst equation (Nernst 1904; Elder et al., 2013):

$$\frac{dC}{dt} = \frac{DA(C_s - C_b)}{h} \tag{15.1}$$

where dC/dt is the dissolution rate, D is the diffusion coefficient of the drug in the solvent system, A is the surface area of the solid exposed to the solvent system, h is the thickness of the stagnant solvent at the interface between the solid surface and the bulk of the solvent system, C_s is the solubility of the drug in the solvent system, and C_b is the concentration of the drug in the bulk of the solution at time t. If the bulk concentration is very low in comparison to the solubility, this parameter is negligible in comparison to C_s and it can be dropped to simplify the equation.

With passive diffusion as the most common mechanism for drug absorption, the rate of appearance depends on the concentration of the drug dissolved, which in turn is influenced by the physicochemical properties of the drug (Amidon et al., 1995). Although the overall bioavailability of different salts of the same drug is expected to be similar, pharmacokinetic profiles likely reflect physicochemical differences found between salt forms of the same drug (Patel et al., 2009). Bighley et al. (1995) presented a summary of drug salts and the influence the salt form has on bioavailability and pharmacokinetics in general. Physicochemical characteristics that can play a profound role not only in pharmacokinetic and toxicity profiles (Thackaberry, 2012) but also in processing and manufacturing include, but are not limited to, hygroscopicity, the physical stability of the crystal forms particularly under humid conditions, the chemical stability of the salt, and of course the solubility (Morris et al., 1994). Li et al. (2005) considered the biopharmaceutical properties, namely the solubility and the dissolution rate, to be just as critical in salt selection as the physicochemical properties such as crystallinity, hygroscopicity, and chemical stability. Salt formation is considered the most practical approach to maximizing the bioavailability of a poorly soluble drug (Huang and Tong, 2004).

In the case of metoprolol succinate and metoprolol fumarate, the maximum drug concentration in the plasma (C_{max}) and the area under the plasma drug concentration–time curve were statistically equivalent, based on a 90% confidence interval (Sandberg et al., 1993), indicating comparable *in vivo* performances. With fenoprofen, the C_{max} following administration of its calcium salt was reached somewhat later than the C_{max} associated with the sodium form (Rubin et al., 1971). This was attributed to the slower dissolution rate for the calcium salt. Bioavailability and the measured distribution and elimination parameters, however, were reported to be similar. It has been suggested that a pharmacokinetic study needs to be performed to allow selection of the ideal salt when two or more salt forms exhibit similar solid state characteristics (Saxena et al., 2009).

INORGANIC SALTS

It has been confirmed that the solubility of the salt depends largely on the counterion. The hydrophobicity of the counterion and the melting point of the salt both play a role in the solubility of the salt form (Anderson and Conradi, 1985). The hydrophobicity of the counterion is most often reflected in the melting point and enthalpy of fusion, in that a hydrophobic counterion is more likely to engage in weaker intermolecular bonds limited to van der Waals forces. Crystal lattice energy, solvation energy, the common ion effect, the hydrated state, and other factors also influence the solubility of a drug salt (Serajuddin and Pudipeddi, 2002). Crystal lattice and hydration energies are expected to increase with an increase in the cation or anion charge, and they should also increase with an increase in the charge density.

The most common method to produce salts involving inorganic counterions is to expose a weak base drug to an inorganic acid, or a weak acid drug to the hydroxide form of the desired counterion. Examples of inorganic acids include phosphoric, sulfuric, nitric, or hydrochloric acid (Dittert et al., 1964). Anderson and Flora (1996) pointed out that the pK_a of that acid should be lower than the pK_a of the conjugate acid formed by the protonation of the base drug. Wells (1988) and Tong and Whitesell (1998) recommended that this difference between pK_a values be at least two units.

Sodium is the most common counterion for salts of acidic drugs. It has even been successfully used in the preparation of an amorphous form of furosemide to achieve pharmaceutical objectives (Nielsen et al., 2013). Diclofenac is marketed as three different salt forms, namely its sodium, potassium, and diethylamine salt. The low solubility of the parent drug (about 0.02 mg/mL) necessitated the preparation of salt forms. Each of the three salts improved the solubility of diclofenac, with 9.7 and 4.6 mg/mL reported for the sodium and potassium salts, respectively (Kumar et al., 2007).

The weakly acidic drug *para*-aminosalicylic acid (PAS) is available as sodium, calcium, or potassium salt. The reported aqueous solubilities of the nonionized and salt forms, in terms of available PAS, are 1 g/600 mL for the nonionized form, 1 g/10 mL for the potassium salt, 1 g/7 mL for the calcium salt, and 1 g/2 mL for the sodium salt. Since the poorly soluble nonionized form of PAS passes through the gastrointestinal tract without being absorbed, it is not surprising that each of the salt forms was able to enhance the oral bioavailability of the parent drug (Wan et al., 1974). However, the bioavailability of the drug from tablets using each of the three salts was considered comparable. The anti-inflammatory properties of fenoprofen were investigated using the sodium salt, but the calcium salt was later considered because it was found to be more stable than the sodium salt (Rubin et al., 1971). The sodium salt became amorphous and darkened in certain formulations. The counterion, therefore, affects the solubility, but could also affect the chemical stability of the salt form. In preformulation studies, the stability and potential formulation issues must be considered before the final salt selection is made.

The phosphate ion and various sulfonates have proved useful for basic drugs. However, hydrochloride salts are by far the most common choice for basic drugs, far outweighing the sulfates, the nearest in frequency (Berge et al., 1977). Bromide and iodide salts of drugs are not as common because their halide counterions are not pharmacologically inert and because they are more expensive. Ionic fluorine appears only in its inorganic form as a prophylactic against dental caries (Miller and Heller, 1975).

Due to the weakening of the crystal lattice strength by the use of a hydrophobic organic counterion, there is an increased chance of formation of amorphous forms. Black et al. reported 25 different salts of ephedrine using organic and inorganic acids. Most of the salts formed using organic acids were either temporarily or permanently amorphous in nature. The recrystallization of certain organic salts is definitely an issue of physical stability and is not ideal for pharmaceutical applications (Black et al., 2007). Therefore, the use of a polymer to stabilize such amorphous forms has been suggested to overcome the problems associated with recrystallization (Kesisoglou and Wu, 2008).

ORGANIC SALTS

At one time, it was believed that the solubility of a salt form could be enhanced by selecting a counterion that is itself more hydrophilic. For diclofenac, an increase in the number of hydroxyl groups in the counterion failed to support this relationship between solubility and the hydrophilicity of the counterion (Fini et al., 1996; Parshad et al., 2004). Indeed, a reduction in the polarity of the counterion was able to enhance the solubility of benzylamine derivatives by reducing the strength of the lattice energy, reflected by a decrease in the melting point (Parshad et al., 2004). Choosing an organic species to react with a drug to develop an organic salt has the potential to provide advantages including lower toxicities and, perhaps surprisingly, a higher aqueous solubility than an inorganic counterion can provide. Triamterene (2,4,7-triamino-6-phenylpteridine) is a diuretic that, despite three amino groups (Figure 15.1), is only weakly monobasic. Most attempts to form classic salts have failed. Acetic acid, however, was shown to form a salt with triamterene that has a higher solubility than the phosphoric, sulfuric, nitric, or hydrochloric acid salts (Dittert et al., 1964). The ammonium and ethanolamine salts of para-aminosalicylic acid were each shown to have a higher aqueous solubility than the potassium, sodium, calcium, or magnesium salts of the same drug (Forbes et al., 1995).

Formation of the hydrochloride salt of the antimalarial agent α-(2-piperidyl)β-3,6-*bis*(trifluoromethyl)-9-phenanthrenemethanol approximately doubles its solubility in water, as shown in Table 15.1. To investigate the ability of an organic counterion to improve the aqueous solubility, various organic acid salts of the antimalarial agent were prepared. Results suggest that a significant increase in solubility can be achieved with the proper choice of the salt form. For example, the lactate salt is approximately 200 times as soluble as the hydrochloride salt (Agharkar et al., 1976).

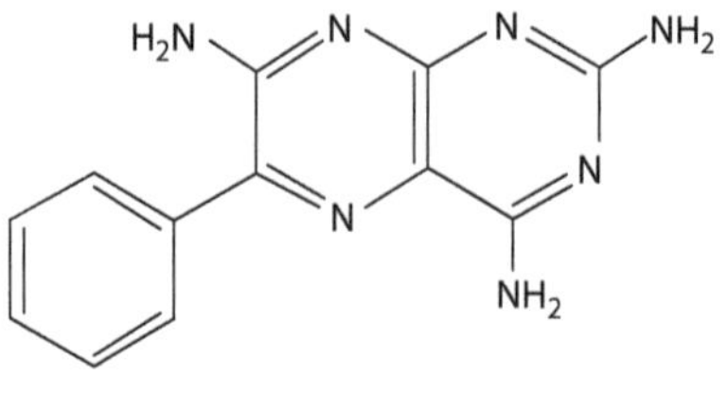

FIGURE 15.1 The chemical structure of triamterene.

TABLE 15.1

Melting Point and Solubility of Salts of an Antimalarial Drug
α-(2-Piperidyl)-3,6-bis(Trifluoromethyl)-9-Phenanthrenemethanol

Chemical	Melting Point (°C)	Solubility (mg/L)[a]
Free base	215	7
Hydrochloride	331	12
d,l-Lactate	172, dec.[b]	1800
l-Lactate	192, dec.	900
2-Hydroxyethane-1-sulfonate	250, dec.	620
Methanesulfonate	290, dec.	300
Sulfate	270, dec.	20

Source: From Agharkar, S. et al., Enhancement of solubility of drug salts by hydrophilic counterions: Properties of organic salts of an antimalarial drug. *J. Pharm. Sci.* 1976. 65. 747–749. Copyright Wiley-VCH Verlag GmbH & Co. KGaA. Reproduced with permission.

[a] Apparent solubility in water at 25°C.

[b] dec. indicates the solid decomposed on melting.

This enhanced aqueous solubility was attributed in part to the decrease in crystal lattice energy as attested by the reduction in melting point between the hydrochloride salt and the lactate salt (Motola and Agharkar, 1984). This has proved true in other studies comparing physicochemical properties of salts with inorganic counterions with those of salts formed using organic counterions (Creasey and Green, 1959). The enthalpies of fusion, however, were not investigated to support this hypothesis.

On the contrary, Surov et al. (2015) reported a lower solubility for the adipate, maleate, and fumarate salts of ciproflaxicin in acidic pH when compared to the hydrochloride salt of the antibiotic. This has been attributed to the differences in their lattice energies due to the formation of hydrates and the type of hydrate formed. When methanedisulfonate, ethanedisulfonate, or camphorsulfonate is employed as the counterion, the product is referred to as a mesylate, edisylate, or camsylate salt, respectively (Miller and Heller, 1975). Miller and Heller (1975) concluded combinations with monocarboxylic acids are usually poorly soluble in water, whereas those of dicarboxylic acids above oxalic acid, which itself is considered toxic, can be water soluble if one carboxylic acid group is still free to dissociate. Examples of di- and tricarboxylic acids that have been used in marketed products include citric, tartaric, succinic, and glutamic acids (Berge et al., 1977; Fiese and Hagen, 1986).

The aqueous solubility of the salt of a drug has also been considered a function of the acid–base strength and aqueous solubility of the counterion employed in the salt formation (Nelson, 1957). As an example, choline itself is considered strongly basic because of the hydroxide counterion, and choline salts of acidic drugs can be readily prepared. The choline cation, being a quaternary amine,

TABLE 15.2

Thermal Properties and Aqueous Solubility of Naproxen, Tolmetin, and Their Salts

Chemical	Melting Point (°C)	Enthalpy of Fusion (kJ/mole)	Solubility (mg/mL)[a]
Naproxen	157	24.8	0.07
Naproxen sodium	261, dec.[b]	35.8, dec.	266
Naproxen choline	146	30.2	472
Tolmetin	162. dec.	47.2, dec.	0.10
Tolmetin sodium	314, dec.	54.7, dec.	163
Tolmetin choline	143	19.7	795

Source: Data from Murti, S. K., On the preparation and characterization of water-soluble choline salts of carboxylic acid drugs, PhD dissertation, University of Missouri–Kansas City, 1993. Reprinted with permission of the author.

[a] Solubility is based on apparent solubility in water at 25°C.
[b] dec. indicates that the solid decomposed on melting.

is insensitive to pH effects on solubility, and is considered highly water soluble. Short-chain (up to C16) monoalkyl quaternaries (the nitrogen bearing one alkyl chain and three methyl groups) and ethoxylated quaternaries of even greater chain lengths are water soluble in general, whereas most dialkyl and trialkyl quaternary ammonium compounds are water dispersible at best (Juczyk et al., 1991). When the nitrogen bears four aliphatic groups, the cation is soluble in water except when two or more of the groups contain more than eight carbons (Shibe and Hanson, 1964).

The choline salts of naproxen and tolmetin yielded marked solubility enhancements, even over that of the sodium salts. The aqueous solubility of the choline salt of naproxen was 6700 times the solubility of naproxen and almost twice that of naproxen sodium. The choline salt of tolmetin was almost 8000 times as soluble as the parent drug and almost 5 times as soluble as its sodium salt (Murti, 1993). Table 15.2 shows that the melting point and the enthalpy of fusion are both affected by the formation of the choline salt, and in fact, the choline salt proved to be more thermally stable.

Quaternary ammonium salts of dantrolene and clodanolene have been prepared, and the effect of the organic cation on the aqueous solubility has been reported (Ellis et al., 1980). It was reasoned that since the hydantoin moiety in each drug is weakly acidic, a strong base should be found for salt formation. The 13 different quaternary ammonium compounds were therefore used in the hydroxide salt form. The acid–base reaction proceeded rapidly, and the salt products were stable during recrystallization steps. Of the four salts for clodanolene, the aqueous solubilities ranged from 2- to 100-fold that of clodanolene sodium, on a mass basis. Of the 11 salts for dantrolene, the benzyltrimethyl ammonium salt exhibited comparable solubility to that of dantrolene sodium. Among the other 10 salts were several examples that yielded enhanced solubilities of up to 1000-fold that of the sodium salt. Twelve of the 15 salts successfully demonstrated muscle relaxant activity when administered orally.

Tris(hydroxymethyl)aminomethane (THAM) has been used to form salts with drugs that bear a carboxylic acid group. Gu and Strickley (1987) reported that, for ketorolac and two investigational nonsteroidal anti-inflammatory drugs, the solubility of the THAM salt was greater than the solubility of the parent acid by about four orders of magnitude. In the case of naproxen, however, the THAM salt was more soluble than the parent acid by three orders of magnitude, and it was less soluble than the sodium salt by one order of magnitude.

The appropriate choice of organic counterion can result in reduced salt toxicity. There is evidence that salicylates may accumulate with chronic administration, which can be compounded if renal function is below normal (Lasslo et al., 1959). The nature and degree of absorption of tartrate from the human intestine has been questioned (Underhill et al., 1931; Pratt and Swartout, 1933), but the fact that several tartrates are reported to possess cathartic activity argues against substantial absorption from the intestinal tract (Lasslo et al., 1959).

Since chemicals commonly found in food and drink are considered nontoxic, it is not surprising that salts employing natural products such as choline (Duesel et al., 1954), ascorbic acid (Alves et al., 1958), and pantothenic acid (Keller et al., 1956a, b; Osterberg et al., 1957) have proved to be less toxic than the parent drug or an inorganic salt form of the same drug. A series of soluble amino acid salts of dihydrostreptomycin was prepared, and the acute toxicity in each case was found to be lower than that of the sulfate or glucuronate salt (Alves et al., 1958). The salt form of aspartic acid, an essential amino acid that is an example of a dicarboxylate ion, has been employed as the counterion in an erythromycin salt to yield an aqueous solubility five times that of the parent drug (Fabrizio, 1973; Windholz et al., 1983). The salt proved to have low toxicity, good compatibility, and durable activity (Fabrizio, 1973). The phosphate salts of the antimalarial drugs of the quinoline and acridine type are favored because of greater tolerance and efficacy (Miller and Heller, 1975). If a particular salt form cannot be isolated owing to its very high solubility, the desired aqueous solubility can be achieved by *in situ* salt formation. This is accomplished by using the appropriate acid or base to adjust the pH while formulating the drug solution (Motola and Agharkar, 1984; Tong and Whitesell, 1998). The *in situ* salt formation method can be effective even if a desired salt form cannot be isolated. This method might appear attractive for injectable formulations, but the formulator must be aware that the solubility of the salt is unknown because it has not been isolated.

POLYMERIC AND MACROMOLECULAR SALTS

In early studies, interactions between cationic drugs and water-soluble polyelectrolytes in solution were characterized as arising not only from Donnan equilibria but also from other interactions that are difficult to rigorously define (Kennon and Higuchi, 1956). Although the interaction was not considered strong, the binding could be extensive. Results indicate that half of the carboxylate groups present in polyacrylate can bind a cationic drug (Kennon and Higuchi, 1957). However, two disadvantages were evident. The first is that ions from dissolved salts can compete effectively with the drug for binding sites. The second is that some anionic polyelectrolyte–cationic drug complexes are sufficiently insoluble that they either precipitate or aggregate to the point of being visible (Kennon and Higuchi, 1957). Poorly soluble polymeric salts have often been employed in sustained release formulations, including the classic example of alginate salts of pilocarpine (Loucas and Haddad, 1972). Tannic acid with acidic phenol groups, and pectic acid with carboxylic acid groups, have been employed in the preparation of sparingly soluble salts of diltiazem (Shah, 1992). Although it is reasonable to assume that some of the complexes formed remained as ions in solution, a precipitate defeats the purpose of using a polyelectrolyte to improve the solubility of a poorly soluble drug.

Macromolecules and colloidal particles have a particular affinity for the lymphatic system and are returned to the vascular compartment through the thoracic duct (Málek et al., 1958). The use of water-soluble macromolecular and colloidal salts has been investigated, and they have been found to provide slow delivery of antibiotics, even with a high concentration of the salt in the lymphatic system, because the only port of entry into the vascular compartment is through lymph channels. In this case, the depot effect is not due to the low solubility of the salt, but rather due to slow absorption. Málek et al. (1958) also reported that the acute toxicity of antibiotics was markedly decreased by the formation of macromolecular salts. For example, the acute LD50 in rats and mice was 5 times greater with streptolymphin and 10 times greater with neolymphin, which are macromolecular salts of streptomycin and neomycin, respectively (Málek et al., 1958).

SALT-SELECTION PROCESS

The approach to salt selection should obtain the most information using the smallest amount of drug material. Selection of the optimum salt form does not involve simply choosing the salt with the highest solubility, but includes consideration of the physicochemical properties of the salt candidates (Elder et al., 2013). The approach must provide analysis and then elimination of salt candidates that fail in the tests (Ware and Lu, 2004). Appropriate tests include powder X-ray diffraction and differential scanning calorimetry to assess crystallinity, melting point, enthalpy of fusion, and polymorphism. Particle size, surface area assessment, hygroscopicity, and possibly vapor sorption analysis together can predict susceptibility to moisture adsorption and the potential for hydrate formation. Ultimately, the solubility of the salt in aqueous media, including water and aqueous media buffered at various pH, is critical. Some assess the bulk and tapped density of the powdered salt to predict compressibility (Ware and Lu, 2004).

The pharmaceutical literature includes several reports on the importance of selecting the optimal salt form for a drug at the initial stage of drug development (Berge et al., 1977; Gould, 1986; Morris et al., 1994; Bighley et al., 1995). A change in the salt form might require repeating many of the typical studies conducted on a new drug candidate, some of which are costly in terms of time and resources, including toxicological, formulation, and stability studies. A method that can provide salt solubility information with a minimal effort would be beneficial.

A salt-selection process for drugs described by Gould (1986) was based on the melting point, solubility, stability, and wettability of the various salt forms. Gould acknowledged desirable characteristics that are less critical and that are usually dependent on processing conditions, as well as the desired biological performance and dosage form. Ideally, the salt should be chemically stable, not hygroscopic, exhibit no processing problems, and dissolve readily (Gould, 1986).

Morris et al. (1994) pointed out that this selection approach could be improved if the salt-selection process involved a decision, in the case of each salt form under consideration, to pursue further studies after the generation of data for each type of parameter. In that way, a salt form that has failed in a test that requires little time or salt sample can be eliminated from further consideration before the expense of time and effort is incurred in the generation of extensive physicochemical data for a salt form that cannot be seriously considered.

Morris et al. (1994) suggested several tiers in the selection process on the basis of the salt samples undergoing progressively more time-consuming and labor-intensive experiments with each set of subsequent experiments. The parameters to be studied and the limits for acceptability of each criterion were set. In the first tier, each salt form that was crystalline was tested for hygroscopicity. High moisture sorption could result in handling and manufacturing difficulties such as a change in the true density or flow behavior. Salt forms that proved to be hygroscopic were eliminated from further consideration. In the second tier, changes in crystal structure under extremes of humidity were studied using powder X-ray diffraction and thermal analysis. This would indicate any proclivity for polymorphic or pseudopolymorphic changes. The second tier also included a determination of the aqueous solubility of the salt forms, to assess potential dissolution or bioavailability problems, and to evaluate whether a solution dosage form is feasible. Salt forms that have passed tier 2 move on to tier 3 where the salt is subjected to accelerated thermal stability and photostability screening. Compatibility with selected excipients can also be conducted at this tier. Placing these experiments at the highest tier results in the fewest number of salt forms considered in these studies that are time consuming and that require much effort. This salt-selection process is reported to be completed in 4–6 weeks.

The use of 96-well plates was suggested as a means to prepare the salt form of trazodone, a weak base drug, with 13 different acids yet using little drug mass (Ware and Lu, 2004). In its base form, trazodone was dissolved in acetone and then added to an acetone solution of the acid, with the exceptions of citric and tartaric acids in water and pamoic acid in dimethyl sulfoxide. Ultimately, only 5 mg of trazodone base was added to each well. Evaporation of the solvent encouraged precipitation of the salt. Petroleum ether was added to wash away excess acid and to act as a nonsolvent if necessary to force salt precipitation. Automated systems have been proposed as a means to provide high throughput experimentation in salt selection (Ware and Lu, 2004; Kumar et al., 2007).

A microfluidization platform was proposed as a means to profoundly reduce the mass of drug employed in the study of salt formation and selection (Thorson et al., 2011). Nucleation and particle growth are induced and encouraged in various solvents by mixing the active with material that provides the potential counterion. Crystals formed by this process were examined by brightfield and polarized light microscopy. Further characterization by Raman spectroscopy enabled selection of five ephedrine and four naproxen salt forms.

An *in situ* pharmaceutical salt-selection process was first reported by Shanker et al. (1994). Good correlation between the solubility of the *in situ* salt and the solubility of the synthesized salt was reported, but the details of the technique have not been published. Tong and Whitesell (1998) presented an *in situ* salt screening technique for basic drugs without the need to make the salts. This technique provides immediate evidence of insoluble salts and can therefore conserve time and resources. In addition, the formulation scientist obtains the maximum amount of information from the smallest amount of compound. The screening technique involves (1) selecting the acids to study, (2) conducting the solubility study using 0.1 M solutions of the respective acid, (3) characterizing the solid residue from the solubility study, and (4) calculating the solubility product and solubility of the salts. The acids selected should have a pK_a that is at least 2 pH units below the pK_a of the conjugate acid of the basic drug. The base is then exposed to 500 μL or 1 mL of the 0.1 M solution of the respective acid in a constant temperature shaker bath. The basic drug, therefore, is in equilibrium with a solution containing the proposed counterion in excess. A direct evaluation of the solubility is not possible, then, because of the common ion effect on the solubility of the proposed salt form. Using the solubility product allows estimation of the aqueous solubility of the salt that would be the product of the reaction of the basic drug with the respective acid. The means by which to arrive at the solubility estimation is described below. An aliquot of the solution is drawn after 1 week and after 2 weeks, filtered, and assayed for drug content. The solubility results can also provide useful information regarding buffer selection for an injectable formulation. For example, the hydrochloride salt might be incompatible with a phosphate or citrate buffer if the solubility of the phosphate or citrate salt, respectively, is less soluble. The residual solid in the solubility study is characterized by hot-stage microscopy, powder X-ray diffraction, and differential scanning calorimetry or thermogravimetric analysis to ensure that the solid exposed to the solution has changed from the base form of the drug to its salt form.

Bowker (2002) provides an extensive discussion of a procedure for salt selection and optimization. Issues presented in that discussion include the choice of the counterion, scale-up of the preparation method, making the decision as to which form to develop, and negative aspects to salt formation. Stahl (2003) discusses practical considerations for preparation of salts. In particular, he notes that the salt form of a drug cannot be isolated under conditions where it is fully ionized. For that reason, organic solvents that suppress dissociation are used to separately dissolve the base and the acid that constitute the salt form. The two solutions are mixed and supersaturation is encouraged if the drug salt fails to precipitate. Stahl notes that techniques such as cooling the mixture, evaporation of the solvent, or the slow addition of a miscible antisolvent can encourage supersaturation and drive the precipitation of the salt form.

The solubility product and solubility of the *in situ* salts are calculated as follows. The amount of precipitated drug in the solubility study, B in g, is converted to B_p, the moles of the base form of the drug precipitated, by using MW, the molecular weight of the base form of the drug:

$$B_p = \frac{B}{MW} \tag{15.2}$$

The moles of precipitated drug can be calculated using:

$$B_p = B_i - (B_s V) \tag{15.3}$$

where B_i in moles is the amount of solid base added; B_s in moles/L is the concentration of the drug in the acid solution, assumed to be the base form of the drug since the molecular weight of the acid form and the base form of the drug differ by 1 g/mole; and V in L is the volume of the solution. Assuming that the precipitate exposed to the saturated solution is composed solely of the 1:1 salt formed by the interaction of the acid with the base drug, that is, A^-BH^+, the molar concentration of the acid remaining in the solution saturated with drug, $[A_s]$, is given by

$$[A_s] = [A] - \frac{B_p}{V} \tag{15.4}$$

where $[A]$ is the original concentration of the acid in moles/L. Using the acid dissociation constant of the acid, K_a, and the pH of the saturated solution, the concentration of the acid in its ionized form remaining in solution, $[A_{ionized}]$, can be calculated as follows:

$$[A_s] = [A_{ionized}] + [AH_s] \tag{15.5}$$

where $[AH_s]$ is the uncharged, acid form of the acid in solution. The acid dissociation constant gives

$$K_a = \frac{[H^+][A_{ionized}]}{[AH_s]} \tag{15.6}$$

Rearranging Equation 15.6 gives

$$\frac{[AH_s]K_a}{[H^+]} = [A_{ionized}] \tag{15.7}$$

Substituting for $[AH_s]$ using Equation 15.5:

$$\frac{([A_s] - [A_{ionized}])K_a}{[H^+]} = [A_{ionized}] \tag{15.8}$$

Collecting common $[A_{ionized}]$ terms:

$$\frac{[A_s]K_a}{[H^+]} = [A_{ionized}] + \frac{[A_{ionized}]K_a}{[H^+]} \tag{15.9}$$

Isolating the molar concentration of the ionized form of the acid in solution:

$$\frac{[A_s]K_a}{[H^+]} = [A_{ionized}]\left(1 + \frac{K_a}{[H^+]}\right) \tag{15.10}$$

$$[A_s]K_a = [A_{\text{ionized}}]\left([H^+] + \frac{[H^+]K_a}{[H^+]}\right) \tag{15.11}$$

$$[A_s]K_a = [A_{\text{ionized}}]\left([H^+] + K_a\right) \tag{15.12}$$

$$\frac{[A_s]K_a}{\left([H^+] + K_a\right)} = [A_{\text{ionized}}] \tag{15.13}$$

The intrinsic solubility of the charged form of an organic compound is governed by its solubility product, K_{sp}, described here (Anderson and Conradi, 1985) for a 1:1 salt of a monoprotic acid, HA, and the base drug in its protonated form:

$$K_{sp} = [BH^+][A^-]\gamma_+ \gamma_- \tag{15.14}$$

where the activity coefficients, γ_i, acknowledge the influence of ionic content in the solution on the activity of each ion which in turn affects the molar concentration in real solutions. For future equations, the activity coefficients will not appear in order to keep the equations uncluttered and ideal behavior in these solutions will be assumed. For salts of the sort $A_a B_b$, the reader is directed to a thorough discussion of this parameter (Amis, 1983).

Acknowledging that $[BH_s^+]$ essentially defines the molar concentration of the base drug in the acid solution, the solubility product of the salt form, K_{sp}, can be calculated:

$$K_{sp} = [A_{\text{ionized}}]\left[BH_s^+\right] \tag{15.15}$$

The solubility product presents the limit to the concentrations achieved by the ions in the saturated solution. Still assuming the 1:1 salt, the molar solubility of the salt is S_{salt}:

$$S_{salt} = \left[A^-BH^+\right] = [A_{\text{ionized}}] = \left[BH_s^+\right] = \sqrt{K_{sp}} \tag{15.16}$$

and the molar solubility of the salt is the square root of the solubility product. The solubility of the salt in mg/mL is given by $MW_{salt}S_{salt}$ where

$$MW_{salt}S_{salt} = MW_{salt}\sqrt{K_{sp}} \tag{15.17}$$

and MW_{salt} is the molecular weight of the particular salt form of the drug.

One must acknowledge, however, that the relationship between the solubility and the solubility product depends on the stoichiometry of the cation and anion in the salt. For an a:b salt, such as A_aB_b, the charge on the A ion would be $^{+b}$ and that on the B ion would be $^{-a}$. Each A_aB_b salt form dissociates on dissolution into ^{a} molecules of A and ^{b} molecules of B:

$$A_aB_b \leftrightarrow aA^{+b} + bB^{-a} \tag{15.18}$$

For a saturated solution of this a:b salt, assuming the molar solubility of the salt is S_{salt}, there would be $a(S_{salt})$ moles/liter of A ions and $b(S_{salt})$ moles/liter of B ions and $[B] = (b/a)[A]$. The solubility product also reflects this stoichiometric relationship in the A_aB_b salt form presented in Equation 15.17 and Equation 15.14 becomes

$$K_{sp} = [A]^a[B]^b \tag{15.19}$$

Substituting the relative molar concentration of the B ion to the A ion into Equation 15.18 gives

$$K_{sp} = [A]^a \left(\frac{b}{a}[A] \right)^b \qquad (15.20)$$

Rearranging to isolate the concentration of A gives

$$[A] = \sqrt[a+b]{\frac{K_{sp}}{(b/a)^b}} \qquad (15.21)$$

Since S_{salt} equals $(1/a)[A]$ or $(1/b)[B]$, Equation 15.21 can be modified to reflect this:

$$S_{salt} = (1/a)[A] = (1/a)\sqrt[a+b]{\frac{K_{sp}}{(b/a)^b}} \qquad (15.22)$$

Taking the (1/a) inside the radical gives

$$S_{salt} = \sqrt[a+b]{\frac{K_{sp}}{(a)^{a+b}(b/a)^b}} = \sqrt[a+b]{\frac{K_{sp}}{(a)^a(b)^b}} \qquad (15.23)$$

$$K_{sp} = a^a b^b (S_{salt})^{a+b} \qquad (15.24)$$

PREDICTABILITY OF SOLUBILITY

It is evident from numerous reports that prediction of the solubility outcome of a change in the counterion of a salt is not simple. Even the rank order of the solubility of inorganic salts of the same drug is apparently not predictable. The order of decreasing molar aqueous solubility for *para*-aminosalicylic acid salts would be $Na^+ > Ca^{2+} > K^+$, but for naproxen it would be $K^+ > Na^+ > Mg^{2+} > Ca^{2+}$ (Chowhan, 1978). Interestingly, when the solubility of the *para*-aminosalicylic acid salts were considered (Forbes et al., 1995), the order of decreasing aqueous solubility was $K^+ > Na^+ > Ca^{2+}$ (low hydrate) $> Ca^{2+}$ (trihydrate) $= Mg^{2+}$. Chowhan (1978) also investigated the solubility for salts of 7-methylsulfinyl-, and of 7-methylthio-2-xanthonecarboxylic acid, and found the order of decreasing aqueous solubility to be $K^+ > Na^+ > Ca^{2+} > Mg^{2+}$, and $Na^+ > K^+ > Ca^{2+} = Mg^{2+}$, respectively. Typically, however, the monovalent cation salt is more soluble in water than the divalent cation salt.

The solid state structure can profoundly influence the physicochemical properties of chlordiazepoxide salts (Singh et al., 1992). Single crystal structures revealed that the base in the mesylate (Singh et al., 1992), tosylate (Singh et al., 1992), and hydrochloride salts (Herrnstadt et al., 1979) was able to dimerize in the crystalline form through hydrogen bonds between the N-oxide oxygen and the hydrogen of the secondary amine. The sulfate salt did not follow this pattern because the counterion itself was capable of hydrogen bonding with the base at the dimerization sites (Singh et al., 1992). This serves as an example of how a difference in solid state structure results in dissimilar physicochemical behavior, although that has not as yet been confirmed for the drug chlordiazepoxide.

A phase solubility method was described by Dittert et al. (1964) to generate data that demonstrate the sensitivity of solubility to pH which is exhibited by weak acid and weak base drugs. Kramer and Flynn (1972) presented equations that define the aqueous solubilities of organic hydrochlorides. At low pH, the solubility, S, is the sum of the concentration of the organic base, [B], and the intrinsic solubility of its protonated form, $[BH^+]_0$, is described in the following equation:

$$S_{pH<pH_{max}} = [B] + [BH^+]_0 = [BH^+]_0 \left(\frac{K_{a,BH^+}}{[H^+]} + 1 \right) \qquad (15.25)$$

where the protonated form has an acid dissociation constant K_{a,BH^+}. The activity of the proton will change in response to both the pH and the ionic strength of the dissolution medium, and this is relevant since the molar concentration of the protons serves as an estimate of the activity of the protons in the aqueous medium. It is the intrinsic solubility of the charged form that can be enhanced by proper salt formation. The subscripted expression, $pH < pH_{max}$, emphasizes that there is a pH maximum below which the solubility remains essentially constant at the intrinsic solubility of the protonated form, $[BH^+]_o$, that is limited by the solubility product, K_{sp}.

In their discussion of dibasic drugs, Lakkaraju et al. (1997) first presented the solubility of the monovalent salt form. As the pH is lowered further than pH_{max}, the solubility can be further enhanced by formation of the divalent salt in solution. S would then be described as

$$S_{pH<pH_{max}} = [B] + [BH^+]_o + [BH^{++}] \quad \text{(dibasic drugs)} \quad (15.26)$$

Since $[B]$ is likely to be negligible in comparison to $[BH^+]_o$ in this pH range, this equation can be reduced to

$$S_{pH<pH_{max}} = [BH^+]_o + [BH^{++}] \quad \text{(dibasic drugs)} \quad (15.27)$$

Substituting for $[BH^{++}]$ based on K_{a2} gives

$$S_{pH<pH_{max}} = [BH^+]_o + \frac{[H^+][BH^+]}{K_{a2}} = [BH^+]_o \left(1 + \frac{H^+}{K_{a2}}\right) \quad (15.28)$$

A single pH_{max} is suggested in Equation 15.25, and a second pH_{max} is observed at a pH below the first pH_{max} when it is appropriate to use Equation 15.26. An example of the effect of divalent salt formation on solubility is provided by a lysine derivative of an antitumor agent 2-(4-aminophenyl) benzothiazole, with pK_{a1} and pK_{a2} of about 7.5 and 10.2, respectively. The deprotonated nature of the lysine counterion provides a solubility of more than 53 mg/mL at pH 5.0, whereas the solubility drops to 7.0 mg/mL at pH 6.3 and to 0.39 mg/mL at pH 7.4. When the pH limits the derivative to a single protonated site, the solubility is less than 0.075 mg/mL (Hutchinson et al., 2002).

The pH-solubility profiles of naproxen and its sodium, potassium, calcium, and magnesium salts were generated by Chowhan (1978), and revealed that at a pH below the pK_a, the solubility is largely limited to the solubility of the uncharged form, with the contribution from the ionized form diminishing as the pH decreases. Indeed, the salt forms can improve the aqueous solubility only in the region where the ionized form of the drug would constitute the major fraction of drug present in solution. It was found that each salt of this carboxylic acid has a characteristic maximum pH (i.e., pH_{max}) above which the solubility of the salt is established by the solubility of the ionized form. It has been suggested that this is the pH at which the ionized and unionized species are simultaneously saturated (Ledwidge and Corrigan, 1998).

Chowhan (1978) generated the appropriate equations to describe the solubility of a weak acid and its salts as a function of pH. At low pH, the nonionized form limits the solubility, S, which can be expressed as the sum of the intrinsic solubility of the uncharged form, $[HA]_o$, and the variable concentration of the salt form, $[A^-]$:

$$S_{pH<pH_{max}} = [HA] + [A^-] = [HA]_o \left(1 + \frac{K_a}{[H^+]}\right) \quad (15.29)$$

where the acid dissociation constant is given by K_a. In this case, the pH_{max} refers to the pH *above* which the solubility remains essentially constant as defined by the intrinsic solubility of the salt

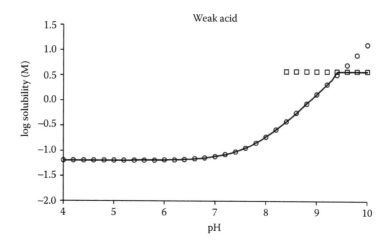

FIGURE 15.2 Effect of pH on the solubility of a weak acid and its salt form where $[HA]_o$ equals 0.064 M, $[A^-]_o$ is 3.8 M, and the pK_a of this weak acid is 7.7. Circles represent Equation 15.29; squares are for Equation 15.30. The continuous curve in the plot is the solubility curve for this weak acid.

form of the acid, $[A^-]_o$. At higher pH, then, the intrinsic solubility of the salt form, $[A^-]_o$, defines the solubility of the two forms:

$$S_{pH>pH_{max}} = [HA] + [A^-] = [A^-]_o \left(\frac{[H^+]}{K_a} + 1 \right)$$
(15.30)

In actuality, Equations 15.29 and 15.30 describe independent curves, and it is the superposition of the two curves that defines a pH-solubility profile for a weak acid. An example is given in Figure 15.2 for a weak acid with a pK_a of 7.7, and an intrinsic solubility of 0.064 M for the weak acid form and 3.8 M for the salt form. The curve defined by the circles results from solubility calculated using Equation 15.29, and the nearly horizontal curve defined by the squares was generated using Equation 15.30. The pH-solubility profile is represented by the continuous curve and reveals that the solubility of the organic acid below the pH_{max} is defined by the intrinsic solubility of the uncharged form. Although modification of the counterion in the salt will not alter the curved portion of the profile, the improved solubility of the salt can result in an elevated solubility in the range above pH_{max} that is governed by the intrinsic solubility of the salt form.

Superposition of the curves for an organic base and its salt form yields a similar profile, essentially a mirror image of an organic acid profile, as shown in Figure 15.3.

The intrinsic solubility of the anion, A^-, of a weak acid salt is governed by the solubility product, K_{sp}, described here (Anderson and Conradi, 1985):

$$K_{sp} = [M^+]\gamma_+ [A^-]\gamma_-$$
(15.31)

where γ represents the activity coefficient for use with molar concentrations, and (+) and (−) subscripts refer to the cation and the anion, respectively. The influence of the counterion, M, and the solubility product on the intrinsic solubility of this salt are shown here:

$$[A^-]_o = \frac{K_{sp}}{[M^+]_{\gamma^+\gamma^-}}$$
(15.32)

The activity coefficients account for effects caused by the solvent and the ionic strength of the solvent system. (As before, it is acknowledged that the activity coefficients allow the use of molar

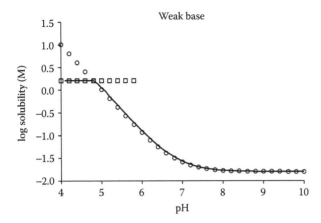

FIGURE 15.3 Effect of pH on the solubility of a weak base and its salt form where $[B]_o$ is 0.016 M and $[BH^+]_o$ is 1.6 M with a pK_a of 6.8 for BH^+. Circles represent Equation 15.25 and squares are at the log of the solubility of the ionized form of the base. The continuous curve in the plot is the solubility curve for this weak base.

concentrations instead of activities to describe nonideal situations. However, to keep equations as simple as possible, molar concentrations will be used in place of molar concentrations with activity coefficients.) For $A_m B_n$ salts, the reader is directed to a more thorough discussion of the parameter (Amis, 1983). The relationship presented in Equation 15.32 also reveals why the common ion effect can profoundly affect the solubility of the drug provided in a salt form. The chloride ion present in solution or in the gastric environment limited the solubility of hydrochloride salts (Lin et al., 1972; Miyazaki et al., 1975, 1980; Serajuddin and Jarowski, 1985). A salt form prepared without using chloride as the counterion is not susceptible to the chloride common ion effect in gastric fluid, unless the salt form is converted to the hydrochloride salt form owing to the overabundance of chloride ion (Li et al., 2005) and the hydrochloride salt form comes out of solution. Similarly, sodium ion can offer a common ion effect to limit the solubility and dissolution rates of sodium salts of drugs (Serajuddin et al., 1987; Ledwidge and Corrigan, 1998).

Positive or negative deviations from expected pH profiles near the pH_{max} can exist under several circumstances. It has been suggested that supersaturation of the drug owing to self-association was believed to cause positive deviations from expected profiles. Self-association, perhaps even to the point of micelle formation, can certainly give the appearance that the solubility was improved (Ledwidge and Corrigan, 1998). Although supersaturation is a thermodynamically unstable condition, formation of the crystal nucleus and subsequent crystal growth are kinetic processes (Ledwidge and Corrigan, 1998), and immediate crystallization might not be observed. Other causes for deviation include the common ion effect or the precipitation of a less soluble polymorphic or solvated form, which can lead to apparent reduced solubility (Ledwidge and Corrigan, 1998).

Anderson and Conradi (1985) reported that attempts to prepare a salt solution at a concentration below the solubility defined by the solubility product might be unsuccessful owing to precipitation of the free acid. They state that this is more likely to occur with salts formed by the reaction of a weak acid with a weak base. To further understand this phenomenon, they defined the *stoichiometric solubility* as the maximum concentration of the 1:1 salt of a carboxylic acid that could be dissolved in pure water without precipitation of the free acid. When very small amounts of the salt of a weak carboxylic acid and a weak organic amine have been added to pure water, the salt is completely dissolved and the pH is given by

$$pH = \frac{1}{2}\left(pK_{a,1} + pK_{a,2}\right)$$

(15.33)

where $K_{a,1}$ and $K_{a,2}$ are the acid dissociation constants of the acid and the protonated base, respectively. This applies up to the point where the free carboxylic acid in the solution reaches its solubility. Upon reaching the solubility of the acid, the concentration of the 1:1 salt in this solution is at the stoichiometric solubility because no more can be dissolved without free acid precipitation. For moderately soluble salts, the stoichiometric solubility would equal the solubility as defined earlier in Equation 15.29, and the activity of the proton is given by the antilog of the negative of both sides of Equation 15.33:

$$a_{H^+} = 10^{-\frac{1}{2}(pK_{a,1}+pK_{a,2})}$$ (15.34)

If additional salt is added to yield a total molar concentration, C_{total}, such that the free acid precipitates, the pH of the solution increases owing to protons being removed from the solution. By utilizing the mass balance and the charge balance equations for the solutions, they derived an expression for the proton activity:

$$a_{H^+} = \frac{K_{a,1}[HA]_o + \sqrt{\left(K_{a,1}[HA]_o\right)^2 + 4C_{total}K_{a,1}K_{a,2}[HA]_o}}{2C_{total}}$$ (15.35)

This predicts that the proton activity is reduced as more salt is added. The pH from this equation allows calculation of the stoichiometric solubility using Equation 15.29.

As more salt is added, excess salt is present in the solid phase and the solution composition is invariant. Therefore, the pH is constant and the product of the cation and anion activities equals the solubility product, as defined in Equation 15.31, in the absence of cation or anion from other sources including molecular complex forms (Amis, 1983). At this point, more salt will not dissolve, and the salt concentration represents the solubility of the drug in the specific salt form. To confirm that the salt solubility has been reached, it should be verified (Anderson and Conradi, 1985) that the solid salt phase in equilibrium with the solution has not been contaminated with the uncharged form precipitate.

There is an intuitively attractive notion that higher solubility can be achieved by selection of a more hydrophilic counterion. This reasoning ignores the probability that stronger interactions are likely in the crystal state when the counterions are increasingly polar, and in fact, the increase in the crystal interaction energies may be the dominant factor in reducing solubility (Anderson, 1985). Dissolution in an aqueous medium requires the energy to hydrate the cation and the anion, and results in the subsequent release of lattice energy. This has been expressed mathematically (Chowhan, 1978) as

$$\Delta G_{solution} = \Delta G_{hx^-} + \Delta G_{hc^+} - \Delta G_{lattice}$$ (15.36)

where $\Delta G_{solution}$ is the change in the Gibbs energy for the process of dissolving a solid in an aqueous solution, G_{hx^-} is the change in the Gibbs energy for hydration of the anion, ΔG_{hc} is the change in the Gibbs energy for hydration of the cation, and $\Delta G_{lattice}$ is the change in the Gibbs energy for the formation of the crystal lattice. For a monovalent organic salt, increasing the radius of the cation, with a constant anion radius, decreases both the hydration and lattice energies (Chowhan, 1978). The difference in solubility, then, depends on the relative magnitudes of these changes. As an example, for a larger decrease in the hydration energies than in the lattice energy, a solubility decrease results (Amis, 1983). For salts where the decrease in lattice energy is much greater than the decrease in the hydration energies, the solubility increases. This last concept is most readily apparent in modifications of salts that result in a decrease in the melting point and the subsequent achievement of an improved solubility.

The relative size of the counterion plays an important role in solubility. The following principles were outlined by Amis (1983) for 1:1 salts, which include most salt forms of drugs:

1. For a salt containing a small cation and a small anion, using a cation of a larger radius with the same anion increases the solubility of the salt. Using an anion of a larger radius with the same cation increases the solubility of the salt.
2. For a salt consisting of a small cation and a large anion, increasing the cation radius with the same anion decreases the solubility. An increase in the radius of the anion with the same cation increases the solubility.
3. For a salt with a large cation and a small anion, increasing the cation radius with the same anion increases the solubility, but increasing the anion size with the same cation would decrease the solubility.
4. For a large cation and large anion salt, an increase in either ionic radius would have little effect on the solubility.

In general, then, the larger the discrepancy in ion size, the greater would be the solubility improvement. In the case of the large cation and large anion, the salt is probably poorly soluble, and a decrease in the size of the drug's counterion would be the direction leading to improved solubility.

FORMULATION CONSIDERATIONS

Salts are frequently chosen on the basis of convenience in the synthetic method and the resultant yield (Gould, 1986). However, the cost of raw materials, ease of crystallization, stability, and physical factors such as hygroscopicity and flow characteristics should also be considered (Miller and Heller, 1975). Toxicologists will be concerned with the chronic and acute dosing of the drug and its conjugate acid or base (Gould, 1986). One of the reasons why lithium carbonate was preferred over the citrate, sulfate, monoglutamate, and acetate salts was the simple fact that the carbonate anion provided the lowest equivalent weight, such that the salt had the highest ratio of lithium per unit weight (Greene, 1975). This results in the smallest mass requirement for a capsule or a tablet.

The salt form will influence a number of physicochemical properties, which can then affect the availability and formulation characteristics of the drug. Preformulation studies must therefore include an extensive evaluation of the physicochemical properties of each salt deemed suitable for clinical trials. These studies should include an evaluation not only of the hygroscopicity but also of the dissolution rate and the equilibrium solubility in appropriate solvent systems. The chemical and physical stability of the salt form must be considered in both preformulation and formulation efforts. A systematic investigation of the salt alone and in the presence of typical excipients should be conducted to determine thermal stability, light sensitivity, solution stability, and the pH influence on solution stability. An interesting case was the effect of sodium chloride on the solubility properties of salts of the serotonergic agonist 2,3,4,5-tetrahydro-8-(methylsulfonyl)-1H-3-benzazepin-7-ol (Rajagopalan et al., 1989). Acetate, hydrochloride, and mesylate salts were prepared and characterized. Although the mesylate salt possessed the highest water solubility (441.3 mg/mL), addition of sodium chloride to the aqueous solution caused a dramatic decrease in the solubility. It was found that the high concentration of chloride ion prompted the precipitation of the hydrochloride salt form of the agonist, which has a solubility of only 1.0 mg/mL. This would preclude the use of sodium chloride as an osmotic agent in parenteral formulations and the use of saline solution as a diluent for clinical use. Both of these problems could be overcome by employing mannitol as the osmotic agent and 5% dextrose as the diluent (Rajagopalan et al., 1989).

A program has been presented that can provide insight into the physical characteristics of a salt before the choice of a candidate for a tablet dosage form for oral administration, when the supply of the substance may still be limited to only 10–15 g (Graffner et al., 1985). Particle size, particle shape, the surface area of the powder, surface color, solubility, lipophilicity, hygroscopicity, and light stability are all measured before development of potential formulations. Physicochemical interactions with typical excipients should be evaluated at this stage of the investigation. Using results from force displacement curves, differences in compaction properties were evident in the different salt forms, including the hydrochloride, methanesulfonate, oxalate, and tartrate salts, of S (−)-*N*-[(1-ethyl-2- pyrrolidinyl)methyl]-2-hydroxy-, 3,5-diethyl-, 6-methoxysalicylamide (Graffner et al., 1985). The oxalate and methanesulfonate salts, for example, exhibited a higher elasticity. The methanesulfonate salt did not form coherent compacts. Results indicated that the methanesulfonate salt was far more hygroscopic than the oxalate salt, and yet each demonstrated reversible water sorption. The difference could not be explained in terms of surface area exposed because the oxalate salt possessed the greater surface area.

Different salts can impart different stability characteristics depending on the degradation mechanism. Differences in hygroscopicity, for example, will largely influence the salt choice for a drug that degrades by hydrolysis. Hygroscopicity can also result in handling and flow problems (Morris et al., 1994). Lithium chloride is an example of a salt that is too hygroscopic to allow tableting (Greene, 1975).

The influence of pH on salt solubility has already been discussed in the previous section. Since the salt forms of drugs involve the ionized form of the drug, the pK_a will largely determine the incidence of precipitation of uncharged drug. The pH of an aqueous medium, then, will be critical to drug solubility (Amidon, 1981; Anderson and Conradi, 1985). Bioavailability of salt forms, then, will depend on the absorption rate for the unionized form from a solution that has a high ionized form reserve present in it. The pH of the medium and the pK_a of the parent drug will determine the ratio of ionized and unionized form concentrations present in the solution at any time, is given by

$$\frac{\left[A^-\right]}{\left[HA\right]}=10^{pH-pK_a} \tag{15.37}$$

and

$$\frac{\left[B\right]}{\left[BH^+\right]}=10^{pH-pK_a} \tag{15.38}$$

for acidic and basic drugs, respectively. As the unionized form of the drug is absorbed, its concentration drops and the charged form generates the uncharged form by acceptance or release of a proton to increase the concentration of the uncharged form in an attempt to reestablish equilibrium between the two forms.

For many poorly soluble drugs, the dissolution rate best reflects the bioavailability of the salt (Juncher and Raaschou, 1957; Berge et al., 1977). Indeed, solubility might affect absorption only to the extent that it affects the dissolution rate. Since absorption is a dynamic process, the solubility of a drug might be of limited consequence if the absorption rate is so rapid that solubility is not attained in the fluid from which the drug is absorbed. The dissolution rate in this instance would be critical since it could establish the effective absorption rate (Berge et al., 1977).

Fortunately, in most cases, the salt form under serious consideration exhibits a faster dissolution rate than the corresponding parent drug at an equivalent pH. This dissolution phenomenon can be explained in light of the parameters that govern the dissolution rate, as found in the diffusion layer model of Brunner (1904):

$$\frac{dM}{dt}=\frac{DS}{h}\left(C_s-C_b\right) \tag{15.39}$$

where dM/dt is the dissolution rate representing the mass of drug, M, dissolved in a period of time, t, from a solid dosage form possessing a surface area of S, where the drug has a diffusivity D in the dissolving fluid and a solubility C_s in the dissolution medium, and the drug concentration in the bulk of that medium at time t is C_b. The parameter h refers to the thickness of a stagnant diffusion medium layer at the surface of the solid, where the drug concentration reaches C_s at steady-state dissolution. Indeed, it is preferable to consider C_s to be the solubility of the drug in the diffusion layer, since it is the maximum concentration possible in that layer that controls the dissolution rate. Nevertheless, on the basis of this equation, it can still be seen that if the solubility in the dissolution medium was increased, the dissolution rate would also increase.

It is also acknowledged that the dissolving solid might act as its own buffer in this stagnant medium (Benet, 1973). This is likely to be the case when the salt is formed by the reaction of a weak acid with a weak base. The cation and anion employed in salt formation can often modify the dissolution rate by acting as buffer components in the stagnant layer found at the solid surface, establishing a pH different from that found in the bulk dissolution medium, which in turn effectively increases or decreases C_s found in Equation 15.39 (Berge et al., 1977). This was believed to be the underlying cause of differences in dissolution rates seen with salts of nonsteroidal anti-inflammatory drugs, including alclofenac, diclofenac, fenbufen, ibuprofen, and naproxen (Fini et al., 1985). In each case, the salt form was able to improve the dissolution rate, and for each drug, the effect of the cation in promoting dissolution was sodium > N-(2-hydroxyethyl)piperazinium > N-methylglucosammonium > argininium. In the case of the weak base salts, dissolution depends on the acidity of the counterion that can influence the pH of the microenvironment at the solid surface.

A drug dissolution rate effect as a result of deposition of insoluble particles or a film on the solid surface of a tablet has been observed in at least three cases, aluminum acetylsalicylate (Levy and Sahli, 1962), benzphetamine pamoate (Higuchi and Hamlin, 1963), and tolazamide (Higuchi et al., 1965). As a representative example to explain this phenomenon, the precipitation of the weak acid, pamoic acid, employed as the source of the counterion, slowed the release rate of benzphetamine in acidic media from a bead containing the weak acid salt of the drug (Higuchi and Hamlin, 1963). A mathematical analysis was presented and applied to release of drug from benzphetamine pamoate pellets. When the acid coat forms, the dissolution rate can be reduced essentially to that of the poorly soluble acid (Higuchi et al., 1965).

The improved thermal stability of naproxen and tolmetin as a result of formation of the choline salt has already been noted. Stability studies of lincomycin as its hydrochloride or cyclamate salt revealed that the cyclamate counterion provided an enhanced thermal stability to the antibiotic without compromising the aqueous solubility (Neville and Ethier, 1971; Neville et al., 1971).

CONCLUSIONS

In conclusion, then, the aqueous solubility of a poorly soluble drug can be improved by the selection and preparation of an appropriate salt. The formulation scientist must then determine the resulting physicochemical properties and assess the sensitivity of the product to the environmental and chemical conditions likely to be encountered in handling and storage. In addition, formation of the salt may also reduce the toxicity and modify the pharmacological activity of the drug. Therefore, it is recommended that salt forms be screened early in the preformulation investigations to allow clinical evaluation of those candidates deemed suitable by virtue of their physicochemical properties. The reader is directed to reviews and discussions regarding various salt forms currently in use in pharmaceutical products, including parenterals (Berge et al., 1977; Motola and Agharkar, 1984; Fiese and Hagen, 1986; Bighley et al., 1995; Wermuth and Stahl, 2002; Paulekuhn et al., 2007; Serajuddin, 2007; Guerrieri et al., 2010; Thackaberry, 2012).

REFERENCES

Aakeröy, C. B., M. B. Fasulo, and J. Desper. 2007. Cocrystal or salt: Does it really matter? *Mol. Pharm.* 4: 317–322.
Agharkar, S., S. Lindenbaum, and T. Higuchi. 1976. Enhancement of solubility of drug salts by hydrophilic counterions: Properties of organic salts of an antimalarial drug. *J. Pharm. Sci.* 65: 747–749.

Alves, F. A., M. G. C. A. N. Graca, and H. L. Baptista. 1958. A new class of antibiotic salts of reduced toxicity. *Nature* 181: 182–183.

Amidon, G. L. 1981. Drug derivatization as a means of solubilization: Physicochemical and biochemical strategies. In *Techniques of Solubilization of Drugs*, Yalkowsky, S. H. (Ed.), pp. 183–211. New York: Marcel Dekker.

Amidon, G. L., H. Lennernas, V. P. Shah, and J. R. Crison. 1995. A theoretical basis for a biopharmaceutics drug classification: The correlation of in vitro drug product dissolution and in vivo bioavailability. *Pharm. Res.* 12: 413–420.

Amis, E. S. 1983. Solubility. In *Treatise on Analytical Chemistry, Part 1. Theory and Practice*, Vol. 3, Kolthoff, I. M. and Elving, P. J. (Eds.), pp. 151–267. New York: Wiley.

Anderson, B. D. 1985. Prodrugs for improved formulation properties. In *Design of Prodrugs*, Bundgaard, H. (Ed.), pp. 243–269. New York: Elsevier Science.

Anderson, B. D. and R. A. Conradi. 1985. Predictive relationships in the water solubility of salts of a nonsteroidal anti-inflammatory drug. *J. Pharm. Sci.* 74: 815–820.

Anderson, B. D. and K. P. Flora. 1996. Preparation of water soluble compounds through salt formation. In *The Practice of Medicinal Chemistry*, Wermuth, C. G. (Ed.), pp. 739–754. London: Academic Press.

Ando, H. Y. and G. W. Radebaugh. 2000. Preformulation. In *Remington, the Science and Practice of Pharmacy*, 20th ed., Gennaro, A. R. (Ed.), pp. 700–720. Philadelphia, PA: Lippincott, Williams & Wilkins.

Ansel, H. C., N. G. Popovich, and L. V. Allen. 1995. *Pharmaceutical Dosage Forms and Drug Delivery Systems*, 6th ed., pp. 108–109. Philadelphia, PA: Williams and Wilkins.

Benet, L. Z. 1973. Biopharmaceutics as a basis for the design of drug products. In *Drug Design*, Vol. 4, Ariens, E. J. (Ed.), pp. 1–35. New York: Academic Press.

Berge, S. M., L. D. Bighley, and D. C. Monkhouse. 1977. Pharmaceutical salts. *J. Pharm. Sci.* 66: 1–19.

Bighley, L. D., S. M. Berge, and D. C. Monkhouse. 1995. Salt forms of drugs and absorption. In *Encyclopedia of Pharmaceutical Technology*, Vol. 13, Swarbrick, J. and Boylan, J. C. (Eds.), pp. 453–499. New York: Marcel Dekker.

Bergström, C. A. S., C. M. Wassvik, K. Johansson, and I. Hubatsch. 2007. Poorly soluble marketed drugs display solvation limitation limited solubility. *J. Med. Chem.* 50: 5858–5862.

Bhattachar, S. N., L. A. Deschenes, and J. A. Wesley. 2006. Solubility: It's not just for physical chemists. *Drug Discov. Today* 11: 1012–1018.

Black, S. N., E. A. Collier, R. J. Davey, and R. J. Roberts. 2007. Structure, solubility, screening, and synthesis of molecular salts. *J. Pharm. Sci.* 96: 1053–1068.

Bowker, M. J. 2002. A procedure for salt selection and optimization. In *Handbook of Pharmaceutical Salts: Properties, Selection, and Use*, Stahl, P. H. and Wermuth, C. G. (Eds.), pp. 161–189. New York: Wiley-VCH.

Brunner, E. 1904. Reaktiongeschwindigkeit in heterogenen systemen. *Z. Phys. Chem.* 47: 56–102.

Chowhan, Z. T. 1978. pH-solubility profiles of organic carboxylic acids and their salts. *J. Pharm. Sci.* 67: 1257–1260.

Creasey, N. H. and A. L. Green. 1959. 2-Hydroxyiminomethyl-*N*-methylpyridinium methanesulfphonate (P2S), an antidote to organophosphorus poisoning. Its preparation, estimation and stability. *J. Pharm. Pharmacol.* 11: 485–490.

David, S. E., P. Timmins, and B. R. Conway. 2012. Impact of the counterion on the solubility and physicochemical properties of salts of carboxylic acid salts. *Drug Dev. Ind. Pharm.* 38: 93–103.

Davies, G. 2001. Changing the salt, changing the drug. *Pharm. J.* 266: 322–323.

Dittert, L. W., T. Higuchi, and D. R. Reese. 1964. Phase solubility technique in studying the formation of complex salts of triamterene. *J. Pharm. Sci.* 53: 1325–1328.

Duesel, B. F., H. Berman, and R. J. Schachter. 1954. Substituted xanthines. I. Preparation and properties of some choline theophyllinates. *J. Am. Pharm. Assoc., Sci. Ed.* 43: 619–622.

Elder, D. P., R. Holm, and H. Lopez de Diego. 2013. Use of pharmaceutical salts and cocrystals to address the issue of poor solubility. *Int. J. Pharm.* 453: 88–100.

Ellis, K. O., R. L. White, G. C. Wright, and F. L. Wessels. 1980. Synthesis and skeletal muscle relaxant activity of quaternary ammonium salts of dantrolene and clodanolene. *J. Pharm. Sci.* 69: 327–331.

Fabrizio, G. 1973. Erythromycin aspartate salt. U.S. Patent 3,764,595.

Fiese, E. F. and T. A. Hagen. 1986. Preformulation. In *The Theory and Practice of Industrial Pharmacy*, Lachman, L., Lieberman, H. A., and Kanig, J. L. (Eds.), pp. 171–196. Philadelphia, PA: Lea & Febiger.

Fini, A., G. Feroci, and G. Fazio. 1996. Effects of the counterions on the properties of diclofenac salts. *Int. J. Pharm. Adv.* 1: 269–284.

Fini, A., V. Zecchi, and A. Tartarini. 1985. Dissolution profiles of NSAID carboxylic acids and their salts with different counterions. *Pharm. Acta Helv.* 60: 58–62.

Forbes, R. T., P. York, and J. R. Davidson. 1995. Dissolution kinetics and solubilities of *p*-aminosalicylic acid and its salts. *Int. J. Pharm.* 126: 199–208.

Gould, P. L. 1986. Salt selection of basic drugs. *Int. J. Pharm.* 33: 201–217.

Graffner, C., M. E. Johansson, M. Nicklasson, and H. Nyqvist. 1985. Preformulation studies in a drug development program for tablet formulations. *J. Pharm. Sci.* 74: 16–20.

Greene, D. S. 1979. Preformulation. In *Modern Pharmaceutics*, Banker, G. S. and Rhodes, C. T. (Eds.), pp. 211–225. New York: Marcel Dekker.

Greene, R. J. 1975. Clinical pharmaceutical aspects of lithium therapy. *Drug Intell. Clin. Pharm.* 9: 17–25.

Gu, L. and R. G. Strickley. 1987. Preformulation salt selection. Physical property comparisons of the tris(hydroxymethyl)aminomethane (THAM) salts of four analgesic/antiinflammatory agents with the sodium salts and the free acids. *Pharm. Res.* 4: 255–257.

Guerrieri, P., A. C. F. Rumondor, T. Li, and L. S. Taylor. 2010. Analysis of relationships between solid-state properties, counterion, and developability of pharmaceutical salts. *AAPS Pharm. Sci. Tech.* 11: 1212–1222.

Herrnstadt, C., D. Mootz, and H. Wunderlich. 1979. Protonation sites of organic bases with several nitrogen functions: Crystal structures of salts of chlordiazepoxide, dihydralazine, and phenformin. *J. Chem. Soc., Perkin Trans.* 2: 735–740.

Higuchi, W. I. and W. E. Hamlin. 1963. Release of drug from a self-coating surface. *J. Pharm. Sci.* 52: 575–579.

Higuchi, W. I., N. A. Mir, A. P. Parker, and W. E. Hamlin. 1965. Dissolution kinetics of a weak acid, 1,1-hexamethylene *p*-tolylsulfonylsemicarbazide, and its sodium salt. *J. Pharm. Sci.* 54: 8–11.

Huang, L.-F. and W.-Q. Tong. 2004. Impact of solid state properties on developability assessment of drug candidates. *Adv. Drug Del. Rev.* 56: 321–334.

Hutchinson, I., S. A. Jennings, B. R. Vishnuvajjala, A. D. Westwell, and M. F. G. Stevens. 2002. Antitumor benzothiazoles. 16. Synthesis and pharmaceutical properties of antitumor 2-(4-aminophenyl)benzothiazole amino acid prodrugs. *J. Med. Chem.* 45: 744–747.

Juczyk, M. F., D. R. Berger, and G. R. Damaso. 1991. Quaternary ammonium salt: Applications in hair conditioners. *Cosmet. Toiletries* 106: 63–68.

Juncher, H. and F. Raaschou. 1957. The solubility of oral preparations of penicillin V. *Antibiot. Med. Clin. Ther.* 4: 497–507.

Keller, H., W. Krüpe, H. Sous, and H. Mückter. 1956a. Versuche zur toxizitätsminderung basicher *Streptomyces*-antibiotica. *Arzneim. Forsch.* 6: 61–66.

Keller, H., W. Krüpe, H. Sous, and H. Mückter. 1956b. The pantothenates of streptomycin, viomycin, and neomycin: New and less toxic salts. In *Antibiotics Annual, 1955–1956*, Welch, H. and Marti-Ibañez, F. (Eds.), pp. 35–38. New York: Medical Encyclopedia.

Kennon, L. and T. Higuchi. 1956. Interaction studies of cationic drugs with anionic polyelectrolytes. I. Sodium carboxymethylcellulose. *J. Am. Pharm. Assoc., Sci. Ed.* 45: 157–160.

Kennon, L. and T. Higuchi. 1957. Interaction studies of cationic drugs with anionic polyelectrolytes. II. Polyacrylic and styrene polymers. *J. Am. Pharm. Assoc., Sci. Ed.* 46: 21–27.

Kesisoglou, F. and Y. Wu. 2008. Understanding the effect of API properties on bioavailability through absorption modeling. *AAPS J.* 10: 516–525.

Khankari, R. K. and D. J. W. Grant. 1995. Pharmaceutical hydrates. *Thermochim. Acta* 248: 61–79.

Kramer, S. F. and G. L. Flynn. 1972. Solubility of organic hydrochlorides. *J. Pharm. Sci.* 61: 1896–1904.

Kumar, L., A. Amin, and A. K. Bansal. 2007. An overview of automated systems relevant in pharmaceutical salt screening. *Drug Discov. Today.* 12: 1046–1053.

Lakkaraju, A., H. Joshi, S. Varia, and A. T. M. Serajuddin. 1997. pH-solubility relationship of avitriptan, a dibasic compound, as a function of counterion. *Pharm. Res.* 14: S–228.

Lasslo, A., C. C. Pfeiffer, and P. D. Waller. 1959. Salts of *p*-acetamidobenzoic acid. *J. Am. Pharm. Assoc., Sci. Ed.* 48: 345–347.

Ledwidge, M. T. and O. I Corrigan. 1998. Effects of surface active characteristics and solid state forms on the pH solubility profiles of drug-salt systems. *Int. J. Pharm.* 174: 187–200.

Levy, G. and B. A. Sahli. 1962. Comparison of the gastrointestinal absorption of aluminum acetylsalicylate and acetylsalicylic acid in man. *J. Pharm. Sci.* 51: 58–62.

Li, S., S.-M. Wong, S. Sethia, H. Almoazen, Y. M. Joshi, and A. T. M. Serajuddin. 2005. Investigation of solubility and dissolution of a free base and two different salt forms as a function of pH. *Pharm. Res.* 22: 628–635.

Lin, S.-L., L. Lachman, C. J. Swartz, and C. F. Huebner. 1972. Preformulation investigation. I. Relation of salt forms and biological activity of an experimental antihypertensive. *J. Pharm. Sci.* 61: 1418–1422.

Loucas, S. P. and H. M. Haddad. 1972. Solid-state ophthalmic dosage systems in effecting prolonged release of pilocarpine in the cul-de-sac. *J. Pharm. Sci.* 61: 985–986.

Málek, P., J. Kolc, M. Herold, and J. Hoffman. 1958. Lymphotrophic antibiotics—"Antibiolymphins," In *Antibiotics Annual, 1957–1958*, Welch, H. and Marti-Ibañez, F. (Eds.), pp. 546–551. New York: Medical Encyclopedia.

Miller, L. C. and W. H. Heller. 1975. Physical and chemical considerations in the choice of drug products. In *Drugs of Choice 1974–1975*, Modell, W. C. (Ed.), pp. 20–29. St. Louis, MO: Mosby.

Miyazaki, S., M. Nakano, and T. Arita. 1975. A comparison of solubility characteristics of free bases and hydrochloride salts of tetracycline antibiotics in hydrochloric acid solutions. *Chem. Pharm. Bull.* 23: 1197–1204.

Miyazaki, S., M. Oshiba, and T. Nadai. 1980. Unusual solubility and dissolution behavior of pharmaceutical hydrochloride salts in chloride-containing media. *Int. J. Pharm.* 6: 77–85.

Morris, K. R., M. G. Fakes, A. B. Thakur, A. W. Newman, A. K. Singh, J. J. Venit, C. J. Spagnuolo, and A. T. M. Serajuddin. 1994. An integrated approach to the selection of optimal salt form for a new drug candidate. *Int. J. Pharm.* 105: 209–217.

Motola, S. and S. Agharkar. 1984. Preformulation research of parenteral medications. In *Pharmaceutical Dosage Forms: Parenteral Medications*, Vol. 1, Avis, K. E., Lachman, L., and Lieberman, H. E. (Eds.), pp. 89–138. New York: Marcel Dekker.

Murti, S. K. 1993. On the preparation and characterization of water-soluble choline salts of carboxylic acid drugs, PhD dissertation, University of Missouri–Kansas City.

Nelson, E. 1957. Solution rate of theophylline salts and effects from oral administration. *J. Am. Pharm. Assoc., Sci. Ed.* 46: 607–614.

Neville G. A. and J. C. Ethier. 1971. Preparation and characterization of lincomycin cyclamate. *J. Pharm. Sci.* 60: 497–499.

Neville, G. A., J. C. Ethier, N. F. H. Bright, and R. H. Lake. 1971. Characterization of some lincomycin and cyclamate salts by thermal analysis and infrared spectroscopy. *J. Assoc. Off. Anal. Chem.* 54: 1200–1210.

Nielsen, L. H., S. Gordon, R. Holm, A. Selen, T. Rades, and A. Mullertz. 2013. Preparation of an amorphous sodium furosemide salt improves solubility and dissolution rate and leads to a faster Tmax after oral dosing to rats. *Eur. J. Pharm. Biopharm.* 85(3 Pt B): 942–951.

Osterberg, A. C., J. J. Olsen, N. N. Yuda, C. E. Rauh, H. G. Parr, and L. W. Will. 1957. Cochlear, vestibular, and acute toxicity studies of streptomycin and dihydrostreptomycin pantothenate salts, In *Antibiotics Annual, 1956–1957*, Welch, H. and Marti-Ibañez, F. (Eds.), pp. 564–573. New York: Medical Encyclopedia.

Parshad H., K. Frydenvang, T. Liljefors, H. O. Sorensen, and C. Larsen, 2004. Aqueous solubility study of salts of benzylamine derivatives and p-substituted benzoic acid derivatives using X-ray crystallographic analysis. *Int. J. Pharm.* 269: 157–168.

Patel, A., S. A. Jones, A. Ferro, and N. Patel. 2009. Pharmaceutical salts: A formulation trick or a clinical conundrum? *Brit. J. Cardiol.* 16: 281–286.

Paulekuhn, G. S., J. B. Dressman, and C. Saal. 2007. Trends in active pharmaceutical ingredient salt selection based on analysis of the orange book database. *J. Med. Chem.* 50: 6665–6672.

Pratt, O. B. and H. O. Swartout. 1933. Tartrate metabolism. *J. Lab. Clin. Med.* 18: 366–370.

Rajagopalan, N., C. M. Dicken, L. J. Ravin, C. S. Randall, and R. Krupinski-Olsen. 1989. Solubility properties of the serotonergic agonist 2,3,4,5-tetrahydro-8-(methylsulfonyl)-1H-3-benzazepin-7-ol. *Drug Dev. Ind. Pharm.* 15: 489–497.

Ravin, L. J. and G. W. Radebaugh. 1990. Preformulation. In *Remington's Pharmaceutical Sciences*, 18th ed., Gennaro, A. R. (Ed.), pp. 1435–1450. Easton, PA: Mack Publishing.

Rubin, A., B. E. Rodda, P. Warrick, A. Ridolfo, and C. M. Gruber. 1971. Physiological disposition of fenoprofen in man. I. Pharmacokinetic comparison of calcium and sodium salts administered orally. *J. Pharm. Sci.* 60: 1797–1801.

Sandberg, A., B. Abrahamsson, A. Svenheden, B. Olofsson, and R. Bergstrand. 1993. Steady-state bioavailability and day-to-day variability of a multiple-unit (CR/ZOK) and a single-unit (OROS) delivery system of metoprolol after once-daily dosing. *Pharm. Res.* 10: 28–34.

Saxena, V., R. Panicucci, Y. Joshi, and S. Garad. 2009. Developability assessment in pharmaceutical industry: An integrated group approach for selecting developable candidates. *J. Pharm. Sci.* 98: 1962–1979.

Schoenwald, R. D. 2002. *Pharmacokinetics in Drug Discovery and Development*, Boca Raton, FL: CRC Press.

Serajuddin, A. T. M. 2007. Salt formation to improve drug solubility. *Adv. Drug Del. Rev.* 59: 603–616.

Serajuddin, A. T. M. and C. I. Jarowski. 1985. Effect of diffusion layer pH and solubility on the dissolution rate of pharmaceutical bases and their hydrochloride salts. I. Phenazopyridine. *J. Pharm. Sci.* 74: 142–147.

Serajuddin, A. T. M. and M. Pudipeddi. 2002. Salt-selection strategies. In *Handbook of Pharmaceutical Salts: Properties, Selection and Use*, Stahl, P. H. and Wermuth, C. G. (Eds.), pp. 135–160. New York: Wiley-VCH.

Serajuddin, A. T. M., P.-C. Sheen, and M. A. Augustine. 1987. Common ion effect on solubility and dissolution rate of the sodium salt of an organic acid. *J. Pharm. Pharmacol.* 39: 587–591.

Shah, K. P. 1992. Use of sparingly soluble salts to prepare oral sustained release suspensions. PhD dissertation, University of Missouri–Kansas City.

Shanker, R. M., K. V. Carola, P. J. Baltusis, R. T. Brophy, and T. A. Hatfield. 1994. Selection of appropriate salt form(s) for new drug candidates. *Pharm. Res.* 11:S–236.

Shibe, W. J. and D. H. Hanson. 1964. New approach to quaternary ammonium compounds. *Soap Chem. Spec.* 40: 83–89.

Singh, D., P. York, L. Shields, and P. V. Marshall. 1992. Structural and physicochemical characterization of chlordiazepoxide salts. Poster presentation at the AAPS Seventh Annual Meeting and Exposition, San Antonio, TX, November 16.

Stahl, P. H. 2003. Preparation of water-soluble compounds through salt formation. In *The Practice of Medicinal Chemistry*, 2nd ed., Wermuth, C. G. (Ed.), pp. 601–615. New York: Academic Press.

Surov, A. O., A. A. Manin, A. P. Voronin, K. V. Drozd, A. A. Simagina, A. V. Churakov, and G. L. Perlovich. 2015. Pharmaceutical salts of ciprofloxacin with dicarboxylic acids. *Eur. J. Pharm. Sci.* 77: 112–121.

Thackaberry, E. A. 2012. Non-clinical toxicological considerations for pharmaceutical salt selection. *Expert Opin. Drug Metab. Toxicol.* 8: 1419–1433.

Thorson, M. R., S. Goyal, B. R. Schudel, C. F. Zukoski, G. G. Z. Zhang, Y. Gong, and P. J. A. Kenis. 2011. A microfluidic platform for pharmaceutical salt screening. *Lab Chip* 11: 3829–3837.

Tong, W.-Q. and G. Whitesell. 1998. *In situ* salt screening—A useful technique for discovery support and preformulation studies. *Pharm. Dev. Technol.* 3: 215–223.

Underhill, F. P., F. I. Peterman, T. C. Jaleski, and C. S. Leonard. 1931. Studies on the metabolism of tartrates. III. The behavior of tartrates in the human body. *J. Pharmacol. Exp. Therap.* 43: 381–398.

Wagner, J. G. 1961. Biopharmaceutics: Absorption aspects. *J. Pharm. Sci.* 50: 359–387.

Wan, S. H., P. J. Pentikainen, and D. L. Azarnoff. 1974. Bioavailability of aminosalicylic acid and its various salts in humans. III. Absorption from tablets. *J. Pharm. Sci.* 63: 708–711.

Ware, E. C. and D. R. Lu. 2004. An automated approach to salt selection for new unique trazodone salts. *Pharm Res.* 21: 177–184.

Wells, J. I. 1988. *Pharmaceutical Preformulation: The Physicochemical Properties of Drug Substances.* Chichester, UK: Ellis Horwood.

Wermuth, C. G. and P. H. Stahl. 2002. Selected procedures for the preparation of pharmaceutically acceptable salts. In *Handbook of Pharmaceutical Salts: Properties, Selection, and Use*, Stahl, P. H. and Wermuth, C. G. (Eds.), pp. 249–263. New York: Wiley-VCH.

Windholz, M., S. Budavari, R. F. Blumetti, and E. S. Otterbein. 1983. *Merck Index*, 10th ed., p. 532. Rahway, NJ: Merck.

16 Prodrugs for Improved Solubility in Water

Steven H. Neau, Nikhil C. Loka, and Kalyan K. Saripella

CONTENTS

INTRODUCTION

Prodrug is a term used by Adrien Albert to describe a chemical that must undergo bioconversion before exerting its pharmacological effect (Albert, 1958, 1964). The term, as it is applied here, will refer to a drug with a covalently bound, inactive moiety (the promoiety) that provides or enhances the desired physicochemical properties, where the promoiety must be removed upon administration to regenerate the parent drug (Stella et al., 1985; Kumar and Singh, 2013). Prodrugs are typically pharmacologically inert; enzymatic or chemical processes are necessary for removal of the inactive moiety to return the active parent drug (Ettmayer et al., 2004; Stella et al., 2007; Rautio et al., 2008; Huttunen et al., 2011). Their successful use is evident when one realizes that 33% of small molecule drugs approved in 2008 were actually prodrugs (Rautio, 2010, Stella, 2010; Huttunen et al., 2011).

The chemical or enzymatic processes that restore the parent drug might guide or limit the selection of the promoiety. As an example, esterases are present throughout the body and can be utilized in the hydrolysis of an ester functional group in a prodrug (Andurkar, 2007; Bai et al., 2014) for a drug bearing a carboxylic acid or an alcohol group (Colaizzi and Pitlick, 1982). The reconversion of the prodrug to the parent drug by enzymatic means requires that the enzyme be capable of catalyzing the reaction that cleaves the promoiety-drug linkage. Prodrugs, especially those intended for parenteral use, should exhibit a long shelf life in aqueous media and yet be rapidly reconverted to the parent drug under physiological conditions (Lallemand et al., 2005b). Chemical reversal *in vivo* should demonstrate less intersubject variability than would biochemical pathways to accomplish such reversal (Notari, 1985).

Following chemical modification of the parent drug, physicochemical properties are expected to change, including solubility, stability, and sometimes the organoleptic properties (Stella, 1975; Stinchcomb et al., 1995; Peng et al., 2010; Domião et al., 2014). The advent of property-based drug design provided numerous approaches to design and develop prodrugs to achieve improved characteristics over those of the parent drug (van de Waterbeemd et al., 2001). However, modifications to generate prodrugs can positively or negatively alter the pharmacokinetics of the parent drug by affecting absorption, distribution, metabolism, and excretion (Notari, 1973; Stella, 1975; Huttunen et al., 2011). The improvement in aqueous solubility, for example, can yield improved bioavailability;

the use of certain promoieties can markedly enhance solution stability (Sinkula, 1977). The influence that the prodrug approach has on biopharmaceutical properties has been reviewed (Sinkula, 1975; Sinkula and Yalkowsky, 1975; Sinkula, 1977; Peng et al., 2010; Domião et al., 2014) and will be discussed briefly later.

To take advantage of the prodrug approach, the drug must bear a functional group capable of being derivatized by covalent attachment to the promoiety. The number of functional groups that have proved to be useful in the generation of biologically labile derivatives is now fairly large, and examples of typical functional groups, including esters, thioesters, amides, acetals, and ketals, have been compiled (Charton, 1977, 1985). Of equal importance is that the prodrug must revert to the drug at an appropriate rate and time (Krise et al., 1999c) to deliver the intact parent drug to the site of action. The prodrug to drug conversion can therefore take place before absorption, as in hydrolysis of an ester or peptide linkage in the gastrointestinal tract catalyzed by intestinal enzymes (Simmons et al., 1995); during absorption, as in hydrolysis by esterases found in the skin (Roy and Manoukian, 1994) or in the brush border membrane (Schmidt et al., 1972; Hirano et al., 1977); after absorption, such as taking advantage of phosphomonoesterases in plasma (Melby and St. Cyr, 1961); or even at the site of action, for example, utilization of β-glucuronidase for reconversion at tumor tissues (Watanabe et al., 1981), depending on the goal for which the prodrug was developed (Bundgaard, 1985a). If a prodrug was designed to improve solubility in water to allow the drug to be administered as an injectable solution, it should be converted back to the drug as soon as possible following injection. The rate of conversion must yield a concentration of the parent drug above the minimum effective level at the site of action (Stella, 1975). Any prodrug found in the blood circulation would be considered drug unavailable for pharmacological activity (Bundgaard, 1985a). Ideally, then, the prodrug should possess adequate solubility in the desired dissolution medium, chemical stability to provide an appropriate shelf life for the product, and the ability to convert rapidly *in vivo* to the parent drug. A suitable prodrug and the promoieties themselves must also prove to be nontoxic (Cho et al., 1986).

Although the use of prodrugs has proved to be a convenient way to deal with solubility, some consider this approach to be *an act of desperation* when problems with a drug candidate appear to be insurmountable (Huttunen et al., 2011). One of the key issues hindering the overwhelming adoption of this approach by the pharmaceutical industry is that the Food and Drug Administration (FDA) requires submission of evidence that both the drug and prodrug candidate are safe, efficacious, and well tolerated (Stella et al., 2007; Pevarello 2009; May and Kratochvil, 2010; Sofia 2014). There is an underlying risk regarding the prodrug approach, as in the case of acyclovir S-acylthioethyl esterification, that the prodrugs could have greater toxicity than the parent drug (Hecker and Erion, 2008; Huttunen and Rautio, 2011). Nevertheless, prodrugs with reduced toxicity and equal or improved efficacy have been reported (Nudelman et al., 2001; Huo et al., 2015; Kaul et al., 2015; Phillips et al., 2015). Using a prodrug approach, it should now be possible to appropriately modify physicochemical properties of a drug candidate to obtain desirable absorption, distribution, metabolism, and excretion characteristics (Huttunen et al., 2011). Indeed, it has been recommended that prodrug forms should be considered early in preclinical studies because it is easier to modify the properties of a drug candidate than to search for a new chemical entity with the desired properties (Huttunen et al., 2011).

This chapter focuses on modification approaches that have been adopted to generate prodrugs primarily for the purpose of improved solubility in water, although there are certainly other purposes for which prodrugs are produced. It will be discovered that dramatic changes in the physicochemical properties can be observed upon minor chemical modifications. Successful prodrug design should involve the simplest chemical modification possible that still achieves the desired property modifications (Anderson, 1985). With the advent of molecular modeling in the prediction of solubility and high throughput screening in drug design, it is possible to identify functional groups responsible for poor solubility and to replace them or alter them with functional groups that can increase solubility without adversely affecting the efficacy or toxicity of the parent drug.

MODIFICATIONS EMPLOYING HYDROPHILIC FUNCTIONAL GROUPS

A common strategy employed to increase aqueous solubility is the introduction of an ionic or ioniz-able group. Common esters employed to increase the aqueous solubility of drugs bearing a hydroxyl group are hemisuccinates, phosphates, dialkylaminoacetates, and amino acid esters. For drugs that have a carboxylic acid group, ester formation with the alcohol of choline or β-dimethylaminoethanol, or amide formation with the amine of an α-amino acid, has been successful in the preparation of prodrugs possessing an enhanced solubility (Amidon, 1981).

The phosphate group is acknowledged as the most commonly used promoiety to increase solu-bility. For example, clindamycin hydrochloride has a solubility of 3 mg/mL, while clindamycin-2-phosphate has a solubility in excess of 150 mg/mL and is hydrolyzed *in vivo* with a reaction half-life of only 10 min (Amidon et al., 1977). The disodium salts of monophosphate deriva-tives at the 2′- or 7-positions of Taxol yielded prodrugs with a solubility greater than 10 mg/mL, compared to 0.25 μg/mL for the parent drug (Vyas et al., 1993). Entacapone is a 3,4-dihydroxy-5-nitrobenzylidine derivative that is a potent inhibitor of catechol-*O*-methyltransferase. When entacapone was reacted with phosphorous oxychloride in dry pyridine to produce its phosphate prodrug, the aqueous solubility increased more than 1700- and 20-fold at pH 1.2 and 7.4, respec-tively (Leppanen et al., 2000). In addition, the prodrug demonstrated stability toward chemical hydrolysis (a $t_{1/2}$ of 2227 h at pH 7.4) and quantitative release of the parent drug due to enzyme-catalyzed hydrolysis in liver homogenate. One of the most dramatic improvements in solubility was seen with the mono- and diphosphate esters of 2-arachidonyl glyceryl ether (i.e., noladin ether), where the phosphate esters increased the solubility more than 40,000-fold, showed high chemical stability in various buffer systems, and were rapidly converted through enzymatic hydrolysis to the parent drug (Juntunen et al., 2003).

Phosphate esters have the desirable qualities of both chemical stability (Flynn and Lamb, 1970) and biological lability (Amidon et al., 1977; Amidon, 1981). There is evidence that the soluble phosphate ester is enzymatically hydrolyzed to the active agent in the body (Melby and St. Cyr, 1961; Hare et al., 1975; Amidon et al., 1977; Miyabo et al., 1981; Varia and Stella, 1984; Leppanen et al., 2000). An abundance of phosphomonoesterases in plasma, for example, was noted by Melby and St. Cyr (1961); the presence of alkaline phosphatase in the brush border membrane was also reported some time ago (Schmidt et al., 1972; Hirano et al., 1977). As a result, bioactivation of the phosphate prodrug can be rapid, as in the case of methylprednisolone (Mollmann et al., 1989).

Phosphate esters are usually freely water soluble and are sufficiently stable that solutions with practi-cal shelf lives can be prepared (Flynn and Lamb, 1970; Hong and Szulczewski, 1984; Kwee and Stolk, 1984; Varia et al., 1984b). In contrast to phosphate monoesters of primary alcohols, the phosphomono-esters of sterically hindered aromatic (Williams and Naylor, 1971), secondary (Kearney and Stella, 1992; Sadafi et al., 1993), and tertiary alcohols (Sadafi et al., 1993; Bentley et al., 2002) experience a slow rate of bioconversion. The incorporation of a spacer group between the alcohol and the phosphate groups was able to enhance the bioconversion rate for sterically hindered alcohols (Kearney and Stella, 1992; Sadafi et al., 1993). On dephosphorylation, however, the spacer group must also degrade or be metabolized to regenerate the parent drug (Varia et al., 1984b). A prodrug of cyclosporine A has been prepared where the ionized phosphate group attached to a sarcosine-serine-(acyloxy)alkyloxycarbonyl group provides the solubilizing component of the promoiety (Lallemand et al., 2005b). One issue with orally administered prodrugs based on a phosphate ester is that, once an enzyme has regenerated the parent drug, the solubility of the parent drug might be exceeded. Precipitation of parent drug can occur, depending on the supersaturation level, drug dose, and solubility of the parent drug, as well as the level of solubilization possible by the prodrug itself or its cleaved promoiety (Heimbach et al., 2003).

Acknowledging that the triphosphate ester of nucleosides is the active form, it was discovered that their poor chemical stability and high ionic state effectively block their oral bioavailability (Pradere et al., 2014). Preparation of the monophosphate ester with a protecting group on the phosphate moiety enabled permeability across the intestinal wall (Sofia 2013), with enzymatic or chemical removal of the protecting group intracellularly. Once the parent monophosphate ester is returned, cellular nucleoside monophosphate kinases can modify the monophosphate ester to the active form (van Rompay et al., 2000).

The use of succinate esters also constitutes a common strategy for solubilization. Chemical stability appears to be poor to satisfactory, and their biological lability is not as good as that of phosphate monoesters. Succinate esters in general are not good substrates for esterases (Amidon et al., 1977; Bundgaard, 1987), and these prodrugs may be eliminated from the body at a rate comparable to the hydrolysis rate, or they may undergo other metabolic pathways before ester hydrolysis (Melby and St. Cyr, 1961; Melby and Silber, 1981). Blood levels of corticosteroids were higher after intravenous (IV) or intramuscular (IM) administration of the phosphate esters, when compared to the succinate esters (Melby and St. Cyr, 1961). Slow and incomplete hydrolysis *in vivo* was experienced by the succinate esters of acetaminophen and 3-hydroxymethylphenytoin (Williams et al., 1983). The succinate ester of chloramphenicol also appears to undergo slow, variable bioconversion (Kauffman et al., 1980; Burke et al., 1982; Ambrose, 1984; Kramer et al., 1984), adding an additional and unpredictable element to chloramphenicol dosing (Glazko et al., 1977; Strebel et al., 1980). An exception would be succinate esters of curcuminoids that proved to be more stable in phosphate buffer than curcumin itself, were readily hydrolyzed in human plasma, and possessed anti-cancer activity (Wichitnithad et al., 2011).

Succinate esters serve as examples of derivatives that exhibit less than optimal pH-hydrolysis rate behavior owing to their increased reactivity in water as a result of intramolecular catalysis of hydrolysis by the terminal carboxylic acid functionality (Anderson and Taphouse, 1981; Anderson et al., 1984; Damen et al., 2000). Since intramolecular catalytic effects are quite sensitive to geometric factors and distances separating the interactive groups (Anderson and Conradi, 1987), intramolecular catalysis by a terminal functional group should be easily controlled by varying the alkyl chain length. With adipate esters at the 21-hydroxyl group of methylprednisolone, no intramolecular catalysis is observed. Decreasing the chain length to succinate or malonate resulted in rate enhancements of 100- and 7700-fold, respectively, at a pH near 5.

It was reasoned that malic acid could be considered an appropriate replacement for succinic acid in the formation of prodrugs because the additional hydroxyl group should improve the stability of the ester by forming an intramolecular hydrogen bond with the carbonyl (Damen et al., 2000). This hydrogen bond was expected to result in conformational rigidity that would also retard hydrolysis. 2'-Malyl paclitaxel was prepared by condensing Taxol (generic name paclitaxel) with protected malic acid (as (*S*)-1,2-*O*-isopropylidene-malic acid) followed by deprotection. 2',7-Dimalyl paclitaxel was prepared under essentially the same reaction conditions except that the protected malic acid was in excess. 7-Malyl paclitaxel was synthesized from baccatin III by reaction with protected malic acid and then the side chain was introduced using the oxazolidine method (Damen et al., 1998). These three derivatives had 20 to 60 times the solubility of paclitaxel in water. They were considered stable in phosphate-buffered saline at pH 7.4 for 48 h at 37°C since no liberated paclitaxel was detected by high-performance liquid chromatography (HPLC). When incubated in human plasma, the parent drug was released from the 2'-malyl derivative but not from the 7-malyl or the 2',7-dimalyl derivatives. This was not surprising since many 2'-acyl taxol derivatives hydrolyzed fairly rapidly to Taxol (Mellado et al., 1984; Magri and Kingston, 1988), and the 7-ester derivatives did not interact with esterases (Vyas et al., 1993). The hydrolysis rate with the prospective 2'-malyl prodrug form was considered promising, and it showed similar activity when compared to that of the parent drug (Damen et al., 2000). It is interesting to note that derivatization at the 2'-hydroxyl group results in a loss of pharmacological activity (Deutsch et al., 1989; Mathew et al., 1992). The 2'-malyl derivative, then, is the only one of the three that could be considered a prodrug.

Sulfate ester prodrugs, which can be prepared using drugs bearing alcohol or phenol groups, have been useful in preparing stable injectable formulations of corticosteroids (Sinkula, 1975). Unfortunately, there are examples where these esters are resistant to hydrolysis *in vivo* and would not constitute suitable prodrugs (Miyabo et al., 1981; Williams et al., 1983). For example, intravenously administered dexamethasone-21-sulfate provided essentially no parent dexamethasone in the plasma or urine, but was instead excreted unchanged in the urine (Miyabo et al., 1981). Oral administration of a prednisolone-21-sulfate prodrug as its sodium salt achieved colon-specific delivery of the parent glucocorticoid, in addition to improving its solubility in water (Doh et al., 2003). The prodrug proved to be chemically stable in pH 1.2 and 6.8 buffer, as well as in the contents of the stomach and small intestine. When incubated with cecal contents, the prodrug was reduced to 9.6% of its original amount in 10 h, presumably owing to the hydrolytic action of a sulfatase from a bacterial source that prompted release of prednisolone.

Two independent methods were used to prepare sulfonate prodrugs of Taxol (Zhao et al., 1991). As seen earlier with other Taxol prodrug reactions, the 2′-position was the preferred position at which to bind the promoiety. The first approach, then, was to prepare the amide derivative of the 2′-succinyl derivative with the organic-soluble tetrabutylammonium salt of taurine or its homolog 3-amino-1-sulfopropionic acid using the mixed anhydride method in tetrahydrofuran. The tetrabutylammonium salts were converted to the sodium salts by ion exchange. The second approach involved the preparation of 2′-acryloyltaxol by the mixed anhydride method and then taking advantage of the nucleophilicity of sodium bisulfite in a Michael reaction in aqueous isopropyl alcohol. Michael addition to the α,β-unsaturated ester occurred readily to yield the desired sodium sulfonate derivative.

A simple method to modify promoiety acidity or basicity is to select other more acidic or basic ionizable functional groups. Convenient solubilizing moieties for ester prodrugs where the formulation pH should be between 3.5 and 5 would be those containing either sulfonic acid ($pK_a < 2$) or tertiary amine ($pK_a > 8$) functionalities. Quaternary ammonium-containing moieties, such as the choline esters mentioned earlier, would also be excellent choices for water-soluble derivatives if solubility was the only consideration (Anderson and Conradi, 1987).

Morpholinoalkyl esters (see Figure 16.1 for chemical structures) of the potent nonsteroidal anti-inflammatory agent, diclofenac, were prepared and characterized regarding solubility and hydrolysis reaction rates (Tammara et al., 1994). The alkyl group provides a spacer between the carboxylic acid of diclofenac and the morpholine moiety, which is the site of protonation to yield an ionized prodrug. Alkyl groups consisting of two, three, and four methylene groups were included in the study, and it was found that increasing the chain length improved the stability in pH 7.4 phosphate buffer, but decreased the stability in simulated gastric fluid. In each case, the solubility was improved at least 2000-fold in simulated gastric fluid and in pH 7.4 phosphate buffer. Experimental partition coefficients between 1-octanol and pH 7.4 phosphate buffer demonstrated that the derivatization also markedly improved the lipophilicity. Although stable in the solid state, the hydrolysis rates in simulated gastric fluid or pH 7.4 phosphate buffer indicate that these prodrugs could be formulated only as dry mixtures to be reconstituted as solutions before use.

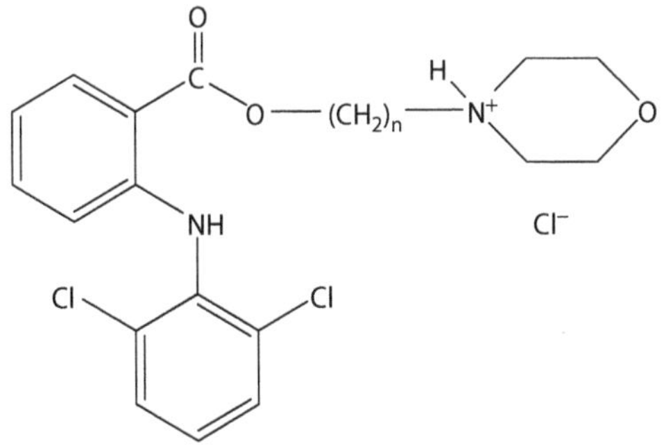

FIGURE 16.1 Chemical structure of water-soluble morpholinoalkyl ester prodrugs of diclofenac. The subscript n equals 2, 3, or 4.

The formation of hydrophilic, but not necessarily ionizable, glycolamide esters has been utilized by Bundgaard and Nielsen (1987, 1988) to generate prodrugs of carboxylic acid-bearing agents, including nonsteroidal anti-inflammatory drugs. The esters possess a high susceptibility to enzymatic hydrolysis and a high stability in aqueous media. *N,N*-disubstituted 2-hydroxyacetamide is the promoiety that is readily cleaved at 37°C in 80% human plasma in pH 7.4 phosphate buffer. The two substituents on the amide nitrogen are the most important structural features for rapid hydrolysis by plasma enzymes, but it is also these substituents that can allow the desired solubility or lipophilicity to be readily achieved. When this approach was taken with furosemide, the hydrolysis rate in human plasma was slow (Mørk et al., 1990). The authors suggest that the furfuryl amino group in the *ortho*-position of these furosemide esters could be contributing steric hindrance to enzymatic approach. Interestingly, esters of naproxen demonstrating different solubility and lipophilicity characteristics were each hydrolyzed with a half-life of less than 2 min in human plasma (Bundgaard and Nielsen, 1988). Preliminary studies have also revealed that the glycolamide esters of naproxen are completely absorbed following oral administration, and yet only the parent drug is detected in the plasma (Bundgaard and Nielsen, 1987).

Water-soluble intermediates to prodrugs of paclitaxel were prepared by transacylation reactions with divinyl adipate at the 2′-hydroxyl that were regioselectively catalyzed by thermolysin, since no other hydroxyl group on paclitaxel was esterified (Khmelnitsky et al., 1997). The vinyl group of this intermediate was then hydrolyzed in acetonitrile containing 1% water using *Candida antarctica* lipase to yield paclitaxel 2′-adipic acid (Table 16.1). Alternatively, the intermediate was used as the acyl donor in a dry reaction with glucose in acetonitrile, again catalyzed by *Candida antarctica* lipase, to yield paclitaxel 2′-adipoylglucose. It was assumed that the glucose was derivatized at the primary alcohol since enzymes of this sort have shown a high degree of selectivity for the primary alcohol of monosaccharides in such transesterification reactions (Therisod and Klibanov, 1986; Martin et al., 1992). Paclitaxel 2′-adipoylglucose and paclitaxel 2′-adipic acid exhibited markedly enhanced solubility that are, respectively, 58- and 1625-fold the solubility of paclitaxel itself (<4 µg/mL) (Khmelnitsky et al., 1997).

Since the sensitivity of the promoiety to acid conditions can be enhanced to effectively target drugs to solid tumors (Niethammer et al., 2001), an acid-sensitive paclitaxel prodrug was prepared. By taking advantage of the 2′ and 7 hydroxyl groups, a bifunctional carbonate intermediate could be formed by condensation with 2,2′-dimethyl-1,3-dioxolane-4-methanol chloroformate (the so-called solketal chloroformate). The intermediate was hydrolyzed to remove the 2′-carbonate and open the acetal ring to form a 7-(2″,3″-dihydroxypropyl carbonoxy) paclitaxel. Carbonates of paclitaxel with hydrophilic functional groups were reported to be more soluble in water and inert to tubulin (Nicolaou et al., 1993). This prodrug is activated under acidic conditions by hydrolytic cleavage of the carbonate to produce paclitaxel, carbon dioxide, and dihydroxypropanol. The prodrug solubility was tested by sonication in room temperature water for 15 min, and proved to be 8.7×10^{-4} M, which is 58 times the 1.5×10^{-5} M solubility of paclitaxel. In addition, the prodrug was found to be chemically stable for at least 24 h at ambient temperature in its proposed formulation for IV infusion, with less than 5% degradation after 48 h (Niethammer et al., 2001). A recent review of acid-sensitive anticancer drug–polymer conjugates includes a discussion of advances in the development and study of macromolecular drug delivery systems, ranging from simple polymer–drug conjugates to site-specific antibody-targeted conjugates (Ulbrich and Subr, 2004).

Replacement of an acidic NH proton with a methyl group is not an acceptable means to produce a prodrug because it is a permanent modification, and it can significantly affect the pharmacological properties of the parent drug (Bansai et al., 1981b). It has been recommended that the NH proton be replaced by a hydroxymethyl group by a simple and facile reaction with formaldehyde. The hydroxymethyl group is readily cleaved in water to return formaldehyde as a product (Alexander et al., 1988). (The positioning of a similar functional group at that site can be achieved by reaction of the parent drug with an appropriate aldehyde.) The hydroxymethyl group, of course, then offers the opportunity for ester prodrug development by reaction with a carboxylic acid-bearing promoiety,

TABLE 16.1
Taxol, Its Reactant Form, and the Possible Products from Reactions Catalyzed by *Candida Antarctica* Lipase

Substance	R Group
Taxol	H —
Modified Taxol as a reactant	
Potential adipic acid product	
Potential adipolyglugose product	

keeping in mind that following hydrolysis of the ester, the hydroxymethyl group is rapidly hydrolyzed in aqueous media to yield the parent drug and formaldehyde. Formaldehyde toxicity does not appear to be a concern at the low levels expected with the use of prodrugs because pivampicillin and methenamine, each of which are marketed as safe drugs, also release formaldehyde on administration (Bansai et al., 1981b). Formaldehyde toxicity, however, will depend on the dose, the dosing frequency, and the duration of the therapy. The *N*-hydroxymethyl derivative usually demonstrates a higher aqueous solubility and dissolution rate, attributed to a lower melting point because hydroxymethylation interferes with hydrogen-bonding capability with the nitrogen in the crystalline state (Bansai et al., 1981a,b).

For drugs that possess an acidic NH functionality, such as amides, imides, carbamates, hydantoins, and urea derivatives, as well as for drugs that have aliphatic and aromatic amines, water-soluble

$$R\text{--}CONH_2 + CH_2O + HNR_1R_2 = R\text{--}CONH\text{--}CH_2\text{--}NR_1R_2 + H_2O$$

FIGURE 16.2   Schematic for preparation of *N*-Mannich base prodrugs.

derivatives can be developed by means of *N*-Mannich base formation, as described in the scheme presented in Figure 16.2. By selecting an appropriate amine component, it is possible to obtain a prodrug with the desired lability, lipophilicity, solubility, and dissolution rate (Bundgaard, 1985a). The bases do not rely on enzymatic hydrolysis and therefore identical decomposition rates are observed in solution with or without human plasma present (Johansen and Bundgaard, 1981a; Bundgaard and Johansen, 1982). *N*-Mannich bases prepared from secondary amines can have a high solubility in the salt form; *N*-Mannich bases derived from primary amines did not demonstrate an improved solubility even when presented as salts. This was attributed to the potential for intramolecular hydrogen bonding, as shown in Figure 16.3.

An example is the *N*-Mannich base of tetracycline and pyrrolidine, rolitetracycline, which returns tetracycline quantitatively in neutral aqueous solution with a half-life of 40 min at 37°C (Vej-Hansen and Bundgaard, 1979; Johansen and Bundgaard, 1981a). Water-soluble prodrugs of carbamazepine with a solubility up to 2800 times that of the parent drug have been prepared for parenteral administration by generation of the hydrochloride salt of the *N*-Mannich bases (Bundgaard et al., 1982). *N*-Mannich bases of theophylline and the morpholino *N*-Mannich base of 5-fluorouracil were prepared for delivery of the drugs transdermally. These prodrugs exhibited enhanced aqueous and lipid solubility, probably owing to the decreased crystal lattice energies, as reflected in the lower melting points (Sloan et al., 1984). The *N*-Mannich base of a benzamide, PC190723, proved to be approximately 100 times more soluble than its parent drug in the pH 2.6, 10 mM citrate buffer chosen for oral administration (Kaul et al., 2013). At physiological pH, the *N*-Mannich base behaves as a prodrug with a conversion half-life of 18.2 min. Intravenous administration in mice allowed calculation of elimination half-lives of 0.26 and 0.96 h for the prodrug and its parent drug, respectively, indicating rapid conversion of the prodrug *in vivo*. In addition, the *N*-Mannich base demonstrated oral bioavailability and widespread distribution. In a mouse model of systemic infection with methicillin-sensitive *Staphylococcus aureus* or methicillin-resistant *S. aureus*, the orally administered prodrug proved to be effective, whereas the parent PC190723 was not (Kaul et al., 2013).

N-acyloxyalkylation of various amides, imides, hydantoins, and uracils, as well as tertiary- and *N*-heterocyclic-amines, has been conducted to generate promising prodrugs (Bodor, 1981; Bundgaard, 1982, 1986). These prodrug types can be obtained by esterification of the intermediate *N*-hydroxyalkyl derivative or, more often, by reacting the NH-acidic drug with an α-acyloxyalkyl halide (Bundgaard and Johansen, 1984). By selecting the appropriate acyl portion of the derivatives, it is possible to modify the drug regeneration rate, solubility, and lipophilicity. The derivatives are, in general, stable in aqueous media, but are readily cleaved *in vivo* by enzyme-mediated hydrolysis. The most common acyloxymethyl derivatives are those resulting in formaldehyde as a hydrolysis product due to employing a hydroxymethyl moiety as the link between the nitrogen and the acyl group. The drug regeneration is assumed to be a two-step process, with enzymatic cleavage of the ester as the first step (Figure 16.4) followed by decomposition of the *N*-hydroxyalkyl derivative to

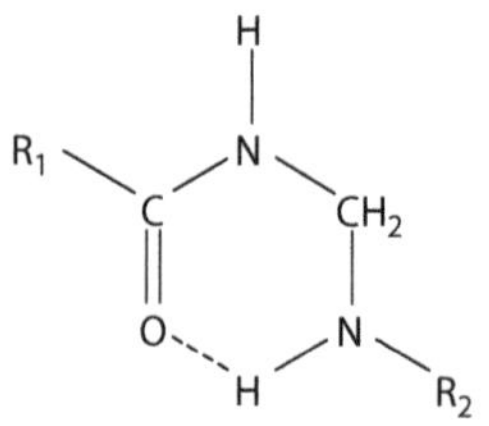

FIGURE 16.3   Potential intramolecular hydrogen bonding with *N*-Mannich bases.

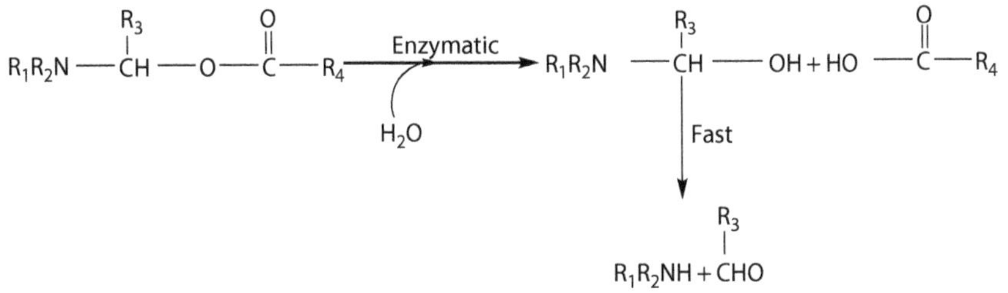

FIGURE 16.4 Drug regeneration from an *N*-Mannich base prodrug by a two-step process.

the corresponding aldehyde and the NH-acidic parent drug. The enzymatic hydrolysis step, then, is the only opportunity to control the drug regeneration rate. Enzymatic hydrolysis can be slowed by steric and electronic factors derived from the carboxylic acid and the R_3 group involved.

An example of a successful prodrug prepared by this method is the hydrochloride salt of the *N*-(*N'*,*N'*-dimethylglycyloxymethyl) derivative of chlorzoxazone (Johansen and Bundgaard, 1981b) that improved the solubility of the parent drug 1000-fold. *N*-acyloxymethyl derivatives of phenytoin, where the acyl group bears an amine group, possess greatly enhanced solubility relative to the parent drug (Varia et al., 1984a). The solubility and the lipophilicity could be modified by the hydrophilic or hydrophobic nature of the acyl moiety. The *N*-acyloxyalkylation can also diminish intermolecular hydrogen bonding in the crystal lattice. It should be noted that formation of the acyloxymethyl prodrugs of phenytoin, where the acyl group had no ionizable functional groups, should also cause diminished hydrogen bonding in the crystal, and indeed these prodrugs possessed a lower melting point, but also a lower solubility in water (Stella et al., 1998).

A second example is allopurinol, a poorly soluble drug, which is also poorly soluble in organic solvents owing to its high melting point (Windholz et al., 1983; Bundgaard and Falch, 1985b). It was found that hydrogen bonding exists between the N_1-H of one molecule and the N_8 of another molecule, and between the N_3 of one and the hydrogen of the N_9-H group of another (Prusiner and Sundaralingam, 1972). *N*-acyloxymethylation blocks intermolecular hydrogen bonding, which can subsequently decrease the melting point and increase both water solubility and lipophilicity (Bundgaard and Falch, 1985a,b; Bundgaard et al., 1990). In particular, the *N*,*N*-dimethyl- and *N*,*N*-diethyl-glycyloxymethyl derivatives demonstrated dramatically enhanced solubility and provided a greater partition coefficient over those of the parent drug.

The *N*-butanoyloxymethyl derivative of bupivacaine exhibited pH-independent solubility in excess of 1 g/mL, that is, a 10,000-fold increase in water solubility compared to the parent drug in its base form (Nielsen et al., 2005). Chemical hydrolysis over a pH range of 0.1–9.8 at 37°C followed first-order kinetics and the pH-stability profile was U-shaped. At neutral to slightly alkaline pH, hydrolysis resulted not only in bupivacaine, but also in an aromatic imide that was believed to be formed by an intramolecular acyl transfer involving nucleophilic attack of the amide nitrogen atom on the ester carbonyl carbon. Since this prodrug and other derivatives described in this report were poor substrates for plasma enzymes, the authors tested and confirmed their susceptibility to pancreatic enzymes. The prodrugs possessed sufficient stability in the gastric environment that the authors noted their potential to enhance oral bioavailability of tertiary amines that have pK_a values below about 6 and an intrinsic solubility in the low micromolar range.

A novel technique to prepare water-soluble prodrugs of drugs bearing a tertiary amine group involves a nucleophilic substitution reaction between the amine and di-*tert*-butyl chloromethyl phosphate, resulting in formation of the quaternary ammonium salt (Krise et al., 1999c). The tertiary butyl group is readily removed under acidic conditions using trifluoroacetic acid, giving the *N*-phosphonooxymethyl prodrug in the free phosphoric acid form. This can be subsequently converted to the desired salt form. Included in the studies were quinuclidine, cinnarizine, loxapine, and amiodarone (Krise et al., 1999b,c). The prodrugs would undergo a two-step bioreversion process.

The rate-limiting step would be dephosphorylation catalyzed by alkaline phosphatase (Krise et al., 1999a), followed by spontaneous breakdown of the *N*-hydroxymethyl intermediate that yields the parent drug. Formation of the phosphonooxymethyl prodrug of loxapine improved the solubility by a factor of 15,000, and provided a chemically stable derivative at neutral pH. Krise et al. (1999a) anticipate that the shelf life of a parenteral formulation of loxapine could be close to 2 years at pH 7.4 and 25°C.

Phenytoin is a drug exhibiting low aqueous solubility and low lipid solubility. A class of lipid conjugates has been synthesized to improve the oral bioavailability by employing triglycerides with 3-hydroxymethylphenytoin covalently bound to the 2-position, or use of position 1 of a glyceride with succinic acid as a linking agent to 3-hydroxymethylphenytoin (Scriba, 1993). Hydroxymethyl-phenytoin itself behaves as a prodrug that decomposes in aqueous solution at physiological pH to yield phenytoin and formaldehyde. The deacyl derivatives of the triglycerides exhibited improved solubility and proved to be the best substrates for hydrolysis by human enzymes (Table 16.2). The pH-rate profiles for these chemicals revealed pseudo-first-order kinetics typical of specific acid- and specific base-catalyzed hydrolysis, with a minimum reaction rate in the range of pH 3–6. The reaction rate constants indicate that solution formulations with an adequate shelf life should be possible in that pH range.

TABLE 16.2

Physicochemical Properties and Hydrolysis Rates for Phenytoin–Lipid Conjugates

R	Melting Point (°C)	Phenytoin Equivalent	Solubility in Water (mg/mL)	Hydrolysis Half-Life in Human Plasma (min)
H—	295	1	0.03	—
	—[a]	0.55	2.26	371
	—[a]	0.55	2.16	—[b]
	116	0.66	2.38	112

Source: With kind permission from Springer Science + Business Media: *Pharm. Res.*, Phenytoin-lipid conjugates: Chemical, plasma esterase-mediated, and pancreatic lipase-mediated hydrolysis *in vitro*, 10, 1993, 1181–1186, Scriba, G. K. E.

[a] These two conjugates were obtained as hygroscopic foams that could not be crystallized.

[b] This conjugate was not considered in the hydrolysis study.

A novel prodrug type was developed for drugs bearing a hydroxyl or an NH-acidic group (Bundgaard et al., 1989, 1991). For the cases involving an NH-acidic group, the drug must first be converted to the N-hydroxymethyl derivative to provide the alcohol group available for further derivatization. In the promoiety, an ionizable amine is separated by a benzene ring from the carboxylic acid group to be employed in ester derivatization. To achieve an amine pK_a value greater than 6, the amino group was separated from the benzene ring by a methylene group, yielding, in the simplest case, an aminomethylbenzoic acid. It was noted that 4-(aminomethyl)benzoic acid has been used as an antifibrinolytic agent, suggesting that this particular cleaved promoiety is not pharmacologically inactive. Other alkylated amines were investigated because N-substituted 4-(aminomethyl)benzoic acids, such as 4-(N,N-dimethylaminomethyl)benzoic acid, do not possess the antifibrinolytic or trypsin-inhibiting effect. Prodrugs with the aminomethyl or another amino group at the 3- or 4-position of the benzene ring show promise of being useful prodrugs since they are able to improve drug solubility and stability in aqueous media. Maximal stability occurred in the pH 3–5 range where shelf lives of up to 14 years were achieved. In pH 7.4 phosphate buffer at 37°C, half-lives in excess of 200 h were obtained. In the presence of 80% human plasma at 37°C, the prodrugs were readily hydrolyzed to quantitatively yield the parent drug.

Some studies have shown that a correlation might not always exist between solubility and the hydrophilicity of the promoiety. For example, the incorporation of polar, hydrogen-bonding substituents in a series of prostaglandin derivatives resulted in an increase in both crystalline interaction energies and hydration energies, and therefore the solubility in water did not increase (Anderson and Conradi, 1980). Predicting an increase in solubility as a result of an increase in the hydrophilicity of a promoiety is considered unreliable (Anderson and Conradi, 1987).

Promoieties employing ionizable acid or base functional groups to accomplish an enhanced solubility in water yield prodrugs where a pH effect on the solubility profile will be evident. Thirteen derivatives of the semisynthetic surfactant 24,25-dihydrofusidic acid have been synthesized and their solubility characterized (Lee et al., 1992). The derivatives were prepared using promoieties employing carboxylic acids, phosphates, sulfates, and primary, tertiary, and quaternary amines. As expected, the carboxylic acids and phosphates contributed to the solubilizing effect when the pH was increased; the amines, with the exception of the quaternary amines, improved solubility when the pH was lowered. Sulfates and the quaternary amines were ionized over the pH ranges studied, and no solubility enhancement due to pH modification was observed.

MODIFICATIONS EMPLOYING AMINO ACIDS

Amino acid esters have been recommended as potentially useful progroups (Kovach et al., 1975; Amidon et al., 1977) in that they provide the carboxylic acid group for reaction with an alcohol or phenol to form an ester prodrug, an ionizable amine as a side group, and the potential for another ionizable side group in certain amino acids. In general, esters employing amino acids, or related short-chain aliphatic amino acids, are rapidly hydrolyzed by plasma enzymes (Bundgaard et al., 1984b), and offer the potential advantage of enhanced absorption from the small intestine due to the presence of amino acid and peptide transporters in the brush border membrane (Majumdar et al., 2004; Dobson and Kell, 2008). Unfortunately, some amino acid prodrugs exhibit poor stability in aqueous solutions, as evidenced by acetaminophen (Kovach et al., 1975), hydrocortisone (Johnson et al., 1985; Fleisher et al., 1986), metronidazole (Bundgaard et al., 1984a), and Taxol (Deutsch et al., 1989) esters. One reason offered for the instability of these esters in aqueous media is the strongly electron-withdrawing effect of the protonated α-amine that makes the ester linkage susceptible to nucleophilic attack (Bundgaard et al., 1989; Zhao et al., 1991). This was supported by the improved stability of the 2′-β-alanyl taxol derivative (Zhao et al., 1991) that, although structurally similar to the 2′-glycyl derivative (Magri, 1985), minimized the effect of the protonated amine by shifting its position one carbon further away. Improved solubility and stability was also observed with the β-alanyl prodrug of bromhexine (Aggarwal and Gupta, 2012). The γ-aminobutyryl taxol derivative was believed to be unstable owing to intramolecular displacement of the 2′-acyl group through a five-membered ring intermediate (Zhao et al., 1991). Thus, of the glycyl, β-alanyl, and γ-aminobutyryl derivatives, the β-alanyl derivative proved to be the most stable because it was able to minimize both of these effects (Zhao et al., 1991). This was seen again with amino acid ester prodrugs of estradiol, where the 3-N,N,N-trimethylaminobutyl ester iodide was more stable than the 3-N,N-dimethylamino butyl ester hydrochloride (the half-life for the pseudo-first-order reaction was 34 h and 5.6 min, respectively) in pH 7.4, 0.05 M phosphate buffer at 37°C because the former could not involve the promoiety nitrogen in the formation of a stable transition state for hydrolysis (Al-Ghananeem et al., 2002). Even cyclic amino acids have been employed as the promoiety with success (Altomare et al., 2003).

Another means to eliminate the influence of the protonated α-amine is to use the amino acid in a peptide component of a promoiety. Lallemand et al. (2005a,b) included the dipeptide sarcosine–serine or sarcosine–lysine in the promoiety of a cyclosporine A prodrug where a phosphate ester or a protonated amine in a side chain provided the solubilizing moiety and not the α-amine of an amino acid. The phenylalanine–alanine prodrug of primaquine was prepared to provide an improved pharmacokinetics profile. The prodrug was successful at preventing malaria, and it proved to be less cytotoxic and caused less hemolysis than did the parent drug (Devanço et al., 2014).

Amino acids combine low toxicity with a wide range of other properties. For example, among the amino acid and dipeptide prodrugs of daunorubicin, the L-leucyl derivative proved to be four times less toxic than daunorubicin, but equally potent against L-1210 leukemia in mice (Baurain et al., 1980). In general, the hydrophilic, acidic, and basic amino acids produced less toxic derivatives than did the more hydrophobic amino acids, such as alanine and leucine. Variations in toxicity and the therapeutic index of these amino acid derivatives were attributed to differences in tissue distribution, rates of cellular uptake, and patterns of intracellular localization (Jones, 1985). Biological reversion can be quite efficient through protease activity when covalent linkages mimic peptide bonds (Amidon et al., 1977). L-Lysyl- and L-alanyl-amide prodrugs of antitumor benzothiazoles demonstrated solubility in somewhat acidic water of a pH around 5 and chemical stability at 25°C in pH 4.5 buffer, with conversion to the free base *in vivo* (Hutchinson et al., 2002).

Acyclovir, because of its poor physicochemical properties, is difficult to formulate for ocular and dermal delivery. Colla et al. (1983) have described highly water-soluble prodrugs, including amino acid esters that may prove useful in the development of solution formulations. The esters were as active as, or only slightly less active than, the parent drug in the inhibition of herpes simplex virus type 1 or type 2. The antiviral activity suggests that the esters are readily hydrolyzed to regenerate the parent drug.

Shen et al. (2009a) report the preparation of the 5′-O-D- and L-amino acid derivatives of adenine 9-beta-D-arabinofuranoside (vidarabine) for use as prodrugs. In addition, the 5′-O-D- and L-amino acid methylester phosphoramidate derivatives were prepared. The researchers reported that some were equally or more potent against pox viruses. Of interest is that the uptake by cultured cells was enhanced in comparison to vidarabine itself. Further research on the 5′-O-valyl ester of vidarabine focused on its synthesis and physicochemical properties (Shen et al., 2009b).

When amino acid ester prodrugs of acetaminophen were prepared (Kovach et al., 1975; Pitman, 1976), the hydrobromide salt of the glycine ester showed enhanced solubility in water, but the hydrochloride salt of the β-aspartic acid ester exhibited a solubility lower than that of the parent drug. The enhanced solubility resulted from the formation of a salt, while the parent drug is a weakly acidic phenol and behaves as essentially a neutral molecule in solution. The reduced solubility in the case of the β-aspartic acid ester resulted from ionization of the terminal carboxylic acid, which, with the protonated amine, gives a zwitterion. The zwitterion behaved as a molecule with an overall neutral character, as is commonly observed with zwitterion behavior in aqueous media, but its larger size resulted in a reduced solubility.

Bundgaard et al. (1984a,b) prepared eight amino acid esters of metronidazole and then evaluated their potential for use in parenteral dosage forms. By generating the hydrochloride salt of the α-amine of each ester, they were able to achieve a solubility greater than 20% w/v only in each case, but the susceptibility to enzymatic hydrolysis varied widely. They have judged the N,N-dimethylglycinate ester to be the most promising candidate on the basis of its excellent solubility of greater than 50% w/v, its rapid hydrolysis rate *in vivo* (12-min half-life) in comparison to the rate in phosphate buffer at physiological temperatures (250-min half-life), and the ease with which it can be synthesized and purified (Bundgaard et al., 1984b). Unfortunately, the instability in solution demands that this prodrug be supplied as a formulation to be reconstituted as a solution just before use.

When the solubilizing promoiety approach is applied to drugs intended to be administered orally, the desired increase in aqueous solubility may be coupled with a dramatic decrease in the intestinal wall–water partition coefficient, and hence a reduced effective membrane permeability (Amidon et al., 1980). If the reconversion to poorly soluble drug is rapid in the gut lumen, either by chemical or enzymatic means, the reduction in membrane permeability by prodrug formation is of no consequence. Nevertheless, the concentration gradient that drives the diffusive transport of the drug would then be limited by its low solubility. The new strategy described by Amidon et al. was to prepare derivatives of insoluble chemicals that are substrates for enzymes found in the brush border region of the mucosal cells located at the inner wall of the small intestine (Amidon et al., 1980; Fleisher et al., 1985). Following cleavage of the promoiety, the more nonpolar parent drug would be located immediately adjacent to the membrane for which it has a high partition coefficient. Theoretically, the membrane would behave as a nonpolar sink for the parent drug. Estrone-lysine and *p*-nitroaniline-lysine demonstrated not only improved solubility, but also an intestinal membrane permeability 5–10 times greater than that of the parent drugs.

The use of amino acids, such as lysine or its analog, ε-aminocaproic acid, as solubilizing promoieties demonstrates that they are particularly effective (Radhakrishnan, 1977). Table 16.3 shows the aqueous solubility of the esters of estrone to be three to five orders of magnitude larger than that of the parent drug. They are also excellent substrates for digestive enzymes (Radhakrishnan, 1977). In addition to the wide selection of possible amino acid (or analog) promoieties to obtain a desired physical property, biochemical reversion has a potential advantage over chemical reversion in that the prodrug may be chemically stable in the formulation but biochemically labile upon administration.

TABLE 16.3
Solubility of Estrone and Estrone Ester Prodrugs

Chemical	Aqueous Solubility (M)	Reference
Estrone	2.96×10^{-6}	Hurwitz and Lin (1977)
Estrone-3'-aminocaproate	0.005	Amidon (1981)
Estrone-3'-lysine ester	0.3	Amidon (1981)[a]

[a] Reprinted from Amidon, G. L., Drug derivatization as a means of solubilization: Physicochemical and biochemical strategies, in *Techniques of Solubilization of Drugs*, Yalkowsky, S. H. (Ed.), p. 203, New York, Marcel Dekker, 1981. Courtesy of Marcel Dekker, Inc.

TABLE 16.4

Solubility, Partition Coefficients, and Regeneration Half-Lives for Menahydroquinone-4 Ester Prodrugs

Derivative	Solubility in Water (mM)[a]	Log P[b]	Hydrolysis Half-Life in Rat Plasma (min)	Hydrolysis Half-Life in Buffer[c] (min)
R_1: $(CH_3)_2NCH_2CO-$ R_2: $H-$	24	4.56	3.01	3410
R_1: $H-$ R_2: $(CH_3)_2NCH_2CO-$	5.7	4.67	2.90	2350
R_1: $(CH_3)_2NCH_2CO-$ R_2: $(CH_3)_2NCH_2CO-$	~50	3.66	15.0	1390

Source: With kind permission from Springer Science + Business Media: *Pharm. Res.*, Vitamin K prodrugs. 1. Synthesis of amino acid esters of menahydroquinone-4 and enzymatic reconversion to an active form, 12, 1995a, 18–23, Takata, J.

[a] Solubility of the hydrochloride salt of the prodrug at room temperature.

[b] Log of the partition coefficient between 1-octanol and pH 7.4 phosphate buffer.

[c] Buffer is pH 7.4 phosphate buffer at 37°C.

Aminoalkanecarboxylic acid ester prodrugs of vitamins K (Takata et al., 1995a) and E (Takata et al., 1995b) exhibit considerable solubility in water and possess a high susceptibility to hydrolysis by liver esterase. Vitamin E prodrugs include primary (glycinate), secondary (sarcosinate), and tertiary aminoacetic acid (*N,N*-dimethylglycinate) ester derivatives. Monoesters and a diester of menahydroquinone-4 (Table 16.4) were prepared using *N,N*-dimethylglycine to improve the solubility and esterase lability of the parent drug (Takata et al., 1995a). Cleavage to regenerate menahydroquinone-4 under conditions similar to those found *in vivo*, which could be described by apparent first-order kinetics, confirms that they act as true prodrugs. The dramatic difference between the *in vitro* and *in vivo* rates of hydrolysis suggests that stable solution dosage forms could be prepared with rapid bioconversion possible on administration.

N-Acylation of amines to provide amide prodrugs has limited application because amides, in general, are relatively stable *in vivo* (Bundgaard, 1987). Certain amides formed with amino acids, however, may be susceptible to enzymatic cleavage. Examples are γ-glutamyl derivatives of dopamine, l-dopa, and sulfamethoxazole, which are hydrolyzed by γ-glutamyl transpeptidase. The use of γ-glutamyl derivatives as kidney-specific prodrugs has been recommended on the basis of their preferential bioactivation in the kidney (Wilk et al., 1978; Orlowski et al., 1979). Various amino acid derivatives of benzocaine have proved to be highly water soluble and were rapidly cleaved not only in the presence of enzymes found in human serum but also by certain proteolytic enzymes (Zlojkowska et al., 1982). Dipeptide prodrugs of 5-fluorouracil were prepared that allowed a comparison of the sensitivity to chemical and enzymatic hydrolysis (Nichifor and Schacht, 1997). It was found that the stability depended on the *N*-terminal amino acid, the configuration of the *C*-terminal substituted glycine (characterized by optical rotation), and the presence of substituents on the dipeptides. Chemical hydrolysis rates were decreased with an increase in the hydrophobicity of the *N*-terminal amino acid. Hydrolysis rates were much lower for dipeptides with free carboxyl end groups than for dipeptides in the ethyl ester form. The prodrug derivatives with the lowest chemical stability possessed dipeptides with amino and ethyl ester end groups, owing to their internal cyclization to the very chemically labile diketopiperazines. The sensitivity of these prodrugs to aminopeptidase and endopeptidase activity was also tested. Aminopeptidase-catalyzed hydrolysis rates were higher for dextrorotatory dipeptides and decreased in the order Ala > Leu > Phe > Gly as the N-terminal amino acid. Endopeptidase activity was higher toward levorotatory dipeptides and decreased in the order Ala > Gly > Phe ≈ Leu at the N-terminus. The presence of a free carboxyl instead of an ethyl ester end group at the C-terminus had little influence on aminopeptidase activity, but suppressed the endopeptidase activity.

MODIFICATIONS EMPLOYING HYDROPHOBIC FUNCTIONAL GROUPS

A high melting point reflects high crystal lattice energy in a solid. A high melting point and a high enthalpy of fusion lead to poor solubility in any solvent. In particular, preferential hydrogen bonding is responsible for high melting points and can actually fix the spatial configuration in the crystalline state. One prodrug approach to improve solubility is to reduce the melting point and enthalpy of fusion by interfering with the stronger interactions that can exist between drug molecules in the crystal framework.

An application of this approach was employed in the preparation of prodrugs of vidarabine. Vidarabine has a solubility of only 0.5 mg/mL, which is due at least in part to a melting point of about 260°C (Windholz et al., 1983) that is attributed to intermolecular hydrogen bonding in the crystalline lattice. When esterification at the 5'-hydroxyl group eliminated the potential for this intermolecular interaction, the melting point was lowered (Repta et al., 1975). By employing an acyl group that is only slightly lipophilic, the formyl group, a vidarabine prodrug with greatly enhanced solubility was obtained. The 5'-formate ester is rapidly hydrolyzed in human blood and has the potential for use in parenteral administrations (Repta et al., 1975). The ethyl ester of levodopa proved to be a highly water-soluble prodrug of levodopa and provided more rapid absorption across biological membranes (Djaldetti et al., 2002), presumably by offering both a higher concentration gradient and a higher partition coefficient. A longer alkyl chain length can lead to a lower melting point (Stinchcomb et al., 1995), but likely also a higher lipophilicity that counters any improvement in solubility achieved by the lower melting point.

Diester and triester prodrugs of the antiviral agent, 6-methoxypurine arabinoside, were prepared because the parent drug has an unfavorable metabolic profile (Jones et al., 1992). The triacetate was able to enhance bioavailability in the rat, as measured by the appearance of the parent drug in the urine. The lower solubility of the longer chain aliphatic or the aromatic triesters was assumed to be the underlying cause of the reduced bioavailability of those derivatives. In contrast, the diesters, in particular the diacetates, significantly enhanced systemic availability, probably resulting from the higher solubility and enhanced partition coefficient found with these prodrugs. These, then, are examples of the phenomenon of improved solubility and improved lipophilicity present in the same prodrug. It would have been worthwhile to conduct an investigation of the melting points and enthalpies of fusion to confirm that the improvements were a result of reduced crystal lattice energy brought about by blocking hydrogen bonding in the crystal state.

With 5-fluorouracil, the N_1 and N_3 sites are each available for acylation reactions. When various N_1- or N_3-acyl derivatives were prepared, they proved to be readily hydrolyzed in aqueous buffer solutions to quantitatively yield the parent drug (Buur and Bundgaard, 1984a, 1984b). The N_1-acyl derivatives were found to be highly unstable; the N_3-derivatives proved to be more stable. Blocking the N_3-position diminished the opportunities for hydrogen bonding in the crystal lattice, resulting in a lower melting point and higher solubility (Table 16.5). The selection of the acyl group influenced the hydrolysis rate under conditions approaching those found *in vivo*, as well as the physicochemical properties of the derivative, such as solubility and lipophilicity. Preparation of the 1-alkylcarbonyloxymethyl prodrugs of 5-fluorouracil was accomplished by reacting the appropriate alkylcarboxymethyl chloride with 5-fluorouracil in 1-methylpyrrolidine and acetonitrile (Taylor and Sloan,

TABLE 16.5

Effect of *N*-Acylation on the Melting Point, Solubility, Partition Coefficient, and Hydrolysis Rate for 5-Fluorouracil

Drug or Derivative	Melting Point (°C)	Solubility (M)[a]	log *P*[b]	Hydrolysis Half-Life in Buffer (min)	Hydrolysis Half-Life in 80% Plasma (min)
5-Fluorouracil (5-FU)	280	0.085	−0.83	—	—
3-Acetyl-5-FU	116	0.249	−0.34	43	4.6
3-Propionyl-5-FU	113	0.190	0.19	50	20
3-Butyryl-5-FU	132	—	0.67	58	28
3-Benzoyl-5-FU	172	0.006	0.80	2900	110

Source: Reprinted from *Int. J. Pharm.*, 21, Buur, A. and Bundgaard, H., Prodrugs of 5-fluorouracil. I. Hydrolysis kinetics and physicochemical properties of various *N*-acyl derivatives of 5-fluorouracil, 349–364. Copyright 1984a. With permission from Elsevier. Reprinted from *Arch. Pharm. Chem. Sci. Ed.*, Buur, A. and Bundgaard, H., Prodrugs of 5-fluorouracil. II. Hydrolysis kinetics, bioactivation, solubility and lipophilicity of *N*-alkoxycarbonyl derivatives of 5-fluorouracil, 37–44. Copyright 1984b. With permission Elsevier.

[a] Solubility in pH 4.0 acetate buffer.

[b] Partition coefficient between 1-octanol and pH 4.0 acetate buffer.

1998). Only two of these prodrugs, the 1-acetyloxymethyl- and the 1-propionyloxymethyl-5-fluorouracil proved to be more soluble in water than the parent drug. Longer alkyl chains resulted in reduced solubility. Hydrolysis of the ester function on the promoiety results in the formation of the labile 1-hydroxymethyl derivative of 5-fluorouracil, which undergoes a rapid loss of formaldehyde to yield the parent drug.

Bioreversible derivatives of thiabendazole (Table 16.6) were generated by *N*-acylation of the benzimidazole moiety (Nielsen et al., 1992). The solubility in water was increased up to 12 times that of the parent drug. The improved solubility, adequate lipophilicity, and chemical stability, along with facile enzymatic hydrolysis, make these derivatives promising prodrugs.

Highly water-soluble lipophilic prodrugs of 2′, 3′-dideoxycytidine were prepared by placing a lipophilic substituent on the exocyclic amine group (Kerr and Kalman, 1992). It was again anticipated that the loss of the NH_2 group as a donor of two intermolecular hydrogen bonds would improve the solubility in water. The parent drug was condensed with an excess of the desired formamide dimethyl acetal to provide derivatization of the N_4 group to the (*N,N*-dimethyl-, (*N,N*-diethyl-, (*N,N*-di-*n*-propyl-, and (*N,N*-diisopropyl-amino)methylene derivatives. In addition, they studied the piperidino-, morpholino-, and pyrrolidino-methylene derivatives. The parent drug is returned by spontaneous first-order hydrolysis that involves an N_4-formyl intermediate. The diisopropyl derivative appears to be the best candidate overall, with at least a threefold improvement in solubility and the longest half-life in 37°C, pH 7.4 phosphate buffer (47.5 h) of the derivatives. The half-life in diluted human serum was the same or longer than in phosphate buffer, indicating that it is unlikely that an enzyme-catalyzed reaction occurs to release the parent drug. Indeed, the authors observed a longer half-life as the serum content was increased, which they believed was indicative of serum protein binding, affording protection from hydrolysis.

Each *N*-alkoxycarbonyl mebendazole prodrug exhibited an enhanced solubility in pH 5.0 acetate buffer, as much as 20 times that of the parent drug (Nielsen et al., 1994). Interestingly, no ionizable

TABLE 16.6

Effect of the Acyl Group on the Melting Point, Solubility, Partition Coefficient, and Hydrolysis Rate of Thiabendazole

Drug or Ester Functional Group (-R)	Melting Point (°C)	Solubility[a] (mM)	Log P[b]	Hydrolysis Half-Life in Buffer (min)	Hydrolysis Half-Life in 80% Plasma (min)
–H	304	0.094	2.47	—	—
—COOCH$_3$	123	0.77	2.05	1620	8
—COOCH$_2$CH$_3$	84	1.2	2.51	2940	24
—COOCH$_2$CH$_2$CH$_3$	68	0.30	2.98	3240	24
—COOCH$_2$CH(CH$_3$)$_2$	72	0.067	3.46	3420	22

Source: Data from Nielsen, L. S., Bundgaard, H., and Falch, E., *Acta Pharm. Nord.*, 4, 43–49, 1992.

[a] Solubility in 0.02 M pH 6.0 phosphate buffer at 21°C.

[b] Partition coefficient between 1-octanol and 0.02 M pH 6.0 phosphate buffer at 21°C.

functional groups were included in the promoieties. The higher solubility was believed to be due to a decrease in the crystal lattice energy, resulting from replacement of the NH proton in the benzimidazole moiety with an alkoxycarbonyl group. The reduced lattice energy was again reflected in the dramatically lower melting points.

MODIFICATIONS INVOLVING POLYMERS AND MACROMOLECULES

Prodrugs consisting of drugs covalently linked to polymeric or macromolecular carriers have been recommended to (1) prolong pharmacological activity, (2) minimize undesirable side effects or toxicity, (3) reduce the required dose by more efficient drug delivery, (4) accomplish site-specific delivery, and (5) increase the solubility of drugs (Filipovic-Grcic et al., 1995; Smith et al., 2014). Water-soluble polymers are especially attractive as the promoiety because many are biocompatible (Liu et al., 2008; Wu et al., 2013), the polymer–drug conjugate can result in an improved solubility (Di Meo et al., 2015), and they can be used to extend the biological drug half-life by preventing enzymes from attacking the parent drug (Caprariis et al., 1994). Macromolecules have served as the promoiety to alter the tissue localization of a carrier-linked drug, the localization largely dictated by the properties of the macromolecule itself (Sezaki and Hashida, 1984). Linear polysaccharides, being water soluble, are particularly suitable as drug carriers; their own solubility properties, and therefore parenteral applicability, are contributed to the resulting prodrug (Molteni, 1982). High molecular weight vinyl polymers are not considered in current investigations because they are known to accumulate in the body (Schacht et al., 1984). Biodegradable polymers, such as polysaccharides or vinyl polymers containing biodegradable linkages, are of greater interest.

Dextran has been selected as a carrier because of its excellent physicochemical properties and pharmacological tolerance (Schacht et al., 1984; Sezaki and Hashida, 1984; Sezaki, 1989). Dextran-nalidixic acid ester was prepared with varied degrees of substitution (DS) to be used as a colon-specific prodrug form (Lee et al., 2001). Solubility of the prodrug in water depended on the DS (i.e., mg of nalidixic acid per 100 mg of dextran-nalidixic acid ester), with 57.6, 0.53, and 0.03 mg/mL possible with DS of 7, 19, and 32. No nalidixic acid was detected after 6 h of incubation of the dextran prodrug in pH 1.2 hydrochloric acid buffer or pH 6.8 phosphate buffer. Nalidixic acid was not detected after incubation of the prodrug in the homogenate of tissue and contents of the small intestine. However, when the dextran prodrug with a DS of 7 or 17 was incubated in rat cecal contents at 37°C, 41 or 32% of the nalidixic acid, respectively, was released within 24 h.

Several amino acids, including phenylalanine, glycine, and leucine, as well as the dipeptide, glycylglycine, and the dicarboxylic acid, succinic acid, were each employed as a spacer to link metronidazole with the dextran backbone (Vermeersch et al., 1990) to prepare water-soluble ester prodrugs with *in vitro* stability and *in vivo* antitrichomonal activity. Succinic or glutaric acid spacers were employed to link methylprednisolone or dexamethasone to dextran for potential colon-specific delivery (McLeod et al., 1993). Little drug was released during incubation with small intestine contents, but faster release rates were observed with cecum and colon contents. Slow hydrolysis rates in pH 6.8 phosphate buffer at 37°C, along with the observed selective enzyme-mediated hydrolysis, and the long residence time in the human colon indicate that these prodrugs indeed have the potential for successful targeted delivery of these glucocorticoids.

A polymeric prodrug was prepared by appending 5-iodo-2′-deoxyuridine (IDU) to poly(d, l-lactic acid) (PLA) using succinic acid as a linker (Rimoli et al., 1999). The IDU loading was consistent with the carboxylic acid endgroups (about 0.024 mEq/g of PLA). The conjugate was chemically stable toward hydrolysis in pH 7.4 phosphate buffer, but was susceptible to enzymatic degradation in biological media containing esterases.

Cyclodextrin has shown promise as a polymeric promoiety. A 5-aminosalicylic acid (5-ASA) prodrug was prepared (Zou et al., 2005) by refluxing 5-ASA and formic acid for 30 min, followed by addition of cold distilled water, to generate 5-formylaminosalicylic acid (5-fASA). 5-fASA was then dissolved in DMF and carbonyldiimidazole was added. α-, β-, or γ-cyclodextrin, dissolved in DMSO, was slowly added, and then triethylamine was added. The mixture was stirred for 24 h, and then an excess of HCl or acetone was used to precipitate the 5-formyl version of the prodrug. 5-ASA-appended cyclodextrin prodrug was prepared from the precipitate by hydrolysis of the formyl group. Chemical stability at pH 1.2, 6.8, and 7.5 at 37°C for 6 h was demonstrated for prodrugs with the ratio of cyclodextrin to 5-ASA up to 1:10. Prodrugs with 1:1 or 1:2 ratios provided substantially higher solubility in 25°C, 0.05 M acetic acid solution (91.8–720 g/L) in comparison to that of 5-ASA itself (1.0 g/L), but this low degree of drug loading would result in a high mass to properly dose the patient. After incubation of the prodrugs with the contents of various regions of the gastrointestinal tract of rats, 5-ASA was liberated slowly in the small intestine, with more rapid release in cecal or colonic mixtures, as desired.

Since hyaluronic acid (HA) receptors are overexpressed in transformed human breast epithelial cells and other cancers (Culty et al., 1992), selectivity for cancer cells can be enhanced by appending antitumor agents to HA. In addition to improving the solubility in water, coupling these drugs to biopolymers in general has provided advantages in terms of chemical stability, localization, and controlled release (Maeda et al., 1992). HA is a linear polysaccharide with alternating glucuronic acid and N-acetyl-glucosamine residues (Figure 16.5). It is one of the glycosaminoglycan components of the extracellular matrix, the synovial fluid in joints, and the scaffold that comprises cartilage

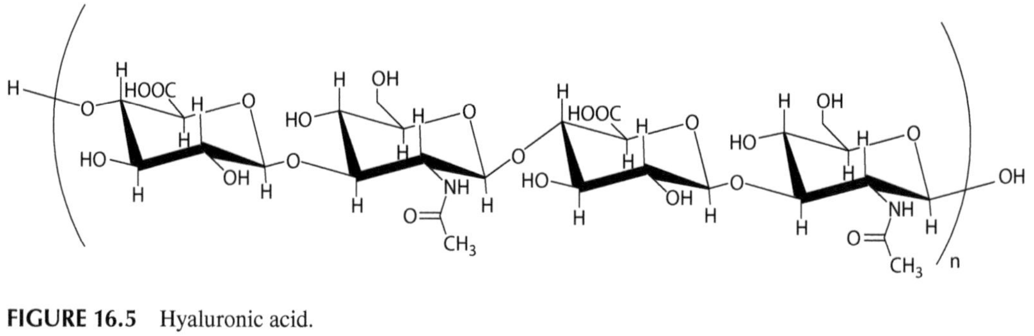

FIGURE 16.5 Hyaluronic acid.

(Laurent et al., 1995). Its immunoneutrality makes it an excellent polymer on which to develop biocompatible and biodegradable drug delivery systems (Freed et al., 1994; Prestwich et al., 1998; Vercruysse and Prestwich, 1998). Luo and Prestwich (1999) reported the preparation of such drug-HA conjugates wherein HA, modified with adipic dihydrazide (ADH), was coupled to Taxol-2'-hemisuccinate NHS ester to give prodrugs with a variety of ADH and Taxol loadings (Table 16.7).

N-(2-hydroxypropyl)methacrylamide (HPMA) has a history of use in the preparation of soluble polymer-drug conjugates to be used as targetable drug carriers (Rihova et al., 1986; Duncan et al., 1987; Kopecek, 1991; Kopecek et al., 2000; Vartikovski et al., 2001; Wohl et al., 2014; Smith et al., 2015). There are at least five polymer–drug conjugates that entered Phase I/II clinical trials as

---

TABLE 16.7

Taxol, Its 2′-Hemisuccinate NHS Intermediate, and Its HA Prodrug Form

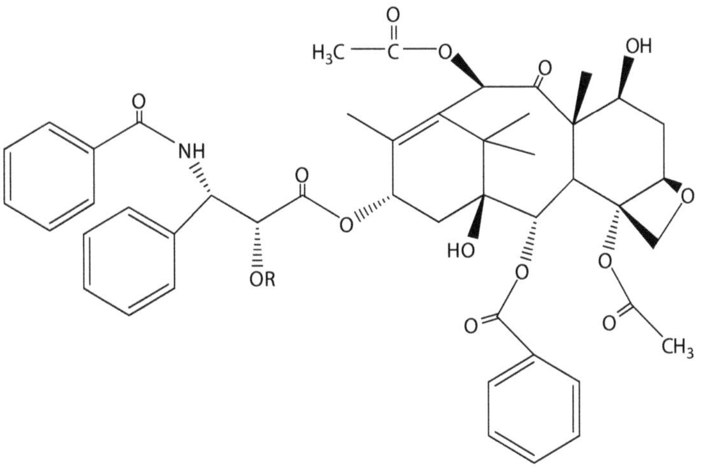

Substance	R Group
Taxol	H-
2′-Hemisuccinate NHS Intermediate	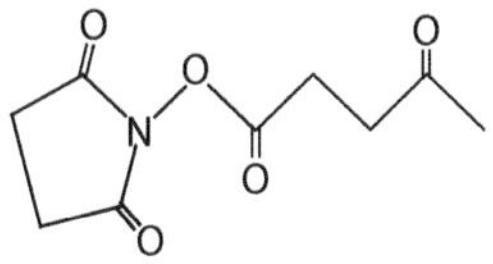
Hyaluronic Acid Adduct	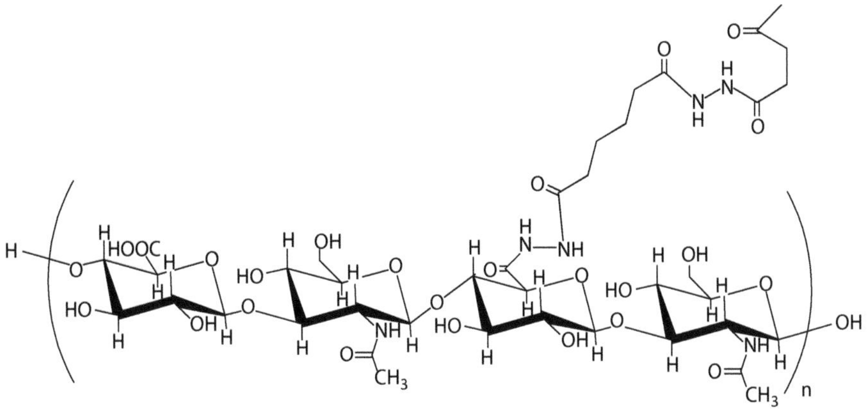

anticancer agents that involved HPMA as the polymer (Duncan et al., 2001). They are HPMA copolymer–doxorubicin, HPMA copolymer–paclitaxel, HPMA copolymer–camptothecin, HPMA copolymer–platinate, and an HPMA copolymer–doxorubicin conjugate that also bore galactosamine. Galactosamine was included to target the conjugate to the liver (Duncan et al., 1986) in order to treat primary and secondary liver cancer (Duncan et al., 2001).

Polymer prodrugs of ribavirin have been prepared to test the effect of the polymer promoiety on inhibition of nitric oxide and to seek evidence of a reduction in hemolytic activity. There was concern that the polymer could interfere with inhibition of nitric oxide synthase (the therapeutic basis of ribavirin activity as an anti-inflammatory agent), and anemia proved to be a serious side effect with ribavirin (Guo et al., 2015). HPMA (Wohl et al., 2014; Smith et al., 2015), polyvinylpyrrolidone (PVP; Kryger et al., 2014; Wohl et al., 2014), polymethacrylic acid (PMAA; Wohl et al., 2014), and polyacrylic acid (PAA; Kryger et al., 2013, 2014; Wohl et al., 2014) were included in these studies. Although HPMA demonstrated the lowest toxicity, HPMA and PAA both reduced cytotoxicity. PVP was the only polymer in these studies that blocked inhibition of nitric oxide synthase. PAA exhibited no hemolytic effect (Kryger et al., 2013, 2014) and proved to be the most effective of these polymeric prodrugs.

Among the water-soluble synthetic polymeric materials employed in the covalent modification of drugs, polyethylene glycols (PEGs) are preferred for their biocompatibility and their lack of antigenicity and toxicity (Weiner and Zilkha, 1973; Zalipsky et al., 1983; Dal Pozzo and Acquasaliente, 1992; Li et al., 2014). In addition, these polymers are soluble in water and organic solvents (Weiner and Zilkha, 1973), and they are commercially available in fractions with well-defined molecular weights (Cecchi et al., 1981). PEG prodrugs have two distinct disadvantages. Esters formed with PEG as the source of the alcohol group would possess an electron-withdrawing group in the α-position of the ester that can assist in the rapid chemical hydrolysis of the ester bond (Chung and Cho, 2004). The PEG component in the prodrug is not biodegradable (Zalipsky et al., 1983), which limits the routes of administration available to these prodrugs.

Mattarei et al. (2015) utilized PEG of short chain length with only three, four, or six repeated units in the preparation of N-monosubstituted methoxy-oligo(ethylene glycol) carbamate ester prodrugs of resveratrol. The use of oligo(ethylene glycol) instead of poly(ethylene glycol) made it possible to maintain a low molecular weight and to allow a higher drug-loading potential, yet provide the desirable physicochemical properties observed with PEG derivatives. The shorter chain length of the oligo(ethylene glycol), though still not biodegradable, also offered the possible use of conventional routes of administration.

Potential indomethacin (Caprariis et al., 1994) and ibuprofen (Cecchi et al., 1981) prodrugs have been prepared by generating the ester between the terminal hydroxyl of various low molecular weight PEGs and the carboxylic acid of the drug. Indomethacin prodrugs demonstrated rapid reconversion in 80% human plasma in isotonic pH 7.4 phosphate buffer. In the absence of enzymes, in pH 2 or 7.4 buffer, the hydrolysis rate was approximately 200 times slower than observed in the presence of enzymes. Preliminary experiments with porcine esterase indicate that enzymatic hydrolysis was probably catalyzed by esterases, and that the hydrolysis can regenerate the parent drug directly. The tetraethylene glycol–ibuprofen derivative was a viscous oil that was poorly soluble in water. However, a PEG of high molecular weight, consisting of approximately 45 monomeric units and corresponding to a molecular weight of 2000, was esterified at both ends and was still found to be freely soluble.

PEG derivatives of paclitaxel (Greenwald et al., 1996; Nam et al., 2014), camptothecin (Greenwald et al., 1998), and doxorubicin (Rodrigues et al., 1999) have been prepared. It was noted that the molecular weight of the PEG must be "of such magnitude so as to maintain a $t_{1/2}$ (circulation) > $t_{1/2}$ (hydrolysis)" (Greenwald et al., 1996). In the case of camptothecin derivatives, PEG with a molecular weight ≥ 20,000 g/mole allowed the bifunctional PEG to be derivatized at both ends and still remain soluble in water (Greenwald et al., 1998). Doxorubicin-polyethylene glycol prodrugs were synthesized in aqueous media by reacting three different maleimide derivatives of doxorubicin with α-methoxypolyethylene glycol (mPEG)-thiopropionic acid amide of 20,000 molecular weight, α, ω-*bis*-thiopropionic acid amide polyethylene glycol of 20,000 molecular weight, or α-*tert*-butoxy-polyethylene glycol-thiopropionic acid amide of 70,000 molecular weight. The thiol group adds to the double bond of the maleimide group in a rapid and selective manner to form a stable thioether bond (Rodrigues et al., 1999). The derivative involving the 70,000 molecular weight PEG was found to possess good chemical stability in pH 7.4 buffer, with less than 10% drug released after 48 h in the medium, but more rapid release at pH 5.0, indicating an acid-sensitive degradation.

Because of its poor solubility in water, tacrolimus, a potent immunosuppressant, was derivatized with mPEG by initially acylating the drug at the 24-, 32-, or 24,32-positions using iodoacetic acid in the presence of dicyclohexylcarbodiimide as a coupling reagent with dimethylaminopyridine as a base (Chung and Cho, 2004). After separation of the three types of iodoacetate esters, reaction of this intermediate ester with the thiol of 5 kDa mPEG-SH, in the presence of sodium bicarbonate as a base, yielded the desired prodrugs. These derivatives proved to be soluble in water and could be converted into tacrolimus using liver homogenates. The half-lives are approximately 10 min in the homogenate, indicating their potential as prodrugs for the immunosuppressant. The half-life in pH 7.4 phosphate buffer at 37°C was 20 h, indicating sufficient chemical stability that solutions of these products could be reconstituted by simple dissolution in water without concern for chemical degradation.

N-hydroxymethylphenytoin, a prodrug in its own right as described earlier, was linked to mono- and polyfunctional polyethylene glycols bearing ionizable and nonionizable end groups (Dal Pozzo and Acquasaliente, 1992). In each of the six derivatives, *N*-hydroxymethylphenytoin was linked to the terminal hydroxyl group of the PEG using a succinic acid spacer. At the opposite end of the PEG chain was a hydroxy, a methoxy, a sodium succinate, or the disodium salt of a more complex dicarboxylate group. Each of the prodrugs, with the exception of the derivative involving a methoxy-capped PEG of only three monomeric units, was freely and rapidly soluble in water in all proportions and demonstrated stability in water for 1 month at room temperature. In undiluted plasma, hydrolysis was too rapid to be characterized. The half-life in 10% diluted plasma exhibited pseudo-first-order kinetics with a half-life of about 3 h. The half-life in isotonic phosphate buffer was 150 h, indicating that these prodrugs possess the *in vivo/in vitro* conversion rate ratio desired of superior prodrugs.

A series of zero generation polyamidoamine dendrimer-based prodrugs were prepared in an attempt to improve the solubility and bioavailability of poorly soluble naproxen (Freeman et al., 2005). Dendrimers are branched molecules with multiple end groups, and typically a drug molecule is covalently bound to an end group of the dendrimer (De Groot et al., 2003). The dendrimer used with naproxen, (G0) PAMAM, was linked through formation of an amide (Figure 16.6). Alternatively, one of two linking chemicals, either lactic acid or diethylene glycol, was attached to the dendrimer, and then naproxen was esterified with the free alcohol group of the linking chemical to form this type of prodrug. In each of the three cases, the water-soluble dendrimer provided a prodrug form that was more hydrophilic than naproxen. Hydrolysis of the prodrug was evaluated at 37°C in pH 1.2 hydrochloric acid buffer, in pH 7.4 phosphate buffer, in pH 8.5 borate buffer, and in 80% human plasma. In the buffer systems, each of the three prodrugs was chemically stable over the

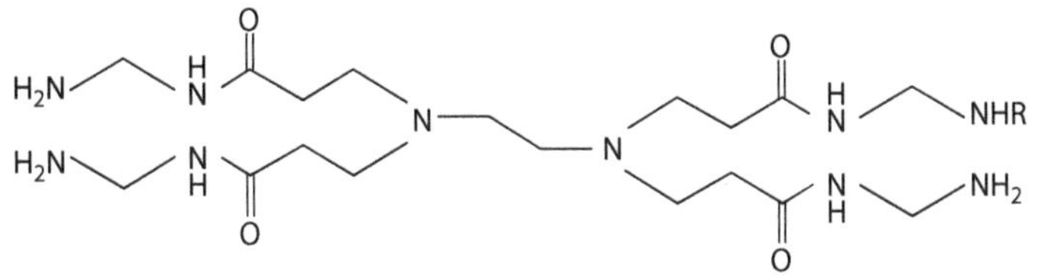

FIGURE 16.6 Dendrimer (G0) PAMAM linked through an amide bond.

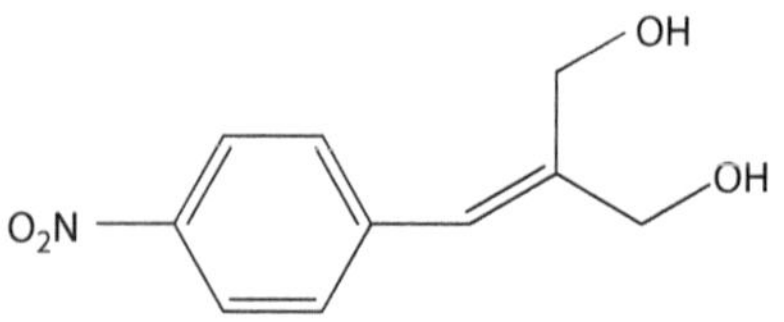

FIGURE 16.7 Double release nitrodiol as the base for prodrug dendrimer development.

course of the 48 h evaluation. In the plasma system, naproxen was released from each of the ester prodrugs through pseudo-first-order kinetics. It was released slowly from the lactic acid ester, with only 25% released in 24 h, and quickly from the diethylene glycol ester, with a half-life of 51 min. It is not surprising that the direct amide linkage to naproxen resulted in a product that was considered unsuitable as a prodrug owing to high stability against enzyme-catalyzed hydrolysis.

Two issues with typical dendrimer prodrugs have been presented by De Groot et al. (2003). First, each single drug molecule must be independently cleaved from the end group in order to be released. Second, the dendrimer itself is not usually completely degraded. To circumvent these issues, they developed a *cascade-release dendrimer* wherein the dendrimer completely and rapidly dissociates into its building blocks when it experiences a single triggering event, and this process also induces release of the drug molecules that were bound to the end groups. The triggering can even be tuned to provide site-specific release. These cascade-release dendrimers possess two or more generations of branched self-elimination linkers, each of which releases multiple leaving groups on activation. Cleavage of the bond between the dendrimer and any linker moiety also results in release of the parent drug with its regained activity. Proof of concept was provided using a double release nitrodiol (Figure 16.7) wherein the nitro group acts as a masked amine group. Reduction of the nitro group to an amine would act as the trigger for the self-eliminations. The nitrodiol was activated using 4-nitrophenyl chloroformate to produce the *bis*(4-nitrophenyl carbonate) derivative, which was then coupled to two equivalents of poorly soluble paclitaxel to yield the desired dendron. At 0°C, paclitaxel reacts with the carbonates at its most reactive 2′-hydroxy group. When the nitro function was reduced under mild conditions, using zinc and acetic acid, complete disappearance of the starting dendron and release of the paclitaxel were observed, and these results were supported by thin layer chromatography studies. Proton-NMR confirmed these results and demonstrated complete release of the paclitaxel molecules. NMR spectra of paclitaxel derivatives can be complicated, but the 2′-H signal of the paclitaxel in the dendron, representing a hydroxyl group bound to an alkyloxy-carbonyl group, is a distinguishable signal ($\delta = 5.46$ ppm). This signal disappears completely and the corresponding 2′-H signal of paclitaxel itself ($\delta = 4.74$ ppm) appears over the course of the decomposition of the dendron.

CHEMICAL AND ENZYMATIC LABILITY OF THE PROMOIETY

Most prodrugs are biologically inactive (Sinkula and Yalkowsky, 1975), and therefore, an important feature in the design of a prodrug is the sensitivity of the modification to cleavage through chemical or enzymatic means to release the promoiety and return the pharmacologically active agent. It should be possible to predict the *in vitro* lability because suitable models for nonenzymatic hydrolysis have been developed for many promoieties of interest (Charton, 1977). A method for predicting *in vitro* reactivity by energy measurements has been recommended (Charton, 1977), although it might not be possible to predict the actual hydrolysis rate, even under *in vitro* conditions, since drugs are generally too complex to allow accurate calculations of rates. Nevertheless, the method could be useful in preliminary screening of potential promoieties meant to undergo rapid enzymatic hydrolysis in blood (Notari, 1985), and in interpolations of chemical or enzymatic labilities within a homologous series of chemicals. Unless one conducts exhaustive animal or human pharmacokinetic studies, however, it is difficult to prove conclusively that a prodrug is indeed rapidly and quantitatively converted *in vivo* to the parent drug (Cho et al., 1986). Results from *in vitro* studies are therefore most useful in screening a series of prodrugs to determine the promising candidates for further study.

Anderson and Conradi (1987) point out that "while coupling of a drug and a solubilizing moiety in a bioreversible manner may indeed constitute the synthesis of a water-soluble prodrug, this is not prodrug design. Prodrug design entails the optimization of the physical and chemical properties of the prodrug so that its effectiveness as a delivery system for the parent drug is also optimized." If intended for parenteral use, the prodrug should be sufficiently stable *in vitro* to allow the development of a ready-to-inject solution. For example, a disadvantage to dicarboxylate hemiesters as a prodrug form is that their solubility is usually limited at the pH optimum for solution stability (Anderson et al., 1985).

Water-soluble prodrugs that are unstable in solution may be prepared as a lyophilized mixture to be reconstituted before use, although this adds significantly to the production cost, and proves to be an inconvenience to those responsible for administration. Ideally, a water-soluble prodrug product in aqueous solution should have a shelf life of 2 years or more at room temperature, in which case the half-life *in vitro* should be at least 13 years. If the only purpose of prodrug formation is to improve the solubility of the parent drug, then bioconversion *in vivo* should be extremely rapid. If it is assumed that more than 90% of the prodrug is converted to the parent drug within 30 min of the injection, the *in vivo* half-life should be 10 min or less. Ideal water-soluble prodrug design therefore requires an *in vivo/in vitro* lability ratio of nearly 10^6. This can be readily achieved only if the bioconversion is enzyme-catalyzed (Anderson and Conradi, 1987).

Three general principles that are valuable in the design of solution-stable prodrugs are that 1. pH-solubility behavior is an important determinant of solution stability, 2. pH-degradation rate profiles can be optimized by considering the effects of neighboring substituents on hydrolysis rates, and 3. building micelle-forming properties into a prodrug can be advantageous in improving stability and solubilizing otherwise insoluble degradation products (Anderson, 1985; Anderson and Conradi, 1987). Many prodrug design problems require the simultaneous application of all three principles to achieve the necessary degree of stability improvement.

With regard to the first principle, the formulation pH can be a major influence on the rate of acid- or base-catalyzed reactions, especially hydrolysis. The above-mentioned discussion of the pH effect on the solubility of prodrugs that were derived using promoieties possessing different ionizable groups serves as a simple illustration of how the selection of the pH and the ionizable functional group can be critical to solubilization. Nevertheless, solution stability of the prodrug must also be considered. Achieving high solubility in the region of optimum solution stability might require selection of an ionizable promoiety with a pK_a far removed from the pH-degradation rate minimum. For example, it has been recommended that the investigator select a sulfonate- or an amine-bearing promoiety, with pK_a values of approximately 1.5 and 9.0, respectively, for a prodrug with a pH-degradation minimum at 3.5–5 (Anderson, 1985).

In the investigations applying the second principle, it has been found that acid-catalyzed hydrolysis is relatively insensitive to polar substituent effects; it is primarily influenced by steric effects. Hydroxide-catalyzed reactions, on the other hand, are sensitive to both steric and electronic effects (Anderson, 1985). In the case of esters of methylprednisolone, by using a nonpolar spacer to increase the distance between the ionizable group of the disposable moiety and the ester function, it was possible to effectively reduce the hydroxide-ion-catalyzed hydrolysis rate. Sterically hindered promoieties were employed to reduce the hydrolysis rates of hemiesters of hydrocortisone, which therefore proved to be more stable than hydrocortisone hemisuccinate (Garrett and Royer, 1962). However, since enzymatic hydrolysis is clearly hindered by steric effects, and since rapid conversion is usually desirable if the prodrug goal is improved solubility alone, deliberate increases in steric bulk should not be pursued (Anderson, 1985).

Dicarboxylic acid hemiesters of methylprednisolone illustrate the third principle since they were shown to undergo micellization in aqueous solution (Anderson et al., 1983). This self-stabilizing

TABLE 16.8

Specific Delivery to Systems or Organs by Targeting Enzymes

Organ or System	References
Cancer	Niculescu-Duvaz et al. (1998); de Groot et al. (2003); Bagshawe et al. (2004); Sharma et al. (2004); Dachs et al. (2005); Rautio et al. (2008); Huttunen and Rautio (2011); Zawilska et al. (2013)
Central nervous system	Anderson (1996); Rautio et al. (2008); Huttunen and Rautio (2011); Zawilska et al. (2013)
Colon	Friend and Chang (1985); McLeod et al. (1993, 1994); Sinha and Kumria (2001); Rautio et al. (2008); Huttunen and Rautio (2011)
Eye	Järvinen and Järvinen (1996); Rautio et al. (2008)
Kidney	Wilk et al. (1978); Orlowski et al. (1979); Hwang and Elfarra (1989); Huttunen and Rautio (2011); Zhou et al. (2014)
Liver	Erion et al. (2004, 2005, 2006); Kumpulainen et al. (2006); Rautio et al. (2008); Huttunen and Rautio (2011); Guo et al. (2015)
Skin	Sloan and Wasdo (2003); Majumdar and Sloan (2006); Sloan et al. (2006); Rautio et al. (2008)
Transporters in the intestinal wall	Han and Amidon (2000); Heimbach et al. (2003); Rautio et al. (2008); Zawilska et al. (2013)

process was not surprising since the prodrugs are amphiphilic, surfactant-like chemicals. Increasing the chain length lowered the critical micelle concentration, and also improved their stability. The major advantage of the micellar prodrug approach is that slightly soluble degradation products, including the poorly soluble parent drug, are solubilized. The core of the micelles, formed by the surfactant-like prodrugs, should behave as an ideal environment for the parent drug since it utilizes the parent drug as the more hydrophobic portion of the molecule. Anderson (1985) also notes that since *in vivo* hydrolysis would destroy the surfactant properties of the micellar prodrugs, they should be better tolerated than the more stable commercial surfactants.

Due to the importance of enzyme systems in the biodegradation of prodrugs, Liederer and Borchardt (2006) have presented a compilation of enzymes that can be targeted to accomplish metabolism of ester prodrugs to their parent drugs. The design of prodrugs by considering the target enzyme system has been discussed in detail (Sinkula and Yalkowsky, 1975; Amidon et al., 1977; Radhakrishnan, 1977; Banerjee and Amidon, 1985; Fleisher et al., 1985; Liederer and Borchardt, 2006; Rautio et al., 2008; Huttunen and Rautio, 2011; Bai et al., 2014). In addition, there are descriptions of enzymes that might be generally useful to facilitate targeting cancer, the central nervous system, the colon, the eye, the kidney, the liver, the skin, or the transporters in the intestinal wall, and to serve as catalysts for reconversion of prodrugs to parent drugs (Table 16.8). In addition, it has been recommended that the kinetic and binding specificity of the enzyme system, the type of reaction to be catalyzed, the enzyme distribution and concentration, and the role of the enzyme in cellular biochemistry should be known (Notari, 1973, 1985).

FURTHER READING

A number of reviews and discussions of prodrugs exist in the literature (Harper, 1959, 1962; Albert, 1964; Ariens, 1966; Digenis and Swintowsky, 1975; Sinkula, 1975; Stella, 1975; Sinkula, 1977; Anderson, 1980; Ettmayer et al., 2004; Huttunen et al., 2011), along with several books that have been cited earlier. The reader will discover that these reviewers approach the prodrug topic from different viewpoints, although some discussion overlap does exist. Reviews have been offered dealing with esters and amides as prodrug types (Digenis and Swintowsky, 1975; Huttunen and Rautio, 2011), antibiotic prodrugs (Notari, 1973), or nucleotide prodrugs (Jones and Bischofberger, 1995), or that include various other prodrug types (Sinkula, 1975; Bodor, 1981, 1982; Bundgaard, 1982, 1985b; Huttunen and Rautio, 2011). The reader is also directed to reviews and discussions that have approached prodrug design by the various functional groups found in the drugs to be modified (Bundgaard, 1982, 1985a, 1986, 1987; Rautio et al., 2008) or generated (Sinkula, 1975; Anderson et al., 1985; Anderson and Conradi, 1987; Rautio et al., 2008; Huttunen and Rautio, 2011).

REFERENCES

Aggarwal, A. K. and M. Gupta. 2012. Solubility and solution stability studies of different amino acid prodrugs of bromhexine. *Drug Dev. Ind. Pharm.* 38: 1319–1327.

Albert, A. 1958. Chemical aspects of selective toxicity. *Nature* 182: 421–423.

Albert, A. 1964. *Selective Toxicity*, pp. 57–63. New York: Wiley.

Alexander, J., R. Cargill, S. R. Michelson, and H. Schwam. 1988. (Acyloxy)alkyl carbamates as novel bioreversible prodrugs for amines: Increased permeation through biological membranes. *J. Med. Chem.* 31: 318–322.

Al-Ghananeem, A. M., A. A. Traboulsi, L. W. Dittert, and A. A. Hussain. 2002. Targeted brain delivery of 17β-estradiol via nasally administered water soluble prodrugs. *AAPS PharmSciTech* 3: E5.

Altomare, C., G. Trapani, A. Latrofa, M. Serra, G. Biggio, and G. Liso. 2003. Highly water-soluble derivatives of the anesthetic agent propofol: *In vitro* and *in vivo* evaluation of cyclic amino acid esters. *Eur. J. Pharm. Sci.* 20: 17–26.

Ambrose, P. J. 1984. Clinical pharmacokinetics of chloramphenicol and chloramphenicol succinate. *Clin. Pharmacokin.* 9: 222–238.

Amidon, G. L. 1981. Drug derivatization as a means of solubilization: Physicochemical and biochemical strategies. In *Techniques of Solubilization of Drugs*, Yalkowsky, S. H. (Ed.), pp. 183–211. New York: Marcel Dekker.

Amidon, G. L., G. D. Leesman, and R. L. Elliott. 1980. Improving intestinal absorption of water-insoluble compounds: A membrane metabolism strategy. *J. Pharm. Sci.* 69: 1363–1368.

Amidon, G. L., R. S. Pearlman, and G. D. Leesman. 1977. Design of prodrugs through consideration of enzyme-substrate specificities. In *Design of Biopharmaceutical Properties through Prodrugs and Analogs*, Roche, E. B. (Ed.), pp. 281–315. Washington, DC: American Pharmaceutical Association.

Anderson, B. D. 1980. Thermodynamic considerations in physical property improvement through prodrugs. In *Physical Chemical Properties of Drugs*, Yalkowsky, S. H., Sinkula, A. A., and Valvani, S. C. (Eds.), pp. 231–266. New York: Marcel Dekker.

Anderson, B. D. 1985. Prodrugs for improved formulation properties. In *Design of Prodrugs*, Bundgaard, H. (Ed.), pp. 243–269. New York: Elsevier Science.

Anderson, B. D. 1996. Prodrugs for improved CNS delivery. *Adv. Drug Del. Rev.* 19: 171–202.

Anderson, B. D. and R. A. Conradi. 1980. Prostaglandin prodrugs. VI. Structure–thermodynamic activity and structure–aqueous solubility relationships. *J. Pharm. Sci.* 69: 424–430.

Anderson, B. D. and R. A. Conradi. 1987. Application of physical organic concepts to *in vitro* and *in vivo* lability design of water soluble prodrugs. In *Bioreversible Carriers in Drug Design: Theory and Application*, Roche, E. B. (Ed.), pp. 121–163. New York: Pergamon Press.

Anderson, B. D., R. A. Conradi, and K. Johnson. 1983. Influence of premicellar and micellar association on the reactivity of methylprednisolone 21-hemiesters in aqueous solution. *J. Pharm. Sci.* 72: 448–454.

Anderson, B. D., R. A. Conradi, and K. E. Knuth. 1985. Strategies in the design of solution-stable, water-soluble prodrugs. I. A physical-organic approach to pro-moiety selection for 21-esters of corticosteroids. *J. Pharm. Sci.* 74: 365–374.

Anderson, B. D., R. A. Conradi, and W. J. Lambert. 1984. Carboxyl group catalysis of acyl transfer reactions in corticosteroid 17- and 21-monoesters. *J. Pharm. Sci.* 73: 604–611.

Anderson, B. D. and V. Taphouse. 1981. Initial rate studies of hydrolysis and acyl migration in methylprednisolone 21-hemisuccinate and 17-hemisuccinate. *J. Pharm. Sci.* 70: 181–186.

Andurkar, S. V. 2007. Chemical modifications and drug delivery. In *Gibaldi's Drug Delivery Systems in Pharmaceutical Care*, Desai, A. and Lee, M. (Eds.), pp. 123–134. Bethesda, MD: American Society of Health-Care Pharmacists.

Ariens, E. J. 1966. Molecular pharmacology, a basis for drug design. *Progr. Drug Res.* 10: 429–529.

Bagshawe, K. D., S. K. Sharma, and R. H. Begent. 2004. Antibody-directed enzyme prodrug therapy (ADEPT) for cancer. *Exp. Opin. Biol. Ther.* 4: 1777–1789.

Bai, A., Z. M. Szulc, J. Bielawski, J. S. Pierce, B. Rembiesa, S. Terzieva, C. Mao, et al. 2014. Targeting (cellular) lysosomal acid ceramidase by B13: Design, synthesis and evaluation of novel DMG-B13 ester prodrugs. *Bioorg. Med. Chem.* 22: 6933–6944.

Banerjee, P. K. and G. L. Amidon. 1985. Design of prodrugs based on enzyme-substrate specificity. In *Design of Prodrugs*, Bundgaard, H. (Ed.), pp. 93–134. New York: Elsevier Science.

Bansai, P. C., I. H. Pitman, and T. Higuchi. 1981a. *N*-Hydroxymethyl derivatives of nitrogen heterocycles as possible prodrugs. II. Possible prodrugs of allopurinol, glutethimide, and phenobarbital. *J. Pharm. Sci.* 70: 855–857.

Bansai, P. C., I. H. Pitman, J. N. S. Tam, M. Mertes, and J. J. Kaminski. 1981b. *N*-Hydroxymethyl derivatives of nitrogen heterocycles as possible prodrugs. I. *N*-Hydroxymethylation of uracils. *J. Pharm. Sci.* 70: 850–854.

Baurain, R., M. Masquelier, D. Deprez-De Campeneere, and A. Trouet. 1980. Amino acid and dipeptide derivatives of daunorubicin. 2. Cellular pharmacology and antitumor activity on L1210 leukemia cells *in vitro* and *in vivo*. *J. Med. Chem.* 23: 1171–1174.

Bentley, A., M. Butters, S. P. Green, W. J. Learmonth, J. A. MacRae, M. C. Morland, G. O'Connor, and J. Skuse. 2002. The discovery and process development of a commercial route to the water soluble prodrug, fosfluconazole. *Org. Proc Res. Dev.* 6: 109–112.

Bodor, N. 1981. Novel approaches in prodrug design. *Drugs Future* 6: 165–182.

Bodor, N. 1982. Novel approaches in prodrug design. In *Optimization of Drug Delivery*, Bundgaard, H., Hansen, A. B., and Kofod, H. (Eds.), pp. 156–174. Copenhagen: Munksgaard.

Bundgaard, H. 1982. Novel bioreversible derivatives of amides, imides, ureides, amines and other chemical entities not readily derivatizable. In *Optimization of Drug Delivery*, Bundgaard, H., Hansen, A. B., and Kofod, H. (Eds.), pp. 178–197. Copenhagen: Munksgaard.

Bundgaard, H. 1985a. Design of prodrugs: Bioreversible derivatives for various functional groups and chemical entities. In *Design of Prodrugs*, Bundgaard, H. (Ed.), pp. 1–92. New York: Elsevier Science.

Bundgaard, H. 1985b. Formation of prodrugs of amines, amides, ureides, and imides. In *Methods in Enzymology*, Vol. 112, Part A, Widder, K. J. and Gree, R. (Eds.), pp. 347–359. New York: Academic Press.

Bundgaard, H. 1986. Design of prodrugs: Bioreversible derivatives for various function groups and chemical entities. In *Design of Prodrugs*, Bundgaard, H. (Ed.), pp. 1–92. Amsterdam: Elsevier Biomedical Press.

Bundgaard, H. 1987. Design of bioreversible drug derivatives and the utility of the double prodrug concept. In *Bioreversible Carriers in Drug Design: Theory and Application*, Roche, E. B. (Ed.), pp. 13–94. New York: Pergamon Press.

Bundgaard, H. and E. Falch. 1985a. Allopurinol prodrugs. II. Synthesis, hydrolysis kinetics and physico-chemical properties of various *N*-acyloxymethyl allopurinol derivatives. *Int. J. Pharm.* 24: 307–325.

Bundgaard, H. and E. Falch. 1985b. Allopurinol prodrugs. III. Water-soluble *N*-acyloxymethyl allopurinol derivatives for rectal or parenteral use. *Int. J. Pharm.* 25: 27–39.

Bundgaard, H., E. Falch, and E. Jensen. 1989. A novel solution-stable, water-soluble prodrug type for drugs containing a hydroxyl or an NH-acidic group. *J. Med. Chem.* 32: 2503–2507.

Bundgaard, H., E. Jensen, and E. Falch. 1991. Water-soluble, solution-stable, and biolabile *N*-substituted (aminomethyl)benzoate ester prodrugs of acyclovir. *Pharm. Res.* 8: 1087–1093.

Bundgaard, H., E. Jensen, E. Falch, and S. B. Pedersen. 1990. Allopurinol prodrugs. V. Water-soluble *N*-substituted (aminomethyl)benzoyloxymethyl allopurinol derivatives for parenteral or rectal delivery. *Int. J. Pharm.* 64: 75–87.

Bundgaard, H. and M. Johansen. 1982. Kinetics of hydrolysis of plafibride (An ureide *N*-Mannich base with platelet antiaggregant activity) in aqueous solution and in plasma. *Arch. Pharm. Chem., Sci. Ed.* 10: 139–145.

Bundgaard, H. and M. Johansen. 1984. Hydrolysis of *N*-(α-hydroxyalkyl)benzamide and other *N*-(α-hydroxyalkyl)amide derivatives: Implications for the design of *N*-acyloxyalkyl-type prodrugs. *Int. J. Pharm.* 22: 45–56.

Bundgaard, H., M. Johansen, V. Stella, and M. Cortese. 1982. Pro-drugs as drug delivery systems. XXI. Preparation, physicochemical properties and bioavailability of a novel water-soluble pro-drug type for carbamazepine. *Int. J. Pharm.* 10: 181–192.

Bundgaard, H., C. Larsen, and E. Arnold. 1984a. Prodrugs as drug delivery systems. XXVII. Chemical stability and bioavailability of a water-soluble prodrug of metronidazole for parenteral administration. *Int. J. Pharm.* 18: 79–87.

Bundgaard, H., C. Larsen, and P. Thorbek. 1984b. Prodrugs as drug delivery systems. XXVI. Preparation and enzymatic hydrolysis of various water-soluble amino acid esters of metronidazole. *Int. J. Pharm.* 18: 67–77.

Bundgaard, H. and N. M. Nielsen. 1987. Esters of *N,N*-disubstituted 2-hydroxyacetamides as a novel highly biolabile prodrug type for carboxylic acid agents. *J. Med. Chem.* 30: 451–454.

Bundgaard, H. and N. M. Nielsen. 1988. Glycolamide esters as a novel biolabile prodrug type for non-steroidal anti-inflammatory carboxylic acid drugs. *Int. J. Pharm.* 43: 101–110.

Burke, J. T., W. A. Wargin, R. J. Sherertz, K. L. Sanders, M. R. Blum, and F. A. Sarubbi. 1982. Pharmacokinetics of intravenous chloramphenicol sodium succinate in adult patients with normal renal and hepatic function. *J. Pharm. Biopharm.* 10: 601–614.

Buur, A. and H. Bundgaard. 1984a. Prodrugs of 5-fluorouracil. I. Hydrolysis kinetics and physicochemical properties of various *N*-acyl derivatives of 5-fluorouracil. *Int. J. Pharm.* 21: 349–364.

Buur, A. and H. Bundgaard. 1984b. Prodrugs of 5-fluorouracil. II. Hydrolysis kinetics, bioactivation, solubility and lipophilicity of *N*-alkoxycarbonyl derivatives of 5-fluorouracil. *Arch. Pharm. Chem. Sci. Ed.* 12: 37–44.

Caprariis, P. D., F. Palagiano, F. Bonina, L. Montenegro, M. D'Amico, and F. Rossi. 1994. Synthesis and pharmacological evaluation of oligoethylene ester derivatives as indomethacin oral prodrugs. *J. Pharm. Sci.* 83: 1578–1581.

Cecchi, R., L. Rusconi, M. C. Tanzi, F. Danusso, and P. J. Ferruti. 1981. Synthesis and pharmacological evaluation of poly(oxyethylene) derivatives of 4-isobutylphenyl-2-propionic acid (ibuprofen). *J. Med. Chem.* 24: 622–625.

Charton, M. 1977. The prediction of chemical lability through substituent effects. In *Design of Biopharmaceutical Properties through Prodrugs and Analogs*, Roche, E. B. (Ed.), pp. 228–280. Washington, DC: American Pharmaceutical Association.

Charton, M. 1985. Prodrug lability prediction through the use of substituent effects. In *Methods in Enzymology*, Vol. 112, Part A, Widder, K. J. and Gree, R. (Eds.), pp. 323–340. New York: Academic Press.

Cho, M. J., V. H. Sethy, and L. C. Haynes. 1986. Sequentially labile water-soluble prodrugs of alprazolam. *J. Med. Chem.* 29: 1346–1350.

Chung, Y. and H. Cho. 2004. Preparation of highly water soluble tacrolimus derivatives: Poly(ethylene glycol) esters as potential prodrugs. *Arch. Pharm. Res.* 27: 878–883.

Colaizzi, J. L. and W. H. Pitlick. 1982. Oral drug-delivery systems for prescription pharmacy. In *Pharmaceutics and Pharmacy Practice*, Banker, G. S. and Chalmers, R. K. (Eds.), pp. 184–237. Philadelphia, PA: J. B. Lippincott.

Colla, L., E. De Clercq, R. Busson, and H. Vanderhaeghe. 1983. Synthesis and antiviral activity of water-soluble esters of acyclovir [9-[(2-hydroxyehtoxy)methyl]guanine]. *J. Med. Chem.* 26: 602–604.

Culty, M., H. A. Nguyen, and C. B. Underhill. 1992. The hyaluronan receptor (CD44) participates in the uptake and degradation of hyaluronan. *J. Cell Biol.* 116: 1055–1062.

Dachs, G. H., J. Tupper, G. M. Tozer. 2005. From bench to bedside for gene-directed enzyme prodrug therapy of cancer. *Anticancer Drugs* 16: 349–359.

Dal Pozzo, A. and M. Acquasaliente. 1992. New highly water-soluble phenytoin prodrugs. *Int. J. Pharm.* 81: 263–265.

Damen, E. W. P., L. Braamer, and H. W. Scheeren. 1998. Lanthanide trifluoromethanesulfonate catalysed selective acylation of 10-deacetylbaccatin III. *Tetrahedron Lett.* 39: 6081–6082.

Damen, E. W. P., P. H. G. Wiegerinck, L. Braamer, D. Sperling, D. de Vos, and H. W. Scheeren. 2000. Paclitaxel esters of malic acid as prodrugs with improved water solubility. *Bioorg. Med. Chem.* 8: 427–432.

de Groot, F. M. H., A. Carsten, R. Koekkoek, P. H. Beusker, and H. W. Scheeren. 2003. Cascade-release dendrimers liberate all end groups upon a single triggering event in the dendritic core. *Angew. Chem. Int. Ed.* 42: 4490–4494.

Deutsch, M., J. A. Glinski, M. Hernandez, R. D. Haugwitz, V. L. Narayanan, M. Suffness, and L. H. Zalkow. 1989. Synthesis of congeners and prodrugs. 3. Water-soluble prodrugs of taxol with potent antitumor activity. *J. Med. Chem.* 32: 788–792.

Devanço, M. G., A. C. Aguiar, L. A. Dos Santos, E. C. Padilha, M. L. Campos, C. R. de Andrade, L. M. da Fonseca, et al. 2014. Evaluation of antimalarial activity and toxicity of a new primaquine prodrug. *PLoS One* 9: e105217.

Digenis, G. A. and J. V. Swintowsky. 1975. Drug latentiation. *Handbook Exp. Pharmacol.* 28: 86–112.

Di Meo, C., F. Cilurzo, M. Licciardi, C. Scialabba, R. Sabia, D. Paolino, D. Capitani, et al. 2015. Polyapartamide-doxorubicin conjugate as potential prodrug for anticancer therapy. *Pharm. Res.* 32: 1557–1569.

Djaldetti, R., R. Inzelberg, N. Giladi, A. D. Korczyn, Y. Peretz-Aharon, M. J. Rabey, Y. Herishano, S. Honigman, S. Badarny, and E. Melamed. 2002. Oral solution of levodopa ethylester for treatment of response fluctuations in patients with advanced Parkinson's disease. *Mov. Disord.* 17: 297–302.

Dobson, P. D. and D. B. Kell. 2008. Carrier-mediated cellular uptake of pharmaceutical drugs: An exception or the rule? *Nat. Rev. Drug Discov.* 7: 205–220.

Doh, M. J., Y. J. Jung, I. Kim, H. S. Kong, and Y. M. Kim. 2003. Synthesis and *in vitro* properties of prednisolone 21-sulfate sodium as a colon-specific prodrug of prednisolone. *Arch. Pharm. Res.* 26: 258–263.

Domião, M. C., K. F. Pasqualoto, M. C. Polli, and R. P. Filho. 2014. To be drug or prodrug: Structure-property exploratory approach regarding oral bioavailability. *J. Pharm. Pharm. Sci.* 17: 532–540.

Duncan, R., S. Gac-Breton, R. Keane, R. Musila, Y. N. Sat, R. Satchi, and F. Searle. 2001. Polymer-drug conjugates, PDEPT and PELT: Basic principles for design and transfer from the laboratory to clinic. *J. Control. Rel.* 74: 135–146.

Duncan, R., P. Kopeckova-Rejmanova, J. Strohalm, I. Hume, H. C. Cable, J. Pohl, J. B. Lloyd, and J. Kopecek. 1987. Anticancer agents coupled to *N*-(2-hydroxypropyl)methacrylamide copolymers. I. Evaluation of daunomycin and puromycin conjugates *in vitro*. *Br. J. Cancer* 55: 165–174.

Duncan, R., L. C. Seymour, L. Scarlett, J. B. Lloyd, P. Rejmanova, and J. Kopecek. 1986. Fate of *N*-(2-hydroxypropyl)methacrylamide copolymers with pendent galactosamine residues after intravenous administration to rats. *Biochim. Biophys. Acta* 880: 62–71.

Erion, M. D., D. A. Bullough, C. C. Lin, and Z. Hong. 2006. HepDirect prodrugs for targeting nucleotide-based antiviral drugs to the liver. *Curr. Opin. Investig. Drugs.* 7: 109–117.

Erion, M. D., K. R. Reddy, S. H. Boyer, M. C. Matelich, J. Gomez-Galeno, R. H. Lemus, B. G. Ugarkar, T. J. Colby, J. Schanzer, and P. D. van Poelje. 2004. Design, synthesis, and characterization of a series of cytochrome P(450) 3A-activated prodrugs (HepDirect prodrugs) useful for targeting phosph(on)ate-based drugs to the liver. *J. Am. Chem. Soc.* 126: 5154–5163.

Erion, M. D., P. D. van Poelje, D. A. Mackenna, T. J. Colby, A. C. Montag, J. M. Fujitaki, D. L. Linemeyer, and D. A. Bullough. 2005. Liver-targeted drug delivery using HepDirect prodrugs. *J. Pharmacol. Exp. Ther.* 312: 554–560.

Ettmayer, P., G. L. Amidon, B. Clement, and B. Testa. 2004. Lessons learned from marketed and investigational prodrugs. *J. Med. Chem.* 47: 2393–2404.

Filipovic-Grcic, J., D. Maysinger, B. Zorc, and I. Jalsenjak. 1995. Macromolecular prodrugs. IV. Alginate-chitosan microspheres of PHEA-l-dopa adduct. *Int. J. Pharm.* 116: 39–44.

Fleisher, D., K. C. Johnson, B. H. Stewart, and G. L. Amidon. 1986. Oral absorption of 21-corticosteroid esters: A function of aqueous stability and intestinal enzyme activity and distribution. *J. Pharm. Sci.* 75: 934–939.

Fleisher, D., B. H. Stewart, and G. L. Amidon. 1985. Design of prodrugs for improved gastrointestinal absorption by intestinal enzyme targeting. In *Methods in Enzymology*, Vol. 112, Part A, Widder, K. J. and Gree, R. (Eds.), pp. 360–381. New York: Academic Press.

Flynn, G. L. and D. J. Lamb. 1970. Factors influencing solvolysis of corticosteroid-21-phosphate esters. *J. Pharm. Sci.* 59: 1433–1438.

Freed, L. E., G. Vunjak-Novakovic, R. J. Biron, D. B. Eagles, D. C. Lesnoy, S. K. Barlow, and R. Langer. 1994. Biodegradable polymer scaffolds for tissue engineering. *Bio/Technol.* 12: 689–693.

Friend, D. R. and G. W. Chang. 1985. Drug glycosides: Potential prodrugs for colon-specific drug delivery. *J. Med. Chem.* 28: 51–57.

Garrett, E. R. and M. E. Royer. 1962. Prediction of stability in pharmaceutical preparations XI. *J. Pharm. Sci.* 51: 451–455.

Glazko, A. J., W. A. Dill, A. W. Kinkel, J. R. Goulet, W. J. Holloway, and R. A. Buchanan. 1977. Absorption and excretion of parenteral doses of chloramphenicol sodium succinate (CMS) in comparison with peroral doses of chloramphenicol (CM). *Clin. Pharm. Ther.* 21: 104.

Greenwald, R. B., C. W. Gilbert, A. Pendri, C. D. Conover, J. Xia, and A. Martinez. 1996. Drug delivery systems: Water soluble taxol 2′-poly(ethylene glycol) ester prodrugs and *in vivo* effectiveness. *J. Med. Chem.* 39: 424–431.

Greenwald, R. B., A. Pendri, C. D. Conover, Y. H. Choe, C. W. Gilbert, A. Martinez, J. Xia, H. Wu, and M. Hsue. 1998. Camptothecin-20-PEG ester transport forms: The effect of spacer group on antitumor activity. *Bioorg. Med. Chem.* 6: 551–562.

Guo, H., S. Sun, Z. Yang, X. Tang, and Y. Wang. 2015. Strategies for ribavirin prodrugs and delivery systems for reducing the side-effect hemolysis and enhancing their therapeutic effect. *J. Control. Release.* 209: 27–36.

Han, H.-K. and G. L. Amidon. 2000. Targeted prodrug design to optimize drug delivery. *AAPS PharmSci.* 2: Article 6.

Hare, L. E., K. C. Yeh, C. A. Ditzler, F. G. McMahon, and D. E. Duggan. 1975. Bioavailability of dexamethasone. II. Dexamethasone phosphate. *Clin. Pharm. Ther.* 18: 330–337.

Harper, N. J. 1959. Drug latentiation. *J. Med. Pharm. Chem.* 1: 467–500.

Harper, N. J. 1962. Drug latentiation. *Prog. Drug Res.* 4: 221–294.

Hecker, S. J. and M. D. Erion. 2008. Prodrugs of phosphates and phosphonates. *J. Med. Chem.* 51: 2328–2345.

Heimbach, T., D. M. Oh, L. Y. Li, N. Rodriguez-Hornedo, G. Garcia, and D. Fleisher. 2003. Enzyme-mediated precipitation of parent drugs from their phosphate prodrugs. *Int. J. Pharm.* 261: 81–92.

Hirano, K., M. Sugiura, K. Miki, S. Iino, H. Suzuki, and T. Uda. 1977. Characterization of tissue-specific isoenzyme of alkaline phosphatase from human placenta and intestine. *Chem. Pharm. Bull. (Tokyo).* 25: 2524–2529.

Hong, W.-H. and D. H. Szulczewski. 1984. Stability of vidarabine-5′-phosphate in aqueous solutions. *J. Parent.Sci. Technol.* 38: 60–64.

Huo, M., Q. Zhu, Q. Wu, T. Yin, L. Wang, L. Yin, and J. Zhou. 2015. Somatostatin receptor-mediated specific delivery of paclitaxel prodrugs for efficient cancer therapy. *J. Pharm. Sci.*104: 2018–2028.

Hurwitz, A. R. and S. T. Liu. 1977. Determination of aqueous solubility and pK_a values of estrogens. *J. Pharm.Sci.* 66: 624–627.

Hutchinson, I., S. A. Jennings, B. R. Vishnuvajjala, A. D. Westwell, and M. F. G. Stevens. 2002. Antitumor benzothiazoles. 16. Synthesis and pharmaceutical properties of antitumor 2-(4-aminophenyl)benzothiazole amino acid prodrugs. *J. Med. Chem.* 45: 744–747.

Huttunen, K. M. and J. Rautio. 2011. Prodrugs—An efficient way to breach delivery and targeting barriers. *Curr. Top. Med. Chem.* 11: 2265–2287.

Huttunen, K. M., H. Raunio, and J. Rautio. 2011. Prodrugs—From serendipity to rational design. *Pharm. Rev.* 63: 750–771.

Hwang, I. Y. and A. A. Elfarra. 1989. Cysteine S-conjugates may act as kidney-selective prodrugs: Formation of 6-mercaptopurine by the renal metabolism of S-(6-purinyl)L-cysteine. *J. Pharm. Exp. Ther.* 251: 448–454.

Järvinen, T. and K. J. Järvinen. 1996. Prodrugs for improved ocular drug delivery. *Adv. Drug Del. Rev.* 19: 203–224.

Johnson, K., G. L. Amidon, and S. Pogany. 1985. Solution kinetics of a water-soluble hydrocortisone prodrug: Hydrocortisone-21-lysinate. *J. Pharm. Sci.* 74: 87–89.

Johansen, M. and H. Bundgaard. 1981a. Decomposition of rolitetracycline and other *N*-Mannich bases and of *N*-hydroxymethyl derivatives in the presence of plasma. *Arch. Pharm. Chem. Sci. Ed.* 9: 40–42.

Johansen, M. and H. Bundgaard. 1981b. Pro-drugs as drug delivery systems. XVI. Novel water-soluble prodrug types for chlorzoxazone by esterification of the *N*-hydroxymethyl derivative. *Arch. Pharm. Chem. Sci. Ed.* 9: 43–54.

Jones, G. 1985. Decreased toxicity and adverse reactions via prodrugs. In *Design of Prodrugs*, Bundgaard, H. (Ed.), pp. 199–241. New York: Elsevier Science.

Jones, R. J. and N. Bischofberger. 1995. Minireview: Nucleotide prodrugs. *Antiviral Res.* 27: 1–17.

Jones, L. A., A. R. Moorman, S. D. Chamberlain, P. de Miranda, D. J. Reynolds, C. L. Burns, and T. A. Krenistky. 1992. Di- and triester prodrugs of the Varicella-Zoster antiviral agent 6-methoxypurine arabinoside. *J. Med. Chem.* 35: 56–63.

Juntunen, J., J. Vepsalainen, R. Niemi, K. Laine, and T. Järvinen. 2003. Synthesis, *in vitro* evaluation, and intraocular pressure effects of water-soluble prodrugs of endocannabinoid noladin ether. *J. Med. Chem.* 46: 5083–5086.

Kauffman, R. E., J. N. Miceli, L. Strebel, J. A. Buckley, A. K. Done, and A. S. Dajani. 1980. Pharmacokinetics of chloramphenicol (CAP) and chloramphenicol-succinate (CAP-Succ) in infants and children. *Clin. Pharm. Ther.* 27: 288–289.

Kaul, M., L. Mark, Y. Zhang, A. K. Parhi, E. J. LaVoie, and D. S. Pilch. 2013. An FtsZ-targeting prodrug with oral anti-staphylococcal efficacy *in vivo*. *Antimicrob. Agents Chemother.* 57: 5860–5869.

Kaul, M., L. Mark, Y. Zhang, A. K. Parhi, Y. L. Lyu, J. Pawlak, S. Saravolatz. et al. 2015. TA709, an FtsZ-targeting benzamide prodrug with improved pharmacokinetics and enhanced in vivo efficacy against methicillin-resistant staphylococcus aureus. *Antimicrob. Agents Chemother.* 59: 4845–4855.

Kearney, A. S. and V. J. Stella. 1992. The *in vitro* enzymatic labilities of chemically distinct phosphomonoesters prodrugs. *Pharm. Res.* 9: 497–503.

Kerr, S. G. and T. I. Kalman. 1992. Highly water-soluble lipophilic prodrugs of the anti-HIV nucleoside analogue 2′,3′-dideoxycytidine and its 3′-fluoro derivative. *J. Med. Chem.* 35: 1996–2001.

Khmelnitsky, Y. L., C. Budde, J. M. Arnold, A. Usyatinsky, D. S. Clark, and J. S. Dordick. 1997. Synthesis of water-soluble paclitaxel derivatives by enzymatic acylation. *J. Am. Chem. Soc.* 119: 11554–11555.

Kopecek, J. 1991. Targetable polymeric anticancer drugs. Temporal control of drug activity. *Ann. NY Acad. Sci.* 618: 335–344.

Kopecek, J., P. Kopeckova, T. Minko, and Z. Lu. 2000. HPMA copolymer-anticancer drug conjugates: Design, activity, and mechanism of action. *Eur. J. Pharm. Biopharm.* 50: 61–81.

Kovach, I. M., I. H. Pittman, and T. Higuchi. 1975. Amino acid esters of phenolic drugs as potentially useful prodrugs. *J. Pharm. Sci.* 64: 1070–1071.

Kramer, W. G., E. R. Rensimer, C. D. Ericson, and L. K. Pickering. 1984. Comparative bioavailability of intravenous and oral chloramphenicol in adults. *J. Clin. Pharm.* 24: 181–186.

Krise, J. P., W. N. Charman, S. A. Charman, and V. J. Stella. 1999a. A novel prodrug approach for tertiary amines. 3. In vivo evaluation of two N-phophonooxymethyl prodrugs in rats and dogs. *J. Pharm. Sci.* 88: 928–932.

Krise, J. P., S. Narisawa, and V. J. Stella. 1999b. A novel prodrug approach for tertiary amines. 2. Physicochemical and *in vitro* enzymatic evaluation of selected *N*-phosphonooxymethyl prodrugs. *J. Pharm. Sci.* 88: 922–927.

Krise, J. P., J. Zygmunt, G. I. Georg, and V. J. Stella. 1999c. Novel prodrug approach for tertiary amines: Synthesis and preliminary evaluation of *N*-phosphonooxymethyl prodrugs. *J. Med. Chem.* 42: 3094–3100.

Kryger, M. B., A. A. Smith, B. M. Wohl, and A. N. Zelikin. 2014. Macromolecular prodrugs for controlled delivery of ribavirin. *Macromol. Biosci.* 14: 173–185.

Kryger, M. B., B. M. Wohl, A. A. Smith, and A. N. Zelikin. 2013. Macromolecular prodrugs of ribavirin combat side effects and toxicity with no loss of activity of the drug. *Chem. Commun.* 49: 2643–2645.

Kumar, P. and C. Singh. 2013. A study on solubility enhancement methods for poorly water soluble drugs. *Am. J. Pharmacol. Sci.* 1: 67–73.

Kumpulainen, H., N. Mähönen, M. L. Laitinen, M. Jaurakkajarvi, H. Raunio, R. O. Juvonen, J. Vepsäläinen, T. Järvinen, and J. Rautio. 2006. Evaluation of hydroxyimine as cytochrome P450-selective prodrug structure. *J. Med. Chem.* 49: 1207–1211.

Kwee, K. S. L. and L. M. L. Stolk. 1984. Formulation of a stable vidarabine phosphate injection, *Pharm. Weekblad, Sci. Ed.* 6: 101–104.

Lallemand, F., O. Felt-Baeyens, S. Rudaz, A. R. Hamel, F. Hubler, R. Wenger, M. Mutter, K. Besseghir, and R. Gurny. 2005a. Conversion of cyclosporine A prodrugs in human tears vs. rabbits tears. *Eur. J. Pharm. Biopharm.* 59: 51–56.

Lallemand, F., P. Perottet, O. Felt-Baeyens, W. Kloeti, F. Philippoz, J. Marfurt, K. Besseghir, and R. Gurny. 2005b. A water-soluble prodrug of cyclosporine A for ocular application: A stability study. *Eur. J. Pharm. Sci.* 26: 124–129.

Laurent, T. C., U. B. G. Laurent, and J. R. E. Fraser. 1995. Functions of hyaluronan. *Ann. Rheum. Dis.* 54: 429–432.

Lee, J. S., Y. J. Jung, M. J. Doh, and Y. M. Kim. 2001. Synthesis and properties of dextran-nalidixic acid ester as a colon-specific prodrug of nalidixic acid. *Drug Dev. Ind. Pharm.* 27: 331–336.

Lee, W. A., H. F.-L. Lu, P. W. Maffuid, M. T. Botet, P. A. Baldwin, T. A. Benkert, and C. K. Klingbeil. 1992. The synthesis, characterization and biological testing of a novel class of mucosal permeation enhancers. *J. Control. Rel.* 22: 223–237.

Leppanen, J., J. Huuskonen, J. Savolainen, T. Nevalainen, H. Taipale, J. Vepsalainen, J. Gynther, and T. Järvinen. 2000. Synthesis of a water-soluble prodrug of entacapone. *Bioorg. Med. Chem. Lett.* 10: 1967–1969.

Li, M., Z. Liang, X. Sun, T. Gong, and Z. Zhang. 2014. A polymeric prodrug of 5-fluorouracil-1-acetic acid using a multi-hydroxyl polyethylene glycol derivative as the drug carrier. *PLoS One* 9: e112888.

Liederer, B. M. and R. T. Borchardt. 2006. Enzymes involved in the bioconversion of ester-based prodrugs. *J. Pharm. Sci.* 95: 1177–1195.

Liu, Z., J. T. Robinson, X. Sun, and H. Dai. 2008. PEGylated nanographene oxide for delivery of water-insoluble cancer drugs. *J. Am. Chem. Soc.* 130: 10876–10877.

Luo, Y. and G. D. Prestwich. 1999. Synthesis and selective cytotoxicity of a hyaluronic acid-antitumor bioconjugate. *Bioconjugate Chem.* 10: 755–763.

Maeda, H., L. Seymour, and Y. Miyamoto. 1992. Conjugates of antitumor agents and polymers: Advantages of macromolecular therapeutics *in vivo*. *Bioconjugate Chem.* 3: 351–362.

Magri, N. F. 1985. Modified taxols as anticancer agents. PhD dissertation, Virginia Polytechnic Institute and State University, Blacksburg.

Magri, N. F. and D. G. I. Kingston. 1988. Modified taxols. 4. Synthesis and biological activity of taxols modified in the side chain. *J. Nat. Prod.* 51: 298–306.

Majumdar, S., S. Duvvuri, and A. K. Mitra. 2004. Membrane transporter/receptor-targeted prodrug design: Strategies for human and veterinary drug develoment. *Adv. Drug Deliv. Rev.* 56: 1437–1452.

Majumdar, S. and K. B. Sloan. 2006. Synthesis, hydrolysis and dermal delivery of N-alkyl-N-alkyloxy-carbonylaminomethyl (NANAOCAM) derivatives of phenol, imide and thiol containing drugs. *Bioorg. Med. Chem. Lett.* 16: 3590–3594.

Martin, B. D., S. A. Ampofo, R. J. Linhardt, and J. S. Dordick. 1992. Biocatalytic synthesis of sugar-containing polyacrylate-based hydrogels. *Macromolecules* 25: 7081–7085.

Mathew, A. E., M. R. Mejillano, J. P. Nath, R. H. Himes, and V. J. Stella. 1992. Synthesis and evaluation of some water-soluble prodrugs and derivatives of taxol with antitumor activity. *J. Med. Chem.* 35: 145–151.

Mattarei, A., M. Azzolini, M. Zoratti, L. Biasutto, and C. Paradisi. 2015. N-Monosubstituted methoxy-oligo(ethylene glycol) carbamate ester prodrugs of resveratrol. *Molecules* 20: 16085–16102.

May, D. E. and C. J. Kratochvil. 2010. Attention-deficit hyperactivity disorder: Recent advances in paediatric pharmacotherapy. *Drugs* 70: 15–40.

McLeod, A. D., D. R. Friend, and T. N. Tozier. 1993. Synthesis and chemical stability of glucocorticoid-dextran esters: Potential prodrugs for colon-specific delivery. *Int. J. Pharm.* 92: 105–114.

McLeod, A. D., D. R. Friend, and T. N. Tozier. 1994. Synthesis and chemical stability of glucocorticoid-dextran conjugates as potential prodrugs for colon-specific delivery: Hydrolysis in rat gastrointestinal tract contents. *J. Pharm. Sci.* 83: 1284–1288.

Melby, J. C. and R. H. Silber. 1981. Clinical pharmacology of water-soluble corticosteroid esters. *Am. Pract.Digest* 12: 156–161.

Melby, J. C. and M. St. Cyr. 1961. Comparative studies on absorption and metabolic disposal of water-soluble corticosteroid esters. *Metabolism* 10: 75–82.

Mellado, W. F., N. F. Magri, D. G. I. Kingston, R. Garcia-Arenas, G. A. Orr, and S. B. Horwitz. 1984. Preparation and biological activity of taxol acetates. *Biochem. Biophys. Res. Commun.* 124: 329–336.

Miyabo, S., T. Nakamura, S. Kuwazima, and S. Kishida. 1981. A comparison of the bioavailability and potency of dexamethasone phosphate and sulphate in man. *Eur. J. Clin. Pharmacol.* 20: 277–282.

Mollmann, H., P. Rhodewald, J. Barth, M. Verho, and H. Derendorf. 1989. Pharmacokinetics and dose linearity testing of methylprednisolone phosphate. *Biopharm. Drug Dispos.* 10: 453–464.

Molteni, L. 1982. Effects of the polysaccharidic carrier on the kinetic fate of drugs linked to dextran and inulin in macromolecular compounds. In *Optimization of Drug Delivery*, Bundgaard, H., Hansen, A. B., and Kofod, H., (Eds.), pp. 285–300. Copenhagen: Munksgaard.

Mørk, N., H. Bundgaard, M. Shalmi, and S. Christensen. 1990. Furosemide prodrugs: Synthesis, enzymatic hydrolysis and solubility of various furosemide esters. *Int. J. Pharm.* 60: 163–169.

Nichifor, M. and E. H. Schacht. 1997. Chemical and enzymatic hydrolysis of dipeptide derivatives of 5-fluorouracil. *J. Control. Rel.* 47: 271–281.

Nicolaou, K. C., C. Riemer, M. A. Kerr, D. Rideout, and W. Wrasidlo. 1993. Design, synthesis and biological activity of protaxols. *Nature* 364: 464–466.

Niculescu-Duvaz, I., R. Spooner, R. Marai, and C. J. Springer. 1998. Gene-directed enzyme prodrug therapy of cancer. *Bioconjug. Chem.* 9: 4–22.

Nielsen, A. B., A. Buur, and C. Larsen. 2005. Bioreversible quaternary N-acyloxymethyl derivatives of the tertiary amines bupivacaine and lidocaine—synthesis, aqueous solubility and stability in buffer, human plasma and simulated intestinal fluid. *Eur. J. Pharm. Sci.* 24: 433–440.

Nielsen, L. S., H. Bundgaard, and E. Falch. 1992. Prodrugs of thiabendazole with increased water-solubility. *Acta Pharm. Nord.* 4: 43–49.

Nielsen, L. S., F. Sløk, and H. Bundgaard. 1994. N-Alkoxycarbonyl prodrugs of mebendazole with increased water solubility. *Int. J. Pharm.* 102: 231–239.

Niethammer, A., G. Gaedicke, H. N. Lode, and W. Wrasidlo. 2001. Synthesis and preclinical characterization of a paclitaxel prodrug with improved antitumor activity and water solubility. *Bioconjugate Chem.* 12: 414–420.

Notari, R. E. 1973. Pharmacokinetics and molecular modification: Implications in drug design and evaluation. *J. Pharm. Sci.* 62: 865–881.

Notari, R. E. 1985. Theory and practice of prodrug kinetics. In *Methods in Enzymology*, Vol. 112, Part A, Widder, K. J. and Gree, R. (Eds.), pp. 309–323. New York: Academic Press.

Nudelman, A., E. Gnizi, Y. Katz, R. Azulai, M. Cohen-Ohana, R. Zhuk, S. R. Sampson et al. 2001. *Eur. J. Med. Chem.* 36: 63–74.

Orlowski, M., H. Mizoguchi, and S. Wilk. 1979. *N*-Acyl-γ-glutamyl derivatives of sulfamethoxazole as models of kidney-selective prodrugs. *J. Pharm. Exp. Ther.* 212: 167–172.

Peng, C., C. Liu, and X. Tang. 2010. Determination of physicochemical properties and degradation kinetics of triamcinolone acetonide palmitate in vitro. *Drug Dev. Ind. Pharm.* 36: 1469–1476.

Pevarello, P. 2009. Recent drug approvals from the US FDA and EMEA: What the future holds. *Future Med. Chem.* 1: 35–48.

Phillips, A. M. F., F., Noqueira, F. Murtinheira, and M. T. Barros. 2015. Synthesis and antimalarial evaluation of prodrugs of novel fosmidomycin analogues. *Bioorg. Med. Chem. Lett.* 25: 2112–2116.

Pitman, I. H. 1976. Three chemical approaches towards the solubilisation of drugs: Control of enantiomer composition, salt selection, and pro-drug formation. *Austr. J. Pharm. Sci.* NS5:17–19.

Pradere, U., E. C. Garnier-Amblard, S. J. Coats, F. Amblard, and R. F. Schinazi. 2014. Synthesis of nucleoside phosphate and phosphonate prodrugs. *Chem. Rev.* 114: 9154–9218.

Prestwich, G. D., D. M. Marecak, J. F. Marecek, K. P. Vercruysse, and M. R. Ziebell. 1998. Chemical modification of hyaluronic acid for drug delivery, biomaterials, and biochemical probes. In *The Chemistry, Biology, and Medical Applications of Hyaluronan and Its Derivatives*, Laurent, T. C. (Ed.), pp. 43–65. London: Portland Press.

Prusiner, P. and M. Sundaralingam. 1972. Stereochemistry of nucleic acids and their constituents XXIX. Crystal and molecular structure of allopurinol, a potent inhibitor of xanthine oxidase. *Acta Cryst.* B28: 2148–2152.

Radhakrishnan, A. N. 1977. Intestinal dipeptidases and dipeptide transport in the monkey and in man. In *Peptide Transport and Hydrolysis*, Ciba Foundation Symposium, pp. 37–59. New York: Elsevier Science.

Rautio, J. 2010. Prodrug strategies in drug design. In *Prodrugs and Targeted Delivery: Towards Better ADME Properties*, Rautio, J. (Ed.), pp. 1–30, Weinheim, Germany: Wiley-VCH Verlag GmbH.

Rautio, J., H. Kumpulainen, T. Heimbach, R. Oliyai, D. Oh, T. Järvinen, and J. Savolainen. 2008. Prodrugs: Design and clinical applications. *Nat. Rev. Drug Discov.* 7: 255–270.

Repta, A. J., B. J. Rawson, R. D. Shaffer, K. B. Sloan, N. Bodor, and T. Higuchi. 1975. Rational development of a soluble prodrug of a cytotoxic nucleoside: Preparation and properties of arabinosyladenine 5'-formate. *J. Pharm. Sci.* 64: 392–396.

Rihova, B., J. Kopecek, P. Kopeckova-Rejmanova, J. Strohalm, D. Plocova, and H. Semoradova. 1986. Bioaffinity therapy with antibodies and drugs bound to soluble synthetic polymers. *J. Chromatogr.* 376: 221–233.

Rimoli, M. G., L. Avallone, P. de Caprariis, A. Galeone, F. Forni, and M. A. Vandelli. 1999. Synthesis and characterization of poly(*d,l*-lactic acid)-idoxuridine conjugate. *J. Control. Rel.* 58: 61–68.

Rodrigues, P. C. A., U. Beyer, P. Schumacher, T. Roth, H. H. Fiebig, C. Unger, L. Messori, et al. 1999. Acid-sensitive polyethylene glycol conjugates of doxorubicin: Preparation, *in vitro* efficacy and intracellular distribution. *Bioorg. Med. Chem.* 7: 2517–2524.

Roy, S. D. and E. Manoukian. 1994. Permeability of ketorolac acid and its ester analogs (prodrug) through human cadaver skin. *J. Pharm. Sci.* 83: 1548–1553.

Sadafi, M., R. Oliyai, and V. J. Stella. 1993. Phosphoryloxymethyl carbamates and carbonates—Novel water-soluble prodrugs for amines and hindered alcohols. *Pharm. Res.* 10: 1350–1355.

Schacht, E., L. Ruys, J. Vermeersch, and J. P. Remon. 1984. Polymer-drug combinations: Synthesis and characterization of modified polysaccharides containing procainamide moieties. *J. Control. Rel.* 1: 33–46.

Schmidt, U., U. C. Dubach, I. Bieder, and B. Funk. 1972. Alkaline phosphatase: A marker enzyme for brush border membrane. *Experientia* 28: 385–386.

Scriba, G. K. E. 1993. Phenytoin-lipid conjugates: Chemical, plasma esterase-mediated, and pancreatic lipase-mediated hydrolysis *in vitro*. *Pharm. Res.* 10: 1181–1186.

Sezaki, H. 1989. Biopharmaceutical aspects of a chemical approach to drug delivery: Macromolecule-drug conjugates. *Yakugaku Zasshi* 109: 611–621.

Sezaki, H. and M. Hashida. 1984. Macromolecule-drug conjugates in targeted cancer chemotherapy. *CRC Crit.Rev. Ther. Drug Carrier Syst.* 1: 1–38.

Sharma, S. K., K. D. Bagshawe, and R. H. Begent. 2004. Antibody-directed enzyme prodrug therapy (ADEPT) for cancer. *Curr. Opin. Investig. Drugs* 6: 611–615.

Shen, W., J. S. Kim, P. E. Kish, J. Zhang, S. Mitchell, B. G. Gentry, J. M. Breitenbach, J. C. Drach, and J. Hilfinger. 2009a. Design and synthesis of vidarabine prodrugs as antiviral agents. *Bioorg. Med. Chem. Lett.* 19: 792–796.

Shen, W., J. S. Kim, S. Mitchell, P. Kish, P. Kijek, and J. Hilfinger. 2009b. 5′-O-D-valyl ara A, a potential prodrug for improving oral bioavailability of the antiviral agent vidarabine. *Nucleos. Nucleot. Nucleic Acids.* 28: 43–55.

Simmons, D. M., G. A. Portmann, and V. R. Chandran. 1995. Danazol amino acid prodrugs *in vitro* and *in situ* biopharmaceutical evaluation. *Drug Dev. Ind. Pharm.* 21: 687–708.

Sinha, V. R. and R. Kumria. 2001. Colonic drug delivery: Prodrug approach. *Pharm. Res.* 18: 557–564.

Sinkula, A. A. 1975. Prodrug approach in drug design. In *Annual Reports in Medicinal Chemistry*, Vol. 10, Heinzelman, R. V. (Ed.), pp. 306–316. New York: Academic Press.

Sinkula, A. A. 1977. Perspective on prodrugs and analogs in drug design. In *Design of Biopharmaceutical Properties through Prodrugs and Analogs*, Roche, E. B. (Ed.), pp. 1–17. Washington, DC: American Pharmaceutical Association.

Sinkula, A. A. and S. H. Yalkowsky. 1975. Rationale for design of biologically reversible drug derivatives: Prodrugs. *J. Pharm. Sci.* 64: 181–210.

Sloan, K. B., S. A. M. Koch, and K. G. Siver. 1984. Mannich base derivatives of theophylline and 5-fluorouracil: Syntheses, properties and topical delivery characteristics. *Int. J. Pharm.* 21: 251–264.

Sloan, K. B. and S. Wasdo. 2003. Designing for topical delivery: Prodrugs can make the difference. *Med. Res. Rev.* 23: 763–793.

Sloan, K. B., S. Wasdo, and J. Rautio. 2006. Design for optimized topical delivery: Prodrugs and a paradigm change. *Pharm. Res.* 23: 2729–2747.

Smith, A. A., B. M. Wohl, M. B. Kryger, N. Hedermann, C. Guerrero-Sanchez, A. Postma, A. N. Zelikin. 2014. Macromolecular prodrugs of ribavirin: Concerted efforts of the carrier and the drug. *Adv. Healthc. Mater.* 3: 1404–1407.

Smith, A. A. A., K. Zuwala, M. B. L. Kryger, B. M. Wohl, C. Guerrero-Sanchez, M. Tolstrup, A. Postma, and A. N. Zelikin. 2015. Macromolecular prodrugs of ribavirin: Towards a treatment for co-infection with HIV and HCV. *Chem. Sci.* 6: 264–269.

Sofia, M. J. 2013. Nucleotide prodrugs for the treatment of HCV infection. *Adv. Pharm.* 67: 39–73.

Sofia, M. J. 2014. Beyond sofosbuvir: What opportunity exists for a better nucleoside/nucleotide to treat hepatitis C? *Antiviral Res.* 107: 119–124.

Stella, V. 1975. Pro-drugs: An overview and definition. In *Pro-drugs as Novel Drug Delivery Systems*, Higuchi, T. and Stella, V. (Eds.), pp. 1–115. Washington, DC: American Chemical Society.

Stella, V. J. 2007. A case for prodrugs. In *Prodrugs: Challenges and Rewards: Parts 1 and 2*, Stella, V., Borchardt, R. Hageman, M., Oliya, R., Maag, H., and Tilley, J. (Eds.), pp. 3–33. New York: Springer Science + Business Media.

Stella, V. J. 2010. Prodrugs: Some thoughts and current issues. *J. Pharm. Sci.* 99: 4755–4765.

Stella, V. J., W. N. A. Charman, and V. H. Naringrekar. 1985. Prodrugs: Do they have advantages in clinical practice? *Drugs* 29: 455–473.

Stella, V. J., S. Martodihardjo, K. Terada, and V. M. Rao. 1998. Some relationships between the physical properties of various 3-acyloxymethyl prodrugs of phenytoin to structure: Potential *in vivo* performance implications. *J. Pharm. Sci.* 87: 1235–1241.

Stinchcomb, A. L., R. Dua, A. Paliwal, R. W. Woodard, and G. L. Flynn. 1995. A solubility and related physicochemical property comparison of buprenorphine and its 3-alkyl esters. *Pharm. Res.* 12: 1526–1529.

Strebel, L., J. Miceli, R. Kauffman, R. Poland, A. Dajani, and A. Done. 1980. Pharmacokinetics of chloramphenicol (CAP) and chloramphenicol-succinate (CAP-Succ) in infants and children. *Clin. Pharmacol. Ther.* 27: 288–289.

Takata, J., Y. Karube, M. Hanada, K. Matsunaga, Y. Matsushima, T. Sendo, and T. Aoyama. 1995a. Vitamin K prodrugs. 1. Synthesis of amino acid esters of menahydroquinone-4 and enzymatic reconversion to an active form. *Pharm. Res.* 12: 18–23.

Takata, J., Y. Karube, Y. Nagata, and Y. Matsushima. 1995b. Water-soluble prodrugs of vitamin E. 1. Preparation and enzymatic hydrolysis of aminoalkanecarboxylic acid esters of d-α-tocopherol. *J. Pharm. Sci.* 84: 96–100.

Tammara, V. K., M. M. Narurkar, A. M. Crider, and M. A. Khan. 1994. Morpholinoalkyl ester prodrugs of diclofenac: Synthesis, *in vitro* and *in vivo* evaluation. *J. Pharm. Sci.* 83: 644–648.

Taylor, H. E. and K. B. Sloan. 1998. 1-Alkyloxymethyl prodrugs of 5-fluorouracil (5-FU): Synthesis, physicochemical properties, and topical delivery of 5-FU. *J. Pharm. Sci.* 87: 15–20.

Therisod, M. and A. M. Klibanov. 1986. Facile enzymatic preparation of monoacylated sugars in pyridine. *J. Am. Chem. Soc.* 108: 5638–5640.

Ulbrich, K. and V. Subr. 2004. Polymeric anticancer drugs with pH-controlled activation. *Adv. Drug Deliv. Rev.* 56: 1023–1050.

van de Waterbeemd H., D. A. Smith, K. Beamont, and D. K. Walker. 2001. Property-based design: Optimization of drug absorption and pharmacokinetics. *J. Med. Chem.* 44: 1313–1333.

van Rompay, A. R., M. Johansson, and A. Karlsson. 2000. Phosphorylation of nucleosides and nucleoside analogs by mammalian nucleoside monophosphate kinases. *Pharmacol. Ther.* 87: 189–198.

Varia, S., S. Schuller, K. B. Sloan, and V. J. Stella. 1984a. Phenytoin prodrugs. III. Water-soluble prodrugs for oral and/or parenteral use. *J. Pharm. Sci.* 73: 1068–1073.

Varia, S. A., S. Schuller, and V. J. Stella. 1984b. Phenytoin prodrugs. IV. Hydrolysis of various 3-(hydroxy-methyl)phenytoin esters. *J. Pharm. Sci.* 73: 1074–1080.

Varia, S. A. and V. J. Stella. 1984. Phenytoin prodrugs. VI. *In vivo* evaluation of a phosphate ester prodrug of phenytoin after parenteral administration to rats. *J. Pharm. Sci.* 73: 1087–1090.

Vartikovski, L., Z. R. Lu, K. Mitchell, I. de Aos, and J. Kopecek. 2001. Water-soluble HPMA copolymer-wortmannin conjugate retains phosphoinositide 3-kinase inhibitory activity *in vitro* and *in vivo*. *J. Control. Rel.* 74: 275–281.

Vej-Hansen, B. and H. Bundgaard. 1979. Kinetics of degradation of rolitetracycline in aqueous solutions and reconstituted formulation. *Arch. Pharm. Chem. Sci. Ed.* 7: 65–77.

Vercruysse, K. P. and G. D. Prestwich. 1998. Hyaluronate derivatives in drug delivery. *Crit. Rev. Ther. Drug Carrier Syst.* 15: 513–555.

Vermeersch, H., J. P. Remon, D. Permentier, and E. Schacht. 1990. *In vitro* antitrichomonal activity of water-soluble prodrug esters of metronidazole. *Int. J. Pharm.* 60: 253–260.

Vyas, D. M., H. Wong, A. R. Crosswell, A. M. Casazza, J. O. Knipe, S. W. Mamber, and T. W. Doyle. 1993. Synthesis and antitumor evaluation of water soluble taxol phosphates. *Bioorg. Med. Chem. Lett.* 3: 1357–1360.

Watanabe, K. A., A. Matsuda, M. J. Halat, D. H. Hollenberg, J. S. Nisselbaum, and J. J. Fox. 1981. Nucleosides. 114. 5′-*O*-Glucuronides of 5-fluorouridine and 5-fluorocytidine. Masked precursors of anticancer nucleosides. *J. Med. Chem.* 24: 893–897.

Weiner, B.-Z. and A. Zilkha. 1973. Polyethylene glycol derivatives of procaine. *J. Med. Chem.* 16: 573–574.

Wichitnithad, W., U. Nimmannit, S. Wacharasindhu, P. Rojsitthisak. 2011. Synthesis, characterization and biological evaluation of succinate prodrugs of curcuminoids for colon cancer treatment. *Molecules* 16: 1888–1900.

Wilk, S., H. Mizoguchi, and M. Orlowski. 1978. γ-Glutamyl dopa: A kidney-specific dopamine precursor. *J. Pharm. Exp. Ther.* 206: 227–232.

Williams, A. and R. A. Naylor. 1971. Evidence for SN 2(P) mechanism in the phosphorylation of alkaline phosphatase by substrate. *J. Chem. Soc. B* 1973–1979.

Williams, D. B., S. A. Varia, V. J. Stella, and I. H. Pitman. 1983. Evaluation of the prodrug potential of the sulfate esters of acetaminophen and 3-hydroxymethyl-phenytoin. *Int. J. Pharm.* 14: 113–120.

Windholz, M., S. Budavari, R. F. Blumetti, and E. S. Otterbein. (Eds.). 1983. *Merck Index*, 10th ed. Rahway, NJ: Merck.

Wohl, B. M., A. A. Smith, B. E. Jensen, A. N. Zelikin. 2014. Macromolecular (pro)drugs with concurrent direct activity against the hepatitis C virus and inflammation. *J. Control. Release*. 196: 197–207.

Wu, D. C., C. R. Cammarata, H. J. Park, B. T. Rhodes, and C. M. Ofner, 2013. Preparation, drug release, and cell growth inhibition of a gelatin: Doxorubicin conjugate. *Pharm. Res.* 30: 2087–2096.

Zalipsky, S., C. Gilon, and A. Zilkha. 1983. Attachment of drugs to polyethylene glycols. *Eur. Polym. J.* 19: 1177–1183.

Zawilska, J. B., J. Wojcieszak, and A. B. Olejniczak. 2013. Prodrugs: A challenge for the drug development. *Pharmacol. Rep.* 65: 1–14.

Zhao, Z., D. G. I. Kingston, and A. R. Crosswell. 1991. Modified taxols. 6. Preparation of water soluble prodrugs of taxol. *J. Nat. Prod.* 54: 1607–1611.

Zhou, P., X. Sun, and Z. Zhang. 2014. Kidney-targeted drug delivery systems. *Acta Pharm. Sinica B*. 4: 37–42.

Zlojkowska, Z., H. J. Krasuka, and J. Pachecka. 1982. Enzymatic hydrolysis of amino acid derivatives of benzocaine. *Xenobiotica* 12: 359–364.

Zou, M. J., G. Cheng, H. Okamoto, X. H. Hao, F. An, F. D. Cui, and K. Danjo. 2005. Colon-specific drug delivery systems based on cyclodextrin prodrugs: *In vitro* evaluation of 5-aminosalicylic acid from its cyclodextrin conjugates. *World J. Gastroenterol.* 11: 7457–7460.

17 Particle Size Reduction

Robert W. Lee, James McShane, J. Michael Shaw, Ray W. Wood, Dinesh B. Shenoy, Xiang (Lisa) Li, and Zhanguo Yue

CONTENTS

INTRODUCTION

Nanotechnology and nanotechnology-enabled product development is a rapidly growing new frontier, with increasing industrial demand for smaller and smaller particle sizes. The smaller particle sizes may translate to easier particle manipulation and may be instrumental for the creation of advanced materials. In the pharmaceutical and biotechnology industry in particular, nanoengineering has made its mark and is influencing every segment and subspecialty. Particle size reduction (or often referred to as micronization) offers a significant opportunity for formulators to solve the product development hurdles inherent with poorly water-soluble active pharmaceutical ingredients (APIs).

In the case of formulations intended for oral administration, poorly water-soluble APIs typically suffer from an inadequate or highly variable rate and/or extent of drug absorption (sometimes as a function of food in the stomach, i.e., fed/fasted variability). Particle size reduction of the API before formulating will significantly increase the specific surface area and subsequently the rate of dissolution of the drug in the gut milieu. Therefore, in the case of poorly water-soluble APIs for which absorption is dissolution limited, particle size reduction may result in significant improvement in the rate and extent of drug absorption such that the bioavailability requirements of the drug are met.

In the case of formulations intended for intravenous administration, size reduction of APIs to nanometer-sized particles render a sterile, aqueous dispersion of such particles infusible. Indeed, particle size reduction methodologies have advanced to the point where nanometer-sized crystalline API particles can be realized. This size reduction approach provides a valuable formulation alternative to the traditional formulation approach of ensuring that a drug is solubilized before intravenous administration. It alleviates the potential issues associated with utilizing high concentrations of aqueous compatible cosolvents and surfactants to solubilize the drug.

In addition, size reduction can also enhance delivery of poorly water-soluble APIs to the respiratory tract. Specifically, aerosolized particles should have aerodynamic diameters in the range of 1–5 μm. With larger particles, deposition occurs primarily on the back of the throat, which can lead to systemic absorption and undesired side effects.

This chapter will provide a theoretical basis for the use of size reduction techniques to solve the formulator's challenge with poorly water-soluble APIs. It will also describe various methodologies available for size reduction, and will outline capabilities and limitations of each. Finally, several examples will be presented where size reduction techniques to nanoparticle sizes have been successfully applied to poorly water-soluble APIs. These examples will include drugs intended for oral and parenteral administration.

THEORY

There are a number of physicochemical properties of an API that are impacted upon size reduction, which need to be considered while resolving pharmaceutical problems related to solubility limitations. Clearly, dissolution rate and its dependence upon particle size reduction is one of those critical properties (Ross and Morrison, 1988; Rabinow, 2004; Kocbek et al., 2006). For example, in the case of oral administration of a poorly water-soluble API, the increase in dissolution rate attendant with size reduction provides for more drug in solution, and available for absorption, during its gastrointestinal transit (Chaumeil, 1998; Merisko-Liversidge et al., 2003; Patravale et al., 2004; Pouton, 2006). In the case of intravenous administration, the dissolution rate will, to a large extent, determine the distribution kinetics and hence availability of drug to interact with pharmacological receptors at the molecular level. Therefore, dissolution phenomena and its dependence on particle size are critical to understanding the value of size reduction to pharmaceutical applications (Setnikar, 1977; Rasenack and Muller, 2002; Merisko-Liversidge et al., 2003; Mosharraf and Nystrom, 2003). This section will focus on and review the theoretical aspects of dissolution, crystal growth, and solubility of crystalline APIs with an emphasis on how these properties are affected by particle size diminution (Noyes and Whitney, 1897; Brunner and Tolloczko, 1900; Nernst, 1904; Hixson and Crowell, 1931; Tawashi, 1968; Anderson, 1980; Cammarata et al., 1980; Valvani and Yalkowsky, 1980; Braun, 1983; Greco Macie and Grant, 1986; Zipp and Rodriguez-Hornedo, 1989; Abdou, 1990; Grant and Higuchi, 1990; Sokoloski, 1990; Grant and Chow, 1991; Ragnarsson et al., 1992; Canselier, 1993; Lu et al., 1993; Yao and Laradji, 1993; Yonezawa, 1994, 1995; Lindfors et al., 2006a, b). The relevance of particle size reduction of crystalline APIs to the improvement of bioavailability (Moschwitzer and Muller, 2006) will also be addressed.

DISSOLUTION PHENOMENA

The dissolution rate of a drug is usually determined experimentally. However, there is an abundance of theoretical and quantitative structure–activity relationship (QSAR) models (Grant and Higuchi, 1990) that provide estimates of the dissolution rates. The mass of the solute (m) at any given time can be defined as

$$m = V c_t \tag{17.1}$$

where V is the volume of the bulk solution and c_t is the concentration of the solute at time t. It follows that

$$\frac{dm}{dt} = V\left(\frac{dc_t}{dt}\right) \tag{17.2}$$

where dm/dt is the rate of dissolution.

If one assumes that a given solid material is thoroughly wetted, it is known that the dissolution rate is strictly proportional to the specific surface area (S) of the dissolving solid, that is,

$$\frac{dm}{dt} \propto S \tag{17.3}$$

The dependence of dissolution rate to specific surface area is the basis for pursuing particle size reduction as a method of increasing the bioavailability of poorly water-soluble drugs.

The dissolution rate per unit surface area is referred to as the *intrinsic dissolution rate* or *mass flux* (J), and is given as

$$J = \left(\frac{dm}{dt}\right)\left(\frac{1}{S}\right) \tag{17.4}$$

The observed dissolution rate may be thought of as being composed of both transport and surface reaction processes. This being the case, then the observed rate constant (k_1) can be expressed as follows:

$$\frac{1}{k_1} = \frac{1}{k_T} + \frac{1}{k_R} \tag{17.5}$$

where k_T is the rate constant describing transport phenomena and k_R is that for reaction. Equation 17.5 can be rewritten as

$$k_1 = \frac{k_T k_R}{k_T + k_R} \tag{17.6}$$

When transport is rate-limiting, $k_T \ll k_R$, and Equations 17.5 and 17.6 reduce to

$$k_1 \sim k_T \tag{17.7}$$

When the surface reaction is rate-limiting, $k_R \ll k_T$, and Equations 17.5 and 17.6 reduce to

$$k_1 \sim k_R \tag{17.8}$$

Two of the simplest theories to explain the dissolution rate of solutes are the interfacial barrier model and the diffusion-layer model (Figures 17.1 and 17.2).

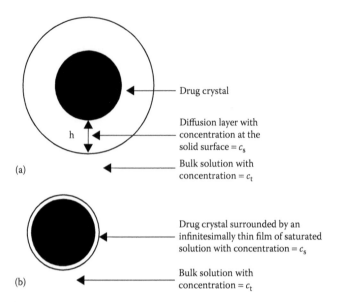

FIGURE 17.1   (a) Diffusion-layer model of dissolution. (b) Interfacial barrier model of dissolution.

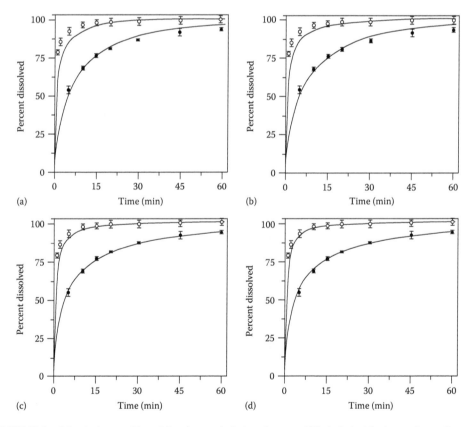

FIGURE 17.2   Dissolution profiles of fine (open circles) and coarse (filled circles) hydrocortisone (Lu et al., 1993). Simulated curves were drawn using spherical geometry without (a) and with (b) a time-dependent diffusion-layer thickness and cylindrical geometry without (c) and with (d) a time-dependent diffusion-layer thickness. Error bars represent 95% CI ($n = 3$). (Reprinted from Lu, A. T. K. et al. *Pharm. Res.*, 10, 1308–1314, 1993, Copyright 1993. With permission from Kluwer Academic Plenum Publishers.)

Both of these theories make the following two assumptions:

1. The solid–liquid interface consists of an infinitesimally thin film (h) of saturated solution that is in intimate contact with the solid.
2. The bulk of the solution is assumed to be well mixed and the concentration of the dissolving solid in the bulk at any given time is c_t.

Interfacial Barrier Model

According to this model, the intrinsic dissolution rate (J) is controlled by the surface reaction between the solute and solvent. If this reaction is first-order, then

$$J = \left(\frac{dm}{dt}\right)\left(\frac{1}{S}\right) = k_R\left(c_s - c_t\right)$$ (17.9)

where k_R is the first-order rate constant for the interfacial reaction and c_s is the concentration of solute at saturation. In this model, transport is not rate-limiting; therefore, the solute concentration gradient ($c_s - c_t$) can be quite large over an infinitesimal distance. For organic substrates, there are not many cases for which the interfacial barrier model applies. The dissolution of gallstones is one example.

Diffusion-Layer Model

One of the earliest theoretical treatments describing dissolution phenomena is attributed to Noyes and Whitney for their investigation of the dissolution of benzoic acid and lead chloride in water (1897). These solutes, because of their low aqueous solubility, were chosen to minimize the change in surface area as the solutes dissolved. As mentioned earlier, it was assumed that an *indefinitely* thin layer of saturated solution was formed instantly around the solute, followed by diffusion of the solute into the bulk solution. Since the first step is fast compared to the second, diffusion into the bulk was taken as the rate-limiting step. The dissolution rate was then modeled using Fick's second law of diffusion and the concentration gradient of the solute. This led to the following first-order equation:

$$\frac{dc}{dt} = k\left(c_s - c_t\right)$$ (17.10)

where dc/dt refers to the dissolution rate of the substance in terms of concentration, and k is a dissolution constant.

Permutations of Diffusion-Layer Model

In order to extend the range of Equation 17.10 from sparingly soluble to more soluble substances, Brunner and Tolloczko (1900) modified Noyes and Whitney's model to account for the changing surface area with time:

$$\frac{dc}{dt} = k_1 S\left(c_s - c_t\right)$$ (17.11)

where k_1 is the dissolution rate constant that takes into account the specific surface area. Note that k_1 is equivalent to the transport rate constant, k_T. It was also pointed out that the rate of dissolution depended on the temperature, structure of the crystal surface, rate of stirring, and arrangement of the experimental apparatus.

A more general theoretical approach for dissolution modeling called the *Film-Model Theory* was postulated by Nernst (1904) and expanded upon by Brunner (1904) in an effort to deconvolute the components of the dissolution constant, k. Both Nernst and Brunner made the following assumptions:

1. The mass flux, that is, intrinsic dissolution rate, is governed by Fick's first law of diffusion:

$$J = \frac{dm}{dt}\left(\frac{1}{S}\right) = -D\left(\frac{dc}{dx}\right)$$ (17.12)

   where dc/dx is the solute concentration gradient and D is the diffusivity (diffusion coefficient), and

2. The concentration gradient within the diffusion layer is constant, thus,

$$\frac{dc}{dx} = \frac{(c_t - c_s)}{h}$$ (17.13)

   where h is the thickness of the stagnant diffusion layer.

Substitution of Equation 17.13 into Equation 17.12 gives

$$J = \left(\frac{dm}{dt}\right)\left(\frac{1}{S}\right) = \frac{D(c_s - c_t)}{h}$$ (17.14)

This led to the following equation:

$$\frac{dc}{dt} = k_2\left(\frac{DS}{Vh}\right)(c_s - c_t)$$ (17.15)

where k_2 is the intrinsic dissolution rate constant.

Sink Conditions

Sink conditions refer to a special case where there is essentially no buildup of the solute, which is assumed to be the case for the absorption of a drug from the gastrointestinal tract. Two ramifications for this special case are that the concentration gradient $(c_s - c_t)$ described in Equation 17.9 is not rate-limiting under any conditions and, if the surface area of the solute is kept constant, the rate of dissolution will follow zero-order kinetics. *In vivo* sink conditions can be approximated *in vitro* by ensuring that the concentration of the solute does not exceed 5%–10% of its solubility. In practice, this is accomplished by either using a large volume of the dissolution medium or continuously replenishing the dissolution medium under carefully controlled conditions. Under sink conditions, $c_s \gg c_t$, and Equation 17.15 can be rewritten as the limiting case:

$$\left(\frac{dc}{dt}\right)_{t \to 0} = k_2\left(\frac{DS}{Vh}\right)c_s$$ (17.16)

Since D, c_s, and k_2 are constants for a given solute, they can be combined into k_3, and Equation 17.16 can be further simplified into

$$\frac{dc}{dt} = k_3\left(\frac{S}{Vh}\right)$$ (17.17)

If one then assumes that the solute surface area (S) and the volume of dissolution medium (V) remain constant, Equation 17.17 can be rewritten as

$$\frac{dc}{dt} = K \tag{17.18}$$

This explains the observance of zero-order kinetics under sink conditions.

Hixson and Crowell's Cubic Root Law

To account for cases where the surface area is changing during the course of the dissolution process, such as for solute crystals and traditional solid dosage forms, Hixson and Crowell developed the *cubic root law*. Instead of modeling on the basis of the rate of change in the concentration of a solute, they sought to describe dissolution in terms of the rate of change in weight of the solute. This was accomplished by multiplying both sides of Equation 17.11 by the volume of the dissolution medium (V), which yields

$$\frac{dw}{dt} = K_2 S \left(c_s - c_t \right) \tag{17.19}$$

where dw/dt is the rate of change in weight of the solute, K_2 is $k_1 V$, and w is the weight of undissolved crystal at time t. Note that in this equation, the surface area (S) is no longer constant but is now variable.

Provided that there is no change in the shape of the drug crystal as it dissolves, its surface varies as the two-thirds power of its volume (v), that is,

$$S \propto v^{2/3} \tag{17.20}$$

Since $v = w/d$, where d is the density of the solute, then

$$S = k_4 w^{2/3} \tag{17.21}$$

where k_4 takes into account the density of the solute and contains a shape constant that is dependent on crystal morphology. Substitution for S in Equation 17.19 gives

$$\frac{dw}{dt} = K_2 \left(k_4 w^{2/3} \right) \left(c_s - c_t \right) \tag{17.22}$$

For the special case where the change in concentration is negligible, ($c_s - c_t$) is constant, and therefore, the rate of dissolution is dependent on surface area alone and Equation 17.19 can be rewritten as

$$\frac{dw}{dt} = k_3 w^{2/3} \tag{17.23}$$

Since the change in solute concentration is negligible, w can be approximated by w_0, the weight of undissolved solute crystals at time 0. This is a reasonable approximation when the initial amount of solute is less than one-twentieth (1/20) of its solubility. Integration of Equation 17.23 under these conditions gives the cubic root law, which can be written as follows:

$$K_4 t = w_0^{1/3} - w^{1/3} \tag{17.24}$$

Under conditions where the initial amount of solute approaches the amount needed to produce a saturated solution (w_s), that is, when $w_s = w_0$, Hixson and Crowell derived the *negative two-thirds law*, which is given as follows:

$$K_5 t = v\left(w^{-2/3} - w_0^{-2/3}\right) \tag{17.25}$$

Dissolution of Monodisperse Systems (z-Law) under Nonsink Conditions

Yonezawa et al. (1994, 1995) derived a model on the basis of the Nernst equation to describe the rate of dissolution of a monodisperse system that can account for various initial amounts of solute, as long as it is less than that needed to saturate the solution. The z-law equation was derived from the Hixson–Crowell treatment under nonsink conditions. The general form of the z-law equation can be expressed as follows:

$$\left(\frac{M}{M_0}\right)^z = 1 - zk_z c_s St \tag{17.26}$$

where M_0 is the initial amount of solute for a monodisperse system, M is the amount at time t, $z = (1/3 - M_0/M_s)$, M_s is the amount of solute at saturation, and k_z is the dissolution rate constant. The cube root law Equation is obtained when M_0 is extremely small, and the negative two-thirds law is obtained in the case when $M_0 = M_s$.

Effect of Particle Size on Rate of Dissolution: Dissolution of Polydisperse Systems

Lu et al. (1993) developed refinements of the Noyes–Whitney-type equations, which included a time-dependent diffusion layer and also accounted for nonspherical particle geometry. Their program simulated initial particle size distributions on the basis of the log normal probability density function. The most accurate simulations were obtained by assuming cylindrical geometry with and without a time-dependent diffusion-layer thickness for fine (calculated mean particle size of 10.9 μm) and coarse (calculated mean particle size of 38.7 μm) hydrocortisone, respectively. The dissolution profiles for fine and coarse hydrocortisone are shown in Figure 17.2.

Other Factors Influencing Dissolution

1. The solubility of the drug will influence the rate of dissolution by determining the magnitude of the drug's concentration gradient ($c_s - c_t$).
2. Crystal morphology dictates the rate of dissolution along the different crystallographic axes. This dissolution anisotropy can be found in all but cubic crystals, which are isotropic.
3. Crystal defects and imperfections influence the crystal lattice energy. These defects, including dislocations, give rise to increased surface energy and may be a major factor in improving dissolution performance of poorly water-soluble, crystalline substances.
4. Polymorphism, where solute molecules crystallize in more than one form, with the polymorphs possessing different energies, will most likely give rise to different dissolution and solubility profiles. Polymorphs that have greater thermodynamic activity will dissolve faster than more stable ones, and this property has been exploited in the pharmaceutical industry in an attempt to increase therapeutic blood levels of insoluble or sparingly soluble drugs. In some instances, new polymorphs have been observed following size reduction processes.
5. Impurities (including surfactants, hydrates, solvates, complexes, and reactive additives) can greatly influence the rate of dissolution by modifying the crystal habit or by interfering with the interfacial transport of solute from the crystal to the bulk solution.
6. Physicochemical properties, such as density, viscosity, and wettability, influence ensemble properties (flocculation, flotation, and agglomeration), which in turn influence dissolution by perturbing the effective specific surface area.

SOLUBILITY

The aqueous solubility of APIs plays a central role in drug formulation. If the given drug substance is sufficiently soluble in water and stable in solution, formulation should proceed in a straightforward fashion. However, if the drug substance is insoluble or sparingly soluble in aqueous medium, this presents a much more difficult challenge in formulation development. The formulator may have to resort to addition of solubilizing agents or organic cosolvents. Particle size also affects the solubility of the compound itself since the free energy of the system increases with decreasing particle size.

The specific surface, which is defined as the surface divided by volume, increases dramatically with decreasing particle size. Figure 17.3 shows the specific surface of spherical particles as a function of diameter. Solubility is defined as the capacity of two or more substances to form spontaneously, one with the other, without chemical reaction, a homogeneous solution (Mader, 1971). One can further classify solubility into *macroscopic* and *microscopic* solubility (Braun, 1983). These two terms are discussed in the following. Note that the solubility of a solute in solvent at equilibrium is independent of particle size *except* for colloidal systems, which are nonequilibrium systems.

Macroscopic Solubility

Macroscopic solubility can be thought of as the usual thermodynamic solubility behavior of dispersions of particles down to a few micrometer in size. A broad definition of solubility was given earlier. Of more interest to us is a more restricted definition for solubility, which refers to the saturation concentration of solutions, that is, the maximum ratio of dissolved matter to solvent under given conditions. An important consideration in terms of thermodynamics is the link between solubility of a solid and the term phase, a phase by Gibbs' definition being a part of a system that is physically and chemically homogeneous in itself. According to Gibbs, the term phase only applies to situations where the number of interfacial molecules is negligible with respect to the number of bulk molecules, that is, if the interfacial energy is negligible compared with the chemical potential of the bulk such that $\gamma_S = \gamma_L$ in mixed phase.

Microscopic Solubility

Microscopic solubility refers to the *solubility* of colloidal systems, which is not strictly defined and depends on many factors. In colloidal systems, the number of interfacial molecules is not negligible with respect to the number of bulk molecules. This attribute is the basis for the special

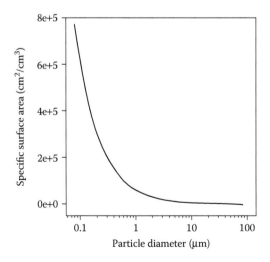

FIGURE 17.3 Specific surface area as a function of particle size.

properties of colloidal systems. Colloidal systems are unstable, and their particle size distribution and solubility are constantly changing. One may assume that the solubility equilibrium of such a system is rapidly established, with the resulting equilibrium solubility existing with the smallest solid particles. However, as mentioned earlier, these systems are not stable and the smallest particles preferentially dissolve giving rise to a new equilibrium based on a coarser particle size distribution with correspondingly lower solubility (Ostwald ripening). As long as the length of time to reach equilibrium is sufficiently longer than the product shelf life, the slow rate of ripening may be inconsequential.

The solubility behavior of the macroscopic system given earlier can be described using the Gibbs–Kelvin equation:

$$\ln\left(\frac{S_r}{S_\infty}\right) = \frac{2V_m\gamma}{RT_r} \tag{17.27}$$

where S_r is the solubility of a crystal of radius r, S_∞ is the solubility of an infinitely large crystal, V_m is the molar volume of the solute, γ is the surface energy of the crystal in contact with the solution (interfacial tension), R is the gas constant, and T is the absolute temperature.

Particles with $r < 1$ μm possess significantly greater solubility than in the case of larger particles. This difference in solubility may be attributed to the greater specific surface area and higher surface free energy for fine particles compared to their larger counterparts. There is a tendency for the finer particles to dissolve and recrystallize on the larger particles. The basis for this is seen in Equation 17.27 and is called *Ostwald ripening*. This will produce a shift in particle size distribution toward larger sizes until the equilibrium solubility of the system is reached.

Ostwald–Freundlich Equation

Ostwald (1900) was the first person to attempt to correlate particle size and solubility. This treatment was amended in 1909 by Freundlich and is written as

$$\ln\left(\frac{S_{r1}}{S_{r2}}\right) = \frac{2M_w\gamma}{RTr}\left(\frac{1}{r_1} - \frac{1}{r_2}\right) \tag{17.28}$$

where S_{r1} and S_{r2} are the solubilities of particles of radius r_1 and r_2, M_w is the molecular weight of the solute, and r is the crystal density. Table 17.1 lists the surface free energies per unit area of some

TABLE 17.1
Values of γ_{sv} for Solids of Varying Polarity

Solid	γ_{sv} (dynes/cm)
Teflon	19.0
Paraffin	25.5
Polyethylene	37.6
Polymethyl methacrylate	45.4
Nylon	50.8
Indomethacin	61.8
Griseofulvin	62.2
Hydrocortisone	68.7
Sodium chloride	155
Copper	1300

common solid–air interfaces (Zografi et al., 1990). Equation 17.28 can be expressed in terms of the molar volume, V_m, of the solute:

$$\ln\left(\frac{S_{r1}}{S_{r2}}\right) = \left(\frac{2V_m\gamma}{RT}\right)\left(\frac{r_2 - r_1}{r_1 r_2}\right) \tag{17.29}$$

The above-described systems are by definition metastable and are affected by temperature fluctuations. Two other factors influencing solubility are the effect of change in crystal morphology and the creation of a higher-energy surface on particles by mechanical stress (grinding).

CRYSTAL GROWTH

Following a size reduction procedure, it is critical that the size is retained during the shelf life of the product; otherwise, the beneficial attributes associated with size reduction will not be realized. Therefore, an understanding of crystal growth phenomena is critical to successful pharmaceutical formulation.

Drug crystals grow via phase transition of a liquid or semisolid material into a solid crystalline form. This process can be described as three discrete steps:

1. Achievement of supersaturation
2. Formation of crystal nuclei
3. Crystal growth

In the context of this chapter, our interest lies in step 3. This section consists of a brief description of the first two steps, followed by a more in-depth treatment of crystal growth.

Supersaturation

The term *supersaturate* was coined in 1788 and was defined as *to add to a solution beyond saturation*. The state of supersaturation may be obtained through cooling, evaporation, or as a result of a chemical reaction between two homogeneous phases. In addition, in the case of drug solutions, supersaturation may be reached through dissolution of

1. A metastable and more thermodynamically energetic polymorph of the drug
2. An amorphous form of the drug
3. Crystals rendered metastable through mechanical means, which increase the surface free energy

The definition of supersaturation is as follows:

$$\sigma = \left(\frac{c_t - c_s}{c_s}\right) \tag{17.30}$$

where σ is the degree of supersaturation.

Although a supersaturated system may remain in this state for an appreciable length of time, it will eventually reach thermodynamic equilibrium through crystallization of excess solute.

Nucleation

This phenomenon is not fully understood; however, it may be described as the formation of minute particles of the solute, which act as nuclei for further deposition of the solute from a supersaturated solution. The probable mechanism is bimolecular addition of drug molecules, X, and may be represented as follows:

$$X + X \rightleftharpoons X_2 \qquad (17.31)$$

$$X_2 + X \rightleftharpoons X_3 \qquad (17.32)$$

$$X_{(n-1)} + X \rightleftharpoons X_n \qquad (17.33)$$

When X_n reaches a threshold value, a nucleus is created. Owing to the movement of solute molecules in solution, clusters containing varying numbers of molecules are produced. These growing crystals may redissolve or grow further, and on reaching a critical size, their solubilities equal that of a supersaturated solution (S_r). This behavior was described by the Gibbs–Kelvin equation (Equation 17.27) and the Ostwald–Freundlich equation (Equation 17.28) given in the previous section.

The systems described earlier are by definition metastable and are affected by temperature fluctuations. The solubility of the solute crystals will be affected as these temperature fluctuations produce periods of undersaturation interspersed with periods of supersaturation. These fluctuations enhance the dissolution of fine particles with concomitant growth of large particles. This crystallization process is driven by thermodynamics and can be described by an equation of the classical free energy change:

$$\Delta G^\theta = -RT \ln C \gamma_a \qquad (17.34)$$

where ΔG^θ is the molar free energy of the dissolved drug with respect to the standard state of the drug in solution, γ_a is the activity coefficient of the dissolved solute, and C is the concentration of the drug in solution (analogous to c_t in the case of dissolution phenomena). For dilute solutions, γ_a is unity. One interpretation of Equation 17.34 is that the higher the drug concentration in solution the greater the driving force to establish a state of equilibrium. The investigation of nucleation phenomena is nontrivial since it is experimentally difficult to produce a system that is free from impurities that interfere with nucleation processes.

Crystal Growth Process

The process of crystal growth is thought to occur in three steps:

1. Diffusion of the drug molecules from the bulk solution to the solid–crystal interface
2. Incorporation of the drug molecule into the crystal lattice, with concomitant release of heat of crystallization
3. Conductance of the heat of crystallization into the bulk solution

Each of these steps is influenced by temperature, rate of stirring, presence of impurities, degree of supersaturation, and the diffusivity of the molecules in solution, which is in turn dependent on the viscosity of the system.

The rate at which crystals grow is defined as the change in linear size per unit time and is given as

$$G = \left(\frac{dL}{dt} \right) \qquad (17.35)$$

where G is the linear growth rate, L is the crystal length, and t is time. There are four models that describe crystal growth, which are based on which step is considered as rate-limiting:

1. Solute transport within the bulk solution phase to the crystal surface
2. Uniform attachment of growth units (i.e., solute molecules) to a surface that is rough on a molecular scale
3. Nucleation of two-dimensional clusters on the surface, which expand and merge to form new layers
4. Spreading of layers from a screw-lattice dislocation that acts as a continuous source of steps

Diffusion-Controlled Crystal Growth Theory

If the equilibrium at the crystal face is established rapidly so as not to be rate-limiting, the crystallization process would be controlled by solute transport, which is proportional to the solute concentration gradient across the stagnant layer $(c_t - c_s)$. The rate of crystallization could be modeled using Ficks' law of diffusion and is given by

$$G = \left(\frac{DV_m (c_t - c_s)}{h} \right)$$ (17.36)

where the terms of the equation were defined earlier in the section on dissolution phenomena. Note that the form of the equation describing diffusion-controlled crystal growth is analogous to the equation describing dissolution phenomena, except for inversion with respect to the direction of the solute concentration gradient. It has been shown that the width of the diffusion layer, h, is essentially nonexistent in well-stirred solutions and that the bulk of the solution in contact with the growing crystal face is not saturated but supersaturated. This would imply the presence of at least two mechanisms: diffusion across the boundary layer and reorganization of the encroaching molecule into the proper orientation for incorporation into the growing crystal lattice. As pointed out by Greco Macie and Grant (1986), the molecular mechanism is more complex than a two-stage process. However, the usefulness of this theory of crystal growth lies in the capability for measuring and reporting crystal growth rates using diffusional and mass transfer equations.

Adsorption-Layer Theory

The other three models differ in mechanism; however, they share common assumptions. Molecules arriving from the bulk solution to the crystal interface retain sufficient energy, allowing them to migrate over the crystal face. Equilibrium is established between the bulk and this loosely adsorbed layer of molecules at the surface, analogous to that found in the interfacial barrier model of dissolution. These molecules will eventually integrate into the crystal lattice in such a way so as to minimize the free energy of the system, that is, where the attractive forces are maximal. The sites of integration and the surface texture are those that differentiate the three models and will be discussed now in more detail.

Uniform attachment of growth units mechanism: This mechanism refers to the situation where there is a discontinuous process of layer-by-layer adsorption of molecules onto a crystal surface that is rough on a molecular scale. This surface roughness provides numerous nuclei for attachment of solute molecules. The crystal growth rate is proportional to the driving force:

$$G = k_5 c_t \ln\left(\frac{c_t}{c_s} \right)$$ (17.37)

with

$$k_5 = \frac{DV_{\mathrm{m}}}{d}$$ (17.38)

where k_5 is a constant that determines the maximum growth rate for a given system and d is the molecular diameter. This mechanism of crystal growth gives rise to rounded crystal surfaces.

Nucleation of two-dimensional clusters mechanism: In cases where the crystal face is smooth, growth can occur by either a two-dimensional nucleation mechanism or by a spiral-growth mechanism. For two-dimensional nucleation, growth occurs by attachment of molecules to the edge of a nucleus on the surface. Under ideal conditions, the growing step on a crystal surface will advance across the crystal face until that particular layer is complete. Before another layer starts, a center of crystallization has to form via surface nucleation. The growth rate for this mechanism is exponentially dependent on the driving force:

$$G = k_6 c_{\mathrm{t}}^{1/3} \left[\ln\left(\frac{c_{\mathrm{t}}}{c_{\mathrm{s}}} \right) \right]^{5/6} \exp\left[-\left(\frac{\pi\gamma^2}{3(k_{\mathrm{B}}T)^2} \right) \ln\left(\frac{c_{\mathrm{t}}}{c_{\mathrm{s}}} \right) \right]$$ (17.39)

with

$$k_6 = \left(\frac{2\pi}{3} \right)^{1/3} \left[\frac{2D_{\mathrm{s}} n_{\mathrm{s}} V_{\mathrm{m}}}{\lambda\alpha} \right]$$ (17.40)

where k_{B} is Boltzmann's constant, D_{S} is the surface diffusion coefficient, n_{S} is the surface solute density, λ is the mean diffusion distance, and α is the lattice spacing.

Spiral-growth mechanism: Another model to describe crystal growth in the presence of smooth crystal faces is the spiral-growth mechanism. The presence of screw-lattice dislocations acts as a continuous source of steps. Surface nucleation is therefore not necessary, and the crystal can grow as if covered with kinks. Under these conditions, there is never a flat face, and growth proceeds at the maximum theoretical rate for the particular level of supersaturation. This model was developed by Burton et al. (1951). It describes the situation where crystal growth occurs via addition of growth units to kink sites for a series of equidistant steps. The curvature of the ensuing spiral is related to the spacings of the successive turns and to the degree of supersaturation. The growth rate is given as follows:

$$G = k_7 c_{\mathrm{t}} \left[\ln\left(\frac{c_{\mathrm{t}}}{c_{\mathrm{s}}} \right) \right]^2$$ (17.41)

with

$$k_7 = \frac{0.05 D k_{\mathrm{B}} T}{\gamma}$$ (17.42)

At low supersaturation, Equation 17.41 predicts that the rate of crystal growth will be proportional to the square of the driving force, which was found to hold experimentally for many systems. At high supersaturation, the rate is predicted to be proportional to the driving force.

By use of the proper experimental conditions and fitting the four models described earlier, it may be possible to arrive at a reasonable mechanistic interpretation of the experimental data. As an example, the crystal growth kinetics of theophylline monohydrate was studied by Rodriguez-Hornedo and Wu (1991). Their conclusion was that the crystal growth of theophylline monohydrate is controlled by a surface reaction mechanism rather than by solute diffusion in the bulk. Further, they found that the data was described by the screw-dislocation model and by the parabolic law, and they concluded that a defect-mediated growth mechanism occurred rather than a surface nucleation mechanism.

Impurities and Crystal Growth

The addition of foreign agents (dispersing agents, growth inhibitors, surface active agents, etc.) to a system before or during crystallization can profoundly influence or interfere with the nucleation processes and with the diffusion of molecules to the surface of the growing crystal. Very small quantities of additives may adsorb into the growing crystal lattice and alter the character of the crystal surface by any one or combinations of the following mechanisms:

1. Changing the properties of the formulation (i.e., surface tension, ionic strength, or the macroscopic solubility, c_s)
2. Altering the adsorption layer at the solid–liquid interface, therefore affecting the integration of growth units
3. Undergoing selective adsorption onto the crystal face, exerting a blocking effect
4. Being adsorbed onto growth steps, disrupting the flow of growth layers across the surface
5. Being adsorbed at kinks on the crystal face, causing rough faces to flatten out
6. Altering the surface energy of a crystal face, which may change its degree of solvation

Since many undesirable changes in pharmaceutics arise from nucleation and crystal growth, impurities (either added intentionally or inadvertently) can modulate or suppress these processes. This may give rise to inhibition of crystal growth in suspensions, emulsions, and ointments, and may also inhibit polymorphic transitions.

PARTICLE SIZE REDUCTION METHODS

There has been a long history of the use of particle size reduction and deaggregation techniques in the pharmaceutical industry, and extensive reviews of these techniques and their theories have been provided previously (Parrot, 1974; Chaumeil, 1998; Merisko-Liversidge et al., 2003; Patravale et al., 2004; Rabinow, 2004; Rasenack and Muller, 2004; Moschwitzer and Muller, 2006). The size reduction processes of interest here are mechanical in nature and capable of reducing drug particle size into the ultrafine range (particle diameter <10 μm).

Particle size reduction can be achieved by two methods:

1. Precipitation—substance is dissolved in appropriate solvent.
2. Mechanical methods—mechanical force is introduce by using different kind of equipments (mills), which is commonly used in the pharmaceutical industry.

There are multitudes of milling techniques/equipment available for the reduction of drug particles into the ultrafine range (Moschwitzer and Muller, 2006). All the techniques fall under two broad categories: dry milling (the size reduction is carried out in the dry state of the particle) and wet milling (size reduction is carried out with the particles being suspended in a liquid medium). A brief discussion of four such techniques (fluid energy milling, ball milling, media milling, and Microfluidizing®) follows. Besides these techniques, modern methods such as those that use supercritical fluids in the micronization process are getting increasingly popular. The most widely applied techniques of this category include the rapid expansion of supercritical solutions (RESS) process, the supercritical antisolvent (SAS) method, and the particles from gas-saturated solutions (PGSS) method. Discussion of these techniques would be out of the scope of this chapter.

FLUID ENERGY MILLING

This is a dry milling technique and represents one of the most efficient, scalable, and industrially popular size reduction techniques. The principal mode of particle reduction is via particle-to-particle collisions with a limited contribution from metal-to-product contact. One type of fluid energy mill, also called an air jet mill or air classifying mill, consists of a circular grinding chamber into which the drug material is fed. Air enters the grinding chamber at a high velocity through a number of jets on the periphery of the chamber. The orifices of the jets are aligned so as to affect rotation of the drug material about the center of the chamber. Comminution of the drug occurs primarily near the outlets of the jets via collisions between the drug particles. The drug particles exit the grinding chamber at its center through an outlet coupled to a receiving vessel. The geometry of the grinding chamber, the position of the outlet, and the alignment of the jets cause the drug particles to follow a spiral course within the chamber. The centrifugal action causes the larger particles to move toward the outer walls of the chamber and the finer particles to move toward the center and through the chamber outlet. Particle comminution for a given mill is a function of the feed rate and nozzle pressure. Increasing the nozzle pressure and decreasing the feed rate affect a greater extent of particle size reduction.

Fluid energy mills are capable of producing ultrafine particles in significant quantities. Particle sizes of milled product from 1 to 30 µm are readily obtained. Fluid energy mills are capable of output rates in the 10–100s of kg/h (McDonald, 1971).

Fluid energy milling has several attractive features from a pharmaceutical processing perspective as it forms an efficient, effective one-step grinding and classifying operation. Fluid energy mills are simple, straightforward designs with no moving parts, and can be readily taken apart for cleaning and sterilizing. The milling process does not introduce any contamination (media, lubricant, etc.) into product from the mill. There is no significant heat generation coupled with micronization process, which makes it more amenable for thermosensitive compounds. In addition, the milled product is discharged directly into a receiving vessel, avoiding handling procedures associated with harvesting of the product from the mill.

Currently, besides catering to the pharmaceutical industry, fluid energy milling is employed for size reduction of agricultural chemicals, carbon black, ceramics, cosmetics, pigments, precious metals, propellants, resins, and toner materials.

BALL MILLING

A ball mill consists of a cylindrical vessel with a port for adding and discharging drug materials and grinding media. The vessel is made to rotate about its principal axis causing the grinding media to move up with the vessel wall and cascade down. The cascading action of the grinding media affects particle size reduction via attrition, impact, and compression caused by the cascading effect. The milling operation can be carried out under dry conditions or wet conditions using suitable media. Typical operating parameters of a ball mill for ultrafine grinding are as follows:

Media charge: 50% of vessel volume
Material charge: 25% of vessel volume
Rotational speed: 50%–85% of critical speed

The critical speed is the speed at which the grinding media cease to cascade owing to the centrifugal force imparted by the rotating vessel. The critical speed can be estimated by employing the following relationship (Lantz, 1990):

$$\text{Critical speed}(\text{rpm}) = 54 \div \sqrt{r_{ft}} \qquad (17.43)$$

where r_{ft} is the vessel diameter measured in feet.

As the rotational speed is decreased, attrition plays a greater role in particle size reduction relative to impaction and compression, yielding a finer grind at the expense of longer processing times.

Some characteristics of the grinding media that affect processing in a ball mill are shape, density, size, and hardness. Increasing the density and hardness of the grinding media increases the rate and extent of size reduction. Decreasing the media size tends to increase the rate and extent of size reduction. The grinding media for generating ultrafine product is typically spherical in shape and composed of ceramic, flint pebbles, or steel. The size of the final product is certainly dependent on the size of the grinding media used (smaller ball size resulting in smaller final product diameter). There are sophisticated versions of the ball mill—pearl mill, bead mill, and sand mill—that use finer grinding media, as the name suggests (Stehr and Schewdes, 1983; Stehr, 1988; Czekai and Seaman, 1999; Muller et al., 1999; Blanton et al., 2002). Ball milling could be conducted as a batch operation or in the contiguous feed mode, making it an attractive technique for specialized applications. Fine grindings with a particle size of 100 ~ 5 mm can be obtained.

Ball milling in water with the presence of surfactants or water-soluble polymers extends the applicability of ball milling poorly water-soluble compounds into the submicron range (Ikekawa, 1971). Particle size distributions with the median particle diameter below 200 nm can be achieved. Figure 17.4 shows the particle size distribution of an aqueous dispersion of a steroid processed in a ball mill. The steroid was milled with polyvinyl alcohol as a stabilizer using 1 mm zirconium silicate beads at 50% of the critical speed. Figure 17.5 shows a scanning electron micrograph of steroid crystals comminuted in a wet ball mill to submicron dimensions.

MEDIA MILLING

Media milling, also called stirred ball milling, is a classical wet milling technique wherein a sufficiently concentrated dispersion of solids within a suitable liquid medium (aqueous/nonaqueous) is subjected to traditional ball milling operation (Merisko-Liversidge et al., 2003; Patravale et al., 2004). Media mills are designed in the horizontal or vertical orientation. The cylindrical grinding chamber contains a shaft coincident with its principal axis. Several disks are mounted along the shaft.

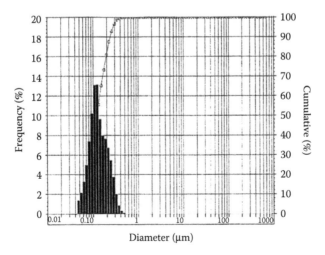

FIGURE 17.4 Particle size distribution of a steroid processed in a wet ball mill as measured by light scattering. (Data generated by NanoSystems, Elan Drug Technologies, a member of the Elan Corporation, plc.)

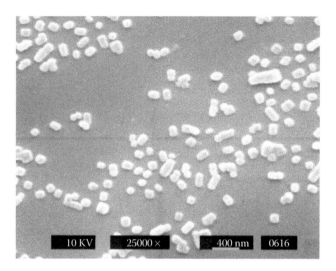

FIGURE 17.5 Scanning electron micrograph of steroid crystals comminuted in a wet ball mill to submicron dimensions. (Data generated by NanoSystems, Elan Drug Technologies, a member of the Elan Corporation, plc.)

The chamber is charged with grinding media to approximately 80% of its volume. The grinding media is typically glass, ceramic, zirconium or plastic of spherical shape with diameter of approximately 0.2–4 mm. The shaft is made to rotate at a high velocity, approximately 20,000 rpm, and the suspension of material is pumped through the grinding chamber to effect size reduction of the suspended material.

Particle comminution occurs owing to a compression–shear action produced by the rotating disks and grinding media.

The liquid medium used for suspending the particles can serve special purposes—such as lubrication and coating of newly formed particles through various physicochemical interactions (electrostatic, hydrophobic, etc.) (Verhoff et al., 2003; Moschwitzer and Muller, 2006).

MICROFLUIDIZATION

Microfluidization is a process involving a high-pressure fluids processor that delivers unique product capabilities, including particle size reduction to nanosized particles for dispersions, emulsions, and liposomes. Microfluidizer processors overcome limitations of conventional processing technologies by utilizing high-pressure streams that collide at ultrahigh velocities in precisely defined microchannels. Combined forces of shear and impact act upon products to create finer, more uniform dispersions and emulsions than can be produced by any other means.

Particle size reduction of a material suspended in a liquid medium can be affected by a Microfluidizer® processor (Microfluidics Corp., Newton, MA, http://www.microfluidicscorp.com/processors.html). A schematic of a Microfluidizer processor is presented in Figure 17.6. In a Microfluidizer processor, a liquid stream is bifurcated and the two streams are directed upon each other under pressures as high as 40,000 psi. Particles suspended in the liquid are reduced in size by forces of shear and cavitation. Suspensions can be prepared with the Microfluidizer processor with mean particle sizes in the micron to submicron range.

The Microfluidizer high shear processor technology is widely used in the pharmaceutical, biotechnology, digital ink, microelectronics, food, chemical, and personal care industries.

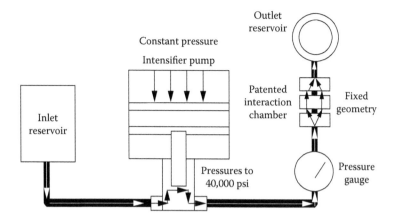

FIGURE 17.6 Schematic of a Microfluidizer® materials processor. (Reprinted from *Innovation through Microfluidizer Processor Technology*, MFIC Corporation, Newton, MA, 2005. With permission.)

STABILIZATION

Particle size reduction involves input of energy that gets disseminated during micronization process, along with formation of smaller particles having new surfaces. With an enormous increase in surface area, the newly formed particles need to be stabilized—to prevent subsequent agglomeration induced by interparticulate interactions and maintain their existence as individual nanoentities.

The particle size distribution of an ultrafine material may increase spontaneously if measures are not taken to stabilize the particles. Particle size growth can occur via agglomeration or crystal growth. This particle size increase will result in a decrease of the available surface area, and hence a decrease of the dissolution rate, potentially lowering drug bioavailability.

Electrostatic repulsion and steric stabilization are two available mechanisms for stabilizing dispersions with respect to particle agglomeration. Electrostatically stabilized dispersions require a surface charge and associated electric double layer. Typically, particles dispersed in water obtain a negative surface charge due to preferential adsorption of anions from solution. Ionizable groups, that is, $RCOOH + H_2O \rightarrow RCOO^- + H_3O^+$ and $R_3N + H_2O \rightarrow R_3NH^+ + OH^-$, may result in $\pm$ surface charge. In general, the degree of stabilization increases with increasing surface potential and thickness of the electric double layer. The surface potential may be altered by changing the pH of the medium or by adsorption onto the particle surface of a charged species (e.g., an ionic surfactant). The thickness of the electric double layer can be increased by lowering the ionic strength of the medium. Figure 17.7 shows the effect of electrolyte concentration on the interaction potentials for electrostatically stabilized dispersions.

Dispersions can also be stabilized by steric stabilization. Steric stabilization is accomplished by partially adsorbing a polymer to the particle surface. Generally, it is important for the polymer to be amphiphilic so that portions of the molecule have an affinity for the particle surface and other portions have an affinity for the water. Figure 17.8 illustrates the adsorption of a sterically stabilizing polymer to a particle surface. The adsorbed polymers on two such particles interpenetrate as the particles approach. The interpenetration of the adsorbed polymers results in a decrease in entropy by restricting the available polymer chain configurations. This interpenetration also results in an increase in the local osmotic pressure of the solution between the two particles. The repulsive force arises as water moves into the intervening space to counter these energetically unfavorable events and drives the particles apart. Pharmaceutical excipients such as poloxamers and polyvinylpyrrolidone (PVP) have been found to be effective for stabilizing a wide range of poorly soluble drugs as

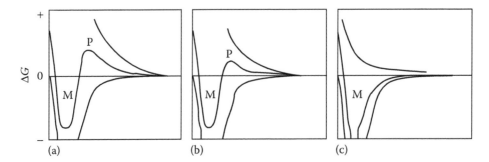

FIGURE 17.7 Effect of electrolyte concentration on the interaction potential of electrostatically stabilized dispersions: (a) At low electrolyte concentration, a high energy barrier, P, prevents particle agglomeration; (b) as the electrolyte concentration decreases, the barrier is lowered; and (c) at high electrolyte concentration, the barrier is removed and the particles agglomerate. (From Meyers, D.: *Surfaces, Interfaces, and Colloids.* 1991. Copyright Wiley-VCH Verlag GmbH & Co. KGaA. Reproduced with permission.)

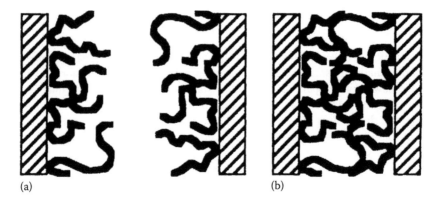

FIGURE 17.8 Illustration of adsorption of a polymer at the solid–liquid interface, inhibiting particle agglomeration via a steric barrier: (a) Adsorbed polymer on the surface of two particles; (b) interpenetration of the adsorbed layers as the particle surfaces approach is energetically unfavorable owing to osmotic and entropic phenomena. (From Meyers, D.: *Surfaces, Interfaces, and Colloids.* 1991. Copyright Wiley-VCH Verlag GmbH & Co. KGaA. Reproduced with permission.)

colloidal dispersions. Electrostatic forces are present along with steric forces and may contribute to the stabilization of a *sterically* stabilized dispersion. A polyelectrolyte such as gelatin is an example where both mechanisms can provide significant contributions toward dispersion stabilization. A polyelectrolyte can increase the electrostatic potential near the particle surface and also provide for stabilization via a steric barrier.

Crystal growth of an API dispersion may occur via Ostwald ripening (see the section titled Microscopic Solubility). The driving force for particle size growth through ripening is the differential solubility between smaller and larger crystals. Ostwald ripening can be inhibited by crystal growth modifiers. These substances undergo strong adsorption at the crystal–solution interface and inhibit deposition of additional molecules to the crystal lattice. PVP, casein, and polyvinylalcohol are examples of substances that have been shown to be inhibitors of crystal growth. Figure 17.9 shows inhibition of both dissolution and crystallization of sulfathiazole suspensions by PVP.

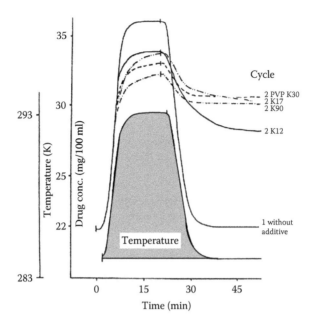

FIGURE 17.9 Inhibition of dissolution and recrystallization of sulfathiazone by PVP. Temperature cycling of 2% sulfathiazole suspensions demonstrating the effect of PVP on dissolution and recrystallization. (From Ziller, K. H. and Rupprecht, H. H. *Pharm. Ind.*, 52, 1017–1022, 1990. With permission.)

PHARMACEUTICAL APPLICATIONS OF SIZE REDUCTION TECHNOLOGY

ORAL AND RESPIRATORY APPLICATIONS

There are numerous examples where size reduction techniques have been applied to poorly water-soluble compounds in order to increase their dissolution rate and improve bioavailability following oral administration (Levy et al., 1963; Hintz and Johnson, 1989; Chaumeil, 1998; Rasenack and Muller, 2002; Kayser et al., 2003; Kocbek et al., 2006; Pouton, 2006). Size reduction, particularly at the submicron dimension, represents a valuable means of improving oral absorption of poorly water-soluble compounds. As shown in Figure 17.10, the increase in dissolution rate from solid (x) with size reduction provides more drug in solution (x) available for absorption during gastrointestinal transit.

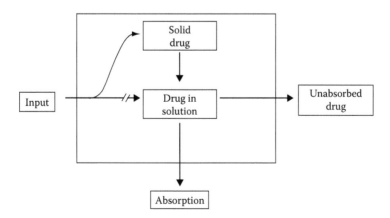

FIGURE 17.10 Intestinal drug absorption events.

TABLE 17.2
Pharmacokinetic Parameters Following Oral and Intravenous Administration of Danazol Formulations to Fasted Male Beagle Dogs ($n = 5$)

Formulation	C_{max} (µg/mL)	T_{max} (hr)	AUC[a] (µg/mL·hr)	Absolute Bioavailability
Cyclodextrin oral	3.94 ± 0.14	1.2 ± 0.2	20.4 ± 1.9	106.7 ± 12.3
Nanoparticle dispersion	3.01 ± 0.80	1.5 ± 0.3	16.5 ± 3.2	82.3 ± 10.1
Conventional dispersion	0.20 ± 0.06	1.7 ± 0.4	1.0 ± 0.4	5.1 ± 1.0
Cyclodextrin IV			19.8 ± 0.6	100

Source: Data generated by NanoSystems, Elan Drug Technologies, a member of the Elan Corporation, plc.
[a] Based on NONLIN 84 AUC values normalized to a dose of 20 mg/kg.

Therefore, the fraction of unabsorbed drug decreases as overall bioavailability increases. Nanoparticles in particular provide for a large surface area available for dissolution since sizes are generally <1000 nm in diameter and *in vivo* agglomeration is minimized by particle stabilization. Table 17.2 illustrates the absolute oral bioavailability of several Danazol formulations: nanoparticle dispersion, solubilized cyclodextrin oral formulation, and conventional suspension. Danazol represents a poorly water-soluble compound (10 µg/mL) whose oral bioavailability is dissolution limited. The results indicated that size reduction of Danazol crystals from 10 µm as conventional suspension to sizes less than 200 nm nanoparticle dispersion resulted in approximately a 16-fold increase in absolute bioavailability (Liversidge and Cundy, 1995). Studies with an oral phenytoin nanoparticle dispersion indicated increases in absorption of nearly threefold when administered to healthy volunteers as compared to an aqueous suspension of micronized drug substance (Wood et al., 1995). For the anti-inflammatory agent naproxen, it has been demonstrated in the rat that size reduction of naproxen from 20–30 µm to 270 nm led to results indicating decreased gastric irritation following oral administration as well as a fourfold increase in the rate of absorption (Liversidge and Conzentino, 1995). Furthermore, in human clinical trials, the time to onset of action of a nanoparticle oral suspension of naproxen reached significant plasma levels (*t*90) in less than 20 min, which was 12-fold faster than commercial formulations of larger particle size (Figure 17.11).

Nanoparticle technology provides for stable solid-in-liquid dispersions of drug with particle sizes generally <1000 nm, thus making an ideal medium for aerosol delivery of poorly water-soluble drugs to the nasal cavity or pulmonary region (Ostrander et al., 1999; Jacobs and Muller, 2002; Rasenack et al., 2003; Irngartinger et al., 2004; Hernandez-Trejo et al., 2005; Gonda, 2006). Surface area coverage by nanoparticle aerosols can be markedly increased relative to micron-sized particles. For example, the theoretical surface area covered by 50 µL of spray volume at a drug concentration of 0.5 mg/mL with particles ~5 µm apart can be calculated to be 0.095 cm2 for 5 µm particles, but increases to 1493 cm2 for 0.2 µm particles. Nebulization studies using a cascade impactor have been performed with nanoparticle dispersions of beclomethasone diproprionate (BDP) of mean particle size 260 nm as compared to an aqueous suspension of BDP having a particle size of 10.5 µm (Ruddy and Eickhoff, 1996; Wiedmann et al., 1996). The cumulative mass fraction of BDP obtained from the cascade impactor was recorded as a function of the cutoff diameter of the impactor stage (i.e., aerosol size in µm). The data suggested that ~80% of nanodispersion formulations reaching the impactor could be found in the <2.5 µm aerosol droplets and represented *respirable* particles. In contrast, the larger micronized BDP formulation, that is, mean diameter ~10.5 µm, showed <40% of the particles to be present in the <2.5 µm aerosol droplets with rapid falloff to only ~10% particles in the 1.25 µm aerosol droplets. In conclusion, size reduction to nanoparticles improved the delivery efficiency of BDP by nebulization as compared to micronized suspensions.

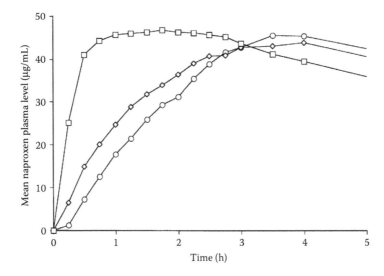

FIGURE 17.11   Influence of formulation on absorption of naproxen (500 mg) in humans (fed); mean plasma data from clinical trials ($n = 23$). Plasma levels of naproxen (mg/mL) are plotted as a function of time (h) where (D) is Naproxen NanoCrystal® dispersion, (♦) is Naproxyn® suspension, and (o) is Anaprox® tablet. (Data generated by NanoSystems, Elan Drug Technologies, a member of the Elan Corporation, plc.)

Particle size reduction of API to nanometer scope can also eliminate the food effect of some water-insoluble drug. For example, The absorption of fenofibrate is increased when administered with food. With micronized fenofibrate, the absorption is increased by approximately 35% under fed as compared to fasting conditions; but exposure to fenofibric acid in plasma, as measured by C_{max} and area-under-the-curve (AUC), is not significantly different (about 95%) when a single dose of fenofibrate with nanoparticle technology is administered under fasting or non-fasting conditions.

INTRAVENOUS APPLICATIONS

Poor water solubility severely limits the ability to deliver APIs by injection. Concerns for patient safety arise, particularly with respect to intravascular administration. Risks of precipitation of drug, vascular occlusion, or excessive uptake of precipitated drug by the liver may result in undesirable effects on hepatic function. To address this need, poorly water-soluble APIs are often administered intravenously with large volumes of vehicle, in the presence of cosolvents and surfactants, or by using delivery systems consisting of polymeric particles (Rao and Geckeler, 2011; Yue, 2011), liposomes (Allen and Cullis 2013), or microemulsions (Solanki et al., 2012). Size reduction to nanoparticles offers an alternative for the intravenous delivery of poorly water-soluble molecules, significantly relaxing the aqueous solubility requirements for safe administration and permitting direct vascular injection (Peters et al., 2000; Moschwitzer et al., 2004; Aramwit et al., 2006).

Historically, the administration of crystalline APIs has mainly found use in parenteral applications associated with intramuscular and subcutaneous injections as well as topical applications of suspensions containing micronized APIs. Commercially marketed pharmaceuticals categorized as suspensions for parenteral administration are illustrated in Table 17.3. Many of these products utilize drug substance size reduction in order to promote dissolution following administration. The degree of success associated with the intravenous administration of crystalline nanoparticles of poorly water-soluble therapeutics largely depends on a thorough understanding of

1. Nanoparticle size and morphology
2. Surface characteristics afforded by the stabilizer
3. Dissolution kinetics

TABLE 17.3

Commercially Marketed Parenteral Suspensions[a]

Drug	Brand Name	Administration/Dosage
Aurothioglucose	Solganal®	IM, 50 mg/mL
Betamethasone (sodium phosphate and acetate salt)	Celestone®, Soluspan®	IM, 6 mg/mL
Colfosceril palmitate	Exosurf Neonatal®	IT, 13.5 mg/mL
Cortisone acetate	Cortone®	IM, 50 mg/mL
Triamcinolone diacetate	Artisocort® Forte	IM, 40 mg/mL
Triamcinolone hexacetonide	Aristospan®	IL, 5 mg/mL IA, 20 mg/mL
Beractant	Survanta®	IT, 25 mg/mL
Dexamethasone acetate	Decadron-LA®	IM, 8 mg/mL
Methylprednisolone acetate	Depo-Medrol®	IM, IS, IL, ST 20, 40 and 80 mg/mL
Medroxyprogesterone acetate	Depo-Provera®	IM, 400 mg/mL
Hydrocortisone acetate	Hydrocortone	IA, IL, ST 25 and 50 mg/mL
Insulin, zinc suspension (pork or human source)	Humulin® L, U, R, and N Iletin® I and II, Lente®, Iletin® Novolin® L, N, and R	SC, 100 units/mL
Prednisolone tebutate	Hydeltra-T.B.A.®	IA, IL, and ST 20 mg/mL

[a] Suspensions listed in reference, Physicians Desk Reference 1996. Does not include ophthalmic, otic, or nasal suspensions. IA = intraarticular; IL = intralesional; ST = soft tissue injection; IM = intramuscular; IT = intratracheal; SC = subcutaneous; and IS = intrasynovial.

Nanoparticle size, as accomplished by size reduction techniques, has been an area of focus using wet milling comminution processes to achieve submicron particle sizes <500 nm (Liversidge et al., 1992; Kondo et al., 1993). The size reduction process from macrocrystalline to nanocrystalline drug substance for poorly water-soluble agents is illustrated in the scanning electron micrographs of Figure 17.12 for drugs of interest in cancer therapy (Merisko-Liversidge et al., 1996). The micrographs demonstrate size reduction from a variety of different macrocrystalline drugs of varied crystal habit and morphology. Noncomminution techniques such as controlled precipitation also provide for characteristic crystal morphologies of drug particles to be prepared (Chan and Gonda, 1994).

Historically, nano- and microparticulates administered intravenously are well known to rapidly clear from the blood to reticuloendothelial organs, mainly the liver (Juliano, 1988; Wattendorf and Merkle, 2008). Large microparticulates of individual or agglomerated particles usually greater than 4–7 μm can also become entrapped within lung capillaries (Gesler and Garvin, 1973). Furthermore, in specific animal species such as the dog, particulate and/or associated surfactant stabilizer materials can lead to marked shifts in hemodynamic parameters (Garavilla et al., 1996). Prolonged circulation times of nanoparticles in the blood pool can usually be achieved by reducing the particle size to <200 nm with the goal of preparing relatively homogeneous nanoparticles of mean diameter in the <100 nm range (Tomlinson, 1987; Mayer et al., 1989; Forssen and Ross, 1994). In combination with size reduction, it is important to stabilize the nanoparticle surface with stabilizers such as select nonionic surfactants that aid in biodistribution away from reticuloendothelial organs such as the liver, spleen, and bone marrow (Illum et al., 1987; Troster et al., 1990). For example, some noncrystalline liposome and polymeric matrix nanoparticles have been surface grafted with 6–10 unit segments of polyethylene glycol chains resulting in prolonged half-lives in the circulation with marked shifts in pharmacokinetic profiles and distribution to tissues (Allen, 1994; Gref et al., 1994). The ability of particles to avoid or prolong capture by the macrophage-type cells of reticuloendothelial organs is thought to be a process akin to *opsonization* with decreased interaction of particle surfaces via complement protein fragments, therefore providing for reduced recognition/uptake by

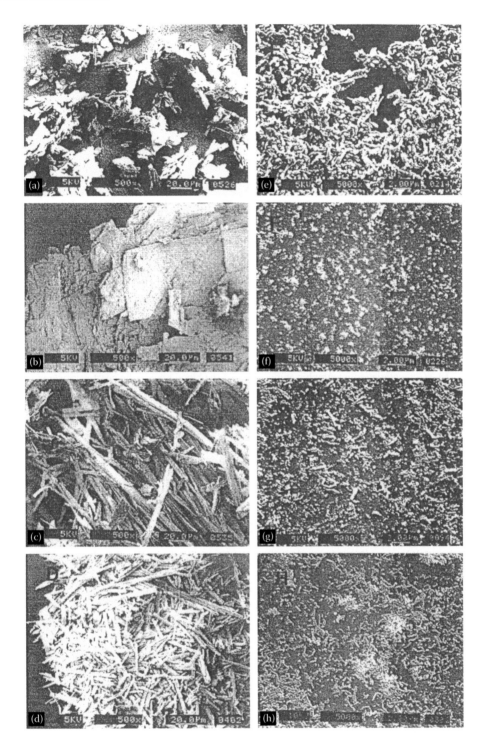

FIGURE 17.12 Nanocrystalline drug suspensions of cytotoxic anticancer agents prepared by wet milling comminution and analyzed using scanning electron microscopy (SEM). Unmilled drug substance at 500× magnification and illustrated on the left-side of the figures: (a) piposulfan, (b) camptothecin, (c) etoposide, and (d) paclitaxel. Corresponding nanocrystalline suspensions at 5000× magnification, and illustrated on the right side of the figures: (e) nanopiposulfan, (f) nanocamptothecin, (g) nanoetoposide, and (h) nanopaclitaxel. (From Merisko-Liversidge, E. et al., *Pharm. Res.*, 13: 272–278, 1996. With permission.)

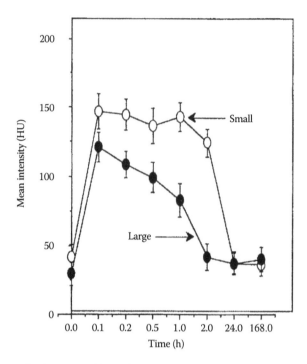

FIGURE 17.13 Computerized tomographic angiography of the blood pool in the heart ventricle of the rabbit following intravenous administration of small 90 nm (s) or large 190 nm (l) nanocrystalline particles of a triiodinated X-ray contrast agent stabilized with Pluronic F-108. Times are indicated following postinjection of the formulation in the ear vein of the rabbit. Techniques and presentation from references: Wolf and Gazelle (1993); Liversidge et al. (1994); Ruddy et al. (1995). (Data generated by NanoSystems, Elan Drug Technologies, a member of the Elan Corporation, plc.)

such organs (Borchard and Kreuter, 1993). The biological importance of both surface stabilization and size for nanocrystalline particles is illustrated in Figure 17.13. *In vivo* studies were performed in rabbits with nanoparticles of a poorly water-soluble triiodinated X-ray agent (Ruddy et al., 1995). A select surfactant, nonionic Pluronic F-108, was utilized in the stabilization of either smaller ~90 or larger ~200 nm nanoparticles of the X-ray agent crystalline core. The smaller-size particles of diagnostic X-ray agent enabled the blood pool compartment in the heart ventricle of the rabbit to be imaged for up to 2 h with a much higher mean intensity than comparable, but larger 200 nm particles that began to decay from the blood pool within 10 min.

All formulations to be administered intravenously must meet strict guidelines on their sterility assurance before any clinical studies in humans (USP 26/NF 21, 2003). Nanoparticulates present unique challenges, and consequently, studies to identify conditions for sterilization (Akers et al., 1987; Marino, 1993; Schwarz et al., 1994) or aseptic processes utilizing barrier technology (Wilkins, 1995) should be incorporated during early phases of development. Ideally, the physicochemical character of the nanoparticulate formulation should be compromised to a minimum during steps that employ steam sterilization, sterile filtration, use of preservatives, freeze drying, gamma irradiation, and procedures associated with aseptic fill. Size reduction processes that achieve a median ranging between 200 and 300 nm diameter of particles can be relatively routine (Liversidge et al., 1992; Liversidge and Cundy, 1995), but this particle size range is not amenable to sterile filtration via 0.2 μm filters. To achieve <100 nm nanocrystalline particles by wet milling processes, optimized milling designs are required with choice drug substances, select surfactant stabilizers, and novel milling media. Furthermore, ultracentrifugation techniques may be required to fractionate out monodisperse subpopulations of <100 nm diameter nanoparticles.

Capillary hydrodynamic fractionation analysis is a useful analytical tool for monitoring dispersity profiles of nanoparticle dispersions before and after differential ultracentrifugation. Small nanoparticles of median ~100 nm or less with 90% of the particles <200 nm can be filtered with good recovery via 0.2 μm sterile filters and has been demonstrated for a number of therapeutic and diagnostic imaging agents (Zheng and Bosch, 1995).

Steam sterilization is routinely performed as the preferred methodology for the terminal sterilization of heat-stable injectable products (PDR, 2007). Nanocrystalline and other suspension particles present special challenges such as solubilization/recrystallization during the heat process leading to particle size growth (Harwood et al., 1993). Furthermore, since surfactant stabilizers are utilized for nanoparticle surface stabilization, it is important that the surfactant being utilized in the formulation has a *cloud point* above the ~121°C temperature utilized during autoclaving. The nonionic, polyoxyethylated Pluronic-type surfactants described earlier develop cloudiness owing to self-association and loss of the water of hydration and will precipitate above a certain temperature, known as the *cloud point* (Hunter, 1992). In nanoparticulate formulations destined for a terminal steam sterilization process, it is critical to include an excipient in the formulation that raises the *cloud point* of the surfactant. This use of *cloud-point* elevation avoids agglomeration of nanoparticles and results in less change in the particle size (Na and Rajagopalan, 1994). The phenomenon illustrated in Figure 17.14 utilizes the cloud-point modifier, sodium lauryl sulfate, at 0.01%.

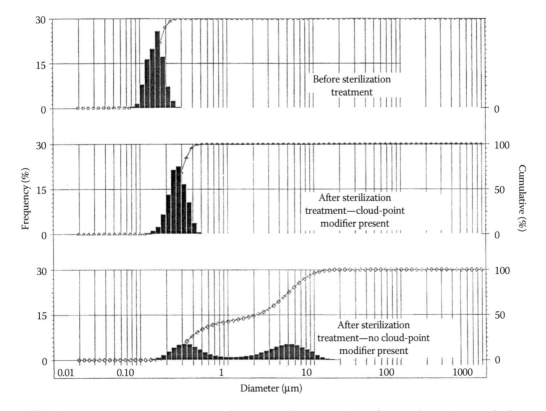

FIGURE 17.14 Particle size distribution of nanocrystalline dispersions of a proprietary therapeutic drug, Pluronic F-68, stabilizer formulation before and after steam sterilization at 122°C with a sterilization cycle exposure time of 12.5 min. The studies were performed in the presence or absence of a small percentage (0.01%) of sodium lauryl sulfate as cloud-point modifier. Particle sizes were measured using a Horiba LA-910 Laser Scattering Particle Size Distribution Analyzer. (From Na, G. C. and Rajagopalan, N., Use of nonionic cloud-point modifiers to minimize nanoparticle aggregation during sterilization, US Patent 5,346,702, 1994.)

TABLE 17.4

List of FDA Approved NanoCrystal® Technology Products

Brand Name	Active Ingredients	Approve Date	Dosage Form/Route	Company
Rapamune	Sirolimus	August 25, 2000	Tablet; oral	Pf Prism Cv
Tricor	Fenofibrate	November 5, 2004	Tablet; oral	Abbvie
Megace Es	Megestrol Acetate	July 5, 2005	Suspension; oral	Endo Pharms Inc
Emend	Fosaprepitant Dimeglumine	January 25, 2008	Powder; intravenous	Merck
Invega Sustenna	Paliperidone Palmitate	July 31, 2009	Suspension, extended release; intramuscular	Janssen Pharms
Invega Trinza	Paliperidone Palmitate	May 18, 2015	Suspension, extended release; intramuscular	Janssen Pharms

In summary, the goal with respect to size reduction of particles for intravenous usage is to provide an acceptable size range with balance in the desired therapeutic efficacy, safety, and formulation shelf life. Poorly water-soluble crystalline APIs are becoming increasingly good candidates for the micronization process in the preparation of biocompatible and pharmaceutically acceptable nanoparticulate formulations.

COMMERCIALIZED PRODUCTS

There have been significant resources spent on micronization technologies. These efforts have resulted in a number of commercially successful products based on effective particle size reduction principles for improving oral bioavailability of the poorly water-soluble drugs and/or to reduce variation in oral bioavailability in the fed and fasted states. Leading drug delivery technologies employing proprietary milling processes (coupled with steric stabilization techniques) that have produced nanotechnology-enabled products are NanoCrystal® technology from Elan Drug Technologies, now owned by Alkermes, (http://www.alkermes.com/), Insoluble Drug Delivery (IDD®) technology from Skye Pharma (www.skyepharma.com/solubilization_idd.html), Biorise® technology from Eurand (www.eurand.com), and NanoEdge® technology from Baxter BioPharma Solutions (www.baxterbiopharmasolutions.com). The NanoCrystal technology has been the forerunner that forms the technology platform for six marketed products in United States (Table 17.4), and SKYPHARMA AG also market the product with nanotechnology, Triglide®.

REFERENCES

Abdou, H. M. (1990) Dissolution, In *Remington's Pharmaceutical Sciences* (Gennaro, A. R., Ed.), pp. 589–602, Mack Publishing, Easton, PA.

Akers, M. J., A. L. Fites, and R. L. Robison. (1987) Formulation design and development of parenteral suspensions, *J. Parenter. Sci. Technol.*, 41: 88–96.

Allen, T. M. (1994) Long circulating (sterically stabilized) liposomes for targeted drug delivery, *TIPS*, 15: 215–220.

Allen, T. M. and P. R. Cullis. (2013) Liposomal drug delivery systems: From concept to clinical applications, *Adv. Drug Delivery Rev.*, 65: 36–48.

Anderson, B. D. (1980) Thermodynamic considerations in physical property improvement through prodrugs, In *Medicinal Research Series, Vol. 10: Physical Chemical Properties of Drugs* (Yalkowsky, S. H., Sinkula, A. A., and Valvani, S. C., Eds.), pp. 231–266, Marcel Dekker, New York.

Aramwit, P., T. Kerdcharoen, and H. Qi. (2006) *In vitro* plasma compatibility study of a nanosuspension formulation, *PDA J. Pharm. Sci. Technol.*, 60: 211–217.

Blanton, T. N., D. K. Chatterjee, and D. Majumdar. (2002) Process for milling compounds, US Patent 6,491,239.

Borchard, G. and J. Kreuter. (1993) Interaction of serum components with poly(methyl methacrylate) nanoparticles and the resulting body distribution after intravenous injection in rats, *J. Drug Target.*, 1: 15–93.

Braun, H. (1983) Particle size and solubility of disperse dyes, *Rev. Prog. Coloration*, 13: 62–72.

Brunner, E. (1904) Reaktionsgeschwindigkeit in heterogenen Systemen, *Z. Phys. Chem.*, 47: 56–102.

Brunner, L. and S. Tolloczko. (1900) Uber die Auflosungsgeschwindigkeit fester Korper, *Z. Phys. Chem.*, 35: 283–290.

Burton, W. K., N. Cabrera, and F. C. Frank. (1951) The growth of crystals and the equilibrium structure of their surfaces, *Phil. Trans. Roy. Soc.*, 243A: 299–358.

Cammarata, A., J. H. Collett, and E. Tobin. (1980) Simultaneous determination of the solubility parameter, δ, and molar volume, V, for some para-substituted acetanilides in water, In *Medicinal Research Series, Vol. 10: Physical Chemical Properties of Drugs* (Yalkowsky, S. H., Sinkula, A. A., and Valvani, S. C., Eds.), pp. 267–276, Marcel Dekker, New York.

Canselier, J. P. (1993) The effects of surfactants on crystallization phenomena, *J. Disp. Sci. Technol.*, 14: 625–644.

Chan, H. K. and I. Gonda. (1994) Shape modification of drug particles by crystallization, *Proceedings of First International Particle Technology Forum*, Vol. 3, pp. 174–179, August 17–19, 1994, American Institute of Chemical Engineers, Denver, NY.

Chaumeil, J. C. (1998) Micronization: A method of improving the bioavailability of poorly soluble drugs, *Methods Find. Exp. Clin. Pharmacol.*, 20: 211–215.

Czekai, D. A. and L. P. Seaman. (1999) Method of grinding pharmaceutical substances, US Patent 5,862,999.

Forssen, E. A. and M. E. Ross. (1994) Daunoxome registered treatment of solid tumors: preclinical and clinical investigations, *J. Liposome Res.*, 4: 481–512.

Garavilla, L. D., N. Peltier, and E. Merisko-Liversidge. (1996) Controlling the acute hemodynamic effects associated with IV administration of particulate drug dispersions in dogs, *Drug Dev. Res.*, 37: 86–96.

Gesler, R. M. and P. J. Garvin. (1973) The biological effects of polystyrene latex particles administered intravenously to rats, a collaborative study, *Bull. Parent. Drug Assoc.*, 27: 101–113.

Gonda, I. (2006) Systemic delivery of drugs to humans via inhalation, *J. Aerosol. Med.*, 19: 47–53.

Grant, D. J. W. and A. H. L. Chow. (1991) Crystal modifications in acetaminophen by growth from aqueous solutions containing *p*-acetoxyacetanilide, a synthetic impurity, *AIChE Symp. Ser.*, 284: 33–37.

Grant, D. J. W. and T. Higuchi. (1990) Solubility behavior of organic compounds, In *Techniques of Chemistry, Vol. XXI* (Saunders, W. H. and Weissberger, A. Eds.), Wiley-Interscience Publication, New York.

Greco Macie, C. M. and D. J. W. Grant. (1986) Crystal growth in pharmaceutical formulation, *Pharm. Int.*, 233–237.

Gref, R., Y. Minamitake, M. T. Peracchia, V. Trubetskoy, V. Torchilin, and R. Langer. (1994) Biodegradable long-circulating polymeric nanospheres, *Science*, 263(5153): 1600–1603.

Harwood, R. J., J. B. Portnoff, and E. W. Sunbery. (1993) The processing of small volume parenterals and related sterile products, In *Pharmaceutical Dosage Forms: Parenteral Medications* (Avis, K. E., Lieberman, H. A., and Lachman, L., Eds.), Vol. 2, pp. 42–51, Marcel Dekker, New York.

Hernandez-Trejo, N., O. Kayser, H. Steckel, and R. H. Muller. (2005) Characterization of nebulized buparvaquone nanosuspensions—effect of nebulization technology, *J. Drug Target*, 13: 499–507.

Hintz, R. J. and K. C. Johnson. (1989) The effect of particle size distribution on dissolution rate and oral absorption, *Int. J. Pharm.*, 51: 9–17.

Hixson, A. W. and J. H. Crowell. (1931) Dependence of reaction velocity upon surface and agitation, *Ind. Eng. Chem.*, 23: 923–931.

Hunter, R. J. (1992) *Foundations of Colloid Science*, Vol. I, pp. 570–571, Oxford University Press, Oxford.

Ikekawa, A., K. Imagawa, T. Omori, and N. Kaneniwa. (1971) Influence of physicochemical properties on ball-milling of pharmaceutical powders, *Chem. Pharm. Bull.*, 19: 1027–1031.

Illum, L., S. S. Davis, R. H. Muller, E. Mak, and P. West. (1987) The organ distribution and circulation time of intravenously injected colloidal carriers sterically stabilized with a block copolymer-polyoxamine 908, *Life Sci.*, 40: 367–374.

Irngartinger, M., V. Camuglia, M. Damm, J. Goede, and H. W. Frijlink. (2004) Pulmonary delivery of therapeutic peptides via dry powder inhalation: Effects of micronisation and manufacturing, *Eur. J. Pharm. Biopharm.*, 58: 7–14.

Jacobs, C. and R. H. Muller. (2002) Production and characterization of a budesonide nanosuspension for pulmonary administration, *Pharm. Res.*, 19: 189–194.

Juliano, R. L. (1988) Factors affecting the clearance kinetics and tissue distribution of liposomes, microspheres and emulsions, *Adv. Drug Deliv. Rev.*, 2: 31–54.

Kayser, O., C. Olbrich, V. Yardley, A. F. Kiderlen, and S. L. Croft. (2003) Formulation of amphotericin B as nanosuspension for oral administration, *Int. J. Pharm.*, 254: 73–75.

Kocbek, P., S. Baumgartner, and J. Kristl. (2006) Preparation and evaluation of nanosuspensions for enhancing the dissolution of poorly soluble drugs, *Int. J. Pharm.*, 312: 179–186.

Kondo, N., T. Iwao, H. Masuda, K. Yamanouchi, Y. Ishihara, N. Yamada, T. Haga, Y. Ogawa, and K. Yokoyama. (1993) Improved oral absorption of a poorly water-soluble drug, HO-221, by wet-bead milling producing particles in submicron region, *Chem. Pharm. Bull.*, 41: 737–740.

Lantz, R. J. (1990) Size reduction. In *Pharmaceutical Dosage Forms: Tablets, Vol. 2* (Lieberman, H. A., Lachman, L., and Schwartz, J. B., Eds.), pp. 107–200, Marcel Dekker, New York.

Levy, G., J. M. Antkowiak, J. A. Procknal, and D. C. White. (1963) Effect of certain tablet formulation factors on dissolution rate of the active ingredient. II. Granule size, starch concentration, and compression pressure, *J. Pharm. Sci.*, 52: 1047–1051.

Lindfors, L., S. Forssen, P. Skantze, U. Skantze, A. Zackrisson, and U. Olsson. (2006a) Amorphous drug nanosuspensions. 2. Experimental determination of bulk monomer concentrations, *Langmuir*, 22: 911–916.

Lindfors, L., P. Skantze, U. Skantze, M. Rasmusson, A. Zackrisson, and U. Olsson. (2006b) Amorphous drug nanosuspensions. 1. Inhibition of ostwald ripening, *Langmuir*, 22: 906–910.

Liversidge, G. G. and P. Conzentino, (1995) Drug particle size reduction for decreasing gastric irritancy and enhancing absorption of naproxen in rats, *Int. J. Pharm.*, 125(2): 309–313.

Liversidge, G. G., E. R. Cooper, J. M. Shaw, and McIntire, G. L. (1994) X-ray contrast compositions useful in medical imaging, US Patent 5,318,767.

Liversidge, G. G. and K. C. Cundy. (1995) Particle size reduction for improvement of oral bioavailability of hydrophobic drugs: I. Absolute oral bioavailability of nanocrystalline danazol in beagle dogs, *Int. J. Pharm.* 125: 91–97.

Liversidge, G. G., K. C. Cundy, J. F. Bishop, and D. A. Czekai. (1992) Surface modified drug nanoparticles, US Patent 5,145,684.

Lu, A. T. K., M. E. Frisella, and K. C. Johnson. (1993) Dissolution modeling: Factors affecting the dissolution rates of polydisperse powders, *Pharm. Res.*, 10: 1308–1314.

Mader, G. (1971) Determination of solubility, In *Physical Methods in Chemistry Part V* (Weissberger, A. and Bryant, W., Eds.), p. 259, Wiley-Interscience Publication, New York.

Marino, F. J. (1993) Pharmaceutical suspensions, Chapter 8, In *Pharmaceutical Dosage Forms: Parenteral Medications* (Avis, K. E., Lieberman, H. A., and Lachman, L., Eds.), Vol. 2, pp. 187–189, Marcel Dekker, New York.

Mayer, L. D., L. C. Tai, S. C. Ko, D. Masin, R. S. Ginsberg, P. R. Cullis, and M. B. Bally. (1989) Influence of vesicle size, lipid composition, and drug-to-lipid ratio on the biological activity of liposomal doxorubicin in mice, *Cancer Res.*, 49: 5922–5930.

McDonald, D. P. (1971) Micronization, *Manuf. Chem. Aerosol News*, 42: 39–40.

Merisko-Liversidge, E., G. G. Liversidge, and E. R. Cooper. (2003) Nanosizing: A formulation approach for poorly-water-soluble compounds, *Eur. J. Pharm. Sci.*, 18: 113–120.

Merisko-Liversidge, E., P. Sarpotdar, J. Bruno, S. Hajj, L. Wei, N. Peltier, J. Rake, et al. (1996) Formulation and antitumor activity evaluation of nanocrystalline suspensions of poorly soluble anticancer drugs, *Pharm. Res.*, 13: 272–278.

Meyers, D. (1991) *Surfaces, Interfaces, and Colloids*, VCH Publishers, New York.

Microfluidics (2005) *Innovation through Microfluidizer® Processor Technology*, MFIC Corporation, Newton, MA.

Moschwitzer, J., G. Achleitner, H. Pomper, and R. H. Muller. (2004) Development of an intravenously injectable chemically stable aqueous omeprazole formulation using nanosuspension technology, *Eur. J. Pharm. Biopharm.*, 58: 615–619.

Moschwitzer, J. and R. H. Muller. (2006) New method for the effective production of ultrafine drug nanocrystals, *J. Nanosci. Nanotechnol.*, 6: 3145–3153.

Mosharraf, M. and C. Nystrom. (2003) Apparent solubility of drugs in partially crystalline systems, *Drug Dev. Ind. Pharm.*, 29: 603–622.

Muller, R. H., R. Becker, B. Kruss, and K. Peters. (1999) Pharmaceutical nanosuspensions for medicament administration as systems with increased saturation solubility and rate of solution, US Patent 5,858,410.

Na, G. C. and N. Rajagopalan. (1994) Use of non-ionic cloud point modifiers to minimize nanoparticle aggregation during sterilization, US Patent 5,346,702.

Nernst, W. (1904) Theorie der Reaktionsgeschwindigkeit in heterogenen Systemen, *Z. Phys. Chem.*, 47: 52–55.

Noyes, A. A. and W. R. Whitney. (1897) The rate of solution of solid substances in their own solutions, *J. Am. Chem. Soc.*, 19: 930–934.

Ostrander, K. D., H. W. Bosch, and D. M. Bondanza. (1999) An *in vitro* assessment of a nanocrystal beclomethasone dipropionate colloidal dispersion via ultrasonic nebulization, *Eur. J. Pharm. Biopharm.*, 48: 207–215.

Ostwald, W. (1900) Über die vermeintliche Isomerie des rotten und gelben Quecksilberoxyds und die Oberflächenspannung fester Körper, *Z. Phys. Chem.*, 34: 495–503.

Parrot, E. L. (1974) Milling of pharmaceutical solids, *J. Pharm. Sci.*, 63: 813–829.

Patravale, V. B., A. A. Date, and R. M. Kulkarni. (2004) Nanosuspensions: A promising drug delivery strategy, *J. Pharm. Pharmacol.*, 56: 827–840.

PDR (2007) Physicians' desk reference, 61st ed., *Product Information on Injectables*, pp. 401–3534, Thompson PDR, Montvale, NJ.

Peters, K., S. Leitzke, J. E. Diederichs, K. Borner, H. Hahn, R. H. Muller, and S. Ehlers. (2000) Preparation of a clofazimine nanosuspension for intravenous use and evaluation of its therapeutic efficacy in murine mycobacterium avium infection, *J. Antimicrob. Chemother.*, 45: 77–83.

Pouton, C. W. (2006) Formulation of poorly water-soluble drugs for oral administration: Physicochemical and physiological issues and the lipid formulation classification system, *Eur. J. Pharm. Sci.*, 29: 278–287.

Rao, J. P. and K. E. Geckeler. (2011) Polymer nanoparticles: Preparation techniques and size-control parameters, *Prog. Polym. Sci.*, 36: 887–913.

Rabinow, B. E. (2004) Nanosuspensions in drug delivery, *Nat. Rev. Drug Discov.*, 3: 785–796.

Ragnarsson, G., A. Sandberg, M. O. Johansson, B. Lindstedt, and J. Sjogren. (1992) *In vitro* release characteristics of a membrane-coated pellet formulation—influence of drug solubility and particle size, *Int. J. Pharm.*, 79: 223–232.

Rasenack, N. and B. W. Muller. (2002) Dissolution rate enhancement by *in situ* micronization of poorly water-soluble drugs, *Pharm. Res.*, 19: 1894–1900.

Rasenack, N. and B. W. Muller. (2004) Micron-size drug particles: Common and novel micronization techniques, *Pharm. Dev. Technol.*, 9: 1–13.

Rasenack, N., H. Steckel, and B. W. Muller. (2003) Micronization of anti-inflammatory drugs for pulmonary delivery by a controlled crystallization process, *J. Pharm. Sci.*, 92: 35–44.

Rodriguez-Hornedo, N. and H.-J. Wu. (1991) Crystal growth kinetics of theophylline monohydrate, *Pharm. Res.*, 8(5): 643–648.

Ross, S. and I. D. Morrison. (1988) *Colloidal Systems and Interfaces*, John Wiley & Sons, New York.

Ruddy, S. B. and W. M. Eickhoff. (1996) Isolation of ultra small particles, US Patent Number 5,503,723.

Ruddy, S. B., E. Merisko-Liversidge, S. M. Wong, W. M. Eickhoff, M. E. Roberts, G. G. Liversidge, N. Peltier, et al. (1995) *Conference on Pharmaceutical Science and Technology*, Fine Particle Society Meetings, August 24, Chicago, IL.

Schwarz, C., W. Mahnert, J. S. Lucks, and R. H. Muller. (1994) Solid lipid nanoparticles (SLN) for controlled drug delivery I. Production, characterization and sterilization, *J. Control. Rel.*, 30: 83–96.

Setnikar, I. (1977) Micronization in pharmaceutics and in specifications of pharmacopoeas, *Boll. Chim. Farm.*, 116: 393–401.

Solanki, S. S., B. Barkar, R. K. Dhanwani. (2012) Microemulsion drug delivery system: For bioavailability enhancement of ampelopsin (2012) *ISRN Pharmaceutics*, 2012

Sokoloski, T. D. (1990) Solutions and phase equilibria, In *Remington's Pharmaceutical Sciences* (Gennaro, A. R., Ed.), pp. 207–227, Mack Publishing, Easton, PA.

Stehr, N. (1988) Recent developments in stirred ball milling, *Int. J. Mineral Process.*, 22: 431–444.

Stehr, N. and J. Schewdes. (1983) Investigation of the grinding behavior of a stirred ball mill, *Ger. Chem. Eng.*, 6: 337–343.

Tawashi, R. (1968) The dissolution rates of crystalline drugs, *J. Mond. Pharm.*, 4: 371–379.

Tomlinson, E. (1987) Biological opportunities for site-specific drug delivery using particulate carriers, Chap. 2, In *Drug Delivery Carriers* (Johnson, P. and Lloyd-Jones, J. G., Eds.), pp. 32–66, Ellis Horwood, Chichester, England.

Troster, S. D., U. Muller, and J. Kreuter. (1990) Modification of the body distribution of poly(methylmethacrylate) nanoparticles in rats by coating with surfactants, *Int. J. Pharm.*, 61: 85–100.

USP 26/NF 21 (2003) *The United States Pharmacopeia*, pp. 1963–1966, United States Pharmacopeial Convention, Rockville, MD.

Valvani, S. C. and S. H. Yalkowsky. (1980) Solubility and partitioning in drug design, In *Medicinal Research Series, Vol. 10: Physical Chemical Properties of Drugs* (Yalkowsky, S. H., Sinkula, A. A., and Valvani, S. C., Eds.), pp. 201–230, Marcel Dekker, New York and Basel.

Verhoff, F. H., R. A. Snow, and G. W. Pace. (2003) Media milling, US Patent 6,604,698.

Wattendorf, U. and H. P. Merkle. (2008) PEGylation as a tool for the biomedical engineering of surface modified microparticles, *J. Pharm. Sci.* 97: 4655–4669.

Wiedmann, T. S., R. W. Wood, and L. Decastro. (1996) Aerosols containing beclomethasone nanoparticle dispersions, WO/1996/025919, PCT/US1996/002347.

Wilkins, J. (1995) Aseptic filling in a rigid isolator at evans medical, Chap. 15, In *Isolator Technology* (Wagner, C. M. and Akers, J. E., Eds.), pp. 293–301, Interpharm Press, Inc, Buffalo Grove, IL.

Wolf, G. L. and G. S. Gazelle. (1993) Current status of radiographic contrast media, *Invest. Radiol.*, 28: S2–S4.

Wood, R. W., W. Clemente, H. Lambert, and J. McShane. (1995) *Single Dose Pharmacokinetic Comparison of Oral Phenytoin Administered as a Novel Nanocrystal Dispersion*, Dilantin-125 Suspension or Dilantin Kapseals, 24th Annual Meeting ACCP.

Yao, J. H. and M. Laradji. (1993) Dynamics of ostwald ripening in the presence of surfactants, *Phys. Rev. E.*, 47: 2695–2701.

Yonezawa, Y., S. Kawase, M. Sasaki, I. Shinohara, and H. Sunada. (1995) Dissolution of solid dosage form. V. New form equations for non-sink dissolution of a monodisperse system, *Chem. Pharm. Bull*, 43: 304–310.

Yonezawa, Y., I. Shinohara, M. Sasaki, A. Otsuka, and H. Sunada. (1994) Dissolution of solid dosage form. IV. Equation for non-sink dissolution of a monodisperse system, *Chem. Pharm. Bull*, 42: 349–353.

Yue, Z., W. Wei, P. Lv, H. Yue, L. Wang, Z. Su, and G. Ma. (2011) Surface charge affects cellular uptake and intracellular trafficking of chitosan-based nanoparticles, *Biomacromolecules*, 12: 2440–2446.

Zheng, J. and H. W. Bosch. (1995) Sterile filtration of nanoparticulate drug formulations, *37th Annual Int. Industrial Pharmaceutical Research and Development Conference*, June 5–9, Merrimac, WI.

Ziller, K. H. and H. H. Rupprecht. (1990) Control of crystal growth in drug suspensions, *Pharm. Ind.*, 52: 1017–1022.

Zipp, G. L. and N. Rodriguez-Hornedo. (1989) Determination of crystal growth kinetics from desupersaturation measurements, *Int. J. Pharm.*, 51: 147–156.

Zografi, G., H. Schott, and J. Swarbrick. (1990) Disperse systems, In *Remington's Pharmaceutical Sciences* (Gennaro, A. R., Ed.), pp. 257–309, Mack Publishing, Easton, PA.

18 Development of Solid Dispersion for Poorly Water-Soluble Drugs

Madhav Vasanthavada, Simerdeep Singh Gupta, Wei-Qin (Tony) Tong, and Abu T. M. Serajuddin

CONTENTS

INTRODUCTION

WHAT IS SOLID DISPERSION?

As early as in 1961, Sekiguchi et al. (1961, 1964) developed the concept of solid dispersion to enhance absorption of poorly water-soluble drugs. It involved formation of eutectic mixtures of drugs with water-soluble carriers by melting their physical mixtures, and once the carriers dissolved, the drug precipitated in a finely divided state in water. Later, Goldberg et al. (1966a,b) demonstrated that a certain fraction of the drug may also be molecularly dispersed in the matrix, forming solid solutions, while other investigators (Mayersohn and Gibaldi 1966; Chiou and Riegelman 1969) reported that the drug may be embedded in the matrix as amorphous materials. On the basis of these considerations, Chiou and Riegelman (1971) defined solid dispersion as "the dispersion of one or more active ingredients in an inert excipient or matrix, where the active ingredients could exist in finely crystalline, solubilized, or amorphous states." Advantage of a solid dispersion as compared to a conventional capsule or tablet formulation is shown schematically in Figure 18.1 (Serajuddin 1999).

Particle size reduction often leads to improvement in the dissolution rate of poorly soluble drugs through an increase in effective surface area. However, for practical purposes, it is difficult to reduce

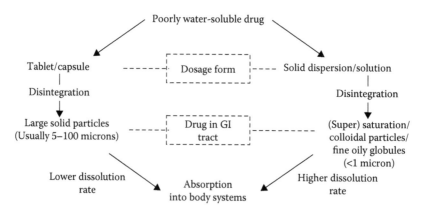

FIGURE 18.1 Advantages of a solid dispersion formulation, as compared to conventional capsule or tablet formulations, for enhancing dissolution rate, and consequent bioavailability of poorly water-soluble drugs. (From Serajuddin, A. T. M., *J. Pharm. Sci.*, 88, 1058–1066, 1999. With permission.)

particle sizes of drug in capsules or tablets to below the 2–5 μm range, while significantly higher particle size is generally preferred during drug product development for ease of handling, formulating, and manufacturing. Solid dispersion, in contrast, could dissolve a portion of the drug immediately upon contact with the gastrointestinal (GI) fluid, resulting in a saturated or supersaturated solution for rapid absorption, and the excess drug could precipitate in the GI fluid in a very finely divided state. These characteristics often result in substantially improved drug absorption from a solid dispersion as compared to a conventional tablet or capsule formulation that uses crystalline drug substance. The literature on the application of solid dispersion in improving dissolution rate and oral bioavailability of poorly water-soluble drugs has been reviewed by Leuner and Dressman (2000).

IMPORTANCE OF SOLID DISPERSION

Although the solid dispersion technology has been studied for over half a century, its application in drug development has attained greater importance since the early 1990s owing to the widespread application of combinatorial chemistry and high-throughput screening (HTS) in drug discovery that favors the selection of poorly water-soluble new chemical entities (NCEs) (Pudipeddi 2006). NCEs with aqueous solubility of less than 10 μg/mL were practically unheard of until around late 1980s; two of the compounds with solubility less than 10 μg/mL that came in the market at this time were lovastatin and simvastatin with the solubility of approximately 7 μg/mL (Serajuddin et al. 1991). Most compounds that were considered to be very poorly soluble during that time, such as prednisolone, phenytoin, digitoxin, digoxin, griseofulvin, chlorthalidon, and so forth, had solubilities between 10 and 100 μg/mL. However, it has been the experience of present authors that almost one-thirds of the compounds that are now emerging from the discovery pipeline have aqueous solubility of less than 10 μg/mL, and two-thirds of the compounds have solubility less than 100 μg/mL. Common strategies such as particle size reduction, salt formation, solubilization in organic solvents, and so forth, are not always successful at achieving the desired extent of dissolution and absorption enhancement for such compounds. There are practical limitations to the degree of particle size reduction achievable by conventional means, which limits the usefulness of this technique. Salt formation, which requires an ionizable functional group on the pharmacophore, may not be feasible for very weakly acidic or basic compounds. Even when a salt is formed, it may prove ineffective to achieve the desired absorption enhancement owing to pH-mediated precipitation of the drug in the gastrointestinal tract (GIT) following initial dissolution (Serajuddin et al. 1986). Solubilized systems, which are typically liquid in nature, rely on micellar or solvent/cosolvent solubilization techniques, formation of oil-in-water emulsion, pH adjustment, or the use of complexing agents. However, the usefulness of these formulations can be limited by their inability to solubilize the entire drug dose in the volume of a single gelatin capsule suitable for oral administration. Solid dispersion formulations, which may not require full solubilization of the drug in the excipient matrix, can provide highly effective oral formulations of poorly water-soluble drugs when the aforementioned options fail.

In addition to the aforementioned formulation options, dissolution rate for a poorly water-soluble drug can be enhanced by converting the drug into its amorphous form (Hancock and Parks 2000). Such an amorphous drug, however, is thermodynamically unstable, and under certain levels of heat and humidity, could crystallize into a more stable, poorly water-soluble form (Matsuda and Kawaguchi 1986). Solid dispersion formulations, by stabilizing amorphous drugs, can provide significant advantages.

EVALUATING THE NEED FOR SOLID DISPERSION

Compared to conventional tablet and capsule dosage forms, solid dispersion formulations are relatively complex drug delivery systems, requiring a substantially greater commitment of time, effort, and resources for development. Therefore, whether there is a need for solid dispersion and whether the desired bioavailability enhancement will not be achieved by other relatively less complex techniques such as particle size reduction or salt formation, should be assessed by careful *in vitro* assessment of the NCE's biopharmaceutical properties and the relevance of these findings to the projected *in vivo* formulation performance (Li et al. 2005). Horter and Dressman (1997), defined a poorly water-soluble drug as one for which the dissolution time of a single dose in the GI fluids exceeds the normal transit time through the absorptive regions of the GIT. Hence, the absorption of poorly water-soluble compounds is dose- dependent and controlled by the dissolution rate in the GIT and solubility in GI fluids. The fraction of the dose absorbed will decrease with an increase in the dose size if the drug particle size or surface area is held constant, while, on the other hand, if the dose size is held constant, the fraction of the dose absorbed will increase with a reduction in particle size or an increase in the particle surface area. If it is determined that complete absorption of the dose might be obtained by reducing the particle size, for instance, to approximately 2–5 μm (within the range of standard manufacturing capability), a conventional tablet or capsule dosage form may still be feasible. However, if it is determined that particle size reduction to the submicron range is necessary, a solid dispersion may provide a viable alternative. *In silico* absorption modeling with software packages, such as GastroPlus® (SimulationsPlus, Lancaster, California), has demonstrated utility in determining the impact of particle size reduction on drug absorption (Dannenfelser et al. 2004).

CHALLENGES IN DEVELOPMENT OF SOLID DISPERSION

Despite its importance and potential advantage in the development of poorly water-soluble drugs, solid dispersion had limited application in pharmaceutical dosage form development for commercial use. By reviewing the literature on solid dispersion, Serajuddin (1999) reported in 1999 that only two solid dispersion products were introduced in the market during the first four decades of the availability of this technology (Gris-PEG®, Novartis, Cesamet®, Lilly). Various issues that impeded the commercial development of solid dispersions include (a) inability to scale benchtop formulations to manufacturing-sized batches, (b) difficulty in controlling physicochemical properties, (c) difficulty in delivering solid dispersion formulations as tablet or capsule dosage forms, and (d) physical and chemical instability of the drug and/or the formulation itself (Serajuddin 1999). In addition, a fundamental knowledge of solid dispersion principles that could lead to successful products was also inadequate. In the present chapter, the theoretical basis for the development of solid dispersions will be discussed, and then attempts will be made to discuss various practical approaches to the formulation of solid dispersions for poorly water-soluble drugs.

PHYSICOCHEMICAL BASIS OF PHARMACEUTICAL SOLID DISPERSION

Since both drug and carrier coexist in solid dispersion, the following questions generally arise: How does solid dispersion form and how is it different from a physical mixture? What is a solid solution? Why do solid dispersion and solid solution demonstrate significantly higher dissolution rate than their corresponding physical mixtures? The answers to these questions are important in understanding the physicochemical basis of formulating solid dispersion dosage forms for pharmaceuticals.

SOLID DISPERSION VERSUS PHYSICAL MIXTURE

A physical mixture, as referred to in this chapter, is a simple blend of two components obtained by traditional blending techniques. A solid dispersion, on the other hand, is a physical mixture that undergoes, either partly or completely, a molecular-level mixing during its formation. Such a molecular mixing results in enhanced drug surface area, and consequently enhanced dissolution rate. In some instances, solid dispersion formation might result in converting the drug in its amorphous state, which would offer higher dissolution rate owing to its higher thermodynamic activity. Molecular-level mixing, which is observed in solid dispersions, is practically impossible to achieve through traditional milling and blending techniques that are used to prepare physical mixtures, thereby making solid dispersions a preferred approach. Moreover, when the right polymer is chosen, solid dispersion can minimize the molecular mobility of drug by increasing the drug's glass transition temperature (T_g), consequently improving physical stability of the drug. However, solid dispersions are complex systems, and there are many factors that influence their formation and physicochemical properties. These factors are discussed in a greater detail in the following sections.

STRUCTURE OF SOLID DISPERSION

A knowledge of the structure of solid dispersion and, particularly, how the drug exists in a carrier matrix, is of critical importance in understanding the performance of solid dispersions. When a solid dispersion is prepared, for instance, by solidifying a comelt of two components A and B, the components may be completely miscible in their melt, but on solidification, the drug could remain trapped molecularly in the solid carrier, or precipitate either as a separate amorphous or crystalline phase. Often, it is a combination of the above-mentioned three scenarios. If the drug is converted to an amorphous form, it will result in higher dissolution rate; however, any subsequent conversion of the amorphous form to its crystalline form during storage could result in slower dissolution rate and consequently lead to decreased bioavailability. Moreover, since crystallization is a highly variable phenomenon, it may be difficult to predict batch failures and loss in product performance during shelf life. It is, therefore, important to understand the thermodynamic and kinetic factors governing the structure of solid dispersions and how they could be helpful in developing a better product.

The core steps involved in the formation of solid dispersion between a drug and polymer are as follows:

1. Transforming drug and polymer from their solid state to fluid or fluid-like state through processes such as melting, dissolving in solvent or cosolvent, or subliming—a process that is not so commonly used.
2. Mixing the components in their fluid state.
3. Transforming the fluid mixture into solid phase through processes such as congealing, solvent removal, and condensation of sublimed mixture.

Although the above is clearly an oversimplified version of solid dispersion formation, it serves as the basis for the present discussion of the thermodynamic aspects governing solid dispersion formation. A physical mixture differs from solid dispersion in that the former would not experience the aforementioned steps, and consequently its components are in native physical state. When a physical mixture converts to solid dispersion, its physical–chemical properties would differ from those of physical mixture, depending on steps 2 and 3, that is, extent of drug–polymer molecular mixing (or molecular miscibility) and the rate of solidification of fluid mixture. The performance of above-mentioned steps may often depend on carriers used; while an acceptable solid dispersion may be formed with one carrier, it may not be the case with another. The following questions arise: Why do different mixtures behave differently? What happens during the mixing process and the subsequent conversion of a fluid mixture to the solid form? What governs the physical structure of drug in solid dispersion?

THERMODYNAMIC PERSPECTIVE OF MISCIBILITY AND PHASE SEPARATION IN SOLID DISPERSION

During the first stage of solid dispersion formation, energy is taken up by the system to overcome drug–drug and polymer–polymer interactions. The amount of energy consumed by the system during this process can be determined calorimetrically by measuring, for example, heat of fusion, heat of solution, heat of sublimation, or a combination of two of these processes (e.g., when drug dissolves in a melting polymer). During the second stage, drug–polymer mixing occurs with relative ease owing to the fluid nature of components. However, two components would molecularly mix only if their free energy of mixing (ΘG_m), as discussed in the following section, is negative. Obviously, for systems involving ternary agents (e.g., plasticizers, surfactants, cosolvent), mixing phenomenon gets further complicated and is beyond the scope of current purpose. Assuming that the mixing is complete, the structure of drug in solid dispersion would depend on the rate of congealing or solvent removal or condensation. In systems that undergo congealing, either a crystalline or partly crystalline drug may precipitate, depending on whether the rate of cooling of fluid mixture is less than the rate of drug crystallization. Similarly, in systems with common cosolvents (e.g., spray drying or SCF process), solvent removal might induce phase separation from a miscible solution.

Free Energy of Mixing (ΘG_m)

One of the obvious criteria for drug and polymer to mix with each other is to have negative free energy of mixing. Whether a given drug will be miscible with a polymer at a specific drug–polymer ratio or not can be identified using the Flory–Huggins model (Flory 1953). The Flory–Huggins model has been extensively applied to study solution behavior of polymers in organic solvents, which are typically small molecules. The model may be extrapolated to pharmaceutical solid dispersions by considering the organic solvent to represent drug substance. Since the model is more applicable to concentrated polymer solutions, it may be well applicable to understand the mixing behavior in pharmaceutical solid dispersions.

The free energy of mixing per mole of drug–polymer mixture can be calculated as follows:

$$\Theta G_m = RT[n_{drug} \ln \varphi_{drug} + n_{polymer} \ln \varphi_{polymer} + n_{drug} \varphi_{polymer} \chi_{drug-polymer}] \tag{18.1}$$

where n_{drug} and $n_{polymer}$ are the number of moles of drug and polymer, φ_{drug} and $\varphi_{polymer}$ are the volume fractions occupied by drug and polymer, R is the gas constant, T is the absolute temperature, and $\chi_{drug-polymer}$ is the Flory–Huggins interaction parameter that accounts for the energy of the interdispersing drug and polymer molecules. The interaction parameter $\chi_{drug-polymer}$ can be experimentally determined using the Hilderbrand solubility parameter, as follows (Hilderbrand and Scott 1950):

$$\chi_{drug-polymer} = \frac{V}{RT}\left(\delta_{drug} - \delta_{polymer}\right)^2 \tag{18.2}$$

where V is the volume occupied by polymer segment, and δ_{drug} and $\delta_{polymer}$ are the Hilderbrand solubility parameters of drug and polymer, respectively. The closer the solubility parameters of drug and polymer are to each other, the smaller will be the interaction parameter and better will be the drug–polymer miscibility. It should be noted here that the $\chi_{drug-polymer}$ term is fairly independent of changes in drug–polymer ratio, and is applicable to mixtures exhibiting very weak drug–polymer interactions. For mixtures with stronger specific interactions (e.g., hydrogen bonding), Equation 18.1 gets further complicated. Interested readers are referred to the work in this area by Coleman et al. (1991).

The free energy of mixing can alternatively be described by using Equation 18.3, which is obtained by rearranging and combining terms from Equation 18.1.

$$\Theta G_m = \Theta H_m - T\Theta S_m \tag{18.3}$$

where ΘH_m is the enthalpy of mixing, ΘS_m is the entropy of mixing, and T is the absolute temperature.

From Equation 18.3, it is inferred that mixing between two components is governed by the competing effects of enthalpy and entropy of mixing, with mixing being favored by a loss in enthalpy and a gain in entropy. In other words, mixing occurs when the free energy of products is less than the free energy of reactants.

Enthalpy of Mixing (ΘH_m)

The term *enthalpy of mixing* generally refers to the net energy gained or lost during the mixing process and is the net result of

1. Positive contribution to the enthalpy of mixing as a result of breaking drug–drug and polymer–polymer interactions
2. Negative contribution to the enthalpy of mixing as a result of forming drug–polymer interactions

Therefore, mixing is favored if heat is liberated (i.e., exothermic process) during bond formation. In other words,

$$\left|\Theta H_{drug-drug}\right| + \left|\Theta H_{polymer-polymer}\right| < \left|2\Theta H_{drug-polymer}\right| \tag{18.4}$$

then, $\Theta H_m < 0$, and the change in enthalpy favors mixing.

Entropy of Mixing (ΘS_m)

The term *entropy of mixing* refers to the level of disorder that is either gained or lost when two components are mixed. For instance, when mixing two large molecules such as a protein and a polymer, the number of confirmations available to the protein and polymer after mixing would be significantly less than that available to neat protein and neat polymer. This leads to $\Theta S_m < 0$, which does not favor mixing. Unless there are strong specific interactions between the protein and polymer that lead to an exothermic mixing (i.e., $\Theta H_m < 0$), which can override the decrease in entropy at the given temperature, molecular mixing of protein and polymer would not be possible. On the other hand, in typical pharmaceutical solid dispersions consisting of a small molecule and a polymer, mixing is mostly due to a large gain in entropy ($\Theta S_m > 0$) resulting from the increased permutation available to the drug dispersed in polymer matrix. If the concentration of drug is increased to a level such that the drug–drug interactions override the drug–polymer interaction or an increase in entropy of mixing, a demixing in the form of two distinct phases, where both components are amorphous or one is crystalline (drug) and the other one is amorphous, could occur. Similarly, if enough molecular mobility exists during storage, then drug–drug interactions and the driving force for crystallization could, for instance, overcome the entropy barrier that drives mixing, and the system could phase separate.

One of the ways to understand the impact of drug composition in phase miscibility of solid dispersions is to calculate the changes in the free energy of mixing (ΘG_m) and plot it against the volume fraction of polymer ($\varphi_{polymer}$), as shown in Figure 18.2.

It should, however, be noted that free energy of mixing as well as strength of hydrogen-bond interactions are dependent on the temperature. Hence, although a drug–polymer mixture is miscible in its fluid state, it could eventually phase separate depending on the molecular mobility and thermodynamic driving force. Such a phenomenon is often the root cause for physical instability, and the consequences of instability will be discussed later. Ternary agents have been added in pharmaceutical systems to promote miscibility. For example, addition of citric acid to solid dispersions of polyvinylpyrrolidone (PVP) and indomethacin enhances the miscibility between drug and polymer (Liu and Zografi 1998). However, ternary agents have also induced phase separation from an otherwise miscible solid dispersion; for example, addition of Myrj 52 to solid dispersions of PVP vinylacetate and itraconazole led to phase separation (Wang et al. 2005).

CLASSIFICATION OF SOLID DISPERSION

A schematic describing the various types of solid dispersion, which is classified on the basis of the solid-state structure of resulting dispersion, is presented in Figure 18.3. Selected types of solid dispersions are discussed.

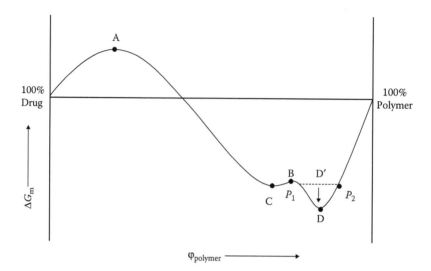

FIGURE 18.2 Hypothetical depiction of drug–polymer miscibility by plotting changes in free energy of mixing (ΔG_m) as a function of volume fraction of polymer ($\varphi_{polymer}$). At composition given by point A, no drug–polymer mixing occurs as $\Delta G_m > 0$. At point B, although drug–polymer mixing occurs, a phase separation into points C and D is possible since composition at these points have lower free energy than at B. Mixture at point D has the lowest free energy than any other points of the same overall composition. If the system hypothetically phase separates into two points (e.g., P_1 and P_2), the composition weighted free energy (given by point D′) is higher than D, hence the system would thermodynamically revert to composition depicted by point D. (Reproduced from Coleman, M. M. et al., *Specific Interactions and the Miscibility of Polymer Blends*, Technomic Publishing Company, Lancaster, PA, 1991.)

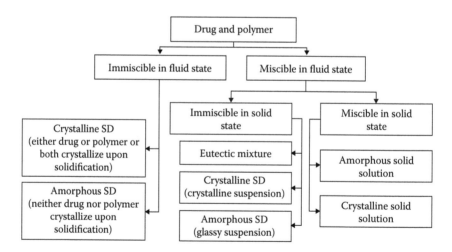

FIGURE 18.3 Flowchart describing the various types of solid dispersions depending on whether the drug and polymer are miscible in their fluid state and solid state.

DRUG AND POLYMER EXHIBITING IMMISCIBILITY IN FLUID STATE

If a drug and polymer are immiscible in their fluid state, it is likely that they would not exhibit miscibility on solidification of the fluid mixture. Such systems may be regarded as similar to their corresponding physical mixtures, although any enhancement in dissolution performance compared to physical mixture may be owing to modification in morphology of drug and/or polymer due to physical transformation (i.e., solid to liquid state and back), intimate drug–polymer mixing, and/or enhanced surface area. Formation of crystalline or amorphous solid dispersions can be influenced by the rate of solidification of mixture and the rate of crystallization of drug, polymer, or both.

DRUG AND POLYMER EXHIBITING MISCIBILITY IN FLUID STATE

If the drug and polymer are miscible in their fluid state, then as discussed in the section titled Thermodynamic Perspective of Miscibility and Phase Separation in Solid Dispersions, the mixture may or may not undergo phase separation during solidification, thereby influencing the structure of solid dispersion.

Eutectic Mixtures

Eutectic mixtures are formed when the drug and polymer are miscible in their molten state, but on cooling, they crystallize as two distinct components with negligible miscibility. When a drug (A) and a carrier (B) are comelted at their eutectic composition defined by point Y, as shown schematically in Figure 18.4, the melting point of the mixture is lower than the melting point of either drug or carrier alone. While some researchers claim eutectics to be an intimate but inert physical mixture of the two components; others claim that the reduction in the melting point of eutectic mixtures is a direct evidence of molecular interaction between the drug and the carrier. At the eutectic composition (Y), both drug and carrier exist in a finely divided state, which results in higher surface area and enhanced dissolution rate of drug. Although not every carrier can form a eutectic with every drug, carriers such as polyethylene glycols (PEG), urea, and polyoxyethylene–polyoxypropylene (Pluronic®) have demonstrated eutectic formation to enhance dissolution rates of many poorly water-soluble drugs (Leuner and Dressman 2000).

Crystalline Solid Dispersion

A crystalline solid dispersion (or suspension) is formed when the rate at which drug crystallizes from drug–polymer miscible mixture is greater than the rate at which drug–polymer fluid mixture solidifies. Such a crystalline solid dispersion may differ from that described in the section titled Drug and Polymer Exhibiting Immiscibility in Fluid State, where even the drug–polymer fluid mixture is not miscible.

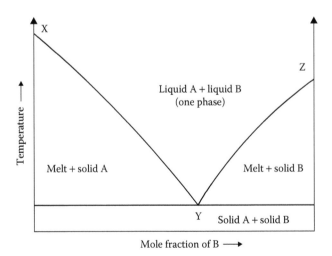

FIGURE 18.4 Phase diagram of a simple eutectic system. At temperatures below curve XY or YZ, either solid A [drug] or solid B [carrier] solidifies first from the molten mixture, respectively. At eutectic composition Y, both drug and carrier solidify simultaneously as a mixture of finely divided crystalline components.

Amorphous Solid Dispersion

If the drug–polymer fluid mixture is cooled at a rate that does not allow for drug crystallization, then the drug is kinetically trapped in its amorphous or a *solidified-liquid* state. Although such systems offer dissolution advantages owing to their higher thermodynamic activity, they also risk the potential for conversion to a more stable and less soluble crystalline form.

Solid Solution

Solid solution is a solid dispersion that is miscible in its fluid as well as solid state. Most pharmaceutical solid solutions are amorphous in nature and can be characterized by studying their composition-dependent changes in single glass transition temperature (T_g). A crystalline solid solution may result when a crystalline drug is trapped within a crystalline polymeric carrier. Crystalline solid solutions are predominant in metallurgy (e.g., alloys), but their possibility in pharmaceutical solid dispersions cannot be ruled out. Poorly soluble drugs have been incorporated in carrier molecules using crystal inclusion and crystal doping techniques (Vishweshwar et al. 2006), although the usage of such technologies has not yet gained widespread application in pharmaceutical product development. Amorphous solid solutions (also termed *amorphous molecular dispersion*) have been shown to enhance the dissolution rate of poorly soluble drugs. As the drug is molecularly dispersed in the carrier matrix, its effective surface area is significantly higher and hence the dissolution rate is increased. In the case of felodipine–PVP solid dispersions, hydrogen-bond interaction between felodipine and PVP has shown to enhance drug dissolution (Karavas et al. 2006). Solid solutions have also improved physical stability of amorphous drugs by inhibiting drug crystallization by minimizing molecular mobility (Yoshioka et al. 1995).

MULTICOMPONENT SOLID DISPERSION

Ternary agents have been added to solid dispersion of two components either to enhance drug dissolution rate or to overcome manufacturing or stability issues. Surfactants have been added to solid dispersions to improve the dissolution rate of poorly water-soluble drugs (Aungs et al. 1977). They have also been used to improve miscibility between drug and polymer or simply to inhibit drug crystallization during storage (Urbanetz 2006). In one study, the miscibility of griseofulvin was increased from 3% w/w to 40% w/w in PEG 6000 by adding 5% w/w of sodium dodecyl sulfate (SDS) (Wulff et al. 1996). Pluronic F-68 was used to increase the solid solubility and dissolution rate of nifedipine from its PEG-based solid dispersion (Mehta et al. 2002). Ternary agents in the form of plasticizers have been used in manufacturing of solid dispersions using the hot-melt extrusion (HME) technique. These agents act by lowering the processing temperature needed to extrude drug–polymer mixture, thereby minimizing potential degradation.

PRODUCT DEVELOPMENT OF SOLID DISPERSION—EXPERIMENTAL PREDICTION OF COMPONENTS

A solid dispersion can be formulated in various ways in order to meet the desired target product profile. The recipe may include one or more polymers, plasticizers, surfactants, release-retarding agents, etc. In order to develop a successful product, formulators should look at the following with an equal eye: (1) expected performance of the product, (2) its physical and chemical stability during processing and on the shelf, and (3) simplicity in commercial manufacturing. Formulating the product with the right ingredients can fulfill these three requirements. There are several companies that sell numerous grades of such excipients, and it gets challenging for formulators to choose the ingredients to make an optimized product. Slight changes in physicochemical properties of the excipients can have detrimental effects on the performance of the product. It is important to find a *sweet spot* in the recipe to obtain a product that fulfills all three product development requirements.

In order to boil down to the potentially correct ingredients that may be compatible to form solid dispersion with the API, there are some theoretically predictive approaches described in the literature. One of the well-known ones is the Hildebrand solubility parameter, which is based on calculating the molar vaporization energies and molar volume of the ingredients (Greenhalgh 1991; Hancock 1997). Greenhalgh and coworkers used ibuprofen and various sugars as model combinations, and studied their miscibility to correlate with the difference in their solubility parameters. It was evident from their investigation that Hildebrand parameters give a prediction of possible incompatibilities between the components of solid dispersion. Hansen modified the Hildebrand solubility parameter to the Hansen solubility parameter, which also included polar and hydrogen-bonding components that were lacking in the previous derivation (Hansen 1996, 2004). The Hansen solubility parameter was more predictive for predicting miscibility of the components of solid dispersions. Even though solubility parameter calculations gave a good direction to the excipients to be used to make a successful solid dispersion product, they still lacked the practical understanding considering the long-term stability and processability of the product. Formulators could get a good target zone to choose the polymers or other excipients, but they still had to prepare the product using all the polymers that fell in that range. Moreover, the solubility parameter calculations did not provide a good understanding of the concentration of the carrier that would keep the product stable. The carriers used in solid dispersions are polymers, which have large and complicated structures, and Hansen and Hildebrand solubility parameters, which were based on the drug solubility in small molecules and solvents, did not make a very promising model to predict drug–polymer miscibility. Surikutchi et al. (2013) made an attempt to explain this misconception in their review. They concluded that even though the concept of solubility parameter is theoretically promising, limited data available on different structural groups in polymers can lead to misleading calculations.

Parikh et al. (2015) introduced a systematic experimental approach to predict miscibility and long-term stability of solid dispersions. They used itraconazole as a model drug that was dissolved and film casted with various concentrations of polymers of different backbones—methacrylate, pyrrolidone, and cellulose. The thinly casted (200 micron) solid dispersions which were also placed at 40°C/75%RH showed instability by physical separation of API, which was analyzed by DSC and p-XRD. Using this technique, a large number of polymers could be screened in a very short period of time to find out the stable combinations. This technique has potential to include other formulation aids such as surfactants to obtain a formulation that had good dispersion property. In conclusion, they did not find a direct correlation between the Hansen solubility parameter values of the components to their practical results. An experimental technique such as film casting is quick and conclusive for the development of solid dispersions. The film casting technique could be taken to the next level by casting the mixture of API, polymer, and a surfactant as well. Gumaste et al. (2016) constructed ternary phase diagrams of itraconazole-poloxamer 188 with Soluplus® and HPMC-AS by film casting to identify physically stable combinations. This technique is one step forward in the direction of product development, where one can know in a very short period of time the ratios that are stable. The combinations are then manufactured by spray drying or melt extrusion to obtain the desired solid dispersions. The product can also be tested for their dispersability and dissolution using the same film casts for in vitro performance evaluation.

In their series of four manuscripts, Serajuddin et al. compiled a list of polymer properties that potentially affect the performance and manufacture of solid dispersions (Gupta et al. 2014, 2016; Meena et al. 2014; Parikh et al. 2014). Physical, thermal, and viscoelastic analyses were performed by his group, which aimed at providing useful information to the formulators to develop solid dispersions. They defined some critical properties of polymers in this database such as glass transition temperature, melt viscosity, tan δ, and molecular weight. Such properties give the information to the formulators to develop desired product, especially when the processing technique is hot-melt extrusion. The viscoelastic properties of polymers not only help to predict the extrusion temperatures and shear rates, but also gives information on miscibility of API in polymer. In their research work, Gupta et al. (2014) demonstrated the use of rheology to predict the extrusion temperature and miscibility of carbamazepine in Soluplus for hot-melt extrusion. They reported that a viscosity range of 1000–10,000 Pa.s is ideal for melt extrusion, and there is a drop in viscosity of the polymer with an increase in temperature.

The drop in viscosity was more prominent in presence of the API, and was concentration dependent. Such an investigation can help formulators to not only estimate the processing temperature to manufacture stable solid dispersion, but also to find out the miscible concentrations.

MANUFACTURING OF SOLID DISPERSION

As reviewed by Serajuddin (1999) in, one of the major hurdles in the development of solid dispersions is the lack of suitable manufacturing techniques that could be scaled up to commercial production. The commercial-scale manufacturing of solid dispersions has received significant attention over the past decade, and various techniques are now available for large-scale manufacturing. When selecting a suitable technique, the following factors have to be considered:

- Physicochemical properties of raw materials
- Ease of manufacturing and scale-up, and the associated cost
- Reproducibility of drug product attributes
- Intellectual property and freedom to operate

Karanth et al. (2006) have reviewed various approaches that may be utilized in the manufacturing of solid dispersions. In this section, selected examples of techniques that have potential for commercial-scale manufacturing of solid dispersions are presented.

HOT-MELT EXTRUSION

Hot-melt extrusion (HME) is a process of converting a raw material into a product of uniform shape and density by forcing it through a die under controlled conditions (Breitenbach 2002). HME involves usage of heat to transform the raw materials into homogenously mixed mass, that is, solid dispersion. While HME has been widely used in the polymer and food industry for more than half-a-century, its ability to operate in a continuous fashion and without the need for organic solvents has made it appealing to the pharmaceutical industry. Over the recent decade, several publications on the pharmaceutical application of HME process to manufacture a variety of solid and semisolid dosage forms have been reported (Choksi 2004).

HME is conducted using a melt extruder. A melt extruder, as shown schematically in Figure 18.5, consists of an opening to feed raw materials, a heated barrel that consists of extruder screws to convey and mix the fed materials, and an exit port, which consists of an optional die to shape the extruding mass. Typically, a physical mixture of drug substance and other ingredients is fed into the heated barrel of extruder at a controlled rate. As the physical mixture is conveyed through heated screws, it

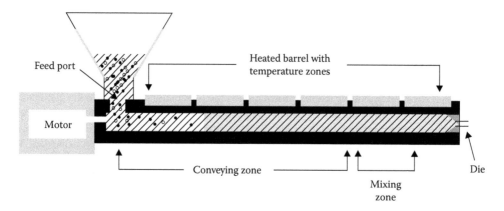

FIGURE 18.5   Schematic showing components of a single-screw melt extruder.

is transformed into its *fluid-like state*, which allows intimate and homogeneous mixing by the high shear of extruder screws. The intimately mixed hot mass, that is, solid dispersion, is extruded through the die opening. The extruded hot strands can either be molded or precisely cut into unit dosage forms using additional accessories named calendaring rolls (Breitenbach 1999). Alternatively, they can be cooled, sized, and either encapsulated or compressed into tablets. Hot-melt extruders are commercially available in different sizes ranging from a benchtop extruder that uses as little as 5 g of material to a commercial-scale extruder that can extrude at rates as high as 120 kg/h.

As the HME process normally involves heating the material to temperatures to or near the melting of drug substance, carriers should be selected such that they do not degrade at such elevated temperatures and pressures. Polymers such as PVP, hydroxypropyl methylcellulose (HPMC), polymethacrylate polymers (e.g., Eudragit EPO), poly(ethyleneoxides) (PEO), HPMC acetate succinate, and so forth, were successfully used during HME to form solid dispersions of itraconazole (Verreck et al. 2003), nicardipine hydrochloride (Nakamichi et al. 2001), nifedipine (Li et al. 2006), indomethacin (Forster et al. 2001), and other model drugs. In some cases, additives such as PEG 6000, Gelucire 44/14, and Sucrosester WE15 have been incorporated as plasticizers in order to lower the processing temperatures (Hulsmann et al. 2000).

When working with limited quantities of material, for instance, during early product development, it is crucial to select suitable carrier(s) while consuming minimal quantities of drug substance. In one study, the authors characterized the rheological and thermal properties of a model drug, indomethacin, along with various polymers and plasticizers, by using very small quantities of ingredients to assess the suitability of melt extrusion and to identify processing conditions (Chokshi et al. 2005). In a different study, optimization of melt extrusion formulation was conducted on a lab-scale extruder by executing a design of experiment using 1 kg batch size. The investigators developed a clear, glassy extrudate by varying the formulation composition in ternary mixtures of itraconazole with hydroxypropyl-β-cyclodextrin (HP-β-CD) and HPMC (Rambali et al. 2003).

Clinical trial materials of itraconazole solid dispersions in HPMC, Eudragit E100, or mixtures of Eudragit E100 and PVPVA64 (70/30% w/w) were manufactured using a corotating twin-screw extruder (Six et al. 2005). Materials were fed at a fixed rate of 1 kg/h with an extruder screw speed of 300 rpm and processing temperature of up to 185°C. The extrudates were cooled, sized, and filled into size 00 capsules for clinical testing at a dose of 100 mg of itraconazole. Results from the study showed that for HPMC formulation, the mean area under the curve (AUC) value of plasma concentrations in eight healthy volunteers was comparable to the comparator's product (Sporanox®), but the values were lower when Eudragit 100 and the Eudragit E100-PVPVA64 mixture were used. The authors concluded that the HME was successfully applied to the manufacture of clinical trial materials.

HOT-MELT ENCAPSULATION

Hot-melt encapsulation is generally suited to formulations that contain solid carriers with melting temperature between 40°C and 70°C. The waxy nature of such carriers limits their sizing into smaller particles, and filling into capsules or compressing as tablets. Using the hot-melt encapsulation technique, such wax-like carriers can be molten and filled directly into capsules, where they solidify. The drug substance is dissolved in the molten carrier, thereby eliminating any content uniformity issues.

Rowley reviewed various developments in filling of liquids and semisolids into hard gelatin capsules (Rowley 2004). Lipid-based carriers and excipients such as PEG, polyoxyethylene–polyoxypropylene (poloxamer), poly(oxyethylene), Gelucires®, lipid surfactants, and so forth, are well suited for this technology. Equipments ranging from benchtop to commercial scale are now available. Volumetric filling of molten mass into hard gelatin capsules and subsequent banding or sealing of filled capsules are carried out in a continuous fashion. While banding is done by applying molten gelatin across the cap–body interface of capsule, sealing is conducted by spraying a hydroalcoholic mixture. Intact capsule seal is obviously necessary to avoid leakage during shelf-life storage as well as to offer consistent capsule disintegration during dissolution process. A capsule-filling machine should possess certain features for successful use during manufacturing. These features include

- Ability to maintain the product in the molten state before dosing
- Accurate dosing of liquid volumes ranging from 0.1 to 1.0 mL
- Surveillance systems to halt dosing when the absence of a capsule body in the die is detected

A successful scale-up of capsule-filling process was demonstrated, for instance, in one study, using a Qualifill semiautomated or H&H capsule filler (Robinson 2001). Gelucire 50/12 or Precirol (a wax comprised of mono-, di-, and triglycerides of palmitostearic acid) was filled into size 2 capsules at a fill weight of 269 mg and at a filling temperature between 50°C and 52°C. Qualifill capsule filler yielded capsules with highly uniform fill weights of less than 1% relative standard deviation.

SPRAY DRYING

Spray drying is a process where a solution of drug substance and carrier is evaporated by spraying the solution as fine droplets into a chamber that is maintained under controlled conditions of heat, humidity, and airflow. The dissolution rate of many poorly water-soluble drugs has been enhanced using spray drying (Sethia and Squillante 2003; Ambike et al. 2005). Organic solvents are normally used during spray-drying process as they are easy to evaporate and possess good solvent capacity for many poorly water-soluble drugs. The morphology form of solid dispersion, and consequently the drug dissolution and stability, can be impacted by the process parameters and geometry of equipment. For instance, the particle size of spray-dried solid dispersion can be controlled by varying the concentration of solute in spray-drying liquid and the droplet size during the spray-drying process (Elversson 2003).

SUPERCRITICAL FLUID TECHNOLOGY

Supercritical fluid (SCF) technology has been successfully applied in particle design engineering of pharmaceuticals, polymer/biomaterials, and chemical compounds (Jung and Perrut 2001). A SCF is a substance that exists above its critical point, which is defined by the conditions of temperature and pressure at which liquid and gaseous states of a substance coexist. When a liquid is heated, its density continues to decrease, while the density of vapor being formed continues to increase. At the critical point, densities of liquid and gas are equal and there is no phase boundary, as shown in Figure 18.6. Above the critical point, that is, in the supercritical region, the fluid possesses the penetrating power typical of a gas and the solvent power typical of a liquid.

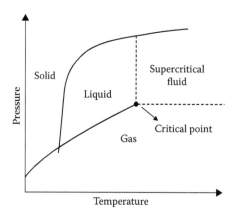

FIGURE 18.6 Supercritical region of a hypothetical compound. The solid lines represent phase boundaries between solid–liquid, liquid–gas, and solid–gas phases. Supercritical region is the region indicated by the dotted line.

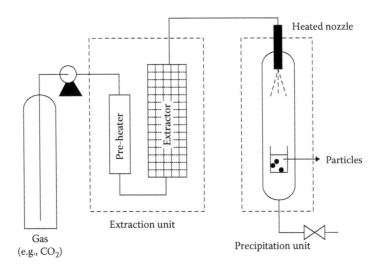

Gas
(e.g., CO_2)

FIGURE 18.7 Schematic of the RESS apparatus. (From Subramanian, B. et al.: 1997. *J. Pharm. Sci.* 1997. 86. 885. Copyright Wiley-VCH Verlag GmbH & Co. KGaA. Reproduced with permission.)

SCF such as supercritical CO_2 has been widely used in the pharmaceutical field owing to its relatively low critical point (304 K and 7.38 Mbar), which can be easily achieved, and the fluid's ability to dissolve most pharmaceutical compounds. One application of the SCF process is the rapid expansion of supercritical solutions (RESS) (Subramanian et al. 1997). During the RESS process, the SCF is diffused through a bed of solid solute (i.e., extractor), as shown schematically in Figure 18.7. As the fluid diffuses through the bed, the solid solute dissolves in it. The fluid solution is then depressurized in a separate chamber, causing an extremely rapid nucleation and precipitation of high-energy solids. How the solids are precipitated depends on factors such as thermodynamic conditions before and after fluid expansion as well as geometry of the equipment being used (Palakodaty and York 1999). RESS has been applied in enhancing dissolution rate of poorly water-soluble compounds through techniques including solid dispersion formation (Sethia 2002; Gong et al. 2005), micro- or nanoparticle formation (Turk et al. 2002), and crystal doping or solid solution formation (Vemavarapu 2002). Drug substances such as indomethacin, nifedipine, carbamezapine, naproxen, and nitrendipine have been processed using this technology to generate drug products with highly reproducible physicochemical properties (Ting et al. 1993; Knez et al. 1995; Subramanian et al. 1997). As a continuous process with no necessity for use of organic solvent, the RESS process is valuable in commercial manufacturing of solid dispersions.

SCFs have also been used in conjunction with organic solvents to generate particles of desired morphology and attributes (Foster et al. 2003). One intrinsic limitation of SCFs is their inability to dissolve moderate to highly polar compounds. Such compounds can be easily dissolved in suitable organic solvents, and SCFs can be used as antisolvents to precipitate the solids. This procedure has been termed *solution-enhanced dispersion by supercritical fluids* (SEDS). Depending on the method by which solution and SCF are introduced and mixed into each other, different applications have been described. These include:

1. Gas Antisolvent (GAS) or Supercritical Antisolvent (SAS) Recrystallization: In this process, SCF is filled into a chamber and a batch of solution is introduced later. The SCF penetrates into the solution and expands it, thereby decreasing the solvent power and resulting in microparticles of precipitating solid mixture. In one study, solid dispersions of felodipine in HPMC and surfactants, such as poloxamer 188, poloxamer 107, and polyoxyethylene hydrogenated castor oil, were prepared using the GAS technique. The resulting solid dispersions had a mean particle size of 200–250 nm and demonstrated higher aqueous solubility and comparable dissolution rate compared to solid dispersions prepared through conventional solvent evaporation (Won et al. 2005).

2. Aerosol Solvent Extraction System (ASES): Here, the solution is sprayed through the atomization nozzle into a chamber filled with SCF. Expansion of solution occurs within the fine droplets of solvent being sprayed, thus creating supersaturation and precipitation of solids as fine particles.

3. Precipitation with Compressed Antisolvent (PCA): The PCA differs from the GAS process in that much higher mass transfer rate and efficient crystallization are achieved by supplying compressed antisolvent into solution being sprayed (Fusaro et al. 2005). In one study, the authors used supercritical CO_2 as the antisolvent to prepare solid dispersions of phenytoin and PVP K30 from their solutions in acetone or acetone/ethanol mixture by using PCA and conventional spray-drying process. A comparison of intrinsic dissolution rates revealed that solid dispersions prepared using the PCA technique had 68% higher dissolution rate when compared to spray-dried solid dispersions (Muhrer et al. 2006). Process parameters of GAS and PCA techniques have also been manipulated to obtain desired morphology and polymorphs of pharmaceutical actives (Edwards et al. 2001; Jahrmer et al. 2005; Muhrer et al. 2006).

FUSION

Hot-melt extrusion has proven to be a commercially feasible technique, but its application may be limited for processing thermolabile drugs. Even though the extrusion shear rate could be increased to decrease the viscosity of most polymers, high temperatures and long residence time could be detrimental to the product. McGinity and coworkers introduced to a fusion technique called Kinetisol® dispersion, which involved use of a custom built compounder by DisperSol Technologies, LLC (Austin, TX) (DiNunzio et al. 2010b,c). The technique involves the use of impact shear along with heat to manufacture solid dispersion in a very short period of time. A premix of drug and polymer was charged into the compounder, and processing parameters such as maximum rotational speed, ejection temperature, and processing time were studied. All the batches using itraconazole and Kollidon® L100-55 were manufactured at not more than 177°C and 14.1 seconds. The material was quench pressed and milled after discharge. From this study, they concluded that it was possible to manufacture solid dispersions without the use of plasticizers in a very short time. In their following work, they demonstrated that the manufacture of temperature-sensitive compound hydrocortisone was possible using this technique (DiNunzio et al. 2010a).

EXAMPLES OF SOLID DISPERSIONS

As summarized in Table 18.1, FDA has approved approximately 17 products based on solid dispersion technology. Here we will discuss several examples of these.

SURFACTANT AND LIPID-BASED SOLID DISPERSIONS

Fusion and solvent evaporation are most commonly used techniques to prepare solid dispersions in the laboratory scale. As reported by Serajuddin (1999), these methods have practical limitations in the scale to commercial production. Even methods such as HME, spray drying, and SCF technique described earlier have many challenges. For example, the drug and/or the carrier may not be stable at the high temperature needed for melt extrusion, a common solvent to dissolve both the relatively hydrophobic drug and the relatively hydrophilic carrier for the purpose of spray drying may not be available, and the SCF technology may not be amenable and cost efficient in most cases. The introduction of surface-active and self-emulsifying excipients that are solid at room temperature represents a breakthrough in commercial development of solid dispersions. It has been reported that formulations incorporating these new excipients may not only increase dissolution rates of poorly water-soluble drugs, but they may also be filled as their molten mass directly into hard gelatin capsules, thus eliminating the need for additional unit operations such as milling, blending, sieving, and so forth. Vasanthavada and Serajuddin (2007) recently reviewed the application of surfactants and

TABLE 18.1
List of FDA Approved Solid Dispersion Products

Brand Name	Active Ingredients	Approve Date	Carrier Material	Manufacturing Method
Gris-PEG	Griseofulvin	April 16, 1975	PEG	Hot-Melt
Isoptin	Verapamil Hydrochloride	March 8, 1975 (Discontinued)	HPC/HPMC	Hot-Melt Extrusion
Cesamet	Nabilone	December 12, 1985	PVP	/
Sporanox	Itraconazole	November 9, 1992	HPMC	Spray Drying
Prograf	Tacrolimus	April 8, 1994	HPMC	Spray Drying
Rezulin	Troglitazone	January 29, 1997	PVP	Hot-Melt Extrusion
Afeditab CR	Nifedipine	March 10, 2000	Poloxamer/PVP	Hot-Melt Encapsulation
Kaletra	Lopinavir; Ritonavir	September 15, 2000	PVP/VA	Hot-Melt Extrusion
Fenoglide	Fenofibrate	August 10, 2007	PEG/Poloxamer	Hot-Melt Encapsulation
Intelence	Etravirine	January 18, 2008	HPMC	Spray Drying
Norvir	Ritonavir	February 2, 2010	PVP/VA	Hot-Melt Extrusion
Zortress	Everolimus	April 20, 2010	HPMC	Spray Drying
Onmel	Itraconazole	April 29, 2010	HPMC	Hot-Melt Extrusion
Incivek	Telaprevir	May 23, 2010 (Discontinued)	HPMCAS	Spray Drying
Zelboraf	Vemurafenib	August 17, 2011	HPMCAS	Coprecipitation
Kalydeco	Ivacaftor	January 31, 2012	HPMCAS	Spray Drying
Noxafil	Posaconazole	November 25, 2013	HPMCAS	Hot-Melt Extrusion

surface-active lipids in the development of solid dispersions. In the opinion of the present authors, such solid dispersion systems will continue to play major roles in the future in the development of bioavailable dosage forms for poorly water-soluble drugs. The advantages of some of the solid dispersion systems are described in this section in relation to the carriers used.

Gelucires®

Gelucire® 44/14 (Gattefossé Corp., St. Priest, France) is a mixture of glyceryl and PEG 1500 esters of long-chain fatty acids and is listed in the European Pharmacopoeia as laurylmacrogolglycerides and in the US Pharmacopoeia as lauroylpolyoxyglycerides. It is a self-emulsifying excipient that is waxy and semisolid at ambient temperature; the suffixes, 44 and 14, in its trade name refer to its melting point and hydrophilic–lipophilic balance (HLB), respectively. It has extensively been investigated as carrier for solid dispersions. Serajuddin et al. (1988) prepared different solid dispersion formulations of a poorly water-soluble basic drug, REV5901, by dissolving the drug in molten PEG 1000, PEG 1450, PEG 8000, or Gelucire® 44/14, and then filling the molten solutions into size 0 hard gelatin capsules in amounts that contained 100 mg of REV5901 and 450 mg of the excipient per capsule. On congealing the formulations to ambient temperature, the incorporated drug existed as either a molecular dispersion (solution) or in the amorphous state within the excipient matrix. When dissolution of the formulations was tested under sink conditions in the 900 mL volume of simulated gastric fluid USP (without enzyme), dissolution from all of the PEG-based solid dispersions was incomplete whereas Gelucire® 44/14 provided complete dissolution (Figure 18.8). Even when water was used as the dissolution medium, where the compound was practically insoluble, the Gelucire® 44/14–based solid dispersion completely released the drug in the dissolution medium, forming a milky dispersion of the free drug as fine, metastable oily globules, while no such release of drug in water from any of the PEG-based formulations was observed. This study demonstrated the advantages of surface-active carriers in drug release from solid dipersions. Similar advantages of Gelucire 44/14® and other surfactants have been reported by many different investigators (Aungst et al. 1977; Al-Razzak et al. 1997; Barker et al. 2003; Nulifer et al. 2003; Vippagunta et al. 2003; He et al. 2005; Soliman and Kohn 2005).

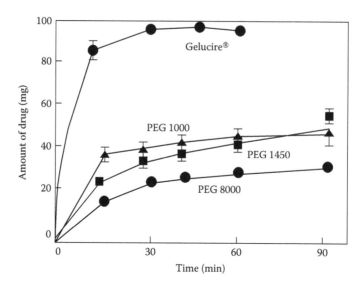

FIGURE 18.8 Relative dissolution rates of REV5901 from solid dispersion formulations of various polyethylene glycols (PEG) and Gelucire® 44/14 in 0.1 M HCl. Each capsule contained 100 mg of drug in a total fill weight of 550 mg. Capsules were prepared by filling with the molten formulations. (From Serajuddin, A. T. M. et al., *J. Pharm. Sci.*, 77, 414–417, 1988. With permission.)

PEG–Polysorbate 80 Mixtures

As reported earlier, the drug release from a PEG-based solid dispersion may be incomplete when the drug solution in molten PEG is filled directly in hard gelatin capsules and allowed to solidify. Serajuddin et al. (1990) demonstrated that this shortcoming of PEG may be overcome by incorporating polysorbate 80 with PEG; solid dispersion formulations prepared from mixtures of PEG and polysorbate 80 may perform similar to Gelucire® 44/14. Another advantage of the system is that although polysorbate 80 is liquid at room temperature, a semisolid matrix is formed when it is mixed with PEG (Figure 18.9), since polysorbate 80 was incorporated within the amorphous region of the PEG solid structure (Morris et al. 1992).

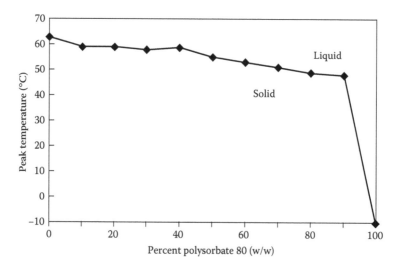

FIGURE 18.9 Phase behavior of PEG 8000 and polysorbate 80 mixtures. Mixtures of PEG 8000 containing up to 90% of polysorbate 80 remain in the solid state at room temperature. (From Morris, K. R. et al., *J. Pharm. Sci.*, 81, 1185–1188, 1992. With permission.)

Joshi et al. (2004) demonstrated that the bioavailability of a weakly basic drug in dogs from a solid dispersion in 3:1-PEG–polysorbate 80 mixture was 21-fold higher than that of a capsule containing micronized bulk drug blended with lactose and microcrystalline cellulose. Similarly, Dannenfelser et al. (2004) reported a 10-fold bioavailability of a highly permeable, poorly water-soluble (aqueous solubility ~0.17 µg/mL at 25°C), neutral compound in dogs from a PEG 3350–polysorbate 80 (3:1) solid dispersion as compared to a conventional capsule formulation containing the micronized drug substance. Other reports also confirm enhanced dissolution (Veiga et al. 1993b) and bioavailability (Sheen et al. 1995) of drugs from PEG–polysorbate mixtures.

Tocopheryl Polyethylene Glycol 1000 Succinate

Another surface-active carrier useful for preparing solid dispersion formulations is tocopheryl polyethylene glycol 1000 succinate (TPGS) or d-α-tocopheryl PEG 1000 succinate (Eastman Chemical, TN). Because of its relatively low melting point (~40°C), TPGS may be filled in its molten form in hard and soft gelatin capsules; however, hard gelatin capsules may require band sealing to prevent leakage of the contents. TPGS is used in the soft gelatin capsule formulation of aprenavir (Agenerase®, GSK, NC) to enhance its bioavailability through a combination of increased solubility and permeability enhancement due to excipient-mediated P-glycoprotein efflux inhibition (Yu et al. 1999). Koo et al. (2000) reported that a solid dispersion of an antimalarial drug, halofantrine, provided 5–7 times higher bioavailability than a conventional tablet formulation. In another study conducted in rats, the effect of TPGS on the solubility and permeability of paclitaxel was demonstrated by improving the bioavailability by 4- to 6-fold by coadministration with TPGS as compared to a formulation without TPGS (Varma et al. 2005). Other investigators also reported similar beneficial influences of TPGS on dissolution and absorption of poorly water-soluble drugs (Boudreaux et al. 1993; Sokol et al. 1993; Chang et al. 1996; Wu 1998).

Block Copolymers

There has also been increased focus on the application of block copolymers in solid dispersion formulations of poorly water-soluble drugs (Suni and Cho 1997; Ho et al. 2000; Passerini et al. 2003; Chen et al. 2004; Yin et al. 2005). Various grades of block copolymers are commercially available as poloxamers (Pluronics). Drugs may be formulated by dissolving them in molten block copolymers and filling the liquid in hard gelatin capsules; the molten mass solidifies at ambient room temperature. Recently, Yin et al. (2005) reported a process where a water-insoluble drug, BMS-347070, and a block copolymer, Pluronic F-127, were dissolved in acetone or methylene chloride and then spray dried to form a dispersion of nanosized crystalline drug material within a crystalline, water-soluble matrix. It was hypothesized that the PEO segments of Pluronic F-127 crystallized while the polypropylene oxide segments of the excipient remained amorphous, creating a size-restricted domain in which the drug substance formed physically stable nanocrystals.

Glycerides

Thixotropic gels (TPGS) of mono- and diglycerides have been used as carriers for solid dispersions. In the development of a hard gelatin capsule formulation of a poorly water-soluble drug, propantheline bromide, the drug substance was first dissolved in Miglyol 829 and the solution was then converted to a semisolid form by incorporating colloidal silicon dioxide to increase the viscosity of the fill material. In another study, colloidal silicon dioxide was used as a thickening agent for the mixture of an oil (diesters of caprylic/capric acids; Captex 200), a surfactant (polysorbate 80), and a cosurfactant (C8/C10 mono-/diglycerides; Capmul MCM) (Patil et al. 2004).

PVP AND CELLULOSE-BASED SOLID DISPERSIONS

Water-soluble synthetic polymers such as polyvinylpyrrolidone (PVP) and cellulose-based polymers such as HPMC have been commonly used to enhance the dissolution rate of poorly water-soluble drugs. PVP has been used extensively not only to enhance the drug dissolution rate

(Bates 1969; Simonelli et al. 1969; Itai et al. 1985; Tantishaiyakul et al. 1999), but also to inhibit crystallization of amorphous drugs from solid dispersions (Simonelli et al. 1969; Doherty and York 1989; Yoshioka et al. 1995). In one study (Perng et al. 1998), solid dispersion of SB-210661 was prepared with PEG 8000 or PVP because addition of surfactants to the drug formulation did not improve its dissolution rate. Following storage of solid dispersions at 25°C/60% RH for 1 year, there was no significant change in the dissolution profile for the PVP dispersion, whereas the PEG dispersion showed as much as 50% decrease in the drug release. Further characterization led to the conclusion that PVP was able to retain the amorphous structure of drug through hydrogen bonding, which was lacking in PEG-based solid dispersions.

HPMC has also been often used to improve drug dissolution rate. In one study, HPMC was used to improve the dissolution rate and bioavailability of albendazole, a poorly water-soluble drug, in beagles (Kohri et al. 1999). In another study, solid dispersion of HPMC with nifedipine showed a higher nifedipine dissolution rate when compared to solid dispersions prepared with methylcellulose and hydroxypropyl cellulose (HPC) (Sugimoto et al. 1982). HPMC, HPC, and PVP showed an inhibitory effect on precipitation of RS-8359 from its supersaturated solution, with the cellulose polymers showing better inhibition than PVP. It was hypothesized that these polymers inhibit crystallization not only by increasing solution viscosity, but also by interacting with the dissolved drug (Usui et al. 1991). More recently, HPMC acetate succinate (HPMC AS) has been shown to offer superior ability to inhibit drug crystallization in both solution and solid state (Shanker 2005). HPMC AS provides functionalities that enable hydrophobic interactions, hydrogen bonding, and electronic interactions with drugs. Unlike PVP and HPMC, HPMC AS exhibits minimal tendency to absorb water and possesses relatively high T_g. In one study, the authors compared the ability of polymers such as PVP, HPMC, HPMC phthalate, and HPMC AS in inhibiting crystallization of nifedipine from its supersaturate solution (pH 6.8) (Figure 18.10) (Tanno et al. 2004). HPMC AS clearly showed superior

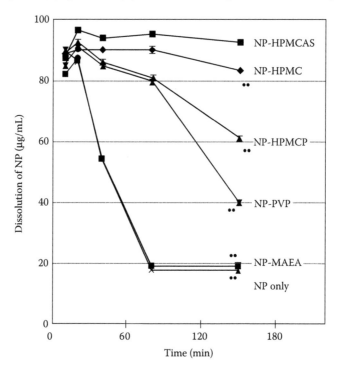

FIGURE 18.10 Inhibitory effect of polymers on recrystallization of nifedipine (NP) from a supersaturated solution at pH 6.8. HPMCAS, hydroxypropyl methylcellulose acetate succinate; HPMC, hydroxypropylmethyl cellulose; HPMCP, hydroxypropylmethyl pthate; PVP, polyvinyl pyrrolidone; MAEA, methacrylic acid ethyl acrylate copolymer. (From Tanno, F. et al., *Drug Dev. Ind. Pharm.*, 30, 13, 2004. With permission.)

ability in maintaining drug supersaturation. Such a supersaturation can result in enhanced absorption of drugs that exhibit solubility-limited absorption (Shanker 2005).

CHARACTERIZATION OF SOLID DISPERSION

Various techniques available for characterization of solid-state properties of raw materials and finished solid dispersions are presented in this section. In most cases, solid dispersions are processed into finished dosage forms using conventional approaches such as tabletting, encapsulation, and so forth, and the characterization of such finished dosage formulations are not presented here.

MODULATED DIFFERENTIAL SCANNING CALORIMETRY

The differential scanning calorimetry (DSC) works on a technique that detects physicochemical transition in a system by measuring the amount of heat absorbed or released as the sample is heated across its suspected transition range. The heat absorbed or released from a sample of known mass is compared with that of an empty reference pan. Modulated differential scanning calorimetry (mDSC) works on an advanced technology version of DSC, where the signal quality has been improved using a mathematical function built in the software. Calorimetric approach provides valuable information to evaluate the structure of the dispersion using sample size as low as 10–20 mg. However, one disadvantage of DSC is that the method is destructive in nature, and may possess certain artifacts. For instance, when DSC was used to characterize the structure of oxidipine and griseofulvin solid dispersion in PEG 6000, it was observed that the endotherm attributed to melting of drug was undermined because the drug was dissolving in the molten carrier when the sample was heated in DSC (Veiga et al. 1993a).

POWDER X-RAY DIFFRACTION

Powder X-ray diffraction (PXRD) is a noninvasive technique that measures the diffraction pattern of drug and/or polymer with sample size as low as 200 mg. A detectable diffraction phenomenon occurs when a crystalline material, owing to its structural periodicity, scatters X-ray. Each crystalline ingredient possesses an X-ray pattern, which is specific to the manner in which the packing occurs. An X-ray pattern of solid dispersions typically reveals loss in crystalline structure and changes in crystal packing (i.e., polymorphism or formation of crystalline solid solution). A major disadvantage of X-ray is its inability to differentiate between amorphous components, as amorphous materials generate a characteristic halo. Several advanced versions of X-ray diffraction are now available such as wide-angle X-ray scattering, X-ray equipped with relative-humidity control, high-temperature X-ray, and so forth, which have rendered solid-state characterization easier.

HOT-STAGE MICROSCOPY

Hot-stage microscopy (HSM) is a valuable technique that often complements DSC measurements by providing a visual assessment of solid dispersion structure. It is more suited to crystalline solid dispersions than to amorphous ones, as the latter lacks the birefringence needed for its visual detection. While thermal analysis could undermine the physical structure of drug in a solid dispersion by dissolving it in the molten polymer, HSM can determine physical structure of drug by characterizing as low as ~2% w/w of crystalline drug in a polymer with low melting point. In one study, HSM was successfully applied to detect crystalline felodipine and hesperetin in PEG matrix, which could not be detected using DSC (Bikiaris et al. 2005). The disadvantage of thermal analysis in characterizing the drug dispersed in polymer with low melting point can alternatively be overcome by using microthermal analysis (µTA). µTA technique combines microscopy and thermal analysis, and can locally heat the mixture to melt only the drug without melting the lower melting point excipient (Galop 2005).

THERMALLY STIMULATED CURRENT

Thermally stimulating current (TSC) is a very sensitive technique that detects the molecular mobility by recording the current generated when the molecules orient in the presence of an electric field. A thermally stimulated depolarization current is obtained by heating the molecules to a temperature above their transition temperature and orienting them or their polar groups to a high-voltage electric field. The molecular orientation is kinetically frozen by rapidly cooling the material to very low temperatures, where molecular motion is negligible. The frozen material is then gradually heated in the absence of electric field, and molecular mobility is detected as the oriented polar groups disorient or relax and generate a depolarization current. TSC is valuable in investigating weak T_g, drug–polymer miscibility, and molecular mobility at sub-T_g conditions. In one study, the molecular mobility of an amorphous chemical entity, LAB687, along with its solid dispersion of PVP K30 was determined using TSC and conventional DSC. While it was complicated to characterize drug–polymer miscibility using DSC, it was easier to characterize such miscibility and T_g using TSC (Shmeis et al. 2004). In another study, the molecular motion of PVP K30 was characterized using TSC, and molecular mobility at temperatures below T_g could be detected (Figure 18.11) (Vasanthavada et al. 2002). mDSC, on the other hand, was unable to detect any such sub-T_g molecular motion.

SPECTROSCOPY

Fourier transform infrared (FTIR) and nuclear magnetic resonance (NMR) spectroscopy have been used frequently to characterize drug–polymer interactions in solid dispersions. Using FTIR, a spectrum of solid dispersion and that of its corresponding physical mixture is compared. A specific interaction, for example, hydrogen bonding, is said to have occurred when the wave number of the functional group involved in the interaction is lowered. In one study, FTIR was used to differentiate hydrogen-bond interaction between PVP–indomethacin and the dimer formation of indomethacin–indomethacin. The presence of molecularly dispersed PVP was able to break the dimer formation and inhibit drug crystallization (Taylor 1997). Solid-state NMR has also proved to be valuable in probing the structural and dynamic properties of drug substance, and in studying drug–polymer interactions. In one study, solid-state NMR could detect the degree of mixing in solid dispersions of Eudragit RL-100 with ibuprofen free acid and sodium salt. The ibuprofen free acid was seen to have much stronger interactions with the polymer than its sodium salt

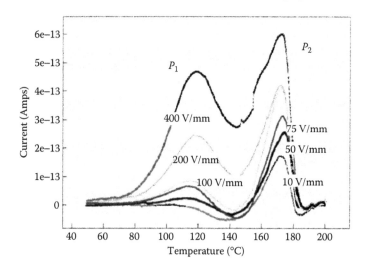

FIGURE 18.11 Thermally stimulated depolarization currents of PVP K30 demonstrating two different global relaxation peaks: P_1 is the β-relaxation peak (representing molecular motion below T_g), and P_2 is the α-relaxation peak (representing mobility at T_g).

(Geppi et al. 2005). Similarly, drug–polymer miscibility was ascertained in ketoprofen and PEO blends by characterizing drug–polymer interactions (Schachter et al. 2004).

DRUG RELEASE

Drug release mechanism from solid dispersions is complex and is largely dependent on the nature of drug dispersed in the carrier matrix (Craig 2002). As a result of such complexity, the development of a biorelevant *in vitro* dissolution testing method becomes even more difficult. The variability in physiological factors, along with the dosage form variability, makes establishment of *in vitro/in vivo* correlation (IVIVC) rather complicated.

In order to assess *in vivo* performance of solid dispersions, Serajuddin et al. (1988) and Dannenfelser et al. (2004) developed a dispersibility test where they determined not only the dissolution rate of drug, but also the particle size of released but undissolved drug in the dissolution media. The hypothesis was that although the drug does not completely dissolve initially from solid dispersion, the undissolved drug particles, if dispersed well, could dissolve, during GI transit, and enhance the bioavailability. In one study (Joshi et al. 2004), the solid dispersion of a weakly basic, poorly water-soluble drug was prepared in a mixture of PEG 3350 and polysorbate 80. During *in vitro* dissolution testing of the solid dispersions, it was observed that part of the drug dissolved rapidly and the remaining undissolved drug was dispersed as submicron particles. Dissolution from capsules containing micronized drug (5–10 μm) did not show complete *in vitro* release either. However, when the solid dispersion formulation was tested in dogs against capsule formulation containing micronized drug and an oral solution of drug in a mixture of PEG 400, polysorbate 80, and water, the relative bioavailability of the solution, the solid dispersion, and the capsule was determined as in the ratio 60:36:1.7. Such a 21-fold superiority in bioavailability of solid dispersion as compared to micronized drug was attributed to the differences between effective particle size of the drug dispersed as submicron particles from solid dispersions and particle size of micronized drug from capsules during *in vivo* dissolution.

Solid dispersions may create, in some cases, supersaturated solutions; however over time, drugs could precipitate from such supersaturated solutions. If the drug precipitates as very fine particles it could redissolve during GI transit, leading to enhanced bioavailability. Determining the nature of the precipitated drug, that is, its morphology and physical form, should be helpful when assessing the *in vivo* performance of solid dispersion. When choosing dissolution media, either simulated gastric or simulated intestinal fluid (whichever has the lower solubilization capacity for the drug) should be selected for testing the particle size of the released drug, with purified water serving as a third, suitable alternative. Although the drug would not dissolve in such a dissolution medium, the concentration and particle size of the released drug (unfiltered suspension or emulsion) would be indicative of *in vivo* performance of the formulation (Dannenfelser et al. 2004).

EVALUATION OF STABILITY

Both chemical and physical stability must be assured in the development of solid dispersions. Since the drug is either molecularly dispersed or intimately mixed with the carrier, there is potential for greater chemical interaction between them. Any physical instability that leads to phase transformations may result in poor performance of dosage forms, including changes in dissolution rates and oral bioavailability.

CHEMICAL INSTABILITY

A suitable drug–excipient compatibility screening technique such as the one developed by Serajuddin et al. (1999) may be applied to identify any potential incompatibility between drug and carrier or any other agents used in the formulation. When the processing of solid dispersion requires high temperature, as in melt extrusion and hot-melt encapsulation, the method may be modified to expose mixtures of drugs and excipients at appropriate high temperatures for a definite period of time. When one of the components convert to liquid at the high temperature, it might not be necessary to add water to the mixture to enable intimate mixing.

One common chemical stability problem encountered with solid dispersion is the formation of reactive intermediates (e.g., peroxides) secondary to excipient degradation (Chen and Hao 1998; Johnson et al. 1994). In one instance, the degradation of a guanine derivative compound was attributed to the generation of formaldehyde owing to oxidation of PEG 400 (Bindra et al. 1994). Peroxides and formaldehydes are also formed owing to the oxidation of polyoxyethylene surfactants under stressed conditions (Frontini et al. 1995; Bergh et al. 1998a,b), and both of them are capable of leading to gelatin cross-linking in capsule shells resulting in a slower dissolution rate (Chen et al. 1998). These instances indicate that careful monitoring of the stability of not only the drug but also of the carriers used in solid dispersion is needed during stressed stability studies to ensure adequate drug stability and reproducible performance of product during shelf life.

Physical Instability

Improving physical instability of solid dispersions has been a subject of discussion for many years (Chiou and Riegelman 1971; Ford 1986). Physical instability in solid dispersions is usually manifested by a decrease in drug dissolution rate; such a decrease is primarily attributed to drug crystallization during storage (Chiou 1977). As discussed in an earlier section under Structure of Solid Dispersion, drug and polymer could be completely miscible in their fluid state during the preparation of solid dispersion, but on solidification, drug could convert to different forms, such as a supersaturated solid solution phase, a distinct amorphous phase, a crystalline phase, or a combination of two or more of these phases. The supersaturated and amorphous phases may subsequently convert to the thermo-dynamically stable, poorly water-soluble crystalline phase, resulting in a decreased drug dissolution rate. Such drug crystallization is more prominent in the presence of moisture, which enhances the molecular mobility (Guillaume and Guyot-Hermann 1992; Suzuki and Sunada 1998). Liu et al. (2006) demonstrated that the dissolution rate of cyclosporine A in water from polyoxyethylene stearate solid dispersions was unaltered when the formulation was stored at 30°C/60% RH (6 months) and 25°C/60% RH (1 year) when packed in aluminum–polyethylene laminated bags. However, the percent release reduced from 87% to 5% at 45 min, when stored at 40°C/75% RH condition for 1 month. The drop in dissolution was attributed to drug crystallization and lump formation in the powder.

With the ultimate objective being to stabilize amorphous systems, several investigators studied the structural and dynamic properties of neat amorphous drugs and their pharmaceutical solid dispersions. Yoshioka et al. (1995) demonstrated that the presence of molecularly mixed PVP inhibits indomethacin crystallization. They postulated the mechanism of drug stabilization to be owing to (a) minimization of molecular mobility of the mixture at intended storage temperature, through elevation of the T_g, of the mixture (i.e., antiplasticizing effects) and/or (b) inhibition of drug crystallization through specific drug–polymer interactions, for example, hydrogen bonding. Several other investigators have delineated the stabilizing ability of polymer to a decrease in molecular mobility (Hancock and Shamblin 2001), decrease in free volume (Shamblin et al. 1988), increase in glass transition temperature (Craig et al. 1994), disruption of drug–drug interactions (Taylor and Zografi 1997), and formation of drug–polymer interactions (Khougaz et al. 2000).

Although the previous findings provide a better understanding of stability of miscible mixtures of amorphous drugs and excipients, the potential for crystallization of drugs still exists, and the prediction of timescale for drug crystallization (i.e., shelf life) from such systems remains elusive. It is very difficult to predict such timescale because of the complex relationship between temperature and molecular mobility of amorphous drug in solid dispersion. For instance, in liquid state, a molecule of less than 10 Å in diameter would take only seconds or minutes to reorient at temperatures near T_g, however, it could take hundreds of hours to reorient at temperatures below T_g (Chang et al. 1994). In addition to the molecular mobility of neat amorphous component, the impact of polymer on the molecular mobility and kinetics of the crystal nucleation of the amorphous drug should be considered when predicting timescale for drug crystallization (Marsac et al. 2006). Therefore, the prediction of shelf life becomes complicated owing to (a) the complex effect of time and temperature fluctuations on the enthalpy and entropy of aging systems, (b) the impact of moisture on phase separation and crystallization, (c) the impact of viscosity changes on the nucleation and crystal growth rate, and (d) the variability in physicochemical properties of dosage form. However, in the recent years, many studies have been conducted to predict crystallization of amorphous materials at temperatures below T_g by extrapolating parameters from molecular relaxation time constants of amorphous phase at temperatures above T_g (Zhou et al. 2002; Johari et al. 2005; Bhugra et al. 2006; Gunawan et al. 2006; Zhou et al. 2007). This is clearly an area of much value to the development of physically stable solid dispersions.

ESTIMATION OF SOLID SOLUBILITY

Depending on their hygroscopic nature, amorphous miscible solid dispersions can absorb water, which can lubricate or plasticize the solid dispersion and enhance its molecular mobility. Such a plasticizing effect is usually manifested by a decrease in T_g. In the presence of water, the drug–drug interaction (i.e., negative enthalpy) could override the breakage of drug–polymer and drug–water–polymer interactions, and any positive entropy effect could result in phase separation and drug crystallization. In such instances, it becomes important to identify the concentration of drug in polymer, that is, solid solubility limit, below which, no phase separation or crystallization should occur.

Quantitative PXRD and thermal analysis have been used to determine solid solubility of drugs in polymeric carrier (Vasanthavada et al. 2004, 2005; Weuts et al. 2005). When phase separation occurs in solid dispersion, it results in formation of a drug-rich phase and a polymer-rich phase. The polymer-rich phase could retain, either by restricting molecular mobility or by interacting with the drug, a certain portion of drug within its matrix. The portion of drug that remains trapped within the polymer may be estimated by measuring the T_g of the polymer-rich phase. In instances where T_g of the polymer-rich phase is similar to that of neat polymer, a complete phase separation may be assumed. In other instances, the differences in T_g values could be a result of the miscible drug in the polymer. mDSC has been used to measure such changes in the T_g to determine solid solubility of drug in polymer. As shown in Figure 18.12, phase separation of trehalose was observed from dextran solid dispersions in the 4-day and 34-day samples. However, a certain fraction of trehalose

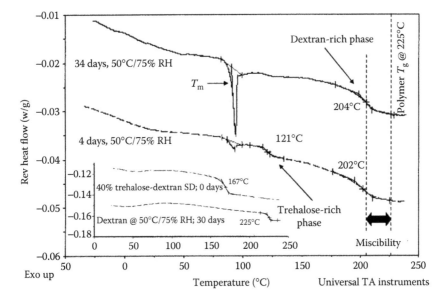

FIGURE 18.12 mDSC scans of 40% solid dispersion of trehalose in dextran when stored at 50°C/75% RH open conditions. Phase separation is seen in 4-day and 34-day samples, as indicated by the two T_{gs} and dehydration of trehalose dehydrate (T_m). The T_g of dextran-rich phase remains at ~20°C below the T_g of neat dextran (inset), indicating trehalose solubility in dextran at 50°C/75% RH.

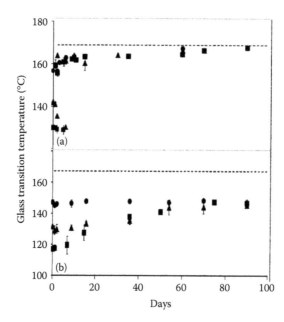

FIGURE 18.13 Changes in the T_g of 30% w/w (•), 20% w/w (_.), and 10% w/w (•) solid dispersions of PVP with (a) griseofulvin and (b) indoprofen, when stored at 40°C/70% RH open conditions. The T_g of different drug-loaded dispersions reached similar values indicating a fully saturated phase. The T_g of solid dispersion was below the T_g of PVP (dotted line) even after 90 days, indicating solid solubility.

remained miscible with dextran as indicated by the substantially low T_g values of dextran-rich phase when compared with T_g of neat dextran (inset). The solid solubility of trehalose was determined to be at 12% w/w at 50°C/75% RH conditions. In another study, changes in the T_g of griseofulvin–PVP and indoprofen–PVP solid dispersions were measured for up to 3 months by storing them at 40°C/70% RH conditions (Figure 18.13). While griseofulvin–PVP system exhibited no miscibility, 13% w/w of indoprofen was found miscible in PVP. It was believed that the presence of hydrogen-bond interaction between indoprofen and PVP, and the absence of such interaction in griseofulvin–PVP dispersion may have contributed to enhanced solid solubility, as determined experimentally. Similar ability of polymer to inhibit drug crystallization in the presence of moisture was observed in the case of solid dispersions of two fragmented molecules of loperamide: F1 and F2. While the crystallization of F1 from its solid dispersion at 52% RH was attributed to increased molecular mobility and lack of drug–polymer hydrogen bonding, the stabilization of F2 from its solid dispersions at similar conditions was believed to be due to drug–polymer hydrogen bonding (Weuts et al. 2005).

SUMMARY

The increasing number of poorly water-soluble compounds entering the pharmaceutical development pipeline in the recent years has triggered the use of several different formulation approaches to enhance the oral bioavailability of such compounds. From salt synthesis, complexation, and nanotechnology to micellar solubilization, microemulsion, and lipid solubilization, every formulation approach possesses its unique set of advantages and limitations. Solid dispersions, in many cases, have clearly demonstrated advantages to enhance drug dissolution rate and absorption. This chapter provides various examples from the literature to underscore the opportunities of using solid dispersions, and discusses as to why, when, and how to develop them. An improved understanding of physical stability of solid dispersions and the ability to prolong drug supersaturation in GI fluids are the two main drivers for increasing future application of solid dispersions. However, the concern over the physical stability of drugs in the solid dispersion still remains the key limiting factor for the routine application of this technique. Perhaps, with further advancement in material science and polymer engineering, and a greater understanding of biopharmaceutical properties governing dosage form selection, solid dispersions technique will be widely applied to develop an oral dosage form of poorly water-soluble drugs.

REFERENCES

Al-Razzak, L. A., L. Dias, D. Kaul, and S. Ghosh. 1997. Lipid based systems for oral delivery: Physiological mechanistic and product development perspectives. *Paper presented at the AAPS Annual Meeting*, Boston, MA. November 2–6, 1997.

Ambike, A. A., K. R. Mahadik, and A. Paradkar. 2005. Spray-dried amorphous solid dispersions of simvastatin, a low Tg drug: *In vitro* and *in vivo* evaluations. *Pharm. Res.* 22: 990–998.

Aungst, B. J., N. H. Nguyen, N. J. Rogers, S. M. Rowe, M. A. Hussain, S. J. White, and L. Shum. 1977. Ampiphilic vehicles improve the oral bioavailability of a poorly soluble HIV protease inhibitor at high doses. *Int. J. Pharm.* 156: 79–88.

Barker, S. A., S. P. Yap, K. H. Yuen, C. P. McCoy, J. R. Murphy, and D. Q. M. Craig. 2003. An investigation into the structure and bioavailability of α-tocopherol dispersions in Gelucire 44/14. *J. Controlled Release* 91: 477–488.

Bates, T. R. 1969. Dissolution characteristics of reserpine-polyvinylpyrrolidone co-precipitates. *J. Pharm. Pharmacol.* 21: 710–712.

Bergh, M., K. Magnusson, J. Lars, G. Nilson, and A. T. Karlberg. 1998a. Formation of formaldehyde and peroxides by air oxidation of high purity polyoxyethylene surfactants. *Contact Dermatitis* 39: 14–20.

Bergh, M., L. P. Shao, G. Hagelthorn, E. Gafvert, J. L. G. Nilsson, and A. T. Karlberg. 1998b. Contact allergens from surfactants. Atmospheric oxidation of polyoxyethylene alcohols, formation of ethoxylated aldehydes, and their allergenic activity. *J. Pharm. Sci.* 87: 276–282.

Bhugra, C., R. Shmeis, S. L. Krill, and M. J. Pikal. 2006. Predictions of onset of crystallization from experimental relaxation times I—correlation of molecular mobility from temperatures above the glass transition to temperatures below the glass transition. *Pharm. Res.* 23: 2277–2290.

Bikiaris, D., G. Z. Papageorgiou, A. Stergiou, E. Pavlidou, E. Karavas, F. Kanaze, and M. Georgarakis. 2005. Physicochemical studies on solid dispersions of poorly water-soluble drugs. Evaluation of capabilities and limitations of thermal analysis techniques. *Thermochimica Acta* 439: 58–67.

Bindra, D. S., T. D. Williams, and V. J. Stella. 1994. Degradation of O-6-benzylguanine in aqueous polyethylene glycol 400 (PEG 400) solutions: Concerns with formaldehyde in PEG 400. *Pharm. Res.* 11: 1060–1064.

Boudreaux, J. P., D. H. Hayes, S. Mizrahi, P. Maggiore, J. Blazek, and D. Dick. 1993. Use of watersoluble liquid Vitamin E to enhance cyclosporine absorption in children after liver transplant. *Transplant Proc.* 25: 1875–1881.

Breitenbach, J. 2002. Melt extrusion: From process to drug delivery technology. *Eur. J. Pharm. Biopharm.* 54: 107–117.

Breitenbach, J., W. Schrof, and J. Neumann. 1999. Confocal Raman spectroscopy: Analytical approach to solid dispersion and mapping of drugs. *Pharm. Res.* 16: 1109–1113.

Chang, I., F. Fujara, B. Geil, G. Heuberger, T. Mangel, and H. J. Sillescu. 1994. Translational and rotational molecular motion in supercooled liquids studies by NMR and forced Rayleigh scattering. *J. Non Crys. Solids* 172: 248–255.

Chang, T., L. Z. Benet, and M. F. Hebert. 1996. The effect of water-soluble vitamin E on cyclosporine pharmacokinetics in healthy volunteers. *Clin. Pharmacol. Ther.* 59: 297–303.

Chen, G. L. and W. H. Hao. 1998. Factors affecting zero-order release kinetics of porous gelatin capsules. *Drug Dev. Ind. Pharm.* 24: 557–562.

Chen, Y., G. G. Z. Zhang, J. Neilly, K. Marsh, D. Mawhinney, and Y. D. Sanzgiri. 2004. Enhancing the bioavailability of ABT-963 using solid dispersion containing Pluronic F-68. *Int. J. Pharm.* 286: 69–80.

Chiou, W. L. 1977. Pharmaceutical applications of solid dispersions: X-ray diffraction and aqueous solubility studies on griseofulvin-poly(ethylene glycol) 6000 systems. *J. Pharm. Sci.* 66: 989–991.

Chiou, W. L. and S. Riegelman. 1969. Preparation and dissolution characteristics of several fast-release solid dispersions of griseofulvin. *J. Pharm. Sci.* 58: 1505–1509.

Chiou, W. L. and S. Riegelman. 1971. Pharmaceutical application of solid dispersion systems. *J. Pharm. Sci.* 60: 1281–1302.

Chokshi, R. J., H. K. Sandhu, R. M. Iyer, N. H. Shah, A. W. Malick, and H. Zia. 2005. Characterization of physico-mechanical properties of indomethacin and polymers to assess their suitability for hot-melt extrusion process as a means to manufacture solid dispersion/solution. *J. Pharm. Sci.* 94: 2463–2474.

Choksi, R. and H. Zia. 2004. Hot-melt extrusion technique: A review. *Iran J. Pharm. Res.* 3: 107–117.

Coleman, M. M., J. F. Graf, and P. C. Painter. 1991. *Specific Interactions and the Miscibility of Polymer Blends.* Lancaster, PA: Technomic Publishing Company.

Craig, D. Q. M. 2002. The mechanism of drug release from solid dispersions in water-soluble polymers. *Int. J. Pharm.* 231: 131–144.

Craig, D. Q. M., P. G. Royall, V. L. Kett, and M. L. Hopton. 1999. The relevance of the amorphous state to pharmaceutical dosage forms: Glassy drugs and freeze dried systems. *Int. J. Pharm.* 179: 179–207.

Dannenfelser, R. M., H. He, Y. Joshi, S. Bateman, and A. T. M. Serajuddin. 2004. Development of clinical dosage forms for a poorly water soluble drug I: Application of polyethylene glycol-polysorbate 80 solid dispersion carrier system. *J. Pharm. Sci.* 93: 1165–1175.

DiNunzio, J.C., C. Brough, J. R. Hughey, D. A. Miller, R. O. Williams, and J. W. McGinity. 2010a. Fusion production of solid dispersions containing a heat-sensitive active ingredient by hot melt extrusion and KinetisolR dispersing. *Eur. J. Pharm. Biopharm.* 74: 340–351.

DiNunzio, J. C., C. Brough, D. A. Miller, R. O. Williams, and J. W. McGinity. 2010b. Applications of KinetiSolR dispersing for the production of plasticizer free amorphous solid dispersions. *Eur. J. Pharm. Sci.* 40: 179–187.

DiNunzio, J. C., C. Brough, D. A. Miller, R. O. Williams, and J. W. McGinity. 2010c. Fusion processing of itraconazole solid dispersions by KinetiSolR dispersing: a comparative study to hot melt extrusion. *J. Pharm. Sci.* 99: 1239–1253.

Doherty, C. and P. York. 1989. Accelerated stability of an x-ray amorphous furesemide polyvinyl pyrrolidone solid dispersions. *Drug Dev. Ind. Pharm.* 15: 1969–1987.

Edwards, A. D., B. Y. Shekunov, A. Kordikowski, R. T. Forbes, and P. York. 2001. Crystallization of pure anhydrous polymorphs of carbamezapine by solution enhanced dispersion with supercritical fluids (SEDS). *J. Pharm. Sci.* 90: 1115–1124.

Elversson, J., A. Millqvist-Fureby, G. Alderborn, and U. Elofsson. 2003. Droplet and particle size relationship and shell thickness of inhalable lactose particles during spray drying. *J. Pharm. Sci.* 92: 900–910.

Flory, P. J. 1953. *Principles of Polymer Chemistry.* New York: Cornell University Press.

Ford, J. L. 1986. The current status of solid dispersions. *Pharm. Acta Helv.* 61: 69–88.

Forster, A., J. Hempenstall, and T. Rades. 2001. Characterization of glass solutions of poorly watersoluble drugs produced by melt extrusion with hydrophilic amorphous polymers. *J. Pharm. Pharmacol.* 53: 303–315.

Foster, N., R. Mammucari, F. Dehghani, A. Barrett, K. Bezanehtak, E. Coen, G. Combes, L. Meure et al. 2003. Processing pharmaceutical compounds using dense gas technology. *Ind. Eng. Chem. Pres.* 42: 6476–6493.

Frontini, R. and J. B. Mielck. 1995. Formation of formaldehyde in polyethyleneglycol and in poloxamer under stress conditions. *Int. J. Pharm.* 114: 121–123.

Fusaro, F. M., M. Hanchen, M. Mazzotti, G. Muhrer, and B. Subramaniam. 2005. Dense gas anti-solvent precipitation: A comparative investigation of the GAS and PCA techniques. *Ind. Eng. Chem. Res.* 44: 1502–1509.

Galop, M. 2005. Study of pharmaceutical solid dispersions by microthermal analysis. *Pharm. Res.* 22: 293–302.

Geppi, M., S. Guccione, G. Mollica, R. Pignatello, and C. A. Veracini. 2005. Molecular properties of ibuprofen and its solid dispersions with Eudragit RL 100 studies by solid-state nuclear magnetic resonance. *Pharm. Res.* 22: 1544–1555.

Goldberg, A. H., M. Gibaldi, and J. L. Kanig. 1966a. Increasing dissolution rates and gastrointestinal absorption of drugs via solid solutions and eutectic mixtures. II. Experimental evaluation of eutectic mixture: Urea-acetaminophen system. *J. Pharm. Sci.* 55: 482–487.

Goldberg, A. H., M. Gibaldi, and J. L. Kanig. 1966b. Increasing dissolution rates and gastrointestinal absorption of drugs via solid solutions and eutectic mixtures. III. Experimental evaluation of griseofulvin-succinic acid solution. *J. Pharm. Sci.* 55: 487–492.

Gong, K., R. Viboonkiat, I. U. Rehman, G. Buckton, and J. A. Darr. 2005. Formation and characterization of porous indomethacin-PVP coprecipitates prepared using solvent-free supercritical fluid processing. *J. Pharm. Sci.* 2583–2590.

Greenhalgh, D. J., A. C. Williams, P. Timmins, and P. York. 1999. Solubility parameters as predictors of miscibility in solid dispersions. *J. Pharm. Sci.* 88: 1182–1190.

Guillaume, F. and A. M. Guyot-Hermann. 1992. Elaboration and physical study of an oxodipine solid dispersion in order to formulate tablets. *Drug Dev. Ind. Pharm.* 18: 811–829.

Gumaste, S.G., S. S. Gupta, and A. T. Serajuddin. 2016. Investigation of polymer-surfactant and polymer-drug-surfactant miscibility for solid dispersion. *AAPS J.* 18: 1131–1143.

Gunawan, L., G. P. Johari, and R. M. Shanker. 2006. Sructural relaxation of acetaminophen glass. *Pharm. Res.* 23: 967–979.

Gupta, S.S., A. Meena, T. Parikh, and A. T. Serajuddin. 2014. Investigation of thermal and viscoelastic properties of polymers relevant to hot melt extrusion, I: Polyvinylpyrrolidone and related polymers. *J. Excip. Food Chem.* 5: 32–45.

Gupta, S.S., N. Solanki, and A. T. Serajuddin. 2016. Investigation of thermal and viscoelastic properties of polymers relevant to hot melt extrusion, IV: Affinisol™ HPMC HME polymers. *AAPS Pharm. Sci. Tech.* 17: 148–157.

Gupta, S.S., T. Parikh, A.K. Meena, N. Mahajan, I. Vitez, and A.T. Serajuddin. 2015. Effect of carbamazepine on viscoelastic properties and hot melt extrudability of SoluplusR. *Int. J. Pharm.* 478: 232–239.

Hancock, B. C. and M. Parks. 2000. What is the true solubility advantage for amorphous pharmaceuticals? *Pharm. Res.* 17: 397–404.

Hancock, B. C. and S. L. Shamblin. 2001. Molecular mobility of amorphous pharmaceuticals determined using differential scanning calorimetry. *Thermochimica Acta.* 380: 95–107.

Hancock, B. C., P. York, and R. C. Rowe. 1997. The use of solubility parameters in pharmaceutical dosage form design. *Int. J. Pharm.* 148: 1–21.

Hansen, C. M. 1969. The universality of the solubility parameter. *Ind. Eng. Chem. Pro. RD* 8: 2–11.

Hansen, C. M. 2004. 50 Years with solubility parameters—past and future. *Pro. Org. Coat* 51: 77–84.

He, Y., J. L. H. Johnson, and S. H. Yalkowsky. 2005. Oral formulation of a novel antiviral agent, PG301029, in a mixture of Gelucire 44/14 and DMA (2:1, wt/wt). *AAPS PharmSci. Tech.* 6: 1–5.

Hilderbrand, J. and R. Scott. 1950. *The Solubility of Non-Electrolytes*, 3rd ed. New York: Reinhold.

Ho, H. O., C. N. Chen, and M. T. Sheu. 2000. Influence of pluronic F-68 on dissolution and biavailability characteristics of multiple-layer pellets of nifedipine for controlled release delivery. *J. Control Release* 68: 433–440.

Horter, D. and J. B. Dressman. 1997. Influence of physicochemical properties on dissolution of drugs in the gastrointestinal tract. *Adv. Drug. Delivery Rev.* 25: 3–14.

Hulsmann, S., T. Backensfeld, S. Keitel, and R. Bodmeier. 2000. Melt extrusion—an alternative method for enhancing the dissolution rate of 17-estradiol hemihydrate. *Eur. J. Pharm. Biopharm.* 49: 237–242.

Itai, S., M. Nemoto, S. Kouchiwa, H. Murayama, and T. Nagai. 1985. Influence of wetting factors on the dissolution behavior of flufenamic acid. *Chem. Pharm. Bull.* 33: 5464–5473.

Jarmer, D. J., C. S. Lengsfeld, K. S. Anseth, and T. W. Randolph. 2005. Supercritical fluid crystallization of griseofulvin: Crystal habit modification with a selective growth inhibitor. *J. Pharm. Sci.* 94: 2688–2702.

Johari, G. P., S. Kim, and R. M. Shanker. 2005. Dielectric studies of molecular motions in amorphous solid and ultraviscous acetaminophen. *J. Pharm. Sci.* 94: 2207–2223.

Johnson, D. M. and W. F. Taylor. 1984. Degradation of feprostalene in polyethylene glycol 400 solution. *J. Pharm. Sci.* 73: 1414–1417.

Joshi, H. N., R. W. Tejwani, M. Davidovich, V. P. Sahasrabudhe, M. Jemal, M. S. Bathala, S. A. Varia, and A. T. M. Serajuddin. 2004. Bioavailability enhancement of a poorly water-soluble drug by solid dispersion in polyethylene glycol-polysorbate 80 mixture. *Int. J. Pharm.* 269: 251–258.

Jung, J. and M. Perrut. 2001. Particle design using supercritical fluids: Literature and patent survey. *J. Supercrit. Fluids* 20: 179–219.

Karanth, H., V. S. Shenoy, and R. P. Murthy. 2006. Industrially feasible alternative approaches in the manufacture of solid dispersions: A technical report. *AAPS Pharm. Sci. Tech.* 7: 87–96.

Karavas, E., G. Ktistis, A. Xenakis, and E. Georgarakis. 2006. Effect of hydrogen bonding interactions on the release mechanism of felodipine from nanodispersions with polyvinylpyrrolidone. *Eur. J. Pharm. Biopharm.* 63: 103–114.

Khoo, S. M., C. J. H. Porter, and W. N. Charman. 2000. The formulation of halofantrine as either non-solubilising PEG6000 or solubilising lipid based solid dispersion: Physical stability and absolute bioavailability assessment. *Int. J. Pharm.* 205: 65–78.

Khougaz, K. and S. D. Clas. 2000. Crystallization inhibition in solid dispersions of MK-0591 and poly(vinylpyrrolidone) polymer. *J. Pharm. Sci.* 89: 1325–1334.

Knez, Z., M. Skerget, P. Sencar-Bozic, and A. Rizner. 1995. Solubility of nifedipine and nitrendipine in supercritical CO2. *J. Chem. Eng. Data.* 40: 216–220.

Kohri, N., Y. Yamayoshi, H. Xin, K. Iseki, N. Sato, S. Todo, and K. Miyazaki. 1999. Improving the oral bioavailability of albendazole in rabbits by the solid dispersion technique. *J. Pharm. Pharmacol.* 51: 159–164.

Leuner, C. and J. Dressman. 2000. Improving drug solubility for oral delivery using solid dispersions. *Eur. J. Pharm. Biopharm.* 50: 47–60.

Li, L., O. Abu Baker, and Z. J. Shao. 2006. Characterization of poly(ethyleneoxide) as a drug carrier in hot-melt extrusion. *Drug Dev. Ind. Pharm.* 32: 991–1002.

Li, S., H. He, L. J. Parthiban, H. Yin, and A. T. M. Serajuddin. 2005. IV-IVC considerations in the development of immediate-release oral dosage form. *J. Pharm. Sci.* 94: 1396–1417.

Liu, C., J. Wu, B. Shi, Y. Zhang, T. Gao, and Y. Pei. 2006. Enhancing the bioavailability of cyclosporine A using solid dispersion containing polyoxyethylene (40) stearate. *Drug Dev. Ind. Pharm.* 32: 115–123.

Liu, Q. and G. Zografi. 1998. Phase behavior of binary and ternary amorphous mixtures containing indomethacin, citric acid, and PVP. *Pharm. Res.* 15: 1202–1206.

Marsac, P. J., H. Konno, and L. S. Taylor. 2006. A comparison of the physical stability of amorphous felodipine and nifedipine systems. *Pharm. Res.* 23: 2306–2316.

Matsuda, Y. and S. Kawaguchi. 1986. Physicochemical characterization of oxyphenbutazone and solidstate stability of its amorphous form under various temperature and humidity conditions. *Chem. Pharm. Bull.* 34: 1289–1298.

Mayersohn, M. and M. Gibaldi. 1966. New method of solid dispersion for increasing dissolution rates. *J. Pharm. Sci.* 55: 1323–1324.

Meena, A., T. Parikh, S. S. Gupta, and A. T. Serajuddin. 2014. Investigation of thermal and viscoelastic properties of polymers relevant to hot melt extrusion, II: Cellulosic polymers. *J. Excip. Food Chem.* 5: 46–55.

Mehta, K. A., M. S. Kislalioglu, W. Phuapradit, W. A. Malik, and N. H. Shah. 2002. Multi-unit controlled release systems of nifedipine and nifedipine: PluronicR F-68 solid dispersion. *Drug Dev. Ind. Pharm.* 28: 275–285.

Morris, K. R., G. T. Knipp, and A. T. M. Serajuddin. 1992. Structural properties of poly(ethylene glycol)-polysorbate 80 mixture, a solid dispersion vehicle. *J. Pharm. Sci.* 81: 1185–1188.

Muhrer, G., U. Meier, F. Fusaro, S. Albano, and M. Mazzotti. 2006. Use of compressed gas precipitation to enhance the dissolution behavior of a poorly water-soluble drug: Generation of drug microparticles and drug-polymer solid dispersions. *Int. J. Pham.* 308: 69–83.

Nakamichi, K., H. Yasuura, H. Fukui, M. Oka, and S. Izumi. 2001. Evaluation of a floating dosage form of nicardipine hydrochloride and hydroxypropylmethylcellulose acetate succinate prepared using a twin-screw extruder. *Int. J. Pharm.* 218: 103–112.

Nilufer, Y., K. Aysegul, O. Yalcin, S. Ayhan, A. O. Sibel, and B. Tamer. 2003. Enhanced bioavailability of piroxicam using Gelucire 44/14 and Labrasol: *In vitro* and *in vivo* evaluation. *Eur. J. Pharm. Biopharm.* 235: 247–265.

Palakodaty, S. and P. York. 1999. Phase behavioral effects on particle formation process using supercritical fluids. *Pharm. Res.* 16: 976–985.

Parikh, T., S. S. Gupta, A. Meena, and A. T. Serajuddin. 2014. Investigation of thermal and viscoelastic properties of polymers relevant to hot melt extrusion, III: Polymethacrylates and polymethacrylic acid based polymers. *J. Excip. Food Chem* 5: 56–64.

Parikh, T., S. S. Gupta, A. K. Meena, I. Vitez, N. Mahajan, and A. Serajuddin. 2015. Application of filmcasting technique to investigate drug–polymer miscibility in solid dispersion and hot-melt extrudate. *J. Pharm. Sci.* 104: 2142–2152.

Passerini, N., B. Albertini, and M. L. Gonzalez-Rodriguez. 2002. Preparation and characterization of ibuprofen-poloxamer 188 granules obtained by melt granulation. *Eur. J. Pharm. Sci.* 15: 71–78.

Patil, P., J. Joshi, and P. Paradkar. 2004. Effect of formulation variables on preparation and evaluation of gelled self-emulsifying drug delivery systems (SEDDS) of ketoprofen. *AAPS Pharm. Sci. Tech.* 5: 1–8.

Perng, C. Y., A. S. Kearney, K. Patel, N. R. Palepu, and G. Zuber. 1998. Investigation of formulation approaches to improve the dissolution of SB-210661, a poorly water soluble 5-lipoxygenase inhibitor. *Int. J. Pharm.* 176: 31–38.

Pudipeddi, M., A. T. M. Serajuddin, and D. Mufson. 2006. Integrated drug product development—From lead candidate selection to life-cycle management. In *The Process of New Drug Discovery and Development*, C. G. Smith and J. T. O'Donnell (Eds.), 2nd ed. 15–51. New York: Informa Healthcare.

Rambali, B., G. Verreck, L. Baert, and D. L. Massart. 2003. Itraconazole formulation studies of the melt extrusion process with mixture design. *Drug Dev. Ind. Pharm.* 29: 641–652.

Robinson, L. 2001. Physical characterization and scale-up manufacture of Gelucire 50/13 based capsule formulations. *Bulletin Technique Gattefosse* 97: 97–111.

Rowley, G. 2004. Filling of liquids and semi-solids into hard two-piece capsules. In *Pharmaceutical Capsules*, F. Podczeck, and B. E. Jones (Eds.). 2nd ed. 169–194. Abingdon, OX: The Batch Press.

Schachter, D. M., J. Xiong, and G. C. Tirol. 2004. Solid-state NMR perspective of drug-polymer solid solutions: A model system based on poly (ethyleneoxide). *Int. J. Pharm.* 281: 89–101.

Sekiguchi, K. and N. Obi. 1961. Studies on absorption of eutectic mixture. I. A comparison of the behavior of eutectic mixture of sulfathiazole and that of ordinary sulfathiazole in man. *Chem. Pharm. Bull.* 9: 866–872.

Sekiguchi, K., N. Obi, and Y. Ueda. 1964. Studies on absorption of eutectic mixture. II. Absorption of fused conglomerates of chloramphenicol and urea in rabbits. *Chem. Pharm. Bull.* 12: 134–144.

Serajuddin, A. T. M. 1999. Solid dispersion of poorly water-soluble drugs: Early promises, subsequent problems, and recent breakthroughs. *J. Pharm. Sci.* 88: 1058–1066.

Serajuddin, A. T. M., P. C. Sheen, and M. A. Augustine. 1986. Preformulation study of a poorly watersoluble drug, α-pentyl-3-(2-quinolinylmethoxy) benzenemethanol: Selection of base for dosage form design. *J. Pharm. Sci.* 75: 492–496.

Serajuddin, A. T. M., P. C. Sheen PC, and M. A. Augustine. 1990. Improved dissolution of a poorly water-soluble drug from solid dispersions in poly(ethylene glycol)-polysorbate 80 mixtures. *J. Pharm. Sci.* 79: 463–464.

Serajuddin, A. T. M., P. C. Sheen, D. Mufson. D. F. Bernstein, and M. A. Augustine. 1988. Effect of vehicle amphiphilicity on the dissolution and bioavailability of a poorly water-soluble drugs from solid dispersions. *J. Pharm. Sci.* 77: 414–417.

Serajuddin, A. T. M., A. B. Thakur, R. N. Ghoshal, M. G. Fakes, S. A. Ranadive, K. R. Morris, and S. A. Varia. 1999. Selection of dosage form composition through drug-excipient compatibility testing. *J. Pharm. Sci.* 88: 696–704.

Serajuddin, A. T. M., S. Ranadive, and E. M. Mahoney. 1991. Relative lipophilicities, solubilities and structure-pharmacological considerations of HMG-CoA reductase inhibitors pravastatin, mevastatin, lovastatin and simvastatin. *J. Pharm. Sci.* 80: 830–834.

Sethia, S. and E. Squillante. 2002. Physicochemical characterization of solid dispersions of carbamazepine formulated by supercritical carbon dioxide and conventional solvent evaporation method. *J. Pharm. Sci.* 91: 1948–1957.

Sethia, S. and E. Squillante. 2003. Solid dispersions: Revival with greater possibilities and applications in oral drug delivery. *Crit. Rev. Ther. Drug Carrier Syst.* 20: 215–247.

Shamblin, S. L., L. S. Taylor, and G. Zografi. 1998. Mixing behavior of colyophilized binary systems. *J. Pharm. Sci.* 87: 694–701.

Shanker, R. M. 2005. Current concepts in the science of solid dispersion, *2nd Annual Simonelli Conference in Pharmaceutical Sciences*, June 9, Long Island University, Brookville, NY.

Sheen, P. C., V. K. Khetarpal, C. M. Cariola, and C. E. Rowlings. Formulation studies of a poorly watersoluble drug in solid dispersions to improve bioavailability. *Int. J. Pharm.* 18: 221–227.

Shin, S. C. and C. W. Cho. 1997. Physicochemical characterization of piroxicam-poloxamer solid dispersion. *Pharm. Dev. Technol.* 2: 403–407.

Shmeis, R. A., Z. Wang, and S. L. Krill. 2004. A mechanistic investigation of an amorphous pharmaceutical and its solid dispersion, Part I: A comparative analysis by thermally stimulated depolarization current and differential scanning calorimetry. *Pharm. Res.* 21: 2025–2030.

Simonelli, A. P., S. C. Mehta, and W. I. Higuchi. 1969. Dissolution rates of high energy polyvinylpyrrolidone (PVP)-sulfathiazole coprecipitates. *J. Pharm. Sci.* 58: 538–549.

Simonelli, A. P., S. C. Mehta, and W. I. Higuchi. 1970. Inhibition of sulfathiazole crystal growth by polyvinylpyrrolidone. *J. Pharm. Sci.* 59: 633–638.

Six, K., T. Daems, J. D. Hoon, A. V. Hecken, M. Depre, M. P. Bouche, P. Prinsen et al. 2005. Clinical study of solid dispersions of itraconazole prepared by hot-stage extrusion. *Eur. J. Pharm. Sci.* 24: 179–186.

Sokol, R. J., N. Butler-Simon, C. Connor, J. E. Heui, F. R. Sinatra, F. J. Suchy, M. B. Heyman, J. Perrault, R. J. Rothbaum, and J. Levy. 1993. Multicenter trial of d-α-Tocopheryl Polyethylene Glycol 1000 succinate for treatment of Vitamin E deficiency in children with chronic choleostasis, *Gastroenterology* 104: 1727–1735.

Soliman, M. S. and M. A. Khan. 2005. Preparation and *in vitro* characterization of a semi solid dispersion of flurbiprofen with Gelucire 44/14 and Labrasol. *Pharmazie* 60: 288–293.

Subramanian, B., R. A. Rajewski, and K. Snavely. 1997. Pharmaceutical processing with supercritical carbon dioxide. *J. Pharm. Sci.* 86: 885–890.

Sugimoto, I., K. Sasaki, A. Kuchiki, T. Ishihara, and H. Nakagawa. 1982. Stability and bioavailability of nifedipine in fine granules. *Chem. Pharm. Bull.* 30: 4479–4488.

Surikutchi, B. T., S. P. Patil, G. Shete, S. Patel, and A. K. Bansal. 2013. Drug-excipient behavior in polymeric amorphous solid dispersions. *J. Excip. Food Chem.* 4: 70–94.

Suzuki, H. and H. Sunada. 1998. Some factors influencing the dissolution of solid dispersions with nicotinamide and hydroxypropylmethylcellulose as combined carriers. *Chem. Pharm. Bull.* 46: 1015–1020.

Tanno, F., Y. Nishiyama, H. Kokubo, and S. Obara. 2004. Evaluation of hypromellose acetate succinate (HPMC AS) as a carrier in solid dispersions. *Drug Dev. Ind. Pharm.* 30: 9–17.

Tantishaiyakul, V., N. Kaewnopparat, and S. Ingkatawornwong. 1999. Properties of solid dispersions of piroxicam in polyvinylpyrrolidone. *Int. J. Pharm.* 181: 143–151.

Taylor, L. S. and G. Zografi. 1997. Spectroscopic characterization of interactions between PVP and indomethacin in amorphous molecular dispersions. *Pharm. Res.* 14: 1691–1698.

Ting, S. S. T., S. J. Macnaughtn, D. L. Tomasko, and N. R. Foster. 1993. Solubility of naproxen in supercritical carbon dioxide with and without cosolvents. *Ind. Eng. Chem. Res.* 32: 1471–1481.

Turk, M., B. Helfgen, P. Hils, R. Lietzow, and K. Schaber. 2002. Micronization of pharmaceutical substances by rapid expansion of supercritical solutions (RESS): Experiments and modeling. *Part.Part. Syst. Char* 19: 327–335.

Urbanetz, N. 2006. Stabilization of solid dispersions of nimodipine and polyethylene glycol 2000. *Eur. J. Pharm. Sci.* 28: 67–76.

Usui, F., K. Maeda, A. Kusai, K. Nishimura, and K. Yamamoto. 1991. Inhibitory effects of water-soluble polymers on precipitation of RS-8359. *Int. J. Pharm.* 154: 59–66.

Varma, M. V. and R. Panchagnula. 2005. Enhanced oral paclitaxel absorption with Vitamin E-TPGS: Effect on solubility and permeability *in vitro, in situ* and *in vivo. Eur. J. Pharm. Sci.* 25: 445–453.

Vasanthavada, M. and A. T. M. Serajuddin. Lipid-based self-emulsifying solid dispersions. In *Lipid- Based Formulations for Oral Drug Delivery: Enhancing the Bioavailability of Poorly Water-Soluble Drugs,* D. J. Hauss (Ed.). pp. 149–183. New York: Informa Healthcare.

Vasanthavada, M., W. Tong, Y. Joshi, and M. S. Kislalioglu. 2004. Phase behavior of amorphous molecular dispersions I: Determination of the degree and mechanism of solid solubility. *Pharm. Res.* 21: 1598–1606.

Vasanthavada, M., W. Tong, Y. Joshi, and M. S. Kislalioglu. 2005. Phase behavior of amorphous molecular dispersions II: Role of hydrogen bonding in solid solubility and phase separation kinetics. *Pharm. Res.* 22: 440–448.

Vasanthavada, M., Z. Wang, Y. Joshi, and M. S. Kislalioglu. 2002. Comparison of the utility of thermally stimulated current and modulated differential scanning calorimeter to study sub-glass transition molecular motions of poly (vinylpyrrolidone). *Paper Presented at AAPS Annual Meeting,* Toronto, ON, October 8, 2002.

Veiga, M. D., M. J. Bernard, and C. Escobar. 1993a. Thermal behavior of drugs from binary and ternary systems. *Int. J. Pharm.* 89: 119–124.

Veiga, M. D., C. Escobar, and M. J. Bernard. 1993b. Dissolution behavior of drugs from binary and ternary systems. *Int. J. Pharm.* 93: 215–220.

Vemavarapu, C., M. J. Mollan, and T. E. Needham. 2002. Crystal doping aided by rapid expansion of supercritical solutions. *AAPS Pharm. Sci. Tech.* 3: 1–15.

Verreck, G., K. Six, G. Van den Mooter, L. Baert, J. Peeters, and M. E. Brewster. 2003. Characterization of solid dispersions of itraconazole and hydroxypropylmethylcellulose prepared by melt extrusion— part I. *Int. J. Pharm.* 251: 165–174.

Vippagunta, S. R., K. A. Maul, S. Tallavajhala, and D. J. W. Grant. 2002. Solid-state characterization of nifedipine solid dispersions. *Int. J. Pharm.* 236: 111–123.

Vishweshwar, R., J. A. Mc. Mahon, J. A. Bis, and M. J. Zaworotko. 2006. Pharmaceutical co-crystals. *J. Pharm. Sci.* 95: 499–514.

Wang, X., A. Michoel, and G. Van den Mooter. 2005. Solid state characteristics of ternary solid dispersions composed of PVP VA64, Myrj 52 and itraconazole. *Int. J. Pharm.* 303: 54–61.

Weuts, I., D. Kempen, A. Decorte, G. Verreck, J. Peeters, M. Brewster, and G. Van den Mooter. 2005. Physical stability of the amorphous state of loperamide and two fragment molecules in solid dispersions with the polymers PVP-K30 and PVP-VA64. *Eur. J. Pharm. Sci.* 25: 313–320.

Won, D. H., M. S. Kim, S. Lee, J. S. Park, and S. J. Hwang. 2005. Improved physicochemical characteristics of felodipine solid dispersion particles by supercritical anti-solvent precipitation process. *Int. J. Pharm.* 301: 199–208.

Wu, S. H., 1998. Vitamin E TPGS as a vehicle for drug delivery system. Paper presented at AAPS short course *Formulation with Lipids,* Parsippany, NJ, June 3, 1998.

Wulff, M., M. Alden, and D. Q. M. Craig. 1996. An investigation into the critical surfactant concentration for solid solubility of hydrophobic drug in different polyethylene glycols. *Int. J. Pharm.* 142: 189–198.

Yin, S. X., M. Franchini, J. L. Chen, A. Hsieh, S. Jen, T. Lee, M. Hussain, and R. Smith. 2005. Bioavailability enhancement of a COX-2 inhibitor, BMS-347070, from nanocrystalline dispersion prepared by spray-drying. *J. Pharm. Sci.* 94: 1598–1607.

Yoshioka, M., B. C. Hancock, and G. Zografi. 1995. Inhibition of indomethacin crystallization in poly(vinylpyrrolidone) coprecipitates. *J. Pharm. Sci.* 84: 983–986.

Yu, L., A. Bridgers, J. Polli, A. Vickers, S. Long, A. Roy, R. Winnike, and M. Coffin. 1999. Vitamin-E TPGS increases absorption flux of an HIV protease inhibitor by enhancing its solubility and permeability. *Pharm. Res.* 16: 1812–1817.

Zhou, D., D. J. W. Grant, G. G. Z. Zhang, D. Law, and E. A. Schmitt. 2007. A calorimetric investigation of thermodynamic and molecular mobility contributions to the physical stability of two pharmaceutical glasses. *J. Pharm. Sci.* 96: 71–83.

Zhou, D. G., G. Z. Zhang, D. Law, D. J. W. Grant, and E. A. Schmitt. 2002. Physical stability of amorphous pharmaceuticals: Importance of configurational thermodynamic quantities and molecular mobility. *J. Pharm. Sci.* 91: 1863–1872.

19 Alteration of the Solid State of the Drug Substances

Polymorphs, Solvates, and Amorphous Forms

Paul B. Myrdal, Stephen J. Franklin,
and Michael J. Jozwiakowski

CONTENTS

INTRODUCTION AND OBJECTIVES

In an ideal solution, the maximum solubility of a drug substance is a function of the solid phase in equilibrium with a specified solvent system at a given temperature and pressure. Solubility is an equilibrium constant for the dissolution of the solid into the solvent, and thus depends on the strengths of solute:solvent interactions and solute:solute interactions. Alteration of the solid phase of the drug substance can influence its solubility and dissolution properties by affecting the solute:solute molecular interactions.

A crystal of higher free energy will yield an apparent higher solubility than a lower energy crystal form of the same molecular structure. In the lowest energy solid state, the energetically favorable solute:solute interactions reduce the escaping tendency of the molecules, and thus fewer molecules dissolve in a given solvent under the same set of environmental conditions. Crystalline polymorphs, solvates, hydrates, and amorphous forms of drug substances have been used to change the thermodynamic driving force for dissolution and increase the apparent solubility of poorly soluble drugs.

Traditional solubilization techniques, such as pH adjustment, cosolvent systems, emulsions, micellization, and complexation, modify the nature of the solvent environment. Manipulation of the solid state of the drug substance can afford a transient change in solubility for any system. However, since the solvent and the chemical form are identical, the system will ultimately revert to the lowest energy solid phase in equilibrium with the solvent, with the lowest solubility. Crystal growth and dissolution has been used to assign relative physical stability for polymorphs by observing the direction of the transformation under a microscope under controlled temperature in contact with a solvent. The rate of transformation in contact with a solvent is normally too fast to consider solution or suspension dosage forms of metastable solids. Systems with unusually large energy barriers, slow reversion kinetics, or excipients to retard crystallization can be useful in limited circumstances.

The most practical use of this technique is to alter the solid phase in dry dosage forms, where molecular mobility is greatly reduced. Metastable forms of solid drugs are often stable to physical transformation in the time context required for marketable formulations. Tablets, capsules, lyophilized powders, granules for constitution, and other solid dosage forms are applicable systems for incorporation of metastable solid phases. In most cases, the brief exposure to gastrointestinal (GI) fluids does not result in conversion to the lower solubility form before generating the desired enhanced effect. Solid-state transformations and transformations induced by adsorbed water during long-term storage can still be problematic. Any consideration of formulating metastable solid phases must balance the expected gain in efficacy with the potential for reversion to the less favorable form before patient use. This involves both an understanding of the phase diagrams (which forms are physically stable under which conditions) and the physical principles governing transformation kinetics.

In this chapter, the theoretical and practical considerations for the use of metastable solids in formulations to gain a solubility or dissolution rate advantage are being explored. Experiments that identify the potential solid forms of the drug and elucidate the potential advantages and disadvantages are suggested. Specific examples of the degree of enhancement that can be expected and special considerations for each type of solid will be covered (polymorphs, solvates, and amorphous forms).

THEORETICAL AND PRACTICAL CONSIDERATIONS

IMPORTANCE OF THE SOLID STATE OF THE DRUG

Origin of the Effect of Solid State on Solubility

When a medicinal chemist discovers a new chemical entity (NCE) with a desired pharmacological effect, structure–activity relationships are used to optimize the series for biological activity. Aqueous solubility, partition coefficient, crystallinity, melting point, particle size, and hygroscopicity, all of interest to the formulator, will also vary within the series of drug candidates. Because the biological activity is often estimated by target enzyme binding studies in very dilute media, solubility may not be optimized simultaneously. If an ionizable drug candidate is selected, the choice of free acid/base form versus the salt forms again produces a myriad of possible physical properties. The alteration of solubility by judicious choice of the salt was covered in an earlier chapter in this book as well as in reviews by Morris et al. (1994), Stahl and Wermuth (2002), and Stahl and Sutter (2006). In many cases, the chosen salt or acid/base can crystallize in a variety of possible arrangements, each of which has the possibility of different physical properties. This includes the possibility of polymorphs, solvates, or noncrystalline (amorphous) forms. Thus, the solid phase chosen for development is the third decision made by the pharmaceutical scientists that has a major impact on the ultimate physical properties of the NCE, including the solubility. In a typical development program, the number of candidates decreases at each stage:

Stage I: Selection of best chemical structure (100–1000)
Stage II: Selection of acid/base/salt form (3–25)
Stage III: Selection of solid phase for development (1–3)

Each of these stages produces molecules of varying solubility by virtue of a change in the crystalline lattice, the last stage being the only one in which the chemical identity or counterion identity is unchanged.

Yalkowsky (1981) has developed equations describing water solubility as a function of both hydrophobicity (log P) and crystal lattice forces. Jain and Yalkowsky (2001) have offered a new general solubility equation, where the molar solubility, log S_w, of a nonelectrolyte can be estimated by

$$\log S_w = -0.01(\text{m.p.} - 25^\circ\text{C}) - C \log P + 0.5 \tag{19.1}$$

where the m.p. is the melting point of the compound (in $^\circ$C) and $C \log P$ is the calculated log P. While the general solubility equation incorporates a series of assumptions to facilitate ease of use and general applicability, it clearly illustrates that the solubility of a drug is dependent on the strengths of the solute:solute interactions (through m.p.) and solute:solvent interactions (through log P). Recently Jain et al. (2006) have demonstrated that the general solubility equation is also useful for weak electrolytes.

Investigation of the solute:solute interactions has led to the observation that melting point or heat of fusion, both a function of the strength of forces holding molecules together in the solid state, can correlate with solubility within a homologous series. This is because the disruption of the crystal forces is a necessary prerequisite to the release of individual molecules into the solvent for dissolution. Grant and Higuchi (1990) summarized correlations in the case of diphenylhydantoin derivatives and substituted pteridines in their book on organic compound solubility. Wells (1988) has noted that in the series of hydroxy substituent phenols, the high melting *para*-form (hydroquinone) has a much lower solubility than the *ortho*- or *meta*-derivatives. Morelock et al. (1994) have used melting points and retention times to correlate with aqueous solubility in a series of reverse transcriptase inhibitors. They have found this useful in selecting the drug candidate that can possess optimum biological parameters and guiding the further synthetic effort. The same factors can govern the solubility differences between drug salt forms or solid phases, since fundamentally the change is brought about by a difference in solute:solute forces in each case. Wells (1988) has shown that riboflavin polymorphs follow a similar inverse correlation with melting point. Form III melts at 180°C–185°C and is soluble to greater than 1000 mg/mL in water. Forms I and II melt at 270°C–290°C and have solubilities of less than 100 mg/mL.

The success of altering solubility by manipulating the solid phase of the drug depends on which factor dominates the aqueous solubility behavior, the hydrophobicity (log P) or the lattice forces.

When the molecule is too lipophilic to have adequate aqueous solubility, cosolvents, prodrugs, or emulsions are effective in increasing the solubility. Altering the solid state in this case may have little effect on its solubility, since poor aqueous solubility is due to the molecular lipophilicity. In contrast, cosolvents and emulsions do not have much impact if the reason for low solubility is the stability of the crystal lattice. When a drug has low log P and a high melting point (>250°C), it is likely that disruption of the lattice is needed to increase the effective solubility. This can be done by altering the crystal form (polymorphs or solvates/hydrates), or by producing the amorphous form and stabilizing it to spontaneous crystallization. The effect of altering the salt form of the drug is discussed in Chapter 15, and has also been reviewed by Berge et al. (1977).

Historical Perspective and Definitions

The effect of the solid state on drug solubility has been known for decades, and pioneer articles by Haleblian and McCrone (1969), Shefter and Higuchi (1963), and Higuchi et al. (1963) have formed the basis for further studies in this area. More recent reviews by Shefter (1981), Abdou (1989), Byrn (1982), Wall (1986), Fiese and Hagen (1986), Brittain (1995), Huang and Tong (2004), Pudipeddi and Serajuddin (2005), and Mao et al. (2005) have summarized the effects of polymorphism or solvate formation on drug solubility. The existence of different internal crystalline arrangements for the same chemical structure has been termed *polymorphism*. Verma and Krishna (1966) observed that the great majority of substances seem to be capable of multiple solid states. The work of Kuhnert-Brandstatter on steroids and barbiturates (as reviewed by Haleblian and McCrone, 1969) seems to indicate that simple organic drug molecules with multiple functional groups can arrange into numerous crystal-packing structures. McCrone et al. (1987), Carstensen (1993), and Byrn (1982) have reviewed the seven different crystal systems, which are uniquely identified by the length of the axes and the angles between them in the unit cell. Chen et al. (2005) have illustrated through the persistent evaluation of a given compound that polymorphic forms can be elusive. Indeed, many drugs crystallize into multiple polymorphic forms, especially monoclinic, triclinic, or orthorhombic types (Wall, 1986; Borka and Haleblian, 1990; Giron, 1995). This relatively common diversity in solid forms gives the formulation scientist variations in physical properties to exploit.

In general, the crystalline form with the closest packing (greatest density) and the highest melting point is the stable form. The stable form will have the lowest solubility and lowest free energy of the different solid phases of the drug. All other phases with the same composition are termed *metastable* forms at this temperature and pressure. In practical terms, the energy barrier for conversion to the stable form can be high enough that the metastable forms can be examined and formulated. This is especially true if the free-energy difference is small (leading to a small driving force) or if significant bond breaking, molecular motion, and bond formation are required for transformation.

If the crystals contain solvent molecules within the lattice structure in defined locations and stoichiometry, these are referred to as *solvates* (*hydrates* if the solvent is water). The term *pseudopolymorph* has been used historically, but is not as specific and should be avoided if the composition is known. In most cases, the solvated form of the drug is the least soluble form in that solvent (e.g., hydrates are the low-energy forms in water). Owing to additional mixing terms, solvates are often more soluble in a solvent of different composition than the nonsolvated crystal (Shefter and Higuchi, 1963). The types of solvates that appear in pharmaceutical systems and their properties of interest are covered in the "Solvates and Hydrates of Drugs" section of this chapter.

Amorphous forms can be made for most pharmaceuticals by producing the solid form faster than the molecules can arrange into a crystalline lattice. Noncrystalline solids may have some short-range order but lack the long-range periodicity and regular intermolecular bonding of crystalline solids. Their synthesis and properties differ markedly from their crystalline forms, as will be described in detail in the section on amorphous drugs. In general, amorphous forms are high-energy, low-density solids that can yield transient dissolution rates considerably greater than crystalline solids.

Liquid crystals are an intermediate state in which the molecules in a crystal can undergo a secondary phase transition to a mesophase, which gives them mobility in 1–2 directions. They are birefringent, but possess flow properties like a liquid phase. Lyotropic liquid crystals form on uptake of water into a system that increases its mobility, and thermotropic liquid crystals can be disrupted by heating above a transition temperature. Cromolyn sodium (Cox et al., 1971), the HMG-CoA reductase inhibitor SQ33600 (Brittain et al., 1995), and the leukotriene D4 antagonist L-660,711 (Vadas et al., 1991) are examples of pharmaceuticals that can form liquid crystals.

The crystal *habit* or external shape may differ when drugs are recrystallized from different solvent systems without changing the internal structure. The presence of additives, the rate of cooling, degree of agitation, and the degree of saturation can all affect crystal habit (Byrn, 1982; Byrn et al., 1999). Habit can affect bulk properties such as density and flowability (Carstensen, 1993) or influence the ability to filter crystals during purification. Chow and Grant (1988) have shown that the dissolution rate of acetaminophen can be altered two to three times by modifying the length to width ratio through incorporation of additives. In general, habit effects on solubility are transient and of a magnitude equivalent to particle-size reduction techniques.

In summary, most drugs are developed as crystalline forms, which have the greatest physical and chemical stability, so that their purity can be increased during recrystallization. Knowledge of the potential polymorphic forms may allow the development scientist to find a metastable form with the prerequisite stability and increased dissolution rate to make it the desirable marketed form. Anhydrate forms usually give faster dissolution rates and higher aqueous solubilities than the hydrated form. Other solvates are not commonly used in pharmaceutical systems owing to potential toxicity of the solvent, but may provide additional solubility enhancement. Amorphous forms have the highest free energy, with the greatest degree of solubility enhancement, but are the most difficult to stabilize against transformation to the stable crystal form. The remainder of the chapter describes the advantages and disadvantages of each type of solid and gives numerous examples from the pharmaceutical literature where alteration of the solid form resulted in increased solubility.

Methods to Study the Solid State during Preformulation Screening

After initial selection of the candidate drug and its salt form (if applicable), it is recommended that a purposeful effort be undertaken to examine the solid states available for development consideration. Balbach and Korn (2004) have offered suggestions on how to screen candidates with small quantities of material. In the absence of such programs, new crystalline forms may be discovered by accident from precipitation of less soluble phases or a change in appearance of the bulk drug during scale-up. If sufficient formulation, analytical, and toxicology work has been completed and it becomes necessary to change the solid state, it may significantly delay the development program. If the newly discovered form is the more stable modification, it may be difficult to reproduce the metastable form. Carstensen (1993) noted that the diazepam tablet development program was complicated by the crystallization of a more stable polymorph after clinical trials had begun. A classic example of an unexpected occurrence of an earlier unidentified polymorph is that of Ritonavir. Bauer et al. (2001) have described how Norvir capsules had unknowingly been manufactured at a level that was supersaturated relative to the most stable conformational polymorph. It was not until several lots of the product failed dissolution testing that the new polymorph was identified.

Byrn et al. (1995) have offered strategic approaches for characterizing pharmaceutical solids with specific emphasis on regulatory considerations. The International Conference on Harmonisation (2000) and the FDA (2004) have also presented their guidance for industry on how to address the issues of pharmaceutical polymorphism. In general, the information that is useful at the early development phase includes

- Number of solid phases that exist for this drug
- Relative physical and chemical stability of these phases
- Solubility of each form in relevant media
- Resistance of metastable forms to conversion during processing
- Possible means to stabilize amorphous or metastable forms, if needed

Another major consideration at this point is to decide on the patentability of any new crystal forms discovered to have significant practical advantages over those in the original patent. Byrn and Pfeiffer (1992) have listed more than 350 patents on crystal forms in the pharmaceutical patent literature granted for showing advantages in terms of stability, formulation, solubility, bioavailability, purification, hygroscopicity, preparation/synthesis, recovery, and prevention of precipitation. More recently, patent applications regarding solid-state properties of drugs have prolifically increased. For example, patents relevant to polymorphic forms numbered over 300 from 2003 to 2006. Indeed the pharmaceutical industry has found that patents surrounding solid-state properties are advantageous for the product life-cycle management. Cabri et al. (2007) have presented cefdinir as an interesting case study and outline the strategies utilized by generic manufacturers to circumvent the innovator's solid-state patent position.

Different crystal forms can be sought by recrystallization experiments varying the solvent system, temperature, precipitation method, and level of supersaturation. Precipitation methods may include slow evaporation of the solvent, addition of antisolvents, or saturation at high temperatures followed by cooling. The solvent systems chosen for study are key aspects of these experiments. Water must be included because of its physiological significance. In addition, water tends to *contaminate* other solvents at low levels and it is often a matter of concern during product storage. In certain conditions, the usual recrystallization solvents for the drug synthesis and purification scheme and any alternate systems that may be used for scale-up of this process should also be studied. Mixtures used in the final steps of the synthetic process should be examined, including azeotropes and solvents with small amounts of miscible water. A suggested list for solvents that have been known to produce different crystalline forms is provided in Table 19.1 (Wells, 1988; Byrn and Pfeiffer, 1992; Byrn et al., 1995; Andersen, 2000; Miller et al., 2005). In general, it is prudent to include hydrogen-bond donating solvents, hydrogen-bond accepting solvents, aprotic solvents, hydrocarbon, and chlorocarbon solvents.

Solid forms isolated from these systems should be subjected to characterization techniques such as hotstage, polarized light microscopy, differential scanning calorimetry (DSC), thermogravimetric

TABLE 19.1

Partial List of Solvents Commonly Utilized for Identifying Different Crystal Forms

Water	Methanol
Ethanol	Isopropanol
Acetone	Acetonitrile
Ethyl acetate	Hexane
Dimethylformamide	Methylene chloride
Diethyl ether	Glacial acetic acid

Note: Any other solvents used in the last steps of synthesis. Aqueous mixtures with the above.

analysis (TGA), X-ray powder diffraction (XRD), infrared spectroscopy (IR), FT-Raman spectroscopy, and solid-state nuclear magnetic resonance (NMR). Reviews on characterizing the solid state have been given by Brittain (1999), Byrn et al. (1999), Bugay (2001), Carstensen (2001), Stephenson et al. (2001), Rodriguez-Spong et al. (2004), and Shah et al. (2006). The solubility of each new form isolated should be studied in water or the solvent/solution of pharmaceutical interest. Composition versus vapor pressure data should be obtained to understand the stability of any hydrated forms with respect to the anhydrate and other stoichiometric hydrates. If the transition to the stable form is fast, intrinsic dissolution measurements can be used to estimate the relative solubilities of new crystal forms.

The method used to identify new solid phases depends in part on the expertise of the investigator and availability of equipment, and in part on the properties of the solid phases. Haleblian and McCrone (1969) have demonstrated the power of the polarized light microscope and hotstage microscope in studying the phase relationships between solid forms versus temperature. Byrn (1982), Wall (1986), and Suryanarayanan (1989) have noted that only XRD and single crystal X-ray studies uniquely identify a solid phase unambiguously, since other methods depend on properties that may or may not change with a change in crystal lattice structure. If the new phase is a solvate, additional techniques are needed to identify the solvent of crystallization and its stoichiometry. DSC has been used extensively in polymorph investigations since the melting point is often the first indication of a new crystalline form (Giron, 1995). Other phenomena such as solid-state transitions and water loss in endotherms are often discernible from the thermogram. Lindenbaum and McGraw (1985) have shown how solution calorimetry can be used to assign relative enthalpy differences between polymorphs of drugs. It is best to use a combination of techniques to elucidate the nature of the new crystal forms, as one technique may not be able to differentiate the forms. For example, the two polymorphic forms of amiloride HCl dihydrate could not be distinguished by IR spectra or microscopic morphology (Jozwiakowski et al., 1993), but are easily identified by XRD. If a metastable form is identified that may be needed to produce the desired or optimal pharmacological effect, further studies should be done to define the relative stability of this form and the proper storage conditions to prevent conversion (Vippagunta et al., 2001). A metastable form should not be used when the more stable crystalline form produces the desired effects; in this case, the potential benefits probably do not offset the risk of conversion between production of the drug product and patient use. The stresses during manufacture of the product need to be studied as well, since compression, milling, granulation, and lyophilization can all change the solid state of the drug between synthesis and formulation. In some cases appropriate precautions, resistant packaging, or stabilizing excipients can keep the drug in the optimum form despite its metastability. Once some of these properties are known, a rational decision can be made on whether to proceed with development of a metastable solid based on a therapeutic need.

Properties Dependent on the Solid State

Once the different solid phases have been identified, their physical properties can be compared to find the form that is optimum for drug product development. Verma and Krishna (1966) described polymorphic forms of common substances that illustrated how their physical properties can be quite different. The cubic form of carbon (diamond) is hard, dense (3.5 g/cc), brilliantly clear, and a poor conductor. In contrast, the hexagonal form of the same element (graphite) is soft, less dense (2.2 g/cc), dull in appearance, and a good conductor. Optical properties of different solid forms can change their color; mercuric iodide is red (tetragonal form) or yellow (orthorhombic form). A classic example is ROY (5-methyl-2-[(2-nitrophenyl)amino]-3-thiophenecarbonitrile), which has three polymorphs that are easily identified by their respective colors of red(R), orange(O), and yellow(Y) (Stephenson et al., 1995).

Drug substances, which tend to be larger organic molecules with multiple hydrogen-bonding sites, are especially prone to different crystalline arrangements, which produce variable physical properties. Table 19.2 lists physical and chemical properties of pharmaceuticals that have been cited

TABLE 19.2

Properties of Drug Substances Dependent on the Solid State

Dissolution rate	Solubility
Chemical stability	Bioavailability
Melting point	Flowability
Particle size/shape	Compressibility
Hygroscopicity	Density
Filterability	Suspension viscosity
Tablet hardness	Color

in the literature as depending on the solid state of the drug. Some of these may provide significant advantages in drug development. Form I of celiprol HCl is much less hygroscopic than the form II polymorph (Narurkar et al., 1988). Form A chlorpropamide forms tablets with greater hardness than those of form C under identical compression forces (Matsumoto et al., 1991). Phenobarbitone also has crystalline forms that differ in compressibility profiles (Shell, 1963). The two polymorphs of methylprednisolone have different chemical stability profiles when exposed to identical temperatures and humidities of storage (Munshi and Simonelli, 1970). Crystal size and shape can alter the filterability or syringeability of suspensions, and affect the weight uniformity of tablets and capsules.

While there are numerous examples of miscellaneous physical property differences between different solid phases of the same drug substance, the excess free energy of metastable states is the most important. The higher energy state, a consequence of decreased crystal lattice energy, produces a greater molecular mobility and thermodynamic escaping tendency in metastable solids. This leads to faster dissolution rates and greater solubilities, which can have formulation and therapeutic implications for pharmaceuticals. Drugs with poor aqueous solubility are more likely to show enhanced bioavailability when metastable solids are used, because their oral absorption tends to be dissolution limited.

Advantages of Using Metastable Solids

Dissolution Rate Improvement

The Noyes–Whitney equation for the dissolution of solids into a solvent (Noyes and Whitney, 1897) can be used to calculate the rate of drug concentration (C) increase with time (t):

$$\frac{dC}{dt} = AK(C_s - C_b) \tag{19.2}$$

where A is the surface area of the solid exposed to solvent, C_s is the saturation concentration or apparent solubility, C_b is the bulk solution concentration, and K is a constant including the diffusion coefficient of the solute, the thickness of the unstirred diffusion layer, and the volume of solvent. Rotating die methods have been developed, such as the Wood's die apparatus, which maintain a constant surface area during the initial phase of dissolution experiments. Under sink conditions, where $C_s \gg C_b$, and with constant surface area (A), the intrinsic dissolution rate (IDR) can be obtained. The IDR (units mg/cm²/min) is directly proportional to solubility, and depends on the intrinsic dissolution properties of the drug in the media, not the dissolution method:

$$IDR \approx K(C_s) \tag{19.3}$$

Changes in the solid state can influence dissolution rate through the surface area term or the solubility term. Surface area differences can arise from simple particle-size effects between different crystal forms and also from shape factors. Different crystal habits and shapes can alter the exposed surface area without a change in median particle-size measurements, since these are often calculated by methods that assume spherical shapes. Abdou (1989) has reviewed the effect of crystalline state on the dissolution rate of pharmaceuticals, and how this contributes to bioinequivalence of various forms.

Differences in solubility between different crystal forms alter the driving force for dissolution, controlled by the difference between the solution concentration and the saturation concentration ($C_s - C_b$). Hamlin et al. (1965) have shown that dissolution rate correlates well with solubility for a large number of pharmaceutical compounds varying in solubility from 0.01 to 10 mg/mL at 37°C. Nicklasson and Brodin (1984) have shown that using cosolvent mixtures for drugs with poor aqueous solubility produces a good correlation between dissolution rate and solubility.

The dissolution rate improvement for most metastable solids is only transient; ultimately the excess solid in equilibrium with the solvent converts to the lowest energy phase. Figure 19.1 (Jozwiakowski and Connors, 1985) illustrates a typical dissolution profile for a metastable solid and a stable solid. In this case, β-cyclodextrin dissolution profiles were measured in 40°C distilled water and plotted on a molar basis (where the molecular weight difference is inconsequential). The concentration of the stable form in water at room temperature (a dodecahydrate) gradually increases to the limit of its solubility (0.0298 M). The metastable form (the anhydrate from oven drying) shows a rapid initial dissolution rate over the first 10 min, peaks at less than 30 min, and then declines to the solubility limit as the excess solid converts to the hydrated form, as verified by microscopy. The same behavior is exhibited by metastable and stable polymorphic forms, for example, forms I and II of meprobamate (Clements and Popli, 1973) and forms I and II of gepirone HCl (Behme et al., 1985). Ultimately, the same equilibrium solubility will be reached regardless of the direction of approach, although the kinetics of this transition can vary considerably for different drugs.

Dissolution rate improvement is often characterized by the IDRs or the change in the initial rate, since in many cases the advantage decreases with time. Table 19.3 shows some data from the pharmaceutical literature that indicates the typical dissolution rate increases that can be obtained by altering the solid state of drugs. Dissolution rate improvements of two to three times have been seen with some polymorphic or solvated forms, but typical increases are 20%–50% over the metastable form. Other polymorphs yield similar dissolution rates, such as tegafur (Uchida et al., 1993), disopyramide (Gunning et al., 1976), or amiloride HCl dihydrate (Jozwiakowski et al., 1993).

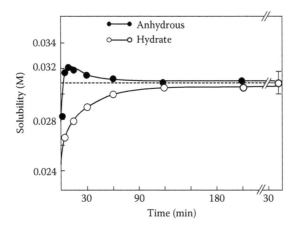

FIGURE 19.1 Dissolution rates for anhydrous and hydrated β-cyclodextrin in water at 40°C. (Reprinted from *Carbohydrate Res.*, 143, Jozwiakowski, M. J. and Connors, K. A., Aqueous solubility behavior of three cyclodextrins, 51–59, Copyright 1985, with permission from Elsevier Science.)

TABLE 19.3

Comparison of Initial Dissolution Rates of Drugs on Alteration of the Solid State

Drug	Solid Form	Relative Rate	Reference
Sulphathiazole	II	2.3	Lagas and Lerk (1981)
	I	1.6	
	III	1.0	
Tegafur	α	1.0	Uchida et al. (1993)
	β	1.2	
	γ	1.0	
Diflunisal	I	1.4	Martinez-Oharriz et al. (1994)
	II	1.4	
	III	1.3	
	IV	1.0	
Iopanoic acid	Amorphate	9.5	Stagner and Guillory (1979)
	II	1.6	
	I	1.0	

The data from Stagner and Guillory (1979) illustrate the larger increases that are often obtained with amorphous forms. The IDR plot for these iopanoic acid forms in pH 6.5 phosphate buffer at 37°C is shown in Figure 19.2. The consequence of this greater effect is the instability of amorphous forms to crystallization, so each system must be studied carefully to evaluate the development potential.

Dissolution rate improvement may be beneficial for producing readily dissolved solids for parenteral or oral administration of drugs subject to hydrolysis. For solid oral dosage forms, the initial rate increase can be sufficient to alter the amount of drug that enters the blood and improve the therapeutic potency. Unlike *in vitro* test systems, the concentration in the GI cavity may never approach

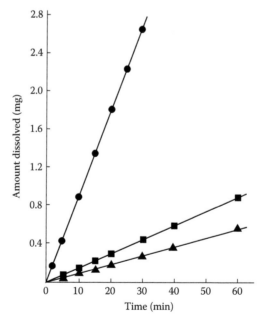

FIGURE 19.2 IDRs for form I (..t), form II (.), and amorphous (•) iopanoic acid in pH 6.5 phosphate buffer at 37°C. (Reproduced from Stagner, W. C. and Guillory, J. K., *J. Pharm. Sci.*, 68, 1005–1009, 1979. With permission from American Pharmaceutical Association.)

the saturation level (C_s), because of the large volume of fluid and the rapid dilution into the bloodstream. This sink effect allows bioavailability increases despite the tendency of these solids to revert to the less soluble form in suspension. Shibata et al. (1983) have shown that faster-dissolving forms of cimetidine are more effective at curing ulcers in the rat than the thermodynamically stable form. Haleblian and McCrone (1969) reported on the adrenal cortex atrophy in rats for a variety of solid forms of fluprednisolone. Doubling the *in vitro* dissolution rate (changing from the α-monohydrate to form I) produced a 50% greater effect of the drug. Amorphous indomethacin provided faster dissolution rates than the crystalline form (Fukuoka et al., 1987) and showed enhanced activity dosed orally in rabbits. Clearly, metastable solids can improve the dissolution rates of poorly soluble drugs and this effect can have therapeutic significance.

Solubility Increases

The solubility of a metastable solid form can be estimated from the maximum in the dissolution rate curve (Shefter and Higuchi, 1963). The accuracy of this determination depends on the rate of transformation versus the rate of dissolution. For systems such as anhydrous/hydrated theophylline in water (Shefter and Higuchi, 1963) that have the general shape given in Figure 19.1, the actual solubility is probably underestimated. The peak of the curve in this case has been described as a steady state involving equal rates of dissolution of the metastable form and conversion to the stable form. Behme et al. (1985) estimated the solubilities of gepirone HCl polymorphs by this method. Chauvet et al. (1992) estimated the solubilities of polymorphs of an anxiolytic agent after 1 h, and obtained linear van't Hoff plots from 30°C to 58°C. Suleiman and Najib (1989) measured the solubility of glibenclamide polymorphs and solvates after 8 h. Kaneniwa et al. (1985) found that the α and γ forms of indomethacin reached plateaus on their respective dissolution–time curves after 8 h, providing accurate estimates of their solubilities. Ghodbane and McCauley (1990) did not see any conversion after 24–72 h in their studies on MK571, which enabled accurate determination of the solubility of both forms in isopropanol and methyl ethyl ketone. Gerber et al. (1991) found that cyclopenthiazide did not convert to its more stable form after 7 days in water or ethanol/water. Hoelgaard and Moller (1983) reported that the aqueous solubility of the anhydrate of metronidazole benzoate could be determined after 48 h without any conversion to the stable monohydrate in the temperature range of 16°C–30°C.

Solubility values based on a plateau in the dissolution rate curve, when dissolution of the metastable form is essentially complete and the system reaches a pseudoequilibrium state before conversion to the stable solid state, are reasonably accurate. Those based on peaks in these curves or obtained by fitting exponential functions to estimate the plateau that might be reached in the absence of conversion should be considered only estimates of the metastable form solubility. The quantitative gain in these systems may be estimated more accurately by comparing initial dissolution rates for the two forms. In most cases, amorphous form solubilities must be estimated by these techniques due to their rapid crystallization when in contact with solvents.

The vitamin riboflavin exists in two polymorphic forms; form II is highly water-soluble and the higher melting form I has poor aqueous solubility (Goyan and Day, 1970). A patent was issued for the more soluble form of riboflavin based on its increased solubility (Biles, 1962). Since then, many examples of solubility differences among crystal forms of the same drug have been cited in the literature. Shefter (1981) compiled a brief list of metastable polymorphs exhibiting a greater solubility than their corresponding stable forms in his review of solubilization by solid-state manipulation. In most cases, the solubility gain was 50%–100%, but chloramphenicol palmitate (3.6 times) and Su-1777DB (4.2 times) showed substantial gains in solubility. Wells (1988) has reported the effect of hydration on the solubilities of ampicillin and glutethimide. The trihydrate form of ampicillin was only 0.75 times as soluble as the anhydrate, and the hydrate of glutethimide was only 0.62 times as soluble as its anhydrate in water. Using the anhydrate forms in dry dosage forms in these cases may impart a transiently higher dissolution rate that can alter the amount absorbed. There are also numerous cases of isoenergetic polymorphs that do not show differences in solubility

(Jozwiakowski et al., 1993; Carstensen and Franchini, 1995). In the latter case, amiloride HCl dihydrate polymorphs A and B showed statistically insignificant differences in solubility over the temperature range of 5°C–45°C in 0.15% NaCl. Given the wide range of behaviors of various drugs, solubility differences between solid phases should be determined experimentally early in the drug development process to identify any potentially useful forms.

Higuchi et al. (1963), in the study of methylprednisolone polymorphs, noted that the ratio of solubility between polymorphs should remain constant regardless of the solvent. This holds true as long as Henry's Law is obeyed, since solvent-dependent terms are cancelled when the temperature dependence of the solubilities is expressed as a ratio. Their resultant expression shows that, when the activity coefficients are 1.0 (dilute solution), the solubility ratio (S_1/S_2) depends only on the enthalpy change for the transition ($\Delta H_{1,2}$), the gas constant (R), and the temperature (T):

$$\frac{d\ln(S_1/S_2)}{dT} = \frac{\Delta H_{1,2}}{RT^2} \qquad (19.4)$$

The magnitudes of the solubility of forms I and II of this drug varied significantly in water, decyl alcohol, and dodecyl alcohol. However, their data showed that the solubility ratio was independent of solvent, but dependent on temperature. Figure 19.3 shows the data for these polymorphs in water. The difference in slopes (indicating a difference in enthalpies of fusion) for the two polymorphs can be used to calculate a transition temperature, where both forms have the same physical stability. The identity of the metastable form and the degree of solubility enhancement both depend on the temperature chosen for comparison.

This constancy of solubility ratio between solvents for two polymorphs at a given temperature does not apply to solvated/nonsolvated pairs, where additional terms arising from the release of the solvate complicate the calculations.

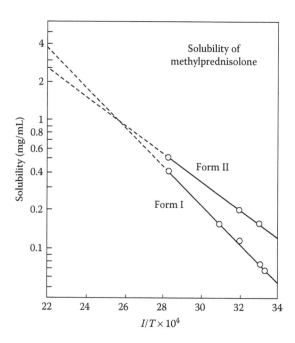

FIGURE 19.3 Water solubility of methylprednisolone polymorphs versus temperature. (Reproduced from Higuchi, W. I. et al. *J. Pharm. Sci.*, 52, 150–153, 1963. With permission from American Pharmaceutical Association.)

Bioavailability Enhancement

An increase in dissolution rate or solubility may allow more convenient formulation of poorly soluble drugs, but the real value in altering the solid state is to improve the therapeutic activity of the drug through enhanced oral bioavailability. Solubility improvement will not increase the bioavailability of all poorly absorbed drugs. Bioavailability problems could be related to rapid metabolism, degradation in the gut, poor intestinal permeability, or low aqueous solubility (Aungst, 1993). Metabolism and chemical degradation can be studied by conventional methods. Intestinal permeability can be assessed by *in vitro* models such as the CACO-2 cell permeability model (Gan et al., 1994). For drugs with poor aqueous solubility owing to their hydrophobic nature, the permeability is often reasonable and the absorption becomes dissolution rate limited. Kaplan (1972) has suggested that an IDR® of greater than 1 mg/min/cm^2 usually indicates a drug that is not dissolution rate limited in oral absorption. A rate of less than 0.1 mg/min/cm^2 almost always indicates a dissolution problem, and intermediate rates are borderline. More recently, a solubility of 0.1 mg/mL or less has been identified as a general rule for ascertaining the importance of dissolution rate in predicting the oral absorption (Dressman et al., 1985).

In order for different solid phases of the same molecule to give higher bioavailability, the rate of transformation to the less available form in the gut needs to be slow compared to the rate of absorption. In most cases for water-insoluble drugs, a significant increase in dissolution rate or solubility will translate into greater oral bioavailability. Polymorphs with melting point differences of less than 1°C are less prone to have energetic differences required to show bioavailability differences, but a very large melting point difference may increase the rate of transformation to the stable form. Normally, a 50% difference in solubility or dissolution rate between two forms is enough to translate into *in vivo* differences in oral dosing.

The bioavailability of various polymorphs of chloramphenicol palmitate has been studied by Aguiar (Aguiar et al., 1967; Aguiar and Zelmer, 1969). They found a linear correlation between the percent polymorph B (in mixtures with polymorph A) and the peak serum levels in humans of chloramphenicol (Figure 19.4). Polymorph B had shown an aqueous solubility at 30°C approximately

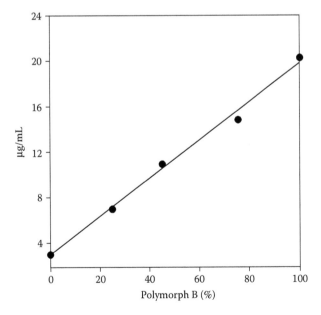

FIGURE 19.4   Peak serum levels of chloramphenicol as a function of the percent of polymorph B (palmitate ester) in mixtures with polymorph A. (Redrawn from Aguiar, A. J. et al., *J. Pharm. Sci.*, 56, 847–853, 1967. With permission from American Pharmaceutical Association.)

twice that of polymorph A. Even with a large particle size, polymorph B still gave better blood levels than polymorph A, showing the relative importance of the solid state. Similar effects have been seen with solvated pharmaceuticals. Abdou (1989) has summarized the work of Poole et al., which shows that ampicillin anhydrate gave higher blood levels in humans compared to ampicillin trihydrate.

There are numerous accounts in the literature of increased bioavailability in animals when changing the solid state. Kato and Kohetsu (1981) showed that form II amobarbital is more rapidly absorbed *in vivo* than form I. Dissolution rate experiments in water at 37°C showed a 1.6 times faster dissolution rate *in vitro* for form II compared to form I. Yokoyama et al. (1981) found that form III of 6-mercaptopurine was 1.5 times as bioavailable in rabbits as form I. It was six to seven times as soluble as the form I polymorph in studies by Kuroda et al. (1982). Kokubu et al. (1987) examined the therapeutic effect of different polymorphs of cimetidine in inhibition of ulcers in the rat. Pharmacokinetic studies found that form C was 1.4–1.5 times as bioavailable as forms A and B. This translated into a greater protection against stress ulceration, as shown in Table 19.4. The effect of form C was significant compared to forms A, B, and D, which were all equivalent.

Other studies have demonstrated that polymorph differences do not always translate into bio-availability differences. Gunning et al. (1976) have published results for disopyramide, an example of a drug that showed similar dissolution rates for both forms (I and II). Bioavailability studies in healthy human volunteers also showed no differences in bioavailability from identical capsule formulations of the two polymorphs. Umeda et al. (1984) reported on the case of benoxaprofen, in which the two forms had no significant differences in bioavailability in rabbits, despite a 1.5 times solubility advantage for form I over form II. Bioavailability differences for solid states need to be verified by *in vivo* studies, and in those cases where there is no advantage, the more stable form should be developed for stability reasons.

Amorphous solids represent an attractive approach for improving the oral bioavailability of poorly soluble drugs. As a result of their higher free-energy state, amorphous solids exhibit higher solubility and faster dissolution than their crystalline forms. These enhanced properties may result in an improved bioavailability if solubility or dissolution of the drug is the limiting step for absorption in the gastrointestinal tract. Kim et al. (2008) found that an amorphous form of atorvastatin calcium, prepared by an antisolvent process, resulted in an increase of 3.4 times for both the intrinsic dissolution rate and apparent solubility in water at 37°C compared to the crystalline form. Similar results were seen with an amorphous atorvastatin solid prepared by a spray-drying method. These increases in dissolution and apparent solubility were enough to increase the bioavailability 2–4 times in rats.

Due to the inherent physical instability of amorphous solids, the majority of *in vivo* studies utilize an amorphous solid dispersion containing a polymer excipient to stabilize the amorphous state.

TABLE 19.4

Comparison of the Four Crystalline Forms of Cimetidine in Their Ulcer Inhibitory Effect in Rats at 12.5 mg/kg

Treatment	Mean Ulcer Area (mm)	Inhibition (%)
Control	22.3 ± 4.3	0
Form A	6.9 ± 2.1	69.1 ± 25.3
Form B	8.7 ± 4.8	60.8 ± 31.1
Form C	2.8 ± 1.7	87.4 ± 26.7
Form D	8.0 ± 2.6	64.1 ± 25.7

Source: Kokubu, H. et al., *Int. J. Pharm.*, 35, 181–183, 1987. With permission.

Miller et al. (2007) demonstrated thatanitraconazole-hydroxypropyl methylcellulose (HPMC) amorphous solid dispersion (1/1) increased the bioavailability 2.48 times compared to the crystalline form in rats. Zerrouk et al. (2001) found that a carbamazepine-PEG6000 amorphous solid dispersion (1/1) increased the bioavailability 1.26 times in rabbits. The use of amorphous solid dispersion technology dates back several decades, including Sugimoto et al. (1980), who showed a nifedipine-PVP amorphous solid dispersion (1/3) led to a 2.92 increase in the bioavailability in dogs.

COMPLICATIONS OF DEVELOPING METASTABLE DRUGS

Solution-Phase Transformations

In contrast to the solubility enhancing effect of metastable solids, there are some potential disadvantages that must be taken into account. In most cases, suspensions of metastable solids are not feasible owing to rapid transformation of the excess solid to the stable (low solubility) form. Shefter and Higuchi (1963) showed that many nonsolvated forms transform to the hydrated form in aqueous suspension within a few hours near ambient temperatures. Haleblian and McCrone (1969) gave some general rules for solution-mediated transformation. The greater the solubility difference, the faster the transition, because of the greater driving force. In addition, higher diffusion rates and dissolution rates lead to faster transitions, as do higher solubilities in the media.

Hoelgaard and Moller (1983) noted that the relative free-energy differences between the two forms will determine the rate of transformation. In the metronidazole benzoate system they studied, with an anhydrate and a monohydrate, the transition temperature (where the free energies of the two forms are equal) was 38°C. In this case, lower temperatures resulted in faster conversion to the monohydrate, because the solubility difference became greater the farther away from the transition temperature. Borka (1971) studied solution-mediated transformations of chloramphenicol palmitate polymorphs. Amorphous drugs converted to the stable α-form in 2 min after it was formed from the melt. Aqueous suspensions of the β-form did not convert to the α-form even after temperature cycling up to 45°C. The transformation occurred readily in isopropanol, which is a better solvent for the drug. This illustrates the role of solubility in determining the rate of conversion.

Clements and Popli (1973) summarized transformation times during dissolution of pharmaceutical compounds from the literature. Their study with meprobamate found that it took 168 h to convert to form I. Other than the example of chloramphenicol palmitate, this was much longer than most systems, which converted to the stable modification in 300 s (theophylline) to 24 h (ampicillin). This is generally slow enough to allow therapeutic advantages to dosing the metastable solid orally, but too rapid to market suspensions of these forms with adequate physical stability.

When a metastable solid dissolves, the solution becomes supersaturated with respect to the stable form. The degree of supersaturation is an important determinant of the tendency to nucleate the stable form. Phase transitions by crystallization of the stable form occur by rearrangement of the molecules in the excess solid or by crystallization of the stable solid from its supersaturated solution. The crystallization process involves nucleation, crystal growth, and Ostwald ripening (dissolution of small crystals and growth of the larger crystals). The nucleation may be either spontaneous (homogeneous) or induced by foreign particles (heterogeneous). Rodriguez-Hornedo et al. (1992) studied the theophylline anhydrate–monohydrate system and concluded that the transformation was solvent-mediated, with the growth rate of the monohydrate crystals dependent on the degree of supersaturation. The anhydrate crystals were acting as heterogeneous nucleation sites for the monohydrate, and kinetic equations were derived showing the relative dissolution rates of the two forms.

Kaneniwa et al. (1988) studied the transformation of phenylbutazone β-form to the α-form in ethanol at 4°C by DSC and XRD. The reaction was essentially complete in 4 days. Kaneniwa et al. (1985) also studied the transformation kinetics of indomethacin polymorphs in ethanol and fit the data to nine different kinetic models. The data fit the Avrami equation best, which assumes two-dimensional nuclear growth. The transformation of the α-form to the γ-form was a function of temperature with an activation energy of 14.2 kcal/mol.

Various techniques have been used to stabilize the metastable form against solution-mediated transformation, with limited success. Ebian et al. (1973) used viscosity-inducing agents such as glycerin, simple syrup, and carboxymethylcellulose to slow the conversion of sulfameter form II to form III. Other structurally related sulfonamides and some surfactants were also able to slow the conversion rate. Otsuka et al. (1994) found that 0.5% gelatin slowed the transformation of phenobarbital polymorphs during dissolution tests. Wall (1986) noted that polyvinylpyrrolidone (PVP), methylcellulose, and sucrose have been used to slow the transformation of sulfamethoxazole to its semihydrate in solution. Shefter (1981) listed other materials that have been used to retard phase transformation by a variety of mechanisms. In addition to those listed earlier, it includes acacia, pectin, sodium alginate, surfactants, and chemically similar materials. In no cases were these agents able to inhibit completely the transition, but retardation of an extremely fast transition may allow practical use of the metastable solid in freshly prepared suspensions or solid forms.

Transformations in the Solid State during Processing

Solid–solid transformations from the metastable state to the stable state are less likely than solution-mediated transformations because of the limited molecular mobility in the solid state. The usual mechanism of these transitions is nucleation and growth of the stable phase within the existing solid. Nucleation often begins at sites of higher free energy, such as crystal defects or regions of disorder, and transformation proceeds to spread across the crystal. Transformation is more likely when the energy difference between the two forms is greater. External forces (heat generated during milling or pressure changes during compression) and the presence of excipients can change the tendency of a metastable solid to undergo solid-state transformation.

Byrn (1982) has stated that polymorphic transformations in the solid state require three steps:

1. Molecular loosening (nucleation by separation from the lattice)
2. Solid solution formation
3. Separation of the product (crystallization of the new phase)

For desolvation reactions, this also involves breaking of the solvent:drug bonds in the solvated crystal. Milling or compression of the solid drug can accelerate the molecular loosening step by the creation of defects and providing energy to overcome the barrier to reaction. Florence and Salole (1976) showed that milling of digoxin, estradiol, and spironolactone induced the formation of amorphous regions into these crystals. Even excipients in the tablet or capsule formulation can become more reactive by this mechanism. York (1983) found that milling caused loss of crystallinity for sucrose, lactose, and microcrystalline cellulose.

Processing stresses can initiate solid-state transformations into the stable modification directly without the formation of amorphous regions. Literature references to changes in the solid state show that milling, compression, fluid-bed granulation, spray drying, and heating can all cause transformation to the stable form during formulation processing. Table 19.5 summarizes some of the drugs for which this has been observed and the process which caused the transition. If the metastable state will be developed to take advantage of its higher free energy, the effect of the expected processing and storage conditions on the physical stability of the drug should be studied.

Particle-size reduction techniques commonly cause solid-state transformations of metastable solids. This may be avoided by crystallizing the drug to the desired particle-size specification, applying cooling devices to the mill, or shortening the milling time by adjusting the feed rate. Amiloride HCl dihydrate transformed from polymorph B to A during ball milling, but did not convert during air impact micronization, which has a shorter contact time (Jozwiakowski et al., 1993).

Compression can cause transformation for many drugs, especially with longer dwell times, higher compressional forces, and defective crystals. Compression studies on drugs alone present a

TABLE 19.5

Examples of Changes in the Solid State of Drugs during Processing

Compound	Process	Reference
Barbitone	Milling	Chan and Doelker (1985)
Caffeine	Milling/compression	Chan and Doelker (1985)
Chlorpropamide	Milling	Chan and Doelker (1985)
Sulfabenzamide	Milling	Chan and Doelker (1985)
Sulfanilamide	Milling	Wall (1986)
Clotrimazole	Milling	Wall (1986)
Digoxin	Milling	Wall (1986)
Amiloride HCl	Milling/compression	Jozwiakowski et al. (1993)
Cephalexin	Milling	Matsumoto et al. (1991)
Fostedil	Milling	Takahashi et al. (1985)
Indomethacin	Compression	Matsumoto et al. (1991)
Piroxicam	Compression	Ghan and Lalla (1992)
Maprotiline HCl	Compression	Chan and Doelker (1985)
Chloroquine diphosphate	Compression	Bjaen et al. (1993)
Chloramphenicol palmitate	Milling	Kaneniwa and Otsuka (1985)
Ranitidine HCl	Milling	Chieng et al. (2006)
Sodium salicylate	Spray drying	York (1983)
Carbamazepine	Fluid-bed granulation	Everz and Mielck (1992)
Chloramphenicol palmitate	Heating	DeVilliers et al. (1991)

worst-case scenario; excipient addition may dilute the effect in actual formulations. Capsule filling uses little to no compression force, depending on the scale and machine design, and can be used when pressure-induced transformations are problematic. Jozwiakowski et al. (1993) calculated the percent conversion of amiloride HCl polymorph B into polymorph A under different compression forces and dwell times using a quantitative XRD method. For this drug, compression force had a greater impact than dwell time, as shown in Table 19.6. The percent conversion was a function of the compression force, but a four times increase in dwell time at the same compression force had no additional impact on the transformation. As expected, there is no change in the stable form (polymorph A) at the highest compression force.

Aqueous granulation in a high shear mixer or a fluid bed can cause hydrate formation, and the subsequent drying can cause desolvation. Carbamazepine was transformed from one anhydrate (form III) to another (form I) through a dihydrate intermediate when both of these processes were used (Everz and Mielck, 1992). The heat of drying can also cause the conversion of one form to another, as seen with chloramphenicol palmitate by DeVilliers et al. (1991).

TABLE 19.6

Transformation of Amiloride HCl Dihydrate Polymorphs during Compression

Initial Polymorph	Compression Variable (Force/Dwell Time)	Conversion (%)
B	1,100 psi/30 s	6
B	3,000 psi/30 s	41
B	3,000 psi/2 min	35
B	12,000 psi/2 min	69
A	12,000 psi/2 min	0

Source: Jozwiakowski, M. J., et al. *Int. J. Pharm.*, 91, 195–207, 1993.

Chemical and Physical Stability Differences for Metastable Forms

Another potential disadvantage of using the metastable solid form is that it can be less chemically and physically stable than the low-energy crystal form. Haleblian and McCrone (1969) reported on a corticosteroid that was more light sensitive in aqueous suspension when one of the two polymorphs was used in the formulation. Haleblian (1975) presented data on the coenzyme form of vitamin B_{12} that had a light-sensitive anhydrate, a light-sensitive hydrate (form B), and a light-stable hydrate (form A). Byrn (1982) studied the four crystal forms of hydrocortisone *t*-butylacetate; forms I and II contain ethanol in the crystal lattice and forms III and IV are nonsolvated. Form I was the only form found to oxidize in the presence of ultraviolet light.

Amorphous forms are generally more reactive than their crystalline counterparts, since they are less dense and have greater molecular mobility. Haleblian and McCrone (1969) noted that penicillin G crystal forms are more stable than the amorphous forms, in both the sodium and potassium salts. Chan and Becker (1988) studied a glycopeptide (a muramyl dipeptide analog) in both the crystalline and amorphous (lyophilized) forms. After 4 days at 80°C and 76% RH, only 5% of the intact amorphous peptide was found by high-performance liquid chromatography (HPLC). A crystalline form was much more stable, showing 83% remaining after the same conditions of storage. Pikal et al. (1978) showed that the chemical stability of cephalothin sodium correlated with the degree of crystallinity (the crystalline form was more stable). Pikal has presented similar data for other members of this drug class; cefamandole nafate and ceftazidime pentahydrate are also much more stable in the crystalline state.

Physical stability differences may also exist among polymorphs, since hygroscopicity is one property that can depend on the solid state. Nonsolvated forms are especially prone to hydrate formation in environments without controlled humidity. Herman et al. (1988) found that theophylline pellet release rates were affected by the transition of anhydrous drug to monohydrate. Matsuda and Tatsumi (1989) concluded that form II furosemide was more stable to heat and moisture than form III. Amorphous oxyphenbutazone (Matsuda and Kawaguchi, 1986) and amiloride HCl anhydrate (Jozwiakowski et al., 1993) also readily transform to hydrated forms unless protected from moderate to high humidity. Not all drugs are susceptible to water uptake and conversion to their hydrated forms; lamivudine does not convert to the 0.2 hydrate at humidities as high as 95% RH (Jozwiakowski et al., 1996).

Solvated forms may desolvate under high temperature or low humidity (hydrates). Byrn (1982) has reviewed the desolvation reaction for caffeine, thymine, theophylline, fenoprofen, and other pharmaceutical hydrates. Factors that have been found to influence this reaction are the appearance of defects, the size of tunnels in the crystal packing arrangement, and the strength of hydrogen bonding between the drug and its solvent of crystallization. For these dehydration reactions, appropriate packaging and manufacturing precautions may be needed to eliminate or reduce the extent of the problem.

SPECIAL CONSIDERATIONS FOR POLYMORPHS

THERMODYNAMIC STABILITY OF POLYMORPHS

Polymorphs, unlike a solvate/nonsolvate pair, have the same composition in the solid state and produce identical solutions on dissolution (below the solubility of the least soluble polymorph). This results in certain thermodynamic relationships between pairs of drug polymorphs that are not applicable to solvated drugs. Giron (1995) and Haleblian and McCrone (1969) have described the different phase diagrams resulting from *monotropic* and *enantiotropic* polymorphs. If the free energies of two polymorphs (or a measure of the free energy such as vapor pressure or solubility) are plotted versus temperature, the curves will intersect owing to a difference in slopes, unless the enthalpy of solution is identical. This point of intersection is the theoretical transition temperature (T_{tr}), which is a constant for the system under constant pressure. If the temperature is fixed, and the free energy is plotted versus pressure, a constant transition pressure would be located. This arises due to the Gibbs phase rule, which specifies the degrees of freedom (F) for a given number of phases (P) and components (C):

$$F = C - P + 2 \qquad (19.5)$$

A pair of polymorphs consists of two phases of one component (the drug), which means that there is only one degree of freedom (Verma and Krishna, 1966).

Enantiotropic polymorphs exhibit this transition temperature below their melting temperature (Figure 19.5), which means that the stable modification depends on the temperature of reference. This temperature represents the point of equal solubility for the two polymorphs, and one will have greater solubility above this temperature, and one below it. These transitions are often reversible, but may be kinetically limited or outside the temperature range studied. Haleblian and McCrone (1969) have cautioned that an enantiotropic relationship cannot be discounted because of the lack of an observed transition point. The transition can be examined microscopically if the crystal habits differ, or by solubility–temperature curves if the metastable form solubility can be measured before transformation.

Monotropic polymorphs have a theoretical transition point above the melting temperature (Figure 19.5); one form is always more stable and the other more soluble. The higher melting form is the least soluble, and the transition to this form is irreversible. In contrast, an enantiotropic transition is often reversible, and can sometimes be observed in both directions under a hotstage microscope by raising and lowering the temperature around T_{tr}. In general, most pharmaceutical polymorphic relationships tend to be monotropic, although enantiotropy is by no means uncommon. This has implications when the formulator must recognize the temperature at which they wish to have increased solubility from the metastable form (often 20°C–25°C for constitution at room temperature or 37°C for faster dissolution in the GI tract).

Giron (1995) has reviewed the general rules for the thermodynamics of polymorphs first published by Burger. If form I is the higher melting form and form II is the lower melting form, the solubility of form I will be higher below T_{tr} and the solubility of form II will be higher above T_{tr} for enantiotropic pairs. Form I will be more dense if the pair is monotropic, or less dense if they are enantiotropic. The heat of fusion for form I will exceed that of form II for monotropic systems, and the reverse is true for enantiotropic systems. Lastly, the transition from form II to form I will be exothermic if the forms are monotropic, and endothermic if they are enantiotropic.

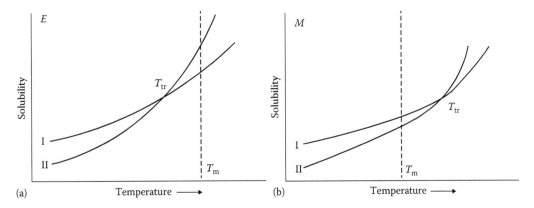

FIGURE 19.5 Solubility/temperature plots for enantiotropic (E) and monotropic (M) polymorphs at a fixed pressure.

The free energy of transition (ΔG_{tr}) between two polymorphs can be expressed as a function of the ratio of their solubilities (Aguiar and Zelmer, 1969; Grant and Higuchi, 1990):

$$\Delta G_{tr} = RT \ln \left[\frac{C_s \text{ polymorph I}}{C_s \text{ polymorph II}} \right] \qquad (19.6)$$

where R is the gas constant and T is the temperature of comparison in degrees Kelvin. The enthalpy difference (ΔH_{tr}) can be calculated from the slopes of the respective van't Hoff plots for each form, and the entropy difference (ΔS_{tr}) can be calculated from these two values through the familiar equation:

$$\Delta S_{tr} = \left[\frac{\Delta H_{tr} - \Delta G_{tr}}{T} \right] \qquad (19.7)$$

If Henry's Law is obeyed (activity can be approximated by molality in dilute solution for poorly soluble drugs), this leads to Equation 19.8:

$$\frac{d \ln(C_s I / C_s II)}{d(1/T)} = -\frac{\Delta H_{tr}}{R} \qquad (19.8)$$

specifying that the solubility ratio of two polymorphs (C_s I/C_s II) depend on the enthalpy difference between them at a given temperature, and not the solvent. At the transition temperature, both forms are in equilibrium with equal solubility, and $\Delta G_{tr} = 0$. Under these conditions, the enthalpy of transition is related to the entropy of transition through the temperature of transition (Grant and Higuchi, 1990):

$$\Delta H_{tr} = T \Delta S_{tr} \qquad (19.9)$$

Behme and Brooke (1991) have derived an equation for estimating the solubility ratio of two polymorphs at a given temperature using DSC data on the enthalpy of fusion (ΔH_f) and the melting temperature (T_m) of each form. The free energy of the transition or the natural logarithm of the solubility ratio multiplied by RT (Equation 19.6) was estimated by the difference between the solubility estimates for each form calculated by Equation 19.10:

$$RT \ln C_s = \frac{\Delta H_f (T_m - T)}{T_m} \qquad (19.10)$$

A ratio of unity (an estimate of the transition temperature) was calculated at 71°C, which closely matched the value from a van't Hoff plot of the two forms (log solubility vs. $1/T$), which intersected graphically at 73°C.

Mao et al. (2005) have developed analogous thermodynamic solubility relationships, providing detailed discussion on appropriate assumptions and models based on limited experimental data.

LITERATURE EXAMPLES OF SOLUBILITY INCREASES WITH POLYMORPHS

Table 19.7 lists a multitude of examples from the pharmaceutical literature where polymorphs of varying solubilities have been reported. In some of these articles, the solubility of each form is listed at multiple equilibration temperatures; in this case, the values closest to room temperature were complied. Only acemetacin, acetohexamide, cyclopenthiazide, and oxyclozamide on this list show solubility ratios (metastable form to stable form) greater than 3.0. Typically, the degree of solubility

TABLE 19.7

Literature Examples of Solubility Increases Using Drug Polymorphs

Drug	Solvent/ Temperature	Polymorphs and Solubilities		Ratio	Reference
Acetohexamide	Distilled water	I	27 µg/mL	II/I = 1.2	Kuroda et al.
	37°C	II	32 µg/mL		(1978)
	0.1NHCl	V	31.4 µg/mL	V/I = 3.7	Graf et al. (1984)
	30°C	IV	16.3 µg/mL	IV/I = 1.9	
		III	10.4 µg/mL	III/I = 1.2	
		I	8.4 µg/mL		
Acemetacin	Butanol	I	9.18 mM	II/I = 1.7	Burger and
	20°C	II	15.33 mM	IV/I = 2.1	Lettenbichler
		IV	19.00 mM	V/I = 2.8	(1993)
		V	25.65 mM	III/I = 4.7	
		III	43.44 mM		
Albendazole	Methanol	I	1.45 mg/mL	I/II = 2.0	Pranzon et al.
	25°C	II	0.72 mg/mL		(2010)
Auranofin	25% aq. PEG200	A	0.55 mg/mL	B/A = 2.5	Lindenbaum et al.
	37°C	B	1.35 mg/mL		(1985)
Benoxaprofen	pH 7 phosphate	I	230 µg/mL	I/II=1.5	Umeda et al.
	buffer 25°C	II	150 µg/mL		(1984)
Buspirone HCl	Isopropanol	I	0.5 g/100g	II/I = 1.7	Sheikhzadeh et al.
	25°C	II	0.84 g/100g	II/I = 2.6	(2007)
	55° C	I	4.77 g/100g		
		II	12.49 g/100g		
Carbamazepine	2-Propanol	I	11.16 mg/mL	I/II = 1.2	Behme and
	26°C	II	9.27 mg/mL		Brooke (1991)
Curcumin	Ethanol	I	6.05 g/kg	III/I = 1.1	Liu et al. (2015)
	25°C	III	6.48 g/kg		
Cyclopenthiazide	Distilled water	II	61.8 µg/mL	II/III = 3.6	Gerber et al.
	37°C	I	34.7 µg/mL	I/III = 2.0	(1991)
		III	17.2 µg/mL		
DifenoxinHCl	1% aq. tartaric acid	I	4.5 mg/100 mL	I/II=1.5	Walking et al.
	37°C	II	3.1 mg/100 mL		(1979)
Etoposide	Water 25°C	II	221.0 µg/mL	II/I = 1.9	Shah et al. (1999)
		II	14.5 µg/mL		
Frusemide	pH 5 acetate buffer	I	57.1 mg/100 mL	II/I = 1.6	Doherty and York
	37°C	I	35.2 mg/100 mL		(1988)
Gepirone HCl	n-Pentylalcohol	II	0.01 mg/mL	II/I = 2.6	Behme et al.
	20°C	I	3.79 mg/mL		(1985)
Glibenclamide	Distilled water 37°C	II	1.06 mg/100 mL	II/I = 1.6	Suleiman and
		I	0.66 mg/100 mL		Najib (1989)
Glycine	Deionized water 5°C	α	141.1 g/kg	α/γ = 1.1	Yang et al. (2008)
		γ	127.2 g/kg		
	25°C	α	226.8 g/kg	α/γ = 1.1	
		γ	202.1 g/kg		
	50°C	α	354.2 g/kg	α/γ = 0.9	
		γ	375.6 g/kg		
Indomethacin	Distilled water	α	0.87 mg/100 mL	α/γ = 1.3	Kaneniwa et al.
	35°C	γ	0.69 mg/100 mL		(1985)

(Continued)

TABLE 19.7 (*Continued*)
Literature Examples of Solubility Increases Using Drug Polymorphs

Drug	Solvent/ Temperature	Polymorphs and Solubilities		Ratio	Reference
Lornoxicam	Distilled water	I	4.96 µg/mL	II/I = 3.1	Zhang et al. (2013)
	25°C	II	15.15 µg/mL		
MefloquineHCl	Distilled water	E	5.1 mg/mL	E/D = 1.2	Kitamura et al.
	37°C	D	4.3 mg/mL		(1994)
Meprobamate	Distilled water	II	6.2 mg/mL	II/I = 1.9	Clements and
	25°C	I	3.3 mg/mL		Popli (1973)
MK571	Isopropylalcohol	II	0.390 mg/mL	II/I = 1.7	Ghodbane and
(Leukotrieneantagonist)	25°C	I	0.228 mg/mL		McCauley (1990)
	Methyl ethyl ketone	II	2.40 mg/mL	II/I = 1.9	
	25°C	I	1.24 mg/mL		
Nimesulide	pH 7	I	16.4 mg/L	II/I = 4.3	Sanphui et al.
	37°C	II	71.0 mg/L		(2011)
Nimodipine	Distilled water	I	0.036 mg/100 mL	I/II = 2.0	Grunenberg et al.
	25°C	II	0.018 mg/100 mL		(1995)
Oxyclozamide	0.1% aqueous	III	109 ppm	III/I = 3.9	Pearson and
	Tween80	II	73 ppm	II/I = 2.6	Varney (1973)
	25°C	I	28 ppm		
Phenylbutazone	pH7 phosphate	I	288.7 mg/100 mL	I/IV = 1.4	Ibrahim et al.
	buffer		279.9 mg/100 mL	II/IV = 1.3	(1977)
	36°C		233.6 mg/100 mL	III/IV = 1.1	
			213.0 mg/100 mL		
Phenobarbital	Distilled water 25°C	II-Ba	1.39 mg/mL	II-Ba/	Kato et al. (1984)
		II	1.28 mg/mL	III-Cy = 1.2	
		III-Cy	1.17 mg/mL	II/III-Cy = 1.1	
Piretanide	pH 1.2	B	13.3 mg/100 mL	B/A = 1.6	Chikaraishi et al.
	37°C	A	8.3 mg/100 mL		(1994)
Ritonavir	Ethanol:Water (99:1)	I	90 mg/mL	I/II = 4.7	Bauer et al. (2001)
	5°C	II	19 mg/mL		
Sulfanilamide	Ethanol	Orthorhombic	21.4 g/1000 g	O/M = 1.5	Carstensen (1993)
	39°C–40°C	Monoclinic	14.0 g/1000 g		
Sulfathiazole	Alcohol:Water (95:5)	I	8.15 g/1000 g	II/I = 1.7	Milosovich (1964)
	24°C	II	14.2 g/1000 g		
Tolbutamide	Distilled water	I	14.61 mg/100 mL	I/III = 1.1	Rowe and
	37°C	III	13.03 mg/100 mL		Anderson (1984)
	Octanol	I	23.54 mg/mL	I/III = 1.2	
	30°C	III	19.33 mg/mL		

enhancement which was achieved was 25%–100% more than the lowest solubility polymorph. This results in a free energy of transition (ΔG_{tr}) of 132–410 cal/mol (Equation 19.6). While the magnitudes of the solubilities vary considerably from solvent to solvent, the degree of enhancement does not, because of the independence of the solubility ratio from the solvent identity (Equation 19.8). Therefore, the expected degree of solubility enhancement for a given pair of polymorphs can be estimated by measuring the enthalpy of solution of each form, and calculating the enthalpy of transition from the difference. This may be experimentally accessible when the direct solubility of the metastable form is not, because of rapid transformation in solution.

Pudipeddi and Serajuddin (2005) recently compiled 81 solubility ratios for 55 different drugs. Their results, which parallel those presented here, show most of the solubility ratios were between 1 and 2 (84%); however, 9% of them had ratios greater than 3. Although the relative increase in solubility is modest, for water-insoluble drugs exhibiting dissolution rate limited absorption, this difference can be important for therapeutic activity.

SOLVATES AND HYDRATES OF DRUGS

TYPES OF SOLVATES AND CHARACTERIZATION METHODS

Molecules from the crystallization solvent can become incorporated into the crystalline lattice of drugs during the synthetic process. These solvent molecules may participate in hydrogen bonding with the drug molecules, fill space in the unit cell, and facilitate closest packing arrangements. Hydrates can also form when drugs absorb water vapor from the atmosphere or are exposed to water during processing or when suspended in water.

Solvates are generally discovered by their physical property differences from nonsolvated forms. Buxton et al. (1988) reported a hygroscopic anhydrate and a nonhygroscopic hemihydrate of paroxetine hydrochloride. Techniques like loss on drying or TGA will detect general weight loss on heating a sample, and the solvent may be identified as water by Karl Fisher analysis or as organic solvents by gas chromatographic analysis of the evolved gas. DSC thermograms will typically show an endotherm before melting, owing to loss of the solvent molecules (Giron, 1995). Hotstage microscopy can be used to visualize this solvent loss by examining the sample under silicon oil during heating. Melting point, solubility, tableting behavior, dissolution rates, crystal habit, density, and hygroscopicity can also differ substantially between nonsolvated and solvated forms of the same drug. Khankari and Grant (1995) have reviewed the characterization methods for pharmaceutical hydrates and the physical properties affected by hydrate formation.

Single crystal X-ray analysis can often be used to localize the solvent molecules in the crystal lattice, which may be present in stoichiometric ratios or nonstoichiometrically. Byrn (1982) has classified solvates as polymorphic (desolvate to a new XRD pattern) or pseudopolymorphic (desolvate to a similar X-ray powder pattern). Nonstoichiometric solvates that desolvate to the same X-ray powder pattern are often caused by the presence of *channels* in the crystal that can take up varying amounts of water based on the vapor pressure. SQ33600 (Brittain et al., 1995) and cromolyn sodium (Cox et al., 1971) are examples of this type of solvate.

The majority of characterized solvates are stoichiometric, with either water or organic solvents present in a fixed ratio with the drug molecules. Glibenclamide was isolated as two nonsolvated polymorphs, a pentanol solvate, and a toluene solvate (Suleiman and Najib, 1989). Furosemide could form solvates with dimethylformamide or dioxane (Matsuda and Tatsumi, 1989). Haleblian and McCrone (1969) studied the solid forms of steroids, and found different dissolution rates for two monohydrates of fluprednisolone, a monoethanol and hemiacetone solvate of prednisolone, and two monoethanolates and a hemichloroform solvate of hydrocortisone. Other solvents that have been reported to form solvates with drugs include methyl ethyl ketone, propanol, hexane, dimethyl sulfoxide, acetonitrile, and pyridine. The potential toxicity concerns eliminate most of these from consideration as practical mechanisms of solubility enhancement for human therapeutics.

Stoichiometric hydrates are the most important solvates affecting the solubility of marketed pharmaceuticals. Hemihydrates, monohydrates, and dihydrates are the most common stoichiometric ratios of water incorporated into the crystalline lattice of drugs. Pfeiffer et al. (1970) have shown how different hydrates of cephalosporins could be isolated from solvent systems of varying water activity. Cephalexin has a monohydrate and a dihydrate form, which are stable under different relative humidity conditions. Cefazolin has a monohydrate, a sesquihydrate (1.5 moles water), and a pentahydrate form (Byrn and Pfeiffer, 1992). Jozwiakowski et al. (1996) have found that lamivudine can form a 0.2 hydrate, where only one of five lamivudine molecules in the crystal lattice is associated with a water molecule. Multiple solvates can be formed for the same drug; Stephenson et al. (1994) have shown that dithromycin can crystallize in at least nine solvate forms, including a cyclohexane trisolvate and an acetonitrile trihydrate. Stephenson et al. (1998) describe the formation of isomorphic desolvates, which are defined as a desolvate that retains its three-dimensional order, resulting in a lattice that is in a high-energy state relative to the parent solvate. The formation of an isomorphic desolvate can lead to an increase in hygroscopicity or reduce the chemical stability of the solid. Isomorphic desolvates are often characterized by similarities in X-ray diffraction patterns compared to the parent solvate; however, the physical properties may differ between the two. Byrn et al. (1995) have also highlighted that desolvated forms of some drugs have unique properties that differ from their nonsolvated counterparts.

THERMODYNAMIC EVALUATION OF THE SOLUBILITY OF SOLVATES

Shefter and Higuchi (1963) first described the thermodynamics of the dissolution of solvated drugs in water. The solubility of a hydrated form in water is a special case that follows the relationship:

$$D[xH_2O]_{solid} \xleftrightarrow{K_s} D_{aq} + xH_2O \tag{19.11}$$

where $D[xH_2O]_{solid}$ represents a solid hydrated drug, D_{aq} is the concentration of dissolved drug in the aqueous solution, and K_s is the solubility equilibrium constant for the system. A hydrate is normally less soluble than its anhydrate in water because it is closer in free energy to the dissolved species. By measuring the solubility for the hydrated and anhydrous forms at a given temperature, the free-energy difference (ΔG) can be calculated:

$$\Delta G = RT \ln\left[\frac{K_s(\text{hydrate})}{K_s(\text{anhydrate})}\right] \tag{19.12}$$

When the solvate of an organic solvent is dissolved in water, the appropriate equation is

$$D[nB]_{solid} \xleftrightarrow{K_{sp}} D_{aq} + nB_{aq} \tag{19.13}$$

with $D[nB]_{solid}$ representing a solid solvate of drug D with n molecules of solvent B per molecule of D, D_{aq} and nB_{aq} are the independently dissolved species in water, and K_{sp} is the solubility product that governs the dissolution of the solvate. In general, Equation 19.12 results in a higher free energy of solvation than the analogous nonsolvated solubility equilibrium, resulting in a higher solubility for solvates of organic solvents in water.

Grant and Higuchi (1990) commented on the solution behavior of solvates in their book on the solubility of organic compounds. The hydrated form will be more stable (less soluble) than the anhydrate in the general case. When the solvate is formed from a nonaqueous solvent that is miscible in water, the free energy of solution of the solvent into the water reduces the activity of water and increases the apparent solubility of the solvate. An example is cited in which caffeine hydrate is less soluble in water than the anhydrate, but the solubility order reverses in ethanol.

Shefter and Higuchi (1963) illustrate the solubility enhancement of solvates with data on theophylline (hydrate and anhydrate), glutethimide (hydrate and anhydrate), cholesterol (hydrate and anhydrate), and succinyl sulfathiazole (pentanol solvate, hydrate, and anhydrate). In the latter case, the dissolution rate curves have the general shape of Figure 19.1, with the anhydrate form peaking at a higher concentration (4 mg/mL) than the hydrate (1 mg/mL), then decreasing to the same level as the solid form converts to the hydrate. In addition, the pentanol solvate curve peaks at 8 mg/mL (eight times the solubility of the hydrate) before it similarly converts. Van Tonder et al. (2004) also found the solubility and dissolution rate of the anhydrate of niclosamide to be significantly higher than that of the two monohydrate forms. The transiently higher solubility of the drug in water is due to the negative free energy of mixing of the solvent with water, which results in a more negative free energy of solution.

As with polymorphic forms, the temperature dependence of solvated drugs can be compared to nonsolvated drugs by van't Hoff plots. The point of intersection of the isochores when log solubility is plotted versus $1/T$ (in degrees Kelvin) represents the transition temperature where the solubility of the solvate equals that of the nonsolvate. By this treatment the transition temperature for theophylline was 73°C and for glutethimide was 52°C. Above this temperature, the hydrated form is more soluble and the anhydrate is the physically stable modification. At the transition temperature, the loss of entropy of solvent molecules incorporated into the crystal is exactly compensated by the favorable enthalpy change. Abdallah and El-Fattah (1984) have used this approach to determine the transition temperature for sulfamethoxazole and its hydrate is 70.5°C. As with polymorphic systems, for a given enthalpy difference, the further the temperature of comparison from the transition temperature, the larger the apparent solubility difference will be between the two forms. Table 19.8 illustrates this with the sulfamethoxazole example using data from Abdallah and El-Fattah (1984).

Literature Examples of the Effect of Solvates on Solubility

There are many examples of drugs that show slower dissolution rates, lower solubilities, or less absorption in the hydrated form than the anhydrate. Stoltz et al. (1989) studied the dissolution rate of oxyphenbutazone powder in distilled water at 37°C. The time to dissolve 50% of the powder was only 0.75 min for the anhydrate and 22.9 min for the monohydrate. The IDR of the anhydrate was 1.63 times as fast as the monohydrate when compressed discs were used. Haleblian and McCrone (1969) reported that the dissolution rate of pellets of fluprednisolone depended on the state of hydration of the drug. The β-monohydrate dissolved 10% faster than the α-monohydrate, but the anhydrate polymorph dissolution rates were 1.6 (form I), 1.4 (form III), or 1.3 times (form II) as fast as the α-monohydrate.

Poole et al. (1968) administered ampicillin anhydrate and trihydrate to human subjects as 250 mg doses of the suspension or in capsules. The anhydrate gave higher bioavailabilities as measured by the area under the blood level versus time curves. In suspensions, the area ratio (anhydrate/trihydrate) was 1.21 and in capsules, this ratio was quite comparable at 1.17. The peak in this curve also occurred earlier for the anhydrate. This was expected based on the 20% higher solubility in water at 37°C (10 mg/mL for the anhydrate and 8 mg/mL for the trihydrate). The difference in dogs was more pronounced; suspensions of the anhydrate gave 1.6 times the AUC of suspensions of the trihydrate form.

Table 19.9 lists many examples of equilibrium solubility differences between solvated and nonsolvated forms of pharmaceutically active compounds. The examples of calcium gluceptate

---

TABLE 19.8
Solubility (mg/100 mL) of Sulfamethoxazole Anhydrate (A) and Hydrate (H) in 0.1 N HCl versus Temperature

Temperature (°C)	Solubility (A)	Solubility (H)	Ratio (A/H)
25	119.3	97.5	1.224
30	143.5	120	1.196
44	271	234	1.158
51	335	300	1.117
70.5			

Note: Extrapolated thermodynamic transition temperature.
Source: Abdallah, O. and El-Fattah, S. A., *Pharm. Ind.*, 46:970–971, 1984.

TABLE 19.9

Literature Examples of Solubility Differences Between Drug Solvates and Nonsolvate

Ampicillin	Water 25°C	Anhydrate: 11.3 mg/mL	A/T = 1.4	Zhu and Grant
		Trihydrate: 7.8 mg/mL		(1996)
Calcium Gluceptate	Distilled water 22°C	Anhydrate: 1.3 molal	A/I = 18.6	Suryanarayanan and
		I (3.5hydrate): 0.07 molal		Mitchell (1986)
Carbamazepine	25°C water	Anhydrate: 0.379 mg/mL	A/T = 3.0	Murphy et al.
		Dihydrate: 0.125 mg/mL		(2002)
DMHP (iron chelator)	Distilled water 25°C	DMHP anhydrate: 0.109 M	F/A = 8.2	Ghosh and Grant
		DMHP formate: 0.894 M		(1995)
Fluconazole	Water 25°C	Anhydrate: 4.29 mg/mL	A/M = 1.2	Alkhamis (2002)
		Monohydrate: 3.56 mg/mL		
Furosemide	Water[a] 37°C	Dioxane solvate (X): 25.9 µg/Ml	X/A = 1.3	Matsuda and
		DMF solvate (D): 24.7 µg/mL	D/A = 1.2	Tatsumi (1990)
		Form I anhydrate: 19.8 µg/mL		
Glibenclamide	Distilled water 37°C	Pentanol solvate: 33.7 mg/100 mL	P/II = 31.8	Suleiman and Najib
		Toluene solvate: 2.5 mg/100 mL	T/II = 2.4	(1989)
		Form II nonsolvate: 1.06 mg/100 mL		
Lamivudine	Distilled water 25°C	I (0.2 hydrate): 84.9 mg/mL	II/I = 1.2	Jozwiakowski et al.
	Ethanol 25°C	II (anhydrate): 98.1 mg/mL	I/II = 1.6	(1996)
		I (0.2 hydrate): 18.5 mg/mL		
		II (anhydrate): 11.4 mg/mL		
Myricetin	Water 23°C	I (monohydrate): 0.5 µg/mL	IA/I = 6.4	Franklin and
		IA (anhydrate): 3.2 µg/mL	IIA/II = 1.2	Myrdal (2015)
		II (monohydrate): 0.6 µg/mL		
		IIA (anhydrate): 0.7 µg/mL		
Niclosamide	Water 25°C	Anhydrate: 13.32 µg/mL	A/H$_A$ = 14.0	Van Tonder et al.
		Monohydrate: (H$_A$): 0.95 µg/mL	A/H$_B$ = 21.8	(2004)
		Monohydrate: (H$_B$): 0.61 µg/mL		
Nifedipine	Water 30°C	Anhydrate: 5.42 µg/mL	A/D = 1.8	Boje et al. (1988)
		Dihydrate: 3.01 µg/mL		
Paroxetine HCl	Distilled water 20°C	I (hemihydrate): 4.9 mg/mL	II/I = 1.7	Buxton et al. (1988)
		II (anhydrate): 8.2 mg/mL		
Piroxicam	0.1 NHCl	A (anhydrate): 11.90 mg/L	B/A = 1.0	Kozjek et al. (1985)
	25°C	B (monohydrate): 12.30 mg/LA	B/A = 1.4	
	0.1 NHCl	(anhydrate): 10.58 mg/L		
	30°C	B (monohydrate): 14.64 mg/L		
Sulfamethoxazole	0.1 NHCl	A (anhydrate): 119.3 mg/100 mL	A/B = 1.2	Abdallahand
	25°C	B (monohydrate): 97.5 mg/10 0mL		El-Fattah (1984)
Theophylline	pH 6 phosphate	Anhydrate: 12 mg/mL	A/M = 2.0	Rodriguez-Hornedo
	buffer, 25°C	Monohydrate: 6 mg/mL		et al. (1992)

[a] Extrapolated intrinsic solubility from buffered pH solutions.

(Suryanarayanan and Mitchell, 1986) and glibenclamide (Suleiman and Najib, 1989) illustrate that anhydrate/hydrate differences and solvate/nonsolvate differences in solubility can be more dramatic than with polymorphs. Since most of the solvate forms cannot be used in human therapeutics, the most practical use of this knowledge in formulation is to use anhydrates in dry solid dosage forms when possible. This must be modified when the hygroscopicity of the anhydrate is high and conversion to the hydrate cannot be controlled adequately during manufacture, packaging, and storage.

Piroxicam (Kozjek et al., 1985) is a particularly interesting example in which the transition temperature is 25°C. At physiologically relevant temperatures, the yellow monohydrate triclinic form is actually more soluble than the white monoclinic needle form. The anhydrous needles also show a negative enthalpy of solution (solubility decreases as temperature increases), which is unusual compared to most organic compounds.

Lamivudine is an example of the effect of hydrates in nonaqueous solvents (Jozwiakowski et al., 1996). In distilled water at 25°C, the anhydrate free base (form II) is 1.2 times as soluble as the 0.2 hydrate (form I). In ethanol at 25°C, the hydrate is 1.6 times as soluble as the anhydrate. The maximum solubility in ethanol–water mixtures was found to be at 40%–60% water in ethanol, when form I is the most stable solid phase. The transition composition was with 18%–20% water in ethanol; in binary mixtures with more than 20% water, only the hydrate was found at equilibrium, and with less than 18% water, only the anhydrate was found at equilibrium.

UTILITY OF AMORPHOUS (NONCRYSTALLINE) FORMS

METHODS OF PRODUCING AMORPHOUS DRUGS

Amorphous drugs are formed either by prevention of the crystal lattice formation (rapid solidification or phase separation) or by disruption of an existing crystal structure (processing energy or desolvation). Examples of formation of amorphous sites during processing have already been cited for digoxin, spironolactone, lactose, and other solids.

The production of partially disordered solids by these techniques will generally result in properties intermediate between the pure crystalline and amorphous phases. Florence and Salole (1976) found that the generation of partial amorphous character in digoxin samples by milling resulted in 7%–118% increases in the apparent solubility, depending on the type and comminution.

Small-scale lots of NCEs are often produced in amorphous forms early in the development process, when the bulk drug synthesis is still being refined. Rapid precipitation from solution to gain high yields is often more important at this stage than optimum crystallization. Huang et al. (1991) have noted that the physical properties, including degree of crystallinity, can vary considerably by batch at this early research stage of development. The antipsychotic CI-936 was found to be more than 90% orally available in the dog as an amorphous form, and poorly and unpredictably absorbed as a crystalline form. The IDR of the amorphous form was 1.4–4.4 times as large as either crystalline lot. The effect was greater in phosphate buffer at pH 7.5, where the bulk powder dissolution of the amorphous form was approximately 10 times that of the slowest dissolving crystalline lot.

Purposeful synthesis of amorphous pharmaceuticals often involves lyophilization from solution or spray drying from a volatile solvent. Cooling of the melt can also produce a noncrystalline form if the drug does not decompose during melting. Similar to freeze drying, Overhoff et al. (2007) have described an ultra-rapid freezing (URF) process. In this process a solution of API and polymer are frozen onto a cold solid surface and then lyophilized. Utilizing danazol, this process was shown to produce amorphous material with high surface area and enhanced dissolution rate. The use of metastable amorphous forms may be required to achieve optimum performance of the solid oral dosage form for poorly soluble drugs. Cefuroxime axetil USP used in the marketed tablet formulation is amorphous, and the USP test specifies the lack of birefrigence under the polarized microscope. Numerous lyophilized formulations of antibiotics and peptides are marketed for injectable use; the dry state limits stability and preservative concerns, and the amorphous solids rapidly dissolve on reconstitution.

EXAMPLES OF SOLUBILITY INCREASES OF AMORPHOUS DRUGS

Amorphous solids have a lower density than their crystalline counterparts. This greater free volume results in a higher molecular mobility and a higher free energy, which is the basis for the enhanced dissolution rates, solubility, and bioavailability exhibited by some amorphous drugs. The crystallization of amorphous solids, their greater hygroscopicity, and their reactivity can cause difficulties in developing stable formulations. The increase in water uptake results from the ability of amorphous solids to absorb water into their internal structure, as opposed to the surface adsorption shown by denser crystalline compounds. Ward and Schultz (1995) showed that in milled albuterol sulfate samples, even small increases in the degree of disorder caused significant changes in the water sorption of the drug. Saleki-Gerhardt et al. (1995) showed a linear correlation between the percent amorphous character in raffinose pentahydrate and the weight percent uptake of water. Burger and Ratz (1990) found that amorphous tetracycline could absorb 20% water compared to 2% for the crystalline form. The amorphous form was also more susceptible to degradation under ultraviolet light than the crystalline form, and this was exacerbated by moisture.

Although amorphous forms tend to crystallize rapidly when in contact with a solvent, the solid forms often show enhanced dissolution rates and transient solubility increases that can translate into greater bioavailability. Otsuka and Kaneniwa (1983) studied the solubility of crystalline and amorphous cephalexin. The maximum solubility in water at 10°C was about 60 mg/mL for noncrystalline drug versus 10–11 mg/mL for the crystalline drug. The difference at 35°C appeared to be less owing to a more rapid crystallization rate at this temperature. Chikaraishi et al. (1996) also reported the effects of temperature on solubility and conversion rate for a solution-mediated phase transition of an amorphous form of piretanide to a crystalline form. Apparent solubility of the amorphous solid was 1.5 times greater than the crystalline form at 45°C. Likewise, a 2-fold increase was seen at 30°C. Conversion of the amorphous solid to the crystalline form was determined to occur faster at 45°C compared to 30°C. Imaizumi et al. (1980) showed that the dissolution of amorphous indomethacin was higher than that of the crystalline form for 2 h, after which crystallization caused the two to be equivalent. Fukuoka et al. (1987) estimated that the initial dissolution rate of the amorphous form was four times that of the crystalline form (γ modification) in phosphate buffer (pH 7.2). They demonstrated that this difference caused an increased oral and rectal absorption of indomethacin in rabbits, and a higher maximum peak in the blood level versus time curve.

The magnitude of the amorphous solubility enhancement is generally much greater than that of a metastable polymorph or an anhydrate/hydrate system. Stagner and Guillory (1979) compared the IDRs of amorphous iopanoic acid to that of the commercial crystalline form in pH 6.5 aqueous buffer at 37°C. The amorphous form was about one order of magnitude faster dissolving than the crystalline state (Figure 19.2). Higuchi et al. (1963) estimated that the amorphous form of methylprednisolone was about 20 times as soluble as the crystalline form I. Doherty and York (1989) found that furosemide amorphous solids stabilized by PVP gave 31–36 times the dissolution rate relative to crystalline drug. The amorphous form of novobiocin free acid was found to be 10 times as soluble as the crystalline free acid in 0.1 N HCl at 25°C (Mullins and Macek, 1960). The amorphous form gave equivalent therapeutic blood levels when dosed to dogs (in suspension at 12.5 mg/kg) as the more water soluble calcium salt, yet the crystalline free acid was not absorbed orally at detectable levels.

Hancock and Parks (2000) have critically evaluated the theoretical and practical aspects of utilizing the amorphous state. Theoretically, the gain in solubility though the use of an amorphous was predicted to be between 10- and 1600-fold. However, these elevated solubilities also represent very favorable driving forces for crystallization, and as a result, the realized gains are appreciably less.

PHYSICAL STABILITY OF AMORPHOUS SOLIDS

From the preceding section, it is apparent that the amorphous forms can have significant advantages in oral bioavailability for drugs with poor aqueous solubility. The high free energy, high solubility physical state responsible for this enhanced activity is a metastable state, and crystallization to a lower energy state is likely given the correct conditions. The commercial development of amorphous forms is limited by the ability to predict and control the physical stability of these systems so that the patient can receive the benefit of this enhanced activity.

The molecular mobility of a molecule in an amorphous solid is a function of the storage temperature in relation to the glass transition temperature (T_g). The glass transition is a second-order phase transition with a change in the heat capacity evidenced by a shift in the baseline on a DSC thermogram. The traditional view of amorphous substances is that they are glassy and brittle below T_g and rubbery and mobile above T_g. Hancock et al. (1995) have shown by relaxation time experiments that some molecular mobility can be seen as low as 50°C below the T_g of indomethacin and sucrose amorphous solids. In a practical sense, storage temperatures of 50°C below T_g are normally required to stabilize completely the amorphous solid against spontaneous crystallization (Yoshioka et al., 1995).

Giron (1995) has noted that relatively stable amorphous forms of pharmaceuticals have been reported for numerous drugs, such as ampicillin, bacitracin, betamethasone, erythromycin, imipramine HCl, indomethacin, nystatin, oxyphenbutazone, rifampicin, succinylsulfathiazole, and tetracycline HCl. Table 19.10 lists the glass transition temperatures of pharmaceutical compounds (drugs and excipients) taken from the literature. Fukuoka et al. (1989) have reported that most of these systems follow a general rule for prediction of glass transition temperatures that cannot be measured by thermal analysis. If the melting temperature is expressed in degrees Kelvin, T_g can be estimated as 70%–80% of T_m. This glass transition temperature can then be used to predict the physical stability of the amorphous solid.

The expected crystallization temperature (T_c) on heating an amorphous solid of known glass transition temperature (T_g) and melting temperature (T_m) is given by

$$T_c \approx T_g + \left[\frac{(T_m - T_g)}{2}\right] \qquad (19.14)$$

For amorphous compounds stored isothermally, the time for crystallization generally decreases with an increase in temperature, due to an increase in viscosity (Saleki-Gerhardt and Zografi, 1994). A mixture of two amorphous compounds will exhibit a single glass transition temperature intermediate between the two original components (Hancock and Zografi, 1994). If the densities of the two components are equal, the new value is a weighted average of the reciprocal values (the Fox equation):

$$\left(\frac{1}{T_g}\right)_{mix} = \left(\frac{w_1}{T_{g1}}\right) + \left(\frac{w_1}{T_{g2}}\right) \qquad (19.15)$$

TABLE 19.10
Glass Transition Temperatures (T_g) of Pharmaceutical Compounds

Drug Substance	Glass Transition (°C)	Reference
Aspirin	−30	Fukuoka et al. (1989)
Glutethimide	0	Ford (1987)
Methyltestosterone	−3	Fukuoka et al. (1989)
Sorbitol	−3	Hancock and Zografi (1994)
Progesterone	6	Fukuoka et al. (1989)
Atropine	8	Fukuoka et al. (1989)
Chloramphenicol	28	Ford (1987)
Indomethacin	47	Hancock et al. (1995)
Phenobarbital	48	Fukuoka et al. (1989)
Sulfathiazole	61	Fukuoka et al. (1989)
Lactose	74	Saleki-Gerhardt and Zografi (1994)
Sucrose	77	Hancock et al. (1995)
Griseofulvin	89	Ford (1987)

TABLE 19.11

Glass Transition Temperature (T_g) of Amorphous Sucrose versus Water Content

Absorbed Water (% w/w)	Glass Transition (°C)
0.00	74
0.99	60
1.47	58
1.98	50
3.13	32

Source: Saleki-Gerhardt, A. and Zografi, G. *Pharm. Res.*, 11: 1166–117, 1994.

When a substance lowers the glass transition temperature of another, it is referred to as a plasticizer. Water has a glass transition temperature of −138°C (Sugisaki et al., 1968), which is low enough that it plasticizes pharmaceutical systems. This is a desired effect when the water content of excipients plasticize the material to enhance compressibility. When water is inadvertently introduced to a metastable system containing an amorphous drug, it can reduce the glass transition temperature into the range where the propensity to crystallize is higher. Table 19.11 (Saleki-Gerhardt and Zografi, 1994) shows how small amounts of absorbed water can change the physical stability of amorphous sucrose by lowering the glass transition temperature closer to room temperature. When partially amorphous materials are created by processing energy, nearly all the measured water content is concentrated in the amorphous regions, which can significantly magnify this effect. Chemical instability and crystallization of amorphous forms can be caused by the absorption of small amounts of atmospheric water by this mechanism. Matsuda and Kawaguchi (1986) found that amorphous oxyphenbutazone crystallized much faster when exposed to ambient humidity. In this case, it crystallized as the anhydrate at lower humidity and to the hemihydrate or monohydrate at moderate to high humidities. Strydom et al. (2009) demonstrated this conversion with an amorphous form of stavudine. The transformation from amorphous to hydrate was seen at relatively low relative humidity (>30%). Furthermore, stability studies at elevated temperature (100°C) indicated that the amorphous solid transforms to form III (hydrate) in the presence of moisture or to form II (anhydrous) in the absence of moisture.

To market an orally available dosage form of an amorphous solid, the drug must remain in the noncrystalline state for the shelf life of the product for predictable absorption. Applying the general rule of 50°C below T_g to inhibit molecular mobility, this means the T_g of the system should be more than 70°C–80°C. For solid dosage forms, excipients with higher glass transition temperatures can be added, which result in antiplasticization. This is why coprecipitates (the subject of Chapter 18) containing amorphous drugs and PVP ($T_g = 280°C$) are often physically stable enough for use in dosage forms. Yoshioka et al. (1995) have shown that indomethacin crystallization can be inhibited by the addition of 20% PVP, which raises the glass transition temperature from 50°C to 66°C and the crystallization temperature from 97°C to 135°C. Fukuoka et al. (1989) applied the same principle in using salicin ($T_g = 60°C$) to stabilize phenobarbital ($T_g = 48°C$) and phenobarbital to stabilize antipyrine ($T_g = -17°C$).

Coamorphous binary mixtures of small molecules are a potential strategy to increase the dissolution of a drug substance while simultaneously improving the stability of the amorphous state. Löbmann et al. (2011) investigated a coamorphous combination of naproxen and γ-indomethacin at molar ratios of 2:1, 1:1, and 1:2. Intrinsic dissolution testing showed an increase in dissolution rate for the amorphous indomethacin compared to the crystalline γ-indomethacin and a further increase was seen with its coamorphous forms. Similar results were seen with naproxen and it was found that naproxen could be made amorphous in combination with γ-indomethacin but not as a pure material. Interestingly, the 1:1 coamorphous blend released both drugs in a synchronized manner. The coamorphous systems were stored under dry conditions at 4°C and 25°C for 21 days, following which, only the 1:1 mixture retained the amorphous state. Löbmann et al. (2012) also investigated a coamorphous mixture of simvastatin and glipizide. Once again the coamorphous mixtures showed improved stability compared to the individual amorphous forms; however, improved stability was determined to be a result of glipizide acting as an anti-plasticizer rather than a molecular interaction of the two compounds. Similar studies have been conducted investigating coamorphous systems, including Allesø et al. (2009), who demonstrated that an amorphous mixture of cimetidine and naproxen enhanced the dissolution rate of both drugs and Chieng et al. (2009) who found that a mixture of indomethacin and ranitidine created a highly stable amorphous binary mixture.

Viscosity agents have been added to suspensions to retard crystallization in much the same manner that they are used to prevent crystallization to a more stable polymorph. Mullins and Macek (1960) found that suspensions of amorphous novobiocin lasted 22 days at 37°C and 6 months at 25°C before converting to the crystalline compound. By adding 1% methyl cellulose to the suspension, they were able to extend this to more than 1 year at 37°C, making a viable drug product when stored at room temperature. Amorphous formulations that utilize polymers to improve both solubility and physical stability are still susceptible to recrystallization in the solid dispersion. Yang et al. (2010) has developed a numerical model to predict the recrystallization kinetics of an efavirenz-PVP system.

There are drug substances that have only been isolated in the amorphous state owing to bulky side chains that prevent effective packing into the crystalline lattice. In this case, the danger of crystallization later in development can be minimized by stressing the drug to show that it cannot readily be made to crystallize. The usual situation is that the drug substance can form a low-energy stable crystal form, and in fact, this may be a large contributing factor to its poor aqueous solubility. The use of any amorphous drug requires study and application of the principles outlined earlier so that inadvertent crystallization of the dosage form does not occur between manufacture and patient use.

STRATEGY FOR WATER-INSOLUBLE DRUG FORMULATION USING METASTABLE SOLIDS

The use of alternate solid-state forms (crystalline polymorphs, crystalline solvates, or amorphous states) is a viable means to increase the dissolution rate, apparent solubility, or oral bioavailability of a poorly soluble drug substance. Because of the possibility of conversion to more stable forms, these metastable forms should be used only if sufficient solubility is not obtained with the lowest energy crystalline form. The technique is most useful for solid dosage forms, where the chance of converting to more stable modifications is greatly reduced versus solution dosage forms. The first step in taking advantage of these possibilities is to characterize fully the potential crystal forms of the drug and the glass transition temperature of its amorphous form, if this is being considered. The decision trees presented by Byrn et al. (1995) can be helpful in identifying the types of preformulation studies needed to address adequately the phase purity and the conditions of stability for each form. If the metastable forms give an enhancement of solubility that is therapeutically important, stress testing should be done to understand the rate and conditions required for conversion. Storage temperature/humidity, initial water content, and processing variables should be examined to ensure that the chosen solid form could be reliably made into a stable dosage form. If a stable hydrate exists and this form is acceptable, this should be used to prevent physical changes later when the dosage form encounters water. If required, means of stabilizing the metastable form against crystallization of the stable crystal form can be studied. If these experiments show that the metastable form cannot be prevented from converting over the product shelf life, it is best to utilize one or more of the other techniques in this book for solubility enhancement.

REFERENCES

Abdallah, O. and S. A. El-Fattah. (1984). Thermodynamic properties of two forms of sulfamethoxazole, *Pharm. Ind.*, 46: 970–971.

Abdou, H. M. (1989). *Dissolution, Bioavailability, and Bioequivalence*, pp. 53–72, Mack Printing Company, Easton, PA.

Aguiar, A. J. and J. E. Zelmer. (1969). Dissolution behavior of polymorphs of chloramphenicol palmitate and mefenamic acid, *J. Pharm. Sci.*, 58: 983–987.

Aguiar, A. J., J. Krc, A. W. Kinkel, and J. C. Samyn. (1967). Effect of polymorphism on the absorption of chloramphenicol from chloramphenicol palmitate, *J. Pharm. Sci.*, 56: 847–853.

Alkhamis, K. A., A. A. Obaidat, and A. F. Nuseirat. (2002). Solid-state characterization of Fluconazole, *Pharm. Dev. Technol.*, 7: 491–503.

Allesø, M., N. Chieng, S. Rehder, J. Rantanen, T. Rades, and J. Aaltonen. (2009). Enhanced dissolution rate and synchronized release of drugs in binary systems through formulation: Amorphous naproxen-cimetidine mixtures prepared by mechanical activation, *J. Controlled Release.*, 136: 45–53.

Andersen, N. G. (2000). *Practical Process Research and Development*, Academic Press, New York.

Aungst, B. J. (1993). Novel formulation strategies for improving oral bioavailability of drugs with poor membrane penetration or presystemic metabolism, *J. Pharm. Sci.*, 82: 979–987.

Balbach, S. and C. Korn. (2004). Pharmaceutical evaluation of early development candidates "the 100 mg-approach," *Int. J. Pharm.*, 275: 1–12.

Bauer, J., S. Spanton, R. Henry, J. Quick, W. Dziki, W. Porter, and J. Morris. (2001). Ritonavir: An extraordinary example of conformational polymorphism, *Pharm. Res.*, 18: 859–866.

Behme, R. J. and D. Brooke. (1991). Heat of fusion measurement of a low melting polymorph of carbamazepine that undergoes multiple-phase changes during differential scanning calorimetry, *J. Pharm. Sci.*, 80: 986–990.

Behme, J., D. Brooke, R. F. Farney, and T. T. Kensler. (1985). Characterization of polymorphism of gepirone HCl, *J. Pharm. Sci.*, 74: 1041–1046.

Berge, S. M., L. D. Bighley, and D. C. Monkhouse. (1977). Pharmaceutical salts, *J. Pharm. Sci.*, 66: 1–19.

Biles, J. A. (1962). Crystallography. Part II, *J. Pharm. Sci.*, 51: 601–617.

Bjaen, A., K. Nord, S. Furuseth, T. Agren, H. Tonnesen, and J. Karlsen. (1993). Polymorphism of chloroquine diphosphate, *Int. J. Pharm.*, 92: 183–189.

Boje, K. M., M. Sak, and H.-L. Fung. (1988). Complexation of nifedipine with substituted phenolic ligands, *Pharm. Res.*, 5: 655–659.

Borka, L. (1971). The stability of chloramphenicol palmitate polymorphs, *Acta Pharm. Suecica*, 8: 365–372.

Borka, L. and J. K. Haleblian. (1990). Crystal polymorphism of pharmaceuticals, *Acta Pharm. Jugosl.*, 40: 71–94.

Brittain, H. G. (1995). *Physical Characterization of Pharmaceutical Solids*, Marcel Dekker, New York.

Brittain, H. G. (1999). *Polymorphism in Pharmaceutical Solids*, Marcel Dekker, New York.

Brittain, H. G., S. A. Ranadive, and A. T. M. Serajuddin. (1995). Effect of humidity-dependent changes in crystal structure on the solid-state fluorescence properties of a new HMG-CoA reductase inhibitor, *Pharm. Res.*, 12: 556–559.

Burger, A. and A. Lettenbichler. (1993). Polymorphism and pseudopolymorphism of acemetacin, *Pharmazie*, 48: 262–272.

Bugay, D. E. (2001). Characterization of the solid-state: Spectroscopic techniques, *Adv. Drug Del. Rev.*, 48: 3–65.

Burger, A. and A. W. Ratz. (1990). Physical and chemical stability of amorphous and crystalline tetracycline hydrochloride, *Sci. Pharm.*, 58: 69–75.

Buxton, P. C., I. R. Lynch, and J. M. Roe. (1988). Solid-state forms of paroxetine hydrochloride, *Int. J. Pharm.*, 42: 135–143.

Byrn, S. R. (1982). *Solid-State Chemistry of Drugs*, Academic Press, New York.

Byrn, S. R. and R. R. Pfeiffer, (1992). *Pharmaceutical Solids Short Course*, SSCI, Inc., Washington, DC, October 27–28.

Byrn, S., R. Pfeiffer, M. Ganey, C. Hoiberg, and G. Poochikian. (1995). Pharmaceutical solids: A strategic approach to regulatory considerations, *Pharm. Res.*, 12: 945–954.

Byrn, S., R. Pfeiffer, and J. G. Stowell. (1999). *Solid-State Chemistry of Drugs*, 2nd ed., SSCI, West Lafayette, IN.

Cabri, W., P. Ghetti, G. Pozzi, and M. Alpegiani. (2007). Polymorphisms and patent, market, and legal battles: Cefdinir case study, *Org. Process Res. Dev.*, 11: 64–72.

Carstensen, J. T. (1993). *Pharmaceutical Principles of Solid Dosage Forms*, Technomic Publishing Co., Lancaster, PA, pp. 133–149.

Carstensen, J. T. (2001). *Advanced Pharmaceutical Solids*, Marcel Dekker, New York.

Carstensen, J. T. and M. K. Franchini. (1995). Isoenergetic polymorphs, *Drug Dev. Ind. Pharm.*, 21: 523–536.

Chan, H. and E. Doelker. (1985). Polymorphic transformation of some drugs under compression, *Drug Dev. Ind. Pharm.*, 11: 315–332.

Chan, T. W. and A. Becker. (1988). Formulation of vaccine adjuvant muramyldipeptides (MDP). 1. Characterization of amorphous and crystalline forms of a muramyldipeptide analogue, *Pharm. Res.*, 5: 523–527.

Chauvet, A., J. Masse, J.-P. Ribet, D. Bigg, J.-M. Autin, J.-L. Maurel, J.-F. Patoiseau, and J. Jaud.(1992). Characterization of polymorphs and solvates of 3-amino-1-(*m*-trifluoromethylphenyl)-6-methyl-1H-pyridazin-4-one, *J. Pharm. Sci.*, 81: 836–841.

Chen, S., I. A. Guzei, and L. Yu. (2005). New polymorphs of ROY and new record for coexisting polymorphs o solvated structures, *J. Am. Chem. Soc.*, 127: 9881–9885.

Chieng, N., J. Aaltonen, D. Saville, and T. Rades. (2009). Physical characterization and stability of amorphous indomethacin and ranitidine hydrochloride binary systems prepared by mechanical activation, *Eur. J. Pharm. Biopharm.*, 71: 47–54.

Chieng, N., Z. Zujovic, G. Bowmaker, T. Rades, and D. Saville. (2006). Effect of milling conditions on the solid-state conversion of ranitidine hydrochloride form I, *Int. J. Pharm. Sci.*, 327: 36–44.

Chikaraishi, Y., M. Otsuka, and Y. Matsuda. (1996). Dissolution phenomenon of the piretanide amorphous form involving phase change, *Chem. Pharm. Bull.*, 44: 2111–2115.

Chikaraishi, Y., A. Sano, T. Tsujiyama, M. Otsuka, and Y. Matsuda. (1994). Preparation of piretanide polymorphs and their physicochemical properties and dissolution behaviors, *Chem. Pharm. Bull.*, 42: 1123–1128.

Chow, A. H. L. and D. J. W. Grant. (1988). Modification of acetaminophen crystals. III. Influence of initial supersaturation during solution-phase growth on crystal properties in the presence and absence of *p*-acetoxyacetanilide, *Int. J. Pharm.*, 42: 123–133.

Clements, J. A. and S. D. Popli. (1973). The preparation and properties of crystal modifications of meprobamate, *Can. J. Pharm. Sci.*, 8: 88–92.

Cox, J. S. G., G. D. Woodard, and W. C. McCrone. (1971). Solid-state chemistry of cromolyn sodium (disodium cromoglycate), *J. Pharm. Sci.*, 60: 1458–1465.

DeVilliers, M., J. van der Watt, and A. Lotter. (1991). The interconversion of the polymorphic forms of chloramphenicol palmitate (CAP) as a function of environmental temperature, *Drug Dev. Ind. Pharm.*, 17: 1295–1303.

Doherty, C. and P. York. (1988). Frusemide crystal forms: Solid state and physicochemical analyses, *Int. J. Pharm.*, 47: 141–155.

Doherty, C. and P. York. (1989). Accelerated stability of an x-ray amorphous frusemide-PVP solid dispersion, *Drug Dev. Ind. Pharm.*, 15: 1969–1987.

Dressman, J. B., G. L. Amidon, and D. Fleisher. (1985). Absorption potential: estimating the fraction absorbed for orally administered compounds, *J. Pharm. Sci.*, 74: 588–589.

Ebian, A. R., M. A. Moustafa, S. A. Khalil, and M. M. Motawi. (1973). Effect of additives on the kinetics of interconversion of sulfamethoxydiazine crystal forms, *J. Pharm. Pharmacol.*, 25: 13–20.

Everz, L. and J. Mielck. (1992). Water-induced physical transformation of a crystalline drug in a fluidized bed: pseudopolymorphism—polymorphism of carbamazepine, *Eur. J. Pharm. Biopharm.*, 38: 28S.

Fiese, E. F. and T. A. Hagen. (1986). Preformulation, in *The Theory and Practice of Industrial Pharmacy* (L. Lachman, H. A. Lieberman, and J. L. Kanig, Eds.), Lea and Febiger, Philadelphia, PA, pp. 171–196.

Florence, A. T. and E. G. Salole. (1976). Changes in crystallinity and solubility on comminution of digoxin and observations on spironolactone and estradiol, *J. Pharm. Pharmacol.*, 28: 637–642.

FDA (2004). *Guidance for Industry: ANDAs: Pharmaceutical Solid Polymorphism: Chemistry, Manufacturing and Controls Information*, CDER, Rockville, MD.

Ford, J. L. (1987). The use of thermal analysis in the study of solid dispersions, *Drug Dev. Ind. Pharm.*, 13: 1741–1777.

Franklin, S. J., and P. B. Myrdal. (2015). Solid-state and solution characterization of myricetin, *AAPS Pharm. Sci. Tech.*, 16: 1400–1408.

Fukuoka, E., M. Makita, and S. Yamamura. (1987). Glassy state of pharmaceuticals. II. Bioinequivalence of glassy and crystalline indomethacin, *Chem. Pharm. Bull.*, 35: 2943–2948.

Fukuoka, E., M. Makita, and S. Yamamura. (1989). Glassy state of pharmaceuticals. III. Thermal properties and stability of glassy pharmaceuticals and their binary glass systems, *Chem. Pharm. Bull.*, 37: 1047–1050.

Gan, L., C. Eads, T. Niederer, A. Bridgers, S. Yanni, P. Hsyu, F. Pritchard, and D. Thakker. (1994). Use of CACO-2 cells as an *in vitro* intestinal absorption and metabolism model, *Drug Dev. Ind. Pharm.*, 20: 615–631.

Gerber, J. J., J. G. van der Watt, and A. P. Lotter. (1991). Physical characterisation of solid forms of cyclopenthiazide, *Int. J. Pharm.*, 73: 137–145.

Ghan, G. and J. Lalla. (1992). Effect of compressional forces on piroxicam polymorphs, *J. Pharm. Pharmacol.*, 44: 678–681.

Ghodbane, S. and J. A. McCauley. (1990). Study of the polymorphism of MK571 by DSC, TG, XRPD and solubility measurements, *Int. J. Pharm.*, 59: 281–286.

Ghosh, S. and D. J. W. Grant. (1995). Determination of the solubilities of crystalline solids in solvent media that induce phase changes: solubilities of 1,2-dialkyl-3-hydroxy-4-pyridones and their formic acid solvates in formic acid and water, *Int. J. Pharm.*, 114: 185–196.

Giron, D. (1995). Thermal analysis and calorimetric methods in the characterization of polymorphs and solvates, *Thermochim. Acta*, 248: 1–59.

Goyan, J. E. and R. L. Day. (1970). Solution dosage forms, in *Prescription Pharmacy*, 2nd ed. (J. B. Sprowls, Ed.), J. B. Lippincott Co., Philadelphia, PA, pp. 163–166.

Graf, E., C. Beyer, and O. Abdallah. (1984). On the polymorphism of acetohexamide, *Pharm. Ind.*, 46: 955–959.

Grant, D. J. W. and T. Higuchi. (1990). *Solubility Behavior of Organic Compounds*, John Wiley & Sons, New York, pp. 22–27.

Grunenberg, A., B. Keil, and J.-O. Henck. (1995). Polymorphism in binary mixtures, as exemplified by nimodipine, *Int. J. Pharm.*, 118: 11–21.

Gunning, S. R., M. Freeman, and J. A. Stead. (1976). Polymorphism of disopyramide, *J. Pharm. Pharmacol.*, 28: 758–761.

Haleblian, J. K. (1975). Characterization of habits and crystalline modification of solids and their pharmaceutical applications, *J. Pharm. Sci.*, 64: 1269–1288.

Haleblian, J. and W. McCrone. (1969). Pharmaceutical applications of polymorphism, *J. Pharm. Sci.*, 58: 911–929.

Hamlin, W. E., J. I. Northam, and J. G. Wagner. (1965). Relationship between *in vitro* dissolution rates and solubilities of numerous compounds representative of various chemical species, *J. Pharm. Sci.*, 54: 1651–1653.

Hancock, B. C. and M. Parks. (2000). What is the true solubility advantage for amorphous pharmaceuticals? *Pharm. Res.*, 17: 397–403.

Hancock, B. C., S. L. Shamblin, and G. Zografi. (1995). Molecular mobility of amorphous pharmaceutical solids below their glass transition temperatures, *Pharm. Res.*, 12: 799–806.

Hancock, B. C. and G. Zografi. (1994). The relationship between the glass transition temperature and water content of amorphous pharmaceutical solids, *Pharm. Res.*, 11: 471–477.

Herman, J., J. P. Remon, N. Visavarungroj, J. B. Schwartz, and G. H. Klinger. (1988). Formation of theophylline monohydrate during the pelletization of microcrystalline cellulose—anhydrous theophylline blends, *Int. J. Pharm.*, 42: 15–18.

Higuchi, W. I., P. K. Lau, T. Higuchi, and J. W. Shell. (1963). Polymorphism and drug availability–solubility relationships in the methylprednisolone system, *J. Pharm. Sci.*, 52: 150–153.

Hoelgaard, A. and N. Moller. (1983). Hydrate formation of metronidazole benzoate in aqueous suspensions, *Int. J. Pharm.*, 15: 213–221.

Huang, H.-P., K. S. Murthy, and I. Ghebre-Sellassie. (1991). Effect of the crystallization process and solid state storage on the physico-chemical properties of scale-up lots of CI-936, *Drug Dev. Ind. Pharm.*, 17: 2411–2438.

Huang, L.-F. and W.-Q. Tong. (2004). Impact of solid state properties on developability assessment of drug candidates, *Adv. Drug Rev.*, 56: 321–334.

Ibrahim, H. G., F. Pisano, and A. Bruno. (1977). Polymorphism of phenylbutazone: properties and compressional behavior of crystals, *J. Pharm. Sci.*, 66: 669–673.

Imaizumi, H., N. Nambu, and T. Nagai. (1980). Stability and several physical properties of amorphous and crystalline forms of indomethacin, *Chem. Pharm. Bull.*, 28: 2565–2569.

International Conference on Harmonisation (2000). Guidance for industry, *Q6A Specifications: Test Procedures and Acceptance Criteria for New Drug Substances and New Drug Products: Chemical Substances*. Geneva.

Jain, N. and S. H. Yalkowsky. (2001). Estimation of the aqueous solubility. I. Application to organic non-electrolytes, *J. Pharm. Sci.*, 90: 234–252.

Jain, N., G. Yang, S. G. Machatha, and S. H. Yalkowsky. (2006). Estimation of the aqueous solubility weak electrolytes, *Int. J. Pharm.*, 319: 169–171.

Jozwiakowski, M. J. and K. A. Connors. (1985). Aqueous solubility behavior of three cyclodextrins, *Carbohydrate Res.*, 143: 51–59.

Jozwiakowski, M. J., N.-A. T. Nguyen, J. M. Sisco, and C. W. Spancake. (1996). Solubility behavior of lamivudine crystal forms in recrystallization solvents, *J. Pharm. Sci.*, 85: 193–199.

Jozwiakowski, M. J., S. O. Williams, and R. D. Hathaway. (1993). Relative physical stability of the solid forms of amiloride HCl, *Int. J. Pharm.*, 91: 195–207.

Kaneniwa, N., J.-I. Ichikawa, and T. Matsumoto. (1988). Preparation of phenylbutazone polymorphs and their transformation in solution, *Chem. Pharm. Bull.*, 36: 1063–1073.

Kaneniwa, N. and M. Otsuka. (1985). Effect of grinding on the transformations of polymorphs of chloramphenicol palmitate, *Chem. Pharm. Bull.*, 33: 1660–1668.

Kaneniwa, N., M. Otsuka, and T. Hayashi. (1985). Physicochemical characterization of indomethacin polymorphs and the transformation kinetics in ethanol, *Chem. Pharm. Bull.*, 33: 3447–3455.

Kaplan, S. A. (1972). Biopharmaceutical considerations in drug formulation design and evaluation, *Drug Metab. Rev.*, 1: 15–34.

Kato, Y. and M. Kohetsu. (1981). Relationship between polymorphism and bioavailability of amobarbital in the rabbit, *Chem. Pharm. Bull.*, 29: 268–272.

Kato, Y., Y. Okamoto, S. Nagasawa, and I. Ishihara (1984). New polymorphic forms of phenobarbital, *Chem. Pharm. Bull.*, 32: 4170–4174.

Khankari, R. K. and D. J. W. Grant. (1995). Pharmaceutical hydrates, *Thermochim. Acta*, 248: 61–79.

Kim, J. S., M. S. Kim, H. J. Park, S. J. Jin, S. Lee, and S. J. Hwang. (2008). Physicochemical properties and oral bioavailability of amorphous atorvastin hemi-calcium using spray drying and SAS process, *Int. J. Pharm.*, 359: 211–219.

Kitamura, S., Chang, L.-C., and J. K. Guillory. (1994). Polymorphism of mefloquine hydrochloride, *Int. J. Pharm.*, 101: 127–144.

Kokubu, H., Morimoto, K., T. Ishida, M. Inoue, and K. Morisaka. (1987). Bioavailability and inhibitory effect for stress ulcer of cimetidine polymorphs in rats, *Int. J. Pharm.*, 35: 181–183.

Kozjek, F., L. Golic, P. Zupet, E. Palka, P. Vodopivec, and M. Japelj. (1985). Physico-chemical properties and bioavailability of two crystal forms of piroxicam, *Acta Pharm. Jugosl.*, 35: 275–281.

Kuroda, T., T. Yokoyama, T. Umeda, A. Matsuzawa, K. Kuroda, and S. Asada. (1982). Studies on drug nonequivalence. XI. Pharmacokinetics of 6-mercaptopurine polymorphs in rabbits, *Chem. Pharm. Bull.*, 30: 3728–3733.

Kuroda, T., T. Yokoyama, T. Umeda, and Y. Takagishi. (1978). Studies on drug nonequivalence. VI. Physicochemical studies on polymorphism of acetohexamide, *Chem. Pharm. Bull.*, 26: 2565–2568.

Lagas, M. and C. F. Lerk (1981). The polymorphism of sulphathiazole, *Int. J. Pharm.*, 8: 14–24.

Lindenbaum, S. and S. E. McGraw. (1985). The identification and characterization of polymorphism in drugs by solution calorimetry, *Pharm. Manufact.*, 2: 27–30.

Löbmann, K., R. Laitinen, H. Grohganz, K. C. Gordon, C. Strachan, and T. Rades. (2011). Coamorphous drug systems: Enhanced physical stability and dissolution rate of indomethacin and naproxen, *Mol. Pharmaceutics.*, 8: 1919–1928.

Löbmann, K., C. Strachan, H. Grohganz, T. Rades, and O. Korhonen. (2012). Coamorphous simvastatin and glipizide combinations show improved physical stability without evidence of intermolecular interactions, *Eur. J. Pharm. Biopharm.*, 81: 159–169.

Lindenbaum, S., E. S. Rattie, G. E. Zuber, M. E. Miller, and L. J. Ravin. (1985). Polymorphism of auranofin, *Int. J. Pharm.*, 26: 123–132.

Liu, J., M. Svard, P. Hippen, and A. C. Rasmuson. (2015). Solubility and crystal nucleation in organic solvents of two polymorphs of curcumin, *J. Pharm. Sci.*, 104: 2183–2189.

Mao, C., R. Pinal, and K. R. Morris. (2005). A quantitative model to evaluate solubility relationship of polymorphs from their thermal properties, *Pharm. Res.*, 22: 1149–1157.

Martinez-Oharriz, M. C., C. Martin, M. M. Goni, C. Rodriguez-Espinosa, M. C. Tros de Ilarduya-Apaolaza, and M. Sanchez. (1994). Polymorphism of diflunisal: Isolation and solid-state characteristics of a new crystal form, *J. Pharm. Sci.*, 83: 174–177.

Matsuda, Y. and S. Kawaguchi. (1986). Physicochemical characterization of oxyphenbutazone and solid-state stability of its amorphous form under various temperature and humidity conditions, *Chem. Pharm. Bull.*, 34: 1289–1298.

Matsuda, Y. and E. Tatsumi. (1989). Physicochemical characterization of furosemide polymorphs and their evaluation of stability against some environmental factors, *J. Pharmacobio-Dyn.*, 12:s-38.

Matsumoto, T., N. Kaneniwa, S. Higuchi, and M. Otsuka. (1991). Effects of temperature and pressure during compression on polymorphic transformation and crushing strength of chlorpropamide tablets, *J. Pharm. Pharmacol.*, 43: 74–78.

McCrone, W. C., L. B. McCrone, and J. G. Delly. (1987). *Polarized Light Microscopy*, McCrone Research Institute, Chicago, IL, pp. 108–124.

Miller, D. A., J. T. McConville, W. Yang, R. O. Williams III, J. W. McGinity. (2007). Hot-melt extrusion for enhanced delivery of drug particles, *J. Pharm. Sci.*, 96: 361–376.

Miller, J. M., B. M. Collman, L. R. Greene, D. J. W. Grant, and A. C. Blackburn. (2005). Identifying the stable polymorph early in the drug discovery-development process, *Pharm. Dev. Tech.*, 10: 291–297.

Milosovich, G. (1964). Determination of solubility of a metastable polymorph, *J. Pharm. Sci.*, 53: 484–487.

Morelock, M. M., L. L. Choi, G. L. Bell, and J. L. Wright. (1994). Estimation and correlation of drug water solubility with pharmacological parameters required for biological activity, *J. Pharm. Sci.*, 83: 948–951.

Morris, K. G., M. G. Fakes, A. B. Thakur, A. W. Newman, A. K. Singh, J. J. Venit, C. J. Spagnuolo, and A. T. M. Serajuddin. (1994). An integrated approach to the selection of optimal salt form for a new drug candidate, *Int. J. Pharm.*, 105: 209–217.

Mullins, J. D. and T. J. Macek. (1960). Some pharmaceutical properties of novobiocin, *J. Pharm. Sci.*, 49: 245–248.

Munshi, M. and A. Simonelli. (1970). Presented at the American Pharmaceutical Association Academy of Pharmaceutical Sciences Meeting, Washington, DC.

Murphy, D., F. Rodriguez-Cintron, B. Langevin, R. C. Kelly, and N. Rodriguez-Hornedo. (2002). Solution-mediated phase transformation of anhydrous to dihydrate carbamazepine and the effect of lattice disorder, *Int. J. Pharm.*, 246: 121–134.

Narurkar, A., A. Purkaystha, P. Sheen, and M. Augustine. (1988). Hygroscopicity of celiprol hydrochloride polymorphs, *Drug Dev. Ind. Pharm.*, 14: 465–474.

Nicklasson, M. and A. Brodin. (1984). The relationship between intrinsic dissolution rates and solubilities in the water–ethanol binary system, *Int. J. Pharm.*, 18: 149–156.

Noyes, A. A. and W. R. Whitney. (1897). The rate of solution of solid substances in their own solutions, *J. Am. Chem. Soc.*, 19: 930–934.

Otsuka, M. and N. Kaneniwa. (1983). Hygroscopicity and solubility of noncrystalline cephalexin, *Chem. Pharm. Bull.*, 31: 230–236.

Otsuka, M., M. Onoe, and Y.Matsuda. (1994). Physicochemical characterization of phenobarbital polymorphs and their pharmaceutical properties, *Drug Dev. Ind. Pharm.*, 20: 1453–1470.

Overhoff, K. A., J. D. Engstrom, B. Chen, B. D. Scherzer, T. E. Milner, K. P. Johnston, and R. O. Williams III. (2007). Novel ultra-rapid freezing particle engineering process for enhancement of dissolution rates of poorly water-soluble drugs. *Eur. J. Pharm. Biopharm.*, 65: 57–67.

Pearson, J. T. and G. Varney. (1973). The anomalous behavior of some oxyclozanide polymorphs, *J. Pharm. Pharmacol.*, 25: 62P–70P.

Pfeiffer, R. R., K. S. Yang, and M. A. Tucker. (1970). Crystal pseudopolymorphism of cephaloglycin and cephalexin, *J. Pharm. Sci.*, 59: 1809–1814.

Pikal, M. J., A. L. Lukes, J. E. Lang, and K. Gaines. (1978). Quantitative crystallinity determinations for β-lactam antibiotics by solution calorimetry: Correlations with stability, *J. Pharm. Sci.*, 67: 767–773.

Poole, J. W., G. Owen, J. Silverio, J. N. Freyhof, and S. B. Rosenman. (1968). Physicochemical factors influencing the absorption of the anhydrous and trihydrate forms of ampicillin, *Curr. Therap. Res.*, 10: 292.

Pranzo, M. B., D. Cruickshank, M. Coruzzi, M. R. Caira, and R. Bettini. (2010). Enantiotropically related albendazole polymorphs, *J. Pham. Sci.*, 99: 3731–3742.

Pudipeddi, M. and A. T. M. Serajuddin. (2005). Trends in solubility of polymorphs. *J. Pharm. Sci.*, 94: 929–939.

Rodriguez-Hornedo, N., D. Lechuga-Ballesteros, and H.-J. Wu. (1992). Phase transition and heterogeneous/epitaxial nucleation of hydrated and anhydrous theophylline crystals, *Int. J. Pharm.*, 85: 149–162.

Rodriguez-Spong, B., C. P. Price, A. Jayasankar, A. J. Matzger, and N. Rodriguez-Hornedo. (2004). General principals of pharmaceutical solid polymorphism: a supramolecular perspective, *Adv. Drug Del. Rev.*, 56: 241–274.

Rowe, E. L. and B. D. Anderson. (1984). Thermodynamic studies of tolbutamide polymorphs, *J. Pharm. Sci.*, 73: 1673–1675.

Saleki-Gerhardt, A., J. G. Stowell, S. R. Byrn, and G. Zografi. (1995). Hydration and dehydration of crystalline and amorphous forms of raffinose, *J. Pharm. Sci.*, 84: 318–323.

Saleki-Gerhardt, A. and G. Zografi. (1994). Non-isothermal and isothermal crystallization of sucrose from the amorphous state, *Pharm. Res.*, 11: 1166–1173.

Sanphui, P., B. Sarma, and A. Nangia. (2011). Phase transformation in conformational polymorphs of nimesulide, *J. Pharm. Sci.*, 100: 2287–2299.

Shah, B., V. K. Kakumanu, and A. Bansal. (2006). Analytical techniques for quantification of amorphous/crystalline phases in pharmaceutical solids, *Pharm. Sci.*, 95: 1641–1665.

Shah, J. C., J. R. Chen, and D. Chow. (1999). Metastable polymorph of etoposide with higher dissolution rate, *Drug. Dev. Ind. Pharm.*, 25: 63–67.

Shefter, E. (1981). Solubilization by solid-state manipulation, in *Techniques of Solubilization of Drugs* (S. H. Yalkowsky, Ed.), pp. 159–182, Marcel Dekker, New York.

Shefter, E. and T. Higuchi. (1963). Dissolution behavior of crystalline solvated and nonsolvated forms of some pharmaceuticals, *J. Pharm. Sci.*, 52: 781–791.

Sheikhzadeh, M., S. Rohani, M. Taffish, and S. Murad. (2007). Solubility analysis of buspirone hydrochloride polymorphs: Measurements and prediction, *Int. J. Pharm.*, 338: 55–63.

Shell, J. W. (1963). X-ray and crystallographic applications in pharmaceutical research III. Crystal habit quantitation, *J. Pharm. Sci.*, 52: 100–102.

Shibata, M., H. Kokubu, K. Morimoto, K. Morisaka, T. Ishida, and M. Inoue. (1983). X-ray structural studies and physicochemical properties of cimetidine polymorphism, *J. Pharm. Sci.*, 72: 1436–1442.

Stagner, W. C. and J. K. Guillory. (1979). Physical characterization of solid iopanoic acid forms, *J. Pharm. Sci.*, 68: 1005–1009.

Stahl, P. H. and B. Sutter. (2006). Salt selection, in *Polymorphism in the Pharmaceutical Industry* (R. Hilfiker, Ed.), Wiley-VCH, Weinheim, Germany.

Stahl, P. H. and C. G. Wermuth. (2002). *Handbook of Pharmaceutical Salts; Properties, Selection, and Use*, Wiley-VCH, Zurich, Switzerland.

Stephenson, G. A., T. B. Borchardt, S. R. Byrn, J. Bowyer, C. A. Bunnell, S. V. Snorek, and L. Yu. (1995). Conformational and color polymorphism of 5-methyl-2-[(2-nitrophenyl)amino]-3-thiophenecarbonitrile, *J. Pharm. Sci.*, 84: 1385–1386.

Stephenson, G. A., R. A. Forbes, and S. M. Reutzel-Edens. (2001). Characterization of the solid state: quantitative issues, *Adv. Drug Del. Rev.*, 8: 67–90.

Stephenson, G. A., E. G. Groleau, R. L. Kleemann, W. Xu, and D. R. Rigsbee. (1998). Formation of isomorphic desolvates: Creating a molecular vacuum, *J. Pharm. Sci.*, 87: 536–542.

Stephenson, G. A., Stowell, J. G. Toma, P. H. Dorman, D. E. Greene, J. R. and Byrn, S. R. (1994). Solid-state analysis of polymorphic, isomorphic, and solvated forms of dithromycin, *J. Am. Chem. Soc.*, 116: 1–9.

Stoltz, M., Caira, M. R. Lotter, A. P. and van der Watt, J. G. (1989). Physical and structural comparison of oxyphenbutazone monohydrate and anhydrate, *J. Pharm. Sci.*, 78: 758–763.

Strydom, S., W. Liebenberg, L. Yu, and M. de Villiers. (2009). The effect of temperature and moisture on the amorphous-to-crystalline transformation of stavudine, *Int. J. Pharm.*, 379: 72–81.

Sugimoto, I., Kuchiki, A. Nakagawa, H. Tohgo, K. Kondo, S. Iwane, I. Takahashi, K. (1980). Dissolution and absorption of nifedipine from nifedipine-polyvinylpyrrolidone coprecipitate, *Drug. Dev. Ind. Pharm.*, 6: 137–160.

Sugisaki, M., H. Suga, and S. Seki. (1968). Calorimetric study of the glassy state. 4. Heat capacities of glassy water and cubic ice, *Bull. Chem. Soc. Jap.*, 41: 2591–2599.

Suleiman, M. S. and N. M. Najib. (1989). Isolation and physicochemical characterization of solid forms of glibenclamide, *Int. J. Pharm.*, 50: 103–109.

Suryanarayanan, R. (1989). Determination of the relative amounts of anhydrous carbamazepine and carbamazepine dihydrate in a mixture by powder x-ray diffractometry, *Pharm. Res.*, 6: 1017–1024.

Suryanarayanan, R. and A. G. Mitchell. (1986). Phase transitions of calcium gluceptate, *Int. J. Pharm.*, 32: 213–221.

Takahashi, Y., K. Nakashima, T. Ishihara, H. Nakagawa, and I. Sugimoto. (1985). Polymorphism of fostedil: characterization and polymorphic change by mechanical treatments, *Drug Dev. Ind. Pharm.*, 11: 1543–1563.

Uchida, T., E. Yonemochi, T. Oguchi, K. Terada, K. Yamamoto, and Y. Nakai. (1993). Polymorphism of tegafur: Physicochemical properties of four polymorphs, *Chem. Pharm. Bull.*, 41: 1632–1635.

Umeda, T., A. Matsuzawa, N. Ohnishi, T. Yokoyama, K. Kuroda, and T. Kuroda. (1984). Physico-chemical properties and bioavailability of benoxaprofen polymorphs, *Chem. Pharm. Bull.*, 32: 1637–1640.

Vadas, E. B., P. Toma, and G. Zografi. (1991). Solid-state phase transitions initiated by water vapor sorption of crystalline L-660,711, a leukotriene D4 receptor antagonist, *Pharm. Res.*, 8: 148–155.

Van Tonder, E. C., T. S. P. Maleka, W. Liebenberg, M. Song, D. E. Wurster, and M. M. de Villiers. (2004). Preparation and physicochemical properties of niclosamide anhydrate and two monohydrates, *Int. J. Pharm.*, 269: 417–432.

Verma, A. R. and P. Krishna. (1966). *Polymorphism and Polytypism in Crystals*, John Wiley & Sons, New York, pp. 1–60.

Vippagunta, S. R., H. G. Brittain, and D. J. W. Grant. (2001). Crystalline solids, *Adv. Drug Del. Rev.*, 48: 3–26.

Walkling, W. D., H. Almond, V. Paragamian, N. H. Batuyios, J. A. Meschino, and J. B. Appino. (1979). Difenoxin hydrochloride polymorphism, *Int. J. Pharm.*, 4: 39–46.

Wall, G. M. (1986). Pharmaceutical applications of drug crystal studies, *Pharm. Manufact.*, 3: 33–42.

Ward, G. H. and R. K. Schultz. (1995). Process-induced crystallinity changes in albuterol sulfate and its effect on powder physical stability, *Pharm. Res.*, 12: 773–779.

Wells, J. I. (1988). *Pharmaceutical Preformulation: The Physicochemical Properties of Drug Substances*, Ellis Horwood Ltd., Chichester, UK, 94–95.

Yalkowsky, S. H. (1981). *Techniques of Solubilization of Drugs*, pp. 1–14, Marcel Dekker, New York.

Yang, J., K. Grey, and J. Doney. (2010). An improved kinetics approach to describe the physical stability of amorphous solids, *Int. J. Pharm.*, 384: 24–31.

Yang, X., X. Wang, and C. B. Ching. (2008). Solubility of form α and form γ of glycine in aqueous solutions, *J. Chem. Eng. Data.*, 53: 1133–1137.

Yokoyama, T., T. Umeda, K. Kuroda, T. Kuroda, and S. Asada. (1981). Studies on drug nonequivalence. X. Bioavailability of 6-mercaptopurine polymorphs, *Chem. Pharm. Bull.*, 29: 194–199.

York, P. (1983). Solid-state properties of powders in the formulation and processing of solid dosage forms, *Int. J. Pharm.*, 14: 1–28.

Yoshioka, M., B. Hancock, and G. Zografi. (1995). Inhibition of indomethacin crystallization in poly (vinyl-pyrrolidone) coprecipitates, *J. Pharm. Sci.*, 84: 983–986.

Zerrouk, N., C. Chemtob, P. Arnaud, S. Toscani, J. Dugue. (2001). In vitro and in vivo evaluation of carbamazepine-PEG 6000 solid dispersions, *Int. J. Pharm.*, 225: 49–62.

Zhang, J., X. Tan, J. Gao, W. Fan, Y. Gao, and S. Qian. (2013). Characterization of two polymorphs of lornoxicam, *J. Pharm. Pharmacol.*, 65: 44–52.

Zhu, H., and D. J. W. Grant. (1996) Influence of water activity in organic solvent plus water mixtures on the nature of the crystallizing drug phase. 2. ampicillin, *Int. J. Pharm.*, 139: 33–43.

20 Pharmaceutical Powder Technology—ICH Q8 and Building the Pyramid of Knowledge

Hans Leuenberger, Silvia Kocova El-Arini, and Gabriele Betz

CONTENTS

The majority of newly discovered drugs coming from synthesis and entering development stage are hydrophobic substances with very low aqueous solubility and the development of drug formulation for the commercial market can result in erratic bioavailability, bioinequivalence, and indeed clinical failures.

Solubilization systems are therefore used to improve wettability and enhance solubility of these pharmaceuticals. Strategies such as drug derivatization, use of cosolvents, surfactants, dispersants, and complexation agents have been reported in the literature (Yalkowsky, 1981). Drug–excipient systems employing hydrophilic matrices have also been extensively explored and documented in a large number of publications. For example, studies reported by the authors on drug–polymer matrices described the use of the percolation threshold to explain the changes in these systems which occur at the critical percolation thresholds. The percolation thresholds in the matrices can help identify the range of drug to polymer ratios, where the desired release behavior is attainable (Leuenberger and

Kocova El-Arini, 2000). Particle reduction techniques can enhance greatly the surface area available for dissolution and improve the bioavailability of water-insoluble drugs. Due to the advances in nanoscience it is now possible to manufacture nanoparticles with special physical properties, which can improve dramatically the behavior of water-insoluble compounds (Rocco, 2000).

THE PYRAMID OF KNOWLEDGE AND THE ROAD MAP

Development of a drug product of water-insoluble drugs requires a tremendous effort in order to assure constant quality of the product, that is, its ability to deliver the therapeutic effect for which it was intended.

To prevent a nonrobust formulation from reaching the end of the development process, the Food and Drug Administration (FDA) launched the Process Analytical Technology, or PAT, initiative (http://www.fda.gov/cder/OPS/PAT.htm), and followed with the 2004 white paper "Innovation or Stagnation" (http://www.fda.gov/oc/initiatives/criticalpath/whitepaper.html), identifying three areas of research and development that need to be improved, namely: "Assessing Safety," "Demonstrating Medical Utility," and "Industrialization." The PAT initiative represents a twenty-first-century concept for quality assurance with its focus on creating a foundation of scientifically based decisions for product design. The goal is to *design in* the quality of the product and not to *test in* the quality by eliminating the bad items. Figure 20.1 (Hussain, 2002) illustrate the steps on a pyramid leading to a product and process quality. To move from the state of the art at the bottom of the pyramid of knowledge, Leuenberger and Lanz (2005) suggest a *road map* that can help achieve the top of the pyramid in fastest possible way. The *road map* includes use of multivariate approach in case of complex formulations and processes; taking advantage of artificial intelligence through uses of artificial neural networks; applying the laws of percolation theory in order to challenge critical phenomena in *chaotic* systems; making use of novel processing techniques; and translating the laws of physical chemistry into corresponding laws of pharmaceutical particle technology (Leuenberger and Lanz, 2005). Some aspects of the *road map* useful in attaining the top of the pyramid were illustrated with selected case studies (Leuenberger et al., 2008).

THE ICH Q8 GUIDELINES

The ICH Q8 (ICH Harmonized Tripartite Guideline) is a set of guidelines for pharmaceutical development which were issued with the aim to design a quality product and its manufacturing process to consistently deliver the intended performance of the product. They are extended to all components of drug product and are summarized in the following:

   Drug Substance—The physicochemical and biological properties of the drug substance that can influence the performance of the drug product and its manufacturability. The compatibility of drug substances with each other and with excipients.
   Excipients—The characteristics, functionality, manufacturability, and their compatibility with other excipients should be established.
   Drug Product—Formulation Development—The evolution of the formulation design should be provided, including information on critical or interacting attributes gained from experimental designs (DOE), and on Robust Formulation—which is the aim of formulation development.
   Manufacturing Process Development (MPD)—The ability of the process to reliably produce a product of the intended quality under different operating conditions, at different scales, or with different equipment.

The MPD program should identify any critical process parameters that should be monitored or controlled (e.g., granulation end point) to ensure that the product is of the desired quality (From Q8 Pharmaceutical Development, ICH Step 4, EMEA—European Medicines Agency, London November 14, 2005 [EMEA/CHMP/167068/2004]).

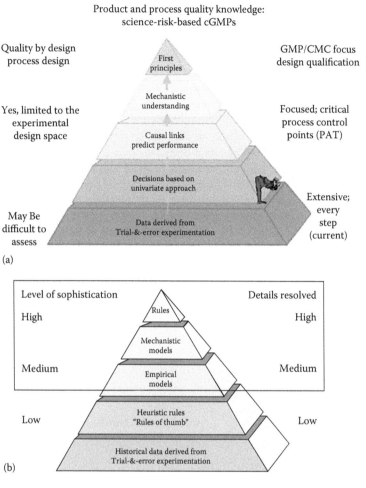

FIGURE 20.1   (a) Product and process quality knowledge. (From Hussain, A. S., FDA.) (b) The pyramid of knowledge for product development. (From Hussain, A. S., *Pharmaceutical Process Scale-Up*, M. Levin (Ed.), New York: Marcel Dekker, 2002. https://www.slideshare.net/a2zpharmsci.)

It is clear from the Q8 guidelines that the science-based approach to a robust pharmaceutical product must extend to all areas of product development.

In this chapter we follow the ICH Q8 recommendations and present a framework of methodologies and advanced tools which can be used to reach the top of the pyramid of knowledge.

IMPLEMENTING THE ICH Q8 RECOMMENDATIONS

SCIENCE-BASED APPROACH TO ROBUST FORMULATION AND PROCESS DEVELOPMENT

The Right, First Time Concept

The application of the *Right, First Time* concept is a major goal of the pharmaceutical industry and is fully supported by FDA (Leuenberger et al., 2013). The goal is to minimize the number of failures creating worldwide annual multibillion dollar losses due to poor pharmaceutical processes and formulations (Benson and McCabe, 2004). This goal can be achieved only by a very rigorous interpretation of *Right, First Time*, that is, the concept should be implemented starting with clinical phase I. However, this is only feasible if the workflow approach of the automotive and aircraft industries is adopted by the pharmaceutical industry, designing first *in-silico* vehicles for drug delivery systems. The *in-silico* design of formulations, for example, with F-CAD (formulation—computer-aided design) or with another suitable software platform is not yet widely used, but will be part of the current digital revolution (Leuenberger and Leuenberger 2016).

For the implementation of the workflow of the automotive and aircraft industries, the use of advanced tools such as F-CAD (more fully explored in the following) is a prerequisite (Leuenberger et al., 2009, 2010, 2011; Puchkov and Leuenberger, 2011; Kimura, 2012; Puchkov et al., 2013). F-CAD corresponds to a straightforward extension of the concept of ICH Q8 (R2) and can be regarded as first principles approach (top of pyramid, Figure 20.1a).

In fact the guidelines of ICH Q8 propose to study critical factors ($n = 2$ or more) within the formulation design space by using experimental design such as 2^n or, for example, a central composite design with $n = 2$ or more factors. The results of the 2^n designs correspond more or less to the behavior of the *tangents* of the *true function* $f(x_1, x_2,....x_n)$, and the result of a central composite design corresponds to an extension of the approximation of the *true function* $f(x_1, x_2,....x_n)$ by adding a quadratic term. Indeed, the result of a central composite design with two factors x_1, x_2: $f(x_1, x_2)$ = $b_0 + b_1 x_1 + b_2 x_2 + b_{12} x_1 x_2 + b_{11} x_1^2 + b_{22} x_2^2$, can be considered as an approximation of the *true function* $f(x_1, x_2)$ by a Taylor series up to the second degree at a specific *working point* $f(0,0)$ within the formulation design space:

$f(0,0) = b_0,$

$$b_1 = \frac{\partial f(x_1, x_2)}{\partial x_1} \text{ (first derivative)}$$

$$b_2 = \frac{\partial f(x_1, x_2)}{\partial x_2} \text{ (first derivative)}$$

$$b_{12} = \frac{1}{2} \frac{\partial \partial f(x_1, x_2)}{\partial x_1 \partial x_2} \text{ (second order derivative)}$$

$$b_{11} = \frac{1}{2} \frac{\partial \partial f(x_1, x_2)}{\partial x_1, \partial x_1} \text{ (second order derivative)}$$

$$b_{22} = \frac{1}{2} \frac{\partial \partial f(x_1, x_2)}{\partial x_2, \partial x_2} \text{ (second order derivative)}$$

A simple example of a Taylor expansion of the true function $f(x) = e^x$ at the site $f(x = 0)$, that is, with one variable x can easily found in textbooks:

$$e^x = 1 + \frac{x}{1!} + \frac{x^2}{2!} + \frac{x^3}{3!} + ..., \quad -\infty < x < \infty$$

It is evident that the true function $e^x = 1 + x/1! + x^2/2!$ with two terms is a second order approximation and only exact within the design space close to $f(x = 0) = 1$, that is, b_0 and in its neighborhood. Thus, the use of experimental design following the guidelines of ICH Q8 yields as an *in-silico* tool the virtual mathematical function, which approximates the true function and can to a certain extent replace the more advanced tool F-CAD. In other words, if F-CAD is not available, which should save laboratory work, as mathematical model the evaluation (*summarizing equation*) of the experimental design can be used. The future will be a virtual tool such as F-CAD or an equivalent tool. However, it is important to keep in mind, that *it is not sufficient to use F-CAD or an equivalent virtual tool for a successful implementation of the automotive and aircraft industry approach by the pharmaceutical industry:*

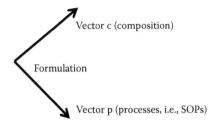

FIGURE 20.2   Simplified illustration (projected on two dimensions) of the formulation design space consisting of the vector composition *c* and of the vector pharmaceutical processes **p**.

It is an absolute necessity to harmonize the pharmaceutical technical equipment to minimize scale-up problems and, last but not least, to interpret rigorously the formulation design space. In accordance with ICH Q8 (ICH harmonized tripartite guidelines, http://www.ich.org) the formulation design space can be defined by two vectors: **c** = composition and **p** = pharmaceutical process (Figure 20.2).

The formulation design space facilitates the application of the *Right, First Time* concept by defining reasonable limits for the product specifications, that is, intermediate products such as granules, and final products such as capsules or tablets. In this context it is important to use the identical formulation design space from the very beginning of any development work up to registration of the medicinal product to be able to use all data. Thus, the classical workflow—starting with a simple capsule formulation as service dosage form for clinical phases I and II and development of the final marketed tablet formulation in clinical phase IIc for clinical phase III, registration and clinical Phase IV—should be replaced by *Right, First Time* workflow starting with the market-ready tablet formulation already at clinical phase I (Table 20.1) (Leuenberger et al., 2013).

Formulation Design Space

The formulation design space can be efficiently described by an experimental design. The number of factors to be evaluated depends on the knowledge and experience of the formulator with the API. It is evident that the formulator needs to know which excipients are chemically compatible with the API. In this context, a suitable factorial design should be used, that will enable the formulator to choose the right excipients showing—in addition—interactions, which may stabilize the API (API–excipient test program, Leuenberger and Becher, 1975). The API should be considered as the primary innovation, that is, as a jewel which needs to be cut and polished by choosing the right excipients to show its brilliance by an excellent bioavailability of the API and by a robust formulation. Thus, during the preformulation work, it may be necessary to perform not only a chemical but also a pharmaceutical-technological API–excipient compatibility program in order to select the optimal excipients for a chemical and technological robust formulation. For this purpose it makes

TABLE 20.1

Conventional Workflow versus *Right, First Time* Workflow

Conventional Workflow	*Right, First Time* Workflow
Clinical Phase I: development of a service dosage form, that is, a *simple* capsule	Clinical Phase I: development of market ready tablet dosage form instead of service form
Capsule redeveloped into a tablet for bioequivalence testing	Small-scale production
Scale-up exercise	Scale-up exercise (computer assisted)
Mass production of final marketed form	Mass production of final marketed form
Two-sigma quality	*Six-sigma* quality

Source: Leuenberger, H. et al., *Swiss Pharma*, 35, 4–16, 2013.

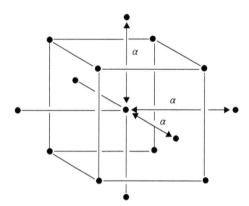

FIGURE 20.3 Central composite design with $n = 3$ factors (From Leuenberger, H., *Pharmazeutische Technologie*, Sucker, H. and Speiser, P. (Eds.), Stuttgart, Germany: Thieme, 1978).

sense to use a mechanical simulator of production high speed tableting equipment, such as the Presster equipment, to test tablet compositions for robustness (Leuenberger, 2013) and for preparing samples for clinical phases I and II (Leuenberger, 2015).

To start already at clinical phase I with the (more or less) final marketed tablet formulation needs a lot of human resources and enough API, as illustrated in the following case study conducted in the former Sandoz (now Novartis) labs (Leuenberger, 1978). To find an optimal formulation it is necessary to choose a central composite design, which is described in Figure 20.3. It is important to use orthogonal designs so that it is still possible to evaluate (at a later stage) an additional factor, which is suspected to be a critical one within the same formulation design space.

The experimental point in the center of the design space is often used to perform 1–3 replicates to get an estimation of the experimental statistical error. The distance α from the center depends on the number of factors n and on the number of confoundings p:

$$\alpha = \sqrt{\frac{\sqrt{2^{n-p}(2^{n-p}+2n+1)}}{2} - 2^{n-p-1}}$$

For $n = 3$ and $p = 0$, $\alpha = 1.215$ (Table 20.2). The number of confoundings p is of special interest to save time and money. In case of a chemical API–excipient compatibility program, a 2^{n-p} factorial design was chosen with $n = 5$ and $p = 1$, which the performance of 16 experiments instead of 32 and to determine the effect of moisture replacing a 4-fold interaction between 4 excipients and the API (Leuenberger and Becher, 1975).

In case of an orthogonal central composite design for $n = 2$ factors $-\alpha = -1$ and $+\alpha = +1$, which leads to a 3×3 design with 3 levels -1, 0, $+1$ and just 9 experiments. To save time and money, that is, for evaluating more than two variables each of the two factors are defined as a ratio of two factors (Leuenberger, 2013).

Case Study of a Tablet Formulation and Its Formulation Design Space

The main goal of this study was as follows: How to design in a reasonable time an optimal tablet formulation taking into account biopharmaceutical and technical issues such as bioavailability and technical robustness, that is, ideal disintegration time, ideal dissolution profile of the API, and sufficient hardness and friability, needed in handling and if necessary coating of the tablets. For obvious reasons it is impossible to test each batch for bioavailability, effectiveness, and side effects, so a choice must be made in advance, depending on the pharmacological profile of the API, whether the API should be released fast or at a controlled rate (Leuenberger and Guitard, 1978). The selection of excipients depends on the results of chemical drug–excipient compatibility program on biopharmaceutical aspects (Biopharmaceutics Classification System), for example, solubility of the API, and on

TABLE 20.2

Central Composite Design for $n = 3$ Factors with No Replicate at the Center Point (0,0,0) with the 5 Coded Levels for Each Factor: $-\alpha, -1, 0, +1, +\alpha$. For $n = 3$ and $p = 0$: $\alpha = 1.215$

Nr.	x_1	x_2	x_3	Nr.	x_1	x_2	x_3
1	−1	−1	−1	9	−α	0	0
2	1	−1	−1	10	α	0	0
3	−1	1	−1	11	0	−α	0
4	1	1	−1	12	0	α	0
5	−1	−1	1	13	0	0	−α
6	1	−1	1	14	0	0	α
7	−1	1	1	15	0	0	0
8	1	1	1				

Source: Leuenberger, H., *Pharmazeutische Technologie*, Sucker, H., Fuchsm, P., and Speiser, P. (Eds.), Stuttgart, Germany: Thieme, 1978.

the results of technological drug–excipient screening program (Leuenberger, 2013). For the study, caffeine anhydrous was used as a drug model. As bioavailability of the API was not tested, the disintegration time was determined and in addition the dissolution profile was characterized by the time point t (in minutes) of 63% API released ($t = t_{63\%}$) by linearization of the profile using Weibull distribution. The Weibull or RRSB (Rosin, Rammler, Sperling, Bennet) distribution is often used to describe the particle size distribution. However, no correlation could be found between the particle size distribution and the dissolution profile of the ensemble of particles (after the disintegration of tablets into particles). In the case of a central composite design with 5 factors, $x_1 =$ filler, $x_2 =$ compression force, $x_3 =$ disintegrant, $x_4 =$ binder, and $x_5 =$ lubricant, it makes sense to reduce the number of trials by confounding the fifth factor with the unlikely 4–fold interaction, that is, $x_5 = x_1 x_2 x_3 x_4$. Thus, a total of 27 experiments are needed (Table 20.3), corresponding to a central composite design with $\alpha = 1.547$ for $n = 5$ factors and $p = 1$ (confounding). The results of this study (Figures 20.4 through 20.6) were published in 1978 by Leuenberger and Guitard, inspired by a publication of Schwartz et al. (1973).

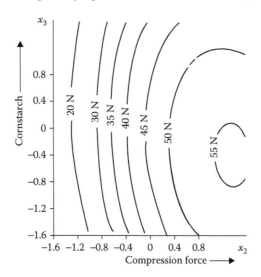

FIGURE 20.4   Contour plot: Tablet hardness [N] as a function of compression force and concentration of corn starch. (From Leuenberger, H., *Pharmazeutische Technologie*, Sucker, H., Fuchs, P., and Speiser, P. (Eds.), Stuttgart, Germany: Thieme, 1978.)

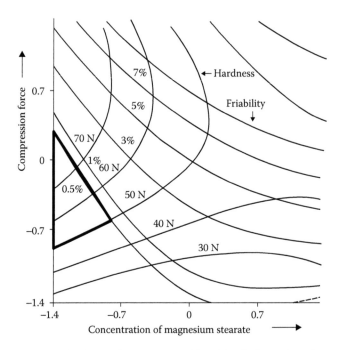

FIGURE 20.5 Contour plots of tablet hardness H (N) and friability F (%) as a function of compression force and concentration of magnesium stearate within the same design space showing the acceptable range H > 50N, F < 0.5% of appropriate formulations. (From Leuenberger, H., *Pharmazeutische Technologie*, Sucker, H., Fuchs, P., and Speiser, P. (Eds.), Stuttgart, Germany: Thieme, 1978.)

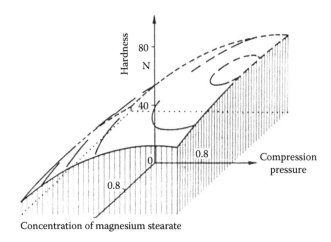

FIGURE 20.6 3D plot of tablet hardness in [N] as a function of magnesium stearate and force. (From Leuenberger, H., *Pharmazeutische Technologie*, Sucker, H., Fuchs, P., and Speiser, P. (Eds.), Stuttgart, Germany: Thieme, 1978.)

The plots of Figures 20.4 through 20.6 are the result of the evaluation of the formulation design space, which can be best described by Table 20.3 showing the central composite design with 5 factors $x_1, x_2,...x_5$. The choice of factors depends on their criticality for the tablet formulation.

For the full exploration of the formulation design space, 27 formulations need to be manufactured in the lab. Subsequently, the quality properties such as dissolution profile, disintegration time, hardness,

TABLE 20.3

Central Composite Design with 5 Factors Describing the Formulation Design Space

Tablet Formulation No.	Factors				
	x_1	x_2	x_3	x_4	x_5
1	−1	−1	−1	−1	+1
2	+1	−1	−1	−1	−1
3	−1	+1	−1	−1	−1
4	+1	+1	−1	−1	+1
5	−1	−1	+1	−1	−1
6	+1	−1	+1	−1	+1
7	−1	+1	+1	−1	+1
8	+1	+1	+1	−1	−1
9	−1	−1	−1	+1	−1
10	+1	−1	−1	+1	+1
11	−1	+1	−1	+1	+1
12	+1	+1	−1	+1	−1
13	−1	−1	+1	+1	+1
14	+1	−1	+1	+1	−1
15	−1	+1	+1	+1	−1
16	+1	+1	+1	+1	+1
17	$-\alpha$	0	0	0	0
18	$+\alpha$	0	0	0	0
19	0	$-\alpha$	0	0	0
20	0	$+\alpha$	0	0	0
21	0	0	$-\alpha$	0	0
22	0	0	$+\alpha$	0	0
23	0	0	0	$-\alpha$	0
24	0	0	0	$+\alpha$	0
25	0	0	0	0	$-\alpha$
26	0	0	0	0	$+\alpha$
27	0	0	0	0	0

Source: Leuenberger, H., *Pharmazeutische Technologie*, Sucker, H., Fuchsm, P., and Speiser, P. (Eds.), Stuttgart, Germany: Thieme, 1978.

and friability of the tablets are determined. At the same time it is possible to establish the summarizing equations for each tablet property, describing the quality of the tablet with a quadratic equation for the property: $Y = b_0 + b_1 x_1 + \dots b_5 x_5 + b_{12} x_1 x_2 \dots b_{45} x_4 x_5 + b_{11} x_1^2 + b_{22} x_2^2 + \dots b_{55} x_5^2$. Table 20.4 shows the different regression coefficients $b_0, b_1 \dots b_{12} \dots b_{11} \dots b_{55}$ for the tablet properties analyzed.

Table 20.5 shows an excellent prediction of the tablet hardness values, as the differences between the experimental and calculated values can be neglected, that is, the residual values are oscillating between −1.9 N and +1.4 N, with 14 values below 0 and 13 values above zero out of a total of 27 values. Thus, there is no systematic trend visible.

Critical Evaluation of the Formulation Design Space and Percolation Theory

The exploration of the formulation design space according to ICH Q 8 is an important step for a systematic and sustainable development of a solid dosage form for originator and for generic pharmaceutical companies. The ICH Q 8 (R2) guidance for industry puts a lot of emphasis on

TABLE 20.4

Regression Coefficients (RC) b_0, $b_1...b_5$, b_{11}, $b_{12}...b_{55}$ of the Quadratic Model Equation as a First Approximation to the Real Behavior of Tablet Hardness, Disintegration Time, Friability, and Dissolution Time t [min] for 63% of API Dissolved

RC	Hardness (N)	Disintegration (s)	Friability (%)	$t_{63\%}$ API Dissolved
b_0	46.36	555.6	2.18	18.8
b_1	1.13	20.0	0.06	0.204
b_2	13.36	153.0	−0.11	4.56
b_3	−0.08	−34.5	0.001	−2.13
b_4	3.52	123.8	−0.766	4.51
b_5	−6.76	85.1	0.210	8.25
b_{11}	0.23	−7.6	−0.479	−1.90
b_{12}	1.50	27.8	0.041	−0.743
b_{13}	0.04	−47.6	−0.131	−2.70
b_{14}	0.28	−2.8	−0.034	1.53
b_{15}	0.06	46.7	−0.052	0.954
b_{22}	−5.08	−1.9	−0.135	0.377
b_{23}	−1.19	−24.2	0.109	1.07
b_{24}	2.01	−40.7	−0.083	−1.55
b_{25}	−5.24	−1.4	0.062	0.225
b_{33}	−2.14	2.9	−0.78	0.874
b_{34}	−1.10	8.7	−0.12	−0.986
b_{35}	0.94	−6.6	−0.05	−0.539
b_{44}	0.11	−43.9	0.97	−2.74
b_{45}	−0.21	7.9	0.07	2.90
b_{55}	2.41	−36.6	−0.82	−0.689

Source: Leuenberger, H., *Pharmazeutische Technologie*, Sucker, H., Fuchsm, P., and Speiser, P. (Eds.), Stuttgart, Germany: Thieme, 1978.

the use of experimental design. The only point not mentioned in the guidelines is the existence of critical concentrations, which are a consequence of percolation theory (Leuenberger et al., 1989a; Bonny and Leuenberger, 1993). Close to critical concentrations, properties that are relevant for the quality of a tablet formulation, such as the dissolution profile (Luginbuehl and Leuenberger, 1994) and disintegration time (Leuenberger et al., 1989a), can show important changes. Figure 20.7 shows the change of the particle size distribution of granules consisting of cornstarch and lactose at the critical concentration, that is, at the percolation threshold of cornstarch in the lactose–cornstarch powder mixture prepared in a fluidized bed. In this context, it is important not to forget the impact of percolation theory, as the resolution of the grid spanning the formulation design space may not be sufficient to detect the effect of critical concentrations or percolation thresholds (Kimura, 2012).

The use of experimental design is a prerequisite for not losing time with a *trial-and-error* approach, which is often the cause of poor formulations and of important financial losses. For originator companies the lack of a sufficient amount of API in an early development stage is a problem for extensive exploration of the formulation design space. In addition, the chemical quality of the API (residual solvents, by-products) may still vary in an early phase. At the same time it has to be kept in mind that in such an early development phase the little amount of API available is very expensive, and a high financial investment in an extensive exploration of the formulation design space with an early prototype of the API may be a risk; for example, in clinical phases

TABLE 20.5
List of Calculated and Experimental Tablet Hardness Values [N]
for 27 Formulations.

Formulation	Hardness (calc.)	Hardness (exp.)	Difference (exp.-calc.)
1	22.62	22.90	0.28
2	26.84	26.70	−0.16
3	59.84	59.60	−0.24
4	40.10	40.20	0.10
5	29.71	30.00	0.29
6	28.87	29.50	0.63
7	35.67	36.20	0.53
8	63.32	63.40	0.08
9	33.48	32.80	−0.69
10	26.74	26.40	−0.34
11	47.64	47.20	−0.44
12	76.58	77.60	−0.98
13	29.81	29.90	0.09
14	30.16	29.80	−0.36
15	67.36	66.90	−0.47
16	49.62	49.50	−0.12
17	45.17	45.40	0.23
18	48.67	49.10	0.43
19	13.52	13.40	−0.08
20	54.88	55.60	0.72
21	41.37	42.70	1.33
22	41.11	40.50	−0.61
23	41.18	40.00	−1.18
24	52.09	54.00	1.91
25	62.60	64.00	1.40
26	41.67	41.00	−0.67
27	46.36	44.50	−1.86

Note: The Quadratic Model Shows an Excellent Fit between Experimental and Calculated Values

Source: Leuenberger, H., *Pharmazeutische Technologie*, Sucker, H., Fuchsm, P., and Speiser, P. (Eds.), Stuttgart, Germany: Thieme, 1978.

I and II in case of small chemical molecules, the attrition rate can be up to 92% (Lowe, 2014; Leuenberger and Leuenberger, 2016). Thus, the market-ready formulation of the dosage form is usually shifted to clinical phase IIc. In case of a generic company, there is enough API available to do such a study.

Substantial savings could be made if the workflow approach of the automotive and aircraft industries is adopted by the pharmaceutical industry. Thus, the first prototype of the drug delivery vehicle could be developed, optimized, and tested *in-silico* and manufactured with a low amount of new API already for clinical phase I, that is, following rigorously the concept and workflow of *Right, First Time*. The adoption of this type of workflow requires a major reorganization of established working units and departments, which may be the reason that so far such a step has not been realized. In addition, the pharmaceutical industry does not seem to be ready yet to use and trust the existing F-CAD technology of CINCAP (Puchkov and Leuenberger, 2011). In this context, it has to be kept in mind that the results of F-CAD are only valid for the *in-silico* formulation, which has

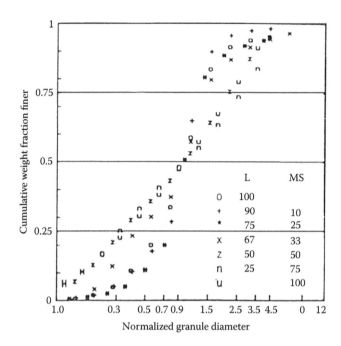

FIGURE 20.7 Cumulative particle size distribution at $p = 0.62$ for different ratios of the binary mixture lactose (L)/cornstarch (MS). The granule diameter is critically linked to the concentration ratio (percolation effect). (From Leuenberger, H. et al., *Boll. Chem. Farm.*, 128, 54–61, 1989b).

been validated in the laboratory formulation design space. Thus, if the *in-silico* formulation was calibrated and validated for a tablet formulation manufactured with a single punch press, the results are only valid for the *in-silico* formulation design space described, for example, by a central composite design of Table 20.3 and by the hidden factors such as the lab SOPs (standard operation procedures) for manufacturing the intermediate products, the lab equipment used for determining the dissolution profile of the API including type of buffer, ionic strength, and so on. Thus, the validated *in-silico* results are not valid for manufacturing the tablets with a rotary press in the production department or by using different SOPs for manufacturing intermediate products, such as granules, with large-scale equipment. For this purpose a harmonization of the equipment is a prerequisite, which is described in Leuenberger and Leuenberger (2016). As mentioned earlier, it is advantageous to establish a technological (galenical) API–excipient compatibility program to avoid poor formulations, in addition to a chemical API–excipient program to avoid chemical degradation of the API of the market-ready tablet formulation (Leuenberger, 2013).

Example of a Technological API–Excipient Screening Program

Table 20.6 shows an example of an experimental design for screening a new API in combination with excipients, which have to be first tested to be chemically compatible. For this screening test it is suggested to use a mechanical simulator of a high-speed tableting press such as the Presster, shown in Figure 20.8 (www.mcc-online.com). The Presster can be also used for manufacturing samples for clinical phases I and II even for high-potent APIs (Levin, 2015). A selection of results for a Paracetamol formulation with a different experimental design is shown in Table 20.7.

The technological screening program uses the Presster as a tool to estimate the likelihood of tableting problems such as sticking in the die leading to a high ejection force (problem of die lubrication) or sticking to the punch surface (high take-off force). It represents a valuable complement to the chemical drug–excipient compatibility tests in the optimal choice of the functional excipients.

TABLE 20.6
Example of a Factorial Design for a Technological Drug–Excipient Screening Program for Optimal Choice of the Functional Excipients. Settings of the Presster according to the Rotary Press in the Production Department to Be Simulated Mechanically Using Low Amount of API

Factor	Level	Conc. (excipient)	Drug Substance (API)
			Strength of API: 10% (w/w) 40% (w/w) 70% (w/w)
A (%, w/w)	−1	Lactose (%)	71 + 10 API 41 + 40 API 11 + 70 API
(Filler + API)	+1	Mannitol (%)	71 + 10 API 41 + 40 API 11 + 70 API
B	−1	Stearic acid	1% (w/w)
(Lubricant)	+1	Magnesium stearate	1% (w/w)
C	−1	Maize starch	15% (w/w)
(Disintegrant)	+1	MCC Sanaq burst*)	15% (w/w)
D	−1	PVP	3% (w/w)
(Binder)	+1	HPC	3% (w/w)
E	−1	Low speed	
(Tableting Speed of Presster)	+1	High speed	

Source: Leuenberger, H., in Process Scale-Up in the Pharmaceutical Industry, workshop, Cologne, October 14–16, 2015.
*Provided by Pharmatrans Sanaq Ltd, Basel, Switzerland.

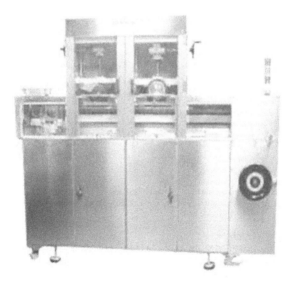

FIGURE 20.8   The Presster equipment. (From Presster, manufactured and distributed by Measurement Control Corporation (MCC), www. mcc-online.com, downloaded 2015.)

Effect of the Tableting Speed

Figures 20.9 and 20.10 show the effect of the tableting speed on the tablet hardness and disintegration time respectively for a low (in gray-color line) speed of 10,800 tablets per hour and for a high (in gray-color dotted line) speed of 108,000 tablets per hour. In the case that the tablet formulation is not sensitive to the tableting speed, the corresponding gray-color line and gray-color dotted lines of the same hardness, respectively, disintegration time will be located at the same site in the formulation design space. For this study an orthogonal 2 × 3 × 3 factorial design was used, which

TABLE 20.7

Results of the Technological Screening Program Using the Presster

Result	D1.2	D1.3	D1.4	D2.2	D2.3	D2.4
UC_{Peak} (kN)	**58.9**	37.1	13.1	39.7	19.1	5.5
LC_{Peak} (kN)	**55.5**	37	14.1	39	19.8	6.2
Peak $_{Ejecti}$ (N)	134.2	78.8	121	**2095.7**	**1306.3**	493.8
Take-off (N)	**2.1**	1.6	1.3	1.1	0.9	0.8
Weight (mg)	504.9	506.2	506.4	504.7	505.2	504.3
Thickness (mm)	4.52	4.58	4.8	3.64	3.82	4.27
Hardness (N)	**>300**	**>300**	**>300**	144	91	**19**
Disint. time (sec)	454	426	174	35	12	6

Source: Leuenberger, H., in Process Scale-Up in the Pharmaceutical Industry, workshop, Cologne, October 14–16, 2015.

TABLE 20.8

Central Composite Design with the Factors A = Ratio Paracetamol/ Lactose and the Ratio B = Granulated MCC Burst 100/ MCC Normal, Keeping Constant the Weight of the Tablet (500 mg) and the Amount of Lubricant (0.5% Magnesium stearate)

Coded Variables		Uncoded Variables	
A	B	Ratio: Paracetamol/Lactose	Ratio: Granulated MCC Sanaq Burst/MCC Normal
0	−1	200 mg P/200 mg L	25 mg MCCbPVP/75 mg MCC
0	1	200 mg P/200 mg L	75 mg MCCbPVP/25 mg MCC
1	0	300 mg P/100 mg L	50 mg MCCbPVP/50 mg MCC
−1	1	100 mg P/300 mg L	75 mg MCCbPVP/25 mg MCC
0	0	200 mg P/200 mg L	50 mg MCCbPVP/50 mg MCC
1	−1	300 mg P/100 mg L	25 mg MCCbPVP/75 mg MCC
−1	−1	100 mg P/300 mg L	25 mg MCCbPVP/75 mg MCC
1	1	300 mg P/100 mg L	75 mg MCCbPVP/25 mg MCC
−1	0	100 mg P/300 mg L	50 mg MCCbPVP/50 mg MCC

Source: Leuenberger, H., 9th Scientific and Technical Forum, Basel, Switzerland, May 23–24, 2013.

corresponds to a central composite design with two factors, A and B, at three levels (−1,0 + 1) related to the composition, and factor C = tableting speed at two levels (−1,+1) corresponding to a low (gray-color line) and a high (gray-color dotted line) speed. In order to save time and money for the 3 × 3 experimental design of the composition, the ratios A and B of *auxiliary substances* were chosen instead of single excipients to accommodate more substances in the experimental design (Table 20.8).

F-CAD (Formulation—Computer Aided Design)

The application of F-CAD enables a rigorous implementation of the *Right, First Time* concept and workflow, that is, first to develop and test *in silico* the drug delivery vehicle and to manufacture a market-ready tablet formulation for clinical phase I (Table 20.1).

F-CAD of Cincap is based on the Cellular Automaton (CA) approach (Puchkov and Leuenberger, 2011; Puchkov et al., 2013) which simulates *in silico* the standard operation procedures (SOP)

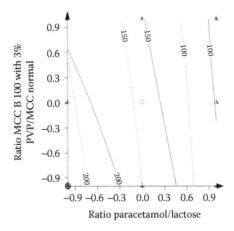

FIGURE 20.9   Effect of the tableting speed on a Paracetamol formulation as a function of the ratio *MCC B 100 granulated with 3% PVP/MCC normal and the ratio Paracetamol/lactose. (From Leuenberger, H., 9th Scientific and Technical Forum, Basel, Switzerland, 2013. www.ifiip.ch/downloads, conference materials.)

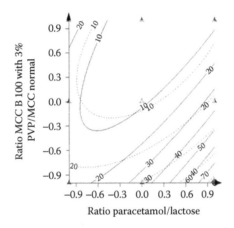

FIGURE 20.10   Tablet disintegration time in sec as a function of the composition (Figure 20.9) and as a function of the tableting speed (Figure 20.9). (From Leuenberger, H., 9th Scientific and Technical Forum, Basel, Switzerland, 2013.)

performed in the laboratory, such as mixing of API with excipient particles, granules growth, compaction of particles, granulates, and so on, and is able to test the API dissolution profile of the respective tablet formulation. Thus, significant financial savings can be realized by replacing expensive lab work with computer simulation. This approach facilitates the exploration of the formulation design space for preparing tablet samples for clinical phase I with a 6σ quality (Figure 20.11). In order to take full advantage of this approach a harmonization of the equipment and of the processes is needed (Leuenberger and Leuenberger, 2016).

CELLULAR AUTOMATON (CA): A FIRST PRINCIPLE APPROACH

The CA approach mimics exactly what happens in reality. Thus, the *in-silico* results have a very high credibility, which is higher than any expert system based on in-house data obtained in the past with similar formulations. Owing to the possibility that the first *in-silico* results can be calibrated with a first lab tablet formulation—that is, performing a *fine-tuning* of the necessary *in-silico*

	Conventional production process	**F-CAD**
Sensitivity of formulation	Experience-based A time-consuming and expensive collection of a huge number of laboratory tests	Calculated by integrated tests during the virtual integrated design
PAT* production process	Risk Any deviation along the PAT registered production process may cause a loss of batch	Flexibility Process variability insignificant for the quality of the final product is defined and registered
Quality	2σ	6σ

FIGURE 20.11 F-CAD approach based on the workflow of the automotive and aircraft industries compared with the current workflow, which leads to a mean quality of 2σ of the final marketed dosage form. Due to a rigorous application of the Right, First Time concept it is possible to achieve a 6σ quality. (From Leuenberger, H. et al., Virtual Design of Tablets, Lörrach 2014). *PAT production process involves a scientific approach and process analytical technology (PAT) tools for process optimization. (From Leuenberger, H. and Lanz, M., *Adv. Powder Technol.*, 16, 1–36, 2005.)

parameters describing the physico-chemical properties of API and excipients—the results of further *in-silico* batches within the defined formulation design space can be trusted. Thus, it is not necessary to explore and validate with lab experiments all cornerstones of its formulation design space.

For simplicity, only the three most important types of physico-chemical behavior of ingredients involved are discussed, that is, API dissolution, excipients which hinder dissolution by their swelling capacity, and hydrophilic excipients such as MCC, which show after a lag time a fast wicking of water similar to disperse SiO_2. Interestingly, for a physico-chemical description of a component such as a water soluble API, a single dimensionless parameter c_1 is needed, which depends on the dynamic API solubility (slope of intrinsic dissolution rate). The parameter c_1 is an estimate at time zero for the number of iterations needed to dissolve an API cell using the CA approach. Thus, a high c_1 value means a low water-soluble drug. For an excipient with swelling capacity, an additional parameter c_2 is needed to describe the swelling process. In general, no more than two parameters are needed per component. Pores of a tablet, that is, the void space, also need a c_1 value, which for a hydrophilic one is equal to zero. For a more refined *in-silico* calculation it is recommended to take care, in addition, of hydrophobic pores of a tablet formulation with poor wettability with c_1 values > 0.

The Diffusion Equation Governing the Dissolution Process

For simplicity the following discussion is limited to the 1D case concerning the differential equation describing the dissolution, which is identical with Fick's law, respectively the 1D heat equation:

$$\frac{\partial}{\partial t}T(\mathbf{r},t) = \kappa \frac{\partial^2}{\partial x^2}T(\mathbf{r},t) \tag{20.1}$$

Row 1 with columns $(i-1),(i),(i+1)$

T_{i-1}	T_i	T_{i+1}

Just imagine a sheet with rows numbered 1, 2, ... 25 and with columns from A to Q. Row number 1 may represent a thin metallic rod consisting of equally sized cubes A to Q, which can be put into a close contact, that heat is easily conducted. At time $t = 0$ the cube (i), which has the temperature T_i is put into close contact with the nearest neighboring cubes H (at the location $i-1$) and J (at the location $i+1$), which have a much lower temperature like the rest of the cubes. Due to the diffusion of heat at time $t = (t + \Delta t)$, the nearest neighboring cubes achieve the temperatures T_{i-1}, respectively, T_{i+1}, which is then described in the next row of this imaginary sheet. Thus, knowing the CA rule set for the 1 D differential Equation 20.1 the time evolution of the heat dissipation can be calculated step by step, that is, row by row. To find a suitable CA rule for the differential Equation 20.1, it is necessary to know the neighborhood and how the heat is transferred in each time step, which was first described by Stephan Wolfram with the rule set 182 and can be found in Wolfram (2002) (Figure 20.12).

This CA rule has many advantages due to the chance to use Boolean logic, that is, only integer values of 0 and 1 are needed, thereby speeding up the calculations and leading to an excellent approximation of the diffusion equation. Solving Equation 20.1 by the finite difference time domain (FDTD) method would first lead to the FDTD code 10210-110, which could be approximated by the CA code 150 mod.2, which leads to less favorable results. The CA rule 182 of Figure 20.12 illustrates the transfer of heat from row (n) to row ($n + 1$), which depends on the neighborhood and can be represented as follows: If both neighboring sites of the central site are occupied => 111 the central site of the next row will be occupied (Figure 20.13).

Figure 20.14 illustrates the heat transfer from row n to row $n + 1$ in case of all possible configurations with 111=> 1, 000=>0, 101=> 1, 010 => 1, which can be understood. The result of the neighborhoods 110 & 011=>0, 100&001=> 1 is a consequence of rule 182 leading to the following pattern of the original imaginary grid sheet (Figure 20.15).

111	110	101	100	011	010	001	000
1	0	1	1	0	1	1	0

FIGURE 20.12   CA rule set for the 1 D heat equation = rule 182 = 10110110 in a binary code. (From Stephan Wofram, *A New Kind of Science*, 2002. See wolframscience.com.)

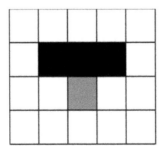

FIGURE 20.13   Central site (dark-gray color) of row $n + 1$: Heat transfer from row n to row $n + 1$ if both neighboring sites of the central site of row n are occupied, which can be well understood.

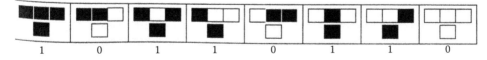

FIGURE 20.14   The effect of updating of row n to become row ($n + 1$) depends on the environment of row n, that is, the first element of row ($n + 1$) becomes occupied (= black = numerically = 1) and the last element (to the most right of the figure) will stay not occupied (= blank = numerically = 0).

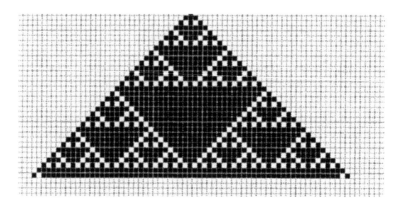

FIGURE 20.15 Pattern of 1 D Cellular Automaton after 32 iterations of the rule 182, keeping in mind that iterations are identical to the updating of the environment, which represents the time evolution of 1 D diffusion equation. (From Puchkov, M. et al., Series in Biomedicine, 2013.)

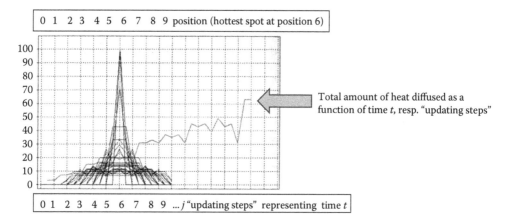

FIGURE 20.16 Numerical solution of the diffusion equation with the 1D CA rule 182 by the updating procedure. The temperature T of the central site decreases with the number of iterations showing a symmetrical heat diffusion to the neighborhood of position 6; the amount of heat transferred is also shown in the figure as evolution of time = x-axis from $t = 0$ to $t = j$ *updating steps*. (From Puchkov, M. et al., Series in Biomedicine, 2013.)

It is important to take into account that with an increasing number of iteration steps (Figure 20.15) a better and better approximation of the diffusion equation with an increasing number of iteration steps is achieved (Figure 20.16).

Figure 20.16 shows the *updating procedure*, that is, the *time evolution*, how the diffusion of a fixed amount of heat is transferred to the neighboring cells, that is, in the neighborhood. At the same time the fixed amount of heat is collected and presented in Figure 20.16 as a separate *cumulative* curve, which corresponds in case of an API, which is dissolving the amount of API dissolved and collected in the recipient (mass instead of heat transfer). At time $t = 0$, the hot metal wire located at position 6 had a temperature of 100°C (could be any temperature above the temperature of the environment, that is, could be at time 0 equal to 100%). At time $(t+\Delta t)$, the temperature at location 6 decreased from 100% to 70% and at time $(t + 2\Delta)$ to approximately 42% and so on, that is, each "updating step with the number $j = 1, 2, 3 \dots$ (see Figure 20.16 with x = time axis regarding the cumulative amount of heat collected)" takes place at a time $(t + j\Delta t)$, that is, equilibrium of the temperature with the environment is reached after $t \rightarrow \infty$, that is, 100% of excess heat is collected, respectively 100% of API is dissolved.

F-CAD is using a 3D-CA approach: With each iteration step, the amount of API dissolved of the API sites is calculated and plotted in a cumulative way to show the API dissolution profile. In the case of a calculation in 1D, a linear function is expected (compare Figure 20.16). In this context the resolution, respectively the overall precision of the model, depends on the number of iterations performed to dissolve 100% of the API, which is taken care of by the parameter c_1 of F-CAD technology in 3D. It is also evident that the resolution depends on the mesh size of the grid. Thus, in 3D the tablet volume needs to be subdivided as much as possible into unit cubes that represent fine particles, a cluster of unit cubes representing coarse particles or dense granules, or void unit cubes representing pores. For this purpose, F-CAD uses the tablet designer module to define first the shape and volume of the tablet, and subsequently to subdivide this volume into a high number of unit cubes with the discretizer module. The higher the number of unit cubes, the higher will be the precision. Thus, a reasonable number of unit cells is in the range of at least 1 million. Another important point is the definition of the environment of a unit cube in 2D (Figure 20.17) respectively in 3D.

F-CAD is using the Moore neighborhood in 3D, which means that the central unit cell C is surrounded by 26 unit cubes as its nearest neighbors. It makes sense to prefer the Moore neighborhood to describe the dissolution process as, in practice, the dissolution starts at the edges of a particle. Figure 20.18 shows the dissolution profile of two caffeine tablet formulations.

The *in-silico* calculation shows (in case of dissolution profile of Formulation B in Figure 20.18) smaller error bars than the experimentally determined error points (Leuenberger et al., 2009). The error bars of the *in-silico* calculations are related to the fact that the caffeine particles are arranged at random within the tablet volume, as it is not possible to distribute the API particles each time in such a way that the particles assume the same location. Thus, if more API particles are located closer to the surface, the API is dissolved faster.

In summary, the rigorous interpretation of the formulation design space (Figure 20.2), the rigorous interpretation of the concept of *Right, First Time*, and the use of percolation theory for process development is most important. To implement the concept of *Right, First Time* in a rigorous way, the pharmaceutical industry needs to adapt the workflow approach of the automotive and aircraft industries for developing and testing first the drug delivery vehicle *in silico*. Applying the first principle approach to obtain a product and process knowledge can help reach the apex of the pyramid of knowledge illustrated in Figure 20.1.

Process Scale—Up in the Pharmaceutical Industry—Harmonization of Equipment

Process scale-up needs to follow the guidelines of ICH Q8 R (2) and should be treated on the same level of sophistication of the knowledge pyramid (Figure 20.1b). Although this statement speaks for itself, it is difficult to realize in practice. Special attention is needed when a simple service dosage form is used during clinical phase I and II with a specified composition since this limits the degree

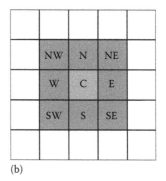

(a)   (b)

FIGURE 20.17   (a) von Neumann neighborhood of cell P. (b) Moore neighborhood of cell C in the center.

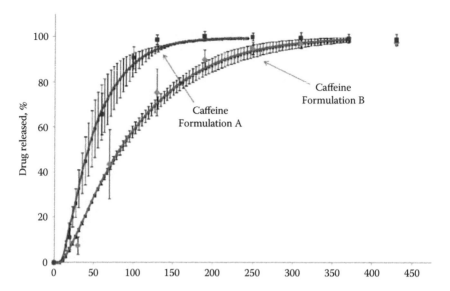

FIGURE 20.18 Dissolution profile of two different caffeine tablet formulations. The time axis represents the number of *updates*, that is, the time evolution (Figure 20.16). (From Krausbauer, E., Contribution to a science based expert system, PhD thesis, University of Basel, Faculty of Science, http://edoc.unibas.ch/diss/DissB_8879, 2009.)

of freedom of the formulation design space in clinical phase III (Leuenberger and Leuenberger 2016). As mentioned earlier the goal of the *Right, First Time* concept is to minimize the number of failures due to poor pharmaceutical processes and formulations. To a large extent this concept is realized in the automotive and aircraft industries, that is, the design and testing of the prototype *in-silico* and manufacture of fully functional vehicles according to the *Right, First Time* approach. However, in case of the pharmaceutical industry, it is not sufficient to apply a software platform such as F-CAD to design and test the drug delivery vehicles. All efforts with F-CAD at an early development stage will not prevent failures if process scale-up issues are neglected. For this purpose, a harmonization of the equipment and of the processes will lead to more important savings than the isolated application of an F-CAD platform to resolve problems of poor formulations. (Leuenberger, 2015). In other words a holistic approach is needed, where it is only possible to contribute to the knowledge on the specific formulation chosen, if all *in-silico* and laboratory experiments are kept within the same formulation design space during the full development from clinical phase I to registration of the formulation. Ideally, all data collected during the early development phases of clinical phases I and II that are part of the road map should also contribute to the knowledge. In this context the application of a fully continuous granulation line needs to be discussed in depth. Large amount of scientific work on continuous pharmaceutical granulation exists in the literature (Vervaet and Remon 2005; Swanborough, 2008; Jarvinen et al., 2012; Dhenge et al., 2013; Parikh, 2016) and there is a trend to implement such a concept in industry (Lee et al., 2015). In the early development phase, however,CS1 maint: Multiple names: authors list (link) there is not enough of the API available for developing and introducing a fully continuous granulation line. For this reason, only a semicontinuous granulation line such as the Glatt Multicell™ concept, as an example, is discussed within the concept of harmonization of the equipment during all clinical phases.

Harmonization of the processes during scale-up must be combined with an intensive use of PAT devices (Leuenberger and Leuenberger, 2016). In this context the PAT power consumption device, which was developed together with Marcel Dürrenberger of the Engineering Department at Sandoz (Novartis), was able to take into account changes in the particle size distribution and of the moisture content of the primary material in order to control the wet agglomeration process (Leuenberger,

TABLE 20.9
Harmonization of the Processes "Wet Agglomeration" and "High Speed Tableting" Thanks to an Intelligent PAT Power Consumption Device That Is Similar to the One Offered by MCC

Type of Mode	% Yield (w/w) 90–710 µm	% Undersize (w/w) < 710 µm	% Undersize (w/w) < 90 µm
Classical mode N = 20 batches (no PAT device)	81.03 ± 2.42	88.30 ± 2.05	6.80 ± 0.51
Automatic control. (with PAT device)	91.45 ± 0.36	96.80 ± 0.31	5.40 ± 0.35

Source: Leuenberger, H., *Pharm. Acta Helv.*, 37, 72–82, 1982a.

1982a). Such a device can take into account the specific properties of the primary material to be processed as an internal reference. Harmonization of the wet agglomeration with the tableting process means that the settings of the high-speed tableting machines can be kept constant from batch to batch. This is possible because the batchtobatch variability of the granule size distribution has been kept at a minimum (Table 20.9). Without the PAT power consumption device, the machine settings have to be adapted from batch to batch in order to get the same properties of the resulting tablets such as hardness and disintegration time.

The harmonization of subsequent processes such as *wet agglomeration process* and *tableting* is as important as the harmonization of the equipment between the development and the production department, which was described in the section on the *API–excipient technological screening program.*

Scale-up in the 4th Dimension and the Glatt Multicell™

In classical scale-up the dimensions of the equipment *x, y, z* are changed and the process time is kept constant. However, in case of the scale-up in the 4th dimension, the size of the equipment is kept constant and the process is repeated in time, thus the time becomes the 4th dimension. The Glatt Multicell™ illustrates the scale-up in the 4th dimension. The optimal harmonization of processes between early development and manufacturing starts with the installation of the same equipment in both departments. Using the Glatt Multicell™ in the production department only without a counterpart in the research and development (R&D) department is completely incorrect as the formulation of the R&D department using different equipment needs to be adapted to the Glatt Multicell™, which was demonstrated by Roche (Basel) and Pfizer (Freiburg, Germany) when H. Leuenberger was consulting the Glatt Group. Only this semi-continuous process offers a real solution to scale-up problems since it uses the same equipment for small- and large-scale production (Leuenberger, 2001; Betz et al., 2003, Werani et al., 2004). The Glatt Multicell™ equipment was developed from the results of the Ph.D. theses of Schade, 1992 and Dörr, 1996 at the University of Basel, Switzerland, and needs to be integrated into the workflow of the R&D and production departments using the same equipment. The quasi-continuous production line entails manufacturing of mini batches in a specially designed high-shear mixer/granulator patented by Glatt AG Pratteln (inventor H. Leuenberger) which is connected to a continuous multi-cell-fluidized bed dryer. A specified amount of powder of the formulation is added to the high-shear mixer and thoroughly mixed. Subsequently, this amount of powder is granulated by continuously adding granulating liquid up to a fixed amount based on the results of a power consumption measurement. The wet granules are then discharged through a screen into the first cell of the fluidized bed dryer unit to avoid any formation of lumps. Thus, the quasi-continuous production of granules can be described as a train of mini-batches passing like parcels through the "dry mixing," "granulation," and "drying" compartments. The multi-cell dryer consists usually of three cells which are designed for different air temperatures, that is, in the first cell the granules are dried at a high temperature, for example, 60°C, and in the last cell ambient air temperature and humidity is used to achieve equilibrium conditions. Thus, a batch defined for quality control purposes consists of a fixed number of mini-batches, and a tight in-process control of the mixing/granulation and drying step that provides an excellent batch record of the quasi-continuous production of granules, as well as an excellent opportunity for a continuous validation of the process and the equipment.

Constant values of the process parameters are important aspects of quasi-continuous granulation. It is well known that certain formulations show an excellent compression profile for small batches but do not keep this property using a larger batch size. To check the compression/hardness profile of a granule batch, different subunits (S) of mini-batches were selected from two formulations and compressed into tablets using different compression forces (Figures 20.19 and 20.20). It shows that in principle the quality of the small batch is not changed by the repetitive procedure.

The above concept preceded the new MODCOS line of the Glatt Group, which is a fully continuous process. However, such a fully continuous process has the disadvantage, that this technique is not suitable for the production of small batches for early clinical trials of Clinical Phase I and Clinical Phase II due to the limited amount of API and its high costs at this early stage.

Q8—IDENTIFYING CRITICAL MATERIAL ATTRIBUTES AND PROCESS PARAMETERS

The ICH Q8 guidelines emphasis on the importance of identifying critical material and process parameters regarding product quality and the PAT initiative focus on critical process control (Figure 20.1) are illustrated with examples in the following case studies.

Critical Material Attributes—Case Study (Carbamazepine)

APIs are routinely assayed at the time of purchase for presence and level of degradation products. However, for many drug substances it is necessary to determine critical properties which may vary as a result of differences in the manufacturing techniques and which, if not monitored, can lead

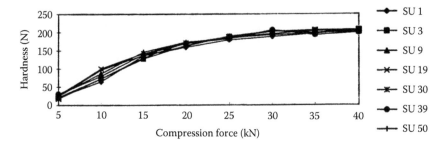

FIGURE 20.19 Compression force/hardness profile (Formulation 1). (From Betz, G. et al., *Pharma. Dev. Technol.*, 8, 289–297, 2003.)

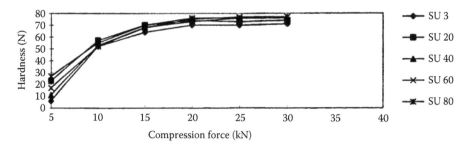

FIGURE 20.20 Compression force/hardness profile (Formulation 2). (From Betz, G. et al., *Pharma. Dev. Technol.*, 8, 289–297, 2003.)

to formulation failure. Furthermore, it is essential that specific tests are adopted to measure these attributes and thus to use them for their monitoring and control. In this case study, an example is given on the use of the slope of the disc intrinsic dissolution rate (DIDR) profile to identify variability in the dissolution property of a water-insoluble drug carbamezapine (CBZ) (Sehic et al., 2010). CBZ undergoes solution-mediated phase transformation during dissolution testing and the kinetics of the transition may differ from one polymorphic form to the other (Rodriguez-Hornedo et al., 2004). Commercial CBZ is available as anhydrous form III which is stable at room temperature (Rustichelli et al., 2000) but in solution the most stable form is the dihydrate. The DIDR profiles of three commercial samples (A, B, and P) exhibited inflection in the curve resulting in two distinct slopes: the initial slope, which describes dissolution of anhydrous phase, and the final slope, which represents the dissolution of dihydrate phase. One-way ANOVA test for the initial 20 min of dissolution showed statistically significant difference between CBZA, B, and P, although the differences were insignificant when compared over the entire 120 min. This indicates that variability in primary CBZ material is expressed in the initial part of dissolution, that is, where anhydrous-dihydrate conversion occurs (Table 20.10). It is also seen in Table 20.10 that, as expected, the DIDR curves of the dihydrates (Da, Db, Dp) prepared from the anhydrous samples did not exhibit inflection points.

Kinetics of phase transformation—Fitting the segments of each profile to a nonlinear model (Systat Software Inc., USA) the estimated times required for conversion of anhydrous CBZ to dihydrate were found to vary between 15 and 25 min. Kobayashi et al. (2000) and Ono et al. (2002) reported that transformation occurs after 5–10 min of intrinsic dissolution test. The discrepancies found in the present work can be explained by the different raw material used. Applying the method of Ono et al. (2002), the dissolution parameters were calculated from the segmented plots using the following equations:

$$\frac{dC}{dt} = k_t C_{SH} \tag{20.2}$$

$$\left(\frac{dC}{dt}\right)_{t=0} = k_t C_{SA} \tag{20.3}$$

$$b = \frac{k_t (C_{SA} - C_{SH})}{k_r} \tag{20.4}$$

where C represents the concentration of carbamazepine in bulk solution (μg/ml); t is the time (min), k_t is the rate constant of the transport process (min), k_r is the rate constant of the phase transformation process (min), C_{SH} is the saturated concentration of dihydrate (μg/ml), C_{SA} is the saturated

---

TABLE 20.10
Dissolution Parameters of Anhydrous CBZ (a, b, p) and the Corresponding Dihydrate Forms

Sample $n = (3)$	Initial Slope (μg/ml min)	Final Slope (μg/ml min)	Intercept (μg/ml)	k_t (per min)	k_r (per min)
A	0.141 ± 0.002	0.098 ± 0.002	0.925 ± 0.130		0.0649 ± 0.016
B	0.152 ± 0.002	0.090 ± 0.001	0.870 ± 0.084		0.0811 ± 0.008
P	0.148 ± 0.002	0.107 ± 0.001	1.137 ± 0.068		0.0583 ± 0.002
Da		0.082 ± 0.000	0.084 ± 0.014	0.00029	
Db		0.082 ± 0.001	0.126 ± 0.029	0.00030	
Dp		0.082 ± 0.001	0.129 ± 0.032	0.00030	

Source: Sehic, S. et al., *Int. J. Pharm.*, 386, 77–90, 2010.

concentration of anhydrous form (μg/ml), and b represents the intercept obtained by the extrapolation of the linear portion of the dissolution curve of the anhydrous form. The parameters k_t, k_r, and C_{SA} were calculated from the above-mentioned equations, and k_t, or the rate constant of the transport process, was calculated from the slope of the dihydrate curve using the solubility value for the respective dihydrate (C_{SH}) obtained from equilibrium solubility testing. C_{SA} was calculated from Equation 20.2 using the estimate of the slope of the initial segment and the k_t value calculated from Equation 20.2. The intercept of the final segment was calculated using Equation 20.4. The results are added in Table 20.10, where it is seen that in addition to the differences in the transition time point, variations in the value for the constant of phase transformation process (k_r) were also observed. The highest k_r value means that the sample has ability to undergo the fastest transformation from anhydrous to dihydrate form, consequently resulting in the highest IDR. In all examined samples, the highest k_r value was observed for CBZB and the lowest one was observed for CBZP. Considering these results, the correlation between the intrinsic dissolution parameters and the rate of transformation is promising and may help to determine the kinetics of transformation for each examined CBZ and eventually can help to predict its behavior in the final formulation by verifying these parameters in the preformulation stage.

The intrinsic dissolution parameters were used to estimate the solubilities of the samples. The calculated solubilities ranked CBZB > CBZP > CBZA and were in agreement with literature data of form III (Kobayashi et al., 2000), but were higher than the experimentally obtained equilibrium solubilities (measured after 72 h) because during the solubility measurements transformation of CBZ anhydrous to CBZ dihydrate took place.

The intrinsic dissolution rates were calculated from the initial part of each profile using Equation 20.5 (Kobayashi et al., 2000, Sethia and Squillante 2004):

$$\text{IDR} = \frac{C}{t} \cdot \frac{V}{S} = k \cdot C_s \tag{20.5}$$

where S is the surface area of the tablet (cm^2), V is volume of test solution (mL), k is intrinsic dissolution rate constant, and C_s represents solubility (mg/mL).

The obtained results have the same ranking as reported in the estimated solubility, that is, IDR CBZB (77.45 ± 2.04) > IDR CBZP (73.92 ± 2.00) > IDR CBZA (69.11 ± 1.96) (μg/min/cm^2). The IDR values of the dihydrates were nearly the same (between 22.43 and 23.09 μg/min/cm^2).

In conclusion, it is important to note that differences in the intrinsic dissolution rates of the samples were relatively small when described by a single value, however, they become important when the intrinsic dissolution behavior is described by a set of kinetic parameters. Considering that carbamazepine has narrow therapeutic index and very narrow dissolution range of acceptance criteria in the USP monograph, the variation in the kinetics of conversion from anhydrate to dihydrate form among different raw material of CBZ is important information. Therefore, the point of transformation as well as the kinetics of the phase transformation may be considered as critical parameters that should be investigated and monitored according to Q8 guidelines for drug substance.

Critical Process Parameters

The wet agglomeration process is the most common process for granulation and tableting of pharmaceutical powders. Conventional wet agglomeration uses a high-shear mixer granulator combined with a fluid-bed dryer or a fluid-bed granulator/dryer. Innovative semicontinuous processes such as the Glatt Multicell™ production line described earlier also use high-shear mixer/granulator in combination with fluid-bed dryer.

To design the process of wet agglomeration in order to limit or eliminate product variability, a mechanistic approach to the critical process parameters is required. A critical process parameter is the process parameter that must be controlled within the design space (i.e., within predetermined limits) to ensure the performance of the product.

The Power Consumption Profile

High-shear granulator—In both the high-shear as well as the fluid-bed granulators, size enlargement and size reduction occur as a dynamic equilibrium. The equilibrium is shifted to a larger granule size due to the addition of granulating liquid. The effect of adding the granulating liquid can be monitored in the high-shear granulator by measuring the power consumption profile, although this is not possible in the fluid-bed granulator.

The power consumption profile of a formulation consisting of 10% starch, 86% lactose, and 4% PVP (w/w) shown in Figure 20.21 exhibits different stages: lag time up to S_2 due to swelling of starch, that is, no formation of granules because the granulating liquid is not available for formation of liquid bridges between particles of the powder; formation of liquid bridges between S_2 and S_3; generation of pharmaceutical granules from S_3 to S_4 (close to S_3 granules of low density are formed, whereas close to S_4 granules of high density are produced); and above S_4 the system is over-wetted (the point of no return). It is apparent from Figure 20.21 that there is no indication of an end point of granulation. But the amount of granulating liquid used in the process may vary between different formulations, and in order to calculate corresponding amounts of granulating liquid in different compositions, a dimensionless amount of granulating liquid (π) is used. The term π defines the degree of saturation of the interparticle void space within the powder bed and is derived from the amount of granulating liquid in liters (S). The power consumption profile is useful as an analytical tool to define S values for different compositions. This enables an unbiased analysis of granules' growth kinetics, since batches are analyzed as a function of the dimensionless term π (Leuenberger 1982a, Betz et al., 2004). For a robust formulation, the granule distribution should not vary from batch to batch and the key factor is the correct amount and type of granulation liquid. The variation in the primary materials (both API and additive) can be compensated by an in-process control based on the power consumption profile. Since there is no granulation end point, the granulation process can be controlled by detection of the turning point of the S-shaped ascent in phase II of the power consumption profile calculated with a computer program based on polynomial function. The peak (= first derivative of the power consumption curve) in Figure 20.22 describes a certain cohesiveness of the moistened powder bed at the beginning of the plateau phase. It is a signal provided by the powder mass and has a self-correcting property as it appears at an earlier time for a slightly coarser starting material, or later for a slightly finer material; as well it takes into account the initial moisture content of the primary material, which depends on seasonal effects. The first derivative of the power consumption profile can thus be used as in-process control for *fine-tuning* the amount of granulating liquid required.

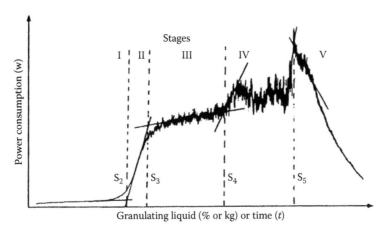

FIGURE 20.21 The division of the power consumption profile. (From Leuenberger, H. and Bier, H. P., *Acta Pharm. Techn.*, 7, 41–44, 1979.)

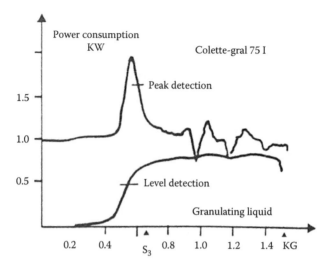

FIGURE 20.22 The peak- or level-detection method can help to find the right amount of granulating liquid. (From Leuenberger, H., *Pharm. Acta Helv.*, 57, 72–82, 1982a.)

UNDERSTANDING POWDER SYSTEMS

Building the pyramid of knowledge is an important stimulus toward development of a solid framework for powder systems. Since the majority of drug delivery systems involve powders, the challenges facing the formulation scientist may be the toughest in the area of powder technology. Pharmaceutical powder technology incorporates many areas (e.g., handling, storage, flow, compression, etc.) where the critical properties of powders must be well defined for the development of a robust formulation and manufacturing process.

Many of the powders used in the manufacture of pharmaceuticals are mixtures. They consist either of one material in a range of sizes, such as milled drugs, or of different materials, such as granules for tablets and capsules, which may include the drug and a number of excipients. The properties of a final product such as a tablet very much depend on the behavior of the powders when subjected to compressional or shearing stresses. Powders can be classified as either *simple* or *complex* depending on whether a single parameter such as the angle of internal friction describes their behavior under normal stress. Lactose, calcium carbonate, and penicillin were described as simple powders, that is, the angle of internal friction was found to be independent of the packing density. Pharmaceutical formulations behave as complex powders and their behavior becomes more difficult to describe with a single parameter due to changes that occur in the interaction forces between particles as the powders are mixed together (Kocova El-Arini and Pilpel, 1974). Leuenberger proposed a model for the estimation of the compressibility and compactibility parameters which can be used to characterize the materials as either plastic or brittle. Its use can be extended both to single powders as well as to mixtures of powders (Leuenberger, 1982b). Obtaining the value of these parameters can help design a robust tablet formulation by maintaining a good balance between plasticity and fragmentation.

CASE STUDY (ROLLER COMPACTION)

This study makes use of compressibility and compactibility parameters to monitor the tensile strength of tablets produced in the roller compactor (Hadzovic et al., 2011). Dry agglomeration by roller compaction is employed when the active ingredient is sensitive to moisture and high temperature or is prone to sticking during tableting. However the roller compaction process can result in tablets with inferior tensile strength (e.g., compared to direct compaction) (Herting and Kleinebudde, 2008) and this loss of tabletability after roller compaction is an example of how the process can affect the performance of formulations. Mixing the drug with excipient is usually the way to improve tablet properties, but the strength of tablets compressed from binary mixtures often cannot be predicted from the compaction properties of the individual materials. In this study we investigate the tensile strength of tablets of mixtures of theophylline (as anhydrate powder [THAP], anhydrate fine powder [THAFP] and monohydrate [THMO]) and microcrystalline cellulose (MCC) produced by roller compaction. In parallel tests, tablets of the same materials were produced by direct compression for comparison. The results of the THAP grade and MCC are compared in Figures 20.23 and 20.24, from which it can be seen that, compared to direct compression, roller compaction decreased the tensile strength of tablets, especially at higher compression pressure (30 bars) and that the decrease was more significant in the MCC tablets. The tensile strengths of tablets of the binary mixtures (100%, 70%, 50%, 30%, and 10% of THAP, and MCC) produced by direct compaction and roller compaction are illustrated in Figure 20.24. Analogous behavior was found with the other grades of theophylline in the mixtures (Hadzovic, 2008). Figure 20.25 shows that the tensile strength of tablets compressed from 100% MCC was higher than the tensile strength of tablets containing 100% THAP. From this result and the fact that after roller compaction the tensile strength of THAP was not decreased significantly, it could be hypothesized that THAP

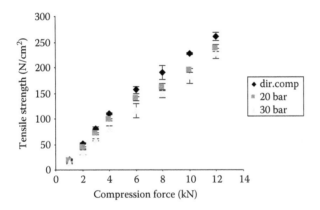

FIGURE 20.23 Tensile strength of tablets of theophylline (THAP) obtained by direct compression and following roller compaction. (From Hadzovic, E. et al., *Int. J. Pharm.*, 416, 97–103, 2011.)

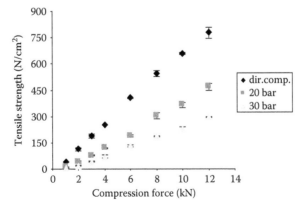

FIGURE 20.24 Tensile strength of tablets of MCC obtained by direct compression and following roller compaction. (From Hadzovic, E. et al., *Int. J. Pharm.*, 416, 97–103, 2011.)

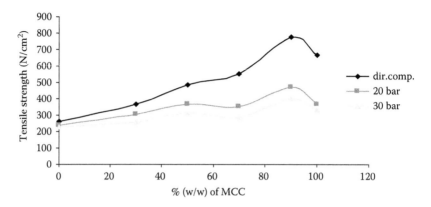

FIGURE 20.25 Tensile strength of theophylline: MCC binary mixtures by direct compression and roller compaction. (From Hadzovic, E. et al., *Int. J. Pharm.*, 416, 97–103, 2011.)

consolidated by fragmentation more than by plastic deformation. Furthermore, it is interesting to note that the mixture of THAP 10% + MCC 90% produced tablets with higher tensile strength than the individual excipient. This phenomenon is characteristic of mixtures of two materials which consolidate by different mechanism (Garr and Rubinstein, 1991). As evident in this study the MCC, as very plastic material, was responsible for mechanical strength of the tablets, whereas theophylline could be considered as being partially fragmentized during compaction. This indicates that it is essential to find an optimum composition for formulation development by roller compaction, which should maintain a good balance between plasticity and fragmentation.

The Leuenberger model—In order to correlate the compressibility of theophylline and MCC with the tensile strength of tablets, we used the Leuenberger equation shown in the following in which the radial tensile strength σ_t at certain forming pressure σ is plotted against the product of the compression pressure and relative density ρ ($\rho = 1 - \varepsilon$, ε = porosity) of tablets (Leuenberger, 1982b):

$$\sigma_t = \sigma_{T\max}(1 - e^{-\gamma\sigma\rho})$$

The parameter $\sigma_{T\max}$ in the Leuenberger equation is the theoretical maximal possible tensile strength for a compact whose porosity is equal to zero, and γ is the compression susceptibility, a constant that describes compressibility. Material with low $\sigma_{T\max}$ show relatively poor compactibilty, and even if high compression pressure is applied this value cannot be exceeded. A high γ value means that at low compression pressure maximal tensile strength could be achieved (Leuenberger, 1982b). Figure 20.26 and Table 20.11 show respectively the plots and the calculated parameters according to Leuenberger equation. It can be seen from Figure 20.26 that theophylline would reach the plateau of the maximal tensile strength at lower compression pressures than MCC, that is, higher compression pressure should be applied to reach maximal tensile strength for MCC. MCC exhibited much higher $\sigma_{T\max}$ values than theophylline and the MCC tablets had higher tensile strength than theophylline tablets (Figures 20.23 and 20.24), which is in agreement with these results.

According to the pressure susceptibility parameter, theophylline will reach maximal tensile strength much faster than MCC. The pressure susceptibility parameter γ for theophylline powders ranged between $8.9 \pm 0.0 \times 10^{-3}$ MPa^{-1} and $12.7 \pm 0.0 \times 10^{-3}$ MPa^{-1}. MCC had much lower γ, that is, $2.5 \pm 0.0 \times 10^{-3}$ MPa^{-1}.

In Figure 20.27 it can be observed that, within the pressure range investigated in this study, even though MCC had a higher maximal tensile strength than the binary mixtures, the mixture of 10% drug and 90% MCC, having high pressure susceptibility value, will reach the maximum tensile strength before MCC. This is because the MCC plot is more linear and it needs higher pressures to reach the plateau.

TABLE 20.11

The Compression Susceptibility Parameter $\gamma \times 10^{-3}(MPa)^{-1}$, and the Maximum Tensile Strength σ_{Tmax} (MPa) of THAP, THAFP, THMO, and MCC by Direct Compression and Roller Compaction

$n = 3 \pm$ s.d.	$\gamma \times 10^{-3}$ [MPa^{-1}]	σ_{Tmax} [MPa]	R^2
THAP powder	8.91 ± 0.1	3.22 ± 0.1	0.999
THAP 20 bars	$7.82 \pm 0,1$	3.94 ± 0.0	0.999
THAP 30 bars	8.25 ± 0.2	2.80 ± 0.1	0.998
THAFP powder	11.78 ± 0.0	3.97 ± 0.1	0.999
THAFP 20 bars	7.33 ± 0.3	3.74 ± 0.1	0.998
THMO powder	12.79 ± 0.0	3.25 ± 0.0	0.999
THMO 20 bars	11.37 ± 0.4	2.11 ± 0.0	0.997
MCC powder	2.45 ± 0.0	29.99 ± 1.8	0.998
MCC 20 bars	5.90 ± 0.2	7.52 ± 0.1	0.999

Source: Hadzovic, E. et al., *Int. J. Pharm.*, 416, 97–103, 2011.

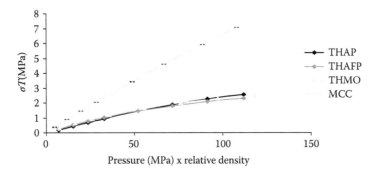

FIGURE 20.26 Tensile strength of theophylline grades and MCC according to Leuenberger. (From Hadzovic, E. et al., *Int. J. Pharm.*, 416, 97–103, 2011.)

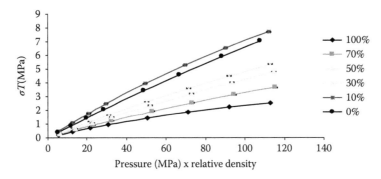

FIGURE 20.27 Tensile strength of THAP and MCC binary mixtures according to Leuenberger equation. (From Hadzovic, E. et al., *Int. J. Pharm.*, 416, 97–103, 2011.)

It appears from Table 20.11 that roller compaction did not significantly change the compressibility and the compactibility of theophylline, but this was not the case with MCC. The maximal tensile strength that a compact could reach when it has zero porosity was largely decreased, and because the pressure susceptibility was increased, tensile strength could be achieved at lower compression pressures.

In conclusion, as the amount of MCC in the binary mixtures increased, the differences in tensile strength of tablets prepared by direct compaction and roller compaction were more prominent. According to the parameters obtained from the Leuenberger equation, theophylline was more compressible, while MCC was the more compactable material. The results of this study show, in an impressive manner, that the choice of the right excipient in the right ratio with the drug plays a major role in the roller compaction process.

Finally, it should be emphasized that with the PAT initiative and the Q8 guidelines being part of the pyramid of knowledge and the first principle approach leading to the top of the pyramid of knowledge, it is possible to improve the performance of the pharmaceutical industry to a six sigma value. This is important for the development of newly discovered drugs, more and more of which are of extremely low water solubility and represent an enormous challenge to formulate into robust dosage forms.

REFERENCES

Benson, R. S. and J. D. J. McCabe. (2004). From good manufacturing practice to good manufacturing performance. *Pharm. Eng.*, 24 (4).

Bonny, J. D. and H. Leuenberger. (1993). Matrix type controlled release systems II: Percolation effects in non swellable matrices. *Pharm. Acta Helv.*, 68: 25–33.

Betz, G., P. Junker Bürgin, and H. Leuenberger. (2003). Batch and continuous processing in the production of pharmaceutical granules. *Pharm. Dev. Technol.*, 8(3): 289–297.

Betz, G., P. Junker Bürgin, and H. Leuenberger. (2004). Power consumption measurement and temperature recording during granulation. *Int. J. Pharm.*, 272: 137–149.

Dhenge, R. M., K. Washino, J. J. Cartwright, M. J. Hounslow, and A. D. Salman. (2013). Twin screw granulation using conveying screws: Effects of viscosity of granulation liquids and flow of powders. *Powder Technol.*, 238: 77–90.

Dörr, B. (1996). *Entwicklung einer Anlage zur quasikontinuierlichen Feuchtgranulierung und Mehrkammer-Wirbelschichttrocknung von pharmazeutischen Granulaten*, dissertation Universitat Basel.

Dörr, B. and H. Leuenberger. (1998). Development of a quasi-continuous production line—A concept to avoid scale-up problems. *European Symposium on Process Technologies in Pharmaceutical and Nutritional Sciences*, PARTEC 98 Nurnberg, Germany (Leuenberger, H. Ed) pp. 247–256.

Garr, J. S. M. and M. H. Rubinstein. (1991). The effect of rate of force application on the properties of microcrystalline cellulose and dibasic calcium phosphate mixtures. *Int. J. Pharm.* 73 (1): 75–80.

Hadzovic, E. (2008). *Roller Compaction of Theophylline*, PhD thesis, University of Basel, Switzerland.

Herting, M. G. and P. Kleinebudde. (2008). Studies on the reduction of tensile strength of tablets after roll compaction/dry granulation. *Eur. J. Pharm. Biopharm.*, 70: 372–379.

Hadzovic, E., G. Betz, S. Hadzidediic, S. Kocova El-Arini, and H. Leuenberger. (2011). Investigation of compressibility and compactibility parameters of roller compacted theophylline and its binary mixtures. *Int. J. Pharm.*, 416: 97–103.

Hussain, A. S. (2002). *Pharmaceutical Process Scale–Up*, M. Levin (Ed.), New York: Marcel Dekker.

ICH Harmonized Tripartite Guideline: Pharmaceutical Development Q8 (R2), Current Step 4 version: http://www.ich.org/fileadmin/Public_Web_Site/ICH_Products/Guidelines/Quality/Q8_R1/Step4/Q8_R2_Guideline.pdf.

Jarvinen, K., M. Toiviainen, M. Jarvinen, and M. Jutti. (2012). Continuous wet granulation process: Granule properties and in-line process monitoring. *American Pharmaceutical Review*, www.americanpharmaceuticalreview.com.

Kimura, G. (2012). Design of pharmaceutical tablet formulation for a low water-soluble drug; search for the critical concentration of starch based disintegrant applying percolation theory and F-CAD (Formulation–Computer Aided Design), Faculty of Science, University of Basel, Switzerland, downloaded from: http://edoc.unibas.ch/diss/DissB_9886.

Kocova ElArini, S. and N. Pilpel. (1974). Shearing and tensile tests on mixtures of pharmaceutical powders. *J. Pharm. Pharmac.*, 26, 11P–15P.

Kobayashi, Y., S. Ito, S. Itai, and K. Yamamoto. (2000). Physicochemical properties and bioavailability of carbamazepine polymorphs and dihydrate. *Int. J. Pharm.*, 193: 137–146

Krausbauer, E. (2009). Contribution to a science based expert system, PhD thesis, University of Basel, Switzerland, Faculty of Science, http://edoc.unibas.ch/diss/DissB_8879.

Krueger, C., M. Thommes, and P. Kleinebudde. (2010). "MCC Sanaq Burst"—A new type of cellulose and its suitability to prepare fast disintegrating pellets. *J. Pharm. Innov.*, 5: 45–57.

Lee, S. L., T. F. O'Connor, X. Yang, C. N. Cruz, S. Chatterjee, R. D. Madurawe, C. M. V. Moore, L. X. Yu, and J. Woodcock. (2015). Modernizing pharmaceutical manufacturing: From batch to continuous production. *J Pharm Innov.*, 10: 191–199.

Leuenberger, H. and W. Becher. (1975). A factorial design for compatibility studies in preformulation work. *Pharm. Acta. Helv.* 50: 88–91.

Leuenberger, H. (1978). Versuchsplanung und Optimierstrategien in *Pharmazeutische Technologie*, H. Sucker, P. Fuchs, and P. Speiser., (Eds.) Stuttgart, Germany: Georg Thieme Verlag, pp. 64–77.

Leuenberger, H. and P. Guitard. (1978). Delivery systems for patient compliance. In *Pharmaceutical Medicine, the Future*, H. Lahon, R. K. Rondel, and K. Kratochvil, (Ed.), 3rd International Meeting of Pharmaceutical Physicians, Brussels, Belgium, October 4–7, pp. 358–372.

Leuenberger, H. and H. P. Bier. (1979). Bestimmung der optimalen Menge Granulierflüssigkeit durch Messung der elektrischen Leistungsaufnahme eines Planetenmischers. *Acta Pharm. Techn.*, 7: 41–44.

Leuenberger, H. (1982a). Granulation–new techniques. *Pharm. Acta Helv.*, 37: 72–82.

Leuenberger, H. (1982b). The compressibility and compactibility of powder systems. *Int. J. Pharma.*, 12 (1): 41–55.

Leuenberger, H., L. Holman, M. Usteri, and S. Winzap. (1989a). Percolation theory, fractal geometry, and dosage form design. *Pharm. Acta Helv.*, 64: 34–39.

Leuenberger, H., L. Holman, M. Usteri, G. Imanidis, and S. Winzap. (1989b). Monitoring the granulation process: Granulate growth, fractal dimensionality and percolation threshold. *Boll. Chem. Pharm.* 128: 54–61.

Leuenberger, H. and S. Kocova El-Arini. (2000). Solubilization systems—The impact of percolation theory and fractal geometry. In *Water-Insoluble Drug Formulation*, Liu, R. (Ed.), Denver, CO: Interpharm Press, pp. 569–608.

Leuenberger, H. (2001). New trends in the production of pharm. Granules: Batch versus continuous processing. *Eur. J. Pharm. Biopharm.*, 52(3): 289–296.

Leuenberger, H. and M. Lanz. (2005). Pharmaceutical powder technology-from art to science: The challenge of FDA's PAT initiative. *Adv. Powder Technol.*, 16: 1–36.

Leuenberger, H., S. Kocova El-Arini, and G. Betz. (2008). Pharmaceutical powder technology—Building the pyramid of knowledge. In *Water-Insoluble Drug Formulation*, 2nd ed., Liu, R. (Ed.), Boca Raton, FL: CRC Press.

Leuenberger, H., M. N. Leuenberger, and M. Puchkov. (2009). Implementing virtual R & D reality in industry: *In silico* design and testing of solid dosage forms. *Swiss Pharma*, 31(7–8): 18–24.

Leuenberger, H., M. N. Leuenberger, and M. Puchkov. (2010). Right, First Time: Computer-aided scale-up for manufacturing solid dosage forms with a shorter time to market. *Swiss Pharma*, 32(7–8), 3–13.

Leuenberger, H., M. N. Leuenberger, and M. Puchkov. (2011). Virtual scale-up of manufacturing solid dosage forms. In *Pharmaceutical Process Scale-up*, 3rd ed., Levin, M. (Ed.). New York and London: Informa Healthcare, Chapter 17.

Leuenberger, H., M. Puchkov, and B. Schneider. (2013). Right. First Time concept and workflow. *Swiss Pharma*, 35: 4–16.

Leuenberger, H. (2013). *Galenical drug-excipient screening program for the development of robust* Six-sigma *quality tablet formulations*, presentation at Pharmatrans Sanaq Forum, 9th Scientific and Technical Forum Basel, Basel, Switzerland. May 23–24.

Leuenberger, H., M. Puchkov, U. Cueni, and G. Sivaraman. (2013). *Virtual Tablet Design*.

Leuenberger, H. (2015). Process Scale-Up in the Pharmaceutical Industry, workshop organized by FlemingEurope. Cologne.

Leuenberger, H. and M. N. Leuenberger. (2016). Impact of the digital revolution on the future of formulation sciences. *Europ. J. Pharm. Sci.*, 87: 100–111.

Levin, M. (2015). Measurement Control Cooperation, New Jersey, personal communication.

Lowe, D. (2014). A new look at clinical attrition, in the pipeline, posted January 10, 2014. http://pipeline.corante.com/archives/2014/01/10/a_new_look_at_clinical_attrition.php, downloaded May 31, 2015.

Luginbuehl, R. and H. Leuenberger. (1994). Use of percolation theory to interpret water uptake, disintegration time and intrinsic dissolution rate of tablets consisting of binary mixtures. *Pharm. Acta. Helv.*, 69: 127–134.

Ono, M., Y. Tozuka, T. Oguchi, S. Yamamura, and K. Yamamoto. (2002). Effects of dehydration temperature on water vapor adsorption and dissolution behavior of carbamazepine. *Int. J. Pharm.*, 239: 1–12.

Parikh, D. M. (2016). Continuous Granulation Technology Trends, Contract Pharma, online features downloaded from: http://www.contractpharma.com/issues/2016-06-01/view_features/continuous-granulation-technology-trends#sthash.mOkMtQvY.dpuf.

Puchkov, M. and H. Leuenberger. (2011). Computer-aided design of pharmaceutical formulations, F-CAD software and a mathematical concept. *Glatt Times*, Nr. 31: 2–6.

Puchkov, M., D. Tschirky, and H. Leuenberger. (2013). 3D Cellular Automata in Computer-aided Design of Pharmaceutical Formulations: Mathematical Concept and F-CAD software in "Formulation Tools for Pharmaceutical Development," Aguilar, J. (Ed.), Woodhead Publishing Series in Biomedicine.

Presster, manufactured and distributed by Measurement Control Corporation, www. mcc-online.com, downloaded October, 14 (2015).

Rocco, M. C. (Ed.). (2000). *Nanotechnology Research Directions: IWGN Workshop Report*, Dordrecht, the Netherlands: Kluwer Academic, p. 360.

Rodriguez-Hornedo, N. and D. Murphy. (2004). Surfactant-facilitated crystallization of dihydrate carbamezapine during dissolution of anhydrous polymorph. *J. Pharm. Sci.*, 93: 449–460.

Rustichelli, C., G. Gamberini, V. Ferioli, M. C. Gamberini, R. Ficarra, and S. Tommasini. (2000). Solid-state study of polymorphic drugs: Carbamazepine. *J. Pharm. Biomed. Anal.*, 23: 41–54.

Schade A. (1992). *Herstellung von pharmazeutischen Granulaten in einem kombinierten Feuchtgranulationsund Mehrkammer-Wirbelschichttrocknungsverfahren*, dissertation, Universitat Basel, Switzerland.

Sehic, S., G. Betz, S. Hadzidedic, S. K. El-Arini, and H. Leuenberger. (2010). Investigation of intrinsic dissolution behavior of different carbamezapine samples. *Int. J. Pharm.*, 386: 77–90.

Sethia, S. and E. Squillante. (2004). Solid dispersion of carbamezapine in PVP K30 by conventional solvent evaporation and supercritical methods. *Int. J. Pharm.*, 272: 1–10.

Schwartz, J. B., J. R. Flamholz and R. H. Press. (1973). Computer optimization of pharmaceutical formulations I, General procedure. *J. Pharm. Sci.*, 62 (7): 1165–1170.

Swanborough, A. (2008). Benefits of continuous granulation for pharmaceutical research, development and manufacture. Thermo Fisher Scientific, UK, Application Note LR-63.

Vervaet, C. and J. P. Remon. (2005). Continuous granulation in the pharmaceutical industry, *Chem. Eng. Sci.*, 60(14): 3949–3957.

Werani, J., M. Grünberg, C. Ober, and H. Leuenberger. (2004). Semi-continuous granulation—The process of choice for the production of pharmaceutical granules? *Powder Technol.*, 140: 163–168.

Wolfram, S. (2002). *A New Kind of Science*, Champaign, IL: Wolfram Media, pp. 1–1197.

Yalkowsky, S. H. (Ed.). (1981). *Techniques of Solubilization of Drugs* (Drugs and the Pharmaceutical Sciences Series), 12, New York: Marcel Dekker.

21 Soft Gelatin Capsules Development

S. Esmail Tabibi, Shanker L. Gupta, and Liangran Guo

CONTENTS

Soft gelatin capsules, also known as *softgels*, are solid capsules consisting of soft shells and liquid/semi-liquid fills. Softgels have numerous advantages over other traditional dosage forms such as tablets and even hard gelatin capsules (Cole et al. 2008). In a review, Jones and Francis (2000) presented results of a consumer survey showing wide acceptability of soft gelatin capsules when compared with other dosage forms. In fact, it is not uncommon for pharmaceutical companies to reformulate marketed solid dosage forms in the form of soft gelatin capsules in order to manage the life cycle or improve consumer acceptability. There are numerous published studies demonstrating improved bioavailability or absorption rate of drugs formulated as soft gelatin capsules (Stella et al., 1978; Sullivan et al., 1986; Savio et al., 1998; Agrosi et al., 2000; Zaghloul et al., 2002; Zuniga et al., 2004; Lissy et al., 2010; Benza et al., 2011; Proietti et al., 2014).

A pharmaceutical scientist will eventually face a task to formulate an oily or an oil-soluble medicament in liquid formulation as a solid dosage form using the soft gelatin capsule, sometimes referred to as *softgel* or *liquigel*™. In the common oral dosage forms, formulators have access to the excipients and processing technologies, thus enabling them to conduct a systematic formulation and process development research and produce an elegant and stable dosage form. On the other hand, owing to its nature, softgel technology has become specialized processing, in which formulators will rely on the others to produce the shell formulation and conduct the shell-content compatibility studies. A suitably formulated medicament is finally encapsulated as the content into a compatible soft gelatin shell.

Because of the highly cost-intensive operation of softgel capsule production, it is not possible for formulation scientists to conduct research on all phases of the formulation and process development of soft gelatin capsules. However, based on the unique advantages and special properties of this type of dosage form, formulators should familiarize themselves with the overall technology and processes involved both in the development and manufacturing aspects.

Softgel capsules have gained popularity in the pharmaceutical industry for human and veterinary use, as an oral dosage form; as suppositories for rectal and vaginal administration; as single-use applicators for ophthalmic, otic, and topical formulations; and as rectal ointments. Their use in cosmetic industry is beyond the scope of this manuscript.

Nomination	Rounds		Ovals		Oblongs		Tubes		Suppositories	
Shape										
	Capsule size	Optimum fill volume (minim)*	Capsule size	Optimum fill volume (minim)	Capsule size	Optimum fill volume (minim)	Capsule size	Optimum fill volume (minim)	Capsule size	Optimum fill volume (minim)
			2	2.3						
	3	3.0	3	3.0						
	4	4.0	4	4.0	3	3.0	3	3.0		
	5	5.0	5	5.0	4	4.0	4	4.0		
	6	6.0	6	6.0	5	5.0	5	5.0		
	7	7.0	$7\frac{1}{2}$	7.5	6	6.0	6	6.0	10	10.0
	9	9.0	10	10.0	8	8.0	8	8.0	17	17.0
	15	15.0	12	12.0	$9\frac{1}{2}$	9.5	$17\frac{1}{2}$	17.5	40	40.0
	20	20.0	16	16.0	11	11.0	30	32.0	80	80.0
	40	40.0	20	20.0	12	12.0	45	45.0		
	50	50.0	30	30.0	14	14.0	65	65.0		
	80	65.0	40	40.0	16	16.0	90	90.0		
	90	80.0	60	60.0	20	20.0	120	120.0		
			80	80.0						
			85	85.0						

* A minim is equal to 0.0616 mL.

FIGURE 21.1 The shapes and sizes of commonly used soft gelatin capsules.

Softgel capsules come in a variety of shapes, sizes, and colors that may be specific to the manufacturer. In Figure 21.1, some representative shapes and sizes are presented. This chapter provides an overview of the manufacturing methods, formulation of the content medicament, composition of the shell, quality control procedures, stability, and shelf-life testing. We also discuss in some detail examples of the products formulated in softgel dosage form.

MANUFACTURING METHODS

PROCESSING EQUIPMENT

An exhaustive discussion on the advantages and disadvantages of different types of machinery used in the production of soft gelatin capsules is beyond the scope of this chapter. Some literature (Stanley, 1986; Reich, 2004; Reddy et al., 2013) describes the manufacturing process and formulation aspects of the softgel technology. A brief description of the various processing technologies follows.

PLATE PROCESS

Historically, the soft gelatin capsules were manufactured by *plate method*, in which elasticized sheets of the formulated gelatin shell were placed on the die plate that contains a number of capsule-shape cavities. By applying vacuum, the gelatin was drawn into the cavities to form capsule wells. The capsule wells were then filled with drug formulation and covered by another sheet of the elasticized gelatin or by folding the gelatin sheet back over the filled wells. The upper plate was then placed on the top of the upper sheet and pressed to form and cut the capsules. These capsules, generally, had one flat side. The major problems with this type of processing were the lack of dosage uniformity, high manufacturing losses, and its labor-/cost-intensiveness. This equipment is no longer available.

ROTARY DIE PROCESS

Robert P. Scherer invented and perfected the *rotary die process* in 1933, according to Ebert (1977), that almost eliminated all the problems associated with the plate process and produced softgel dosage forms with improved uniformity and high standards of accuracy. This is the first continuous process in which the outer faces of two counter-rotating rollers contain precisely machined and aligned die cavities. The die rollers rotate in opposite directions and the matching die cavities from each die roller create the capsule pocket. Figure 21.2 presents a schematic view of the rotary die process.

The process is automatic and produces capsules in various shapes and sizes. In this process, the elasticized shell formulation converts into two ribbons and the formulation of the medicament, either in the liquid or in the paste form, was simultaneously pumped between the rotating rollers. The injection pressure of the formulated content of the capsule causes the gelatin ribbons to swell into the die cavity and fill with the formulation. The convergence between the synchronized counter-rotating rollers hermetically seals and severs the completed capsules from the ribbons. The precise and extremely low clearance of the rotating parts demands continuous lubrication of the machine to avoid even a slight buildup. The lubrication oil should, therefore, be a GRAS—generally recognized as safe—material. Immediately after manufacture, the formed capsules automatically undergo volatile solvent washing to remove any traces of lubricating oil from the exterior of the capsules. The capsules are then conveyed to a drying station and dried on trays, either in air or under vacuum, to equilibrium moisture content with forced conditioned air of 20%–30% relative humidity at 21°C–24°C (Stanley, 1986). The drying technique may proceed with an infrared drying step to speed up the process. At this point, the shell contains 6%–10% moisture based on the gelatin formulation used to produce the shell. The dried capsules will then be transferred to the inspection station and sampled for release, after performing the required quality control tests for sizes sorting, color sorting, and packaging. Branding, if desired, may be done by either heat branding or ink printing at the finishing department. All of these steps may be integrated into a continuous operation by employing proper equipment at each step. Figure 21.3 depicts the schematic presentation of the entire process.

Following the success of rotary die process, in 1949 the Norton Company has announced the development of another continuous soft gelatin capsule processing technology known as *reciprocating die process*.

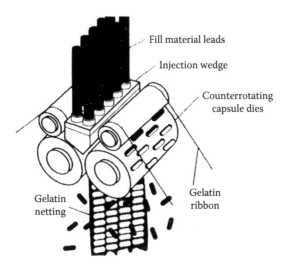

FIGURE 21.2 The rotary die encapsulating machine. (Courtesy of Banner Pharmacaps, Inc.)

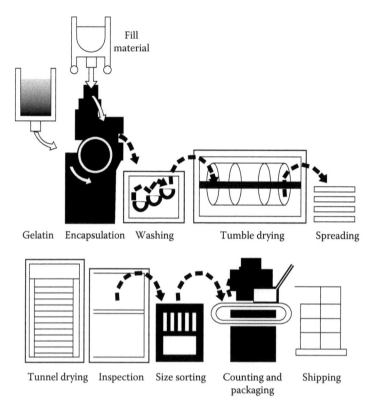

Gelatin   Encapsulation   Washing   Tumble drying   Spreading

Tunnel drying   Inspection   Size sorting   Counting and   Shipping
                                            packaging

FIGURE 21.3 The total production process. From preparation of shell and fill material composition to counting and packaging finished product, the state-of-the-art equipment used for each step of the process. (Courtesy of Banner Pharmacaps)

ACCOGEL PROCESS

Although the rotary die process and reciprocating die process were capable of producing soft gelatin capsules containing oily liquids and pastes, the incorporation of powders into soft gelatin capsules was made possible by the *accogel process* (Augsburger, 1996). Developed in 1949 by Lederle Laboratories, this rotary process is a continuous one that produces softgel capsules containing granules and powders. Briefly, the process involves a *measuring roll* that holds the fill formulation in its cavities under the vacuum and rotates directly above the elasticized sheet of the gelatin ribbon. The ribbon is drawn into the capsule cavities of the *capsule die roll* by vacuum. The measuring rolls empty the fill material into the capsule-shaped gelatin cavities on the die roll. The die roll then converges with the rotating *sealing roll* covered with another sheet of elasticized gelatin. The convergence of two rotary rolls creates pressure to seal and cut the formed capsules.

SEAMLESS PROCESS

Truly seamless one-piece soft gelatin capsules were produced by the Globex Mark II Capsulator. Figure 21.4 schematically shows this process, which does not require dies. In this process, a molten-gelatin stream flows though the outer nozzle of a concentric tube at a constant rate, and precision metering pump dispenses the medicated liquid formulation through the inner orifice. This method is often referred to as a *bubble method* that creates seamless, spherical softgel capsules called pearl. The process uses the pulsating mechanism at the orifice to force the emerging stream to break up into an intermittent but steady flow of uniformly sized, tubular-shaped composite droplets of immiscible cooling oil. The fundamental principle of interface physics—the tendency of liquids to

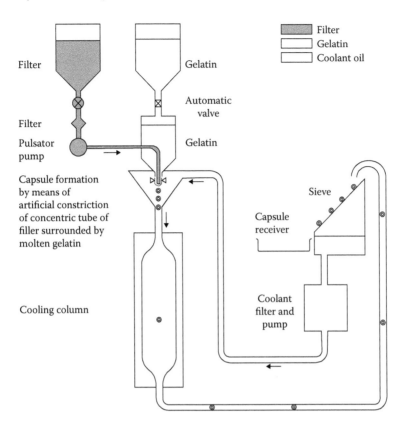

FIGURE 21.4   Schematic presentation of Globex Mark II capsule-filling machine. (Courtesy of Kinematic & Control Corp.)

form spherical drops due to surface tension—transforms tubular shape drops into a spherical shape. The congealed gelatin on cooling envelops the core-medicated formulation with an even shell. The cooling oil quickly carries the formed capsule away from the pulsating nozzle, slowly congeals the gelatin, and automatically ejects the capsules from the system as one-piece soft gelatin capsules (Rakucewicz, 1986; Augsburger, 1996). Unlike the previous methods, the drying in this process involves a cooling step to allow the gelatin shell to congeal (Rakucewicz, 1986). The separated capsules must be thoroughly washed and degreased by a volatile solvent and spread for drying in a suitable dryer (Rakucewicz, 1986; Augsburger, 1996).

FORMULATION CONSIDERATIONS

An important consideration in the development of soft gelatin capsules is the composition of the fill content, be it solution, suspension, or solid. The contents of soft gelatin capsules vary from solids, solid in liquid, solution or suspension, a combination of miscible liquid, or a simple liquid formulation. It is critical that each formulation is carefully developed depending on the physicochemical characteristics of the drug molecule. An optimum formulation consists of a minimum volume or weight that can be filled in the smallest possible capsule for ease of administration and for maximum therapeutic effectiveness. Composition of the capsule content and shell composition of commonly available commercial products are presented in Tables 21.1 and 21.2, respectively.

In recent publications and presentations from Cardinal Health (www.cardinal.com), numerous new formulations of shells containing plant-derived ingredients have been presented. In a presentation by Stroud et al. (2006), semisolid formulations of acetaminophen and ibuprofen were formulated using traditional encapsulation techniques in soft gelatin shell formulations containing polysaccharides.

TABLE 21.1

The Content Composition of Commercially Available Products

Product		Generic Name of Active Ingredients	Content Composition[a]			
			Oils	Water Miscible Solvents	Other Ingredients	Surface Active Agents
Aquasol A		Retinol (Vitamin A)				Polysorbate 80
Depakene		Valproic acid	Corn oil			
VePesid		Etoposide (VP-16)		Polyethylene glycol-400	Citric acid, water	
Lanoxicaps		Digoxin		Propylene glycol, polyethylene glycol 400, and ethanol		
Zantac		Ranitidine HCl	Coconut oil and triglycerides			
Oxsoralen-Ultra		Methoxsalen	Content composition is not available			
Adalat	10 mg	Nifedipine	Peppermint	Polyethylene glycol-400	Na saccharine	
	20 mg					
Norvir		Ritonavir	Caprilic/capric triglycerides	Propylene glycol and ethanol	Citric acid	Polyglycolyzed glycerides, polysorbate 80
Nimotop		Nimodipine	Peppermint oil	Polyethylene glycol 400		
Unisom SleepGel		Diphenhydramine HCl		Propylene glycol and polyethylene glycol[a]		
Procardia	10 mg	Nifedipine	Peppermint oil	Polyethylene glycol 400, glycerin	Na saccharine	
	20 mg					
Accutane	10 mg	Isotretinoin	Soybean oil, beeswax, hydrogenated soybean and vegetable oils		Na edetate and buthylated hydroxy anisole	
	20 mg					
	40 mg					
Marinol	2.5 mg	Dronabinol (δ-9-THC)	Sesame oil			
	5 mg					
	10 mg					
Sandimmune	25 mg	Cyclosporine	Corn oil, Labrafil M 2125 CS	Ethanol		
	50 mg					
	100mg					
Chromogen		Ferrous sulfate, ascorbic acid, cyanocobalamin, and desiccated stomach substance	Content composition is not available			
Doxidan Liqui-Gels		Casanthranol and docusate sodium		Polyethylene Glycol [a]		
Surfak		Docusate calcium	Corn oil			
Ginsana		Standardized ginseng extract	Sunflower oil, beeswax			Lecithin, chlorophyll
Vesanoid		Tretinoin	Beeswax, hyrogenated vegetable oils, hydrogenated soybean oil flakes, and soybean oil		Disodium edetate and buthylated hydroxy anisole	
Correctol Stool Softner		Docusate sodium		Polyethylene glycol - 400,and propylene glycol		
Neoral	25 mg	Cyclosporine	Corn oil	Propylene glycol and ethanol	DL-(alpha) tocopherol	Polyoxyl 40 hydrogenated castor oil
	100 mg					

(Continued)

TABLE 21.1 (*Continued*)

The Content Composition of Commercially Available Products

Product	Generic Name of Active Ingredients	Content Composition[a]			
		Oils	Water Miscible Solvents	Other Ingredients	Surface Active Agents
PhosChol 900	Phosphatidyl-choline	Content composition is not available			
Nytol	Diphenhydramine HCl		Polyethylene glycol*		
Protegra	Antioxidant vitamins and mineral supplement	Cottonseed oil, soybean oil, beeswax		Calcium phosphate	
Alka-Seltzer Plus	Various analgezics and decongestants		Polyethylene glycol*	Potassium acetate and povidone	
One -A-Day Antioxidant Plus	Antioxidant vitamins and mineral supplement	Soybean oil, beeswax, partially hydrogenated vegetable oils			Lecithin
One -A-Day Garlic	Garlic oil macerate			Xylose	
Vicks DayQuil	Various analgesics and decongestants		Propylene glycol and polyethylene glycol*	Povidone	
Vicks NyQuil	Various analgesics and decongestants plus doxylamine succinate		Propylene glycol and polyethylene glycol*	Povidone	
Phayzyme-125	Simethicone	Soybean oil, yellow wax, hydrogenated soybean oil, and vegetable shortening			Lecithin and polysorbate 80
Robitussin Night-Time Cold	Acetaminophen, pseudoephedrine HCl, dextromethorphan HBr, and doxylamine succinate		Propylene glycol and polyethylene glycol*	Povidone, sodium acetate, and	Sorbitan*
Robitussin Severe	Guaifenesin and pseudoephedrine HCl		Propylene glycol and, polyethylene glycol*	Povidone and sodium acetate	Sorbitan*
Robitussin C&C LiquiGels	Guaifenesin, pseudoephedrine HCl, dextromethorphan HBr		Propylene glycol and polyethylene glycol*	Povidone and sodium acetate	Sorbitan*
Robitussin C&C Flu	Acetaminophen, guaifenesin pseudoephedrine HCl, and dextromethorphan HBr		Propylene glycol and polyethylene glycol*	Povidone and sodium acetate	Sorbitan*
Dimetapp Liqui-Gels	Brompheniramine maleate phenylpropanolamine, HCl		Propylene glycol and polyethylene glycol*	Povidone and sodium acetate	Sorbitan*
Dimetapp C&C Liqui-Gels	Brompheniramine Maleate, Phenylpropanolamine HCl, and Dextromethorphan HBr		Propylene glycol and polyethylene glycol*	Povidone and sodium acetate	Sorbitan*
Gas-X	Simethicone				
Sleepinal	Diphenhydramine HCl		Propylene glycol and polyethylene glycol 400	Povidone	
Unique E	Mixed tocopherols				
SuperEPA	Omega-3				
Benadryl Day-Free	Diphenhydramine HCl				
Nutr-E-Sol	Vitamine E				
Breath Plus	Parsley seed oil, peppermint oil, vitamin E, and beta carotene	Sunflower oil		Chlorophyll	

(Continued)

TABLE 21.1 (*Continued*)

The Content Composition of Commercially Available Products

Product		Generic Name of Active Ingredients	Content Composition[#]			
			Oils	Water Miscible Solvents	Other Ingredients	Surface Active Agents
CoQuinone		Coenzyme Q₁₀	Alpha Lipoic acid	The rest of the content composition and entire shell composition are not known		
KALETRA		Lopinavir and ritonavir	Oleic acid	Propylene glycol		Polyoxyl 35 castor oil
TARGRETIN®		Bexarotene		Polyethylene Glycol 400	Povidone butylated hydroxyanisole	Polysorbate 20
Rocaltrol	0.25 mcg	Calcitriol =synthetic vitamin D	Fractionated triglyceride of coconut oil		Butylated hydroxyanisole and butylated hydroxytoluene	
	0.5 mcg					
Prometrium®	100 mg	Micronized progesterone	Peanut oil			Lecithin
	200 mg					
Chromagen®		Ferrochel® (elemental iron)** Ester-C®***, vitamin B₁₂ (cyanocobalamin), and dessicated stomach substance	Soybean oil, yellow beeswax			Lecithin
Chromagen® FA		Ferrochel® (elemental iron)** Ester-C®***, vitamin B₁₂ (cyanocobalamin), and folic acid	Soybean oil, yellow beeswax			Lecithin
Chromagen® FORTE		Ferrochel® (elemental iron)** ferrous fumarate (elemental iron), Ester-C®***, vitamin B₁₂ (cyanocobalamin), and Folic Acid	Soybean oil, yellow beeswax			Lecithin
Hectorol®	0.5 mcg	Doxercalciferol®	Fractionated triglyceride of coconut oil.	Ethanol	Butylated hydroxyanisole	
	2.5 mcg					
Agenerase	50 mg	Amprenavir	D-alpha tocopheryl polyethylene glycol 1000 succinate (TPGS)	Polyethylene Glycol 400 and propylene glycol		
	150 mg					
Primacare®		Omega-3 fatty acids, linoleic acid, linolenic acid, cholecalciferol and dl-alpha-tocopheryl acetate, and calcium carbonate	Natural wax and natural oils,			Other ingredients
PrimaCare® One		Omega-3 fatty acids, linoleic acid, linolenic acid, folic acid, pyridoxine HCl, Ester-C ® ***, cholecalciferol, dl-alpha-tocopheryl acetate, calcium carbonate carbonyl iron	Vegetable shortening, soybean oil, yellow beeswax			Lecithin
Amnesteem®	10 mg	Isotretinoin	Yellow wax, hydrogenated vegetable oil, and soybean oil		Butylated hydroxyanisole, and edetate disodium	
	20 mg					
	40 mg					
Fortovase®		Saquinavir	Medium chain mono- and diglycerides		Povidone and dl-alpha tocopherol	
Avodart™		Dutasteride	Mono-and diglycerides of caprylic/capric acid		Butylated hydroxytoluene	
CM Plex		Proprietary fatty acid blend				
Nephrocaps®		Ascorbic acid, folate, niacinamide, thiamine mononitrate, riboflavin, pyridoxine HCl, cyanocobalamin, calcium pantothenate, and biotin				
Quickgels®		Diphenhydramine hydrochloride		Polyethylene glycol*		
Maximum Strength Gas Aid		Simethicone	Peppermint oil			

(*Continued*)

TABLE 21.1 (*Continued*)
The Content Composition of Commercially Available Products

Product		Generic Name of Active Ingredients	Content Composition*			
			Oils	Water Miscible Solvents	Other Ingredients	Surface Active Agents
Benadryl® Dye-Free Allergy Liqui-Gels®		Diphenhydramine HCl		Polyethylene glycol 400		
Maximum Strength Unisom Sleepgels®		Diphenhydramine HCl		Polyethylene glycol 400 and propylene glycol	Polyvinyl acetate phthalate	
Vicks NyQuil LiquiCaps, Multi-Symptom Cold/Flu Relief		Acetaminophen, dextromethorphan HBr, doxylamine succinate, and pseudoephedrine HCl		Polyethylene glycol and propylene glycol	Povidone	
Vicks DayQuil Multi Symptom Cold/Flu Relief LIQUICAP®		Acetaminophen, dextromethorphan hbr, and pseudoephedrine HCL		Polyethylene glycol and propylene glycol	Povidone	
Alka-Seltzer Plus Cold Liqui-Gels		Acetaminophen, chlorpheniramine maleate, and pseudophedrine HCl		Polyethylene glycol and propylene glycol	Povidone, polyvinyl acetate phthalate, and potassium acetate	
Alka-Seltzer Plus Cold & Cough Liqui-Gels		Acetaminophen, chlorpheniramine maleate, dextromethorphan HBr, and pseudophedrine HCl		Polyethylene glycol and propylene glycol	Povidone, polyvinyl acetate phthalate, and potassium acetate	
Alka-Seltzer Plus Night-Time Cold Liqui-Gels		Acetaminophen, dextromethorphan HBr doxylamine succinate, and pseudophedrine HCl		Polyethylene glycol and propylene glycol	Povidone, polyvinyl acetate phthalate, and potassium acetate	
Phillip's® Liqui-Gels®		Docusate sodium		Polyethylene glycol and propylene glycol	Methylparaben, propylparaben, and shellac	
Dulcolax®		Docusate sodium		Polyethylene glycol and propylene glycol		
Ultra Strength PHAZYME®		Simethicone				
Gas-X Extra Strength		Simethicone				
Gas-X Maximum Strength		Simethicone				
Gas-X with Maalox Extra Strength		Simethicone and calcium carbonate				
Optimum Omega (Pharmanex) Epa and Dha Fish Oils		Marine lipid concentrate, D-alpha tocopherol), and deodorized garlic oil				
Hytrin	1 mg	Terazosin hydrochloride	Mineral oil	Propylene glycol	Povidone	
	2 mg					
	5 mg					
	10 mg					
Alkyrol	250 mg	Aalkylglycerols				
	500 mg					

* Type is not provided.
** Ferrochel® (ferrous *bis*-glycinate chelate) is a registered trademark of Albion International, Inc., Clearfield, Utah.
*** Ester-C® is a patented pharmaceutical grade material consisting of calcium ascorbate and calcium threonate. Ester-C® is a licensed trademark of Zila Nutraceuticals, Inc.
@ synthetic vitamin D_2 analog.

Source: Reproduced from Physicians' Desk Reference, Medical Economics Company, Inc., Montvale, NJ, 2006.

TABLE 21.2

The Shell Composition of Commercially Available Products

Product		Generic Name	Parabens		Gelatin	Glycerin	Color		TiO₂	Others Ingredients
			Methyl	Propyl			FD&C	Others		
Aquasol A		Retinol (Vitamin A)	X	X	X	X	Red #40			Ethy vanillin
Depakene		Valproic acid	X	X	X	X	Yellow #6	Iron oxide	X	
VePesid		Etoposide (VP-16)	X	X	X	X		Iron oxide	X	Sorbitol
Lanoxicaps		Digoxin	X	X	X	X	Blue #1			Sorbitol
Zantac		Ranitidine HCl	X(?)	X(?)			Yellow #6 Blue #1 Red #40		X	Sorbitol
Oxsoralen-Ultra		Methoxsalen	Shell composition is not available							
Adalat		Nifedipine			X	X	Yellow #6	Iron oxide		Inert ingredients
Norvir		Ritonavir	Shell composition is not available							
Nimotop		Nimodipine			X	X			X	
Unisom SleepGel		Diphenhydramine HCl			X	X	Blue #1		X	Sorbitol Pharmaceutical glaze
Procardia		Nifedipine					Yellow #6	Iron oxide		Inert ingredients
Accutane	10 mg	Isotretinoin	X	X	X	X		Iron oxide	X	
	20 mg						Red #3 Blue #1		X	
	40 mg						Yellow #6 and # 10		X	
Marinol	2.5 mg	Dronabinol (δ-9-THC)	X	X	X	X			X	
	5 mg						Yellow #6			
	10 mg						Yellow #6			
Sandimmune	25& 100	Cyclosporine			X	X		Red iron oxide	X	Sorbitol
	50 mg							Yellow iron oxide		
Chromogen		Ferrous sulfate, ascorbic acid, cyanocobalamin, and desiccated stomach substance	Shell composition is not available							
Doxidan Liqui-Gels		Casanthranol and docusate sodium			X	X	Blue #1 Red #40		X	Sorbitol
Surfak		Docusate calcium	X	X	X	X	Blue #1 Red #40			Sorbitol Other ingredients
Atromid-S		Clofibrate			X		Blue #1 Red #28 Red #40 Yellow #6	D&C Red # 28 Red #30 Yellow #10		
Ginsana		Standardized ginseng extract			X	X				Chlorophyll
Vesanoid		Tretinoin	X	X	X	X		Red and yellow Iron oxide	X	

(Continued)

TABLE 21.2 (*Continued*)
The Shell Composition of Commercially Available Products

Product	Generic Name	Parabens Methyl	Propyl	Gelatin	Glycerin	Color FD&C	Others	TiO₂	Others Ingredients
Correctol Stool Softner	Docusate sodium					X	X	Yellow #6 Red #40 D&C Red #33	Sorbitol
PhosChol 900	Phosphatidyl-choline	Shell composition is not available							
Nytol	Diphenhydramine HCl			X	X				Sorbitol Edible ink
Protegra	Antioxidant vitamins and mineral supplement			X	X	Red #40 Blue #1		X	Edible ink (?)
Alka-Seltzer Plus	Various analgezics and decongestants			X	X		Artificial Colors	X	Sorbitol
One -A-Day Antioxidant Plus	Antioxidant vitamin and mineral supplement nutrition facts			X	X	Yellow #5	Artificial Colors	X	
One -A-Day Garlic	Garlic oil macerate			X	X				Sorbitol
Vicks DayQuil	Various analgezics and decongestants			X	X	Red #40 Yellow #6			Sorbitol
Vicks NyQuil	Various analgezics and decongestants plus doxylamine succinate			X	X	Yellow #10 Blue #1			Sorbitol (?)
Phayzyme-125	Simethicone	X	X	X	X	Red #40		X	
Robitussin Night-Time Cold	Acetaminophen, pseudoephedrine HCl, dextromethorphan HBr, and doxylamine succinate			X	X	Green #3 Yellow #6	D&C Green #5 and Yellow #10	X	Mannito, sorbitol Pharmaceutical glaze
Robitussin Severe	Guaifenesin and pseudoephedrine HCl			X	X	Green #3		X	Mannito, sorbitol Pharmaceutical glaze
Robitussin C&C Liqui-Gels	Guaifenesin, pseudoephedrine HCl, dextromethorphan HBr			X	X	Blue #1 Red #40		X	Mannito, sorbitol Pharmaceutical glaze
Robitussin C&C Flu	Acetaminophen, guaifenesin pseudoephedrine HCl, and dextromethorphan HBr			X	X	Red #40 Yellow #10			Mannito, sorbitol
Dimetapp Liqui-Gels	Brompheniramine maleate phenylpropanolamine, HCl			X	X	Red #33		X	Mannito, sorbitol Pharmaceutical glaze
Dimetapp C&C Liqui-Gels	Brompheniramine maleate, phenylpropanolamine HCl, and dextromethorphan HBr			X	X	Red #40		X	Mannito, sorbitol Pharmaceutical glaze
Chromogen Forte	Ferrous fumarate, ascorbic acid, folic acid, and cyanocobalamin	Shell composition is not available							
Chromogen FA	Ferrous fumarate, ascorbic acid, folic acid, and cyanocobalamin	Shell composition is not available							
Neoral	Cyclosporine			X	X		Iron oxide black	X	Other ingredients
Gas-X	Simethicone			X	X	Blue #1 Red #40 Yellow #10		X	Sorbitol Pepermint oil
Correctol Stool Softner	Docusate sodium			X	X	Yellow #6 Red #40	D&C Red #33		Sorbitol

(*Continued*)

TABLE 21.2 (*Continued*)
The Shell Composition of Commercially Available Products

Product	Generic Name	Shell Composition								
		Parabens				Color				
		Methyl	Propyl	Gelatin	Glycerin	FD&C	Others	TiO_2	Others Ingredients	
Sleepinal	Diphenhydramine HCl			X	X	Blue #1 (?) Green #3 (?)	D&C Yellow #10		Sorbitol	
Unique E	Mixed tocopherols	Shell composition is not available								
Nutr-E-Sol	Vitamin E	Shell composition is not available								
SuperEPA	Omega-3	Shell composition is not available								
Benadryl Day-Free	Diphenhydramine HCl			X	X				Sorbitol	
Breath Plus	Sunflower oil, parsley seed oil, peppermint oil, chlorophyll, vitamin E and beta carotene	Shell composition is not available								
CoQuinone	Coenzyme Q_{10}	Shell composition is not available								
KALETRA	Lopinavir and ritonavir			X	X	Yellow No. 6		X	Sorbitol	Water
TARGRETIN®	Bexarotene			X	X			X	Sorbitol	
Rocaltrol 0.25 mcg	Calcitriol/synthetic vitamin D	X	X	X	X	Yellow No. 6		X		
Rocaltrol 0.5 mcg						Yellow No. 6, Red No. 3				
Prometrium® 100 mg	Micronized progesterone			X	X	Yellow No. 10, Red No. 40		X		
Prometrium® 200 mg						Yellow No. 6, Yellow No. 10				
Chromagen®	Ferrochel®(elemental iron) ** Ester-C®***, vitamin B_{12} (cyanocobalamin), and dessicated stomach substance	X	X	X	X	Yellow No. 6, Red No. 40, Blue No. 1		X		
Chromagen® FA	Ferrochel® (elemental iron) ** Ester-C®***, vitamin B_{12} (cyanocobalamin), and folic acid	X	X	X	X	Yellow No.10, Red No. 40, Blue No. 1		X		Black Ferric Oxide
Chromagen® FORTE	Ferrochel® (elemental iron) ** ferrous fumarate (elemental iron), Ester-C®***, vitamin B_{12} (cyanocobalamin), and folic acid	X	X	X	X	Yellow No. 6, Red No. 40, Blue No. 1		X		
Hectorol® 0.5 mcg	Doxercalciferol@			X	X	Yellow No.10		X		
Hectorol® 2.5 mcg						Yellow No.10, Red No. 40,				
Agenerase 50 mg	Amprenavir			X	X			X	Sorbitol and sorbitan solution	
Agenerase 150 mg										
PrimaCare® One	Omega-3 fatty acids, linoleic acid, linolenic acid, folic acid, pyridoxine HCl, ester-C® ***, Cholecalciferol, dl-alpha-tocopheryl acetate, calcium carbonate carbonyl iron	X	X	X	X	Blue No. 1	Red No. 33	X		
Amnesteem® 10 mg	Isotretinoin			X	X					Red iron oxide paste and black ink
Amnesteem® 20 mg								X		Red iron oxide paste, yellow iron oxide paste, and black ink
Amnesteem® 40 mf								X		Red iron oxide paste, yellow iron oxide paste, and black ink
Fortovase®	Saquinavir			X	X			X		Red and yellow iron oxide
Avodart™	Dutasteride			X	X					Ferric oxide (yellow)

(*Continued*)

TABLE 21.2 (*Continued*)
The Shell Composition of Commercially Available Products

Product		Generic Name	Parabens Methyl	Propyl	Gelatin	Glycerin	Color FD&C	Others	TiO$_2$	Others Ingredients	
CM Plex		Proprietary fatty acid blend	Shell composition is not available								
Nephrocaps®		Ascorbic acid, folate, niacinamide, thiamine mononitrate, riboflavin, pyridoxine HCl, cyanocobalamin, calcium pantothenate, and biotin	Shell composition is not available								
Quickgels®		Diphenhydramine hydrochloride			X	X	Red No. 40, Blue No. 1		X	Sorbitol	
Maximum Strength Gas Aid		Simethicone			X	X	Blue No. 1, Red No.40		X		
Benadryl® Dye-Free Allergy Liqui-Gels®		Diphenhydramine HCl			X	X				Sorbitol	
Maximum Strength Unisom Sleepgels®		Diphenhydramine HCl			X	X	Blue No. 1		X	Sorbitol	
Vicks NyQuil LiquiCaps, Multi-Symptom Cold/Flu Relief		Acetaminophen, dextromethorphan HBr, doxylamine succinate, and pseudoephedrine HCl			X	X	Blue No. 1		X	Sorbitol	
Vicks DayQuil Multi-Symptom Cold/Flu Relief LIQUICAP®		Acetaminophen, dextromethorphan HBr, and pseudoephedrine HCl			X	X	Yellow No.6, Red No. 40			Sorbitol	
Alka-Seltzer Plus Cold Liqui-Gels		Acetaminophen, pseudoephedrine Hcl, and dextromethorphan HBr			X	X	Red No. 40		X	Sorbitol	
Alka-Seltzer Plus Cold & Cough Liqui-Gels		Acetaminophen, chlorpheniramine maleate, dextromethorphan HBr, and pseudoephedrine HCl			X	X	Blue No. 1	Red No. 33	X	Sorbitol	
Alka-Seltzer Plus Night-Time Cold Liqui-Gels		Acetaminophen, dextromethorphan HBr doxylamine succinate, and pseudoephedrine HCl			X	X	Blue No. 1	Yellow No.10	X	Sorbitol	
Phillip's® Liqui-Gels®		Docusate sodium	X	X	X	X	Blue No. 2		X	Sorbitol	
Dulcolax®		Docusate sodium			X	X	Red No. 40, Yellow No 6	Yellow No.10		Sorbitol	
Ultra Strength PHAZYME®		Simethicone			X	X	Yellow No 6				
Gas-X Extra Strength		Simethicone			X	X	Blue No. 1, Red No. 40	Yellow No.10	X	Sorbital	
Gas-X Maximum Strength		Simethicone			X	X	Blue No. 1, Red No. 40			Sorbital	
Gas-X with Maalox Extra Strength		Simethicone and calcium carbonate			X	X	Blue No. 1	Red No. 28	X	Sorbital	SiO$_2$
Optimum Omega (Pharmanex) Epa & Dha Fish Oils		Marine lipid concentrate, D-Alpha Tocopherol), and Deodorized Garlic Oil	Shell composition is not available								
Hytrin	1 mg	Terazosin hydrochloride	X	X	X	X		Iron Oxide	X	Vanillin	
	2 mg							D&C Yellow #10			
	5 mg						Red #40	D&C Red #28			
	10 mg						Blue #1				
ALKYROL	250 mg	Alkylglycerols	Shell composition is not available								
	500 mg										

* Type is not provided.

* * Ferrochel® (ferrous *bis*-glycinate chelate) is a registered trademark of Albion International, Inc., Clearfield, Utah.

* * * Ester-C® is a patented pharmaceutical grade material consisting of calcium ascorbate and calcium threonate. Ester-C® is a licensed trademark of Zila Nutraceuticals, Inc.

@ synthetic vitamin D$_2$ analog.

(?) Denotes that the ingredient may exist in the shell composition.

Source: From Physicians' Desk Reference, Medical Economics Company, Inc. Montvale , NJ, 2006.

TABLE 21.3

Solubility of Penclomedine in Various Vehicles at 25°C

Vehicle	Solubility (mg/mL)
0.1 N HCl	<1
0.1 N NaOH	<1
Acetate buffer (pH 4)	<1
Carbonate buffer (pH 9)	<1
Corn oil	174
Neobee M-5[a]	224
Olive oil	163
Tributyrin	289
Peanut oil	165
Safflower oil	186
Soybean oil	177
Soybean oil with 1% tween	172
Sunflower oil	177
Trioctanoin	230
Water	<1

[a] A fractionated coconut oil.

In another study, Tindal and Asgarzadeh (2006) prepared small-scale batches using a proprietary production process to minimize the drug losses that normally result in large-scale batches. Recently, a New Drug Application (NDA) for Rayaldee®, an oral soft capsule, has been approved by the U.S. Food and Drug Administration (FDA). Rayaldee capsules contain vitamin D3 analog and are used for the treatment of secondary hyperparathyroidism in adults. In capsule shells of Rayaldee contain modified starch.

Stella et al. (1978) reported formulation of a hydrophobic amine into a soft gelatin capsule using oleic acid as a solvent. Initially, the solubility of the drug was determined in oleic acid. It was found that the drug was soluble in oleic acid in concentrations up to 23% w/w. The soft gelatin formulation in oleic acid improved bioavailability of this antimalarial drug significantly over the standard hard gelatin capsule formulation. The mean area under the curve (AUC) for hard gelatin capsule formulation was 16% (±10%) of the AUC for soft gelatin capsule formulation in this study conducted in beagle dogs by means of a crossover experimental design (Stella et al., 1978). At the National Cancer Institute, a majority of the molecules under development are hydrophobic in nature (Vishnuvajjala et al., 1994). The solubility and stability of these molecules are determined before dosage form considerations. For example, the solubility of NSC 338720 (Penclomedine) was determined in various vehicles suitable for soft gelatin capsule formulation, which are presented in Table 21.3.

As can be seen, the liquids under consideration are water-immiscible liquids such as vegetable oils (corn oil, peanut oil), long chain triglycerides (trioctanoin), and medium chain triglycerides (Neobee M-5). The solubility of Penclomedine is 150–200 mg/mL in these water-immiscible vehicles, which is convenient for dissolving a maximum amount of drug in minimum amount of vehicle for a given capsule size. A small-scale pilot batch of the product was prepared in representative vehicles—corn oil, trioctanoin, Neobee M-5 in the presence and absence of surfactant Tween 80—and placed on stability at accelerated temperatures. It is possible that there is migration of water from the capsule shell into the cavity during the manufacture of softgel capsules or shelf-life storage, thereby forming a cosolvent containing organic solvent and water resulting in precipitation of a water-insoluble drug in the capsule cavity. The surfactant is sometimes added to aid in the dissolution of active drug in the cosolvent mixture. It also helps in the enhancement of oral bioavailability of the active drug by emulsifying the oil solution in the gastrointestinal tract (Kwong et al., 1994).

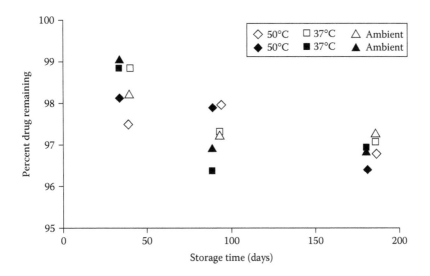

FIGURE 21.5 Long-term stability of concentrated solutions (200 mg/mL) of Penclomedine in Neobee M-5 with (filled symbols) and without 0.5% Tween 80 at various temperatures.

Another important consideration is the stability of the drug at 35°C–40°C because of processing requirements of soft gelatin capsules, fill materials may be heated up to 35°C during encapsulation. The stability data for the pilot scale batch of Penclomedine is presented in Figure 21.5. The data indicate that this drug is fairly stable in various vehicles under consideration. A human Phase I clinical batch in Neobee Oil was produced and its shelf-life surveillance at controlled room temperature has shown 3 years of stability.

Similar developmental studies were conducted for another experimental anti-HIV compound, NSC 629243, a thiocarbamate, by the Developmental Therapeutics Program, NCI (http://dtp.nci.nih.gov). This molecule has very poor water solubility (<1 mg/mL). Solubility studies were conducted to find a suitable solvent for soft gelatin encapsulation. On the basis of the solubility data, sesame oil (64 mg/mL) and Miglyol® (fractionated coconut oil, BP; 140 mg/mL) were chosen for further evaluation. In the case of sesame oil, antioxidants—BHA/BHT mixture and three different concentrations of thioglycolic acids, 0.1%, 0.5%, and 1.0% (v/v)—were evaluated to determine their ability to protect against further degradation of the drug owing to oxidation reaction (Strickley and Anderson, 1993). Similar studies were conducted in Miglyol formulations in the presence of a surfactant and an antioxidant. In these studies, Miglyol formulations did not show any degradation at elevated temperatures when compared with sesame oil formulations. Further studies were performed in actual soft gelatin capsules with two representative formulations—Miglyol alone and sesame oil containing 1.0% (v/v) thioglycolic acid as an antioxidant. In an accelerated stability study conducted for 6 months in soft gelatin capsules formulations, the Miglyol formulation demonstrated superior stability over sesame oil, presumably because it is saturated oil, which affords improved stability against oxidation.

It is also possible to dissolve hydrophobic drugs in water-miscible organic solvents such as polyethylene glycol 400 used with CAI, NSC 609974 (Vishnuvajjala et al., 1994); Gelucire 44/14® (a proprietary solvent that is a mixture of glyceryl and polyethylene glycol 1500 esters of fatty acids); cosolvent mixtures containing various proportions of medium chain triglycerides; polyoxyl 35 castor oil (Cremophor EL®); and polyglycolized glycerides (e.g., commercial formulation of anti-HIV protease inhibitor, ritonavir; PDR 2006). However, some of these excipients can cause migration of water from the soft gelatin capsule shell (water content range 10%–20%) into the capsule cavity, thereby causing precipitation of the active drug substance. Serajuddin et al. (1986) reported that water migration from the shell resulted in crystallization of a water-insoluble drug under development.

One of the solvents commonly used as a pharmaceutical aid for dissolution of hydrophobic drugs is ethanol. However, for drugs to be used in soft gelatin capsules, ethanol cannot be used easily because ethanol diffuses quite readily through soft gelatin films (Moreton and Armstrong, 1995) at a fairly rapid rate. The diffusion is fast enough that most of the ethanol would diffuse out through the drying phase during the manufacture of softgel capsules. Moreton and Armstrong (1998) found that changing the composition of plasticized gelatin gels changes the diffusion coefficient of the gelatin film to ethanol. They showed that replacing glycerol with higher polyols (xylitol or sorbitol) results in substantial reduction in the diffusion coefficient of ethanol. The greatest reduction, 5- to 10-fold, was observed in films with the least amount of moisture.

The compounds that are difficult to formulate in soft gelatin capsules are fairly water-soluble small organic molecules, acids, and bases. These compounds tend to cause migration of water from the shell into the cavity and tend to permeate into the capsule shell, depending on the water content of the shell. Armstrong et al. (1984) studied the aqueous solubility of four different solutes and their relative migration into the capsule shell from an isopropyl myristate formulation. They concluded that with an increase in the aqueous solubility, the fraction of active drug migrating into the capsule shell increased as well. In the case of acids and bases, Patel et al. (1989a, 1989b, 1992) showed that it is possible to neutralize them using a corresponding base or acid. The resulting salt or ester may then be formulated in a hydrophilic solvent such as polyethylene glycol.

In all of the preceding cases, it is apparent that one has to be aware of the dynamic equilibrium that exists between the soft gelatin capsule contents and the capsule shell during the manufacturing process of soft gelatin capsules (e.g., in the drying of capsules) and long-term storage. It is possible for the contents of the formulation to migrate into the shell, and/or water may permeate from the capsule shell into the capsule cavity.

In addition, one may consider the addition of an antioxidant since soft gelatin capsule shell is permeable to oxygen, resulting in oxidation of oxygen-sensitive, active drug substance. However, the oxidation potential should be confirmed in the preformulation *workup* of the molecule. In a study conducted to evaluate the effects of various formulation and environmental parameters on the oxygen permeability of gelatin film, Hom et al. (1975) concluded that relative humidity and plasticizer concentration affect oxygen permeability the most. The oxygen permeability of the gelatin film made with 40%–50% glycerin increased with increasing relative humidity. The oxygen permeability increased 10-fold by raising the relative humidity from 47% to 80% at room temperature. In general, therefore, it is recommended that soft gelatin capsules be stored in a cool, dry place for maximum stability.

CONTROL AND TESTING

Quality control of the in-process and final product is critical for the overall presentation of any dosage form, and production of soft gelatin capsules is no exception.

IN-PROCESS CONTROLS

Some of the in-process controls such as seal tests, shell-thickness checks, fill weights, and shell weights are done during the encapsulation process to decide the fate of the batch and the possibility of taking any corrective action (Stanley, 1986). Weight variation, determination of the content weight (by difference of the gross weight and the weight of the shell), and shell-thickness measurement are among the principal in-process tests.

BATCH-RELEASE TESTS

The quality control release testing of the batch can be divided into physical, chemical, and microbiological tests. Obviously, some of these tests are product specific, such as chemical tests; however, a few tests are performed owing to the nature of the dosage form, for example, microbiological testing of soft gelatin capsule shells. The description of some of these tests is included for information only, because the soft gelatin capsule manufacturers are well equipped and well trained to perform these tests on a regular basis.

A description of appearance that may be an indication of batch-to-batch variability will also provide any indication of change during stability studies, for example, a *dull* versus *shiny*, *polished* versus *unpolished*, or *spotty*, and other characteristics. Determination of *leakers* indicates the physical integrity of the soft gelatin capsules, generally reported as *percent leakers*. A vacuum leakage test determines the seal strength, and it is generally a predictive stress test. In this test, the intact soft gelatin capsules are placed under vacuum for 4 h at room temperature and the number of leakers determined. Depending on the percentage of leakers, the batch will be accepted or rejected.

Another physical test that is routinely performed for soft gelatin capsules is for *firmness*. The test is, usually conducted by trained individuals, involves gently pressing the final dosage form in between the fingers and comparing the resulting deformation with a suitable *control*. This is a qualitative test and subject to interpretation, depending on the training and experience of the individual performing the test. Vemuri (1984), by describing the use of a commercial universal testing machine (Instron Model 1122, Instron Engineering Corporation, Canton, Mass.), concluded that the mechanical strength for soft gelatin capsules stored in polystyrene containers decreases continuously over a 20-weeks storage period as indicated by the decrease in the *deformation force*. Moreover, product stored in polystyrene containers gained about five times as much moisture as product stored in glass containers. This moisture gain resulted in decreased firmness or increased *stickiness* of the capsules. When the data obtained by the testing instrument was analyzed against the sensory evaluation, a poor correlation coefficient was obtained. Therefore, it is recommended that the subjective interpretation be avoided by the use of an appropriate mechanical instrument to measure the capsule firmness initially and during the shelf-life storage.

Hakata et al. (1981, 1994) studied the effect of storage temperature on the physicochemical properties of soft gelatin capsule shells. They concluded that capsules stored at 40°C disintegrated much slower than those stored at 25°C. The prolonged disintegration time was correlated with increase in the gel strength of the shells. It has been shown by other investigators (Khalil et al., 1974; Baes, 1981; Lalla and Bhat, 1995) that when soft gelatin capsules are stored at extreme temperatures, either high or low, the dissolution characteristics change owing to changes in the gel structure of the shell or owing to the interaction of the active drug with the softgel capsule shell. Some of these changes can be averted by judicious selection of fill composition and shell formulation as reported by Shah et al. (1992). By adding as much as 12.5% glycerin to the fill composition along with polyethylene glycol (PEG) 400 and using glycerin and sorbitol as plasticizer in the shell composition, the shell elasticity can be improved remarkably over long-term storage.

Most of the soft gelatin capsules' shell compositions contain parabens as preservatives since gelatin is intrinsically subject to microbial degradation. Wild et al. (1993) have shown that soft gelatin capsules contain low moisture and do not support microbial activity or growth. Their recommendation is that soft gelatin capsules as a dosage form for oral and topical application can be formulated without parabens as a preservative.

In addition to shell elasticity and microbial challenge tests, disintegration and dissolution tests may be performed, depending on the pharmacopoeial requirements for a given product. A disintegration test may have a different meaning with respect to soft gelatin capsules than its definition related to tablets. Since the shell does not bear any medication and most of the content formulations are physically in liquid state, it is our experience that disintegration is defined as *the time to leak the content*. The endpoint for the disintegration test can be set depending on the water miscibility of the formulation vehicle and can be either presence of the oil on the surface of the media or the presence of cloudy medium owing to water immiscibility of the softgel capsule vehicle.

Besides the United States Pharmacopoeia (USP) methods for dissolution, one should be aware of the other methods available for measuring dissolution and correlating it with *in vivo* bioavailability. One such method is the rotating dialysis cell method as reported by Takahashi et al. (1994, 1995). In their studies, rotating dialysis cell method provided a better correlation with *in vivo* blood concentration of a given model drug (ibuprofen) when compared with paddle-dissolution method as given in the Japanese Pharmacopoeia (JP). The paddle method given in JP is similar to the dissolution method given in the USP.

REFERENCES

Agrosi, M., S. Mischiatti, P. C. Harrasser, and D. Savio. 2000. Oral bioavailability of active principles from herbal products in humans. A study on Hypericum perforatum extracts using the soft gelatin capsule technology. *Phytomedicine*, 7(6): 455–462.

Armstrong, N. A., K. C. James, and W. K. L. Pugh. 1984. Drug migration into soft gelatin capsule shells and its effect on *in vitro* availability. *J. Pharm. and Pharm.*, 36: 361–365.

Augsburger, L. L. 1996. Hard and soft shell capsules, in *Modern Pharmaceutics*, 3rd ed. (G. S. Banker and C. T. Rhodes, Eds.), New York: Marcel Decker, pp. 395–440.

Baes, E. A. 1981. Soft shell capsules. *Manuf. Chem.*, 52: 33–34.

Benza, H. I. and W. L. L. Munyendo. 2011. A review of progress and challenges in soft gelatin capsules formulations for oral administration. *Int. J. Pharm. Sci. Rev. and Res.*, 10: 20–24.

Cole, E. T., D. Cadé, and H. Benameur. 2008. Challenges and opportunities in the encapsulation of liquid and semi-solid formulations into capsules for oral administration. *Adv. Drug Del. Rev.*, 60: 747–756.

Developmental Therapeutics Program, National Cancer Institute, National Institutes of Health, http://dtp.nci.nih.gov.

Ebert, W. R. 1977. Soft elastic gelatin capsules: A unique dosage form. *Pharm. Tech.*, 1(10): 44.

Gullapalli, R. P. 2010. Soft gelatin capsules (softgels). *J. Pharm. Sci.*, 99: 4107–4148.

Hakata, T., H. Sato, Y. Watanabe, and M. Matsumoto. 1994. Effect of storage temperature on the physicochemical properties of soft gelatin capsule shells. *Chem. Pharm. Bull.*, 42: 1496–1500.

Hakata, T., K. Yasuda, and H. Okano. 1981. Effect of storage temperature on disintegration time of soft gelatin capsules. *Arch. Pr. Pharm.*, *Yaku.*, 41: 276–281.

Hom, F. S., S. A. Veresh, and W. R. Ebert. 1975. Soft gelatin capsules. 2. Oxygen permeability study of capsule shells. *J. Pharm. Sci.*, 64: 851–857.

Jones, W. J. and J. J. Francis. 2000. Softgels: Consumer perceptions and market impact relative to other oral dosage forms. *Adv. Ther.*, 17(5): 213–221.

Khalil, S. A. H., L. M. M. Ali, and A. M. M. A. Khalek. 1974. Effects of aging and relative humidity on drug release. Part 1. Chloramphenicol capsules. *Pharm. Technol.*, 29: 36–37.

Kwong, E. C., P. L. Lamarche, G. R. Down, S. A. McClintock, and M. L. Cotton. 1994. Formulation assessment of MK-886, a poorly water-soluble drug, in the beagle dog. *Int. J. Pharm.*, 103: 259–265.

Lalla, J. K. and S. U. Bhat. 1995. Protracted disintegration of hematinic capsules in soft gelatin shells. Part 1. Gelatin-mineral interactions. *Ind. Drugs*, 32: 320–327.

Lissy, M., R. Scallion, D. D. Stiff, and K. Moore. 2010. Pharmacokinetic comparison of an oral diclofenac potassium liquid-filled soft gelatin capsule with a diclofenac potassium tablet. *Exp. Op. Pharm.*, 11: 701–708.

Moreton, R. C. and N. A. Armstrong. 1995. Design and use of an apparatus for measuring diffusion through glycerogelatin films. *Int. J. Pharm.*, 122: 79–89.

Moreton, R. C. and N. A. Armstrong. 1998. The effect of film composition on the diffusion of ethanol through soft gelatin films. *Int. J. Pharm.*, 161: 123–131.

Patel, M. S., F. S. Morton, and H. Seager. 1989a. Advances in softgel formulation technology. Part 1. *Man. Chem.*, 60: 26–28.

Patel, M. S., F. S. Morton, and H. Seager. 1989b. Softgel technology. *Man. Chem.*, 60: 47.

Patel, M. S., F. S. Morton, H. Seager, and D. Howard. 1992. Factors affecting the chemical stability of carboxylic acid drugs in enhanced solubility system (ESS) softgel formulations based on polyethylene glycol (PEG). *Drug Dev. Ind. Pharm.*, 18: 1–19.

Proietti, S., G. Carlomagno, S. Dinicola, and M. Bizzarri. 2014. Soft gel capsules improve melatonin's bioavailability in humans. *Ex. Op. Dr. Met. & Tox.*, 10: 1193–1198.

Rakucewicz, J. 1986. *Soft Elastic Gelatin Capsule Manufacturing: The Globex Story.* Dear Park, NY: Kinematics & Control Corp.

Reddy, G., M. Muthukumaran, and B. Krishnamoorthy. 2013. Soft gelatin capsules-present and future prospective as a pharmaceutical dosage forms—A review. *Int. J. Adv. Pharm. Gen Res.*, 1: 20–29.

Reich, G. 2004. Formulation and physical properties of soft capsules, in *Pharmaceutical Capsules*, 2nd ed. (F. Podczek and B. E. Jones Eds.), London: Pharmaceutical Press, pp. 201–212.

Savio, D., P. C. Harrasser, and G. Basso. 1998. Softgel capsule technology as an enhancer device for the absorption of natural principles in humans. A bioavailability cross-over randomised study on silybin. *Arz.-Fors.*, 48: 1104–1106.

Serajuddin, A. T. M., P. C. Sheen, and M. A. Augustine. 1986. Water migration from soft gelatin capsule shell to fill material and its effect on drug solubility. *J. Pharm. Sci.*, 75: 62–64.

Shah, N. H., D. Stiel, M. H. Infeld, A. S. Railkar, and M. Patrawala. 1992. Elasticity of soft gelatin capsules containing polyethylene glycol 400-quantitation and resolution. *Pharm. Tech.*, 16: 126.

Stanley, J. P. 1986. Capsules part two, soft gelatin capsules, in *The Theory and Practice of Industrial Pharmacy*, 3rd ed. (L. Lochman, H. A. Leiberman, and J. L. Kanig, Eds.), Philadelphia, PA: Lea & Febiger, pp. 398–412.

Stella, V., J. Haslam, N. Yata, H. Okada, and S. Lindebaum. 1978. Enhancement of bioavailability of a hydrophobic amine antimalarial by formulation with oleic acid in a soft gelatin capsule. *J. Pharm. Sci.*, 67(10): 1375–1377.

Strickley, R. and B. Anderson. 1993. Solubilization and stabilization of an anti-HIV thiocarbamate, NSC 629243, for parenteral delivery using extemporaneous emulsions. *Pharm. Res.*, 10: 1076–1082.

Stroud, N., K. Tanner, R. Shelley, E. Youngblood, D. Kiyali, and S. McKee. 2006. Development of novel, soft capsules containing semi-solid fill formulations. AAPS Annual Meeting & Expectation, San Antonio, TX, poster presentation.

Sullivan, T. J., J. L. Walter, R. F. Kouba, and D. C. Maiwald. 1986. Bioavailability of a new oral methoxsalen formulation: A serum concentration and photosensitivity response study. *Arch. Derm.*, 122: 768–771.

Takahashi, M., M. Mochizuki, K. Wada, T. Itoh, and M. Goto. 1994. Studies on dissolution tests of soft gelatin capsules. Part 5. Rotating dialysis cell method. *Chem. Pharm. Bull.*, 42: 1672–1675.

Takahashi, M., H. Yuasa, Y. Kanaya, and M. Uchiyama. 1995. Studies on dissolution tests for soft gelatin capsules by the rotating dialysis cell (RDC) method. Part 6. Preparation and evaluation of ibuprofen soft gelatin capsule. *Chem. Pharm. Bull.*, 43: 1398–1401.

Thomson, P. D. R. 2006. *Physicians' Desk Reference*. Montvale, NJ: Thomson Publishing.

Tindal, S. and F. Asgarzadeh. 2006. Laboratory scale softgel encapsulation (Mini-cap). *AAPS Poster Presentation*.

Vemuri, S. 1984. Measurement of soft elastic gelatin capsule firmness with a universal testing machine. *Drug Dev. In. Pharm.*, 10: 409–423.

Vishnuvajjala, B. R., E. Tabibi, D. Lednicer, and R. Varma. 1994. *NCI Investigational Drugs, Pharmaceutical Data*. Bethesda, MD: Pharmaceutical Resources Branch, National Cancer Institute, National Institutes of Health.

Wild, F., D. Vidon, and P. Metziger. 1993. Survival of microorganisms in a soft gelatin capsule shell with and without parabens. *STP Pharm. Sci.*, 3: 346–350.

Zaghloul, A. A., B. Gurley, M. Khan, H. Bhagavan, R. Chopra, and I. Reddy. 2002. Bioavailability assessments of oral coenzyme Q10 formulations in dogs. *Drug Dev. In. Pharm.*, 28(10): 1195–1200.

Zuniga, Z. R., C. L. Phillips, D. Shugars, J. A. Lyon, S. J. Peroutka, J. Swarbrick, and C. Bon. 2004. Analgesic safety and efficacy of diclofenac sodium softgels on postoperative third molar extraction pain. *J. Oral and Max. Surg.*, 62(7): 806–815.

22 Oral Modified-Release Drug Delivery for Water-Insoluble Drugs

Shaoling Li, Nuo (Nolan) Wang, Rong (Ron) Liu, Zhanguo Yue, Zhihong (John) Zhang, and Wei (William) Li

CONTENTS

INTRODUCTION

Over the last several decades, the increasing complexity of drug development has led to a greater appreciation of the potential added value of modified-release (MR) delivery systems, including sustained- and controlled-release dosage forms. MR dosage forms offer a number of possible advantages, such as improved patient compliance by reducing the frequency of dosing, improved safety and efficacy associated with reducing drug peaks and troughs, and increased therapeutic efficacy

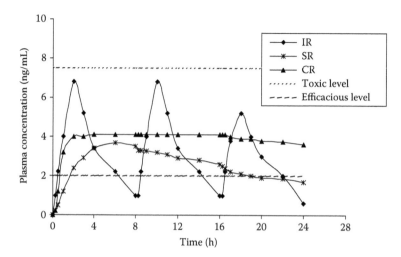

FIGURE 22.1 A typical plasma concentration profile comparing differences between immediate-release (IR), sustained-release (SR), and controlled-release (CR) oral dosage forms.

and effectiveness both by absorption enhancement as well as by focusing drug release at or near its site of action. With an ever-increasing number of water-insoluble or poorly water-soluble compounds discovered as the result of high-throughput screening (HTS), MR drug delivery of water-insoluble drugs is becoming an important product development strategy to maximize utility. In addition, these approaches are useful as a life-cycle extension tool for application to clinically proven drug molecules. In this respect, the development of such a drug delivery product may create greater value in fulfilling unmet medical needs not addressable by the marketed immediate release formulation.

Since more than 80% of candidate drugs have traditionally been developed for oral adminis- tration, this chapter will focus on a discussion of theories, delivery technologies, examples, and future perspectives regarding design of oral MR delivery systems for water-insoluble compounds. Figure 22.1 illustrates one of the classic clinical benefits of applying sustained- and controlled- release dosage forms, that is, improving the safety profile and patient compliance by reducing peak plasma concentration while at the same time providing for prolonged effective drug levels in the blood at levels sufficient for therapy, but below those that provoke unwanted side effects.

In the initial design of an oral MR drug product, a number of parameters often dictate feasibility and as such need to be critically evaluated. These important parameters include

- Physicochemical properties of the drug.
- Biopharmaceutical and pharmacokinetic (PK) information of the drug available after immediate release administration.
- Physiological factors affecting absorption, for example, gastrointestinal (GI) transit time, gastric emptying time, GI content, surface area, pH, enzymatic metabolism, and site- specific absorption.
- Desired therapeutic and PK profile.

FACTORS INFLUENCING ORAL MODIFIED-RELEASE DELIVERY SYSTEM DESIGN AND PERFORMANCE FOR WATER-INSOLUBLE DRUGS

COMPOUND CHARACTERISTICS

Physicochemical properties of the drug, such as ionization constant (pK_a), aqueous solubility, partition coefficient (log P), and chemical stability significantly influence the dosage form design.

Since the drug preferentially transports across biological lipid membrane in a unionized form, the relationship between drug properties such as pK_a, solubility, and the physiological environment of GI tract is of significant importance. In general, the nature of drug solubility is one of the most important factors for the design of the MR dosage forms as it limits the choice of release mechanism available. In some cases, low drug solubility may make some delivery platforms better candidates than others. Application of solubilization techniques enables design and development of oral MR dosage forms for poorly water-soluble drugs and can provide more choices and options in designing such a delivery system.

The biological half-life, $t_{1/2}$, is an important biopharmaceutical parameter quantitatively describing the elimination rate of the drug from the body and is one of the criteria for consideration in MR dosage form design. To maintain plasma levels of a therapeutic agent over a prolonged period of time, the rate of drug absorption must be approximately equal to the rate of drug elimination, which is determined by the $t_{1/2}$. Typically, therapeutic compounds with very short $t_{1/2}$ and high volume of distribution undergo rapid clearance making prolonged delivery and action difficult. On the other hand, the compounds that do have a relatively long $t_{1/2}$ exhibit by definition extended plasma levels. In general, compounds with $t_{1/2}$s shorter than 2 h or greater than 8 h are not good candidates for sustained-release dosage forms. In some unique cases, however, development of a controlled-/sustained-release oral dosage form may be considered for the drugs with $t_{1/2}$ longer than 8 h as the controlled release of these compounds can still offer reduced Cmax, thereby leading to elimination of Cmax associated side effects. For the compounds that show short half-life (<2 h), a MR dosage form design combining an immediate-release (IR) component and a controlled-release portion could mitigate the low bioavailability issue caused by extensive first pass metabolism.

The absorption window and characteristics of a compound also affect the suitability of a drug as a MR candidate. Enzymatic processes in the gut may cause significant drug loss even before the drug is absorbed, and compounds that are poorly metabolized either in the lumen or tissue of the intestine presystemically may not be suitable for MR dosage forms. Designing a once daily, zero-order, controlled-release product, for example, requires the drug to demonstrate good absorption in the lower GI tract, including the ascending colon, since the transit time of a delivery system is very limited at the upper GI tract.

PHYSIOLOGICAL ENVIRONMENT OF GI TRACT

Successful drug release from an oral dosage form, either an immediate release or a MR dosage form, and uptake into the general circulation will be dependent upon several key factors: delivery of the drug to the absorption site, providing a stable solubilized form of the drug, transport of the drug molecule across the membrane of GI tract, and delivery of the drug to its site of action. Notably, the physiological environment of the GI tract plays an important role in determining the solution state and bioavailability of the drug after it is released from the dosage form.

The Biopharmaceutics Classification System (BCS) is a drug development tool that allows estimation of the contribution of three fundamental factors of the drug including dissolution, solubility, and intestinal permeability, which govern the rate and extent of drug absorption from solid oral dosage forms. The dissolution is the process by which the drug is released, dissolved, and becomes ready for absorption. Permeability refers to the ability of the drug molecule to permeate through a membrane into the systemic circulation. According to BCS definition, drugs are classified into four categories: BCS Class I drugs are those with high drug solubility and permeability, BCS Class II drugs are ones having low solubility and high permeability, the BCS Class III drugs have high solubility and low permeability, and BCS Class IV compounds are poorly soluble and permeable. In the case of water-insoluble drugs discussed in this chapter, which are typically BCS Class II compounds, the drug dissolution and solubilization may be a serious limitation to oral drug absorption.

The components and properties of aqueous GI fluids to which a dosage form is exposed are important in determining the rate of dissolution and the level of solubilization, and therefore, the pattern of drug absorption. One important property of GI fluids is pH, which exerts a major influence on the overall absorption process for water-insoluble drugs since most drugs are either weak acids or bases and the drugs have to be in solution before being transported across the GI membrane. The pH of the fluids in the GI tract varies considerably, ranging from very acidic (pH 1) in the stomach to about neutral (pH 6–7) in the small intestine and somewhat basic (pH 8) in the large intestine. The aqueous solubility of acid and basic compounds and, by virtue of the Noyes–Whitney relationship, their dissolution rate from the dosage form is typically pH dependent. The pH of the fluids will have less impact for unionizable drugs. For example, acidic drugs dissolve most readily in alkaline media and, therefore, are expected to have a greater rate of dissolution in intestinal fluid than in gastric fluid. Furthermore, as the major site of drug absorption is the small intestine, it would seem that water-insoluble basic drugs need to dissolve in the acidic gastric fluids and to remain in solution in the intestinal environment to be well absorbed from the intestine. In some cases, however, the water-insoluble drug could be delivered through the unique formulation approaches and stayed as a stable solution or supersaturation form in the GI tract that lead to reasonable fraction absorbed and bioavailability.

Dissolution rate is a function of the drug concentration at the site of absorption, which is directly proportional to the saturation solubility of the drug. For a weakly acidic drug, increasing the pH increases the extent and rate at which the drug dissolves, which in turn can significantly influence the absorption behavior of the drug.

$$AH \overset{K_a}{\longleftrightarrow} A^- + H^+$$

$$K_a = \frac{\left[A^-\right]\left[H^+\right]}{\left[AH\right]} \tag{22.1}$$

At a given pH, the saturation solubility of the drug in the boundary layer is

$$C_h = [AH] + [A^-] \tag{22.2}$$

When the drug is dissolving in an aqueous solution in which the drug is totally unionized, the drug saturation solubility is $C_s = [AH]$. Therefore,

$$C_h = C_s \left(1 + \frac{K_a}{\left[H^+\right]}\right) \tag{22.3}$$

For a weakly basic drug, however, the rate of dissolution decreases as the pH increases.

$$BH^+ \overset{K_b}{\longleftrightarrow} B + H^+$$

$$K_b = \frac{[B]\left[H^+\right]}{\left[AH^+\right]} \tag{22.4}$$

Similarly, at a given pH

$$C_h = [BH^+] + [B] \tag{22.5}$$

The drug saturation solubility is $C_s = [B]$ when the drug is totally unionized in an aqueous solution. Therefore,

$$C_h = C_s \left(1 + \frac{[H]}{K_b} \right)$$
(22.6)

Ideally, the release of an ionizable compound from a sustained-release product should be programmed in accordance with the variation in physiological pH along different segments of the GI tract. Thus, theoretically, the amount of the absorbed (uncharged) species and the plasma concentration can be kept approximately constant throughout the time course of drug release and action.

Another important factor that may influence solubility, dissolution rate, and therefore absorption of water-insoluble compounds is the contents of the GI fluids. The GI fluids contain various materials, such as bile salts, enzymes, and mucin. Bile salts are surface active and as such could potentially enhance the rate or extent of absorption of water-insoluble drugs. Thus, the increased absorption of a water-insoluble compound, griseofulvin (GF), after a fatty meal may be facilitated by bile salt secretion into the gut resulting in solubilization (Crounse 1961; Kraml et al. 1962).

In Vitro and *In Vivo* Evaluations

The rational development of a drug delivery system can be timely and costly. Formulation development and optimization requires a step-wise approach by first screening and evaluating various formulations *in vitro* before one initiates formulations/dosage forms testing *in vivo*.

The drug release or dissolution rate is considered one of the most important *in vitro* characteristics as the *in vivo* absorption for BCS Class II compounds can be significantly affected by these parameters. Identifying a discriminating and predictive *in vitro* dissolution/drug-release test method is important in the cost-effective development of oral solid dosage forms. The ability of using an *in vitro* dissolution test to predict the *in vivo* performance and correlate with the resulting absorption profile, that is, establishment of *in vitro/in vivo* correlation (IVIVC), has been an ongoing industrial effort with the ultimate goal being a validated *in vitro* test and IVIVC model that can be used for multifarious purposes including (Skelly et al. 1990; Food and Drug Administration 1997a, b; Yu et al. 1998; Sunkara and Chilukuri 2003):

- Facilitating screening, monitoring, and optimization of dosage forms
- Providing product quality and process control
- Assisting in certain regulatory determinations and judgments when there are minor formulation and process changes, and sometimes, a change in manufacturing equipment, methods, or sites

Over the last decade, it has been increasingly reliable to use the *in vitro* dissolution or drug release rate test as an indication of the *in vivo* absorption characteristics and PK behavior for the oral solid dosage form based on a well-established IVIVC (Hwang et al. 1995; Food and Drug Administration 1997b; Modi et al. 2000). In particular, the application of IVIVC studies for supporting regulatory submissions is gaining currency. As a result, the Food and Drug Administration (FDA) has published guidance for the industry regarding development, evaluation, and application of IVIVCs for extended-release oral dosage forms (Food and Drug Administration 1997).

In Vitro Methods

Several known *in vitro* dissolution/release-rate test methods have been reported for assessing *in vitro* performance of MR dosage forms. The selection of a particular *in vitro* dissolution test method for a product is often dependent on the type and/or design of the dosage form. These commonly used tests are summarized in the following:

1. USP Apparatus I (basket method): preferred for capsules and dosage forms that tend to float or disintegrate slowly
2. USP Apparatus II (paddle method): preferred for tablets
3. USP Apparatus III (bio-dis dissolution method with reciprocating cylinder): useful for the bead-type dosage forms
4. USP Apparatus IV (flow-through cell method): used for poorly soluble drugs
5. USP Apparatus VII (known as ALZA release rate test method using reciprocating holder): used mainly for osmotically controlled dosage forms

In addition to selection of a suitable type of dissolution apparatus, the dissolution media is another critical element in generating IVIVCs. Besides the compendial dissolution media, proper selection and use of biorelevant dissolution media to mimic GI biological conditions can be of benefit as has been reported, especially for dosage forms containing poorly water-soluble drugs (Galia et al. 1998; Nicolaides et al. 1999; Dressman and Reppas 2000; Sunesen et al. 2005; Vertzoni et al. 2005; Schamp et al. 2006; Wei and Löbenberg 2006). The commonly used dissolution media are

1. Deionized water
2. Buffers over the range of physiologic pH (1 through 7.5)
3. Simulated gastric and intestinal fluids (SGF and SIF)
4. Surfactant-containing dissolution media
5. Biorelevant media, such as FaSSIF and FeSSIF, that model composition of the gastric and intestinal contents before and after meal intake

In Vivo Methods

In vivo evaluations are often conducted in animal models to obtain preliminary information with respect to the *in vivo* absorption characteristics and PK profile of the dosage form. The selection of the test animals is related to a number of factors including convenience, history, and familiarity with the model and the similarity of the selected species to humans with regard to GI and other physiological elements. For oral MR dosage forms, selection of a suitable animal model is not a trivial task owing to the differences in the anatomy and physiology of GI tract between animal species and humans. Dogs have been widely used as an animal model for assessment of the oral absorption and PK profile of oral MR dosage forms due to the similarity of canine anatomy and physiology of the upper GI with that of humans. Having said that, evaluation of the MR dosage forms in dogs and other animal species should be carefully interpreted as dogs typically show a much shorter GI transit time, meaning these data cannot be translated to human *in vivo* performance without some risk (Uchida et al. 1986; Dressman and Yamada 1991; Kararli 1995).

In vivo studies in humans are essential in evaluating and demonstrating PK and pharmacodynamic performance of oral MR dosage forms. The studies required for evaluating MR dosage forms include single and multiple dose assessments as well as randomized, crossover study under fasting and nonfasting conditions. In some cases, the additional studies may be needed to understand and define the cause of the food effect if any.

ORAL MODIFIED-RELEASE PRODUCT DESIGNS FOR WATER-INSOLUBLE DRUGS: MODELS, THEORIES, AND EXAMPLES

To date, the challenges associated with development of an oral MR dosage form for water-insoluble drugs have not been systematically studied and discussed. In many cases, the physicochemical properties of the drug and its sensitivity to the conditions of the GI track make it more difficult to attain the desired absorption and PK profile. This is a clear point of concern in developing a MR product for poorly water-soluble drugs.

Several known mechanism-based approaches, such as dissolution-controlled, diffusion- and/or erosion-controlled, combination of dissolution- and diffusion-controlled, and osmotically controlled systems have been widely used for sustained- or controlled-release delivery of water-soluble compounds. These models, in principle, are also applicable for designing MR delivery systems of water-insoluble drugs in combination with solubility-enhancing technology.

There have been a number of formulation approaches explored and widely practiced in the pharmaceutical industry to improve delivery of poorly water-soluble compounds, especially in development of immediate release dosage forms. These delivery approaches are based on various techniques described as following:

- Increased saturation solubility and as a consequence of the Noyes–Whitney equation (Equation 22.7), dissolution rate of the drug
- Particle size reduction (micronization and nanosization)
- Solid dispersion or solid solution
- Formation of the salt and polymorphs
- Use of co-solvents
- Complexation with the excipients such as cyclodextrins
- Other delivery techniques
- Achieving a sustained solubilization of the drug by
- Use of lipid-based delivery systems
- Use of surfactants to form micelles
- Other techniques

Drug solubilization and the ability to maintain the drug in solution throughout the GI tract, in particular at the site of absorption, become two of the important criteria when a specific, controlled- or sustained-release dosage form is being considered for delivery of a poorly water-soluble drug. Another important feature for such a delivery system is the ability to simultaneously release both drug and solubilization agent(s) throughout the GI tract.

DISSOLUTION-CONTROLLED SYSTEMS

For water-insoluble drugs, dissolution-controlled systems are an obvious choice for achieving sustained-release because of their slow dissolution rate characteristics. Theoretically, the dissolution process at steady state can be described by the Noyes–Whitney equation as shown in Equation 22.7. The rate of dissolution of a compound is a function of surface area, saturation solubility, and diffusion layer thickness. Therefore, the rate of drug release can be manipulated by changing these parameter.

$$\frac{dC}{dt} = \frac{D \times A(C_s - C_t)}{h \times V} \tag{22.7}$$

where dC/dt is the dissolution rate; D is the diffusion coefficient; A is the surface area of drug; C_s is the saturation solubility of the drug; C_t is the concentration at time, t; h the diffusion layer thickness; and V is the volume.

In recent years, nanotechnologies have received a great deal of attention in solving delivery problems of water-insoluble compounds. NanoCrystal® (Elan Drug Delivery, Inc., King of Prussia, PA) dispersions are small crystals of the drug substance, characterized in the submicron domain and often less than 400 nm in diameter. These dispersions are produced by high-energy wet milling (Elan Pharmaceutical 2004) and stabilized against agglomeration through surface adsorption of stabilizers, and have been incorporated into oral dosage forms to produce sustained-release profiles.

Alternatively, nanosized drug delivery particles, such as lipid-based nanoparticles or the nano-structured lipid dispersions, can be produced by dispersing water-insoluble drug in lipid-based excipients to form micron or submicron particles by high-pressure homogenization, microprecipitation, or dispersed-phase technology. In these cases, the drug release can be modified by proper selection of the solubility-enabling carrier(s) and controlling particle size of the final product (Elan Pharmaceutical 2004; Saffie-Siebert et al. 2005). Fine particles, for example, of the poorly water-soluble compounds cholesterol acetate (CA), GF, and megestrol acetate (MA) were produced by extraction of the internal phase of oil-in-water emulsions using supercritical carbon dioxide. Using the supercritical fluid extraction method, particles with mean volume diameter measured by light scattering technique ranging between 100 and 1000 nm were consistently produced. The study showed that emulsion droplet size, drug solution concentration, and organic solvent content in the emulsion were the major parameters responsible for particle size control. The GF and MA nanoparticles produced were crystalline as demonstrated by X-ray powder diffraction and exhibited a 5- to 10-fold increase in the dissolution rate compared with that of micronized powders. Theoretical calculations indicated that dissolution was governed mainly by the surface kinetic coefficient and the specific surface area of the particles produced. The rate of drug release could be manipulated and modified by formation of nanostructured particles by proper control of the particle size.

DIFFUSION- AND EROSION-CONTROLLED SYSTEMS

A diffusion-controlled system is typically based on the drug diffusion through an inert membrane or a drug-carrying matrix. Sustained- or controlled-release of water-insoluble drugs is achieved by a matrix diffusional system, in which the drug is homogeneously dissolved or dispersed throughout a matrix with addition of solubility-enhancing excipients such as lipids, surfactants, and/or a counter-ion for ionizable drugs. The physical form of the drug-carrying matrix may be a liquid, semisolid, or solid, and the finished dosage form may be a soft or hard gelatin capsule, or a tablet.

Matrix System

In a typical diffusion-controlled matrix system, drug in the outside layer of the matrix is exposed to the solution medium and dissolved first; it then diffuses out of the matrix as illustrated in Figure 22.2. The process continues at the interface between the bulk medium and solute and gradually moves toward the interior. In this approach, the dissolution rate of the drug within the matrix must be significantly faster than the diffusion rate of the dissolved drug. The release rate of a drug

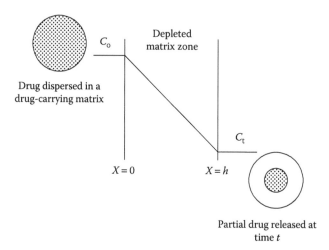

FIGURE 22.2 Schematic illustration of a diffusion-controlled matrix system for which the diffusion process is typically governed by Fick's Law (Equation 22.9).

from a diffusion-controlled system can be mathematically described by a square-root-of-time relationship, as seen in Equation 22.8 that has been widely applied in analyzing release data and fitting the model. A zero-order release cannot be achieved using a diffusion-controlled matrix system.

$$M = kt^{1/2} \tag{22.8}$$

where M is the amount of drug released, k is the constant combining various contributing factors such as drug concentration in the matrix, porosity of the matrix, and so forth.

$$J = -D\frac{dC}{dX} \tag{22.9}$$

where J is the flux, D is the diffusion coefficient of the drug, and dC/dX is the concentration gradient over the distance.

For the matrix system containing dissolved drug, the fractional release M/M_∞ can be described by Equation 22.10 (Good and Lee 1984).

$$\frac{M}{M_\infty} = \left(\frac{4}{\ell}\right)\left[\frac{Dt}{\pi}\right]^{1/2} \tag{22.10}$$

where M is the amount of drug released at time t, M_∞ is the total amount of drug released, ℓ is the thickness of the matrix sheet, and D is the drug diffusion coefficient in the matrix.

For the system containing dispersed drug, where the drug loading per unit volume is greater than the drug solubility in the matrix, the drug release rate can be expressed by the Higuchi Equation (Higuchi 1961):

$$M = [C_s(2A - C_s)Dt]^{1/2} \tag{22.11}$$

where C_s is the drug solubility in the matrix; A is the drug loading per unit volume.

Equation 22.11 was derived based on these assumptions: (1) a pseudosteady state exists, (2) the drug particles are small compared to the average distance of diffusion, (3) the diffusion coefficient is constant, (4) perfect sink conditions exist in the external media, (5) drug release is exclusively through diffusion, (6) the drug concentration in the matrix is greater than the drug solubility in the polymer, and (7) no interaction between drug and matrix takes place. In the case of $A \gg C_s$, Equation 22.11 reduces to

$$M = [2DAC_s t]^{1/2} \tag{22.12}$$

Thus, the amount of drug released is proportional to the square root of time, A, D, and C_s. In some cases, diffusion is not the only pathway by which a drug is released from the delivery system. The erosion of the delivery matrix following relaxation of the polymer and other functional excipient(s) contributes to the overall drug release as well. Examples of the diffusion- and erosion-controlled matrix delivery systems are discussed in the following.

Sustained-Release Liquid-Filled Hard Gelatin Capsules

GPI 1485, an experimental neuroimmunophilin ligand, was in development for the treatment of Parkinson's disease and postprostectomy erectile dysfunction. The compound has a short biological half-life, which makes it a good candidate for an extended-release product that may simplify dosing regimens, improve patient compliance, and make termination of treatment easier. GPI 1485 was formulated in a liquid-filled hard gelatin capsule by using excipients such as Labrafil® and Precirol® A to 5 (Gattefossé Corp., Paramus, NJ) as oil and wax carriers, respectively, as the

TABLE 22.1

Effect of Composition of GPI 1485, Labrafil® and Precirol A to 5® on Time Required for 80% of the Drug to Be Released (T80%)

Composition (%) (GPI 1485/Labrafil®/Precirol A to 5®)	T80% (h)
100:0:0	1.0
75:25:0	4.5
75:20:5	8.0
75:12.5:12.5	8.3
75:5:25	22.0
75:0:25	>24.3

Source: Dordunoo, S. K., *Bull. Techn. Gattefossé*, 29, 29–39, 2004.

principle drug solubilizer and carrier (Dordunoo 2004). The functional excipients selected were either solid or semisolid in nature and capable of solubilizing the poorly water-soluble compound, GPI 1485, and providing sustained-release characteristics. The delivery system was prepared by first melting and dissolving the drug with the lipid at about 100°C, and then cooling the molten material to approximately 75°C to allow filling of the material into an appropriate size of hard gelatin capsule. The ratio of Labrafil to Precirol that significantly impacted the drug-release rate is collected in Table 22.1. Prolonged release of the drug over 24 h was achieved with a formulation containing 75% drug and 25% Precirol. A square root of time plot showed linearity over the first 9 h of the release and, subsequently, a slower rate indicated drug release from the capsule formulated with 75% drug and 1:1 ratio of Labrafil and Precirol was diffusion controlled.

A proprietary matrix delivery system invented by Supernus Pharmaceuticals (Rockville, MD; formerly Shire Laboratories, Inc.) was prepared by incorporating a poorly water-soluble drug (e.g., nifedipine, naproxen, or acyclovir) into particles comprising (1) a core formed from a hydrophobic material, or a hydrophobic emulsion or dispersion; and (2) an alternating layer containing hydrophilic/hydrophobic materials as an interface between the core and each succeeding layer. The drug was released from the system by diffusion and erosion, as well as by enhanced dissolution resulting from the surface-active nature of the interfaces (Belenduik et al. 1995; Supernus Pharmaceuticals 2006). The hydrophobic materials may be selected from a group of medium- or long-chain carboxylic acids such as capric acid, oleic acid, and lauric acid; or from a group of carboxylic acid esters such as glyceryl monostearates and monoglyceride and diglyceride esters; or from a group of long-chain carboxylic acid alcohols, such as lauric acid alcohol and caprylic acid alcohol. A surfactant such as vitamin E tocopherol polyethylene glycol (TPGS), Tween 60 or 80 may be chosen and used to form colloidal emulsion. The formulation matrix or the emulsion core can be processed by heating or melting the drug with the hydrophobic component(s) and hydrophilic component(s) at 70°C–80°C and then cooling them in a spray-drying or *prilling* column to form beads. The emulsion cores/beads can be further coated in a fluidized bed apparatus, alternatively with a surfactant-containing hydrophobic solution and a stable emulsion or dispersion of the drug in a hydrophobic material to provide the multilamellar drug delivery system. The multilamellar particles can be filled into hard gelatin capsules to generate a final dosage form or may be further processed as solid tablets by incorporating other tablet excipients such as disintegrates and lubricants. Depending upon the nature of the drug, particularly the diffusion coefficient of the drug within the matrix system, the release rate can be manipulated and controlled by altering the composition of the functional excipients. Figure 22.3 shows a typical drug-release profile from such a delivery system (Supernus Pharmaceuticals 2006).

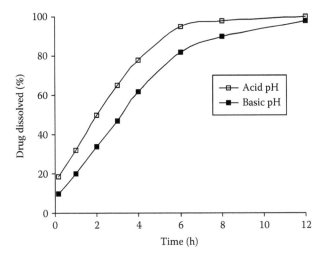

FIGURE 22.3 Drug-release profile from a sustained-release lipid-based matrix system for delivery of poorly water-soluble drugs. (Modified from Technical Technologies Data Sheet published by Supernus Pharmaceuticals, 2006.)

Controlled-Release Microparticles

Felodipine, a poorly water-soluble drug, was formulated with various erodable lipophilic excipients such as stearic acid, Cetanol, Carnauba wax, and Precirol ATO 5 to form solid-dispersion microparticles using a spray chilling method (Savolainen et al. 2002a, b, 2003). The drug was mixed and melted with the excipients, then the melt mixtures were sprayed through a specially constructed pneumatic nozzle into a chilled vessel or bath containing carbon dioxide ice at a temperature of −50°C, the atomization air temperature of 400°C, and the pressure of approximately 7 bar. The resulting microparticles were found to be mostly spherical in shape with a mean diameter of 25–35 μm and could be further processed with other tablet excipients to produce a solid tablet. Studies suggested that the drug release could be manipulated by the choice of the lipid carrier as shown in Figure 22.4.

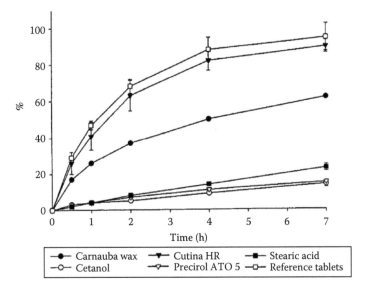

FIGURE 22.4 Comparison of felodipine release rates from difference different lipophilic matrices. (Adapted from Savolainen, M. et al., *Int. J. Pharm.*, 244, 151, 2002b.)

Soft Gelatin-Based Controlled-Release Capsules

Versatrol™ controlled-release softgel technology by Banner Pharmacaps (High Point, NC) uses a standard softgel shell combined with lipid-assisted drug delivery to enhance the absorption of poorly soluble compounds. Depending on the physicochemical properties of the active molecule, an emulsion or a suspension is selected as a matrix to achieve various release patterns such that drug release is mainly diffusion controlled (Banner Pharmacaps 2006). For example, controlled release of a sparingly water-soluble drug was achieved with a wax matrix as the contents and a soft gelatin capsule as the fill carrying body. The release rate could be tailored by modifying the wax matrix components (Hassan et al. 2003).

Controlled-Release Solid-Dispersion/Solution Delivery Systems

Over the last decade, solid-dispersions or solid solutions, high-energy supersaturated systems, have been extensively studied and widely used to enable delivery of water-insoluble compounds (Gruenhagen 1995; Sheen et al. 1995; Serajuddin 1999; Erkoboni and Andersen 2000; Leuner and Dressman 2000; Forster et al. 2001; Vippagunta et al. 2002; Verreck et al. 2003; Chokshi et al. 2005). Combining solid-dispersion (SD) and modified-release (MR) techniques, a novel dissolution and/or diffusion-modulating approach has become increasingly attractive in designing oral modified-release drug delivery systems for poorly water-soluble drugs. Though SD technique has been widely used to achieve immediate release for poorly water-soluble drugs, modified release characteristics can be achieved by properly choosing type and amount of the polymeric materials with controlled-release characteristics (Chiou and Eiegelman 1971; Ford 1986; Craig 1990, 2002; Serajuddin 1999; Tanaka et al. 2005; Reitz et al. 2008). Either by directly modifying the release characteristics of solid dispersion matrix using rate-controlling polymeric materials or combining other modified-release techniques such as membrane coating, the desired drug release profile can be obtained. Such MR dosage forms containing SD provide an immediately available dose for an immediate action followed by a gradual and continuous release of subsequent doses to maintain the plasma concentration over an extended period of time.

To modify the release characteristics of poorly water-insoluble drugs, both hydrophobic polymer and water-insoluble or slower-dissolving carriers can be used. Depending on the physicochemical characteristics of the drug molecule, one could incorporate a soluble polymeric material into a hydrophobic matrix to modulate the release of practically insoluble drugs. Commonly used polymeric materials as the rate-controlling matrix-forming excipients in the modified-release solid-dispersion systems are summarized in Table 22.2. The studies have shown that hydroxypropyl methylcellulose (HPMC) is one of the excipient choices for use in solid dispersion formulation as a drug carrier and precipitation inhibitor. Methacrylate copolymers, such as Eudragit RL® and Eudragit RS®, have been widely used as tablet coatings and as retardants of drug release in sustained-release formulations. The swellability and permeability, pH-independent or -dependent properties, as well as the flexibility for processing enable wide application of the methacrylate copolymers in designing the MR-SD drug delivery systems (Mehta et al. 2001; Wagner and McGinity 2002). Various techniques such as hot-melt extrusion, spray-drying and high pressure homogenization have been used to prepare solid dispersion system, while hot-melt extrusion is one of the mostly practiced techniques (Wagenaar and Müller 1994; Hülsmann et al. 2000, 2001; Ghebremeskel et al. 2006; Wu et al. 2009). The benefits of using hot-melt extrusion over others include fewer unit operations with better content uniformity and an anhydrous process with reduced processing time.

Indomethacin (IMC), a poorly water-soluble drug, was formulated with biocompatible, non-swelling acrylic polymers such as Eudragit RD 100, Eudragit L 100, Eudragit S, or Eudragit RS or RL (Degussa GmbH, Bennigsenplatz, Düsseldorf) to produce a MR matrix system using a thermal treating or hot-melt extrusion process (Azarmi et al. 2002; Zhu et al. 2006). The study showed that IDM was transformed from a crystalline form into an amorphous form in the Eudragit RD 100 granules following hot-melt extrusion. Thermal processing facilitated the formation of a solid solution with a continuous matrix structure. Varying the drug-to-polymer ratio impacted drug-release

TABLE 22.2
Commonly Used Polymeric Materials in Modified-Release Solid-Dispersion Systems

Polymeric Materials	Properties and Applications
Hydrophobic Materials	
Ethylcellulose	Typically combined with hydrophilic polymer to achieve desired release characteristics
Cellulose acetate butyrate (CAB)	Can be combined with hydrophilic polymer to achieve desired release characteristics
Methacrylate copolymers	Good swellability, permeability, and ease of processing
Glycerol distearate (Precirol)	Used with surfactant(s) in the lipid-based, self-emulsifying solid-dispersion matrix
Carnauba wax	Ease of processing at lower temperature
Cellulose acetate phthalate (CAP)	pH-sensitivity, used in the matrix and/or film coating to achieve modified-release characteristics
Polyvinyl acetate (PVA)	Sustained-release characteristics and film former, used in the matrix and/or film coating to achieve modified-release characteristics
Hydrophilic Materials	
Hydroxypropyl methylcellulose (HPMC)	Hydrophilic polymer with varied gelling property based on molecular weight/viscosity of the grade used, re-crystallization inhibition property
Hydroxypropyl cellulose (HPC)	Varied gelling property, can be combined with hydrophobic polymeric materials to achieve release characteristics
Sodium alginate	Good gelling and cross-linking property
Carbopol	Highly efficient gel matrix formers for controlling drug release
Polyethylene oxide (Polyox or PEO)	Varied gelation characteristics based on molecular weight and viscosity of the grade used

characteristics. Inclusion of a plasticizer, such as Pluronic F68 (BASF, Florham Park, NJ), which also behaves as a surface-modifying agent, decreased the glass transition temperature of the solid-solution/solid-dispersion matrix and increased the drug-release rate. Processing conditions, such as heating/melting temperatures and holding time may affect the property of the resulting matrix and, therefore, the drug-release properties. The hot-melt extrudates can be further fabricated to produce capsule-filled granules or solid tablets. Figure 22.5 shows the effect of the temperature on the drug release of IDM from the Eudragit RS matrices.

Hüslmann et al. (2000, 2001) evaluated use of various polymers, PEG 6000, PVP, or a vinyl-pyrrolidone-vinylacetate copolymer as the carrier and Gelucire 44/14 as the functional excipient in a solid-dispersion system prepared by hot-melt extrusion method for solubility and dissolution rate enhancement of a poorly water-soluble drug, 17-estradiol hemihydrate. Ghebremeskel et al. (2006) studied the performance of various solid-dispersion systems prepared by hot-melt extrusion using polyvinylpyrrolidone (PVP)-K30, Plasdone-S630, and HPMC-E5 as the polymeric carriers with the surfactant(s) such as Tween 80 and Docusate Sodium added as a plasticizer. Using a hot-melt extrusion and spheronization process, Young and his coworkers demonstrated the success of preparing the controlled-release dosage forms of theophylline with various polymeric materials and other functional excipients. In one study, theophylline (30%) was mixed with an acrylic copolymer, Eudragit Preparation 4135F (48%), microcrystalline cellulose (15%), and polyethylene glycol 8000 (7%) to prepare the solid-dispersion pellets and achieve the sustained-release characteristics (Young et al. 2002). In a separate study, various theophylline modified-release solid-dispersion systems comprising theophylline (20%), Acryl-EZE, a methacrylic acid copolymer (60%), triethyl citrate (15%) and an optional gelling polymer Methocel K4M Premium (5%) or Carbopol 974P (5%) were

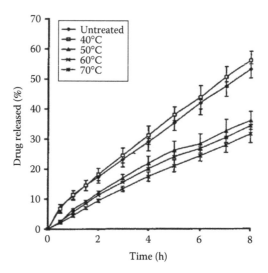

FIGURE 22.5 The effect of the temperature of heat treating on the release of indomethacin from Eudragit RS matrices. (Adapted from Azarmi, S. et al., *Int. J. Pharm.*, 246, 171, 2002.)

prepared and evaluated for the drug release characteristics (Young et al. 2005). The effect of gelling polymer, Methocel K4M Premium (HPMC), and Carbopol 974P (carbomer) on the theophylline release properties were evaluated, respectively. The study showed that the excipient blends were physically and chemically stable during processing, and that the resulting dosage forms exhibited pH-dependent dissolution properties. Hot-melt extrusion matrix containing HPMC or carbomer affected the drug release mechanism and kinetics from the thermally processed dosage forms. At concentration of 5% or below, carbomer was more effective than HPMC at extending the duration of theophylline release from the SD matrix tablets. The influence of HPMC or carbomer on the theophylline release properties of the melt-extruded Acry-EZE tablets are shown in Figures 22.6 and 22.7, respectively.

An example of combining solubility/dissolution rate enhancement by solid dispersion and controlled release by film coating was demonstrated by Young et al. (2007). The authors studied the film coating of melt-extruded beads of guaifenesin with polymer Eudragit L30 D-55 to achieve a pH-dependent release profile. Polyethylene oxide (Polyox or PEO) was blended with other functional excipients to prepare a solid-dispersion matrix by melt extrusion and beads by spheronization process. The guaifenesin containing SD beads were film-coated with a methacrylic acid copolymer in a

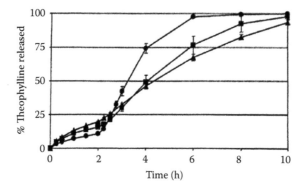

FIGURE 22.6 Influence of Methocel® K4M Premium on the theophylline release properties of melt-extruded Acryl-EZE® tablets (paddle method, 2 h in 0.1 N HCL followed by 8 h in pH 6.8 PBS, 900 ml, 37°C, 50 rom, $n = 6$). Key: (●) 2%; (■) 2.5%; (▲) 5%.

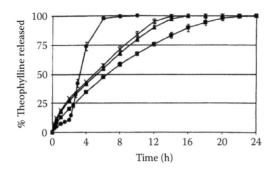

FIGURE 22.7 Influence of Carbopol 974P on the theophylline release properties of melt-extruded Acryl-EZE® tablets (paddle method, 2 h in 0.1 N HCL followed by 22 h in pH 6.8 PBS, 900 ml, 37°C, 50 rom, $n = 6$). Key: (●) 0%; (■) 2.5%; (▲) 5%; (x) 10%.

fluidized bed apparatus to achieve modified-release characteristics. The study showed that addition of ethylcellulose to the extruded powder blend decreased and stabilized the drug release rate from the thermally processed pellets. The study also demonstrated film coating to be an efficient process for providing melt-extruded beads with pH-dependent drug-release properties.

Electrospinning was introduced as a novel technique for preparing a controlled-release (CR) amorphous SD system and polymeric nanofibers for a poorly water-soluble drug, Piroxicam (PRX) (Paaver et al. 2015). In the study, HPMC K100M premium CR was used as an amorphous-state stabilizing polymer carrier in nanofibers. The authors evaluated various drug-polymer (PRX/HPMC) ratios weight by weight (w/w) ranging from 1:1 to 4:1. The study showed that the electrospun CR-SD nanofibers exhibited a short lag time, the absence of initial burse release, and zero-order linear CR release kinetics.

Figure 22.8 illustrates development and fabrication of a typical modified-release solid-dispersion system for poorly water-soluble drugs.

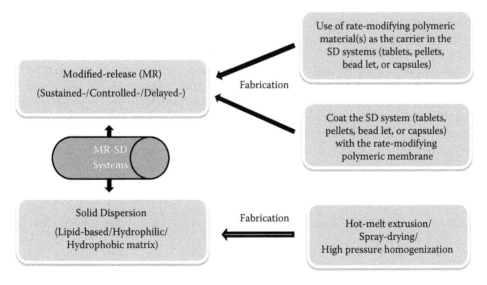

FIGURE 22.8 Development and fabrication of a typical modified-release solid-dispersion (MR-SD) delivery system for poorly water-soluble drugs.

Membrane Reservoir Systems

Sustained or controlled release of water-insoluble drugs can be achieved through another type of diffusion-controlled system: the reservoir. Such systems comprise a drug core and a surrounding polymeric membrane that controls or modifies the drug-release rate. Since drug-release kinetics can be controlled by changing the characteristics of the polymeric material(s) used for the rate-controlling membrane, a zero-order release profile could be attainable with the design. Drug release from such a delivery system is mathematically described by Equation 22.13 for a simple slab-like system, and will vary depending on the geometry of the system (Higuchi 1961; Baker et al. 1974; Flynn et al. 1974; Good and Lee 1984).

$$\frac{dM_t}{dt} = \frac{ADK\Delta C}{d} \tag{22.13}$$

where dM_t/dt is the steady state release rate at time t, A the surface area of the reservoir system, D the diffusion coefficient, K the participant coefficient, ΔC the concentration difference across the membrane, and d is the diffusion layer thickness.

An example of such a reservoir matrix system is a rate-controlling membrane coated solid solution beads comprising: (1) a hydrophobic long-chain fatty acid or ester material; (2) a surfactant; and (3) a therapeutic agent that, in admixture, forms a solid solution at room temperature (Burnside et al. 2004). In this example, the model compound, acyclovir was formulated with the solubility-enhancing agent, Labrasol, and other excipients such as Compritol 888 (Gattefossé Corp., Paramus, NJ) and Talc to prepare granules or bead lets with particle sizes ranging from approximately 150–300 µm using a spray-melt method. The bead let size can be controlled by altering the drug-to-solubilizing agent ratio and/or changing the processing parameters. The acyclovir-containing bead lets were further coated with a rate-controlling polymer solution containing Eudragit L30D, hydroxypropyl methylcellulose acetate succinate (HPMCAS), and other coating additives. The release rate can be controlled by adjusting the composition of the coating formulation.

Osmotically Controlled Systems

In principle, the osmotically controlled system operates by a membrane diffusion-controlled mechanism. The drug release takes place through an orifice in the membrane through an osmotic pumping mechanism, where a semipermeable membrane such as cellulose acetate is utilized to regulate the osmotic permeation of water (Theeuwes 1975, 1980). The osmotically controlled delivery systems are capable of providing not only prolonged zero-order release but also programmable delivery profiles such as delayed, pulsatile, and ascending. The delivery rate from such an osmotically driven system is generally regulated by the osmotic pressure of the drug layer/core formulation with an elementary, single layer design or the osmotic pressure of the push layer with a multilayer design and by the water permeability of the semipermeable membrane. The controlled rate of drug release in the GI tract is independent of posture, pH, GI motility, and fed or fasting conditions. The biologically inert components of the delivery system remain intact during the transit through GI tract and are eliminated in the feces as an insoluble shell. Equation 22.14 can be used to describe and predict release rate from such an osmotic system from which the drug can be delivered in a liquid, solubilized form suspended in high molecular weight polymer, melt, or suspension:

$$\frac{dM}{dt} = \frac{A}{h} k\pi C \tag{22.14}$$

where dM/dt is the delivery rate of the solute (drug), A the membrane area, h the membrane thickness, k the constant, π the osmotic pressure, and C is the concentration of drug in the dispensed mass.

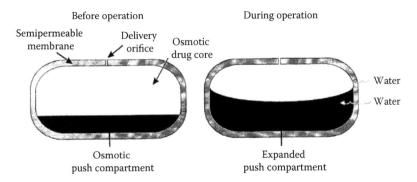

FIGURE 22.9   A cross-section of an OROS® Push-Pull™ bilayer system before and during operation.

OROS® Push-Pull™ Drug Delivery System

Delivery systems that use a multicompartment core can theoretically deliver drugs of any solubility (Wong et al. 1986; Theeuwes et al. 1991). A basic Push-Pull™ system consists of two layers: the first contains the drug, osmotically active hydrophilic polymer(s), and other pharmaceutical excipients; the second layer, often called the *push layer*, contains a hydrophilic expansion polymer, other osmotically active agents, and the excipients, as shown in Figure 22.9. Poorly water-soluble compounds can be delivered using an OROS Push-Pull delivery system by incorporating drug as a micronized form, or as a hot-melt material suspended in a polymer matrix.

The OROS Push-Pull delivery technology was used for successful controlled release of nifedipine, a poorly water-soluble calcium channel blocker. Procardia XL® tablets is a once-daily nifedipine product developed by ALZA Corporation (Mountain View, CA) and marketed by Pfizer (New York City) (Wong et al. 1988, 2003) as an antihypertensive agent. Nifedipine has an elimination half-life of approximately 2 h, and oral absorption is known to be proportional to the dose. Owing to its poor aqueous solubility and the BCS Class II drug characteristics, the compound is usually micronized to increase the specific surface area for an enhanced dissolution rate enabling drug absorption. The controlled-release osmotic pump system for nifedipine consists of an osmotically active drug core tablet surrounded by a semipermeable membrane. The core itself is divided into two layers: (1) an active drug layer comprising 20 wt% nifedipine, 71 wt% poly(ethylene oxide) with a molecular weight of 200,000, 2 wt% potassium chloride, 5 wt% hydroxypropyl methylcellulose, and 2 wt% magnesium stearate; and (2) an osmotic push layer consisting of 68.7 wt% poly(ethylene oxide) with a molecular weight of 5,000,000, 29.3 wt% sodium chloride, and 2% w/w magnesium stearate. The wet granulation method is used to prepare drug layer and push layer granules. The compressed bilayer core is then coated with a semipermeable membrane containing 95 wt% cellulose acetate (CA) with an acetyl content of 39.8% and 5 wt% poly(ethylene glycol) 4000 as a permeation enhancer. An exit orifice on the drug layer side is formed by laser drilling through the semipermeable membrane with an opening of 0.26 mm in diameter. The Procardia XL tablet was designed to release drug at a constant rate over 24 h as shown in Figure 22.10.

Clinical study demonstrated a steady plasma level throughout the day after dosing of a single 60-mg dose with elimination of the rapid rise in plasma concentration seen with IR dosing (20 mg nifedipine administered three times a day) as shown in Figure 22.11. The study also showed that the product was well tolerated with an improved safety profile.

OROS Push-Stick™ Drug Delivery System

The OROS Push-Stick technology is designed to deliver high doses of poorly water-soluble or slowly dissolving drugs at a controlled rate (Wong et al. 2003; Cruz et al. 2005). The basic system consists

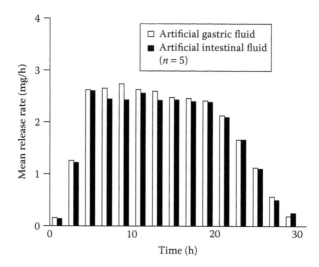

FIGURE 22.10 A zero-order release profile with release duration of 24 h and independent of the pH of the dissolution medium. (Adapted from Wong, P. et al., in *Modified-Release Drug Delivery Technology*, Rathbone, M.J. et al. (Eds.), Osmotically Controlled Tablets, New York: Marcel Dekker, p. 107, 2003.)

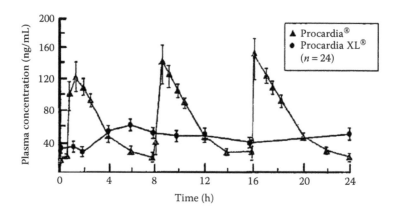

FIGURE 22.11 Steady-state plasma profiles of immediate-release nifedipine (three times a day) and Procardia XL® on day 5. (Adapted from Wong, P. et al., in *Modified-Release Drug Delivery Technology*, Rathbone, M.J. et al. (Eds.), Osmotically Controlled Tablets, New York: Marcel Dekker, p. 107, 2003.)

of two layers, typically in a capsule-shaped tablet surrounded by a semipermeable membrane; however, the system has a much larger exit orifice than the Push-Pull™ systems to allow for delivery of insoluble drug suspended in a hydrophilic polymer. Depending on the physicochemical properties of the drug, a subcoat between the tablet and the semipermeable membrane can be applied to ease and facilitate the optimum delivery. In addition, wetting agent(s) and/or solubilizing agent(s) such as sodium lauryl sulfate (SLS), Poloxamer 188, and Poloxamer 407 (BASF, Florham Park, NJ) can be used to enhance the dissolution rate and, therefore, oral absorption. Such a delivery system containing 85 wt% ibuprofen was prepared by using a similar drug and push layer granulation and compression and coating processes similar to those in the Push-Pull™ delivery system (Cruz et al. 2005).

L-OROS® Drug Delivery System

L-OROS® drug delivery technology, a proprietary controlled-release delivery system invented by ALZA Corporation (Mountain View, CA), combines drug solubilization technology enabling delivery of poorly water-soluble drugs and control delivery for 2–24 h. The solubility-enhancing formulations can be either solution, suspension, or semisolid in nature. One of the primary solubility-enhancing approaches is to dissolve the drug in a lipid-based liquid carrier formulated with a surfactant and/or co-surfactant to form an emulsion or microemulsion *in situ* (also called a self-emulsifying formulation (SEF), or a self-microemulsifying drug delivery system or S(M)EDDS). Other solubilization techniques include using nanosized drug particles stabilized with selective polymer(s) that can be further formulated into a nonaqueous-based nanosuspension and formulating the drug into a high-energy supersaturated delivery system such as solid solution and solid dispersion (Wong et al. 2006).

Various L-OROS delivery platforms provide modified delivery of the drug formulations, such as the L-OROS HARDCAP™ system, L-OROS SOFTCAP™ system, and a delayed bolus delivery system (Wong et al. 1995, 2003). The delivery systems could offer therapeutic advantages by providing various delivery profiles such as continuous and bolus delivery, as well as delayed delivery to a site-specific target in the GI tract. In addition to the controlled-release features that L-OROS delivery systems offer, an enteric coating layer can be applied to any of these dosage forms to prevent drugs that may be adversely affected by pH, from releasing in the stomach, in addition to providing a delayed release for the purpose of site-specific delivery in the lower GI tract.

L-OROS SOFTCAP™ Delivery System

This system is designed to deliver liquid drug formulations with the aim of enabling delivery of insoluble drugs. The L-OROS SOFTCAP system consists of a soft gelatin capsule containing a liquid drug formulation surrounded by a barrier layer, an osmotic push layer, and a semipermeable membrane as shown in Figure 22.12. A delivery orifice is drilled through the three outer layers, but not through the gelatin shell. When the system is administered orally, water permeates through the rate-controlling membrane and activates the osmotic engine that expands, allowing hydrostatic pressure inside the system to build up, and forcing the liquid formulation to release through the hydrated gelatin capsule shell at the delivery orifice (Wong et al. 1995; Dong et al. 2001). The components and excipients, which need to be chemically and physically compatible with the gelatin capsules, include lipids, surfactants, and pharmaceutical solvents that can assist in solubilization and/ or dispersion. Some of the materials used may also protect the drug from enzymatic degradation. Typical liquid formulation types include the SEF or SMEDDS, self-assembly micellar formulation (SAMF), and other lipid-based delivery formulations. Extensive information on the preparation techniques, *in vitro* screening and *in vivo* evaluation, as well as the role of the functional excipients

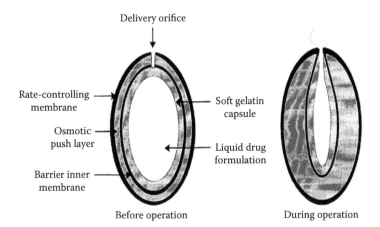

FIGURE 22.12 Configuration of the L-OROS® SOFTCAP™, a cross-sectional view before ingestion and during drug release.

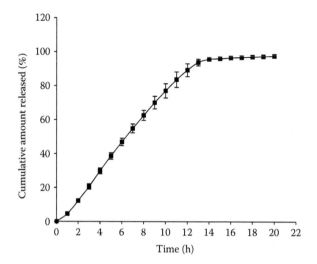

FIGURE 22.13   Controlled release of guaifenesin from a L-OROS® SOFTCAP™ delivery system. (Modified from Li, S. et al., *L-OROS® SOFTCAP™:* Robustness, reproducibility, and stability, published poster, AAPS Annual Meeting, November 2001.)

have been widely studied and reported by pharmaceutical scientists (Constantinides et al. 1996; Khoo et al. 1998; Charman 2000; Kommuru et al. 2001; Porter and Charman 2001a,b; Boyd et al. 2003; Kataoka et al. 2003; Porter et al. 2004; Strickley 2004; Sek et al. 2006).

The robustness of L-OROS SOFTCAP delivery technology was demonstrated using a commercially available soft gelatin capsule product containing guaifenesin (200 mg). The system was coated with three layers to achieve controlled release of the liquid formulation. The first coat was an inner barrier made of an aqueous latex-based suspension that formed a water-impermeable membrane to minimize hydration of the gelatin shell during drug release. The second layer was an osmotic push layer composed of hydrophilic suspending polymers and osmotic agents such as sodium chloride and film-forming polymers suspended in a coating-solvent mixture comprising water and ethanol. The third layer, a rate-controlling membrane typically formed using CA as the main component and a water permeation enhancer as needed, was applied. Finally, an exit orifice was mechanically or laser drilled through the three coating layers but not the gelatin shell. The study showed that such a delivery system provided robust, zero-order rate release of guaifenesin over 12–24 h (Figure 22.13) (Li et al. 2001).

L-OROS HARDCAP Delivery System

The system is designed to deliver liquid drug formulations, especially to accommodate more viscous formulations, such as suspension and semisolid formulation and to allow for higher drug loading (Wong et al. 1995, 2003, 2006; Dong et al. 2001, 2004). The design uses the hard gelatin capsule as a drug formulation carrying body and typically consists of a barrier layer to separate the liquid-containing compartment from the push layer. The barrier layer is formulated by using inert materials that are compatible with the liquid drug formulation and push layer, which is mainly composed of poly(ethylene oxide) with a molecular weight of 5,000,000. The delivery system is surrounded by a semipermeable membrane with a laser-drilled exit orifice on the drug side as shown in Figure 22.14.

MA, a progestogen widely used in the palliative treatment of endometrial carcinoma and breast cancer, is administered orally as a solid dosage form. Owing to its lipophilic nature, the drug is poorly soluble in water and had low oral bioavailability when administered without significant formulation efforts (Farinha et al. 2000; Alakhov et al. 2004; Shekunov et al. 2006). Combining nanoparticle engineering technique enhancing the drug dissolution rate and the osmotically controlled delivery

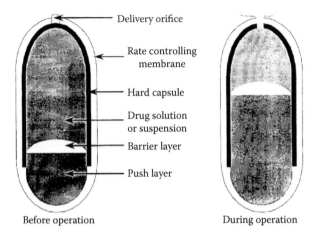

FIGURE 22.14 Configuration of a L-OROS® HARDCAP™ delivery system, a cross-sectional view before ingestion and during drug release.

concept, controlled delivery of MA with enhanced oral absorption could be achieved (Dong et al. 2004; Wong et al. 2006). The drug crystals were first nanosized to a mean particle size of less than 1 micron using a high-energy wet-milling technique. On removal of the water by using freeze-drying process, the freeze-dried powder was suspended in a nonaqueous-based liquid carrier containing lipids such as capric acid and surfactant such as Cremophor EL mixed at a given ratio. The liquid suspension was filled into the hard gelatin capsule body. The liquid formulation containing capsule body was assembled with a barrier layer and push layer for further coating with a semipermeable membrane and laser drilling to form an exit orifice on the drug compartment side. The delivery system provided a constant release of the drug suspension formulation for a duration of 4–24 h.

Progesterone, another poorly water-soluble steroid, was formulated in a self-emulsifying liquid formulation and delivered through a L-OROS HARDCAP delivery system for over 12 h at a zero-order release rate. Figure 22.15 shows a typical zero-order release profile of progesterone from a L-OROS HARDCAP delivery system.

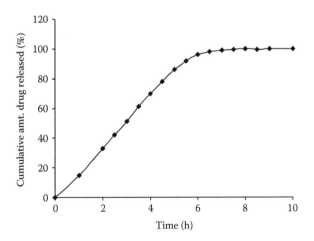

FIGURE 22.15 Controlled-release profile of progesterone from a L-OROS® HARDCAP™ delivery system. (Modified from *Delivery Times*, published by ALZA Corp., Vol. II, Issue 2, 2004.)

Other Osmotically Controlled Delivery Systems

On the basis of the long-standing scientific foundation of the OROS-controlled delivery principles, other osmotically controlled systems have been suggested. Combined with the need to provide adequately bioavailable dosage forms for increasingly difficult-to-formulate drug candidates, some of these innovative ideas have become reality for controlled release of poorly water-soluble drugs.

EnSoTrol® Osmotic Drug Delivery System

EnSoTrol, a proprietary osmotically controlled delivery system invented by Supernus Pharmaceuticals (Rockville, MD: formerly Shire Laboratories, Inc.) comprises a solubility-enabled core with osmotic and wicking agents surrounded by a semipermeable membrane with an exit orifice, which allows release of the solubilized drug (Rudnic et al. 2000, 2004; Flanner et al. 2005; Supernus Pharmaceuticals 2006). The solubility-enabled core typically contains nonswelling solubilization agents such as surfactants (Tween 60 and 80, etc.) as well as materials such as polyethylene-containing surfactants and cyclodextrines that inhibit crystal formation. The inclusion of wicking agents in the formulation can create channels or pores in the drug core, which facilitates the movement of water molecules through the core and creates a network of increased surface area, allowing the drug to diffuse through and to be released. Typical wicking agents include but are not limited to colloidal silicon dioxide, SLS, low molecular weight polyvinyl pyrrolidone, and PEG. When administered orally, the contents of the GI tract induce solubilization of the core contents through fluid uptake across the membrane coat. The solubilized core contents are then released through the laser-drilled exit orifice. The drug release is primarily driven by the osmotic pressure and regulated by water flux through a semipermeable membrane. A typical drug release profile using the EnSoTrol system is shown in Figure 22.16.

Nifedipine, as discussed earlier, a poorly water-soluble compound that has been used to treat hypertension, was formulated with nonswelling solubilizing agents, PEG 8000 and SLS, a wicking agent, Cab-O-Sil. RTM, and osmotic agents, xylitol and sorbitol lactose, to form a drug core using the wet granulation method. Lubricants such as magnesium stearate were used to prevent sticking of the tablet core to the die and to ease the core compression. The tablet was then coated in a pan coater or fluid bed dryer with a solution composed primarily of CA to form a semipermeable rate-controlling membrane. An exit orifice for drug release was formed using the laser drilling method.

Solubility Modulated Drug Delivery System

The proprietary solubility modulated, controlled-release delivery system (Merck & Co., Inc., Rahway, NJ) comprises a core that contains drug and a number of controlled-release solubility modulating units that hold complexing agents or surfactants; these are dispersed in an individual

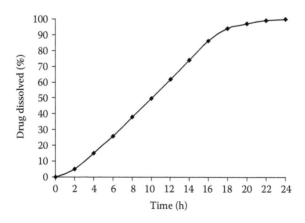

FIGURE 22.16   Drug-release profile through EnSoTrol® osmotic delivery system. (Modified from Technical Data Sheet published by Supernus Pharmaceuticals, 2006.)

matrix substrate or surrounded by a water-insoluble coating with one or more pore-forming agents (McClelland and Zentner 1990). The core is then surrounded with a semipermeable membrane to regulate the drug release.

Simvastatin, a HMG CoA reductase inhibitor, is highly effective in the reduction of blood cholesterol levels in humans and has neither acidic nor basic functionalities. The drug is poorly soluble in water with a value of 30 µg/mL at 20°C. A solubility modulated controlled delivery system was prepared by first preparing a controlled release sodium dodecyl sulfate (SDS) surfactant particles to modulate the drug solubility. The SDS granules were prepared with lactose at a 1:1 ratio in a fluid bed granulator and were coated with a microporous layer that allowed continuous release of SDS over the time. Next, using a wet granulation method, the drug was mixed with controlled-release SDS (C.R. SDS granules) and other excipients to further form drug-containing granules. The dried granules were then compressed into core tablets using a tablet press. A microporous coat containing CA butyrate 318–20 dissolved in an acetone/methanol solvent mixture and a pore former (sorbitol dissolved in a water/methanol solvent blend) was applied to the core tablet to form a membrane of sufficient thickness to provide a continuous release of simvastatin for 4–24 h.

Osmotically Controlled Release of Solid Dispersions

Controlled release of poorly soluble drugs may also be achieved by using solid-solution or solid-dispersion preparation techniques in combination with osmotically controlled release concepts (Appel et al. 2004). These delivery systems consist of a core with an osmotic agent and the drug in the form of a solid dispersion with the major portion of the mixture being amorphous and stabilized with ionizable and nonionizable cellulosic polymers (e.g., carboxymethylcellulose [CMC] and its sodium salt, hydroxypropyl-methylcellulose phthalate [HPMCP], or HPMCAS). A water-permeable membrane is coated onto the drug-containing core with at least one delivery orifice that allows drug release. The amorphous solid dispersion of the drug may be prepared by various techniques, such as hot-melt mixing/extrusion, solvent-based spray drying, and spray coating.

A poorly water-soluble glycogen phosphorylase inhibitor with solubility of about 1 mg/mL was processed into a solid dispersion with 10 wt% drug and 90 wt% HPMCAS using a solvent-based (acetone) spray-drying method. The resulting solid-dispersion particles with a mean diameter of 5–20 microns were shown to be essentially amorphous by a powder X-ray diffraction analysis. The solid-dispersion particles were further processed by mixing with other tablet excipients such as microcrystalline cellulose, poly(ethylene oxide) with a molecular weight of 600,000, and a lubricant; these were compressed into tablets containing 30 wt% of the solid dispersion. The cores were then coated with a water-permeable membrane comprising 70/30 wt% CA and PEG 3350 that was dissolved in 68/22 wt% acetone/water. The coated cores were drilled either mechanically or by laser to form an exit orifice for drug release. The study showed a tenfold increase in the total amount of the drugs available in solution after releasing from an osmotic CR tablet containing solid dispersion as compared to that from an osmotic CR tablet comprising unmanipulated, crystalline drug, as indicated in Table 22.3.

BIOADHESIVE SUSTAINED- AND CONTROLLED-RELEASE DRUG DELIVERY SYSTEMS

Bioadhesive drug delivery systems refer to those delivering drugs through adhesion to physiological surfaces of the body. The bioadhesive sustained- and controlled-release drug delivery systems discussed in this section, however are focused on mucoadhesive or mucosal-adhesive drug delivery systems. Mucoadhesive drug delivery systems have historically been used to deliver drugs locally at sites such as the eye, the oral, and nasal cavities as well as systemically through the GI track (Mathiowitz et al. 1999). Bioadhesives have been increasingly used in the oral sustained/controlled drug delivery systems. The bioadhesive sustained/controlled drug delivery systems can improve drug bioavailability through intimate contact of the dosage forms with mucosal surfaces and as such can increase the duration of action through prolonging the transition time in the GI track (Park and Robinson 1984).

TABLE 22.3

Comparison of Drug Release from an Osmotic Controlled Release Tablet Containing Solid Dispersion as Compared to That from an Osmotic Controlled Release Tablet with Crystalline Drug That Had Not Been Manipulated

	Drug Concentration (µg/mL)	Drug Concentration (µg/mL)
Time (h)	CR w/ Solid Dispersion	CR w/o Solid Dispersion
0	0	0
1	1.3	0
2	12.8	1.8
4	46.5	4.9
8	82.7	7.5
19.5	55.9	7.9

Source: Appel, L. E. et al., Controlled release by extrusion of solid amorphous dispersions of drugs, U.S. Patent 6706283, 2004.

The human GI tract is lined by a layer of *mucus* synthesized by cells that form part of the epithelium. Mucus is composed mostly of water, cross-linked mucins, electrolytes (inorganic salts and carbohydrates), and other substances depending on the location (Marriott and Gregory 1990). Mucins are high molecular weight glycoproteins that have protein backbones covered by covalently bonded oligosaccharide side chains (Longer et al. 1985). Mucin macromolecules form gel-like mucous layers through noncovalent bonding between mucin side chains (Bansil et al. 1995). These oligosaccharide side chains are terminated with sialic acid, which renders a negative charge for mucins in the pH > 3 environment (Bansil et al. 1995). The mucus gel layer is constantly being replaced, and the estimated turnover time of GI mucus layer is believed between 6 and 48 h (Marriott and Hughes 1990; Khanvilkar et al. 2001).

Mucoadhesive drug delivery systems employ natural and synthetic polymers as bioadhesion components. The polymers studied for mucoadhesive drug delivery are summarized in Table 22.4. Most of these polymers are hydrophilic and have similar mechanisms, which provide for their mucosal bioadhesion characteristics. These properties are hydrophilicity (low aqueous surface contact angle), rich in hydrogen bonding groups such as hydroxyl and carboxylic groups (bonding to mucosal surface), and polymer chain flexibility (diffusion and interpenetration of mucosal surface). The most common bioadhesive polymers are synthetic poly(acrylic acid) (PAA), poly(methacrylic acid) (PMA), poly(methyl methacrylate) (PMMA) polymers, and natural polymers such as chitosan and hyaluronic acid and hyaluronan (Ch'ng et al. 1985; Park and Robinson 1987; Lehr et al. 1992; Henriksen et al. 1996; Pritchard et al. 1996). Many efforts have been made to improve the bioadhesive properties of these materials by grafting adhesion promoters such as carbohydrates or PEG onto these polymers (Garcia-Gonzalez et al. 1993; De Ascentiis et al. 1995; Shojaei and Li 1995; Serra et al. 2006). Such modification has produced many PAA, PMA, PMMA, and chitosan derivatives (listed in Table 22.4) for use in mucoadhesive drug delivery. Most of the polymer modifications enhance adhesion of the polymer to mucosal surface through improved wetting, adsorption, interpenetration, and entanglement. In recent years, new bioadhesive polymers containing thiol groups have been produced (Bernkop-Schnurch et al. 1999; Marschütz and Bernkop-Schnürch 2002). These thiolated polymers (thiomers) have strong mucoadhesive properties owing to their ability to form disulfide bonds between the thiomer and cysteine-rich subdomains of the mucus gel layer (Marschütz and Bernkop-Schnürch 2002; Roldo et al. 2004). Thiomers such as thiolated chitosan and PAA exhibited nearly 20- and 140-fold improvements in mucoadhesive properties relative to the nonthiolated ones, respectively (Clausen and Bernkop-Schnürch 2000; Kast et al. 2003).

TABLE 22.4
Polymers Studied for Bioadhesive Drug Delivery

Bioadhesive Polymers

PAA-based polymers
- PAA
- Polycarbophil (copolymer of PAA and divinyl glycol)
- Copolymer of olig(methyl methacrylate) and PAA
- Copolymer of PAA and PEG monoether monomethacrylate (PAA-CO-PEG)
- PAA/chitosan complex
- Pluronic-*g*-polyacrylic acid copolymers

PMMA-based polymers
- PMMA
- PMMA grafted starch

PMA-based polymers
- PMA
- Poly(methacrylic acid—grafted—ethylene glycol)

Thiomers
- Polycarbophil-cysteine
- Chitosan-thioglycolic acid
- PAA-cysteine

Spheromers
- Poly(fumaric acid: sebacic acid) (p[DA:SA])
- Fumaric anhydride oligomer
- L-DOPA-grafted butadiene maleic anhydride (L-DOPA-BMA)

Natural polymers
- Chitosan
- Hyaluronic acid/hyaluronan
- Lectin
- Pectin
- Tragacanth

Other polymers
- Polyanhydride and derivatives
- Sodium carboxymethyl cellulose (Na CMC)
- Polyvinyl alcohol (PVA)
- Polyvinylpyrrolidone (PVP)
- Hydroxypropyl cellulose (HPC)
- Poly(methyl vinyl ether-co-malic anhydride) (PMVEMA)
- Poly(methyl vinyl ether-co-maleic acid) (PMVEMAC)
- Polystyrene

How and why polymers adhere to mucosal surfaces is a topic of great research interest. The topic has been extensively reviewed by Peppas and Sahlin (1996), but it is generally believed that adhesion of polymers to the mucosal surface is the result of several processes related to wetting on the mucosal surface (Kaelbe and Moacanin 1977), electronic transfer between the polymer and glycoprotein network (Derjaguin et al. 1977), adsorption between polymer mucosal surface (hydrogen bonding and Van der Waals forces) (Kinloch 2001), and polymer diffusion (interpenetration) (Voyutskii 1963). Many new polymer derivatives with improved bioadhesion properties are being developed based on manipulating these processes.

Although bioadhesive drug delivery systems have been studied extensively in the past several decades, it is only recently that such systems have been used for delivering water-insoluble drugs. One such system, Spherazole™ CR (Spherics Pharmaceuticals, Inc., Mansfield, MA), has been used for controlled release of the BCS Class II water-insoluble drug itraconazole (Jacob 2005, 2006; Jacob et al. 2005).

A typical Spherazole™ CR system is a tablet that consists of a sandwiched structure as shown in Figure 22.17. Such a system was prepared by the following procedures: The water-insoluble drug itraconazole is layered onto microcrystalline cellulose with Eudragit E100 as a binder to form a granulate. The granulation is blended with spray-dried lactose, hyprom-ellose, and magnesium stearate to form a blend. The blend is compressed to form an inner-core layer. The inner-core layer is sandwiched between two outer bioadhesive layers consisting of poly(fumaric-co-sebacic)anhydride (p[FA:SA] 20:80) with Eudragit RS PO and citric acid by compression.

The Spherazole™ CR tablet is designed to reside in the stomach for more than 6 h to provide enhanced bioavailability, reduced side-effects associated with high C_{max} of a immediate release dosage form, and reduced variability (%CV). The Spherazole™ CR tablet formulations have been studied *in vivo* by comparing with Sporanox® capsule (Janssen, Beerse, Belgium) in a three-way randomized crossover clinical study in eight healthy volunteers. The study results showed that the Spherazole™ CR tablet had improved bioavailability, reduced C_{max}, and prolonged T_{max} as compared to the Sporanox capsule (Figure 22.18). The results also showed that the Spherazole CR tablet had a significantly reduced variability as compared to Sporanox capsule (Figure 22.19).

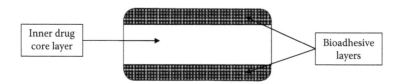

FIGURE 22.17 Schematic illustration of Spherazole™ CR bioadhesive drug delivery system (a cross-sectional view).

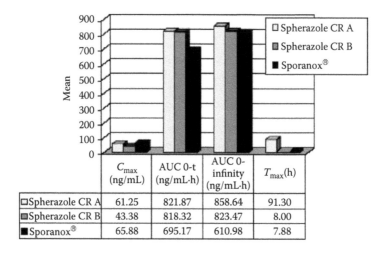

	C_{max} (ng/mL)	AUC 0-t (ng/mL·h)	AUC 0-infinity (ng/mL·h)	T_{max}(h)
☐ Spherazole CR A	61.25	821.87	858.64	91.30
▨ Spherazole CR B	43.38	818.32	823.47	8.00
■ Sporanox®	65.88	695.17	610.98	7.88

FIGURE 22.18 Pharmacokinetic parameters for the Spherazole™ CR tablet, 100 mg, compared with the Sporanox® IR capsule. (Note: Types A and B differed in levels of rate-controlling excipients.) (Adapted from Jacob, J. *Gastroretentive, bioadhesive drug delivery system for controlled release of itraconazole: Pharmacokinetics of Spherazole™ CR in healthy human volunteers*, Controlled Release Society 34th Annual Meeting and Exposition, 2006.)

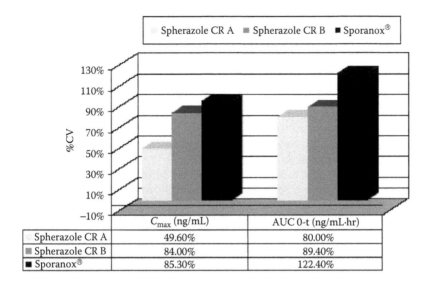

	C_{max} (ng/mL)	AUC 0-t (ng/mL·hr)
Spherazole CR A	49.60%	80.00%
Spherazole CR B	84.00%	89.40%
Sporanox®	85.30%	122.40%

FIGURE 22.19 Calculation of percentage coefficient of variation (% CV) of C_{max} and AUC0-t for Spherazole™ CR tablet, 100 mg, compared with Sporanox® capsule. (Note: Types A and B are differed in levels of rate-controlling excipients.) (Adapted from Jacob, J., *Gastroretentive, bioadhesive drug delivery system for controlled release of itraconazole: Pharmacokinetics of Spherazole™ CR in healthy human volunteers*, Controlled Release Society 34th Annual Meeting and Exposition, 2006.)

FUTURE PERSPECTIVES

Given the abundance of water-insoluble or poorly water-soluble drugs, as well as drugs exhibiting other development challenges such as metabolic and enzymatic instability, the pharmaceutical industry continues to seek solutions to overcome these limitations to develop innovative, clinically safe, and patient-friendly products. As said earlier, MR delivery products offer tremendous advantages with respect to therapeutic indices, pharmacoeconomics, and patient compliance. In addition, the MR products provide prolonged market life and are cited as one of the most important life-cycle management strategies for the innovative, therapeutically effective compounds.

One of the future focuses in research and development of MR oral dosage forms for poorly water-soluble drugs will be to conduct systematic studies to address the challenges associated with the functional parameters, in particular, physicochemical properties of the compound and GI physiological environment and factors that have significant impact on dosage form design. Efforts should also be made to improve the robustness and capability of various delivery designs applicable to poorly water-soluble drugs that have been discussed in this chapter with continuous understanding of delivery mechanism and product performance *in vitro* and *in vivo*.

ACKNOWLEDGMENTS

We are grateful to Dr. M. Brewster and Dr. L. Dong for their critical reading and comments of the manuscript.

REFERENCES

Alakhov, V., G. Pietrzynski, K. Patel, A. Kabanov, L. Bromberg, and T. A. Hatton. (2004). Pluronic block copolymers and Pluronic poly(acrylic acid) microgels in oral delivery of megestrol acetate, *J. Pharm. Pharmacol.*, 56: 1233.

Appel, L. E., W. J. Curatolo, S. M. Herbig, J. A. Nightingale, and A. G. Thombre. (2004). Controlled release by extrusion of solid amorphous dispersions of drugs, US Patent 6706283.

Azarmi, S., J. Farid, A. Nokhodchi, S. M. Bahari-Saravi, and H. Valizadeh. (2002). Thermal treating as a tool for sustained release of indomethacin from Eudragit RS and RL matrices, *Int. J. Pharm.*, 246: 171.

Baker, R. W. and H. K. Lonsdale. (1974). In *Controlled Release of Biologically Active Agents*, A. C. Tanquary, and R. E. Lacey, (Eds.). Advances in Experimental Medicine and Biological Series, No. 47; New York: Plenum Press, 1974, p. 15.

Banner Pharmacaps. (2006). Technologies, Technical Data Sheet.

Bansil, R., E. Stanley, and J. T. LaMont. (1995). Mucin biophysics, *Ann. Rev. Physiol.*, 57: 635.

Belenduik, G. W., E. M Rudnic, and J. A. McCarty. (1995). Multilamellar drug delivery systems, US patent 5447729.

Bernkop-Schnurch, A., V. Schwarz, and S. Steininger. (1999). Polymers with thiol groups; a new generation of mucoadhesive polymers? *Pharm. Res.*, 16: 876.

Boyd, B. J., C. J. Porter, and W. N. Charman. (2003). Using the polymer partitioning method to probe the thermodynamic activity of poorly water-soluble drugs solubilized in model lipid digestion products, *J. Pharm. Sci.*, 92: 1262.

Burnside, B. A., C. M. McGuinness, E. M. Rudnic, R. A. Couch, X. Guo, and A. K. Tustian. (2004). Solid solution beadlet, US Patent, 669267.

Ch'ng, H. S., H. Park, P. Kelly, and J. R. Robinson. (1985). Bioadhesive polymers as platforms for oral controlled drug delivery II: Synthesis and evaluation of some swelling, water-insoluble bioadhesive polymers, *J. Pharm. Sci.*, 74: 399.

Charman, W. N. (2000). Lipids, lipophilic drugs, and oral drug delivery—some emerging concepts, *J. Pharm. Sci.*, 89: 967.

Chiou, W. L. and S. Eiegelman. (1971). Pharmaceutical application of solid dispersions, *J. Pharm. Sci.* 60: 1281–302.

Chokshi, R. J., H. K. Sandhu, R. M. Iyer, N. H. Shah, A. W. Malick, and H. Zia. (2005). Characterization of physico-mechanical properties of indomethacin and polymers to assess their suitability for hot-melt extrusion process as a means to manufacture solid dispersion/solution, *J. Pharm. Sci.*, 94: 2463.

Clausen, A. E. and A. Bernkop-Schnurch. (2000). *In vitro* evaluation of the permeation-enhancing effect of thiolated polycarbophil, *J. Pharm. Sci.*, 89: 1253–1261.

Constantinides, P. P., G. Welzel, H. Ellens, P. L. Smith, S. Sturgis, S. H. Yiv, and A. B. Owen. (1996). Water-in-oil microemulsions containing medium-chain fatty acids/salts: Formulation and intestinal absorption enhancement evaluation, *Pharm. Res.*, 13: 210.

Craig, D. Q. M. (1990). Polyethylene glycols and drug release, *Drug Dev. Ind. Pharm.*, 16: 2501–2526.

Craig, D. Q. M. (2002). The mechanism of drug release from solid dispersions in water-soluble polymers, *Int. J. Pharm.*, 231: 131–44.

Crounse, R. G. (1961). Human pharmacology of griseofulvin. The effect of fat intake on gastrointestinal absorption, *J. Invest. Dermatol.*, 37: 529.

Cruz, E., S. Li, A. D. Ayer, B. J. Pollock, G. C. Ruhlmann, C. Garcia, A. M. Wong, and L. G. Hamel. (2005). Oros Push-Stick for controlled delivery of active agents, US Patent Application 20050089570.

De Ascentiis, A., C. N. Bowman, P. Colombo, and N. A. Peppas. (1995). Mucoadhesion of poly(2-hydroxy-ethyl-methacrylate) is improved when linear poly(ethylene oxide) chains are added to the polymer network, *J. Control Release*, 33: 197.

Derjaguin, B. V., Y. P. Toporov, V. M. Muller, and I. N. Aleinikova. (1977). On the relationship between the electrostatic and the molecular component of the adhesion of elastic particles to a solid surface, *J. Colloid. Interface Sci.*, 58: 528.

Dong, L., K. Shafi, P. Wong, and J. Wan. (2001). L-OROS® SOFTCAP™ for controlled release of nonaqueous liquid formulations, *Drug Deliv. Technol.*, 2: 1.

Dong, L., K. Shafi, A. Yum, P. Wong, C. Dong Liang, and S. L. Wong Patrick. (2004). Controlled release capsule for delivery of liquid formulation, US patent application 20040058000.

Dong, L., P. Wong, and S. Espinal. (2001). L-OROS® HARDCAP™: A new osmotic delivery system for controlled release of liquid formulation, poster presentation, 28th International Symposium of Controlled Release of Bioactive Materials, San Diego, CA.

Dordunoo, S. K. (2004). Sustained release liquid filled hard gelatin capsules in drug discovery and development: A small pharmaceutical company's perspectives, *Bull. Techn. Gattefossé*, 29: 29–39.

Dressman, J. B. and C. Reppas. (2000). *In vitro–in vivo* correlations for lipophilic, poorly water-soluble drugs, *Eur. J. Pharm. Sci.*, 2: S73.

Dressman, J. B. and K. Yamada. (1991). Animal models for oral drug absorption. In *Pharmaceutical Bioequivalence*, P. G. Welling, F. L. Tse, and S. Dighe, (Eds.), New York: Marcel Dekker, p. 235.

Elan Pharmaceutical. (2004). NanoCrystal Technologies, Technical Data Sheet.

Erkoboni, D. and R. Andersen. (2000). Improved aqueous solubility pharmaceutical formulations, PCT Patent Application WO 0056726.

Farinha, A., A. Bica, and P. Tavares. (2000). Improved bioavailability of a micronized megestrol acetate tablet, *Drug Dev. Ind. Pharm.*, 26: 567.

Flanner, H. H., L. C. McKnight, and B. A. Burnside. (2005). System for osmotic delivery of pharmaceutical active agents, US Patent 6838093.

Flynn, G. L., S. H. Yalkowsky, and T. J. Roseman. (1974). Mass transport phenomena and models: Theoretical concepts, *J. Pharm. Sci.*, 63: 479.

Food and Drug Administration. (1997a). *Guidance for Industry*, Extended-release oral dosage forms: Development, evaluation, and application of *in vitro/in vivo* correlations.

Food and Drug Administration. (1997b). *Guidance for Industry*, SUPAC-MR: Modified release solid oral dosage forms: Scale-up and post-approval changes: Chemistry, manufacturing and controls, *in vitro* dissolution testing, and *in vivo* bioequivalence documentation.

Ford, J. L. (1986). The current status of solid dispersions, *Pharm. Acta Helv.*, 61: 69–88.

Forster, A., J. Hempenstall, and T. Rades. (2001). Characterization of glass solutions of poorly water-soluble drugs produced by melt extrusion with hydrophilic amorphous polymers, *J. Pharm. Pharmacol.*, 53: 303.

Galia, E., E. Nicolaides, D. Horter, R. Lobenberg, C. Reppas, and J. B. Dressman. (1998). Evaluation of various dissolution media for predicting *in vivo* performance of Class I and II drugs, *Pharm. Res.*, 15: 698.

Garcia-Gonzalez, N., I. W. Kellaway, H. Blanco-Fuente, S. Anguiano-Igea, B. Delgado-Charro, F. J. Otero-Espinar, and J. Blanco-Mendez. (1993). Design and evaluation of buccoadhesive metoclopramide hydrogels composed of poly(acrylic acid) cross linked with sucrose, *Int. J. Pharm.*, 100: 65.

Ghebremeskel, N. A., C. Vemavarapu, and M. Lodaya. (2006). Use of surfactants as plasticizers in preparing solid dispersions of poorly water soluble API: Stability testing of selected solid dispersions, *Phar. Res.*, 23: 1928–1936.

Good, W. R., and P. I. Lee. (1984). Sustained-release delivery systems. In *Medical Applications of Controlled Release*, R. S. Langer, and D. L. Wise, (Eds.), Boca Raton, FL: CRC Press, pp. 1–10.

Gruenhagen, H. H. (1995). Melt extrusion technology, *Pharm. Manuf. Int.*, 2: 167.

Hassan, E., N. Chidambaram, and M. Price. (2003). Soft gelatin capsule as a drug delivery system: I controlled release profiles of theophylline, *Proceedings*, CRS 30th Annual Meeting, Glasgow, Scotland.

Henriksen, I., K. L. Green, J. D. Smart, G. Smistad, and J. Karlsen. (1996). Bioadhesion of hydrated chitosans: An *in vitro* and *in vivo* study, *Int. J. Pharm.*, 145: 231.

Higuchi, T. (1961). Rate of release of medicaments from ointment bases containing drugs in suspension, *J. Pharm. Sci.*, 50: 874.

Hulsmann, S., T. Backensfeld, and R. Bodmeier. (2001). Stability of extruded 17 ss-estradiol solid dispersions, *Pharm. Dev. Technol.*, 6: 223–229.

Hulsmann, S., T. Backensfeld, S. Keitel, and R. Bodmeier. (2000). Melt extrusion—An alternative method for enhancing the dissolution rate of 17β-estradiol hemihydrate, *Eur. J. Pharm. Biopharm.*, 49: 237–242.

Hwang, S. S., J. Gorsline, J. Louie, D. Dye, D. Guinta, and L. Hamel. (1995). *In vitro* and *in vivo* evaluation of a once-daily controlled release pseudoephedrine product, *J. Clin. Pharmacol.*, 35: 259.

Jacob, J. (2005). *Pharmacokinetics of bioadhesive, gastroretentive, controlled release tablets of itraconazole: (Spherazole CR) in beagle dog model*, Controlled Release Society 33rd Annual Meeting and Exposition, Vienna, Austria.

Jacob, J. (2006). *Gastroretentive, bioadhesive drug delivery system for controlled release of itraconazole: pharmacokinetics of Spherazole™ CR in healthy human volunteers*, Controlled Release Society 34th Annual Meeting and Exposition, Long Beach, California.

Jacob, J., M. Bassett, M. Schestopol, E. Mathlowitz, A. Nangia, B. Carter,, P. Moslemy, Z. E. Shaked, D. Enscore, and C. Sikes. (November 10, 2005). Polymeric drug delivery system for hydrophobic drugs, US patent application 20050249799.

Kaelbe, D. H. and J. Moacanin. (1977). A surface analysis of bioadhesion, *Polymer*, 18: 475.

Kararli, T. T. (1995). Comparison of the gastrointestinal anatomy, physiology, and biochemistry of humans and commonly used laboratory animals, *Biopharm. Drug Dispos.*, 16: 351.

Kast, C. E., D. Guggi, N. Langoth, and A. Bernkop-Schnurch. (2003). Development and *in vivo* evaluation of an oral delivery system for low molecular weight heparin based on thiolated polycarbophil, *Pharm. Res.*, 20: 931.

Kataoka, M., Y. Masaoka, Y. Yamazaki, T. Sakane, H. Sezaki, and S. Yamashita. (2003). *In vitro* system to evaluate oral absorption of poorly water-soluble drugs: Simultaneous analysis on dissolution and permeation of drugs. *Pharm. Res.*, 20: 1674.

Khanvilkar, K., M. D. Donovan, and D. R. Flanagan. (2001). Drug transfer through mucus, *Adv. Drug Deliv. Rev.*, 48: 173.

Khoo, S. M., A. J. Humberstone, C. J. Porter, G. A. Edwards, and W. N. Charman. (1998). Formulation design and bioavailability assessment of lipidic self-emulsifying formulations of halofantrine, *Int. J. Pharm.*, 167: 155.

Kinloch, A. J. (2001). *Adhesion and Adhesives Science and Technology*, 1st ed., Springer.

Kommuru, T. R., B. Gurley, M. A. Khan, and I. K. Reddy. (2001). Self-emulsifying drug delivery systems (SEDDS) of coenzyme Q10: Formulation development and bioavailability assessment, *Int. J. Pharm.*, 212: 233.

Kraml, M., J. Dubuc, and D. Beall. (1962). Gastrointestinal absorption of griseofulvin. I Effect of particle size, addition of surfactants and corn oil on the level of griseofulvin in the serum of rats, *Can. J. Biochem. Physiol.*, 40: 1449.

Lehr, C. M., J. A. Bouwstra, E. H. Schacht, and H. E. Junginger. (1992). *In vitro* evaluation of mucoadhesive properties of chitosan and some other natural polymers, *Int. J. Pharm.*, 78: 43.

Leuner, C. and J. Dressman. (2000). Improving drug solubility for oral delivery using solid dispersion, *Eur. J. Pharm. Biopharm.*, 50: 47.

Li, S. et al. (November 2001). L-OROS® SOFTCAP™: Robustness, reproducibility, and stability, published poster, Annual AAPS Meeting, Denver, Colorado.

Longer, M. A., H. S. Ch'ng, and J. R. Robinson. (1985). Bioadhesive polymers as platforms for oral controlled drug delivery. III. Oral delivery of chlorothiazide using a bioadhesive polymer, *J. Pharm. Sci.*, 74: 406.

Marriott, C. and N. P. Gregory. (1990). Mucus physiology and pathology. In *Bioadhesive Drug Delivery Systems*, Lenaerts, V. and Gurny, R. (Eds.), Boca Raton, FL: CRC Press, p. 1.

Marriott, C. and D. R. L. Hughes. (1990). Mucus physiology and pathology. In *Bioadhesion—Possibilities and Future Trends*, Gurny, R. and Junginger, H. E. (Eds.), Stuttgart, Germany: Wissenschaftliche Verlagsgesellschaft mbH, p. 29.

Marschutz, M. K. and A. Bernkop-Schnurch. (2002). Thiolated polymers: Self-crosslinking properties of thiolated 450 kDa poly(acrylic acid) and their influence on mucoadhesion, *Eur. J. Pharm. Sci.*, 15: 387.

Mathiowitz E., D. E. Chickering III, and C. M. Lehr. (1999). *Bioadhesive Drug Delivery Systems: Fundamentals, novel approaches, and development*, New York: CRC Press, p. 477.

McClelland, G. A. and G. M. Zentner. (1990). Solubility modulated drug delivery system, US Patent 4946686.

Mehta, K. A., M. S. Kislaloglu, W. Phuapradit, A. W. Malick, and N. H. Shah. (2001). Release performance of a poorly soluble drug from a novel Eudragit-based multi-unite erosion matrix, *Int. J. Pharm.*, 213: 7–12.

Modi, N. B., A. Lam, E. Lindemulder, B. Wang, and S. K. Gupta. (2000). Application of *in vitro–in vivo* correlation (IVIVC) in setting formulation release specifications, *Biopharm. Drug Dispos.*, 21: 321.

Nicolaides, E., E. Galia, C. Efthymiopoulos, J. B. Dressman, and C. Reppas. (1999). Forecasting the *in vivo* performance of four low solubility drugs from their *in vitro* dissolution data, *Pharm. Res.*, 16: 1876.

Paaver, U., J. Heinamaki, I. Laidmae, A. Lust, J. Kozlova, E. Sillaste, K. Kirsimae, P. Veski, and K. Kogermann. (2015). Electrospun nanofibers as a potential controlled-release solid dispersion system for poorly water-soluble drugs, *Int. J. Pharm.*, 479: 252–260.

Park K. and J. R. Robinson. (1984). Bioadhesives as platforms for oral controlled drug delivery. *Int. J. Pharm.*, 19: 107.

Park, H. and J. R. Robinson. (1987). Mechanisms of mucoadhesion of poly (acrylic acid) hydrogels, *Pharm. Res.*, 4: 457.

Peppas, N. A. and J. J. Sahlin. (1996). Hydrogels as mucoadhesive and bioadhesive materials: A review, *Biomaterials*, 17: 1553.

Porter, C. J. and W. N. Charman. (2001a). *In vitro* assessment of oral lipid based formulations, *Adv. Drug Deliv. Rev.*, 50: S127.

Porter, C. J. and W. N. Charman. (2001b). Lipid-based formulations for oral administration: Opportunities for bioavailability enhancement and lipoprotein targeting for lipophilic drugs, *J. Recept. Signal Transduct. Res.*, 21: 215.

Porter, C. J., A. M. Kaukonen, A. Taillardat-Bertschinger, B. J. Boyd, J. M. O'Connor, G. A. Edwards, and W. N. Charman. (2004). Use of *in vitro* lipid digestion data to explain the *in vivo* performance of triglyceride-based oral lipid formulations of poorly water-soluble drugs: Studies with halofantrine, *J. Pharm. Sci.*, 93: 1110.

Pritchard, K., A. B. Lansley, G. P. Martin, M. Helliwell, C. Marriott, and L. M. Benedetti. (1996). Evaluation of the bioadhesive properties of hyaluronan derivatives: Detachment weight and mucociliary transport rate studies, *Int. J. Pharm.*, 129: 137.

Reitz, C., C. Strachan, and P. Kleinebudde. (2008). Solid lipid extrudates as sustained-release matrices: The effect of surface structure on drug release properties, *European J. Pharm. Sci.*, 35: 335–343.

Roldo, M., M. Hornof, P. Caliceti, and A. Bernkop-Schnurch. (2004). Mucoadhesive thiolated chitosans as platforms for oral controlled drug delivery: synthesis and *in vitro* evaluation, *Eur. J. Pharm. Biopharm.*, 57: 115.

Rudnic, E. M., B. A. Burnside, H. H. Flanner, S. E. Wassink, R. A. Couch, and J. E. Pinkett. (2000). Osmotic drug delivery system, US Patent 6110498.

Rudnic, E. M., B. A. Burnside, H. H. Flanner, S. E. Wassink, R. A. Couch, and J. E. Pinkett. (2004). Osmotic drug delivery system, US Patent 6814979.

Saffie-Siebert, R., J. Ogden, and M. Parry-Billings. (2005). Nanotechnology approaches to solving the problems of poorly water-soluble drugs, *Drug Discov. World Summer*, 6: 71.

Savolainen, M. et al. (2002a). *Evaluation of controlled-release microparticles prepared by spray chilling*, poster publication, AAPS Annual Meeting, Toronto, Canada.

Savolainen, M., J. Herder, C. Khoo, K. Lovqvist, C. Dahlqvist, H. Glad, and A. M. Juppo. (2003). Evaluation of polar lipid-hydrophilic polymer microparticles, *Int. J. Pharm.*, 262: 47.

Savolainen, M., C. Khoo, H. Glad, C. Dahlqvist, and A. M. Juppo. (2002b). Evaluation of controlled-release polar lipid microparticles, *Int. J. Pharm.*, 244: 151.

Schamp, K., S. A. Schreder, and J. Dressman. (2006). Development of an *in vitro/in vivo* correlation for lipid formulations of EMD 50733, a poorly soluble, lipophilic drug substance, *Eur. J. Pharm. Biopharm.*, 62: 227.

Sek, L., B. J. Boyd, W. N. Charman, and C. J. Porter. (2006). Examination of the impact of a range of pluronic surfactants on the *in vitro* solubilization behavior and oral bioavailability of lipidic formulations of atovaquone, *J. Pharm. Pharmacol.*, 58: 809.

Serajuddin, A. T. M. (1999). Solid dispersion of poorly water-soluble drugs: Early promises, subsequent problems, and recent breakthroughs, *J. Pharm. Sci.*, 88: 1058–1066.

Serra, L., J. Domenech, and N. A. Peppas. (2006). Design of poly(ethylene glycol)-tethered copolymers as novel mucoadhesive drug delivery systems, *Eur. J. Pharm. Biopharm.*, 63: 11.

Sheen, P. C., V. K. Khetarpal, C. M. Cariola, and C. E. Rowlings. (1995). Formulation of a poorly watersoluble drug in solid dispersions to improve bioavailability, *Int. J. Pharm.*, 118: 221.

Shekunov, B. Y., P. Chattopadhyay, J. Seitzinger, and R. Huff. (2006). Nanoparticles of poorly watersoluble drugs prepared by supercritical fluid extraction of emulsions, *Pharm. Res.*, 23: 196.

Shojaei, A. H. and X. Li. (1995). Novel copolymers of acrylic acid and poly ethylene glycol monomethylether monomethacrylate for buccal mucoadhesion: Preparation and surface characterization, *Pharm. Res.*, 12: S210.

Skelly, J. P., G. L. Amidon, W. H. Barr, L. Z. Benet, J. E. Carter, J. R. Robinson, V. P. Shah, and A. Yacobi. (1990). *In vitro* and *in vivo* testing and correlation for oral controlled/modified-release dosage forms, *Pharm. Res.*, 7: 975.

Strickley, R. G. (2004). Solubilizing excipients in oral and injectable formulations, *Pharm. Res.*, 21: 201.

Sunesen, V. H., B. L. Pedersen, H. G. Kristensen, and A. Mullertz. (2005). *In vivo–in vitro* correlations for a poorly soluble drug, danazol, using the flow-through dissolution method with biorelevant dissolution media, *Eur. J. Pharm. Sci.*, 24: 305.

Sunkara, G. and D. Chilukuri. (2003). IVIVC: An important tool in the development of drug delivery systems, *Drug. Del. Tech.*, 3: 52.

Supernus Pharmaceuticals (formerly Shire Laboratories). (2006). Technologies, Technical Data Sheet.

Tanaka, N., K. Imai, K. Okimoto, S. Ueda, Y. Tokunaga, A. Ohike, R. Ibuki, K. Higaki, and T. Kimura. (2005). Development of novel sustained-release system, disintegration-controlled matrix tablet (DCMT) with solid dispersion granules of nilvadipine, *J. Control Release*, 108: 386–395.

Theeuwes, F. (1975). Elementary osmotic pump, *J. Pharm. Sci.*, 64: 1987.

Theeuwes, F. (1980). Osmotic drug delivery. In *Controlled Release Technologies: Methods, Theory and Applications*, Kydonieus, A. F. (Ed.), Boca Raton, FL: CRC Press, p. 195.

Theeuwes, F., P. Wong, and S. Yum. (1991). Drug delivery and therapeutic systems. In *Encyclopedia of Pharmaceutical Technology*, Swarbrick, J. and Boylan, J. (Eds.), Vol. 4, New York: Marcel Dekker, pp. 303–348.

Uchida, T., M. Kawata, and S. Goto. (1986). *In vivo* evaluation of ethyl cellulose microcapsules containing ampicillin using rabbits, beagle dogs and humans, *J. Pharmacobiodyn.*, 9: 631.

Verreck, G., K. Six, G. Van den Mooter, L. Baert, J. Peeters, and M. E. Brewster. (2003). Characterization of solid dispersions of itraconazole and hydroxypropylmethylcellulose prepared by melt extrusion—Part I, *Int. J. Pharm.*, 251: 165.

Vertzoni, M., J. Dressman, J. Butler, J. Hempenstall, and C. Reppas. (2005). Simulation of fasting gastric conditions and its importance for the *in vivo* dissolution of lipophilic compounds, *Eur. J. Pharm. Biopharm.*, 60: 413.

Vippagunta, S. R., K. A. Maul, S. Tallavajhala, and D. J. Grant. (2002). Solid-state characterization of nifedipine solid dispersions, *Int. J. Pharm.*, 236: 111.

Voyutskii, S. S. (1963). *Autohesion and Adhesion of High Polymers*, New York: Interscience.

Wagenaar, B. W. and B. W. Muller. (1994). Piroxicam release from spray-dried biodegradable microspheres, *Biomaterials*, 15: 49–53.

Wagner, K. G. and J. W. McGinity. (2002). Influence of chloride ion exchange on the permeability and drug release of Eudragit RS 30D films, *J. Control Release*, 82: 385–397.

Wei, H. and R. Lobenberg. (2006). Biorelevant dissolution media as a predictive tool for glyburide a class II drug, *Eur. J. Pharm. Sci.*, 29: 45.

Wong, P., B. Barclay, J. C. Deter, and F. Theeuwes. (1986). Osmotic device with dual thermodynamic activity, US Patent 4612008.

Wong, P., B. Barclay, J. Deters, and F. Theeuwes. (1988). Osmotic device for administering certain drugs, US Patent 4765989.

Wong, P., L. C. Dong, R. Zhao, and C. Pollock-Dove. (2006). Controlled release nanoparticle active agent formulation dosage forms and methods, US Patent Application 20060057206.

Wong, P. S., S. K. Gupta, and B. E. Stewart. (2003). Osmotically controlled tablets. In *Modified-Release Drug Delivery Technology*, Rathbone, M. J. et al. (Eds.), New York: Marcel Dekker, p. 107.

Wong, P. S., F. Theeuwes, B. L. Barclay, and M. H. Dealey. (1995). Osmotic dosage system for liquid drug delivery, US Patent 5413572.

Wu, K., J. Li, W. Wang, and D. A. Winstead. (2009). Formation and characterization of solid dispersions of piroxicam and polyvinylpyrrolidone using spray drying and precipitation with compressed antisolvent, *J. Pharm. Sci.*, 98: 2422–2431.

Young, C. R., M. Crowley, C. Dietzsch, and J. W. McGinity. (2007). Physicochemical properties of filmcoated melt-extruded pellets, *J. Microencapsul.*, 24: 57–71.

Young, C. R., C. Dietzsch, M. Cerea, T. Farrell, K. A. Fegely, A. Rajabi-Siahboomi, and J. W. McGinity. (2005). Physicochemical characterization and mechanisms of release of theophylline from meltextruded dosage forms based on a methacrylic acid copolymer, *Int. J. Pharm.*, 301: 112–120.

Young, C. R., J. J. Koleng, and J. W. McGinity. (2002). Production of spherical pellets by a hot-melt extrusion and spheronization process, *Int. J. Pharm.*, 242: 87–92.

Yu, K., M. Gebert, S. A. Altaf, D. Wong, and D. R. Friend. (1998). Optimization of sustained-release diltiazem formulations in man by use of *in vitro/in vivo* correlation, *J. Pharm. Pharmacol.*, 50: 845.

Zhu, Y., N. H. Shah, A. Waseem Malick, M. H. Infeld, and J. W. McGinity. (2006). Controlled release of a poorly water-soluble drug from hot-melt extrudates containing acrylic polymers, *Drug. Dev. Ind. Pharm.*, 32: 569.

23 Scalable Manufacturing of Water-Insoluble Drug Products

Nitin P. Pathak, Richard (Ruey-ching) Hwang, and Xiaohong Qi

CONTENTS

INTRODUCTION

Pharmaceutical companies invest heavily in research and development (R&D) to develop new medicines. Recent data suggest that the overall spending on pharmaceutical R&D is steadily increasing while the approval of new drugs is declining (Venugopal, 2002; Med Ad News, 2003). The pharmaceutical industry spent $1.25 billion for each new molecular entity approved by the Food and Drug Administration (FDA) in 2004 (PAREXEL, 2005/2006). The statistics suggest that the value of the current world pharmaceutical market is an estimated $550 billion, and that worldwide R&D spending in the pharmaceutical industry was $53 billion in 2005 (PAREXEL, 2005/2006). Apart from the growing research spending, the pharmaceutical industry is facing tough challenges in the current business environment (Table 23.1). To compete in today's business environment and operate an effective global pharmaceutical R&D organization, it is imperative that the pharmaceutical development process be a lean operation where controlling cost is as important as efficiency.

When a drug loses patent protection, sales drop sharply. This is a well-researched fact with examples of brand drugs like Lovenox, Prozac, Diflucan, Cipro, Claritin, and so forth, losing about 80% of market share to generics in the first 6 months after patents expired. Recently, patent challenges to successful brands are common examples of intense industry competition and environmental pressure on ethical pharmaceutical companies engaged in drug discovery and development. Legislative

TABLE 23.1

Major Challenges for the Pharmaceutical Industry

Time and resource requirements for discovering and developing new medicines

Competition (generic and other brand companies)

R&D spending

Patent life

Price controls

Government legislation

Regulatory requirements

Managed health care

Cost of new enabling technologies

challenges in drug importation (e.g., Internet pharmacies) and price controls in various markets are drivers that are forcing ethical pharmaceutical companies to change the way that drugs are discovered and developed. The recent withdrawals of previously approved COX-2 selective drugs are an indication of tightened regulatory scrutiny for future drug products by the approving authority.

Figure 23.1 illustrates the regulatory timeline associated with meeting FDA requirements for registering the discovered drug molecule through the sequential development process. Discovering and successfully commercializing a new drug takes years. Ethical pharmaceutical companies have to support discovery and development efforts under intense regulatory requirements for proving the safety and efficacy of new medications. The time and resource consumption required to successfully bring a new drug to market is not sustainable in the current industry environment. The aforementioned external environmental pressures for ethical pharmaceutical companies are drivers for making fundamental changes in how medicines are discovered and developed.

The systematic evaluation of new drugs is a time- and resource-consuming process that requires constant knowledge management. The rate of success in the discovery and eventual commercialization of a pharmaceutical product is very low. The attrition of drugs in early clinical phases (Phases I and II) is high before the drug molecule moves up in the advance phases of studies (Phases III and IV). The probability of successfully discovering and developing a drug molecule in a particular therapeutic category also depends on historical success rates and attrition observed in the category. For these reasons, investing heavily in developing process understanding for scalable manufacturing of drug products in early phases is not advisable.

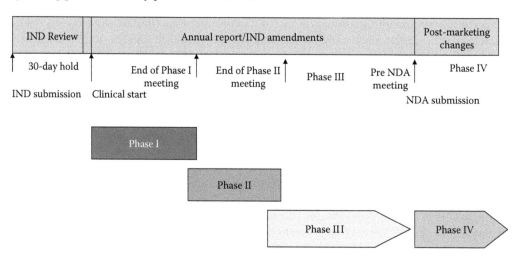

FIGURE 23.1 Regulatory process for new chemical entities approval.

Often, the challenges experienced by an ethical pharmaceutical company in development of water-insoluble drug products revolve around the following factors:

- Active pharmaceutical ingredient (API) development and optimization of synthetic commercial route
- Therapeutic dose determination based on the therapeutic index and effective dose required to mitigate the targeted disease state
- Relatively low upfront investment in time and resources for developing a market image drug product manufacturing process

Because of the limited aqueous solubility of compounds, a small change of API particle size could make slower dissolution from dosage forms, and the increased dosing amount could cause incomplete dissolution after dosing. The altered dissolution characteristics can make systematic exposure of drug after oral administration lower than what we expect. It is important to make appropriate risk analysis when API process changes or dosing amount changes are made. The reasons why this is critical for water-insoluble drugs are that we cannot use the same strategy to bridge formulation and process changes that can be applied for Biopharmaceutics Classification System (BCS) class 1 compounds.

Table 23.2 lists the common challenges for exploratory and full development phases of drug product manufacturing. The API synthesis in early phases of development and the eventual optimization of the synthetic route for large-scale bulk API manufacturing pose numerous challenges in the development of the acceptable market image drug product. The crystalline morphology, API density, particle size, and the evolution of environmental health and safety requirements pose additional challenges to develop process understanding for drug product manufacture. The changes in morphology and particle size have a direct impact on powder flow and other key drug product attributes such as dissolution. The change in bulk density has direct impact on the scale of equipment and preference for enabling technology for successfully developing a drug product. For example, if the density of the API decreases, a large capacity blender, granulator, and so forth, may be required. Similarly, if the enabling technology is a wet granulation process involving fluid-bed technology, then for a low density API, the process may need to be modified to accommodate quick wetting of the API mass initially in the process to keep homogeneous wet granulation process in order to prevent fines during the granulation, which could cause poor powder flow and/or sticking problem. This is generally accomplished by quick wetting of the mass with low air fluidizing volume for enabling powder wetting. It is observed that if high air volumes are applied initially, the powder has a tendency to accumulate in the fluid-bed bags, thus creating undesirable fines in the granulation. However, high air volumes may be necessary if the API bulk density is high. It is necessary to adjust

---

TABLE 23.2
Drug Product Manufacturing Challenges

Early Development Phase (Phases I and II)	Late Development Phase (Phases III and IV)
Dose of drug molecule not known	API scale-up activities have effect on morphology
API morphology keeps changing	Optimization of drug product formulation and manufacturing processes
API synthetic route not finalized (number of synthetic steps not optimized)	Key process parameters and their effects on critical drug product attributes not well defined
Drug product manufacturing process poorly understood	Development of clinical manufacturing process and its alignment with commercial manufacturing
Drug product in-process controls not established	Commercial scale and scale-up challenges of drug products
Attrition rate is high	

inlet air volume according to powder characteristics to process API with different powder character-istics. Alternatively, formulation scientists may have to shift the enabling technology from fluid-bed granulation to something like extrusion-based processing technology. Formulation scientists have to constantly monitor the API changes to develop and optimize manufacturing process.

Therapeutic dose constantly changes as more and more clinical data on safety and efficacy become available. During the Phase I studies in healthy human volunteers, a tolerable dose range is established. The pharmacokinetic profile of the drug in terms of adsorption, distribution, metabo-lism, and excretion (ADME) is also established. This initial read on the dose range provides clues to the possible therapeutic doses. On the basis of this information, a potential strategy to develop a for-mulation and choice of enabling processing technology is conceptualized by the formulator. During the Phase II efficacy trials in the intended patient population, therapeutic dose range-finding studies are conducted, maximum tolerated dose is determined, and minimum effective dose is evaluated. The outcomes of these clinical trials often have significant impact on the effective dose selection. The dose changes at this stage also impact formulation composition and preferred manufactur-ing processes. Some of the complex challenges that a formulation scientist may encounter are low density API obtained during the API optimization process and a high effective dose requirement determined by Phase II studies. In such cases, the formulation scientist has to rethink the strategy for formulation and enabling process technology to successfully manufacture a quality drug product in a reasonable period of time. At this point, the safety profile and, to a large extent, efficacy are established and additional pressures built for a company to either realize commercial potential of the drug in the market or terminate the project.

In the early phases of development, drug product manufacturing is tied to clinical supply require-ments. Drug products are produced in minimal quantities and in customized formats. On the con-trary, in late-stage drug development, the drug product demand increases in volume. In this stage, clinical supply needs and drug product process become more defined with repetitive requirements of drug product manufacturing on a larger scale. Figure 23.2 illustrates the requirements of clinical supplies in early- and late-stage development with emphasis on manufacturing requirements.

The development of the concept *Quality by Design (QbD)* has significantly transformed pharma-ceutical quality regulation from an empirical process to a more scientific and risk-based approach. According to the ICH Q8 guidelines, QbD is a proactive and systematic risk-based approach to phar-maceutical development that begins with predefined objectives and emphasizes product and process understanding and process control based on sound science and quality risk management (Yu, 2008).

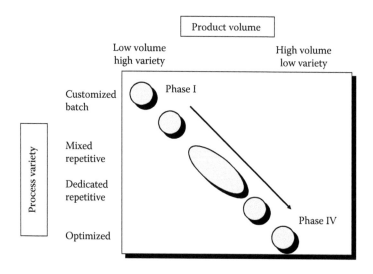

FIGURE 23.2 Clinical supply requirements in different development phases.

The elements of QbD consists of the following parameters:

1. Quality Target Product Profile (QTPP): Include dosage form, delivery systems, dosage strength(s), and so on. It is a prospective summary of quality characteristics of a drug product to be achieved, taking into account dosage strength(s) and container closure system of the drug product, together with the attributes affecting pharmacokinetic characteristics (e.g., dissolution, aerodynamic performance) and drug product quality criteria (e.g., sterility, purity, stability and drug release) appropriate for the intended marketed product.
2. Critical Quality Attributes (CQAs): Include physical, chemical, biological, or microbiological properties or characteristics of an output material including finished drug product. Potential drug product CQAs derived from the QTPP and/or prior knowledge are used to guide the product and process development and they should be within an appropriate limit, range, or distribution to ensure the desired product quality.
3. Critical Material Attributes (CMAs): Include physical, chemical, biological, or microbiological properties or characteristics of an input material. CMAs should be within an appropriate limit, range, or distribution to ensure the desired quality of that drug substance, excipient, or in-process material.
4. Critical Process Parameters (CPPs): Parameters monitored before or in process that significantly influence the appearance, impurity, and yield of final product.

This chapter will focus on technologies and suggest paradigms to broadly accomplish the development of robust solid dosage formulations and process understanding for future generations of new water-insoluble drug products.

PHASE I STRATEGIES FOR DRUG PRODUCT MANUFACTURING OF WATER-INSOLUBLE NEW CHEMICAL ENTITIES

Usually, the goal in the early phase of drug development is to minimize resource commitment and simplify the assessment of new chemical entities (NCEs) in the clinic. The dosage form and manufacturing strategies should support the objective of a minimalistic approach. In this model, the recommendation is to screen as many NCEs as possible, as quickly as possible, with minimal resource. To be successful in achieving this objective, businesses need to dedicate themselves to developing standardized methodologies for developing dosage forms through supporting good manufacturing practices (GMP) procedures for the water-insoluble drugs.

During Phase I studies, healthy volunteers are administered with a single dose of an investigational drug, and each receives only one dose. The study may or may not be placebo controlled. The starting dose is generally a large factor below the expected efficacious dose (i.e., no observable adverse effect level [NOEL] × safety margin). The dose is raised only after ascertaining that no adverse effects are observed. The new dose is generally administered to a different volunteer. The doses are raised until safety becomes an issue. The pharmacokinetic ADME data on the NCE is gathered by determining the plasma levels of drug after administering the dose.

The next stage of assessment is a multidose tolerance (MDT) study. The objective of this study is to assess pharmacodynamic and pharmacokinetic effects and to collect data for any adverse event observed. For this assessment, a range of doses is administered with placebo control to healthy volunteers for 7–14 days. The intention of these studies is to assess any potential saturation of metabolism.

To accomplish the single-dose and MDT studies mentioned earlier, the dosage form selected should encompass the range of doses desired for the duration of study with flexibility required for changing doses. Extemporaneous prescription compounding in clinics is one approach to provide dosing flexibility. This can be achieved through simple compounding of API in the following dosage forms:

- Extemporaneously Prepared Solution/Suspension (EPS)
- Extemporaneous Dispensation of API in a Capsule

EXTEMPORANEOUSLY PREPARED SOLUTION/SUSPENSION

Biopharmaceutical properties like poor solubility and permeability are major development issues hindering bioavailability of the NCEs (Venkatesh and Lipper, 2000). In relative terms, the overall rate of absorption of the NCE is affected more frequently by its solubility than its permeability (Hörter and Dressman, 2001). EPS is simplest dosage methodology that can support Phase I objectives. The water-insoluble drug is individually weighed in bottles or other suitable containers. These preweighed doses are reconstituted in the clinic (with an appropriate vehicle specified in the protocol) and dosed immediately. The vehicle composition may solubilize the drug or act as a suspending vehicle. The administering pharmacist in the clinic can also perform dilutions to achieve desired lower doses for a patient. This is typically done in cases where the drug is solubilized in the enabling vehicle. Vehicles used in such procedures include sterile water for injection, dextrose solution, or purified water. Diluted Tween 80 solution and water are most frequently used as a solution for reconstitution. The buffering system for reconstitution can also be used, when investigational compounds have pH-dependent solubility profile. The solubilization of API can be achieved by utilizing numerous techniques such as cosolvents (Yalkowsky and Roseman, 1981a,b) or complex formation (Gupta and Cannon, 2000). Commonly used solvents available to accomplish solubilization are alcohol USP, propylene glycol USP, polyethylene glycol USP (molecular weight 200 and 600), and glycerine USP. These solvents are generally recognized as safe (GRAS) by the FDA and are miscible with water. The level of precedent use in formulation is available in the inactive ingredient guide (Food and Drug Administration, 2006).

The EPS placebo requirement for clinical studies could become an additional challenge in cases where the NCE is colored, bitter tasting, and so forth. In most cases, the reconstituting vehicle alone can be utilized as a placebo. When this is not feasible, bittering agents, buffer salts, and color additives can be used to meet these challenges. This methodology has the advantage of not requiring additional instructions for the clinical pharmacist to prepare the reconstituted solution/suspension for dosing.

The dosing of the NCE immediately after reconstitution helps avoid the need for extensive stability studies. Typically, 12 h stability in solution/suspension (after reconstitution) needs to be assured. The stability data generated for the GMP batch of bulk API supports the regulatory requirement. The GMP requirement for the API dispensing process is much simpler. The analytical resource requirement is limited to identity testing of dispensed API in a bottle. Dose uniformity for this approach could be assured by monitoring individual filling weight through manufacturing process. Overall, this methodology complies with lean manufacturing principles in reducing cycle time to the clinic.

For water-insoluble drugs requiring MDT studies, the dose requirement could run into thousands of bottles. If the company does not wish to invest resources into developing a solubilizing vehicle, then large numbers of bottles can be dispensed using autodose high-precision dispensing technology (Hariharan et al., 2003; Autodose and Powdernium, 2005). This technology allows for simplicity in reconstituting the entire content of the bottle with an aqueous-based vehicle and dosing the entire content of the bottle.

EXTEMPORANEOUS DISPENSATION OF ACTIVE PHARMACEUTICAL INGREDIENT IN A CAPSULE

Capsule dosage form offers distinct advantages in early phase clinical trials for water-insoluble drugs. The NCE exhibiting color and taste challenges and flexible dosing amount can be easily dispensed in opaque-colored capsules. In the past, use of this dosage form was limited as some level of formulation development work was prerequisite and technologies did not exist to accurately dispense a wide range of API in a capsule.

Capsule shell sizes are generally standardized with finite volumes (Rudnic and Schwartz, 2000; Capsugel, 2006) available for dispensing the API or powder blend. The capsule size selection would depend on the dose and the bulk density of the NCE. Historically, if the doses were within a reasonable range, it was feasible to dispense API directly into the capsule body utilizing manual, semiautomatic, or automatic high-speed encapsulators available for manufacturing.

Recent advances in dispensing technology for a powder into capsules have pushed the threshold, and today's technologies such as Xcelodose™ and autodose high-precision dispensing technology (Hariharan et al., 2003; Autodose and Powdernium, 2005) offer new opportunities with this dosage form. These technologies offer an opportunity to accurately dispense an NCE into a capsule shell with great flexibility in dispensing doses for Phase I trials. The stability studies and potential for interaction with formulation components are minimized using this approach. However, stability data indicating API compatibility with the capsule shell are required. Cross-linking of capsule shell and entrapment of the dispensed dose (e.g., especially low doses, 5 mg or less) are potential concerns, but advances in capsule shell material (e.g., hydroxypropyl methylcellulose [HPMC] capsule shells offered by Capsugel and Shionogi) have reduced this concern. Experience with this technology suggests that to achieve accuracy at low doses one may have to compromise on the throughput. Throughput from these machines also depends on powder flow characteristics. In cases where this technology does not accommodate dispensation owing to flow challenges, alternative approaches require some formulation efforts with one or two excipients to improve flow characteristics of the API (Mouro et al., 2006). In this case, it is necessary to show acceptable dose uniformity of capsule formulations with regular content uniformity testing. The overall distinct advantages this technology offers are reduced analytical resources, reduced formulation requirements, minimal GMP manufacturing resources, and the provision of sound documentation for each capsule produced.

PHASE II STRATEGIES FOR DRUG PRODUCT MANUFACTURING OF WATER-INSOLUBLE NEW CHEMICAL ENTITIES

The objective of Phase II clinical studies is to achieve evidence of efficacy in the target patient population and assess short-term safety. There are two types of Phase II studies: the early Phase II (or proof of concept) study that focuses on confirmation of efficacy and the late Phase II study (dose finding purpose). During the late Phase II studies, therapeutic dose ranges and dosing regimens are defined, and the minimum effective dose and maximum tolerated dose are established.

For clinical supply management, it is a challenge to recommend clinical supplies with doses that could accommodate the low and high end of the regimen. Patient compliance is a critical factor in developing the clinical dosage form. For example, if only the smallest dose is available, the number of doses would increase, and this could potentially cause patient compliance issues. Similarly, if a higher clinical dosage form is selected, this could cause limitations in the dosing regimen. The clinical study planner has to strike a balance between the lowest and highest possible doses to come up with a few doses that will allow for reasonable formulation and manufacturing of dosage form to ensure patient compliance in the clinical setting.

Typical approaches for water-insoluble compounds to make an oral dosage form are

1. to formulate with surface active agent and/or pH-modifying agent to improve aqueous solubility and wettability of the compounds,
2. to introduce micronization or nanotechnology to maximize drug dissolution from the formulation,
3. to utilize amorphous phase of the candidate compounds.

The drug product demand and forecast for conducting studies in Phase II and beyond play a key role in developing strategies for the formulation and manufacturing scale. The data for a molecule in Phase II are suggestive of customized repetitive batches with often slight modifications in batch sizes. The dosing amount and solubility ratio are important factors for deciding the formulation strategy. Combination of the first two approaches given earlier would determine the optimal path for dosage forms.

For this phase of development, Huang (2005) has recommended a standardized approach to developing a tablet and capsule formulation. This approach standardizes the formulation where few compositions are available for scientists to *plug and play* their API and quickly develop a clinical image dosage form. Huang recommends formulation composition with soluble and insoluble types of inert diluents and commonly used disintegrants such as crospovidone, sodium croscarmellose, sodium starch glycolate, and calcium carbonate. For lubrication, Huang recommends magnesium stearate at 0.5% or separate screening studies for other lubricants such as stearic acid (1%), hydrogenated vegetable oil (lubritab, 2%), and sodium stearyl fumerate (1%). Finally, glidant use is recommended as optional with colloidal silicon dioxide as the ingredient of choice. Understanding of API material characteristics (e.g., ductility, brittleness, etc.) also aids in selecting appropriate standardized formulation. The use of these formulations certainly has some distinct advantages at this stage of development. Standard manufacturing process also can be applied to these standardized formulations. These formulations can be evaluated for the two standard processing approaches, namely, dry granulation and wet granulation (Figures 23.3 and 23.4). Process understanding of how a standardized placebo behaves with the two processing techniques provides indications to an optimum processing technique for a formulation. The development time required for further process understanding is relatively low.

Once the standardized formulation composition and preferred processing technology are well understood, plugging in the API and manufacturing the clinical dosage is a relatively low-risk proposition. The impact of API drug load on the standardized formulation is the only risk that one has to manage to successfully manufacture a clinical drug product. If the drug loading in the formulation is high (i.e., >10%), there is higher potential for it to impact the manufacturing process. Understanding of API properties (i.e., morphology, density, flow, particle size, compressibility, cohesivity, etc.) can

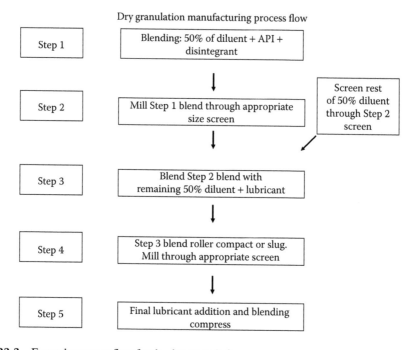

FIGURE 23.3 Example process flow for the dry granulation process.

Scalable Manufacturing of Water-Insoluble Drug Products   **705**

Wet granulation manufacturing process flow

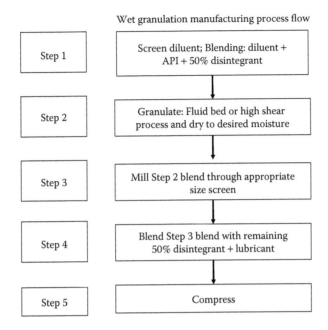

Step 1	Screen diluent; Blending: diluent + API + 50% disintegrant
Step 2	Granulate: Fluid bed or high shear process and dry to desired moisture
Step 3	Mill Step 2 blend through appropriate size screen
Step 4	Blend Step 3 blend with remaining 50% disintegrant + lubricant
Step 5	Compress

FIGURE 23.4   Example process flow for the wet granulation process.

help in assessing this risk and impact. If the drug loading is very low (i.e., <1%), the preferred technology could be wet granulation to ensure content uniformity. Table 23.3 suggests two broad risk factors where variability in dose and drug loading in standard formulations could pose challenges in the clinical manufacturing environment. Also mentioned are the authors' suggested risk mitigation techniques to ensure quality compliance. The processes and the manufacturing scales vary widely, and process validation is nonexistent at this stage in the development. Hence, the obligation for ensuring quality drug product lies solely on the in-process controls and sound understanding of how the API will behave in the standardized formulation during manufacturing. Although specialized

TABLE 23.3
Phase II Clinical Manufacturing Challenges with Standardized Formulations

	Factors	Clinical Manufacturing Challenge	Suggested Risk Mitigation Approaches
1.	Low dose (<1 mg or below 1% drug loading)	Content uniformity	In-process controls such as stratified sampling, process analytical technology (PAT) application, and blend homogeneity. Assess modification of dissolution through optimization of API characteristics and then perform assessment of specialized technologies [hot-melt extrusion (HME), spray-dried dispersion, solid dispersion, etc.] for long-term resolution.
2.	High dose (>10% drug loading)	Potential risk in process ability during manufacture	API material characterization before manufacturing for potential impact assessment. Process understanding and evaluation of specialized technologies [twin-screw wet granulation (TSWG), extrusion, solid dispersion, etc.] for long-term resolution.

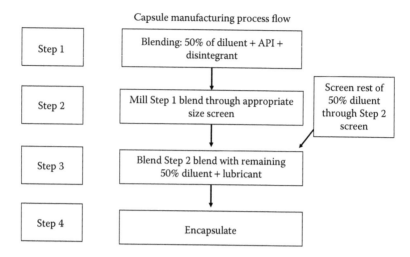

FIGURE 23.5 Example process flow for the encapsulation process.

techniques are available to manage some of the risks, they are best considered long-term strategies to consider these options on case-by-case basis.

Figures 23.3 through 23.5 illustrate the stepwise process flow typically utilized in wet and dry granulation techniques for the manufacture of tablet dosage forms. For capsules, the process tends to be simpler with utilization of first three steps from dry granulation followed by encapsulation in appropriate-size capsule shells. Depending on the batch size, a manual filler (e.g., Bonapace), semi-automatic encapsulator (e.g., Capsugel Ultra 8), or automated encapsulator (Zanasi, Macofar, etc.) could be utilized for manufacturing.

Alexander and Muzzio (2002) suggest that for scale-up of blending operation one must consider the geometry of the blenders, total number of revolutions, fill volume, and total blending time. In theory, blend uniformity is achieved by three essentially independent mechanisms: (1) convection, which causes the large particles to move in the direction of flow owing to blender rotation; (2) dispersion, which considers the random movement of particles due to collision or interparticle motion and generally parallel to the axis of rotation; and (3) shear, which refers to particle separation from large agglomerates. In most tumbling blend operations, the shear involved is relatively minimal, unless an intensifier bar is utilized.

Rekhi and Sidwell (2005) explain the theory of size reduction during the milling operation. The material being milled is subjected to one or more of four forces during milling: (1) shear (cutting forces), (2) compression (crushing forces), (3) impaction (the direct, high-velocity collision force), and (4) tension (forces that elongate or pull particles apart). Cleavage during milling occurs at the weakest point in the granules. The characteristics of the granules after size reduction depend mainly on the type of the mill used, impeller type and speed, screen size, and thickness. Mill selection in turn depends on the material characteristics and classification. Materials can be classified as hard, soft, fibrous, and intermediate on Moh's scale. The important material properties are toughness, brittleness, abrasiveness, cohesive/adhesiveness, melting point, agglomeration tendency, moisture content, flammability, toxicity, and reactivity. These properties must be considered when making a selection between high-energy or low-energy mill. In low-energy mills, the size reduction is accomplished primarily by shear and some attrition whereas in high-energy mills, the size reduction is achieved by high-velocity impact between the rapidly moving impeller/blades and the powder being milled. At times, wet milling of the agglomerates is performed to increase surface area and facilitate efficient drying as well as improve size uniformity and granule formation.

Granulation is a process of agglomeration where significant particle growth is accomplished in a powder blend by the addition of binder solution. The unit operation is intended to ensure content uniformity, improve blend flow, provide narrow particle size distribution, and densify the material. For water-insoluble compounds, the wet granulation process can be the process to modify intrinsic dissolution rates of the compounds. The mechanism to accomplish granulation involves powder mixing, binder addition in solution or liquid, wetting of powder mass and nucleation, growth of the granules, and densification of the powder and granule attrition and breakage. The resulting wet mass is further dried and processed downstream to a finished dosage form (Figure 23.4). Gokhale et al. (2005) classified the granulation process as (1) low-shear (PK blender with intensifier bar, planetary mixer, ribbon blenders, etc.) granulator, (2) moderate-shear granulator (fluid-bed granulation with rotor granulator), and (3) high-shear (HS) granulator (ULTIMAPROTM and GMXTM). The process variables affecting the quality of granules are (1) powder blend load, (2) impeller speed, (3) granulation liquid addition method and rate, (4) chopper speed, and (5) granulation time.

Process factors also need to be considered for this unit operation such as granulation liquid requirement for a particular blend mix. This largely depends on the blend characteristics, but in theory the liquid requirement is generally close to saturation. The saturation requirement largely depends on the blend composition. Lipps and Sakr (1994) concluded in their study that the insoluble fillers like dibasic calcium phosphate (DCP) and some grades of lactose can be granulated well below the 100% liquid saturation level. Physical characteristics of the drug and drug load, type of binder, binder solvent, types of excipients, and quantity play a critical role in overall granule characteristics.

It is important to recognize the differences in utilizing the wet granulation technique for water-soluble and water-insoluble API. Furthermore, concentration of the drug in the blend also plays an important role in these considerations. The water-soluble drugs may have the tendency to become solubilized during the granulation and recrystallize on drying. Hence, the volume of the granulation vehicle required in this case becomes a critical parameter in the development process. This is also important for water-insoluble compounds, as the solubilized compounds should be crystallized into the most stable crystal form that has lower aqueous solubility than the original form. In the case of water-insoluble drugs, controlled particle growth and dissolution profiles with content uniformity are challenging tasks. Chowhan (1998) studied the effect of API physical properties on the wet granulation process and resulting granulation. The change in the particle shape of the API was observed to go from spherical to plate structure resulting in the decreased compressibility of the granulation. In summary, for a wet granulation process the scientist must understand the various formulations, process and equipment variables, and the interdependencies of all variables impacting the downstream processing of the solid dosage forms.

For drying of the granulation in fluid-bed process, inlet air temperature, moisture carrying capacity of the air, air volume and velocity, atomization air pressure, liquid spray rate, product temperature, and exhaust air temperatures are the key process variables that dictate the rate of water removal. Examples of different techniques for drying the wet granulation include tray drying, fluid-bed drying, microwave drying, and radio frequency drying. It is important to recognize that the mechanism and principles for water removal differ from process to process. Tray drying seems to be the slowest process where water is removed from the static bed. This may also lead to migration of drug to the surface and has the potential for recrystallization (O'Connor and Schwartz, 1985). Fluid-bed drying tends to be a very efficient process; however, the process leads to loss of density in dried granulation owing to air fluidization of wet mass. This may be a limitation in high-dose scenario as the size of the tablet would tend to increase.

Schwartz (2002) suggests special consideration for the compression process. Press speed for material that compacts by plastic deformation, overmixing of lubricant in the force feeder, heat buildup on long compressions runs, material abrasiveness, and tooling care are important variables for consideration. Dwell time and compression and ejection forces are other variables identified for monitoring process.

Scientists have successfully utilized the cosolvent approach in developing soft gelatin formulations (Tabibi and Gupta, 2000). When the solubilization of an NCE in a definite concentration is accomplished, soft gelatin capsules can become a dosage form of choice. Once a cosolvent system is developed for a drug, generally the scale-up of this process to a commercial scale can be achieved with relative ease. Equipment for filling liquids in a capsule on both small and large scales is readily available. However, the challenge encountered in this approach is achievement of adequate solubility and stability in the cosolvent system that can be contained in a specified capsule volume. This dosage form also limits the quantity of water as an enabling solvent.

As formulation scientists engage themselves in formulation and process development activities, in-process controls begin to assume major importance for demonstrating quality during the manufacturing process. Current GMPs state that in-process controls must exist to assure batch uniformity and quality of drug product (21 CFR 211.110 and EU GMP Guidelines Annex 13). The in-process controls are to be implemented to monitor and control critical process parameters during manufacturing of drug product. In-process controls assume a greater level of importance in ensuring that each manufactured lot meets all its specifications since limited process validation is available for exploratory clinical lots. In-process controls are dependent on previous experience with the particular dosage form, formulation characteristics, manufacturing process complexity, and batch size.

In-process controls are of two types: (1) in-process *monitoring* during the manufacturing and (2) in-process *testing* of the intermediate material. Monitoring is defined as periodic checks performed during manufacturing to ensure that the process conforms to the preestablished ranges and, if necessary, to adjust the manufacturing parameters before further processing. An example of in-process monitoring would be machine adjustment to ensure that tablet weight or capsule fill weight is maintained in the specified range. In-process testing can be defined as GMP testing performed during manufacturing to assess the performance of key manufacturing steps by ensuring compliance to a specified target range before further processing. An example of the in-process testing would be the verification of blend uniformity for compliance to target acceptance range before an encapsulation or tablet compression step. Authors' suggested examples of common in-process monitoring and testing controls for tablet and capsule dosage forms are listed in Table 23.4.

Blend uniformity testing is intended to demonstrate content uniformity and adequate mixing of ingredients at the blending unit operation. However, research has proven that one cannot rely only on this assurance as segregation of API could happen in the downstream processing during compression and/or encapsulation. Product blend during these processes can be subjected to machine vibration during manufacturing and thus have potential for impacting the overall quality of the drug product. Stratified sampling and testing is an approach to demonstrate that quality (batch uniformity) is maintained throughout the encapsulation or compression run. Stratified sampling is defined as the process

TABLE 23.4

In-Process Monitoring and Testing Controls for Tablet and Capsule Dosage Forms

Unit Process	In-Process Monitoring	In-Process Testing
Blending		Blend uniformity
Compressing	Appearance	Stratified sampling and testing
	Friability	
	Hardness	
	Weight variation	
	Thickness	
Granulation		
Dry granulation	Solid fraction	Compliance to target solid fraction
	Thickness	range
Wet granulation	Moisture assessment	Drying endpoint target (moisture test)
	Granule size	Sieve analysis
Encapsulation	Appearance	Blend uniformity
	Weight variation	Stratified sampling and testing

of sampling and testing dosage units at predefined intervals by collecting representative samples from specifically targeted locations/time points in the compression or filling operations that have the greatest potential to yield extreme highs and lows in test results (Food and Drug Administration, 2003b; Boehm et al., 2003). Stratified sampling and testing during the downstream processing help to demonstrate maintenance of homogeneity throughout the manufacturing process.

The FDA guidance for industry (Food and Drug Administration, 2004) on stratified sampling provides recommendations on how to test and evaluate routine manufacturing batches. It is suggested to correlate stratified sampling data with powder blend data and finished dosage unit data to assess uniformity of content and to monitor during the manufacturing process. The guidance document describes in detail the sampling plans and recommended criteria for demonstrating quality control during manufacturing.

Another way to complement the in-process quality assurance is through application of process analytical technology (PAT). Multivariate analysis of pharmaceutical manufacturing processes equipped with PAT, or process monitoring and real-time product testing, leads to better assessment and understanding of the effect of process parameters on product quality attributes.

Advantages gained by such an approach might include the following:

1. Specifications based on correlations of multiple variables rather than outputs of single variables
2. Specification criteria based on curve fitting factors rather than single output limits
3. The elimination of some end product testing for product release
4. Arrival at a very thorough manufacturing process understanding
5. The refinement of model based specifications by new knowledge gained during the life-cycle of a product

PAT can be described as a system for designing, analyzing, and controlling manufacturing through timely measurements (i.e., during manufacturing process) of critical quality and performance attributes of raw and in-process materials and processes with the goal of ensuring final product quality (Food and Drug Administration, 2004). It is important to note that the term *analytical* in PAT is viewed broadly to include risk analysis as well as chemical, physical, microbiological, and mathematical testing conducted in an integrated manner (Food and Drug Administration, 2003a, 2004). The philosophy of this approach is to build quality into the product during each step in the manufacturing process. FDA guidelines (Food and Drug Administration, 2004) state that the objective of PAT is to enhance understanding and control the manufacturing process, to support the idea that "quality cannot be tested into products; it should be built in or should be by design." The guidelines further describe the concepts of process understanding including (1) identification and explanation of all critical sources of variability, (2) management of process variables, and (3) prediction of quality attributes accurately and reliably through the design space established for materials used, process parameters, manufacturing environment, and other conditions (Food and Drug Administration, 2003a, 2004).

The benefits of PAT application are real-time control over the manufacturing process through in-line, at-line, and online application of PAT tools. In-line measurement can be defined as invasive and noninvasive measurements where the sample is not removed from the process stream. An example of in-line measurement would be the placement of an infrared sensor in close proximity (e.g., on the conveyer belt) to measure content uniformity in the process stream. Similarly, a temperature probe introduced into the process stream to measure the temperature of material at different ports is also an example of in-line measurement. At-line measurement is where a sample is physically removed from the process stream and analyzed in close proximity. At-line measurements are routinely performed during the manufacturing process. Moisture measurement to determine the progress of a drying cycle within the processing room is one good example of at-line measurement. Finally, online measurement involves a sample being initially diverted from the manufacturing process, analyzed, and returned back to the process stream. Online measurements are becoming increasingly common. For instance, tools are now available to measure the particle size of the granules where the granulation stream is diverted for measurement, quickly analyzed, and reintroduced directly back into the process stream.

PAT tools offer manufacturers the ability to perform continuous quality verification. These techniques offer real-time feedback to enhance process intelligence and control. The measurements are typically nondestructive in nature and provide feedback on whether the product's key attributes are within the acceptable working range. The real-time measurement and feedback afford the opportunity to identify and rectify problems and thus effectively mitigate the risk of quality failure. Wide ranges of technologies are currently available to provide real-time quality assessment. These are based on the principles of the following analytical technologies: near infrared, mid-infrared, Raman, UV-visible, acoustic emission spectroscopy, particle sizing, fluorescence, microscopy, chromatography, and mass spectroscopy. It is important to recognize a key distinction that PAT tools act as means for measuring metrics for the key performance parameters identified for a product and process. The scientists have to identify the key process parameters through systematic evaluation of each process and its impact on the desired quality attribute (e.g., dissolution, content uniformity, etc.). Once identified, the rational approach is to monitor only those key process parameters that matter.

For successful application of PAT in increasing process and product understanding, the following three guidelines are helpful:

1. Specify the drug product quality attributes
2. Understand the parameters that will affect the quality attributes
3. Carefully choose a measurement system that is capable of verifying those parameters

In Table 23.5, the authors suggest the PAT application for monitoring and testing of key quality attributes for the tablet and capsule dosage forms that are currently available in the industry.

TABLE 23.5

Process Analytical Technology Application for In-Process Monitoring and Testing of Tablet and Capsule Dosage Forms

Unit Operation	In-Process Monitoring	PAT Application	In-Process Testing	PAT Application
Blending	Appearance	Visual—performed at-line	Blend uniformity	Tools available for online testing
Compression	Friability	Performed at-line	Stratified sampling and testing	Performed offline in analytical labs
	Hardness	Performed at-line		
	Weight variation	Performed at-line or at-line		
	Thickness	Performed at-line		
Granulation				
Dry granulation	Solid fraction	Performed at-line	Compliance to target solid fraction range	Performed at-line
Wet granulation	Moisture assessment	Drying endpoint target (moisture test) and drying cycle	Tools available for online measurement of drying cycle	
Encapsulation	Appearance	Visual—performed at-line	Blend uniformity	Tools available for online testing
	Weight variation	Performed in-line or at-line	Stratified sampling and testing	Performed offline in analytical labs

TABLE 23.6
Examples of Applications of Near Infrared Spectroscopy in Unit Operations

Unit Operation

Powder mixing	Blend uniformity monitoring (Corredor et al., 2015)
Freeze drying	Moisture content analysis (Kauppinen et al., 2014)
Compression	Content uniformity (Sulub et al., 2008)
Hot melt extrusion	Screw design and drug loading (Islam et al., 2014)
Fluidized bed granulation	Determine the moisture content, size distribution, and bulk density (Burggraeve et al., 2013)
Fluid bed coating	Film thickness (Lee et al., 2011)

Temperature measurements during the drying cycle, online particle size analysis, and content uniformity during blending operation are some examples of key measurements that may impact overall quality of the product. PAT tools have been successfully applied in these cases.

Among those PAT tools, near infrared spectroscopy (NIR) has drawn great attention in the pharmaceutical industry. It is a rapid, noninvasive analytical technique with no need for extensive sample preparation. NIR has been described in both the United States and the European Pharmacopeia. It is the most commonly used device in the manufacturing process, and it has been used for the identification and characterization of raw materials and intermediates, analysis of dosage forms manufacturing, and prediction of one or more variables in process streams or final product streams (composition) on the basis of on-line, in-line or at-line spectroscopic measurements (Corredor et al., 2015). Examples using NIR in different unit operations are listed in Table 23.6.

PHASES III AND IV STRATEGIES FOR DRUG PRODUCT MANUFACTURING OF WATER-INSOLUBLE NEW CHEMICAL ENTITIES

The Phase II program generally concludes with findings related to the dose–response characteristics of the drug and the dosing regimen (i.e., frequency of dosing). Positive results from these studies that demonstrate proof of efficacy set the stage for the Phase III clinical trials.

The objective of the Phase III studies is to demonstrate efficacy in a large patient population and gather in-depth understanding of the safety profile. Long-term studies are initiated in this phase to demonstrate safety and to support commercial objectives in marketing and pricing. These are generally placebo-controlled studies and most often utilize one or two doses at the expected therapeutic level. These studies are designed to include an ethnically diverse patient population from both genders. Long-term safety is assessed by utilizing for a period of 1–3 years to reveal any unexpected side effects. At the successful conclusion of Phase III, the company files a new drug application (NDA) with the FDA for marketing approval. Another set of important clinical studies, generally performed in parallel with Phase I and Phase III, are the large dose–response and the proof-of-efficacy studies. The purpose of these studies is to evaluate potential drug–drug interactions with commonly used commercially available drugs. In addition to these, further pharmacokinetics and pharmacodynamics of the drug are also studied in pediatric and geriatric populations. Once the company receives approval from the FDA, the drug enters into the postmarketing Phase IV. The objectives of Phase IV studies are to assess potential new indications and postapproval marketing support.

The transition from Phases II to III for drug product manufacturing is a very critical step as the formulation scientists and the process scientists are diligently working to optimize the composition and the process. The formulation and the process go hand in hand. The clinical supply requests tend to move from customized batches to repetitive batches as the formulation becomes further optimized. The volume of clinical supplies needed at this stage increases radically along with matching placebo requests for blinded studies. Formulators tend to study the standardized formulations to assess scalability. In general, large batches of the standardized formulation support the initial transition from Phase II to Phase III. This is one time when pressure begins to build for quickly developing a market image formulation for filing. It is also important to ascertain that the bioavailabilities of Phases II and III formulations/processes are equivalent; otherwise, there may be a need to re-establish new dosing strategies. The companies are beginning to develop strategies to bridge the gap with methodology for developing a robust formulation in a short period of time. At the same time, companies are beginning to look at ways to manage the risk of failing batches and avoid costly demonstration batches.

We all are familiar with the batch mode of operations utilizing separate unit processes to accomplish value-added staged processing. A *batch* is the finite quantity of finished product resulting from a process that subjects quantities of input materials to an ordered set of processing activities over a finite period of time using one or more pieces of equipment. The term *batch* also implies the "specific quantity of a drug or other material that is intended to have uniform character and quality, within specified limits, and is produced according to a single manufacturing order during the same cycle of manufacture" (International Society for Measurement and Control, 1995; Food and Drug Administration, 2017). Tom and Kovacs (1998) specify that drug products manufactured in a batch mode are dependent on three factors: (1) the order or sequence of the process, (2) the quantity and quality of the material used, and (3) the operating parameters used in executing each unit operation. Changes in any of these three factors can alter the product produced. Unlike continuous processing, extending the run time in the batch process does not produce additional product.

These discrete unit operations in a batch mode have a specific purpose and intention: to run the drug product recipe in a specific and consistently controlled manner. Each process step adds value to the recipe and facilitates the transformation of raw materials to an elegant, finished drug product. The manner in which the company achieves FDA approval for the recipe is by optimizing each unit operation through a systematic design of experiments and demonstrating that if key variables are controlled well in the specified range, a high-quality product can be consistently obtained. In order to achieve FDA approval, companies must demonstrate the optimization of unit process on many scales (e.g., one-tenth scale, commercial scale, etc.). In general, manufacture of the simplest recipe still requires 5–6 unit operations. Demonstrating controlled process at different scales by optimizing each unit operation becomes an extraordinarily time-consuming process, requiring great resources. Individual companies and the industry as a whole need to rethink ways in which the process can be modified to move away from traditional practices and explore ways to simplify the process optimization in the twenty-first century.

Currently, pharmaceutical businesses should not only consider creating value through innovation in discovering and developing new drugs, but also look for ways to bring drugs to market faster and more economically. Value in sustaining growth has to come from the innovation of new products, increasing speed to market (thereby having greater, useful patent life to leverage benefits of innovation), and development of processes that are independent of scale in research and commercial settings. Availability and advancement in science and technology provide opportunities for companies to raise the bar and shift their development paradigm. To sum it all, cost, advancement in technology, more stringent quality and regulatory requirements, efficiency and efficacy requirements, the highly competitive fragmented market, costly patent litigation, and global competition in emerging economies are serving as drivers to integrate process unit operations and simplify manufacturing processes.

Continuous process can be defined as a processing methodology wherein raw materials are constantly fed into the processing train with the yield on the basis of first-in-first-out (FIFO). The processed material is subjected to a consistent process modification environment (e.g., mixing speed, temperature, constant shear forces, etc.) to execute a drug product recipe for successfully manufacturing a quality drug product continuously over a period of time. In this paradigm, the batch size is independent of scale and truly depends on the duration of process run. Continuous processing systems are well established in the liquids manufacturing arena and are especially designed for

TABLE 23.7
Batch versus Continuous Process in Unit Operations and Equipment

Unit Operations Equipment	Processing	Discrete/Continuous Unit Operations
Mixing	PK blender	Batch process
Dry or wet	IBC mixer	Batch process
granulation	HS mixer–granulator	Batch process
	Ribbon mixer	Continuous process
	Twin-screw wet granulator	Continuous process
Milling	High-shear milling (Fitz milling)	Continuous process
	Low-shear delumping (Quadro Comil)	Continuous process
Drying	Fluid-bed dryer	Batch or semicontinuous
	Tray dryer	Batch process
	Convection tunnel dryers	Continuous process
	Radio frequency tunnel dryer	Continuous process
Dry granulator	Roller compaction (TF Mini, Gertis, etc.)	Continuous process
	Slugging	Continuous process
Compression	Rotary presses	Continuous process
Encapsulation	Automated encapsulators (Macofar, Zanasi, etc.)	Continuous process
	Ultra 8	Batch process
	Autodose®/Xcelodose™	Continuous process
	Bonapace	Batch process

Source: Foster, A. et al., *Int. J. Pharm.* 226, 147, 2001.

large-volume product lines. The continuous manufacturing of solid dosage forms is still a challenging concept. If one looks at the individual unit operations in the dry granulation and wet granulation processes (Table 23.7), many processes, although performed in a batch setting, can fit the definition of continuous processing (Lodaya and Mollan, 2004). Another challenge with the continuous process is demonstration of quality and process controls during the start-up and shutdown periods. For the majority of the duration run, the process stays in a steady state. A fixed constant quantity of waste is registered during start-up and shutdown periods. This could be significant if the batch size is small.

One distinct difference between the use of batch mode and continuous mode is that in batch processing, the scale of the equipment typically changes with the batch size. This in turn brings about changes in equipment surface area-to-volume and can have a significant impact on processes and intermediate quality of the processed material. Geometries of research and commercial equipment not equating well add to further ambiguity in successful scale-up of processes. Process-understanding studies in such cases take up significant time and resources. On the other hand, for continuous operating equipment, the size of the equipment does not change significantly, and thus is less prone to impact quality.

Clearly, the advantages of continuous processing through integration and automation of unit processes are numerous. They include scale independence, consistent processing of unit masses, an FIFO philosophy, real-time process performance data to demonstrate quality through the application of PAT tools, minimization of wastage, quickly developed process understanding, and knowledge gained related to products utilizing the previously applied processing methodology. These advantages should eventually lead to economy of scale and help the bottom line financial results.

The challenge of attaining the desired vision in process automation and integration is developing one such system that offers flexibility and is responsive enough to manage process variation in an integrated fashion. Another challenge is to effectively deal with material idiosyncrasies and the ability of the integrated continuous process in managing such issues. Finally, demonstration of quality maintenance from start to finish throughout the manufacturing process poses its own challenges.

Many organizations and scientists have engaged in developing continuous processing systems that integrate several unit operations to minimize the scale impact (Gamlen and Eardly, 1986; Lindberg et al., 1987; Lindberg, 1988; Bonde, 1998; Dorr and Leuenberger, 1998; Silke et al., 1999; Pathak et al., 2000; Keleb et al., 2001; Leuenberger, 2001; Ghebre-Sellassie et al., 2002). Such systems offer distinct advantages in minimizing scale impact and allow for flexibility in running the process, on the basis of realistic commercial demand. Consistent with *lean manufacturing* principles, this can be considered a *pull system* of batch processing rather than a *build-to-stock* approach, as batch size can be customized to market needs. The following are a few examples of concepts that have been implemented to facilitate the manufacture of pharmaceutical products in a continuous fashion.

GLATT MULTICELL™ UNIT

In 1994, Glatt developed the concept of a semicontinuous wet granulation production line. The concept leveraged the knowledge developed in producing granulation in the 5–9 kg scale range in the research environment and provided the capability to sequentially dry the minibatches in continuous manner in a series of fluidized bed dryers. The prototype consisted of HS granulation, screening, and drying in sequential steps. The drying is accomplished in a temperature gradient with the first dryer operating at higher temperature (~60°C) and the third at ambient temperature and humidity conditions. The miniature batches are processed one at a time and transferred to the dryers for further processing. If required, additional dryers can be added to the system.

The HS granulator design allows for high-pressure spraying and a dosing system that provides the capability to induce high energy into the granulator in comparison to the conventional granulators. The design allows for continuous cleaning of the granulator walls and is capable of self-discharging. In this system, the batch quantity of the material is introduced into the granulator, mixed, and granulated. The granulated material is then wet milled before discharge into the three sequential dryers. The dryers operate on the typical fluid-bed principle, and the drying is accomplished in sequential steps to achieve the desired moisture level.

The advantage of this system is that the optimized research-scale batch is leveraged for manufacturing a series of minibatches to meet commercial production requirements. This aspect of the system allows for minimizing the waste associated with costly scale-up studies required before regulatory filing. The granulation is fairly reproducible, provides better control observed on a smaller scale, and is a self-cleaning system. The drying is accomplished in a gentle manner to accommodate temperature-sensitive drugs.

Along with these advantages, this semicontinuous wet granulation production system poses certain challenges as well. This system may not accommodate material with diverse physical properties (e.g., densities). In addition, the granulation and the sequential drying steps timing need to be fairly synchronized to achieve a turnkey, automated, continuous operation without any slack. Of course, equipment breakdown in any system component may jeopardize batch material quality in various stages of processing.

TWIN-SCREW GRANULATION

Twin-Screw Wet Granulation

The twin-screw extrusion (TSE) technology is utilized extensively in the plastics and food industries to complement continuous manufacturing of products. Ghebre-Sellassie et al. (2002) and Keleb et al. (2001) have cited the application of this technology in the continuous production of pharmaceutical products. Commercially available TSE provide the great flexibility required for effective continuous mode of operation. The schematic of such a system is shown in Figure 23.6.

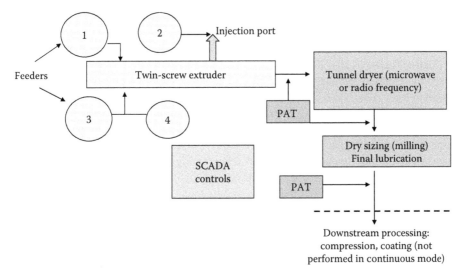

FIGURE 23.6 Process flow schematic based on continuous production of pharmaceutical granulation (From Ghebre-Sellassie, I. et al., U.S. Patent 6,499,984B1, 2002).

The twin-screw extruder provides the following advantages to facilitate scalability and robustness in the wet granulation process:

1. Modular screw design to assist in densification, and distributive and dispersive mixing
2. Efficient granulation endpoint determination
3. Consistent processing of unit mass of material
4. Sustained processing at a steady state for any duration of processing
5. Short residence time, limiting the material's exposure to harsh shear
6. Efficient design to facilitate waste minimization
7. Operation using the FIFO principle
8. Self-cleaning system
9. Flexibility in efficient process optimization

A typical TSE system consists of a feeding port for introducing dry powders into the extruder, a mixing zone where powders are mixed intimately, and a discharge zone for taking the granulation to the next step in the processing. Typically, granulation liquid is also introduced close to the feeding port to allow for sufficient mixing and optimal granule growth. The screw design optimization is a key part of the development activity. The screw design is optimized on the basis of the formulation process requirements.

Dispersive mixing is defined as breakdown of the morphological domains (Manas-Zloczower, 1994). If the active ingredient in the formulation needs to be broken down into smaller-size particles, the screw design needs to include a modular element utilized for dispersive mixing. On the other hand, *distributive* mixing is viewed as a means to achieve blend homogeneity requirements of the process. In this type of mixing, the minor phase (generally active API) gets evenly distributed in the overall mass being processed. To achieve the desired content uniformity, the screw design must include modular elements that will facilitate distribution of the API. The screw design becomes the critical part of process development activity. For formulation with low drug loading, the design will be dominant in screw elements that will facilitate distributive mixing. If the process requires breaking down the API into smaller particles, the design will be dominant in dispersive elements. Formulation and process scientists generally take a balanced approach to achieve the overall quality objective.

Typical screw design is constructed utilizing the functional screw elements (dispersive and distributive types) and conveying screw elements to facilitate forward movement of material in the TSE while subjecting the material mass to effective mixing. The densification of the mass is achieved by carefully selecting the conveying elements with successively narrow pitch. The technique was effectively utilized by scientists in developing a high-dose tablet through densification of the granulation for a low bulk density API (Shah, 2005).

Lodaya et al. (2003) describe a typical process description and process parameters for a Twin-Screw Wet Granulation (TSWG) process. The independent variables in the TSE process are screw design or configuration, screw rpm, temperature, and locations for liquid feed. The granulation characteristics are highly dependent on the screw configuration. Typical key process parameters are powder feed rate, liquid feed rate, and process temperature, and the extruder motor torque is one of useful information to monitor the process consistency. The authors suggest that the process should be run at a steady torque. The maximum torque for any given feed rate, screw design, and rpm should be 80% or below the manufacture-recommended limiting torque.

Figure 23.6 illustrates the schematic of continuous process described in the invention (Ghebre-Sellassie et al., 2002). Ghebre-Sellassie et al. (2002) utilized the TSE capabilities to develop a prototype that integrated the loss-in-weight feeders (Pathak et al., 2000), a TSE, liquid feeders, a wet mill, conveying and leveling devices, a tunnel dryer (radio frequency or microwave drying principle), and a dry milling operation to achieve continuous production of pharmaceutical granulation. Process analytical tools are applied at key steps to ensure that the key process parameters are in control. It is a single-pass, continuous, automated system for producing pharmaceutical granulation. The system incorporates a supervisory control and data assess (SCADA) system that monitors and controls the integrated unit operation. The throughput in such a system can range from a few kilograms to 50 kilograms production of the pharmaceutical granulation per hour. The granulation yield can then be further lubricated if required and compressed or encapsulated as desired.

Multiple loss-in-weight feeders (Pathak et al., 2000) can be utilized to accurately and precisely meter in the raw materials (in particular ratio) into the inlet port of the feeder. The TSE (with optimized screw design) is utilized for mixing and wet granulation with the assistance of the granulation liquid feed introduced into the TSE. The initial screw speed is kept low to quickly determine the water-carrying capacity of the unit mix in the TSE. Slowly, the screw speed is increased along with a simultaneous increase in the feeder metering rate to achieve desired granulation. Once the steady state is achieved, throughput is maintained throughout the process run. The wet granulation is milled through an appropriate-size screen and leveled on the dryer conveyor belt. Radio frequency or microwave drying facilitates the moisture removal along the depth of the granulation bed. The sensors placed at various points in the dryer facilitate the monitoring of the progress in the drying cycle. The PAT tools monitor the inlet and outlet moisture during the drying cycle. Content uniformity is also monitored in a similar manner. Any nonconformity to quality standards is fed back through the SCADA system, and the material is instantly discarded as waste until the automatic adjustments are made to bring quality into control.

HOT-MELT EXTRUSION

Numerous formulation approaches have been published to enhance the solubility of a drug molecule. It is a well-known fact that the amorphous phase of a drug has higher solubility, a higher dissolution rate, and higher bioavailability when compared with the crystalline form of the same drug. Alvarez-Núñez and Leonard (2004) utilized HME followed by milling of the extrudate to create milled solid dispersion (MSD) on the basis of this technique for formulation of amorphous systems. A mixture of a drug compound and polymer that has strong interaction with the drug is heated until homogeneous liquid phase (very likely the polymer starts to melt first, and a drug molecule is dispersed into the polymer matrix) is obtained. The mixture is rapidly cooled down to room temperature to obtain solid dispersion of drug that exists as an amorphous phase. A significant increase in dissolution rate of the otherwise poorly soluble drug was observed in comparison to crystalline form. Furthermore, on assessing the stability on long-term storage, it was observed that the degree of amorphous-to-crystal transformation depended on the drug-to-polymer ratio and the type of polymer used.

HME technology can also utilize TSE for processing materials in a consistent manner. TSE offers processing of unit mass in a controlled-temperature environment. Solid dispersion, solid solutions, eutectics, glass solutions, and suspensions all can be processed in a controlled-temperature environment in a continuous manner. TSE offers ability to dissolve API in a polymer matrix and achieve mixing at a molecular level. TSE has barrels that allow consistent temperature control. The barrels have integrated heating and cooling systems to maintain temperatures in the desired range. The extrudate is passed through a die to yield a desired shape (e.g., spaghetti, tube, etc.) that is quickly cooled to room temperature, and further processed to a finished drug product. The key development activities are (1) selection of polymer and (2) extrusion process parameters. The criteria for polymer selection include a drug–polymer interaction and glass transition temperature (T_g) of potential polymers and final products (Foster et al., 2001; Alvarez-Núñez et al., 2002; Alvarez-Núñez and Leonard, 2004). Extrusion process parameters include twin-screw design, extrusion temperature, and screw rpm. The extrusion temperature is selected on the basis of the drug/polymer's melting point, solubility of API in a polymer, and polymer T_g values.

PROCESS OPTIMIZATION

Process development activities go hand in hand with formulation development activities. The formulation development objectives include preformulation work that entails understanding of solid state of API, preliminary bioperformance, and drug–excipient compatibility studies. The formulation development activities also consist of establishing understanding of physical and chemical characteristics required for the clinical and commercial product, *in vitro* dissolution, formulation variables on bioavailability, key quality attributes or specifications, optimization of formulation, and development of specific test procedures and methods as well as the development of cleaning procedures and testing methodologies.

The goal of process development is to develop a process that meets product specifications and follows current Good Manufacturing Practices (cGMP). The critical process variables or parameters that impact the product quality attributes are identified and, in turn, the in-process specifications and test methods are developed. A process equipment train for manufacturing a particular batch scale of drug product is then identified. The key activities in accomplishing process development include (1) layout of the preferred process flow diagram that identifies the order of addition from the specified formulation recipe, (2) challenging the critical process parameters in the process flow to identify working ranges and alert ranges by measuring response to the product quality attributes, and (3) performing process characterization studies to demonstrate the process control. The product quality attribute is a response that can be measured (e.g., blend uniformity, content uniformity, particle size distribution, dissolution profiles, etc.) and a critical process parameter is defined as a variable that can or should be controlled to comply with quality specifications. Table 23.8 lists the quality attributes and the process parameters for a wet granulation tableting process.

Chao et al. (1993) describe a systematic approach to process optimization through process understanding. They recommend developing a process summary that comprises four basic steps:

1. Manufacturing flow diagram
2. Variables and responses
3. Cause-and-effect diagram
4. Influence matrix

The first step is mainly to put together a plan and describe sequential process activities. For each process in the flow diagram, inputs and outputs are shown with a list of desired quality attributes

TABLE 23.8

List of Quality Attributes and Potential Process Parameters for a Wet Granulation Process

Process Step	Product Quality Attributes	Measure (Units)	Process Parameter (Variables)	Rationale
1. Blending	Blend uniformity	Analytical technique (% rsd)	Blender rpm	Impacts final
	Potency	% theory	Time/revolution	drug product
	Yield	kg	Order of addition	quality
	Specific volume	cc/g	Load size	
2. Milling	Particle size distribution	Sieve analysis (size)	Milling speed	Impacts
	Yield	Loose density	Screen size	dissolution and
	Specific volume	Tap density	Screen type	downstream
	Appearance	kg	Feed rate	processing;
		cc/g		process
		Visual		understanding
3. Granulation	Blend uniformity	Analytical technique (% rsd)	Granulating liquid	Impacts final
	Specific volume	cc/g	addition rate, mix load	drug product
	Particle size distribution	d50, d90, etc.	Wet mass time	quality
	Surface area	m²/g	Quantity of granulating	
	Yield	kg	agent	
			Impeller rpm	
			Chopper speed	
4. Drying	Density	Density	Load size	Impacts final
	Drying endpoint	Moisture content (% LOD)	Initial temperature	drug product
	Throughput	Yield (kg)/unit time	Drying cycle profile	quality and
	Granule flow	% rsd	Air flow/humidity	downstream
	Segregation index	kg	Drying time	processing
	Yield	P-XRD	Cooling time	
	Crystal form			
5. Milling	Particle size distribution	Sieve analysis (size)	Milling speed	Impacts
	Mill choking	Loose density	Screen size	dissolution and
	Yield	Tap density	Screen type	downstream
	Blend uniformity	Buildup	Feed rate	processing;
		kg	Blender rpm	process
		Analytical technique (% rsd)		understanding
6. Blending	Potency	% theory	Time/revolution	Impacts final
	Yield	kg	Order of addition	drug product
	Specific volume	cc/g	Load size	quality
	Blend uniformity	Analytical technique (% rsd)	Blender rpm	
7. Lubrication	Potency	% theory	Time/revolution	Impacts final
	Yield	kg	Order of addition	drug product
	Specific volume	cc/g	Load size	quality
	Powder flow			
8. Compression	Hardness	Tablet hardness tester (kp/KN)	Precompression force or	Impacts final
	Weight variation	Scale (mg)	thickness	drug product
	Friability	%	Compression force or	quality
	Thickness	Inches	thickness	
	Disintegration	Time	Granule feed rate	
	Dissolution	USP %Q in minutes	Penetration depth	
			Compression speed	

(Continued)

TABLE 23.8 (*Continued*)
List of Quality Attributes and Potential Process Parameters for a Wet Granulation Process

Process Step	Product Quality Attributes	Measure (Units)	Process Parameter (Variables)	Rationale
9. Film coating	Appearance	Defect rate—Visual	Weight gain	Impacts final
	Assay	(AQL testing)	Inlet and outlet	drug product
	Water content	Analytical test (mg/g or % LC)	temperatures	quality and
	Mechanical integrity	KF (%)	Spraying rate	regulatory
	Microbial limit test	Defect rate	Inlet air humidity	requirements
		FU/g	Atomizing air pressure	
			Pan speed	
10. Finished tablets	Content uniformity	Analytical technique (% rsd)		Requirement for final drug
	Assay	Analytical technique (mg/g)		product
	Purity	Analytical technique		disposition
	Disintegration	(% impurity)		decision
	Dissolution	Time		
	Appearance	USP %Q in minutes		
	Friability			

and process variables or parameters. Once the entire process diagram is laid out, a systematic approach is utilized to gauge the impact of variables on the product attributes. This is performed by ranking the desired attributes on a scale of 1–10, with 10 being very important to the customer and regulatory agency and 1 important from a process-understanding perspective. Through this exercise, the key product attributes are identified as focal points to measure the impact of various process parameters.

Cause-and-effect diagrams (Food and Drug Administration, 1987; Chao et al., 1993) provide another way of pictorially representing the main processing steps with process parameters that may have an effect on the key product attribute. For example, in a wet granulation step, the load size, impeller rpm and duration, and granulation liquid volume/addition rate may have an effect on the overall content uniformity and dissolution profiles, which is critical for water-insoluble candidates of the dosage form. A cause-and-effect diagram of the entire process provides a guideline and overall understanding of the various key parameters that may impact a common quality attribute such as content uniformity. It is important, however, to understand that not all parameters will have a significant impact on the desired quality attribute. The next step in the process optimization is to determine which parameter influences the quality attributes most, and what would be the acceptable range to control the parameter so as to meet the quality attribute consistently time after time. This systematic analysis is performed to develop an influence matrix and to define the strength of the relationship between variables and response as strong (S), moderate (M), weak (W), or none (N). Construction of such a matrix identifies those variables that have the greatest influence on the desired quality attribute. Design of experiments and statistical analyses of the data are tools available to scientists to determine key process parameters and develop sound understanding of the manufacturing process.

These studies are essential parts of regulatory dossiers, independent of batch or continuous manufacturing.

FUTURE PERSPECTIVE

As one can relate, the manufacturing of solid dosage forms for the water-insoluble drugs can be challenging in the clinical and commercial setting. The authors have attempted to illustrate the challenges and suggest drug development paradigms consistent with regulatory guidelines and *lean manufacturing* principles. Although the focus was primarily on solid dosage forms, the principles can be applied broadly to other dosage form technologies and help in building universal platforms for development. Knowledge is one source of innovation in our industry, and this in combination with developments in other fields inspires the industry leaders to continuously create new value. Seamless transfer of products and processes from research to commercial status is one area where there is room for innovation. In the current industrial environment, it is imperative that companies invest wisely and develop quality drugs with intention of speed to market to benefit patients and sustain business.

ACKNOWLEDGMENT

The authors would like to extend thanks to Mark Aills, MPH, in Pfizer Global R&D, for his valuable comments and suggestions in the preparation of this chapter.

REFERENCES

Alexander, A. W. and F. J. Muzzio, 2002. Batch size increase in dry blending and mixing. In *Pharmaceutical Process Scale-Up*, M. Levine (Ed.), New York: Marcel Dekker, vol. 118, pp. 115–132.

Alvarez-Núnez, F. A. and M. R. Leonard, 2004. Formulation of a poorly soluble drug using hot melt extrusion. The amorphous state as an alternative. *Am. Pharm. Rev.* 7(4), 88–92.

Alvarez-Núnez, F. A., M. R. Leonard, and L. F. Crawford, 2002. Glass transition temperature measurement as predictors of the physical stability of a poorly soluble pharmaceutical agent formulated as solid dispersion. AAPS, Toronto, ON.

Autodose, S. A. and M.T.M. Powdernium, 2005. Expert high-precision powder dispensing technology. https://www.drugdiscoveryonline.com/doc/powdernium-new-technology-for-high-precision-0001

Boehm, G., J. Clark, J. Dietrick, L. Foust, B. Garth, C. Jon, D. John et al. 2003. The use of stratified sampling of blend and dosage units to demonstrate adequacy of mix for powder blends. *PDA J. Pharm. Sci. Technol.* 57, 59–74.

Bonde, M., 1998. Continuous granulation. In *Handbook of Pharmaceutical Granulation Technology*, D. M. Parikh (Ed.), New York: Marcel Dekker, pp. 369–386.

Burggraeve, A., T. Monteyne, C. Vervaet, J. P. Remon, and T. De Beer, 2013. Process analytical tools for monitoring, understanding, and control of pharmaceutical fluidized bed granulation: A review. *Eur. J Pharm. Biopharm.* 83(1), 2–15.

Capsugel, 2006. Capsule sizes and capacities. http://www.capsugel.com/products/vcaps_chart.php

Chao, A. Y., F. F. John, R. F. Johnson, and P. V. Doehren, 1993. Prospective process validation in pharmaceutical process validation. *Drugs Pharm. Sci.* 129, 7–30.

Chowhan, Z. T., 1998. Aspects of granulation scale-up in high shear mixers. *Pharm. Technol.* 12, 26–44.

Corredor, C. C., R. Lozano, X. Bu, R. McCann, J. Dougherty, T. Stevens, D. Both, and P. Shah, 2015. Analytical method quality by design for an on-line near-infrared method to monitor blend potency and uniformity. *J. Pharm. Innov.* 10(1), 47–55.

Dorr, B. and H. Leuenberger, 1998. Development of a quasi-continuous production line—A concept to avoid scale-up problems. Preprints First European Symposium on Process Technologies in Pharmaceutical and Nutritional Sciences, PARTEC 98 Nurnberg, pp. 247–256.

Food and Drug Administration, 1987, May. *Guidelines on General Principles of Process Validation*. Rockville, MD: Division of Manufacturing and Product Quality (HFN-320), Center for Drugs and Biologics.

Food and Drug Administration, 2003a, August. *Guidance for Industry PAT—A Framework for Innovative Pharmaceutical Manufacturing and Quality Assurance*.

Food and Drug Administration, 2003b, October. *Guidelines for the Industry on Powder Blends and Finished Dosage Units—Stratified In-Process Dosage Unit Sampling and Assessment*. Washington, DC: US Department of Health and Human Services, Center for Drug Evaluation and Research (CDER).

Food and Drug Administration, 2004, September. *Guidelines for the Industry on PAT—A Framework for Innovative Pharmaceutical Development, Manufacturing, and Quality Assurance.* Washington, DC: US Department of Health and Human Services, Center for Drug Evaluation and Research (CDER).

Food and Drug Administration, 2006. *Inactive Ingredient Guide.* http://www.accessdata.fda.gov/scripts/cder/iig/index.cfm

Food and Drug Administration, 2017, April. Code of Federal Regulations, Title 21 CFR, Washington, DC.

Foster, A., J. Hempenstall, I. Tucker, and T. Rades, 2001. Selection of excipients for melt extrusion with two poorly water-soluble drugs by solubility parameter calculation and thermal analysis. *Int. J. Pharm.* 226, 147.

Gamlen, M. and C. Eardly, 1986. Continuous granulation using a Baker Perkins MP50 (Multipurpose) extruder. *Drug Dev. Ind. Pharm.* 12, 1710–1713.

Ghebre-Sellassie, I., M. J. Mollan Jr, N. Pathak, M. Lodaya, and M. Fessehaie, 2002. Continuous production of pharmaceutical granulation. U.S. Patent 6,499,984B1.

Gokhale, R., Y. Sun, and A. J. Shukla, 2005. High-shear granulation. In *Handbook of Pharmaceutical Granulation Technology* 2nd ed., D. M. Parikh (Ed.), Boca Raton, FL: Taylor & Francis Group, vol. 154, pp. 191–228.

Gupta, P. K. and J. B. Cannon, 2000. Emulsion and microemulsions for drug solubilization and delivery. In *Water-Insoluble Drug Formulation*, R. Liu (Ed.), Boca Raton, FL: Interpharm/CRC, pp. 169–212.

Gurvinder Singh, R. and R. Sidwell, 2005. Sizing of granulation. In *Handbook of Pharmaceutical Granulation Technology* 2nd ed., D. M. Parikh (Ed.), Boca Raton, FL: Taylor & Francis Group, vol. 154, pp. 491–512.

Hariharan, M., L. D. Ganorkar, G. E. Amidon, A. Cavallo, P. Gatti, M. J. Hageman, I. Choo, J. L. Miller, and U. J. Shah, 2003. Reducing the time to develop and manufacture formulation for first oral dose in humans. *Pharm. Technol.* 27(10), 68–84.

Hörter, D. and J. B. Dressman, 2001. Influence of physicochemical properties on dissolution of drugs in the gastrointestinal tract. *Adv. Drug Deliv. Rev.* 46, 75.

Huang, L. F., 2005, July. Formulation strategies and practices used for water-insoluble drug candidates at early phases of drug development. Pharmaceutical Education Associates Meeting on Water-Insoluble Drug Delivery Conference, Philadelphia, PA.

International Society for Measurement and Control, 1995. Batch control part I: Models and terminology, ISA-S88.01.

Islam, M. T., M. Maniruzzaman, S. A. Halsey, B. Z. Chowdhry, and D. Douroumis, 2014. Development of sustained-release formulations processed by hot-melt extrusion by using a quality-by-design approach. *Drug Deliv. Transl. Res.* 4(4), 377–387.

Kauppinen, A., M. Toivianinen, M. Lehtonen, K. Järvinen, J. Paaso, M. Juuti, and J. Ketolainen, 2014. Validation of a multipoint near-infrared spectroscopy method for in-line moisture content analysis during freeze-drying. *J. Pharm. Biomed. Anal.* 95, 229–237.

Keleb, E. I., A. Vermeire, C. Vervaet, and J. P. Remon, 2001. Cold extrusion as a single-step granulation and tabletting process. *Eur. J. Pharm. Biopharm.* 52, 359–368.

Lee, M. J., D. Y. Seo, H. E. Lee, I. C. Wang, W. S. Kim, M. Y. Jeong, and G. J. Choi, 2011. In line NIR quantification of film thickness on pharmaceutical pellets during a fluid bed coating process. *Int. J. Pharmaceut.* 403(1), 66–72.

Leuenberger, H., 2001. New trends in the production of pharmaceutical granules: Batch versus continuous processing. *Eur. J. Pharm. Biopharm.* 52, 289–296.

Lindberg, N. O., 1988. Some experiences of continuous wet granulation. *Acta Pharm. Suec.* 25, 239–246.

Lindberg, N. O., C. Turfvesson, and L. Olbjer, 1987. Extrusion of an effervescent granulation with a twin screw extruder. *Drug Dev. Ind. Pharm.* 13, 1891–1913.

Lipps, D. and A. M. Sakr, 1994. Characterization of wet granulation process parameters using response surface methodology. 1. Top-spray fluidized bed. *J. Pharm. Sci.* 83, 937.

Lodaya, M. and M. Jr. Mollan, 2004. Continuous processing in pharmaceutical manufacturing. *Am. Pharm. Rev.* 7, 70–75.

Lodaya, M., M. Mollan, and I. Ghebre-Sellassie, 2003. Twin-screw wet granulation. In *Pharmaceutical Extrusion Technology*, I. Ghebre-Sellassie and C. Martin (Eds.), New York: Marcel Dekker, pp. 323–343.

Manas-Zloczower, I., 1994. Dispersive mixing of solid additives. In *Mixing and Continuous Compounding of Polymers*, I. Manas-Zloczower and Z. Tadmor (Eds.), Munich: Carl Hanser Verlag, pp. 55–83.

Med Ad News, February 2003. New Medicines: 78 new medicines approved: Despite fears of an FDA slowdown, the regulatory agency cleared more new medicines for marketing in 2002 than in 2001. (10th Annual Report).

Mouro, D., M. Deanna, N. Robert, M. Bruce, K. Harry, and S. Umang, 2006. Enhancement of XcelodoseTM capsule-filling capabilities using roller compaction. *Pharm. Technol.* 30.

O'Connor, R. E. and J. B. Schwartz, 1985. Spheronization II Drug release from drug-diluent mixtures. *Drug Dev. Ind. Pharm.* 11, 1837–1857.

PAREXEL, 2005/2006. *Pharmaceutical R&D Statistical Sourcebook*, M. P. Mathieu (Ed.), Comparative R&D spending, sales, and product launch trends worldwide: A2005 Analysis, p. 6.

Pathak, N. P., M. Lodaya, M. Moll, I. Ghebre-Sellassie, and C. Conrad, 2000. Performance characteristics of loss-in-weight dry feeders: November 2000, AAPS 2000 Annual Meeting, Indianapolis, IN.

Reich, G. 2005. Near-infrared spectroscopy and imaging: Basic principles and pharmaceutical applications. *Adv. Drug Deliv. Rev.* 57(8), 1109–1143.

Rudnic, E. M. and J. B. Schwartz, 2000. *Oral Solid Dosage Forms in Remington—The Science and Practice of Pharmacy*, 20th ed., Eaton, PA: Mack Publishing, pp. 858–893.

Schwartz, J. B, 2002. Scale-up of the compaction and tablet process. In *Pharmaceutical Process Scale-Up*, M. Levine (Ed.), New York: Marcel Dekker, vol. 118, pp. 221–237.

Shah, U., 2005. Use of modified twin screw extruder. *Pharm. Technol.* 29, 52–66.

Silke, G., A. Knoch, and G. Lee, 1999. Continuous wet granulation using fluidized-bed techniques: I. Examination of powder mixing kinetics and preliminary granulation experiments. *Eur. J. Pharm. Biopharm.* 48, 189–197.

Sulub, Y., R. LoBrutto, R. Vivilecchia, and B. W. Wabuyele, 2008. Content uniformity determination of pharmaceutical tablets using five near-infrared reflectance spectrometers: A process analytical technology (PAT) approach using robust multivariate calibration transfer algorithms. *Analytica Chimica Acta* 611(2), 143–150.

Tabibi, E. S. and S. L. Gupta, 2000. Soft gelatin capsules development. In *Water-Insoluble Drug Formulation*, R. Liu (Ed.), Boca Raton, FL: Interpharm/CRC, pp. 609–633.

Tom, T. H. and K. S. Kovacs, 1998. Batch process automation. In *Automation and Validation of Information in Pharmaceutical Processing*, J. F. deSpautz (Ed.), New York: Marcel Dekker, vol. 90, pp. 417–432.

Venkatesh, S. and R. A. Lipper, 2000. The role of the development scientist in compound lead selection and optimization. *J. Pharm. Sci.* 89, 145.

Venugopal, P. V., 2002, June 3. WIPO Conference on the Intellectual Property and Economic Development, Geneva, Switzerland.

Xcelodose™ precision micro-filling system. https://www.pharmaceuticalonline.com/doc/xcelodose-s-precision-powder-micro-filling-sy-0001

Yalkowsky, S. H. and T. J. Roseman, 1981a. Solubilization of drugs by cosolvents. *J. Pharm. Sci.* 70, 91–134.

Yalkowsky, S. H. and T. J. Roseman, 1981b. *Solubilization of Drugs by Cosolvents; Techniques of Solubilization of Drugs*, S. H. Yalkowsky (Ed.), New York: Marcel Dekker.

Yu, L. X., 2008. Pharmaceutical quality by design: Product and process development, understanding, and control. *Pharm. Res.* 25(4), 781–791.

Index

Note: Page numbers followed by f and t refer to figures and tables respectively.

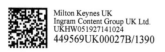

9 781032 339214